CURRENT THERAPY
IN GASTROENTEROLOGY
AND LIVER DISEASE - 2

Current Therapy Series

Bayless:
Current Therapy in Gastroenterology and Liver Disease
Bayless, Brain, Cherniack:
Current Therapy in Internal Medicine
Brain, Carbone:
Current Therapy in Hematology-Oncology
Callaham:
Current Therapy in Emergency Medicine
Cameron:
Current Surgical Therapy
Cherniack:
Current Therapy of Respiratory Disease
Dubovsky, Shore:
Current Therapy in Psychiatry
Ernst, Stanley:
Current Therapy in Vascular Surgery
Foley, Payne:
Current Therapy of Pain
Fortuin:
Current Therapy in Cardiovascular Disease
Garcia:
Current Contraceptive Management
Garcia, Mastroianni, Amelar, Dubin:
Current Therapy of Infertility
Garcia, Mikuta, Rosenblum:
Current Therapy in Surgical Gynecology
Gates:
Current Therapy in Otolaryngology—
Head and Neck Surgery
Glassock:
Current Therapy in Nephrology and Hypertension
Grillo, Austen, Wilkins, Mathisen, Vlahakes:
Current Therapy in Cardiothoracic Surgery
Jeejeebhoy:
Current Therapy in Nutrition
Johnson:
Current Therapy in Neurologic Disease
Kass, Platt:
Current Therapy in Infectious Disease
Krieger, Bardin:
Current Therapy in Endocrinology and Metabolism
Lichtenstein, Fauci:
Current Therapy in Allergy, Immunology and Rheumatology
Long:
Current Therapy in Neurologic Surgery
McGinty, Jackson:
Current Therapy in Orthopaedic Surgery
Nelson:
Current Therapy in Neonatal-Perinatal Medicine
Nelson:
Current Therapy in Pediatric Infectious Disease
Parrillo:
Current Therapy in Critical Care Medicine
Provost, Farmer:
Current Therapy in Dermatology
Resnick, Kursh:
Current Therapy in Genitourinary Surgery
Rogers:
Current Practice of Anesthesiology
Trunkey, Lewis:
Current Therapy of Trauma
Welsh, Shephard:
Current Therapy in Sports Medicine

CURRENT THERAPY IN GASTROENTEROLOGY AND LIVER DISEASE - 2

THEODORE M. BAYLESS, M.D.
Professor of Medicine
The Johns Hopkins University School of Medicine
Physician, The Johns Hopkins Hospital
Director, Meyerhoff Digestive Disease–
Inflammatory Bowel Disease Center
Baltimore, Maryland

1986

B.C. DECKER INC • Toronto • Philadelphia

Publisher

B.C. Decker Inc.
3228 South Service Road
Burlington, Ontario L7N 3H8

B.C. Decker Inc.
P.O. Box 30246
Philadelphia, Pennsylvania 19103

Sales and Distribution

United States and Possessions	**The C.V. Mosby Company** 11830 Westline Industrial Drive Saint Louis, Missouri 63146
Canada	**The C.V. Mosby Company, Ltd.** 5240 Finch Avenue East, Unit No. 1 Scarborough, Ontario M1S 4P2
United Kingdom, Europe and the Middle East	**Blackwell Scientific Publications, Ltd.** Osney Mead, Oxford OX2 OEL, England
Australia	**Holt-Saunders Pty. Limited** 9 Waltham Street Artarmon, N.S.W. 2064 Australia
Japan	**Igaku-Shoin Ltd.** Tokyo International P.O. Box 5063 1-28-36 Hongo, Bunkyo-ku, Tokyo 113, Japan
Asia	**Holt-Saunders Asia Limited** 10/F, Inter-Continental Plaza Tsim Sha Tsui East Kowloon, Hong Kong

Current Therapy in Gastroenterology and Liver Disease - 2   ISBN 0-941158-89-6

© 1986 by B.C. Decker Incorporated under the International Copyright Union. All rights reserved. No part of this publication may be reused or republished in any form without written permission of the publisher.

Library of Congress catalog card number: 85-062984

10   9   8   7   6   5   4   3   2   1

CONTRIBUTORS

JAFFER A. AJANI, M.D.

Assistant Professor of Medicine, Department of Medical Oncology, University of Texas Cancer Center; Anderson Hospital and Tumor Institute, Houston, Texas
Gastric Carcinoma

MARVIN EARL AMENT, M.D.

Professor of Pediatrics, University of California, UCLA School of Medicine; UCLA Medical Center, Los Angeles, California
Gastrointestinal Disorders in the Immunodeficient State

SINN ANURAS, M.D., F.A.C.P.

Professor of Internal Medicine, Texas Tech University Health Sciences Center School of Medicine; Director, Division of Gastroenterology, Texas Tech University Health Sciences Center, Lubbock, Texas
Chronic Intestinal Pseudo-Obstruction

MARK APPLER, M.D.

Fellow in Gastroenterology, University of Pittsburgh School of Medicine, Pittsburgh, Pennsylvania
Liver Transplantation: Gastroenterologic Considerations

FRANCOIS AUCLAIR, M.D.

Research Fellow in Geographic Medicine, Tufts-New England Medical Center, Boston, Massachusetts
Endocarditis Prophylaxis

ARTHUR H. AUFSES Jr., M.D.

Franz W. Sichel Professor and Chairman of Surgery, Mount Sinai School of Medicine of the City University of New York; Director of Surgery, The Mount Sinai Hospital, New York, New York
Crohn's Disease: Surgical Treatment

WILLIAM P. BALDUS, M.D.

Associate Professor, Mayo Medical School; Staff Physician, Department of Internal Medicine, Division of Gastroenterology, Mayo Clinic, Rochester, Minnesota
Hemochromatosis

PETER A. BANKS, M.D.

Associate Professor of Medicine, Tufts University School of Medicine, Lecturer in Medicine, Harvard Medical School; Chief of Gastroenterology, Saint Elizabeth's Hospital, Boston, Massachusetts
Acute Pancreatitis: Medical Considerations

JOHN G. BANWELL, M.D., F.A.C.P.

Professor, Division of Gastroenterology, Department of Medicine, Case Western Reserve University School of Medicine, Cleveland, Ohio
Bacterial Overgrowth Syndrome

RONALD G. BARR, M.A., M.D.C.M., F.R.C.P.(C)

Associate Professor of Pediatrics, McGill University Faculty of Medicine; Director, Developmental Pediatric Clinics, Montreal Children's Hospital, Montreal, Quebec, Canada
Recurrent Abdominal Pain in Childhood and Adolescence

JOHN GILL BARTLETT, M.D.

Professor of Medicine, The Johns Hopkins University School of Medicine; Chief, Division of Infectious Diseases, The Johns Hopkins Hospital, Baltimore, Maryland
Intra-abdominal Sepsis

THEODORE M. BAYLESS, M.D.

Professor of Medicine, The Johns Hopkins University School of Medicine; Physician, The Johns Hopkins Hospital; Director, Meyerhoff Digestive Disease—Inflammatory Bowel Disease Center, Baltimore, Maryland
Idiopathic Inflammatory Bowel Disease and Neoplasia

ROBERT W. BEART Jr., M.D.

Associate Professor of Surgery, Mayo Medical School; Head, Section of Colon and Rectal Surgery, Mayo Clinic and Mayo Foundation, Rochester, Minnesota
Colorectal Carcinoma: Adjuvant Therapy

RICHARD G. BLACK, M.D.

Associate Professor, Department of Anesthesiology and Critical Care Medicine, The Johns Hopkins University School of Medicine, Baltimore, Maryland
Chronic Intractable Abdominal Pain

LAURENCE M. BLENDIS, M.D., F.R.C.P., F.R.C.P.(C)

Professor of Medicine, University of Toronto Faculty of Medicine; Senior Staff Physician, Service Chief, General Medical Floor, Toronto General Hospital, Toronto, Ontario, Canada
Portosystemic Encephalopathy

EDGAR C. BOEDEKER, M.D.

Associate Professor of Medicine, Uniformed Services

University of the Health Sciences, Bethesda, Maryland; Chief, Department of Gastroenterology, Walter Reed Army Institute of Research, Washington, District of Columbia
Traveler's Diarrhea

GAIL L. BONGIOVANNI, M.D.

Assistant Professor of Clinical Medicine, University of Cincinnati College of Medicine; Attending Physician and Director, Digestive Disease Center, University of Cincinnati Medical Center, Cincinnati, Ohio
Acute Infectious Diarrhea

H. WORTH BOYCE Jr., M.D., F.A.C.P.

Professor of Medicine, Director, Division of Digestive Diseases and Nutrition, University of South Florida College of Medicine, Tampa, Florida
Caustic Injury

JAMES L. BOYER, M.D.

Professor of Medicine, Yale University School of Medicine, New Haven, Connecticut
Primary Biliary Cirrhosis

ROBERT A. BRANCH, M.D.

Professor of Medicine and Pharmacology, Vanderbilt University School of Medicine, Nashville, Tennessee
Drug Use in Patients with Hepatic Disease

ANTHONY N. BRANNAN, M.D.

Chief Resident Associate, Section of Colon and Recal Surgery, Mayo Clinic and Mayo Foundation, Rochester, Minnesota
Colorectal Carcinoma: Adjuvant Therapy

GREGORY B. BULKLEY, M.D., F.A.C.S.

Associate Professor of Surgery, Director of Surgical Research, The Johns Hopkins University School of Medicine; Active Staff, The Johns Hopkins Hospital, Baltimore, Maryland
Intestinal Obstruction

DONALD O. CASTELL, M.D.

Professor of Medicine, Bowman Gray School of Medicine of Wake Forest University; Chief of Gastroenterology, North Carolina Baptist Hospital, Winston-Salem, North Carolina
Achalasia

SIDNEY COHEN, M.D.

T. Grier Miller Professor of Medicine, GI Section/Department of Medicine, University of Pennsylvania School of Medicine; Chief, Gastrointestinal Section, Hospital of the University of Pennsylaniva, Philadelphia, Pennsylvania
Diffuse Esophageal Spasm and Related Disorders

ALASTAIR M. CONNELL, M.D.

Professor of Internal Medicine, Virginia Commonwealth University Medical College of Virginia; Vice President for Health Sciences, Virginia Commonwealth University
Constipation

MARC COOPERMAN, M.D.

Associate Professor of Surgery, Ohio State University College of Medicine; Attending Staff, Ohio State University Hospitals, Columbus, Ohio
Intestinal Ischemia

BYRON DeLEMOS, M.D.

Fellow in Gastroenterology, University of Pittsburgh School of Medicine, Pittsburgh, Philadelphia
Liver Transplantation: Gastroenterologic Considerations

TOM R. DeMEESTER, M.D.

Professor of Thoracic and Cardiovascular Surgery, Chairman, Department of Surgery, Creighton University School of Medicine; Chief, Department of Surgery, Saint Joseph Hospital, Omaha, Nebraska
Esophageal Reflux: Surgical Treatment

GILBERT DERAY, M.D.

International Fellow, Merck Sharp and Dohme, Paris, France
Drug Use in Patients with Hepatic Disease

KIERTISIN DHARMSATHAPHORN, M.D.

Associate Professor of Medicine, University of California School of Medicine; Attending Physician, University of California, San Diego Medical Center, San Diego, California
Secretory Diarrhea

JOHN WHITBY DOBBINS, M.D.

Associate Professor of Medicine, Yale University School of Medicine; Attending Physician, Yale-New Haven Hospital, Consultant, West Haven Veterans Administration Hospital, New Haven, Connecticut
Hyperoxaluria and Nephrolithiasis

WILLIAM O. DOBBINS III, M.D.

Professor of Internal Medicine, University of Michigan Medical School; Associate Chief of Staff for Research, Veterans Administration Medical Center, Ann Arbor, Michigan
Whipple's Disease

ADRIAN P. DOUGLAS, M.D., M.R.C.P.

Clinical Associate Professor of Medicine, University of California, UCLA School of Medicine, Los Angeles, California
Celiac Sprue and Related Diseases

VICTOR W. FAZIO, M.B., B.S., F.R.A.C.S., F.A.C.S.

Chairman, Department of Colon and Rectal Surgery, The Cleveland Clinic Foundation, Cleveland, Ohio
Ostomy Care

MARK K. FERGUSON, M.D.

Assistant Professor of Surgery, University of Chicago Pritzker School of Medicine; Attending Thoracic Surgeon, University of Chicago Medical Center, Chicago, Illinois
Cancer of the Esophagus and Cardia: Surgical Treatment

ROBERT S. FISHER, M.D.

Professor of Medicine, Temple University School of Medicine; Chief, Gastroenterology Section, Director, Functional Gastrointestinal Diseases Center, Temple University Hospital, Philadelphia, Pennsylvania
Disorders of Gastric Emptying

JOHN GREGORY FITZ, M.D.

Assistant Professor of Medicine, University of California School of Medicine, San Francisco, California
Cholestasis and Sclerosing Cholangitis

DAVID E. FLEISCHER, M.D.

Associate Professor, Georgetown University School of Medicine, Washington, District of Columbia
Laser Treatment in Gastrointestinal Disease

C. RICHARD FLEMING, M.D.

Associate Professor of Medicine, Mayo Medical School; Consultant in Gastroenterology, Mayo Clinic, Rochester, Minnesota
Parenteral Nutrition

BARRY A. FRANK, M.D.

Clinical Assistant Professor of Medicine, Department of Internal Medicine, University of South Florida College of Medicine, Tampa, Florida
Caustic Injury

HANS FROMM, M.D.

Professor of Medicine, George Washington University School of Medicine and Health Sciences; Director, Division of Gastroenterology, George Washington University Medical Center
Cholelithiasis

THOMAS R. GADACZ, M.D., F.A.C.S.

Associate Professor of Surgery, The Johns Hopkins University School of Medicine; Chief, Surgical Service, Veterans Administration Medical Center, Baltimore, Maryland
Alkaline Reflux Gastritis

JERRY D. GARDNER, M.D.

Chief, Digestive Diseases Branch, National Institute of Arthritis, Diabetes, Digestive and Kidney Diseases, Bethesda, Maryland
Gastrinoma

PAUL E. GARFINKEL, M.D., M.Sc., F.R.C.P.(C)

Professor and Vice-Chairman, Department of Psychiatry, University of Toronto Faculty of Medicine; Psychiatrist-in-Chief, Toronto General Hospital, Toronto, Ontario, Canada
Anorexia Nervosa and Bulimia

JOSEPH E. GEENEN, M.D., F.A.C.P., F.A.C.G.

Clinical Professor of Medicine, Department of Gastroenterology, Medical College of Wisconsin, Milwaukee, Wisconsin; Consultant in Gastroenterology, Froedtert Lutheran Memorial Hospital, Milwaukee, Wisconsin, Saint Luke's Hospital and Saint Mary's Medical Center, Racine, Wisconsin
Endoscopy in Bile Duct Obstruction and Ampullary Dysfunction

ANGELIKI GEORGOPOULOS, M.D.

Assistant Professor, The Johns Hopkins School of Medicine; Active Staff, The Johns Hopkins Hospital, Baltimore, Maryland
Postprandial Hypoglycemia

RALPH A. GIANNELLA, M.D.

Mark Brown Professor of Medicine and Director, Division of Digestive Diseases, University of Cincinnati College of Medicine; Attending Physician, University of Cincinnati Hospitals, Cincinnati, Ohio
Acute Infectious Diarrhea

STANLEY M. GOLDBERG, M.D., F.A.C.S.

Clinical Professor of Surgery, Director and Head, Division of Colon and Rectal Surgery, Department of Surgery, University of Minnesota Medical School, Minneapolis, Minnesota
Anorectal Disorders

ENOCH GORDIS, M.D.

Professor of Clinical Medicine, Mount Sinai School of Medicine of the City University of New York, New York, New York; Director, Alcoholism Treatment Program, City Hospital Center, Elmhurst, New York
Alcoholism

DAVID Y. GRAHAM, M.D.

Professor of Medicine and Virology, Baylor College of Medicine; Chief, Digestive Disease Section, Veterans Administration Medical Center, Houston, Texas
Gastric Ulcer

RICHARD J. GRAND, M.D.

Professor of Pediatrics, Tufts University School of Medicine; Chief, Division of Pediatric Gastroenterology and Nutrition, The Boston Floating Hospital, New England Medical Center, Boston, Massachusetts
Growth Failure in Inflammatory Bowel Disease

JEFFREY GRAY, M.D.

Clinical Assistant Professor, University of Pittsburgh School of Medicine, Pittsburgh, Pennsylvania
Liver Transplantation: Gastroenterologic Considerations

LEONARD L. GUNDERSON, M.D., M.S.

Professor of Oncology, Mayo Medical School; Consultant in Radiation Oncology, Mayo Clinic, Rochester, Minnesota
Intraoperative Irradiation

STEPHEN B. HANAUER, M.D.

Assistant Professor of Medicine, Section of Gastroenterology, University of Chicago Medical Center, Chicago, Illinois
Crohn's Disease of the Small Bowel

JOHN H. HELZBERG, M.D.

Fellow in Digestive Diseases, Yale University School of Medicine, New Haven, Connecticut
Primary Biliary Cirrhosis

THOMAS R. HENDRIX, M.D.

Moses and Helen Golden Paulson Professor of Gastroenterology, The Johns Hopkins University School of Medicine, Baltimore, Maryland
Gastroesophageal Reflux: Medical Treatment

H. FRANKLIN HERLONG, M.D.

Associate Professor of Medicine, The Johns Hopkins University School of Medicine, Baltimore, Maryland
Hepatorenal Syndrome and Ascites

BASIL ISAAC HIRSCHOWITZ, B.Sc., M.B., B.Ch., M.D., F.A.C.P., F.R.C.P.E., F.R.C.P.

Professor of Medicine, Professor of Physiology and Biophysics, Univeristy of Alabama School of Medicine; Director, Division of Gastroenterology, Department of Medicine, University of Alabama School of Medicine; Consultant, Birmingham Veterans Administration Hospital, Birmingham, Alabama
Duodenal Ulcer

JEFFREY S. HYAMS, M.D.

Assistant Professor of Pediatrics, University of Connecticut School of Medicine, Farmington, Connecticut; Director, Division of Pediatric Gastroenterology, Hartford Hospital, Hartford, Connecticut
Gastrointestinal Bleeding in Children

FRANK LYNN IBER, M.D.

Professor of Medicine, University of Maryland School of Medicine; Gastroenterologist, Veterans Administration Medical Center and University of Maryland Hospital, Baltimore, Maryland
Portal Hypertension

DAVID G. JAGELMAN, M.S.(Lond), F.R.C.S.(Eng), F.A.C.S.

Head, Section of Familial Polyposis; Staff Surgeon, Department of Colorectal Surgery, Cleveland Clinic Foundation, Cleveland, Ohio
Familial Polyposis Coli and Hereditary Cancer of the Colon

ROBERT T. JENSEN, M.D.

Senior Investigator Digestive Diseases Branch, National Institute of Arthritis, Diabetes, Digestive and Kidney Diseases, National Institutes of Health, Bethesda, Maryland
Gastrinoma

LAWRENCE F. JOHNSON, M.D., Col., M.C.

Professor of Medicine, Director, Digestive Disease Division, Uniformed Services University of the Health Sciences; Chief, Gastroenterology Service, Walter Reed Army Medical Center, Washington, District of Columbia
Esophageal Stricture

JAMES H. JOHNSTON, M.D.

Clinical Associate Professor of Medicine, University of Mississippi School of Medicine; Staff Physician, Saint Dominic Hospital and Baptist Medical Center, Jackson, Mississippi
Lower Gastrointestinal Bleeding

IAN T. JONES, M.B., B.S., F.R.A.C.S., F.R.C.S.

Clinical Associate Staff, Department of Colon and Rectal Surgery, The Cleveland Clinic Foundation, Cleveland, Ohio
Ostomy Care

PAUL A. KANTROWITZ, M.D.

Assistant Clinical Professor of Medicine, Harvard Medical School, Boston, Massachusetts; Chief of Gastroenterology, Mount Auburn Hospital, Cambridge, Massachusetts
Infectious Esophagitis

STEPHEN L. KAUFMAN, M.D.

Associate Professor of Radiology, The Johns Hopkins School of Medicine, Baltimore, Maryland
Percutaneous Transhepatic Biliary Drainage and Retained Biliary Stone Extraction

RUSSELL D. KEINATH, M.D.

Instructor in Internal Medicine; Fellow in Gastroenterology, University of Michigan Medical School, Ann Arbor, Michigan
Whipple's Disease

KEITH A. KELLY, M.D.

Roberts Professor of Surgery, Mayo Medical School; Head, Section of Gastroenterologic and General Surgery, Mayo Clinic, Rochester, Minnesota
Ileostomy Alternatives

GERALD T. KEUSCH, M.D.

Professor of Medicine, Tufts University School of Medicine; Attending Physician and Chief, Division of Geographic Medicine, Department of Medicine, New England Medical Center, Boston, Massachusetts
Endocarditis Prophylaxis

RAYMOND S. KOFF, M.D.

Professor of Medicine, Boston University School of Medicine; Chief, Hepatology Sections, Boston University Medical Center and Veterans Administration Medical Center, Boston, Massachusetts
Chronic Hepatitis

BURTON I. KORELITZ, M.D.

Clinical Professor of Medicine, New York Medical College, Valhalla, New York; Chief, Section of Gastroenterology, Lenox Hill Hospital, New York, New York
Crohn's Disease of the Colon

GUENTER J. KREJS, M.D.

Professor of Internal Medicine, University of Texas Southwestern Medical School, Dallas, Texas
Functional Diarrhea

JOHN RICHARD LAKE, M.D.

Senior Research Fellow, University of California, San Francisco, California
Cholestasis and Sclerosing Cholangitis

JOHN D. LLOYD-STILL, M.D.

Professor of Pediatrics, Northwestern University Medical School; Head, Division of Gastroenterology, Director, Cystic Fibrosis Center, Children's Memorial Hospital, Chicago, Illinois
Cystic Fibrosis

MAURO MALAVOLTI, M.D.

Visiting Assistant Professor, George Washington University School of Medicine and Health Sciences, Washington, District of Columbia
Cholelithiasis

DANIEL G. MALONE, M.D.

Senior Staff Fellow, Section of Mast Cell Physiology, Laboratory of Clinical Investigation, National Institute of Allergy and Infectious Diseases, National Institutes of Health, Bethesda, Maryland
Allergic Gastroenteropathy

SIMEON MARGOLIS, M.D., Ph.D.

Professor of Medicine and Biological Chemistry, The Johns Hopkins University School of Medicine; Active Staff, The Johns Hopkins Hospital, Baltimore, Maryland
Postprandial Hypoglycemia
Food Fads and Alternatives

RICHARD W. McCALLUM, M.D., F.A.C.P., F.R.A.C.P.(Austral), F.A.C.G.

Professor of Medicine, University of Virginia School of Medicine; Chief of the Division of Gastroenterology, University of Virginia Medical Center, Charlottesville, Virginia
Functional Disorders of the Upper Gastrointestinal Tract

CHARLES E. McQUEEN, M.D.

Assistant Professor of Medicine, Uniformed Services University of the Health Sciences, Bethesda, Maryland; Staff, Department of Gastroenterology, Walter Reed Army Institute of Research, Washington, District of Columbia
Traveler's Diarrhea

DEAN D. METCALFE, M.D.

Senior Investigator; Chief, Section of Mast Cell Physiology, Laboratory of Clinical Investigation, National Institute of Allergy and Infectious Diseases, National Institutes of Health, Bethesda, Maryland
Allergic Gastroenteropathy

ESTEBAN MEZEY, M.D.

Professor of Medicine, The Johns Hopkins University School of Medicine; Staff Physician, Division of Gastroenterology, The Johns Hopkins Hospital, Baltimore, Maryland
Alcoholic Liver Disease

MACK C. MITCHELL, M.D.

Assistant Professor of Medicine, The Johns Hopkins University School of Medicine; Active Staff Physician, The Johns Hopkins Hospital, Baltimore, Maryland
Drug-Induced Liver Damage

KATHLEEN J. MOTIL, M.D., Ph.D.

Assistant Professor of Pediatrics, Baylor College of Medicine; Investigator, USDA/ARS Children's Nutrition Research Center, Physician, Section on Nutrition and Gastroenterology, Texas Children's Hospital, Houston, Texas
Growth Failure in Inflammatory Bowel Disease

GARY A. NEWMAN, M.D.

Assistant Clinical Professor of Medicine, Jefferson Medical College of Thomas Jefferson University; Consultant Gastroenterologist, Lankenau Hospital, Philadelphia, Pennsylvania
Functional Disorders of the Upper Gastrointestinal Tract

SANTHAT NIVATVONGS, M.D., F.A.C.S.

Associate Professor of Surgery, Division of Colon and Rectal Surgery, University of Minnesota Medical School, Minneapolis, Minnesota
Anorectal Disorders

ROY C. ORLANDO, M.D.

Associate Professor of Medicine, University of North Carolina at Chapel Hill School of Medicine, Chapel Hill, North Carolina
Barrett's Esophagus

S. CHRIS PAPPAS, M.D., F.R.C.P.(C)

Assistant Professor of Medicine, University of Toronto Faculty of Medicine; Staff Physician, Liver Disease Program, Division of Gastroenterology, Sunnybrook Medical

Center, Toronto, Ontario, Canada
Fulminant Hepatic Failure

RENE PELEMAN, M.D.

Fellow in Gastroenterology, University of Pittsburgh School of Medicine, Pittsburgh, Pennsylvania
Liver Transplantation: Gastroenterologic Considerations

MARK A. PEPPERCORN, M.D.

Associate Professor of Medicine, Harvard Medical School; Director of Gastroenterology Clinic, Beth Israel Hospital, Boston, Massachusetts
Ulcerative Colitis and Proctitis

JAY A. PERMAN, M.D.

Associate Professor of Pediatrics, The Johns Hopkins University School of Medicine; Director, Pediatric Gastroneterology and Nutrition, The Johns Hopkins Children's Center, Baltimore, Maryland
Carbohydrate Malabsorption

WILLIAM PETERSON, M.D.

Fellow in Gastroenterology, University of Pittsburgh School of Medicine, Pittsburgh, Pennsylvania
Liver Transplantation: Gastroenterologic Considerations

DAVID A. PEURA, M.D., Col., M.C.

Associate Professor of Medicine, Digestive Disease Division, Uniformed Services University of the Health Sciences, Bethesda, Maryland; Director, Clinical Services, Gastroenterology Service, Walter Reed Army Medical Center, Washington, District of Columbia
Esophageal Stricture

J. LOREN PITCHER, M.D., F.A.C.P.

Professor of Medicine, Associate Dean for Clinical Affairs and Medical Director, University of New Mexico School of Medicine and University of New Mexico Hospital, Albuquerque, New Mexico
Acute Upper Gastrointestinal Bleeding

HENRY A. PITT, M.D.

Associate Professor of Surgery, The Johns Hopkins University School of Medicine; The Johns Hopkins Hospital, Baltimore, Maryland
Acute Cholecystitis

THOMAS POZEFSKY, M.D.

Assistant Professor of Medicine, The Johns Hopkins University School of Medicine, Baltimore, Maryland
Obesity

DANIEL H. PRESENT, M.D.

Associate Clinical Professor of Medicine, Mount Sinai School of Medicine of the City University of New York, New York, New York
Fulminant Colitis and Toxic Megacolon

THOMAS C. QUINN, M.D.

Associate Professor of Medicine, The Johns Hopkins University School of Medicine, Baltimore, Maryland; Senior Investigator, Laboratory of Immunoregulation, National Institute of Allergy and Infectious Diseases, Bethesda, Maryland
Parasites of the Small Intestine

WILLIAM J. RAVICH, M.D.

Assistant Professor in Medicine, Gastroenterology Division, Clinical Director, The Swallowing Center, The Johns Hopkins University School of Medicine; Director, Gastrointestinal Lab and Endoscopy Unit, The Johns Hopkins Hospital, Baltimore, Maryland
Pharyngeal Dysphagia

ROLANDO H. ROLANDELLI, M.D.

Research Associate, Harrison Department of Surgical Research, University of Pennsylvania School of Medicine; Fellow in Nutrition and Metabolism, Philadelphia Veterans Administration Medical Center, Philadelphia, Pennsylvania
Enteral Feeding: Liquid Formula Diets

JOHN L. ROMBEAU, M.D., F.A.C.S.

Assistant Professor of Surgery, University of Pennsylvania School of Medicine; Director of Nutritional Support Service, Veterans Administration Medical Center, Philadelphia, Pennsylvania
Enteral Feeding: Liquid Formula Diets

JOEL J. ROSLYN, M.D.

Assistant Professor of Surgery, University of California School of Medicine, UCLA Medical Center, Los Angeles, California
Acute Cholecystitis

JOHN L. SAWYERS, M.D.

Professor of Surgery and Director, Section of Surgical Sciences, Vanderbilt University School of Medicine; Surgeon-in-Chief, Vanderbilt University Medical Center, Nashville, Tennessee
Peptic Ulcer Disease: Surgical Treatment

BRUCE F. SCHARSCHMIDT, M.D.

Professor of Medicine, University of California School of Medicine, San Francisco, California
Cholestasis and Sclerosing Cholangitis

DAVID SCHREIBER, M.D.

Fellow in Gastroenterology, University of Pittsburgh School of Medicine, Pittsburgh, Pennsylvania
Liver Transplantation: Gastroenterologic Considerations

PAUL C. SCHROY III, M.D.

Fellow, Cornell University Medical College; Senior Clinical and Research Fellow, Gastroenterology Service,

Department of Medicine, Memorial Sloan-Kettering Cancer Center, New York, New York
Bone Marrow Transplant: Gastrointestinal Considerations

MARVIN M. SCHUSTER, M.D.

Professor of Medicine and Psychiatry, The Johns Hopkins University School of Medicine; Director, Division of Digestive Diseases, Francis Scott Key Medical Center, Baltimore, Maryland
Irritable Bowel Syndrome

LEONARD B. SEEFF, M.D.

Professor of Medicine, Georgetown University School of Medicine; Chief, Gastroenterology-Hepatology Section, Veterans Administration Medical Center, Washington, District of Columbia
Acute Viral Hepatitis

HARRY S. SHABSIN, Ph.D.

Instructor, Department of Psychiatry and Behavorial Sciences, Division of Behavorial Biology, The Johns Hopkins University School of Medicine; Director, Gastrointestinal Pain Center, Division of Digestive Diseases, Francis Scott Key Medical Center, Baltimore, Maryland
Chronic Abdominal Pain: A Cognitive Behavioral Treatment Approach

SOL SILVERMAN Jr., D.D.S.

Professor and Chairman of Oral Medicine, University of California School of Medicine, San Francisco, California
Painful Mouth

JAMES V. SITZMANN, M.D.

Assistant Professor of Surgery, The Johns Hopkins University School of Medicine, Baltimore, Maryland
High Biliary Stricture

MICHAEL V. SIVAK Jr., M.D.

Head, Section of Gastrointestinal Endoscopy, Department of Gastroenterology, Cleveland Clinic, Cleveland, Ohio
Sclerotherapy of Esophageal Varices

DAVID B. SKINNER, M.D.

Dallas B. Phemister Professor and Chairman of Surgery, University of Chicago, Chicago, Illinois
Cancer of the Esoplhagus and Cardia: Surgical Treatment

ADAM NEIL SMITH, M.D., F.R.C.S.

Reader in Surgery, Department of Surgery/Urology, University of Edinburgh; Consultant Surgeon, Gastrointestinal Unit, University of Edinburgh, Western General Hospital, Edinburgh, Scotland
Diverticular Disease of the Colon

KONRAD H. SOERGEL, M.D.

Professor of Medicine, University of Wisconsin Medical School; Chief, Section of Gastroenterology, Froedtert Memorial Lutheran Hospital, Milwaukee, Wisconsin
Diabetic Diarrhea

NORMAN SOHN, M.D., F.A.C.S.

Clinical Assistant Professor of Surgery, New York Medical College, Valhalla, New York; Associate Surgeon, Lenox Hill Hospital, New York, New York
Rectal Carcinoma: Sphincter Sparing Procedures

PETER SPEELMAN, M.D.

Senior Fellow, Department of Medicine, University of Washington School of Medicine; Infectious Disease Division, Harborview Medical Center, Seattle, Washington
Sexually Transmitted Intestinal Disease

WALTER E. STAMM, M.D.

Associate Professor of Medicine, University of Washington School of Medicine; Head, Infectious Disease Division, Harborview Medical Center, Seattle, Washington
Sexually Transmitted Intestinal Disease

ROBERT G. STRICKLAND, M.D., F.R.A.C.P., F.A.C.P.

Professor of Medicine, Head, Division of Gastroenterology, Department of Medicine, University of New Mexico School of Medicine, Albuquerque, New Mexico
Premalignant Conditions of the Stomach

JOHN R. STROEHLEIN, M.D.

Associate Professor of Clinical Medicine, Baylor College of Medicine; Director, Endoscopy Unit/Digestive Disease Laboratory, The Methodist Hospital, Houston, Texas
Gastric Carcinoma

PAUL H. SUGARBAKER, M.D.

Department of Surgery, National Cancer Institute, National Institutes of Health, Bethesda, Maryland
Hepatic Neoplasia

ALAN G. SUNSHINE, M.D.

Fellow in Gastroenterology, Hospital of the University of Pennsylvania, Philadelphia, Pennsylvania
Diffuse Esophageal Spasm and Related Disorders

FRANCIS JOSEPH TEDESCO, M.D.

Professor of Medicine; Chief, Section of Gastroenterology, Department of Medicine, Vice President for Clinical Activities, Medical College of Georgia School of Medicine, Augusta, Georgia
Parasitic Diseases of the Colon

MARK L. TEITELBAUM, M.D.

Assistant Professor of Psychiatry and Medicine, The Johns Hopkins University School of Medicine; Director, Psychiatric Consultation-Liaison Service, The Johns Hopkins Hospital, Baltimore, Maryland
Hypochondriasis, Hysteria, and Depression

DANIEL W. THOMAS, M.D.

Assistant Professor of Pediatrics, University of Southern California School of Medicine; Attending Gastroenterologist, Children's Hospital of Los Angeles, Los Angeles, California
Protein-Losing Enteropathy

PHILLIP P. TOSKES, M.D.

Professor of Medicine, University of Florida College of Medicine; Director, Division of Gastroenterology, Hepatology and Nutrition, University of Florida College of Medicine and Veterans Administration Medical Center, Gainsville, Florida
Chronic Pancreatitis: Exocrine and Endocrine Insufficiencies

PHILIP A. TUMULTY, M.D.

David J. Carver, Professor Emeritus of Medicine, The Johns Hopkins Hospital, Baltimore, Maryland
Functional Illness

JON A. van HEERDEN, M.B., Ch.B., F.R.C.S.(C), F.A.C.S., M.S. (Surg) (Minn)

Professor of Surgery, Mayo Medical School, Rochester, Minnesota
Pancreatic and Periampullary Neoplasia

DAVID H. VAN THIEL, M.D.

Professor of Medicine, Chief of Gastroenterology, University of Pittsburgh School of Medicine, Pittsburgh, Pennsylvania
Liver Transplantation: Gastroenterologic Considerations

RAMA P. VENU, M.D., F.A.C.P., F.A.C.G.

Associate Clinical Professor of Medicine, Department of Gastroenterology, Medical College of Wisconsin, Milwaukee, Wisconsin; Consultant in Gastroenterology, Froedtert Lutheran Memorial Hospital, Milwaukee, Wisconsin, St. Luke's Hospital and St. Mary's Medical Center, Racine, Wisconsin
Endoscopy in Bile Duct Obstruction and Ampullary Dysfunction

ARNOLD WALD, M.D.

Associate Professor of Medicine, University of Pittsburgh School of Medicine; Head, Gastroenterology Unit, Montefiore Hospital, Pittsburgh, Pennsylvania
Incontinence

JOHN M. WALSHE

Reader in Metabolic Disease, University of Cambridge; Physician, Addenbrooke's Hospital, Cambridge, England
Wilson's Disease

ANDREW L. WARSHAW, M.D.

Associate Professor of Surgery, Harvard Medical School; Visiting Surgeon, Massachusetts General Hospital, Boston, Massachusetts
Pancreatitis: Surgical Considerations

JEROME D. WAYE, M.D.

Clinical Professor of Medicine, Mount Sinai School of Medicine of the City University of New York; Chief, Gastrointestinal Endoscopy Unit, Mount Sinai Hospital and Lenox Hill Hospital, New York, New York
Polyps of the Colon

WILLIAM ALLEN WEBB, M.D.

Associate Professor of Surgery, University of South Alabama College of Medicine, Mobile, Alabama; Head, Endoscopy Section, Surgical Clinic, Opelika, Alabama
Foreign Body Extraction from the Upper Gastrointestinal Tract

JACK D. WELSH, M.D.

Professor of Medicine, University of Oklahoma Health Sciences Center; Oklahoma Memorial Hospital and Veterans Administration Medical Center, Oklahoma City, Oklahoma
Intestinal Gas

ELLIOT WESER, M.D., F.A.C.P.

Professor of Medicine, University of Texas Health Science Center; Chief, Medicine Service, Audie L. Murphy Memorial Veterans Hospital, San Antonio, Texas
Short Bowel Syndrome

SIDNEY J. WINAWER, M.D.

Professor of Clinical Medicine, Cornell University Medical College; Chief, Gastroenterology Service, Department of Medicine, Memorial Sloan-Kettering Cancer Center, New York, New York
Bone Marrow Transplant: Gastrointestinal Considerations

PETER YANG, M.D.

Assistant Professor, Division of Gastroenterology, Department of Medicine, Case Western Reserve University School of Medicine; Director, Gastrointestinal Procedure Unit, University Hospital of Cleveland, Cleveland, Ohio
Bacterial Overgrowth Syndrome

MICHAEL J. ZINNER, M.D., F.A.C.S.

Associate Professor of Surgery, The Johns Hopkins University School of Medicine; The Johns Hopkins Hospital, Baltimore, Maryland
Stress Ulcer and Acute Erosive Gastritis

ALVIN M. ZFASS, M.D.

Professor of Medicine, Director of Endoscopy, Medical College of Virginia of Virginia Commonwealth University, Richmond, Virginia
Constipation

EVA SARA ZINREICH, M.D.

Assistant Professor of Oncology, Radiology and Radiological Sciences, The Johns Hopkins University School of Medicine, Baltimore, Maryland and T-G Mures, Romania
Cancer of the Esophagus: Radiation Treatment

PREFACE

I agreed to edit this text on therapy in digestive diseases feeling that the medical, surgical, and nutritional therapeutic options for these disorders had increased dramatically in the past decade.

Although there are excellent textbooks on the diagnosis and pathophysiology of gastrointestinal and liver diseases, these texts often do not provide specific and detailed guidelines or recommendations for the physician caring for an individual patient. As an alternative, the reader-practitioner may consult reviews of the literature, which often describe the results of well-performed clinical trials, and still be left without the answer to his specific patient care problem. It was this realization—that information on therapy may be hard to extract from the literature—that led to the preparation of *Current Therapy in Gastroenterology and Liver Disease: 1984-1985*.

Sales of the first volume were brisk, and feedback from readers has been gratifying. They appreciated the personalized opinions of the authors and their precise suggestions at various decision points. Reviewers also pointed out that they could quickly find answers to questions that are not covered in many major textbooks. The reviewer in the *New England Journal of Medicine* felt the 1984-1985 book had passed his "ultimate test." It became the most used book on his desk. This praise was echoed both by purchasers and by the authors of the many chapters. I was pleased with the response to that edition.

In this all-new second edition, every chapter has been written by a new author. Ten new subjects have been added, bringing the number of chapters to 108. I have included topics that arose as clinical issues during the past year at the Harvey M. and Lyn P. Meyerhoff Digestive Disease-Inflammatory Bowel Disease Center at The Johns Hopkins Hospital, believing them to be problems faced by gastroenterologists around the country. The authors were chosen because of their knowledge of the specific subject and also, quite importantly, because they are actively caring for patients with the disorders about which they have written. I asked the authors, who represent 72 different medical centers, to give direct advice as if they were providing a consultation when seeing an individual patient. Concise but thorough guidelines to therapy have been provided, with the assumption that the correct diagnosis has been established. Although the use of references has been minimized, authors have tried to give their rationale for particularly controversial opinions. Alternative approaches, potential side effects, and common dosage forms, as well as parameters for monitoring therapy, are provided. On some unsettled issues, advocates from both sides present their views.

While the target audience for this book is the experienced practitioner who is familiar with digestive diseases, I have found that medical and surgical house officers appreciate information from a specific chapter that applies to a patient currently in their care. Even though much of the discussion focuses on adults, ten chapters deal with problems common to children and adolescents. Since there is a close interaction between the medical and the surgical considerations in digestive disease care, both aspects have been stressed in many of the chapters. Twenty-three of the chapters have been written by surgeons. In addition, many of the subjects, such as those concerning nutrition and those focusing on psychologic aspects of care, would be of interest to a variety of health professionals.

Although the nature of the book is opinionated and perhaps dogmatic in areas, it is obvious that modes of therapy will change as new drugs and new procedures are developed and new clinical trials are published. We plan to incorporate such changes in a subsequent edition in two years.

My sincere appreciation is extended to the authors who have shared their expertise and experience with us. Thanks also to my wife and sons; to my secretary, Lois Williams; to our publisher, Brian Decker and his staff for conceiving and providing this excellent and timely series of therapy volumes; and especially to Mary Mansor and her colleagues, who edited the manuscripts.

Theodore M. Bayless

CONTENTS

Esophagus

Painful Mouth 1
  Sol Silverman Jr.

Gastroesophageal Reflux: Medical
Treatment 6
  Thomas R. Hendrix

Esophageal Reflux: Surgical
Treatment 9
  Tom R. DeMeester

Barrett's Esophagus 16
  Roy C. Orlando

Caustic Injury 20
  Barry A. Frank
  H. Worth Boyce Jr.

Esophageal Stricture 25
  David A. Peura
  Lawrence F. Johnson

Laser Treatment in Gastrointestinal
Disease 30
  David E. Fleischer

Diffuse Esophageal Spasm and
Related Disorders 33
  Alan G. Sunshine
  Sidney Cohen

Achalasia 37
  Donald O. Castell

Pharyngeal Dysphagia 39
  William J. Ravich

Foreign Body Extraction from the
Upper Gastrointestinal Tract 44
  William Allen Webb

Sclerotherapy of Esophageal
Varices 48
  Michael V. Sivak Jr.

Cancer of the Esophagus and Cardia:
Surgical Treatment 54
  Mark K. Ferguson
  David B. Skinner

Cancer of the Esophagus:
Radiation Treatment 57
  Eva Sara Zinreich

Infectious Esophagitis 61
  Paul A. Kantrowitz

Stomach and Duodenum

Duodenal Ulcer 66
  Basil Isaac Hirschowitz

Gastric Ulcer 69
  David Y. Graham

Peptic Ulcer Disease:
Surgical Treatment 72
  John L. Sawyers

Gastrinoma 77
  Robert T. Jensen
  Jerry D. Gardner

Acute Upper Gastrointestinal
Bleeding 80
  J. Loren Pitcher

Gastrointestinal Bleeding in
Children 88
  Jeffrey S. Hyams

xv

Stress Ulcer and Acute Erosive
Gastritis 91
  Michael J. Zinner

Alkaline Reflux Gastritis 93
  Thomas R. Gadacz

Disorders of Gastric Emptying 95
  Robert S. Fisher

Functional Disorders of the Upper
Gastrointestinal Tract 100
  Gary A. Newman
  Richard W. McCallum

Obesity 106
  Thomas Pozefsky

Anorexia Nervosa and Bulimia 116
  Paul E. Garfinkel

Gastric Carcinoma 120
  John R. Stroehlein
  Jaffer A. Ajani

Premalignant Conditions of the
Stomach 124
  Robert G. Strickland

Intraoperative Irradiation 129
  Leonard L. Gunderson

Hypochondriasis, Hysteria, and
Depression 134
  Mark L. Teitelbaum

Functional Illness 137
  Philip A. Tumulty

Chronic Abdominal Pain: A Cognitive
Behavioral Treatment Approach 141
  Harry S. Shabsin

Chronic Intractable Abdominal Pain 145
  Richard G. Black

Carbohydrate Malabsorption 149
  Jay A. Perman

Postprandial Hypoglycemia 153
  Angeliki Georgopoulos
  Simeon Margolis

Bacterial Overgrowth Syndrome 156
  John G. Banwell
  Peter Yang

Whipple's Disease 160
  Russell D. Keinath
  William O. Dobbins III

Celiac Sprue and Related Diseases 162
  Adrian P. Douglas

Parasites of the Small Intestine 166
  Thomas C. Quinn

Short Bowel Syndrome 172
  Elliot Weser

Hyperoxaluria and Nephrolithiasis 175
  John Whitby Dobbins

Diabetic Diarrhea 179
  Konrad H. Soergel

Gastrointestinal Disorders in the
Immunodeficient State 181
  Marvin Earl Ament

Bone Marrow Transplant:
Gastrointestinal Considerations 188
  Paul C. Schroy III
  Sidney J. Winawer

Allergic Gastroenteropathy 193
  Daniel G. Malone
  Dean D. Metcalfe

Protein-Losing Enteropathy 197
  Daniel W. Thomas

Parenteral Nutrition 201
  C. Richard Fleming

Enteral Feeding: Liquid Formula
Diets 206
  Rolando H. Rolandelli
  John L. Rombeau

Food Fads and Alternatives 213
   Simeon Margolis

Crohn's Disease of the Small Bowel 216
   Stephen B. Hanauer

Growth Failure in Inflammatory
Bowel Disease 223
   Richard J. Grand
   Kathleen J. Motil

Crohn's Disease: Surgical Treatment 229
   Arthur H. Aufses Jr.

Intestinal Obstruction 232
   Gregory B. Bulkley

Intestinal Ischemia 239
   Marc Cooperman

Secretory Diarrhea 244
   Kiertisin Dharmsathaphorn

Constipation 248
   Alastair M. Connell
   Alvin M. Zfass

Chronic Intestinal
Pseudo-Obstruction 251
   Sinn Anuras

Acute Infectious Diarrhea 253
   Gail L. Bongiovanni
   Ralph A. Giannella

Traveler's Diarrhea 257
   Charles E. McQueen
   Edgar C. Boedeker

Parasitic Diseases of the Colon 262
   Francis Joseph Tedesco

Sexually Transmitted Intestinal
Disease 264
   Peter Speelman
   Walter E. Stamm

Intra-abdominal Sepsis 270
   John Gill Bartlett

Endocarditis Prophylaxis 277
   Francois Auclair
   Gerald T. Keusch

Ulcerative Colitis and Proctitis 279
   Mark A. Peppercorn

Fulminant Colitis and
Toxic Megacolon 284
   Daniel H. Present

Crohn's Disease of the Colon 291
   Burton I. Korelitz

Idiopathic Inflammatory Bowel Disease
and Neoplasia 296
   Theodore M. Bayless

Anorectal Disorders 301
   Santhat Nivatvongs
   Stanley M. Goldberg

Incontinence 307
   Arnold Wald

Ostomy Care 310
   Victor W. Fazio
   Ian T. Jones

Ileostomy Alternatives 314
   Keith A. Kelly

Rectal Carcinoma: Sphincter
Sparing Procedures 318
   Norman Sohn

Colorectal Carcinoma:
Adjuvant Therapy 320
   Anthony N. Brannan
   Robert W. Beart Jr.

Polyps of the Colon 325
   Jerome D. Waye

Familial Polyposis Coli and
Hereditary Cancer of the Colon 328
   David G. Jagelman

Lower Gastrointestinal Bleeding 333
James H. Johnston

Intestinal Gas 340
Jack D. Welsh

Irritable Bowel Syndrome 342
Marvin M. Schuster

Diverticular Disease of the Colon 345
Adam Neil Smith

Recurrent Abdominal Pain in
Childhood and Adolescence 349
Ronald G. Barr

Functional Diarrhea 353
Guenter J. Krejs

LIVER, BILIARY TRACT, AND PANCREAS

Drug Use in Patients with
Hepatic Disease 356
Gilbert Deray
Robert A. Branch

Hepatorenal Syndrome and Ascites 361
H. Franklin Herlong

Portosystemic Encephalopathy 366
Laurence M. Blendis

Alcoholism 369
Enoch Gordis

Alcoholic Liver Disease 374
Esteban Mezey

Portal Hypertension 376
Frank Lynn Iber

Acute Viral Hepatitis 380
Leonard B. Seeff

Fulminant Hepatic Failure 383
S. Chris Pappas

Chronic Hepatitis 387
Raymond S. Koff

Drug-Induced Liver Damage 391
Mack C. Mitchell

Liver Transplantation:
Gastroenterologic Considerations 394
David H. Van Thiel
Mark Appler
David Schreiber
Jeffrey Gray
Rene Peleman
Byron DeLemos
William Peterson

Primary Biliary Cirrhosis 397
John H. Helzberg
James L. Boyer

Cholestasis and Sclerosing
Cholangitis 400
John Gregory Fitz
John Richard Lake
Bruce F. Scharschmidt

Wilson's Disease 406
John M. Walshe

Hemochromatosis 409
William P. Baldus

Hepatic Neoplasia 412
Paul H. Sugarbaker

High Biliary Stricture 418
James V. Sitzmann

Cholelithiasis 422
Hans Fromm
Mauro Malavolti

Percutaneous Transhepatic Biliary
Drainage and Retained Biliary
Stone Extraction 424
Stephen L. Kaufman

Endoscopy in Bile Duct Obstruction
and Ampullary Dysfunction 429
Joseph E. Geenen
Rama P. Venu

Acute Cholecystitis 433
Joel J. Roslyn
Henry A. Pitt

Acute Pancreatitis: Medical
Considerations 437
Peter A. Banks

Pancreatitis: Surgical Considerations 442
Andrew L. Warshaw

Chronic Pancreatitis: Exocrine and
Endocrine Insufficiencies 447
Phillip P. Toskes

Cystic Fibrosis 450
John D. Lloyd-Still

Pancreatic and Periampullary
Neoplasia 455
Jon A. van Heerden

ESOPHAGUS

PAINFUL MOUTH

SOL SILVERMAN Jr., D.D.S.

Oral pain is an extremely common complaint. The source can be local benign traumatic, infectious, inflammatory, or neoplastic disease; the pain can be due to oral manifestations of systemic diseases, such as blood dyscrasias, Crohn's disease, or diabetes mellitus; or it can be a medication-induced symptom. Oral malignancies and neuropathies also are associated with pain. The most frequently encountered pain-associated lesions will be covered in this chapter.

APHTHOUS ULCERS

Aphthous ulcers (canker sores) occur in about 30 percent of the general population. They can appear at any age, and the number of ulcers and the frequency vary widely. While most lesions appear as single, well-circumscribed ulcers less than 6 mm in diameter, with surrounding erythema and accompanying discomfort, they may occur in batches or as large ulcers (major aphthae) exceeding 6 mm in diameter. The latter can be confused with other conditions and will persist for longer than the usual 1 to 2 weeks. The cause remains unknown, although there can be initiating factors, such as trauma or food (e.g., citrus, chocolate, nuts). There appears to be a genetic predisposition, since aphthae are more common when there is a positive family history (Fig. 1–A).

The major histologic defect is a lymphocytic invasion, so it is reasonable that the best and most reproducibly effective management is the use of systemic and/or topical corticosteroids. Lidex ointment (0.05%) mixed with equal parts Orabase applied four to eight times daily is effective. Systemic prednisone in daily doses from 30 to 40 mg will usually control most attacks in less than a week, often in a few days. Use of a larger dose for a short period of time rather than the converse is more efficacious and causes fewer adverse effects. Systemic dosage form is usually preferred (when treatment is indicated) because of the convenience. In the otherwise healthy outpatient the main side effects (seen in fewer than half the patients) are slight bloating, frequency of urination, and insomnia. When treatment is less than a week, tapering the dose is not necessary. Repeated short-term therapy does not appear to incur any long-term adverse effects. Other empiric approaches have not been uniformly effective. Some patients with Crohn's disease and painful aphthous ulcers will improve with swishing of a prednisolone solution.

HERPES

Herpes infections with their associated pain occur in three forms: primary herpetic gingivostomatitis, herpes labialis (cold sore), and recurrent intraoral herpes.

Primary herpes usually occurs in youngsters, but can occur in adults. It is characterized by a sudden onset, oral pain, ulcers, and inflammation; malaise and fever; and lymphadenopathy. Except in the immunocompromised patient, antibodies are developed within a week, and healing is usually complete by the end of the second week. Treatment is supportive, except in the compromised patient, for whom intravenous (5 mg per kilogram body weight every 8 hours) or oral acyclovir (200 mg five to six times daily) must be considered.

Herpes labialis occurs in less than 20 percent of the general population and does not appear related to herpes antibody levels. Management is supportive, since all treatment studies, including acyclovir ointment (Zovirax ointment), have shown them not to be superior to empiric approaches. Corticosteroid ointments are helpful, since this is also an inflammatory lesion.

Recurrent herpes occurs only on keratinized mucosa (gingiva and palate). This is one of the features that aids in the differentiation of the unrelated aphthous ulcer, which occurs almost exclusively on unkeratinized mucosa. This condition is relatively rare and attacks vary in frequency. The attacks do not appear related to circulating antibody levels and are managed by empiric approaches. Since this is an inflammatory lesion and spread of virus has not been a problem, a topical corticosteroid (Lidex in Orabase) has been helpful.

VESICULOEROSIVE DISORDERS

Other benign but painful ulcerative oral mucosal diseases often are included in the differential diagnosis because of confusing signs and symptoms. These include erosive lichen planus (Fig. 1–B), erythema multiforme

(Fig. 1–C), pemphigoid, pemphigus, and lupus erythematosus. All of these conditions can occur without skin lesions and can have overlapping clinical signs and symptoms. The vesiculoerosive diseases can be diagnosed by a combination of clinical findings and biopsy. All are responsive to corticosteroids. Dosages vary considerably, however, depending upon patient response, general health, and side effects. Combination of prednisone (30 to 60 mg per day) with Imuran (50 to 100 mg per day) will often enhance corticosteroid efficacy and even allow a lower than usual prednisone dosage.

CANDIDIASIS

Candidiasis is becoming a more common cause of oral disease and discomfort. In the general population its occurrence as a part of the normal oral flora approximates 40 percent. Antibiotics, xerostomia (disease-, radiation-, or drug-induced), diabetes mellitus, anemia, and immunosuppression are common causes of candidiasis. It occurs commonly in AIDS victims and those at high-risk for AIDS as well as in denture wearers, since the denture material often serves as a reservoir for the fungus. Symptoms are usually those of pain, burning, and "bad taste." Signs include angular cheilitis, inflammation, and/or surface white colonies of fungi. The predominant species is *Candida albicans*.

Treatment includes altering any evident underlying condition, peroxide-saline mouth rinses (3% hydrogen peroxide mixed with equal parts saline), and antifungals. There is a range of antifungal medications: nystatin vaginal troches (100,000 U dissolved orally 3 to 4 times daily), Mycelex oral tablets (clotrimazole, 10-mg tablets dissolved, five times daily), or ketoconazole (Nizoral, 200 mg taken with food once daily). The antifungals are taken for 2 weeks. Some individuals have chronic candidiasis for unknown reasons and treatment may have to be prolonged and/or repeated frequently.

GINGIVITIS

Gingivitis, manifested primarily by erythema, edema, and ulceration, is most often a manifestation of a local irritation or infection (Fig. 1–E). The most common cause is poor hygiene which in turn leads to acute necrotizing ulcerative gingivitis (Vincent's infection). It is associated with pain and possibly bleeding and fever. Principle organisms are usually fusiform and spirochete species. Treatment involves an oxidizing mouth rinse (3% hydrogen peroxide mixed with equal parts warm water), improvement of oral hygiene, and, if the signs and symptoms warrant, an antibiotic (penicillin V, 1,000 to 1,500 mg per day is the first choice, and erythromycin in the same dosage is the second choice).

Care must be exercised, since similar signs and symptoms may be the first evidence of infectious mononucleosis and leukemia. Other conditions that must be included in the differential diagnosis are the vesiculoerosive inflammatory diseases of lichen planus, erythema multiforme, pemphigoid, pemphigus, and herpetic gingivitis. Therefore, biopsy must be considered if initial response fails or the diagnosis remains an enigma.

Gingivitis is often associated with periodontal disease (periodontitis, pyorrhea). This is caused by subgingival infections that lead to loss of supporting alveolar bone. In turn, this bone loss leads to pockets or spaces around the teeth. These pockets serve to accumulate debris, substrate, and bacteria (plaque) which accelerate the process.

Periodontal disease eventually leads to loosening of teeth and pain. In the early stages, however, it is not always apparent. Periodic dental examinations are essential to prevent this infection, which is the most common cause of tooth loss in adults. Office care involving careful subgingival curettage and conscientious home care (brushing, flossing, rinsing) often can prevent or control this process. Plaque-reducing mouth rinses are now becoming available (i.e., Viadent, 10 ml four times daily, held in the mouth 1 minute and then emptied).

GLOSSITIS

Glossitis is relatively common. It can occur as a loss of papillae (filiform) of the dorsal tongue and is usually accompanied by some degree of pain. The glossitis may be associated with an idiopathic transient and partial depapillation (geographic tongue, glossitis migrans [Fig. 1–D]) or may be the manifestation of systemic disease, such as iron deficient or megaloblastic anemias, hyperglycemia, or drug toxicity. It may also be due to xerostomia (drug- or disease-induced), candidiasis, or an allergy. Therefore, control depends upon appropriate testing to identify the cause.

Not too infrequently a patient, often an older female, may present with a normal appearing tongue that burns. This may be related to any of the above considerations or anxiety, and often it can be managed by a tranquilizer type drug or an antidepressant. Two drugs that have been helpful are chlordiazepoxide (5 to 10 mg three times daily) or amitriptyline (25 mg three to six times daily).

CARIES

Caries (dental decay) is commonly associated with spontaneous pain or discomfort in response to a chemical (food) or physical (chewing) irritants. It is well established that three essentials are required to produce the carious lesion: bacteria, a substrate, and a susceptible tooth. Conditions that predispose to xerostomia (e.g., tranquilizers and belladonna type drugs, Sjögren's syndrome, head and neck irradiation) may promote caries.

The diagnosis is based on x-ray examination (radiolucencies of the enamel and dentin) and clinical observation of an area of tooth structure that is soft, necrotic, discolored, and often sensitive. There is no absolute correlation between extent of caries and symptoms (pain).

Treatment includes the following: (1) restorative dentistry to remove decay; (2) proper mouth hygiene to reduce bacterial flora and substrate (frequent brushing

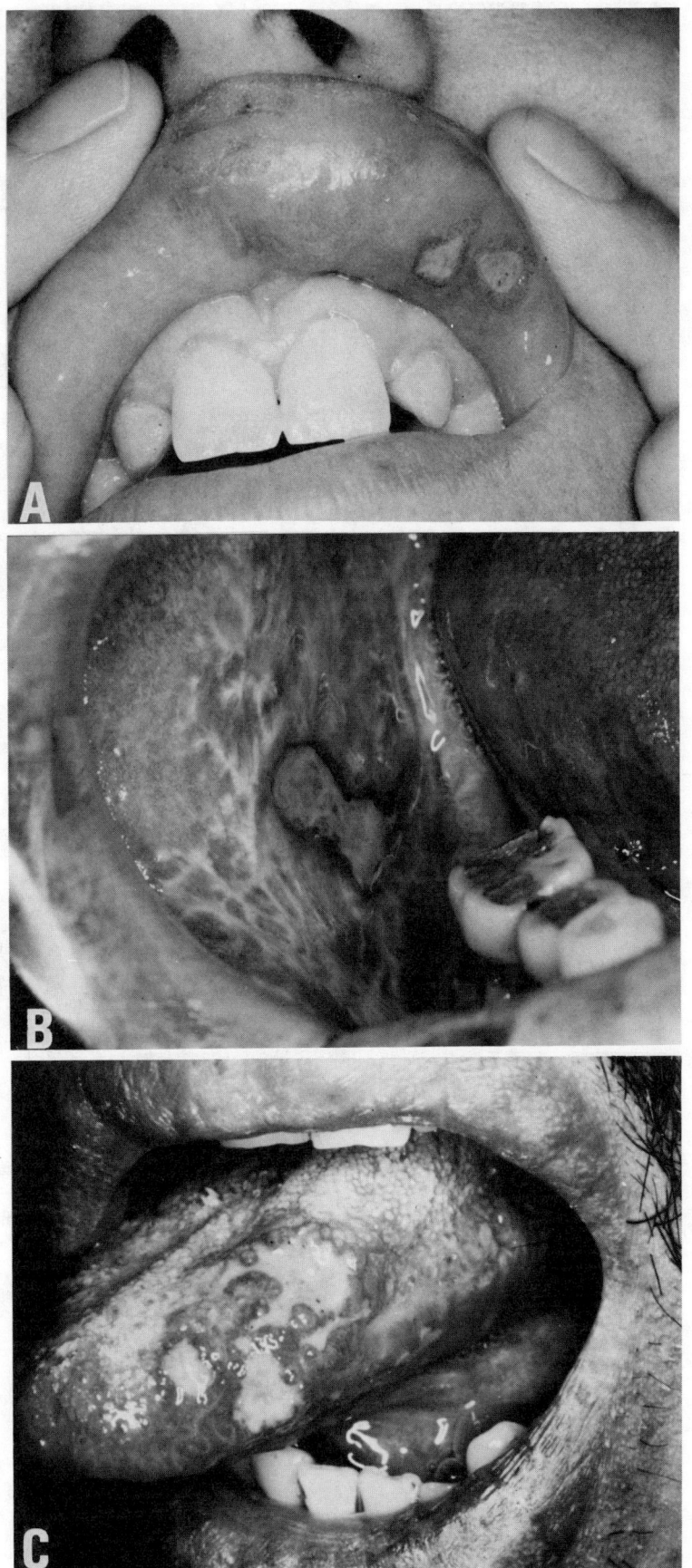

Figure 1 Some oral lesions associated with pain. *A*, Aphthous ulcers present for 1 week. *B*, Erosive lichen planus present for 1 year. *C*, Erythema multiforme present for 4 months.

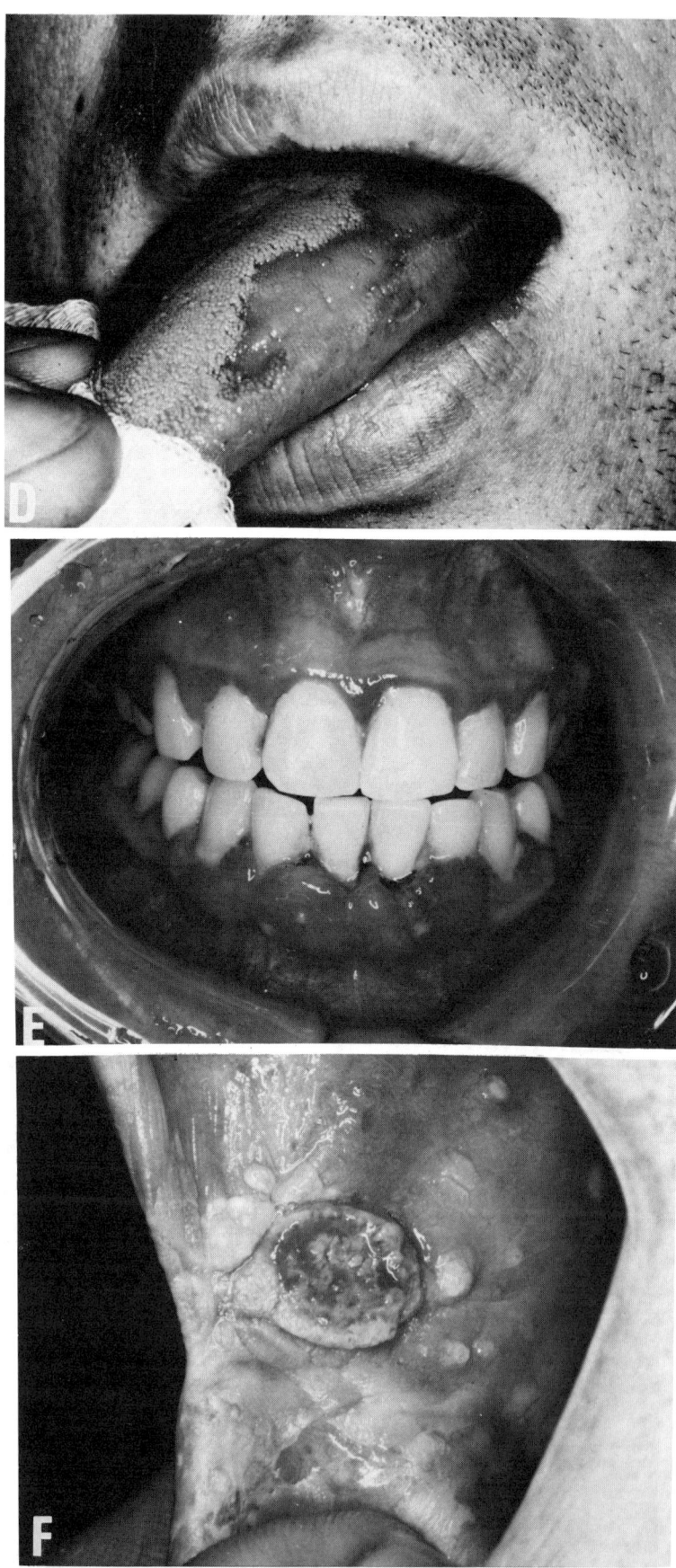

D, Recurrent glossitis migrans present for 2 weeks. *E*, Acute ulcerative gingivitis present for 3 weeks. *F*, Squamous carcinoma associated with buccal leukoplakia.

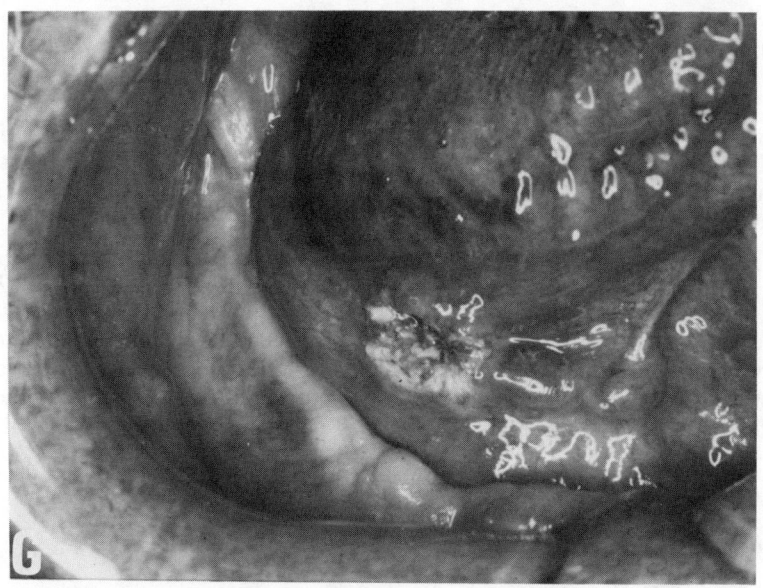

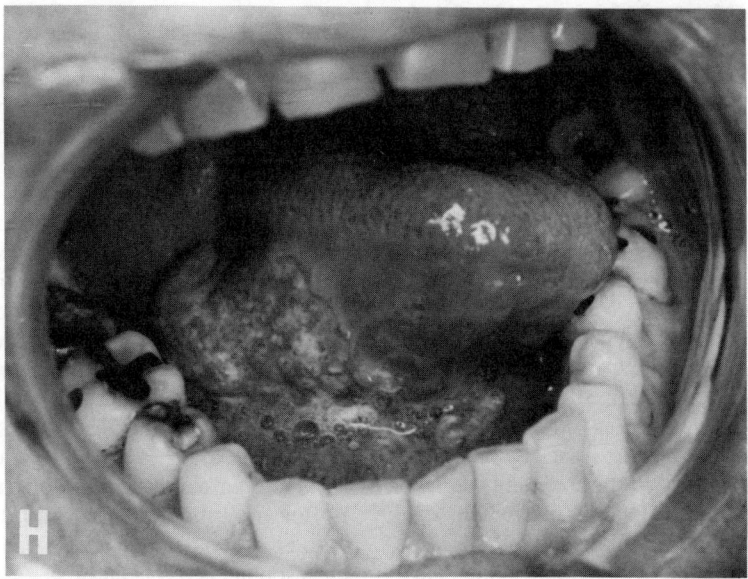

G, Early squamous carcinoma noticed for 1 month. *H*, Advanced squamous carcinoma noticed for 5 months.

with dentifrices and the use of mouth rinses); (3) reduction of carbohydrate (mainly sucrose) and sticky foods (e.g., jams, cookies, foods that tend to adhere to tooth surfaces for prolonged periods); and (4) topical applications of fluoride to form a more acid-resistant tooth structure (fluoroapatite instead of hydroxyapatite). Fluoride also contributes to bacterial control and remineralization.

If the bacteria reach the pulp of the tooth, an abscess will form and pain will increase. There may or may not be swelling. Often this is not localized to the offending tooth. While extraction or endodontia (root canal) is the only definitive treatment form, antibiotics and analgesics are needed in the interim. The antibiotic of choice is penicillin V, 1,000 to 1,500 mg daily, or erythromycin in the same dosage as a penicillin alternative. Tylenol with 30 to 60 mg codeine is usually sufficient for associated pain.

LEUKOPLAKIA

Leukoplakia (white patch) can occur on any mucosal surface (Fig. 1–F). When there is associated pain, it may indicate a dysplastic or malignant (squamous carcinoma) growth (Fig. 1–G, and 1–H). Most oral cancers, even in the very early stages, are associated with pain. The most frequent manifestations are erythema and ulceration (with or without leukoplakia). If such lesions are not reversible within 2 to 3 weeks by reducing trauma or irritation (e.g., tobacco, spicy foods, chemicals, dentures), a biopsy should be performed. It must be remembered that oral cancer accounts for about 4 percent of all cancers each year. The risk increases dramatically in smokers and drinkers.

MUCOSITIS

One of the most severe forms of oral pain is that associated with mucositis (stomatitis) induced by radiation, chemotherapy, and/or bone marrow transplants. Viscous xylocaine is often helpful, particularly before meals to help nutritional intake. Bland, warm mouth rinses may be helpful (baking soda with or without salt). Systemic analgesics are usually required. Because of focal infection, antibiotics must be considered. Clindamycin, 300 mg 4 times a day, is useful because of its broad spectrum and little evidence of developing resistant organisms or allergies. Current evidence implicates a herpetic stomatitis in many of these patients. Therefore, a culture and acyclovir (the equivalent of 5 mg per kilogram body weight every 8 hours) must be included in the management plan. Because of the frequency of candidiasis, antifungal medications (mentioned before) are in order, or amphotericin B if an intravenous route has been established. Fluoride mouth rinses daily are important to reduce the possibility of decay because of concomitant xerostomia.

GASTROESOPHAGEAL REFLUX: MEDICAL TREATMENT

THOMAS R. HENDRIX, M.D.

Gastroesophageal reflux occurs daily in everyone. In most individuals these episodes are asymptomatic, and if symptoms are produced, they usually are not considered as abnormalities requiring medical attention. In a study of hospital staff and employees considered in good health, 7 percent experienced heartburn, the characteristic symptom of gastroesophageal reflux, daily, and more than one-third had the symptom at least once a month. Despite these symptoms, none sought medical advice nor considered they had any dysfunction or disease.

If our discussion is limited to those patients demonstrated to have gastroesophageal reflux in the course of evaluation of their presenting complaints, we find a wide spectrum of symptoms ranging from troublesome heartburn at one extreme to serious damage to the esophageal mucosa at the other. The serious end of the spectrum comprises erosive esophagitis and its sequelae, such as peptic stricture and Barrett's esophagus, a complication of reflux in which the ulcerated squamous mucosa is replaced with columnar mucosa having a considerable potential for malignant transformation. It seems likely that our convention of lumping all of these consequences of gastroesophageal reflux into a single entity, gastroesophageal reflux disease (GERD), obscures important pathophysiologic features which, if better understood, could lead to more rational therapy.

The recognition that there are two, not mutually exclusive, patterns of reflux *postprandial* and *nocturnal*, is an important first step towards making sense of the heterogeneity of GERD. While everyone has some postprandial reflux, nocturnal reflux is not seen in "normal" individuals. Symptomatic postprandial reflux may be merely an exaggeration of a "normal phenomenon," whereas nocturnal reflux is clearly pathologic. Nocturnal reflux is frequently associated with the complications of reflux, i.e., esophagitis, stricture, Barrett's esophagus, and pulmonary aspiration. It is particularly treacherous because: (1) it is less likely to produce symptoms that warn the individual that something is wrong; (2) swallowing is only one-tenth as frequent during sleep as when awake; (3) rate of production of alkaline saliva is reduced during sleep; and (4) gravity does not aid in the clearing of the esophagus. Until we have a better understanding of the factors underlying symptomatic and pathologic reflux, our treatment of necessity must be empiric.

A second important concept in understanding reflux and planning for its treatment is that gastroesophageal reflux causes a vicious cycle which, if not interrupted, leads to progression of symptoms and esophageal damage. Reflux of irritant material into the esophagus interferes with effective peristalsis and leads to delayed clearing of the esophagus. The latter is associated with decreased sphincter tone, thus setting the stage for further reflux, which, if not interrupted, may progress to esophagitis and its complications.

TREATMENT MODALITIES

Treatment is aimed at improving the function of the elements that protect the esophagus from the irritant nature of refluxed gastric contents. These elements are (1) the gastroesophageal reflux barrier, which is primarily the function of the lower esophageal sphincter (ES); (2) the combined effects of peristalsis and gravity to produce rapid clearing of refluxed material from the esophagus; (3) the acid neutralizing capacity of saliva; and (4) the squamous epithelial barrier, which prevents the penetration of noxious material, primarily H^+ ions, into the mucosa. Successful treatment must reduce reflux sufficiently to permit the restoration of the normal squamous epithelial barrier. It is analogous to treating sunburn (damage to another epithelial barrier). If the damaged epithelium is not well protected from the damaging factor, ultraviolet light in the case of sunburn and gastric contents in reflux, healing will not occur.

In practical terms treatment aims at (1) decreasing the frequency and duration of reflux episodes, (2) increasing the rate of clearing of refluxed material from the esophagus, and (3) decreasing the noxious nature of refluxed gastric contents.

Decreasing Frequency and Duration of Reflux Episodes

The frequency and duration of reflux episodes may be decreased by improving LES tone and function, elevating the head of the bed, and weight reduction.

Improving Lower Esophageal Sphincter Function

Sphincter function may be improved by *dietary* and *drug* therapy. Protein meals have been shown to increase sphincter tone, whereas fatty meals decrease it. In addition, chocolate, caffeine, peppermint, and alcohol decrease sphincter tone. Sphincter tone is increased by antacids, cholinergic agents (bethanechol), and metoclopramide. A variety of drugs decrease sphincter tone, including theophylline, anticholinergic agents, calcium channel blocking agents, beta-adrenergic agonists (isoproterenol), alpha-adrenergic antagonists (phentolamine), diazepam, and progesterone containing contraceptives. Smoking also is associated with increased reflux. Gastric distention is associated with decreased sphincter pressure; thus small meals, low in fat, empty promptly, thereby avoiding impairment of the sphincter's barrier function. In addition, since dyspepsia is often associated with delayed gastric emptying, those foods that the patient associates with dyspepsia should be avoided. Finally, bethanechol and metoclopramide increase both the rate of gastric emptying and sphincter tone. Aerophagia and inspiring air into the esophagus lead to gastric distention and eructation, thus interfering with sphincter function.

Elevation of Head and Chest When Reclining

Elevation of the head of the bed on 6-inch blocks has been shown, by continuous intraesophageal pH recording, to decrease the frequency and duration of nocturnal reflux episodes.

Weight Loss

Overweight patients with reflux should be urged to lose weight. Although the reflux symptoms are often increased with increases of 10 or more pounds, and unmanageable reflux symptoms become tractable with weight loss, the mechanisms responsible are poorly understood. Realistically, however, if we had to rely on the patient's ability to lose weight to control reflux symptoms, only a few patients would improve.

Increasing Esophageal Clearing

Effective esophageal clearing of refluxed acid from the stomach depends upon the combined action of effective peristalsis and bicarbonate secretion in saliva. Maneuvers that improve esophageal peristalsis and increase salivary flow improve esophageal clearing. Those factors outlined above which decrease the frequency and duration of reflux episodes are probably the most important in improving esophageal clearing because they interrupt the vicious cycle which perpetuates reflux of irritant gastric contents.

Bethanechol has been shown to improve esophageal clearing. This action is widely attributed to increased amplitude of esophageal peristaltic contractions, but more likely the reason is its cholinergic stimulation of salivary flow. Other means of stimulating salivary flow, such as sucking hard candy or chewing gum, although not formally tested are reported by some patients to be helpful in controlling heartburn. Nocturnal esophageal clearing is facilitated by enlisting the aid of gravity by raising the head of the bed.

Decreasing Irritant Quality and Volume of Gastric Juice

Antacids

Antacids have been the mainstay of dyspepsia and reflux treatment for as long as any of us can remember. Aluminum-magnesium hydroxide antacids taken 1 and 3 hours after meals and at bedtime have been shown to control gastric acidity sufficiently to heal peptic ulcers of the stomach and duodenum. Patients report that antacids of all types give prompt but usually only transient relief of heartburn; hence the large volume of sales of over-the-counter antacid preparations. Calcium carbonate antacids, e.g., Tums, enjoy considerable popularity because of their quick effect. Because they may be sucked, neutralization of the esophageal surface is prolonged and sucking stimulates endogenous "antacid" production by stimulating increased salivary flow.

To prolong the effect of antacid and to decrease the irritant nature of refluxed material, antacids have been mixed with *alginic acid* (Gaviscon), which is supposed to form a viscous antacid foam that floats on top of the gastric contents so that when sphincter failure allows reflux, the material entering the esophagus is not pure gastric juice but rather alginic acid with its associated antacid. In spite of the attractiveness of this approach, Gaviscon's control of reflux symptoms was significantly superior to placebo in only two of four placebo-controlled studies of 244 patients.

Recent preliminary reports of sucralfate "slurry" being helpful in experimental and human esophagitis may lead to an important additional treatment in some patients with resistant esophagitis.

Histamine$_2$ Receptor Antagonists

The introduction of histamine$_2$ receptor antagonists *cimetidine* and *ranitidine* has provided a convenient, acceptable, and effective means of decreasing the volume and acid content of gastric juice. It seems likely that the major contribution of these agents to the treatment of reflux is more effective and longer lasting control of nocturnal acid secretion, which thus provides increased protection of the esophagus in its most vulnerable period which is unattainable with antacids. Doubling the traditional doses of cimetidine to 600 mg, or of ranitidine to 300 mg at bedtime provides even greater suppression of nocturnal acid secretion.

TREATMENT STRATEGIES

Most practitioners advocate a gradual approach in treatment of gastroesophageal reflux. The first step is "lifestyle" modifications, such as elevation of the head of the bed, weight loss, cessation of smoking, eating small meals, avoiding dyspeptic foods, and use of antacids. If these measures fail to produce improvement, then drugs with specific effects on motility, e.g., bethanechol or metoclopramide, and on gastric secretion, e.g., cimetidine or ranitidine, should be added.

There is an old military axiom that you will get on target sooner with less expenditure of ammunition if the first salvo is over the target. This philosophy is also applicable to therapeutics, especially in disorders in which dysfunction is perpetuated by a cycle of events. In addition, if therapy is promptly successful in controlling symptoms, the patient is much more likely to take the physician's advice regarding changes in lifestyle than if control is achieved only after passage through several treatment phases over 1 or 2 months.

My approach to the treatment of gastroesophageal reflux is to institute therapy with an intensive 2-week treatment schedule. The aim is to interrupt the cycle so that a simpler, less demanding schedule may then be followed to maintain control of reflux symptoms. The patient is told that it is a 2-week trial.

The intensive 2-week trial consists of the following:

1. Elevation of head of bed on 6-inch blocks.
2. Small meals with decreased fat intake and avoidance of chocolate, coffee, alcohol, and foods the patient associates with dyspepsia. No food intake after evening meal.
3. Decrease or stop smoking.
4. Histamine$_2$ receptor antagonist—cimetidine, 300 mg 3 times daily before meals and 600 mg at bedtime or ranitidine, 150 mg in the morning and 300 mg at bedtime.
5. Aluminum-magnesium antacid, 30 ml after meals and at bedtime.
6. Bethanechol, 25 mg at bedtime. Metoclopramide is associated with troublesome side effects too frequently to be used in this initial treatment trial.
7. It is possible that a slurry of sucralfate may prove to be useful therapy in some patients.

The sequence of simplifying the regimen in patients who have responded is empiric. Usually the treatment that the patient has found the least tolerable, e.g., elevation of the head of the bed, omission of coffee, or antacids, is the first to be discontinued. The evening dose of histamine$_2$ receptor antagonist is usually maintained for a prolonged period of time.

If treatment fails to improve the patient's symptoms one of the following must be considered: first and most likely, the diagnosis is wrong and symptoms that have been attributed to reflux actually have a different origin; or second, the patient has such severe reflux disease that medical means are inadequate to interrupt the destructive cycle. Failure of medical therapy is often manifested by return of symptoms as the intensive treatment is relaxed to a level compatible with long-term maintenance therapy or by failure of the regimen to heal erosive esophagitis. Regardless of the cause of failure of therapy, diagnostic tests should be performed to establish whether or not the patient has pathologic reflux and whether the reflux episodes are associated with the pain that brought the patient to the physician in the first place. In my experience continuous ambulatory intraesophageal pH recording for 18 to 24 hours is the most direct method of getting the needed information. The patient who has symptoms attributed to reflux but no erosive esophagitis should never be referred for surgical therapy until it is clearly demonstrated that pathologic reflux exists and that reflux is the cause of the patient's pain. Finally, only about 5 percent of reflux patients are candidates for antireflux surgery. The most frequent indication is failure to heal erosive esophagitis or the presence of late complications of esophagitis, e.g., progressive Barrett's esophagus, stricture, or both. The next chapter covers surgical treatment of reflux, and there are separate chapters on *Esophageal Stricture* and on *Barrett's Esophagus*.

ESOPHAGEAL REFLUX: SURGICAL TREATMENT

TOM R. DeMEESTER, M.D.

The primary goal of antireflux surgery is to *reestablish the competency of the cardia by improving its function*. To accomplish this, it is of paramount importance that the surgeon understand the physiology of the cardia, and know how to recognize a mechanically deficient cardia and how the deficiency can be corrected by a surgical procedure. Consequently, antireflux surgery is different from the simple extirpation of a diseased organ whose function is of no concern, since it will be destroyed with its removal. Rather, antireflux surgery is designed to improve the function of an organ that will remain in the patient, and to provide complete and permanent relief of all symptoms and complications of gastroesophageal reflux secondary to an incompetent cardia. Ideally, the reconstructed cardia should permit the patient to swallow normally, belch to relieve gaseous distention, or vomit when it is necessary to do so. The end result should restore the patient to a normal life with no further need for medical, postural, or dietary therapy. The more often antireflux surgery can achieve these goals safely and dependably, the wider the indications for the operation should become.

The persistence of nausea, heartburn, regurgitation, dysphagia, chest pain, or epigastric pain after an antireflux procedure represents a clinically poor result due either to an incorrect initial diagnosis or technical failure. The problem with using symptoms as an indicator of success is that often a patient who has undergone surgery to be freed from his symptoms will not readily admit postoperatively to their presence. Thus, using only the lack of postoperative symptoms as an indication of operative success is not dependable. Similarly, the report of a normal barium swallow cannot be used as a measure of success, since the symptoms of reflux or its complications may be present in a patient who has no radiologic evidence of a hiatal hernia or regurgitation of barium from the stomach into the esophagus. Rather, the success of a procedure depends on (1) relief from symptoms, (2) objective evidence on 24-hour esophageal pH monitoring that reflux has been reduced to physiologic levels, and (3) evidence on esophageal manometry that the mechanical defect of the cardia has been corrected.

PATIENT EVALUATION

To evaluate properly a patient who might be a candidate for an antireflux procedure, it is necessary that the surgeon become familiar with the diagnostic tools used to objectively assess the patient's symptoms. Approximately 10 percent of the patients referred to me because of dissatisfaction with the outcome of a previous antireflux procedure were incorrectly diagnosed prior to their initial operation. An error in diagnosis is usually due to a failure to objectively document increased esophageal acid exposure when it was thought to be present, or to determine the correct cause for the increased exposure when it was known to be present. It is my opinion that an antireflux procedure is indicated *only* when there is *increased esophageal acid exposure due to reflux of gastric contents through a mechanically deficient cardia* (Table 1). To perform an antireflux procedure on a patient with a manometrically normal distal esophageal sphincter makes little sense. An antireflux procedure may stop existing reflux but it is unlikely that the cause of the reflux was a mechanically defective cardia. In such patients, surgery can cause more symptoms than it cures.

On the other hand, a patient who has the proper indication for an antireflux procedure may have a poor surgical result if his surgeon is prone to making modifications in technique without knowing what effect they have on the organ's function. Only recently have we begun to appreciate the fact that when an operation is designed to improve organ function, surgical technique becomes paramount and changes in technique can have a profound effect on postoperative function. No change in technique should be made indiscriminately; changes should be accepted and applied only after their effect on function has been carefully evaluated.

In general, if a surgeon understands the physiology of the cardia and the principles necessary for its reconstruction, and appropriately selects patients by preoperative testing, he or she will collect a group of very gratified patients, relieved of their symptoms and grateful for life. Such a reward makes the time and effort exerted in understanding and applying the science of surgery to gastroesophageal reflux meaningful.

DEFINITION AND RECOGNITION OF A MECHANICALLY DEFECTIVE CARDIA

In man, the antireflux mechanism consists of a valvular cardia and the propulsive pump-like function of the body of the esophagus. Failure of one of these components can usually be compensated for by the other. Failure of both components inevitably leads to abnormal esophageal exposure to gastric juice.

Mechanical failure of the valvular component of the antireflux mechanism is diagnosed by measuring inadequate mechanical characteristics of the sphincter on manometry. Based on our experience correlating esopha-

TABLE 1 Pathophysiologic Indications for Antireflux Surgery

Documented pathologic reflux
Documented mechanically defective cardia
   DES pressure 6 mm Hg or less
   Abdominal length of DES 1 cm or less
   Overall length of DES 2 cm or less

DES = distal esophageal sphincter

geal manometry within 24-hour esophageal pH monitoring in both control subjects and patients, we have defined a mechanically deficient cardia as having (1) an average sphincter pressure of 6 mm Hg or less; (2) an average length of sphincter exposed to the positive pressure environment of the abdomen of 1 cm or less; and/or (3) a sphincter with an average overall resting length of 2 cm or less (Table 1). These values are two standard deviations below the mean measurements in normal control subjects and are associated with an 85 to 90 percent incidence of increased esophageal acid exposure on 24-hour esophageal pH monitoring.

The key factor in the *competency* of the cardia is the *distal esophageal sphincter pressure*, but the efficiency of the pressure can be nullified by *inadequate abdominal length* or an *abnormally short overall resting length of the sphincter*. Patients with a low sphincter pressure, or those with a normal pressure but a short abdominal length, are unable to protect against reflux caused by fluctuations of intra-abdominal pressure that occur with daily activities or changes in body position. Patients with a low sphincter pressure, or those with a normal pressure but a short overall length, are unable to protect against reflux caused by independent increases in gastric pressure over intra-abdominal pressure. In this situation, reflux can occur whenever an increase in gastric pressure exceeds the sphincter pressure necessary to provide competency for the overall length of sphincter present. Gastric distention can cause shortening of the overall length of the sphincter in a manner similar to the shortening of the neck of a balloon on inflation. Thus, reflux is more apt to occur in patients with short sphincters, because with gastric distention the length of the sphincter readily drops below that which is necessary for the sphincter pressure present to maintain competency. Thus, individuals who have a short overall sphincter length on a resting esophageal motility study are at a disadvantage in protecting against reflux caused by normal gastric pressure and dilatation. On the other hand, in individuals who have a normal overall sphincter length on a resting esophageal motility study, it is possible for primary gastric pathologic changes to cause gastric dilatation, shortening of the sphincter length, and reflux of gastric contents through a sphincter which, when the stomach is decompressed, has normal mechanical parameters. The first situation is a form of mechanically incompetent cardia and can be corrected by an antireflux procedure. The second situation may require gastric surgery to correct.

The patient who has, on a resting motility study, a deficiency of one, two, or all three of the components of a competent cardia, i.e., sphincter pressure, abdominal length and overall length, has a mechanically defective cardia as a basis for experiencing the symptoms and complications associated with the regurgitation of gastric contents into the esophagus. Such patients are less apt to receive benefits from medical therapy because their problem is a mechanical deficiency. They have a pathophysiologic defect that a surgical antireflux procedure is designed to correct.

Failures of the *esophageal pump component* of the antireflux mechanism often occur with a mechanical deficiency of the valvular component. This is usually caused by a primary or reflux-induced *motility disorder*, a *hiatal hernia*, or a *myogenic abnormality*. Each of these abnormalities produces inefficiency in the propulsive pumping action of the body of the esophagus and potentiates the effects of a mechanically defective valve. Studies have indicated that surgery can improve the efficiency of the esophageal pump by reducing a hiatal hernia, but it is not effective in improving the other causes of pump failure, with the exception of a reflux-induced motility disorder. The latter, however, is often difficult to differentiate from a primary motility disorder.

Habitual pharyngeal swallowing is an effort to compensate for a mechanically defective valve of the antireflux mechanism and can result in pumping an excessive amount of air into the stomach. This leads to gastric dilatation and repetitive belching with further reflux of gastric contents into the esophagus. Surgical correction of the defective valvular component will usually remove the need for the excessive swallowing and alleviate the symptoms of gastric distention. Other causes for habitual swallowing resulting in excessive air intake, gastric dilatation, and reflux are attempts to compensate for a decreased saliva production, or the loss of secondary peristalsis. A surgical antireflux procedure has no benefit in these situations and may potentiate the gastric dilatation, causing a gas bloat syndrome.

PATIENT SELECTION AND CLINICAL INDICATIONS FOR ANTIREFLUX SURGERY

Prior to undertaking any rational therapy for gastroesophageal reflux, a precise diagnosis as to the cause of abnormal acid exposure of the esophagus is necessary. An antireflux procedure should be considered only for those patients who have a mechanically defective cardia, as defined in Table 1, and one of the clinical indications shown in Table 2. If the cardia is manometrically normal, the patient should be evaluated for a gastric or esophageal cause of the abnormal esophageal acid exposure. If neither is found, the increased acid exposure is probably due to transient spontaneous relaxation of the sphincter. Such patients usually can be managed by medical therapy, but in severe cases an antireflux procedure can be helpful. The clinical indications to proceed with

TABLE 2 Clinical Indications for Antireflex Surgery

Complications of Gastroesophageal Reflux

   Persistent endoscopic esophagitis
   Esophageal stricture
   Barrett's esophagus
   Pulmonary fibrosis from chronic aspiration

Uncontrolled Symptoms

   Heartburn and regurgitation
   Chest pain
   Chronic cough or wheezing
   Dysphagia

an antireflux operation in patients with a mechanically defective cardia are the presence of a complication of reflux, namely, persistent endoscopic esophagitis, esophageal stricture, Barrett's columnar line esophagus, or radiographic evidence of repetitive aspiration pneumonia.

Esophagitis

The development of esophagitis as a complication of gastroesophageal reflux appears to be related to the composition of the refluxed material and the pattern in which it is exposed to the esophageal mucosa. Thus, it is possible to have a mechanically defective cardia and not develop esophagitis. In our clinic this occurs in about 50 percent of symptomatic patients. In my experience, patients with esophagitis and a mechanically defective cardia commonly receive little long-term benefit from medical therapy and will eventually require a surgical antireflux procedure to correct the condition. If severe endoscopic esophagitis is present, surgery should be performed rather quickly in these patients, since strictures can develop while they are receiving medical therapy. If 24-hour esophageal pH monitoring is normal in a patient with unequivocal endoscopic esophagitis, then the possibilities of alkaline, drug-induced, or retention esophagitis should be considered.

Stricture

A benign esophageal stricture, secondary to reflux esophagitis in a patient with a mechanically defective cardia, is a sign of progressive disease and failure of medical management, and an indication for surgical therapy. Prior to surgery, a malignant cause of the stricture should be excluded. This can be difficult and the roentgenographic barium swallow can be misleading. To make this differentiation, several biopsy specimens and brushings from within the lumen of the stricture should be obtained. Rigid endoscopy occasionally may be required to get an adequate biopsy specimen. When a malignant etiology has been excluded, the stricture is progressively dilated up to a No. 60 F bougie prior to surgery. When it is fully dilated, esophageal manometry and 24-hour pH monitoring is performed. *Manometry* is used to determine the adequacy of *peristalsis* in the distal esophagus and the ability of the distal *esophageal sphincter to relax* on deglutition. If either of these measurements is deficient, caution should be exercised in performing an antireflux procedure and serious consideration given to a colon interposition. If increased esophageal acid exposure is documented and the cardia is mechanically deficient, a *transthoracic* antireflux procedure is recommended. I prefer this approach in order to obtain full mobilization of the esophagus to allow placement of the repair in the abdomen without undue tension. Rarely is a Collis gastroplasty necessary to gain added length. If 24-hour esophageal pH monitoring is normal, the cardia is either competent, indicating that the stricture is probably secondary to drug ingestion and dilation may be all that is needed, or pure alkaline reflux is present. See the chapter on *Esophageal Stricture*.

Barrett's Esophagus

It is my belief that Barrett's esophagus is a columnar-lined esophagus acquired as a complication of persistent reflux esophagitis. It is almost always associated with a severe mechanical defect of the cardia, and in my mind, represents end-stage reflux disease. A patient with a Barrett's esophagus is at risk of developing a stricture, hemorrhage from esophageal ulcer, and adenocarcinoma. It is established that control of reflux by an antireflux procedure can avert the complications of bleeding ulceration and stricture, and may, although not proven, protect against the development of adenocarcinoma by causing a reduction in the degree of pleomorphism and anaplasia. The presence of a Barrett's esophagus is an indication for multiple mucosal biopsy. If marked mucosal dysplasia or carcinoma in situ is found, an esophageal resection should be considered. If these changes are not found, I believe an antireflux procedure should be performed. The chapter on *Barrett's Esophagus* provides additional details of management.

Aspiration Pneumonia

Patients with roentgenographic evidence of previous recurrent pneumonias and a history of episodes of nocturnal choking or waking up with gastric contents in the mouth or soilage of the bed pillow may be suffering from repetitive pulmonary aspiration secondary to gastroesophageal reflux. The chest roentgenogram often shows a large hiatal hernia and signs of pleural thickening, bronchiectasis, and pulmonary fibrosis. In such patients, 24-hour pH monitoring should be done to confirm the presence of increased esophageal acid exposure. If this is present, esophageal manometry should be performed and if a mechanical defect of the cardia is found, an antireflux procedure is indicated. In my experience, these patients usually have a nonspecific motility abnormality of the esophageal body which tends to propel the refluxed material toward the pharynx. Other esophageal pathologic conditions that can cause repetitive aspiration are achalasia, a hiatal hernia with a competent sphincter but a narrow diaphragmatic hiatus (see Dysphagia), and a pharyngeal or esophageal diverticulum.

Persistent Reflux Symptoms

The indication for antireflux surgery in a symptomatic patient with a mechanically defective cardia but without reflux complications is his unwillingness to put up with the chronic symptoms that persist despite the best medical therapy. In this situation, it is important to objectively demonstrate the presence of abnormal reflux with 24-hour pH monitoring and a mechanically defective cardia on manometry. If the symptoms have persisted more than four to six months while the patient was receiving medical therapy, or if the patient is tired of the restriction and expense of medical therapy, an antireflux repair can be done. If there are normal mechanical components of the cardia, a gastric or esophageal cause for the increase in esophageal acid exposure should be searched for. If the 24-hour esophageal pH monitoring test is normal, a cause for the symptoms other than reflux should be investigated.

Atypical Chest Symptoms

Chronic atypical symptoms of reflux which can indicate the need for operation in a patient with a mechanically defective cardia are chest pain from a reflux-induced esophageal irritation or spasm, and pulmonary symptoms such as chronic cough, hoarseness, or wheezing. Generally, these atypical symptoms overshadow any gastroesophageal complaints and focus the physician's attention on the heart or lungs. Chest pain indistinguishable from coronary artery disease can be caused by reflux. These patients are usually thought to have coronary artery disease, but they have normal coronary arteries on arteriography or have had a coronary artery bypass procedure without relief of their chest pain. The tip-off that the pulmonary symptoms may be related to reflux is the history of recurrent pneumonias, the presence of chronic interstitial pulmonary fibrosis on the chest roentgenogram, adult onset of asthma, or a chronic cough that eludes all efforts to uncover its cause.

The relationship of the cardiac or pulmonary symptoms to reflux can be clarified with 24-hour esophageal pH monitoring by correlating the timing of the onset of the symptom with a reflux episode. If the symptom occurs during or immediately after a reflux episode and the patient has a mechanically defective cardia but no complication of reflux, medical therapy should be tried. If this therapy fails, an antireflux procedure can be helpful in controlling or abolishing the symptoms. If normal mechanical components of the cardia are found, a search should be made for a gastric or esophageal cause for the increase in esophageal acid exposure. If the 24-hour pH monitoring test is normal, the presence of a motility disorder in the body of the esophagus should be investigated. Attempts to induce esophageal spasm and precipitate an episode of chest pain may be helpful.

Dysphagia

Dysphagia also is an indication for an antireflux procedure. This symptom may be associated with regurgitation or chest pain while eating, which are usually related to the presence of a large paraesophageal hernia, intrathoracic stomach, or a small hiatal hernia with a Schatzki ring or a narrow diaphragmatic hiatus. In the latter condition, the dysphagia and chest pain that occur during eating are due to distention and contraction of the portion of the stomach above the narrow diaphragmatic opening. Occasionally, the contents in the herniated portion of the stomach can be regurgitated back into the eshopagus and, in some patients, up into the pharynx. All of these conditions are easily identified with an upper gastrointestinal roentgenographic barium examination done by a knowledgeable radiologist. A cine- or videoesophagram using thick barium or a barium-coated hamburger can be helpful in identifying the latter two problems when they are not readily apparent on a standard barium study. These patients have little or no heartburn, since the cardia is usually competent and reflux of gastric contents into the esophagus does not occur. The surgical repair of these abnormalities includes an antireflux procedure because of an associated mechanically defective cardia initially or the potential of destroying the competency of the cardia during the repair of the hernia.

Reflux in Infants and Children

In addition to these general indications for antireflux surgery, there are specific clinical situations in which an antireflux procedure is indicated. In children with incompetent cardias, the complications of reflux are esophagitis, recurrent pneumonia, anemia, and failure to thrive. Esophagitis is rapidly progressive in this age group, and a stricture may develop in a matter of weeks, even while the child is undergoing an acceptable form of medical therapy. Consequently, once the complication of esophagitis has been confirmed in a child with documented reflux, the need for a surgical antireflux procedure becomes urgent. In infants, failure to thrive, anemia, and aspiration pneumonia may be the only evidence that reflux is present. Once gastroesophageal reflux is objectively established by 24-hour esophageal pH monitoring, surgical correction should be performed.

Aperistalsis

The presence of endoscopic esophagitis reflux in association with scleroderma or after balloon dilatation for achalasia is an indication for early surgical therapy, since esophagitis in the presence of a severe motility disorder can rapidly progress to stricture formation. The Belsey Mark IV procedure should be done in this situation because its low outflow resistance makes it particularly suitable to an esophageal body that has poor peristaltic activity. Once a stricture has developed under these conditions, esophageal resection and a colon interposition are usually necessary to reestablish alimentation.

Vagotomy or Gastric Disorder

The presence of a mechanically defective cardia after vagotomy and pyloroplasty or gastric resection can allow reflux of gastric and pancreatobiliary secretions into the esophagus. This problem is usually manifested by symptoms of pulmonary aspiration. Endoscopic esophagitis can occur but is usually absent. Medical therapy designed to control both acid and alkaline reflux usually fail, and a bile-diverting procedure, without reconstruction of the cardia, is of little benefit in preventing the symptoms of aspiration. The proper surgical therapy is an *antireflux operation* with the addition of a *bile-diverting procedure* if *symptomatic* alkaline gastritis is present.

Consideration of Bile Gastritis and Esophageal Propulsive Force

Prior to proceeding with a surgical antireflux repair, there are two things a surgeon should do. First, specific queries should be addressed to the patient about complaints of *epigastric pain, nausea, vomiting,* and *loss of appetite*. In the past, we accepted these symptoms as part of the reflux syndrome, but now we realize that they can be due to bile reflux gastritis, which occurs independently or in association with gastroesophageal reflux. As previously mentioned, the problem is usually seen in patients who have had prior upper gastrointestinal surgery, although this is not always the case. The correction of only the incompetent cardia in such patients will result in disgruntled individuals who continue to complain of nausea and epigastric pain on eating. If surgery is necessary to control gastroesophageal reflux and severe duodenogastric reflux is present, consideration should be given to performing a *bile diversion procedure* as well. When bile reflux gastritis is diagnosed after an antireflux repair, *sucralfate* may relieve the persistent complaint of nausea and epigastric pain.

Second, prior to an antireflux repair the surgeon should evaluate the *propulsive force* of the body of the esophagus to determine if there is sufficient power to propel a bolus of food through a newly reconstructed valve. This can be done by esophageal manometry, or better, a radioisotopic measurement of esophageal transit time.

CHOICE OF ANTIREFLUX REPAIR

Currently in the United States, the Belsey partial fundoplication, the Nissen fundoplication, and the Hill posterior gastropexy with calibration of the cardia are the most widely used antireflux repairs. Each of the procedures, based on the reported experience in the literature, provides good to excellent relief of the symptoms of gastroesophageal reflux in 84 to 89 percent of the patients (Table 3).

There has been only one published randomized trial comparing the Nissen, Hill (noncalibrated), and Belsey antireflux procedures in which an attempt was made to compensate for variations in surgical skills and experience. This study showed that the Nissen repair, as opposed to the Belsey and Hill repairs, when done by a surgeon with average skill, resulted in best control of gastroesophageal reflux as assessed objectively with the standard acid reflux test and 24-hour pH monitoring of the distal esophagus. This was accomplished at the expense of a temporary mild postoperative dysphagia and the inability to vomit after the repair. The study was designed to evaluate the degree of technical difficulty of each procedure in constructing a competent cardia. It did not evaluate the durability of the various repairs.

Nissen Fundoplication

Over 10 years of personal experience, I have had several of my patients who had undergone Nissen fundoplication submit voluntarily to postoperative studies consisting of esophageal manometry, 24-hour esophageal pH monitoring, and thorough questioning about their esophageal symptoms. These studies have convinced me of the durability of the Nissen procedure. I have modifed the operation only slightly to reduce the incidence of temporary dysphagia and eliminate any persistent dysphagia associated with the repair. My current technique consists of only minor refinements of the method originally published by Nissen. The operation as initially described consisted of wrapping the stomach 360 degrees around the lower 4 to 5 cm of esophagus. Based on our studies, it became evident that only the fundus of the stomach should be used to construct the gastric wrap. The length of the wrap should be limited to 1.5 cm. It should be constructed over a No. 60 F bougie and held in place with one permanent horizontal reinforced mattress suture as shown in Figure 1.

The Nissen fundoplication can be performed through either an abdominal or thoracic incision. The abdominal

TABLE 3 Results of Primary Surgical Antireflux Repairs for Gastroesophageal Reflux Disease

Repair	No. of Patients	Follow-up Period (yr)	Good Results (%)	Reflux Recurrence (%)	Dysphagia (%)	Gas Bloat (%)	Mortality (%)
Belsey							
Skinner	632	1–5	85	7	—	—	1.3
Orringer	892	3–15	84	11	—	—	1
Hill							
No operative motility	76	8 (mean)	65	12	—	—	—
Operative motility	93	4 (mean)	89	0	—	—	—
Nissen							
5 reports	1,141	1–12	87	7	4/48 8	97/1,115 8	1

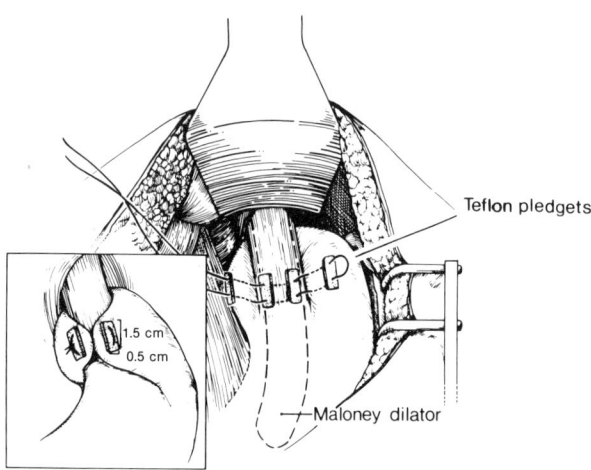

Figure 1 Construction of the fundoplication by the transabdominal approach illustrating the placement of the horizontal mattress stitch and the positions of the pledgets. The wrap is formed over a No. 60 F bougie with enough space left over to allow the passage of an index finger through the wrap adjacent to the bougie. Insert shows the completed fundoplication.

incision is preferred unless the following specific indications for a transthoracic approach exist:

1. Previous hiatal hernia repair. With a transthoracic approach a circumferential incision in the diaphragm can be made for simultaneous exposure of the upper abdomen, allowing dissection of the previous repair from both sides of the diaphragm.
2. Need for a concomitant esophageal myotomy for achalasia or diffuse spasm.
3. Esophageal stricture. In this situation, the thoracic approach is preferred to obtain maximum mobilization of the esophagus for placing the repair, without tension, below the diaphragm.
4. Sliding hiatal hernia that does not drop below the diaphragm during a roentegenographic barium study in the upright position. This can indicate esophageal shortening, and again, a thoracic approach is preferred for maximum mobilization of the esophagus.
5. Associated pulmonary pathologic changes. In this situation, the nature of the pulmonary disorder can be evaluated and the proper pulmonary surgery performed in addition to the antireflux repair.
6. Obesity. In obese patients the thoracic approach gives better exposure and allows for a more precise repair.

The principle *disadvantages* of the *thoracic* approach are (1) the need for a chest tube postoperatively along with its potential risk for infection; (2) greater compromise of respiratory function and higher incidence of postoperative atelectasis and pneumonia; and (3) the develoment of post-thoracotomy pain. The incidence of the latter can be reduced by resecting a short segment of rib posteriorly rather than running the risk of producing a rib fracture, avoiding excessive spreading of the ribs and placing substantial strain on the costicartilage, and avoiding an overtight closure of the inner space and muscle layer.

The principle *disadvantages* of an *abdominal* approach are (1) poor exposure of the distal thoracic esophagus with the inability to mobilize it sufficiently to limit tension on a repair; (2) the risk of splenic injury, and (3) the possibility of an incisional hernia necessitating reoperation.

Belsey Partial Fundoplication

The choice of a Belsey partial fundoplication is influenced by the strength and quality of the peristaltic contractions in the body of the esophagus. The esophagi, having normal motility and strong peristaltic contractions, do well with a complete Nissen fundoplication. Where peristalsis is absent, severely disordered, or of low magnitude (below 20 mm Hg), the Belsey two-thirds partial fundoplication should be done. Similarly, a Belsey partial fundoplication should be used after a myotomy for achalasia or esophageal spasm, or when a repair is done on an emergency basis, such as the closure of an esophageal perforation when the quality and amplitude of the esophageal contractions are unknown.

Hill Procedure

The Hill procedure differs from the Nissen and Belsey operations in that its major component is not a fundoplication but rather a *posterior abdominal gastropexy*. Such operations place the stomach and the esophagus under a great deal of continual tension due to normal respiratory and swallowing movements. Consequently, most of these operations result in dislodgement of the gastropexy and a return of reflux symptoms. With the exception of the Hill procedure, which anchors the gastroesophageal junction posteriorly to the median arcuate ligament, the gastropexy operations did not stand the test of time and were gradually abandoned. Hill currently recommends that his operation be accompanied by *intraoperative manometry* to calibrate the cardia. This is essential, since palpating the degree of imbrication of the posterior and anterior walls of the cardia to the median arcuate ligament cannot be done accurately and carries the risk of leaving the gastroesophageal junction too loose, allowing persistent reflux even though it has been anchored securely into the abdominal environment, or too tight, causing partial or complete esophageal obstruction. The major *disadvantages* of the Hill procedure are the potential for *injury to the celiac axis* and the necessity to be familiar with and have available *intraoperative manometry*. Its *advantage* is that it can be performed on *postgastrectomy patients* in whom the remaining stomach is insufficient for a fundoplication.

Angelchik Prosthesis

Aware of the complications associated with the stan-

TABLE 4 Comparison of Current Antireflux Procedures

Operation	Concept of Function	Ease of Instruction	Effectiveness of the Valve	Outflow Resistance	Toleration of Tension	Best Use
Hill posterior gastroplexy	Complex	Difficult	Dependent on intraoperative manometrics	Dependent on degree of imbrication of cardia	Best	Previous gastric resection
Belsey partial fundoplication	Simple	Most difficult	Effective—patient usually able to belch	Lowest	Poor	Poor esophageal pump
Nissen fundoplication	Simple	Average	Most effective—patient unable to belch	Highest; long and tight wrap can cause permanent dysphagia	Fair	Standard antireflux procedure
Angelchik prosthesis	Poorly understood	Easiest	Appears effective	Average; pseudocapsule can cause permanent dysphagia	Poor?	High-risk patient; short life expectancy

dard antireflux operations, and desiring a procedure that can be performed by less experienced surgeons, Angelchik designed a silicone prosthetic collar that can be easily placed around the abdominal esophagus as an antireflux device. The introduction of the Angelchik prosthesis has been plagued with difficulties not uncommon for prosthetic devices. In the early version of the prosthesis the tabs, which are used to tie the device in place, had a tendency to become unattached. Consequently, the device would migrate throughout the peritoneal cavity and produced various symptoms depending on where it finally came to rest. The tie tabs were therefore changed to a continuous strip of Silastic-impregnated Dacron. This completely encircles the outside of the prosthesis so that detachment is not possible, and the only way that it can become dislodged is for the tabs to break. Since this design change, there have been no reports of displacement. A second problem has been the use of the device in the presence of an esophageal or high gastric suture line or when there has been extensive trauma to the cardia. This has led to the dramatic complication of erosion of the prosthesis into the gastrointestinal tract, with subsequent passage of the device in the feces or endoscopic removal of the device from the stomach. This complication, however, has been reported in fewer than 1 percent of patients. A bizarre complication occurs from puncture of the prosthesis by improper instrumentation during its implantation causing leakage of the Silastic filling into either the mediastinum or the abdomen. Sepsis around the prosthesis has not been a problem, although the device should never be employed in patients with preexisting sepsis or when the gastrointestinal tract has been opened during the procedure. Incidental implantation of the device for a hiatal hernia discovered at the time of another abdominal procedure is especially to be condemned. Currently, the principal difficulty with a prosthesis is transient postoperative dysphagia, which occurs in about 30 percent of the patients following implantation. In about 2 percent of patients, persistence of dysphagia has necessitated removal of the device.

The principal disadvantage of the Angelchik prosthesis is the potential long-term deleterious effect of having an implantable material around the cardia. Although this appears to be minimal, there have been enough long-term problems with Silastic breast implants to suggest that similar problems might occur with the esophageal prosthesis. Since there is no long-term experience with the device comparable to that of other antireflux repairs, the use of the device should be *restricted to high-risk patients* with *short life expectancies*.

As can be concluded from this discussion, each of the antireflux procedures has its particular benefits and optimal conditions for its use, and their characteristics are summarized in Table 4.

INDICATIONS FOR A REPEAT ANTIREFLUX PROCEDURE VERSUS COLON INTERPOSITION

That operative failures should occur is not unreasonable when one considers the possibility of making an error in diagnosis, the change in thought process required to move from extirpative to functional surgery, and the profound effect technique can have on postoperative esophageal function. The pertinent question is: When should one revert to an esophagectomy as the solution instead of making another attempt at an esophageal procedure? There is no absolute course of action in such patients; the decision must be based upon the surgeon's individual experience and a careful preoperative evaluation.

My experience has provided some helpful guidelines. First, when the overriding complaint of a patient who has already undergone multiple esophageal procedures is dysphagia rather than regurgitation or heartburn, extirpation should be seriously considered.

Second, the presence of weak contractions in the body of the esophagus, or failure of the distal esophageal sphincter to relax following a primary peristaltic wave on the motility study, usually indicates extensive scarring of the distal esophagus—and a need for its replacement.

Third, the distention of a balloon in the distal esophagus initiates, through a local reflex arc, a contraction in the body of the esophagus above the balloon that can be felt manually, and a relaxation of the esophagus and distal sphincter below it. This mechanism is responsible for the so-called secondary peristaltic wave of the esophagus, which propels a bolus of food into the stomach which has failed to reach that destination with the primary peristaltic wave. The reflex is commonly damaged by performing multiple surgical procedures on the esophagus, and postoperatively these patients are required to swallow repetitively to induce a primary peristaltic wave in order to push the bolus of food into the stomach.

When *two* of these observations are present, I favor removal of the esophagus over attempting another esophageal procedure with the risk of failure again. Esophagectomy and replacement with an acceptable esophageal substitute can restore reasonable swallowing if properly performed by an experienced surgeon. It is wise, however, to counsel patients who undergo this procedure not to anticipate normal swallowing, lest they expect us to do what we are unable to do.

BARRETT'S ESOPHAGUS

ROY C. ORLANDO, M.D.

Barrett's esophagus is a disorder in which the distal esophagus is lined by columnar epithelium instead of the usual stratified squamous epithelium. While initially believed to be of congenital origin, the presence of columnar epithelium in the distal esophagus is in most cases acquired as a complication of gastroesophageal reflux. Thus, repeated and prolonged exposure of the esophageal lining to gastric contents containing acid, pepsin, and bile results in necrosis of squamous epithelium and subsequent replacement by the more acid-resistant columnar epithelium. At first glance lining of the distal esophagus by columnar epithelium would appear to represent a successful adaptation for protection against continued reflux injury. Unfortunately, the metaplastic columnar lining is unstable as evidenced by studies of tritiated thymidine labeling showing abnormalities in cell proliferation and by its frequent association with adenocarcinoma of the esophagus, an otherwise rare condition. It is this association with esophageal adenocarcinoma that has established the importance of Barrett's esophagus as a recognizable premalignant condition.

DIAGNOSIS

Barrett's esophagus can develop from childhood to late adult life and appears to have no sex predominance. Patients usually present with complaints similar to those seen with reflux esophagitis: heartburn, regurgitation, dysphagia, and/or odynophagia. Other subjects may be asymptomatic and discovered only during evaluation for gastrointestinal bleeding or an unrelated complaint. Since patients with Barrett's esophagus are clinically indistinguishable from those with symptomatic reflux, careful radiologic, endoscopic, and histologic evaluations of the esophagus are necessary for diagnosis.

Radiologic Evaluation

As a first approach, patients with reflux symptoms should have a barium study of the upper gastrointestinal tract. The presence of a mid-esophageal stricture, deep esophageal ulcer, or, with the addition of air contrast, a reticular mucosal pattern is highly suggestive of Barrett's esophagus.[1] These radiologic findings necessitate early endoscopy with biopsy for histologic confirmation. The absence of these findings, however, does not exclude the diagnosis.

Endoscopic Evaluation

Upper endoscopy has both greater sensitivity and specificity than radiologic studies in identifying the type, severity, and extent of reflux-related esophageal mucosal lesions, including Barrett's esophagus. For this reason most patients with persistent symptoms will eventually require endoscopy and biopsies. It is estimated that as many as 10 to 15 percent of subjects with gross esophagitis will have Barrett's esophagus. At endoscopy Barrett's esophagus will be detected by the visualization of a velvety red mucosa in the distal esophagus which contrasts sharply with the lighter pink squamous lining. While it is reliable in adults, a recent report suggests that distinguishing columnar from squamous mucosa by color may be more difficult in children.[2] When visualized, the red columnar epithelium appears in the lower esophagus as either a circumferential lesion or as isolated islands in association with tongues of red mucosa extending orad from the gastroesophageal junction (Fig. 1). Within the circumferential lesions, small islands of squamous mucosa may persist. Although endoscopic observations are generally accurate when circumferential lesions displace the squamocolumnar junction 3 cm or more into the tubular esophagus or when islands of red mucosa are observed above the squamocolumnar junction, the diagnosis must be confirmed by histologic demonstration of columnar epithelium on biopsy specimens from these areas.

While endoscopy with biopsy remains the usual method for diagnosing Barrett's esophagus, errors in over- or underdiagnosis can occur with this technique. This is because of the inability to identify accurately the true esophagogastric junction, thus ensuring an esophageal location of the biopsy site. Underdiagnosis can thus occur in patients with a short segment of Barrett's and overdiagnosis in patients with a hiatal hernia. Since errors in either direction have considerable clinical impact for the patient, it is essential that the diagnosis of Barrett's be

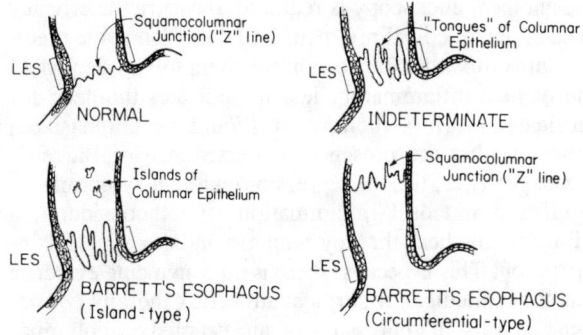

Figure 1 The normal squamocolumnar junction and its relationship to the lower esophageal sphincter (LES) is shown for comparison with that for patients with island-type and circumferential-type Barrett's esophagus. Patients with the indeterminate pattern may represent another form of Barrett's esophagus or a markedly irregular (variant of normal) squamocolumnar junction. (Reprinted with permission from Herlihy KJ, et al. Gastroenterology 1984; 86:436–443.)

accurate and made only when biopsy specimens containing columnar epithelium have clearly been obtained from esophagus and not from stomach. In difficult cases, such as those above, the distinction can best be made by performing manometrically guided Rubin-Quinton tube suction biopsies.[3] This procedure provides assurance that any columnar tissue obtained lies above the lower esophageal sphincter and, therefore, in the esophagus. There is one circumstance, however, in which the need for this approach is obviated and that is whenever endoscopic biopsies from the lower esophagus reveal specialized columnar epithelium (see below).

Histologic Evaluation

Three recognizable types of columnar epithelium have been identified in the esophagus of patients with Barrett's: specialized columnar, atrophic gastric fundic, and junctional. Each type may be found alone or in any combination with the others. Specialized columnar epithelium has a distinctive villiform structure with microvilli and goblet cells. Since tissue with this structure is not found in stomach, its presence in biopsy specimens of the lower esophagus is pathognomonic for Barrett's esophagus. In contrast, both the junctional and atrophic fundic epithelia found in Barrett's resemble tissues found in proximal stomach. Therefore, when these latter types are found on biopsy, a confident diagnosis of Barrett's requires assurance from the endoscopist that biopsies were from esophagus and not from stomach. As noted above, in difficult cases confirmation of the diagnosis should be sought by performing manometrically guided suction biopsies to ensure that all biopsies are obtained above the lower esophageal sphincter.

Additional Techniques

There are three additional techniques that may help make the diagnosis of Barrett's esophagus. The first is instillation of Lugol's solution during endoscopy. By staining black the glycogen-containing squamous mucosa, better discrimination from nonstaining columnar epithelium is provided. The second is scintigraphic scanning with ^{99m}Tc pertechnetate. This may identify columnar epithelium in esophagus because of the ability of ectopic gastric mucosa to selectively pick up and concentrate this material. The third technique, and one found useful at our institution, is measurement of the esophageal transmural electrical potential difference (PD) using a perfused catheter technique that allows simultaneous measurement of pressure.[4] By identifying the lower esophageal sphincter, the pressure tracing establishes the location of the recorded PD. Barrett's esophagus can then be identified by the presence of a high PD (> -25 mV) in the lower esophagus (Fig. 2). This occurs because columnar epithelium has an intrinsically higher PD than that of squamous epithelium.

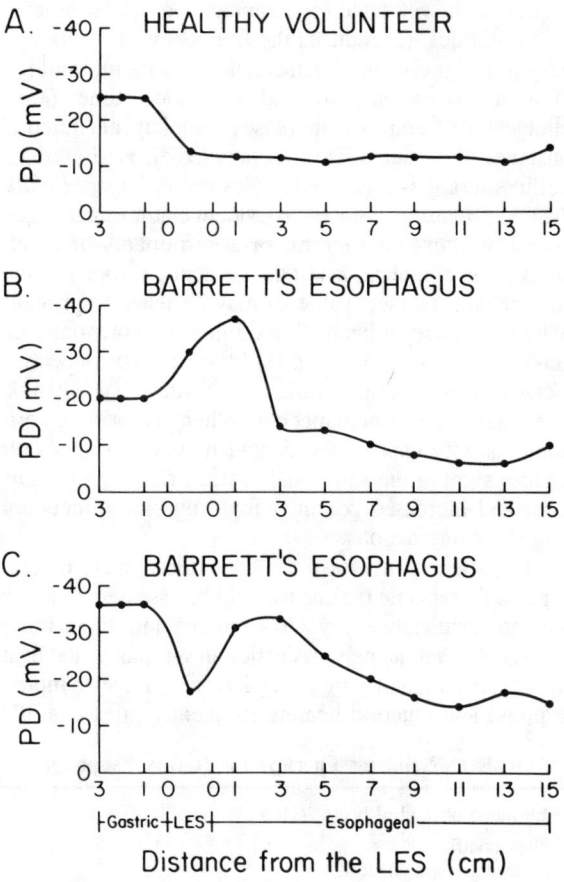

Figure 2 Potential difference profile of a healthy subject (A) is shown for comparison with the two types (B,C) of high potential difference (PD) profiles identified in patients with Barrett's esophagus. In both Barrett's profiles the esophageal PD is increased to > -25 mV. In B, the PD increases to > -25 mV as the probe is pulled through the lower esophageal sphincter (LES) into the esophagus, while in C, the PD falls to a normal value in the LES before increasing to > -25 mV in the lower esophagus. (Reprinted with permission from Herlihy KJ, et al. Gastroenterology 1984; 86:436–443.)

TREATMENT

Since the columnar lining of the lower esophagus (Barrett's esophagus) is acquired by repeated injury to squamous mucosa from gastroesophageal reflux, the cornerstone of treatment is intensive medical or surgical antireflux therapy. Successful antireflux therapy by means of healing inflammatory mucosal lesions and preventing their return halts the progression of disease. This success, however, is not guaranteed despite the good intentions of the patient, physician, and surgeon.

Medical Antireflux Therapy

Medical antireflux therapy usually entails a combination of nondrug and drug therapy. Nondrug therapy (Table 1) is employed in all patients, while drug therapy (Table 2) is tailored to individual patient needs. An ideal drug regimen should include an agent that (1) reduces the potency of the refluxate (e.g., antacids or an H_2 blocker like ranitidine), (2) reduces the frequency of reflux episodes (e.g., gaviscon, bethanechol, or metoclopramide), (3) reduces esophageal acid clearance time (e.g., bethanechol), and (4) increases esophageal mucosal resistance (e.g., sucralfate). (A detailed discussion of antireflux therapy is presented in *Gastroesophageal Reflux: Medical Treatment*.) Since it is evident that no single agent favorably alters all four major determinants of reflux esophagitis, combinations of agents acting through different mechanisms (see Table 2) may be tried empirically to achieve mucosal healing. Examples of potentially effective regimens include an H_2 blocker + bethanechol, sucralfate + bethanechol, or an H_2 blocker + sucralfate + bethanechol. When prescribing combinations with unproven efficacy, however, one should not lose sight of the additional cost, difficulty in compliance, and increased potential for drug side effects and drug-drug interactions.

In patients with Barrett's the effectiveness of each selected therapeutic regimen should be assessed clinically and endoscopically every 2 to 4 months until the primary goal is achieved, namely, reduction in symptoms and healing of inflammatory mucosal lesions. Since symptom response and mucosal healing frequently fail to parallel one another, endoscopy is required to ensure the efficacy of each new medical regimen. Failure of intensive medical antireflux therapy to control symptoms adequately and/or heal inflammatory lesions indicates the need for surgical antireflux therapy. It should be emphasized, however, that the presence or persistence of Barrett's esophagus (i.e., lack of regression) without symptoms or significant mucosal inflammation is not considered a failure of medical therapy which mandates surgical intervention. This is because there is no convincing evidence that either medical or surgical antireflux therapy *consistently* results in regression of an established columnar lining.

Surgical Antireflux Therapy

In many patients with Barrett's esophagus surgical antireflux therapy is a reasonable alternative to intensive medical antireflux therapy. Among the patients who would benefit are those who (1) have failed to improve with intensive medical therapy, (2) relapse rapidly after healing on medical therapy, (3) cannot comply with the medical regimen, (4) have associated aspiration pneumonia or severe bleeding, or (5) prefer the risks and costs of surgery to those of taking multiple medications for prolonged periods. Decisions as to type of surgical antireflux repair are presented in the chapter on *Esophageal Reflux: Surgical Treatment*.

Evaluation of Effectiveness of Therapy

While effective antireflux therapy can prevent progression of Barrett's esophagus, its capacity for inducing regression of the columnar lining and/or reducing the risk of malignant transformation remains unproven. Indeed, a recent case report reemphasizes our lack of understanding of the relationship both between reflux and regression and reflux and malignant transformation of the columnar lining. This report describes a patient with Barrett's esophagus who developed an adenocarcinoma 8 years after surgery (colonic interposition) despite clear documentation by pH probe that reflux had not continued.[5] This case also supports the rationale for judging the success of antireflux therapy, either medical or surgical, by its ability to control symptoms and heal inflammatory lesions rather than by the yet unproven potential for inducing regression of the columnar lining.

SURVEILLANCE

For Esophageal Adenocarcinoma

The prevalence of adenocarcinoma in patients with Barrett's esophagus is approximately 10 percent. A recent report suggests that the incidence (i.e., the rate at which new tumors develop over a specific time period) of this malignancy in Barrett's may be lower.[6] The mean time of follow-up in this series was short, however, and

TABLE 1 Nondrug Therapy for Reflux Esophagitis

Elevation of head of bed 6 inches

Diet modification
  Decrease size of meals
  Decrease fat and increase protein content
  Decrease content of following substances:
    coffee (caffeinated and decaffeinated), tea, cola beverages, alcohol, carminatives (peppermint, spearmint), spices, chocolate, citrus juices, tomato products

Weight reduction (where appropriate)

Modification/cessation of drug intake:
  alcohol, smoking, aspirin, nonsteroidal anti-inflammatory agents, anticholinergics, progesterone, birth control pills, theophylline, tetracycline, beta-adrenergic agonists, Valium, Demerol, morphine, calcium-channel blockers

TABLE 2 Drug Therapy for Reflux Esophagitis

	Dose	Mechanism(s) of Action
Antacid: liquid, e.g., Mylanta II (HCl Neut. capacity 25 mEq/5 ml)*	15 ml q.i.d. 1 hr p.c. and q.h.s. *or* 15 ml 7 times/day 1 hr a.c. and p.c. and q.h.s.	Buffer HCl ↑ LESP
Gaviscon (Al hydroxide, Mg trisilicate, $NaHCO_3$, alginic acid)	2-4 tabs q.i.d. p.c. and q.h.s.	↓ Reflux by viscous mechanical barrier Buffer HCl in esophagus
H_2 receptor antagonists		
Cimetidine (Tagamet)	300 mg q.i.d. p.c. and q.h.s.	↓ HCl secretion ↓ Gastric volume
Ranitidine (Zantac)	150 mg b.i.d. p.c. and q.h.s.	Same as cimetidine
Bethanechol (Urecholine)	25 mg q.i.d. ½ hr a.c. and q.h.s.	↑ LESP ↑ Esophageal acid clearance
Metoclopramide (Reglan)	10 mg q.i.d. ½ hr a.c. and q.h.s.	↑ LESP ↑ Gastric emptying ↓ Duodenogastric reflux
Sucralfate (Carafate)	1 g q.i.d. 1 hr p.c. and q.h.s.	↑ Tissue resistance Buffer HCl in esophagus Bind pepsin/bile salts

* Patients with reflux are not known to be hypersecretors of gastric acid. Therefore therapeutic doses of antacids are based on basal HCl secretion of 1–7 mEq/hr (mean, 2 mEq/hr) and peak meal-stimulated HCl secretion of 10–60 mEq/hr (mean, 30 mEq/hr).

LESP = lower esophageal sphincter pressure

thus the recommendation for long-term close surveillance remains unchanged. The only alternative to continued surveillance for malignancy in this high-risk group is surgical resection of the columnar lining. Since this would require distal esophagectomy, a procedure with significant morbidity and a mortality rate of 2 to 5 percent, its routine use for prophylaxis against cancer is not recommended.

At our institution routine clinical and endoscopic follow up is recommended every 12 months for patients with Barrett's esophagus. Using a standardized report form with its diagram of esophagus and stomach, the endoscopist depicts the extent and pattern of all esophageal abnormalities (e.g., red mucosa, ulcers, erosions, friability, exudate) and site of biopsies. Multiple pinch forceps biopsies and brush cytology are performed in areas known to be or suspected to be Barrett's esophagus. The distance of each biopsy from the mouth and squamocolumnar junction, and/or location with respect to other landmarks is recorded on both specimen containers and record sheet to ensure accurate interpretation of histologic data.

The finding of carcinoma in situ at biopsy of columnar epithelium warrants surgical resection; the esophagectomy should be extended where possible to include all areas lined by columnar mucosa. The finding of marked dysplasia in the columnar lining is more problematic and in the presence of active inflammation possible dysplastic changes may reflect reactive nonmalignant epithelial changes. In this circumstance repeat endoscopy with biopsy and cytology is recommended for confirmation of dysplasia and to rule out a missed malignancy. If dysplasia alone is confirmed, intensification of medical antireflux therapy is indicated with surveillance at closer intervals. Data are currently not available to determine if a prophylactic esophagectomy is warranted in all patients with persistent dysplasia despite intensification of antireflux therapy. This decision is best made on a case-by-case basis after consultation among surgeon, pathologist, endoscopist, primary care provider, and patient.

For Colonic Neoplasms

There have been two recent preliminary reports suggesting that patients with Barrett's esophagus are at increased risk for the development of colonic neoplasms, both adenomas and adenocarcinoma.[7,8] The mean age of the patients with Barrett's discovered to have these abnormalities was 63 and 64 years. This age group, even in the absence of Barrett's, has a relatively high prevalence of colonic neoplasms. Before any firm recommendations can be made, further details will be needed for both patient and control groups, including whether patients had other independent risk factors for colonic neoplasms (e.g., family history). It is not clear from a pathogenetic point of view why a relationship should exist between the two disorders.

In the interim, routine screening with yearly stool guaiac, complete blood count, and sigmoidoscopy may be reasonable. If either a positive stool guaiac or an iron deficiency anemia were discovered and an upper endoscopy (performed yearly for surveillance of esophageal cancer) failed to provide an explanation (such as erosive esophagitis or Barrett's ulcer), then colonoscopy and/or barium enema would be indicated to search for a lesion in the lower gastrointestinal tract.

REFERENCES

1. Levine MS, Kressel HY, Caroline DF, et al. Barrett's esohagus: reticular pattern of the mucosa. Radiology 1983; 147:663–667.
2. Dahms BB, Rothstein FC. Barrett's esophagus in children: a consequence of chronic gastroesophageal reflux. Gastroenterology 1984; 86:318–323.
3. Paull A, Trier JS, Dalton MD, et al. The histologic spectrum of Barrett's esophagus. N Engl J Med 1976; 295:476–480.
4. Herlihy KJ, Orlando RC, Bryson JC, et al. Barrett's esophagus: clinical, endoscopic, histologic, manometric, and electrical potential difference characteristics. Gastroenterology 1984; 68:436–443.
5. Hamilton SR, Hutcheon DF, Ravich WJ, et al. Adenocarcinoma in Barrett's esophagus after elimination of gastroesophageal reflux. Gastroenterology 1984; 86:356–360.
6. Spechler SJ, Robbins AH, Rubins HB. Has the risk of cancer in Barrett's esophagus been exaggerated? Gastroenterology 1984; 86:1262.
7. Sontag SJ, Schnell T, Chintam R. Barrett's esophagus and colonic neoplasia. Gastroenterology 1984; 86:1261.
8. Tripp M, Sampliner RE, Morgan TR. Colonic adenoma and Barrett's esophagus. Clin Res 1985; 33:40A.

CAUSTIC INJURY

BARRY A. FRANK, M.D.
H. WORTH BOYCE Jr., M.D., F.A.C.P.

The ingestion of corrosive chemicals presents a complicated diagnostic and therapeutic challenge to the physician. Though it is a relatively uncommon problem for the average clinician, it is estimated that 5,000 children under 5 years of age accidentally ingest corrosives each year. Other groups at risk include adults under the influence of alcohol and the mentally retarded, psychotic, or depressed (suicidal) patient. Numerous chemicals containing both alkali and acid have been implicated in such ingestion (Table 1).

PATHOLOGY

The pathological changes that ensue after ingestion of these corrosives are variable and depend upon the nature, concentration, and physical state of the agent; the amount ingested; time of exposure ("dwell" time); and the amount of reexposure secondary to vomiting or reflux. Clearly, the ingestion of a large volume of a relatively mild chemical can be just as lethal as a small volume of a more destructive agent. Alkali causes liquefaction (saponification) necrosis which dissolves superficial mucosa and rapidly diffuses into deeper tissues. Blood vessel thrombosis results in further cellular necrosis and degeneration, enhancing the agent's penetration and commonly resulting in full-thickness burns. In older reports, these agents were predominantly in the form of flakes or solid pellets which would adhere to oropharyngeal and esophageal mucosa leading to corrosive injury. Since the mid-1960s, however, the ingestion of liquid agents containing concentrated sodium or potassium hydroxide has led to more extensive damage involving the oropharynx, esophagus, and stomach.

Acid compounds produce a coagulation necrosis of the surface epithelium and usually cause extensive damage to the stomach. Though this coagulum tends to limit penetration into the deeper layers of the gastric wall, pylorospasm leads to pooling of the caustic agent in the antrum where severe changes can occur. The resultant damage can lead to pyloric obstruction, antral stenosis with a "linitis plastica" type of appearance, or an hourglass type of deformity which may develop weeks to months after ingestion. The presence of food tends to limit the changes in the distal stomach, while ingestion on an empty stomach causes more extensive involvement. The esophagus is relatively spared, probably because of the usual rapid transit of the acid through the esophagus, the greater resistance of esophageal squamous epithelium to acid, and the "protection" afforded by the superficial coagulation necrosis which prevents deeper penetration into the tissue. Between 20 and 50 percent of patients ingesting strong liquid acids, however, may have significant esophageal burns.

NATURAL HISTORY

The natural history of corrosive injury is also variable but can be classified into three stages (Table 2). Stric-

TABLE 1 Household Corrosives

Chemicals	Brand Name
Alkali	
Sodium hydroxide	Drano, Easy-Off
Sodium hydrochlorite	Mr. Muscle, Liquid-plumr,
(+KOH, NaOH)	Chlorox
Acid	
Sodium bisulfate	Sani-Flush
Sodium acid sulfate	Vanish
Hydrochloric +NH_4Cl	Lysol
Sulfuric acid	Battery fluid
Drugs	
Potassium Chloride	Slo-K
Quinidine	Quinaglute
Tetracycline	Doxycycline

TABLE 2 Natural History of Corrosive Esophageal Injury

Acute Necrotic Phase (up to 10 days)
  Inflammation, microabscesses, ulceration, edema

Granulation Phase (between 7 and 12 days → 2-4 weeks)
  New blood vessels, fibroblasts → adhesions
  Degeneration of muscle and nerves

Cicatrization (Chronic) Phase (2 weeks → months)
  Contraction, scarring, strictures

---

tures may develop during the cicatrization phase of recovery with approximately 80 percent manifested within the first eight weeks after injury. The development of strictures, however, can occur insidiously over months to many years after the initiating event. Final recovery is marked by regeneration of stratified squamous epithelium which is devoid of glands. A well known "deceptive" period occurs after injury when edema, spasm, and dysphagia begin to subside and swallowing improves (between the second and seventh days) only to be followed by serious "new" symptomatology after the first week. Careful observation and therapeutic measures should not be aborted during this stage of the process.

CLINICAL PRESENTATION

Recent studies have underscored the variability of the clinical presentation in these patients and the difficulty in assessing the degree of injury from the presenting signs and symptoms. In one study of 378 patients by Gaudreault et al, the incidence of mild to severe esophageal injury was similar regardless of the presence of signs or symptoms.[1] In another study by Mansson, corrosive lesions of the pharynx, stagnation of secretions in the hypopharynx, elevated temperature, and leukocytosis were factors suggestive of lesions in the esophagus but none was statistically significant.[2] Both authors concluded that the *presence or absence of signs or symptoms cannot accurately predict the occurrence or severity of gastrointestinal tract injury*. No symptoms may be noted, or mild to moderate signs and symptoms may occur, including increased salivation and drooling, mouth or chest pain, dysphagia, odynophagia, abdominal pain, nausea, vomiting, and hematemesis. With more extensive damage, fever, shock with tachycardia and hypotension, massive hematemesis, and signs of mediastinitis and peritonitis can be seen. Tachypnea, dyspnea, hoarseness, and stridor suggest either associated laryngeal edema or actual epiglottic or laryngeal damage due to aspiration of the corrosive agent. Pneumonia and tracheoesophageal fistula also may ensue.

DIAGNOSIS AND INITIAL THERAPY

Hospitalization is urgently required in all cases of suspected corrosive ingestion. Attempts should be made to identify the nature of the offending agent, though this often is not possible. Because of the large number of possible caustic agents and the marked variability in their formulation, the clinician or an associate should contact a major poison control center for up-to-date product information before accepting or rejecting the possibility of damage from a product that is suspected of having been ingested. An essential caveat is that the patient always should be suspected of ingesting multiple drugs or other substances concomitant with the caustic agent, especially if the intent was suicide.

Careful physical examination should be performed, including inspection of the oral and pharyngeal tissues and auscultation for signs of pneumonitis or signs suggesting a perforated viscus. It is important to note, however, that *the lack of oral or pharyngeal burns does not preclude the possibility of extensive esophageal or gastric pathologic changes*. If the patient is seen within the first hour after ingestion, gastric intubation *preferably under fluoroscopic guidance* and lavage with water should be carried out. Oral intake should be restricted and intravenous fluids started during the initial resuscitative efforts.

Usually by the time these patients present for medical care, most of the chemical tissue damage has been completed. Therefore, neutralization of the offending agent is rarely indicated. As noted above, gastric lavage using water should be performed if the patient is seen during the immediate post injury period. Emetics should be avoided. Ventilatory support should be instituted if indicated and intravenous fluids begun, with the addition of colloids or blood products as necessary. Vital signs should be measured and physical examination performed frequently. Indirect laryngoscopy should be performed early to visualize the hypopharynx and larynx and assess injury in these areas.

Further recommendations concerning diagnostic and therapeutic intervention are controversial, and the literature is lacking in controlled, double-blinded trials assessing the various proposed modalities. Therefore, most recommendations in the literature are anecdotal and difficult to assess because of the lack of control groups or the lack of control over the variables being evaluated.

Therapy in proven cases of ingestion must be individualized and based upon the location and degree of injury as assessed by *endoscopy*. If there was suicidal intent, psychiatric consultation should be obtained immediately. Patients without evidence of oral, pharyngeal, esophageal, or gastroduodenal injury can be reassured and discharged from medical care. Those patients who present with profound shock and evidence of widespread necrosis and perforation require emergent resuscitation and operation. This usually involves cervical esophagostomy, gastrostomy or jejunostomy, and resection with drainage of the affected areas. Between these two extremes, no consensus exists concerning appropriate management.

Radiography

On presentation, all patients should undergo roentgenography including plain films of the neck, chest, and abdomen looking for signs of perforation or pneumonia.

Widening of the mediastinum, with or without free air, pneumoperitoneum, pleural effusion, pericarditis, or abnormal displacement of the pleural reflection all suggest perforation. Contrast radiography is a poor method to determine the degree and location of acute injury. Its importance is in documenting perforation (or changes indicative of impending perforation) and, later in the course, stricture formation. Water-soluble agents are recommended initially because of the significant risk of perforation.

The esophageal findings early after injury include mucosal edema or scalloping with blurred esophageal margins, ulceration, sloughing of the mucosa, intramural collections of contrast indicative of intramural dissection, and decreased or absent peristalsis. Gaseous dilatation with intraluminal retention of contrast material is considered by some a sign of impending perforation similar to the "toxic" dilatation of the colon seen in ulcerative colitis.[3] Later, stenoses and aperistalsis can be seen as indicative of fibrous replacement of the damaged mucosa and deeper layers.

Gastric involvement is divided into three stages. The first is the acute phase, lasting from 1 to 10 days, in which gastric folds are noted to be thickened and ulcerated, the antrum rigid and atonic, and the pylorus dilated. Duodenal involvement may be variable with edema, ulceration, atony, and dilatation. The subacute phase is second, lasting 11 to 16 days and characterized by atony, dilatation, and rigidity of the antrum, pylorus, and duodenum. The third phase is the chronic phase, lasting from 21 days to months after ingestion, during which time antral stenosis and contracture with or without gastric outlet obstruction may occur.

Though contrast radiography is of limited value in assessing the extent of injury acutely, it is a valuable tool especially in patients in whom endoscopic visualization is limited because of impending perforation or severe edema and narrowing. Later it is useful in assessing strictures, scarring, outlet obstruction and in the long-term surveillance for malignancy.

Endoscopy

The use of endoscopy in the diagnosis of caustic injuries has been controversial, but most experts now agree on the need to document the extent of damage with early (within 12 to 24 hours) fiberoptic panendoscopy. The advent of newer, small-caliber forward-viewing flexible endoscopes has facilitated these examinations, reducing the risk of perforation or mucosal injury. We believe that careful fiberoptic panendoscopy is indicated in anyone suspected of ingesting a corrosive substance—regardless of the lack of symptoms or oral burns—in whom injury to the upper gastrointestinal tract is in doubt. Early endoscopy is contraindicated in the presence of shock, suspected perforation, severe hypopharyngeal edema or necrosis, a necrotic epiglottis, severe respiratory distress, or unavailability of an experienced endoscopist. When performed carefully, utilizing direct vision and minimal insufflation during passage, fiberoptic endoscopy is safe and can accurately document the location and degree of injury. An attempt should be made to examine the entire upper gastrointestinal tract to the proximal duodenum whenever feasible.

Grade I (first-degree) injury is characterized by erythematous mucosa with erosions but without ulceration. There is minimal to no loss of mucosa and no hemorrhage. These lesions do not proceed to stricture formation (Table 3). In grade II (second-degree) injury ulceration with more intense erythema and edema are seen. Areas of gray-white exudate and hemorrhage are noted but intervening areas of normal mucosa may be present. Esophageal motility is present, either as peristalsis or tertiary contractions. Grade III (third-degree) injuries reveal extensive ulceration and hemorrhage with a gray to black exudate, mucosal slough, atonic muscle and a dilated lumen. More severe injury may result in gangrene, periesophagitis, and perforation with mediastinitis, peritonitis, tracheoesophageal fistula, or pleural effusion. Such patients may require urgent surgical intervention if they are to survive. Periodic follow-up endoscopy may be necessary to assess new symptoms, the rate of healing, or to examine areas of stenosis. Grade III injury most often leads to stricture formation.

There is some controversy concerning the implications of finding necrotic, black-based ulcers on endoscopic examination. Ulcers with this appearance previously were thought to imply full-thickness gastric wall injury indicative of future perforation. More recent data, however, suggest that the black discoloration is due to hematin formation by acid effects upon erythrocytes and does not necessarily imply full-thickness injury or impending perforation. Several authors have reported successful medical management of patients with black-based, necrotic ulcers.

MANAGEMENT

Further therapeutic intervention is based upon the clinical status of the patient and the degree of injury assessed by radiographs and early fiberoptic panendoscopy. Again, the lack of controlled trials precludes definitive arguments in support of any therapeutic modality. Our recommendations, based upon our experience utilizing these various modalities and a review of the literature, represent a "common sense" approach to the management of these patients.

TABLE 3 Endoscopic Staging of Corrosive Esophageal Injury

Grade I	Erythema, edema
	Erosions and exudate, no ulcers or hemorrhage
Grade II	Intense erythema and edema
	Gray-white exudate with ulcers and hemorrhage
	Loss of mucosa
Grade III	Extensive ulceration and hemorrhage
	Gray-black exudate, mucosal slough
	Dilated, atonic lumen, no peristalsis

Nasogastric Intubation

A soft, Silastic nasogastric tube should be placed, *preferably under fluoroscopic guidance*, to ensure maintenance of a lumen and for gastric access. Emphasis should be placed on utilizing fluoroscopic control for placement of these tubes to prevent inadvertent curling of the tube above the level of injury, to ensure proper placement within the antrum of the stomach, and to reduce the risk of perforation of injured tissues by keeping the tube in the proper axis during passage. Despite the theoretical disadvantage of precipitating further mucosal damage with the tube, it provides several therapeutic functions: (1) in less serious injuries, it allows feeding and hydration while putting the esophagus at rest during the initial days post injury; (2) it helps maintain luminal patency and may reduce adhesions between apposing ulcerations; (3) in more serious cases, it allows decompression of the upper gastrointestinal tract while the patient is observed for complications or prepared for urgent surgery. In less serious cases, the tube can be removed in three to ten days, after the patient is able to swallow liquids and the risk of more severe injury has passed. A soft diet can then be instituted as tolerated.

Total Parenteral Nutrition

In patients with more severe injuries (grade III), early feeding via the nasogastric tube or perorally is contraindicated. In these cases, total parenteral nutrition (TPN) is beneficial in maintaining and improving overall nutrition while allowing the gastrointestinal tract to rest and heal. DiConstanzo and his associates, in a series of 94 patients, have advocated the use of TPN in all patients with grade II or III injuries.[4] Their observations suggest that TPN: (1) protects the burn from surface trauma and infection that may arise from eating; (2) diminishes the frequency of local, mechanical complications and infections; (3) reduces the potential for aspiration pneumonia; (4) reduces the frequency of stenoses by decreasing the stimulus to fibroblastic reaction; (5) promotes a feeling of well-being; and (6) reverses the hypercatabolism associated with the acute injury. These factors, particularly the reduction in the incidence of strictures, have not been evaluated in a controlled fashion and therefore are difficult to endorse. In patients with more severe gastrointestinal tract injury, however, TPN appears useful in supporting nutrition.

Antibiotics and Corticosteroid Therapy

The use of antibiotics and corticosteroids is fraught with controversy in the literature. Antibiotics are purported to combat local and systemic infection, reduce necrosis, inhibit the local stimulating effect of infection on fibroblasts, and cover the increased risk of infection in patients treated with steroids. Corticosteroids are said to reduce inflammation and granulation and thereby reduce the number and/or severity of strictures.

Spain (1950) demonstrated experimentally that mice given steroids 24 hours *before* caustic ingestion had a decreased incidence of strictures while no effect was noted in animals given steroids 48 hours *after* injury. Cardona and Daly (1971) reported 133 patients treated with antibiotics and steroids. In this uncontrolled trial, only 9 percent of patients subsequently developed strictures that required further therapy. They also suggest that the strictures encountered were less dense, more pliable, and yielded to dilation far more readily than in patients treated by other methods. Haller and associates (1971) reported on 235 children after caustic ingestion and noted a 12 percent incidence of strictures. They stated that steroids inhibited granulation and resulted in strictures that were less dense and easier to manage. Again, this study was uncontrolled. Tewfik, in a retrospective, uncontrolled report of 86 cases, also supported the use of antibiotics and steroids noting an 8.8 percent incidence of strictures.[5]

Others have argued against the use of steroids stating that they facilitate infection, are of no proven benefit especially in severe grade II and grade III burns, and cannot be given early enough to be effective. Middlekamp (1969), reporting on 32 patients, found that steroids delayed, but did not prevent, strictures. Webb (1970), evaluating 42 patients, noted a 23 percent incidence of strictures in patients with second degree burns treated with steroids and antibiotics and a 100 percent incidence of strictures in patients with third degree burns treated in this fashion. They concluded that steroids were of no benefit in patients with third degree injuries and that the efficacy of steroids in second degree burns could not be determined from their study. DiConstanzo (1980) stated that "systemic use of steroids and antibiotics is not indicated and, in fact, is dangerous in the way used hitherto." Oakes and his colleagues (1982) in their review of the subject concluded that "after more than 20 years of clinical experience, there are no convincing data to prove that steroid therapy is more effective than nonsteroid therapy in *any* patient, even those with second degree burns." They further state that "in view of the dangers and the lack of proven efficacy, clinicians should not feel compelled to institute steroid therapy for caustic esophagitis simply because it has come to be considered standard therapy."

Because corticosteroids impair wound healing, suppress the body's immune defense mechanisms, and potentially can mask the signs and symptoms of infection or perforation, we do not routinely prescribe them unless the patient is noted to have *laryngeal edema with associated respiratory stridor*. In such cases, 1 to 2 mg per kilogram per day of *prednisone* or its equivalent is prescribed for several days and, thereafter, rapidly tapered. Patients so treated require antibiotic coverage.

Antibiotics are recommended in any patient with proven or suspected infection and in those patients with grade II and III caustic injury. It is not necessary to routinely initiate antibiotic therapy in all patients regardless of the severity of injury. Broad-spectrum coverage with penicillin and aminoglycosides or the newer third-generation cephalosporins alone or in combination would appear to be most appropriate. Other antibiotics, including erythromycin, oxacillin, ampicillin, clindamycin, and chloramphenicol in various combinations have been used effectively.

Peroral Dilation

Peroral esophageal dilation under fluoroscopic guidance is one of the cornerstones of therapy for caustic ingestion and can be begun safely early in the postinjury course. Dilation maintains luminal patency preventing tight stenoses and thereby facilitating nutrition and promoting "well-being." We prefer the tapered-tip Maloney dilators, though others utilize the blunt-tip Hurst bougies. In later stages, the Savary or Eder-Puestow dilators used over guide wires are preferred for treating tight strictures. Whichever equipment is chosen, we stress the importance of *fluoroscopic control* of the procedure to reduce the risk of perforation by a "wayward" tip of the dilator or guide wire. Patients with grade I injuries do not require dilation but should be examined with a barium swallow and a bolus challenge between two and three months after ingestion or sooner if dysphagia occurs. Severe grade III lesions contraindicate early dilation but can usually be dilated safely after endoscopic evidence of mucosal healing is noted. In the remaining patients; i.e., those with grade II injury, early (3 to 7 days after injury), nonforceful dilation can be undertaken to prevent tight stenoses which may develop in anywhere from 4 to 27 percent of these patients. Dilation should be performed cautiously using fluoroscopy, advancing no more than four F units (three dilators) in any one session. We generally begin early dilation with about a No. 40 F dilator or smaller and "sound" the esophagus carefully before using a larger dilator. Furthermore, it is prudent to "overlap" the bouginage sequence, beginning each new session with the last dilator easily passed at the preceding session. Dilation frequency may be varied but usually is repeated every 1 to 3 days during the second and third week after injury.

In patients with grade III injury a dramatic tightening of the stenosis is to be expected between 14 and 21 days after injury when fibroblastic activity reaches its peak. At this stage it may be necessary to temporarily "back off" several dilator sizes or switch to dilation over a guide wire with more rigid dilators (Eder-Puestow or Savary). The main effort should be directed at preventing significant loss of lumen patency. If adequate lumen patency can be maintained at this stage, the operator will find that intervals between dilation gradually can be lengthened. Though some patients may heal without the need for further dilation, some of them will require periodic peroral dilation throughout their lives. The chapter *Esophageal Stricture* provides additional details on dilation.

When early therapy is inadequate or injury is extremely severe, peroral dilation may be impossible or considered too risky because of the degree of stenosis or length of esophageal injury. In such instances, gastrostomy is indicated with placement of an indwelling thread for Tucker retrograde dilation. This approach can be continued indefinitely and may be preferable in some patients to extensive, high-risk surgical procedures.

Esophageal Stents

In 1966, Fell et al described an esophageal splinting technique that prevented stricturing in animal models.[6] Subsequently, Reyes[7] reporting on three patients, and Mills[8] reporting on an additional four patients, refined this technique using it in children and adults. They suggest that the use of an intraluminal esophageal stent would reduce inflammation and granulation, minimize scarring, and prevent fusion of mural ulcers with subsequent obliteration of the lumen by granulation tissue. They propose that stents promote complete epithelialization by providing a clean base of granulation tissue upon which healing can occur. They have fashioned their stents utilizing a modified Silastic tubing which is placed intraoperatively under direct endoscopic control. The results reported in these seven patients are encouraging with no strictures being noted in follow-up between 1 and 20 months. The groups studied are small, however, and further experience with this technique is necessary before it can be recommended. The use of stents in patients with carcinoma of the esophagus is discussed in both the *Esophageal Stricture* and *Cancer of the Esophagus and Cardia: Surgical Treatment* chapters.

Surgery

Specific recommendations concerning the surgical approach to these patients is beyond the scope of this text. Acute surgical intervention is indicated for those patients with grade III lesions who are deteriorating despite intensive medical management, for those patients who present with or develop overt perforation, or for those patients who develop a tracheoesophageal fistula. Generally, diverting procedures utilizing cervical esophagostomy, gastrostomy or jejunostomy, and resection or exclusion of the affected tissues is warranted. Severe gastric lesions with perforation are treated with resection and Billroth I or Billroth II anastomoses or total gastrectomy, depending on the extent of injury. Reconstructive surgery for esophageal lesions is usually performed in a staged fashion after diversion allows time for resuscitation of the patient and adequate healing of the damaged tissues. These procedures usually include either colon interposition or esophagogastrostomy or pharyngogastrostomy. The experience, expertise and clinical judgment of the surgeon will govern the techniques employed and the results obtained.

Patients who are candidates for surgery in the later stages of recovery after caustic ingestion include those who fail to improve with conservative medical management and require too frequent dilation or those who cannot be dilated (patients who have been lost to follow-up and who return with extensive, long strictures of the esophagus in whom wire or string passage has failed); patients who develop a tracheoesophageal fistula; and patients who cannot handle the psychological stresses of long-term dilation therapy. The appropriate procedure will depend upon the extent and location of the injury but usually will include esophagectomy with an esophagogastric or esophagocolic (colon interposition) anastomosis. Obviously, every effort should be made to preserve the intact esophagus using careful dilation by an experienced physician before surgical intervention is contemplated.

COMPLICATIONS

Long-term complications include recurrent or delayed strictures, especially in those patients with grade II and III injuries, and *squamous cell carcinoma* of the esophagus. Various studies have reported a 2 to 5 percent incidence of squamous cell carcinoma after corrosive injury to the esophagus, a risk estimated as approximately one thousand times greater than that of the normal population. The latency period before carcinoma develops varies from 12 to 41 years and is shorter for injuries occurring after childhood. Therefore, these patients require long-term surveillance with careful attention to changes in their symptoms or physical examination. Specific surveillance protocols, however, have not yet been defined.

REFERENCES

1. Gaudreault P, et al. Predictability of esophageal injury from signs and syndromes: A study of caustic injections in 378 children. Pediatrics 1983; 71(5):767–770.
2. Mansson I. Diagnosis of acute corrosive lesions of the esophagus. J. Laryngol Otol 1978; 92:499–503.
3. Martel WM. Radiologic features of esophagogastritis secondary to extremely caustic agents. Radiology 1972; 103:31–36.
4. DiConstanzo J, Nouclere M, Jouglard J, et al. New therapeutic approach to corrosive burns of the upper gastrointestinal tract. Gut 1980; 21:370–375.
5. Tewfik TL, Schloss MD. Ingestion of lye and other corrosive agents—a study of 86 infant child cases. J Otolaryngol 1980; 9:72–77.
6. Fell, SC, Denzie A, Becker NH, et al. The effect of intraluminal splinting in the prevention of caustic stricture of the esophagus. J Thorac Cardiovasc Surg 1966; 52:675–681.
7. Reyes HM, Chung-Yuan L, Schlunk FF, et al. Experimental treatment of corrosive esophageal burns. J Pediatr Surg 1974; 9:317–327.
8. Mills LJ, Estrera AS, Platt MR. Avoidance of esophageal stricture following severe caustic burns by the use of intraluminal stents. Ann Thorac Surg 1979; 28:60–65.

ESOPHAGEAL STRICTURE

DAVID A. PEURA, M.D., Col., M.C.
LAWRENCE F. JOHNSON, M.D., Col., M.C.

Dysphagia, defined as difficulty in swallowing, is an important symptom of esophageal obstruction. It can result from either a fixed stenosis, such as a benign or malignant stricture, or an esophageal motility disorder that impedes the passage of swallowed material. Stenosis of the esophagus usually produces dysphagia once progression of the disease decreases the lumen diameter by 50 percent. Characteristically, dysphagia resulting from stenosis occurs primarily with solid food, whereas the dysphagia from an esophageal motor disorder occurs with liquids alone or with both liquids and solids. Dysphagia should never be considered functional and all patients with this symptom should have a complete evaluation.

Once the cause of the patient's dysphagia has been determined by means of history, physical examination, and appropriate diagnostic studies, the main goal of therapy is the reestablishment and maintenance of a patent lumen. The purpose of this chapter is to discuss the methods utilized to maintain luminal patency in patients with structural esophageal narrowing. Most patients with structural lesions, regardless of the cause, can be safely and effectively managed by nonsurgical methods. Individuals with dysphagia from benign strictures can obtain long-lasting relief of symptoms following peroral bouginage. Lumen patency can be reestablished and maintained in most individuals with malignant strictures by periodic dilation and, when necessary, the nonoperative placement of a prosthetic tube. While surgical management is an acceptable alternative to peroral bouginage, it is rarely required for benign strictures and is usually only palliative for most malignant strictures.

Patients with dysphagia from any cause should be counseled about several nonspecific measures to prevent food impaction at the site of narrowing. They should be advised to (1) chew their food carefully, (2) alter the physical characteristics of their diet as necessary to include such things as pureed foods, (3) drink sufficient fluids with their meals and pills to facilitate passage, and (4) direct particular attention to their dentition. Proper dental occlusion is necessary to ensure thorough mastication of food and uniformity of bolus size prior to swallowing. Poorly fitting dentures should be corrected to prevent malocclusion. Moreover, patients whose hard palates are covered by a dental appliance should be made aware that their sensation of bolus size prior to swallowing will be impaired, and thus, they should consciously chew their food well prior to swallowing. Patients should also avoid drinking alcohol in large quantities before meals, since this may dull their consciousness and make them less aware of bolus size prior to deglutition. If food impaction occurs, patients should be instructed not to induce gagging or retching, since both could potentially cause esophageal mucosal laceration or perforation. They should be counseled to seek medical attention immediately to relieve the impaction. Physicians should be cautioned not to attempt to blindly push impacted material into the stomach nor send patients with impaction home hoping that the material will pass spontaneously. Such treatment could result in esophageal perforation.

INSTRUMENTS FOR PERORAL DILATION

Since the early 1950s, peroral dilation has been performed with *rubber mercury-filled dilators*. These instruments have proven to be both safe and effective and are the most commonly used dilators in clinical practice today. The rounded tip (Hurst) and tapered tip (Maloney) rubber mercury-filled dilators are supplied in sizes 16 to 60 F units (1 mm dilator diameter = 3 F). Each sequentially sized dilator is 2 F units larger than the preceding one. In general, rubber dilators that are smaller than 30 F are so flexible that they tend to bend in the hypopharynx and thus prove ineffective when dilating most stenotic lesions. Because of their tapered tip (14 F for all dilators), Maloney dilators are preferred by most clinicians. This tapered tip is easier to pass through the cricopharyngeus and serves as a guide that allows safe passage of the larger main shaft through tight, angulated, or tortuous strictures. Unfortunately, the tapered tip of the Maloney dilator is flexible and therefore it occasionally curls up in the esophagus and causes perforation as the dilator is advanced. In contrast, while the rounded tip of the Hurst dilator is more difficult to pass through the hypopharynx, it provides a more forceful stretch of an esophageal stricture and may in certain cases provide more effective dilation.

Peroral dilations using *metal dilators* with *guide wires* are best for complex, long, or very tight esophageal strictures. Eder-Puestow metal olive dilators are supplied in sizes 15 to 45 F. The metal olives are attached to a flexible metal rod, and this assembly is passed over the accompanying guide wire that has been previously positioned in the stomach by *fluoroscopy*. This guide wire is a stainless steel piano wire with a flexible distal spring tip (7 F) that bends whenn resistance is met to guard against perforation. In addition, this wire ensures a proper plane of passage for the dilator through both the hypopharyngeal cricopharyngeal region and the esophageal stricture. Because of the added stiffness of the metal rod, more force can be applied during dilation with metal dilators. In addition, no swallowing effort is required by the patient for passage of this instrument.

Recently, *coaxial balloon catheters* have become available for dilating esophageal strictures. Coaxial balloons exert a radial rather than a longitudinal force on the strictured segment. These instruments come in sequential sizes and can be hydrostatically or pneumatically inflated to a predetermined fixed diameter. Coaxial balloon dilation should be performed over a previously positioned guide wire, and position of the instrument during dilation should be monitored by fluorscopy. Alternatively, the instruments may be passed along side or through the biopsy channel of a fiberoptic endoscope, thus allowing visual control of the dilation procedure. Recently, lumen-seeking balloon catheters have become available which not only facilitate dilation of long, tortuous strictures but also facilitate the passage of guide wires over which more conventional dilation instruments may be passed.

Savary dilators are hollow radiopaque bougies made of plastic-coated polyvinyl material. These instruments are supplied in sizes 15 to 45 F and are most often passed over a metal guide wire in the same manner as the Eder-Puestow dilators. Although Savary dilators are relatively new and clinical experience with their use is limited, they have characteristics that in the future may make them preferable to the metal olive instruments. For instance, because of their plastic construction, Savary dilators are better tolerated by the patient and less apt to cause traumatic damage to the teeth and hypopharynx than their rigid metal counterparts. Savary instruments are also tapered so that they lack the abrupt waist of the metal olives. This tapering permits a more gradual but less forceful dilation. In addition, because of their single-piece construction, serial dilation with Savary instruments can be accomplished without the inconvenience of changing olives.

Dilation of strictures should *not* be performed with an endoscope, since fiberoptic instruments are not designed for this purpose. Forcible manipulation through a narrowed area could damage the instrument as well as the esophagus.

PATIENT PREPARATION

All patients should be informed of the indications, techniques, and potential risks associated with esophageal dilation. While bouginage performed by experienced physicians is associated with low risk to the patient, the potential complications of this procedure include bleeding, esophageal perforation, and pulmonary aspiration. Most esophageal dilation can be conducted as an outpatient procedure. Local anesthetic sprays or gargles may be used to desensitize the hypopharynx prior to dilation. After several sessions, however, most patients no longer require any application of anesthetic. In adults, sedation and general anesthesia are not required for dilation and should be avoided, since they interfere with patient observation, cooperation, and proper monitoring both during and after the dilation. While some substernal chest pain may be associated with esophageal dilation, it should quickly subside when the dilation is completed. If this is not the case, or the patient develops odynophagia, back pain, fever, tachycardia, or leukocytosis, then esophageal perforation should be suspected and diagnostic procedures initiated to exclude this possibility.

We use fluoroscopic control for the initial dilation session in all patients. This is primarily to document that the dilator passes through the strictured area and does not curl in the esophagus and merely simulate passage through the narrowed area. Subsequent dilations performed with rubber dilators may be performed without fluoroscopy. We feel, however, that fluoroscopy is mandatory when metal dilators are used, both to document the appropriate positioning of the guide wire in the stomach and to observe the actual dilation procedure. Fluoroscopic or direct endoscopic monitoring of dilation is also necessary with coaxial balloon instruments to ensure proper balloon position. In addition, fluoroscopy should be used in those patients with long, tortuous strictures or those with large hypopharyngeal or esophageal diverticuli, since blind instrumentation could result in perforation caused by trauma to the esophageal wall or inadvertent intubation of the diverticulum.

To minimize the chance of pulmonary aspiration from retained gastric or esophageal contents, patients should be instructed to take nothing orally for at least 6 hours prior to the dilation. Dentures or oral appliances should be removed prior to instrumentation. Individuals who are known to have a dilated esophagus that incompletely empties, such as occurs in achalasia or neoplasms of the gastric cardia, should have the esophagus emptied with a large-bore nasogastric tube prior to any instrumentation. Suction equipment should be available during the procedure to remove any oropharyngeal secretions.

TECHNIQUES OF DILATION

All instruments should be thoroughly cleaned prior to use with an antiseptic solution such as Betadine (povidine-iodine). This helps prevent bacteremia caused by instrument contamination. During dilation, the patient should be comfortably positioned, either sitting in a straight-back chair or lying in the lateral decubitus position with the head slightly elevated. Individuals should not be dilated in a standing position, since a vasovagal reaction could result in a fall with subsequent injuries.

Dilators should be lubricated over their distal tips with a water-soluble jelly. Only a small amount of lubricant should be used, since any excess could be wiped off in the hypopharynx and produce a foreign body sensation, occlude the airway, or be aspirated. Gloves should be worn by the operator to minimize any risk of transmitting or acquiring an infection.

Rubber dilators are passed through the mouth into the midline of the hypopharynx, guided by the second and third fingers of one hand, similar to intubation with a fiberoptic endoscope. The operator must guard against lateral deviation of the dilator into the area of the pyriform sinus during passage. As the tip of the dilator enters the area of the cricopharyngeus (i.e. approximately 15 cm from the incisor teeth), the patient is asked to swallow to relax the upper esophageal sphincter. This allows the dilator to be gently advanced into the body of the esophagus. Forward pressure is then applied to the dilator and the instrument is passed the stricture. The amount of force used to advance a dilator through a stricture is something that must be learned through experience. After it passes through the narrowed area the dilator is quickly withdrawn, and the patient is allowed to clear any oral secretions.

Dilation with Eder-Puestow olives must always be done over a guide wire. Using fluoroscopic control, the wire is passed through the mouth and the stricture and positioned in the stomach. If the wire is difficult to pass, it may be inserted through the biopsy channel of a fiberoptic endoscope and maneuvered through the strictured lumen under direct vision. Care must be taken to ensure that the wire is not placed through the trachea and into a bronchus such that inadvertent bronchial dilation could occur along with a pneumothorax.

Once correct positioning of the guide wire in the body of the stomach is ascertained, the appropriate sized metal olive is attached to the dilator shaft. The olive is lightly lubricated and the assembly passed over the guide wire through the stricture, while the proximal length of the wire is firmly held by an assistant. The proximal tip of the guide wire should be covered with the protective guard supplied with the unit to prevent inadvertent injury to the eyes of the patient, operator, or assistant, since the tip tends to flop about. Because the metal shaft of the dilator assembly permits a more forceful dilation, care must be taken that the operator's hand does not slip and injure the patient's face. During passage of the assembly, force on the dilator shaft should always be directed in the axis of the wire. This minimizes angulation and pressure on the hypopharyngeal area. Care must be taken not to pull the wire back inadvertently as the dilator is advanced; otherwise, the path of the assembly is not guided by the wire. When the metal dilator has been documented to pass through the area of the stricture, it is removed, and an assistant determines fluoroscopically that the guide wire has remained in the stomach so that subsequent dilations can be performed. Following the last dilation, the guide wire is pulled back against the metal dilator shaft and the whole assembly is withdrawn.

The size of the initial dilator is determined by making an esimate of the size of the strictured esophageal lumen. This estimate can be made during endoscopy or based on measurements obtained from a barium esophagram. It is best to start with a dilator smaller than the estimate rather than one too large and risk an esophageal perforation. The number of dilations done per session depends on patient tolerance, the degree of resistance offered by the stricture, and the degree of resistance felt by the operator. A minimum of three progressive-sized dilations usually can be accomplished safely during one session. In patients with erosive hemorrhagic esophagitis, it is not unusual to find a small amount of blood-tinged mucus on the dilator. When necessary, dilations may be performed daily. Usually the last dilator size passed during the previous session is the first dilator size passed at the next session, followed by the next two larger sizes.

The largest dilator size is determined mainly by the cause and nature of the stricture. In general, most uncomplicated peptic strictures can be gradually dilated to a size 50 F with minimal risk. Chronic longstanding strictures with thick, rigid, fibrotic walls, such as those caused by radiation or caustic injury or scleroderma, should not be dilated to this extent becuase of the increased risk of perforation. These patients should be dilated to a size 40 F, since at this luminal diameter most individuals will be able to eat a regular diet if cautioned to chew their food well.

As with any peroral instrumentation, there is a potential risk associated with esophageal dilation. Allergic reaction to topical anesthetic spray, bleeding from esophageal laceration, esophageal perforation, and pulmonary aspiration are all potential but rare complications associated with bouginage. Nevertheless, patients should be counseled about these complications prior to dilation while informed consent is obtained.

TREATMENT OF SPECIFIC LESIONS

Peptic Strictures

Strictures caused by gastroesophageal reflux are usually short and located at the gastroesophageal junction. When associated with a Barrett's esophagus, however, these strictures may be more proximally located. Peptic strictures are best treated using progressive dilation with either Maloney or Hurst dilators. These strictures can be dilated once or twice a week until a lumen size of 50 F is achieved. Once this has been achieved, luminal patency can be maintained with a single infrequent passage of a large diameter dilator. Vigorous treatment of the underlying gastroesophageal reflux will retard the recurrence of peptic strictures and decrease future requirements for dilation. Often, a single series of dilations is sufficient to relieve dysphagia from a peptic stricture permanently, provided medical or surgical antireflux measures are concomitantly employed. Some strictures will recur, however, and these will require chronic dilation. Following successful dilation of a peptic stricture, the patient should be counseled to return for reevaluation and repeat dilation as soon as dysphagia returns. A "benign peptic stricture" that requires frequent dilation to relieve recurrent dysphagia suggests the presence of an underlying malignant process.

Long Segment Strictures

Long segment strictures are caued by severe gastroesophageal reflux, prior caustic ingestion, or prolonged nasogastric intubation. They may occur at any level of the esophagus and are quite tortuous and sometimes difficult to manage. Careful, slowly progressive, fluoroscopically controlled dilation of these strictures is necessary to minimize the risk of perforation of the fibrotic esophageal wall. These strictures often require metal dilators or coaxial balloon dilators passed over guide wires for optimal management. Long segmental strictures should be dilated only to 40 F or less for reasons previously discussed.

Rings and Webs

Dysphagia caused by a lower esophageal ring (Schatzki's or "B" ring) can usually be effectively treated with a single passage of a larger diameter rubber dilator (50 F). If symptoms recur they usually respond well to repeat dilation.

Esophageal webs can occur at any level but are typically found in the cervical esophageal area. Webs rarely cause significant dysphagia, but if symptomatic, they can be effectively treated with a single dilation using a large diameter rubber bougie.

Malignant Strictures

Dilatation. Dysphagia due to narrowing of the esophageal lumen caused by carcinoma of the esophagus can be effectively treated with peroral bouginage with minimal risk. In those patients who receive primary radiotherapy for their tumors, dilation should be begun before radiation and continued during and after radiation as necessary to ensure esophageal patency. While it has been said that dysphagia from esophageal cancer cannot be palliated with dilation during radiotherapy for fear of esophageal perforation, two studies from our institution have shown this not to be the case. If clinically needed, we perform esophageal dilation during radiotherapy.

While most malignant strictures respond to conventional rubber dilators, on occasion far advanced malignant strictures require dilation with metal olives or coaxial balloon instruments. Because malignant strictures are often irregular, shelved, and tortuous, fluoroscopic control of dilation is often necessary to facilitate dilation and prevent perforation.

Dysphagia from adenocarcinoma of the cardioesophageal junction does not respond well to bouginage, since it is difficult to dilate and maintain patency of the gastric cardia. Similarly, dysphagia caused by extrinsic compression by malignancies of the lung or mediastinal lymph nodes does not respond well to bouginage, since the extrinsic lesion quickly compresses the esophageal lumen again when the dilator is removed.

Esophageal dilation is effective in palliating dysphagia that results from anastomotic strictures after surgical therapy for esophageal cancer. These strictures and those that occur following radiation of esophageal malignancies should be dilated cautiously to a size not greater than 40 F, since perforation of the fibrotic esophageal wall is a potential problem.

Prosthetic tubes. Dysphagia secondary to intraluminal cancer that does not respond to periodic dilation may be treated with a nonoperatively placed *polyvinyl prosthetic tube* to ensure continued lumen patency. In a similar manner, these prosthetic tubes can palliate the incessant coughing that results from aspiration caused by a malignant tracheoesophageal fistula. While placement of these tubes may improve the patient's quality of life, they do not appear to prolong life, nor do they prevent the known late complications of the disease, such as malnutrition, aspiration, and hemorrhage. The tubes also are not without risk, since they may erode through the esophageal wall into an organ or a major blood vessel. Therefore, we use them only in those patients whose life expectancy is short and who have one of the above two indications.

Even though various types of prosthetic tubes are commercially available, we choose to make our own

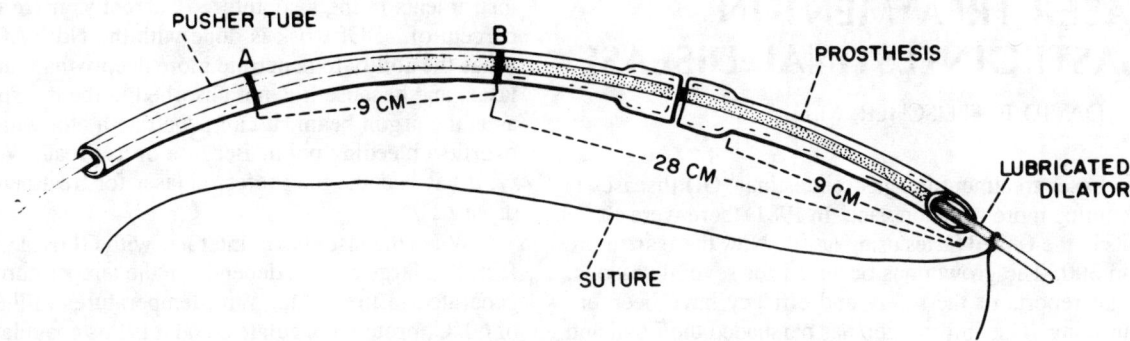

Figure 1 A prosthesis designed for a 5-cm tumor with a 2-cm flange and 4-cm distal extension to prevent occlusion. B indicates the level from the incisor teeth at which the prosthesis enters the tumor and A the level at which the prosthesis flange rests on the oral tumor margin. (From Peura et al. Esophageal prosthesis in cancer. Am J Dig Dis 1978; 23:798.)

prostheses, tailored to meet an individual patients' needs. Tygon (Norton Plastics, Akron, OH) polyvinyl tubing for the prosthesis comes in three sizes (10 mm, 12 mm, 17 mm). A 10-mm prosthesis will accommodate liquids and pureed food, while a 17-mm tube will accommodate a well masticated regular diet. In preparation for tube placement, a patient should be progressively dilated to accommodate a size 50 F dilator. This permits placement of the largest diameter (17 mm) prosthesis. In addition, the patient should undergo endoscopy to determine the upper and lower limits of the tumor as measured from the incisor teeth. These measurements are important in manufacturing the prosthesis.

In preparing a tube, it is important that sufficient length of polyvinyl tubing be used so that the prosthesis length exceeds tumor length by 6 to 7 cm. This additional length allows for a 2- to 3-cm flange to anchor the prosthesis above the tumor and a 4-cm extension below the tumor to prevent tube occlusion by caudad tumor growth. The prosthesis should not touch the cricopharyngeus because this causes discomfort for the patient and prosthesis instability. The prosthesis should not extend across the gastroesophageal junction, since this could permit gastroesophageal reflux. In addition, the distal end of the tube lying free in the stomach prevents stable prosthesis seating and has been associated with gastric perforation.

To facilitate prosthesis placement in the patient, a second tube (pusher tube) is cut of sufficient length to extend from the orad tumor margin 8 to 10 cm beyond the incisor teeth. The distal end of the prosthetic tube should be beveled to facilitate passage through the tumor. Both the pusher tube and beveled flanged protheses are placed over a small caliber rubber dilator which acts as a guide for esophageal intubation.

Prior to prosthesis placement, the patient is counseled regarding the indications and potential complications. Local anesthesia is applied to the hypopharynx and mild sedation is given. The prosthesis assembly (pusher tube, prosthesis, and dilator held in place by a silk thread, Fig. 1) is passed through the mouth under fluoroscopic control so that the prosthesis flange rests at the orad tumor margin. At this point the silk thread is released, the dilator removed, and the prosthesis is seated into the tumor mass by gentle, twisting caudad pressure on the pusher tube. The pusher tube is then removed. A barium swallow is performed immediately after placement to ensure proper positioning of the prosthesis in the tumor and patency of the lumen prior to oral feeding. On the following day the patient again has a radiographic study to ensure that proper prosthesis position has been maintained.

All patients with a prosthesis are counseled to chew their food well and drink a large glass of water with each meal to rinse away adherent debris. When a 17-mm diameter prosthetic tube is employed, there is no need for special mechanical preparation of food other than careful mastication. Should a tube become obstructed, the patient is counseled to seek medical attention so that disimpaction may be undertaken by direct vision endoscopy.

Other Palliative Modalities

Recently, endoscopic laser therapy of nonresectable esophageal tumors has been shown to reestablish lumen patency and palliate dysphagia. In a similar manner, treatment with commercially available bipolar electrodes has been shown to have palliative benefit. While experience with destruction and desiccation of an intraluminal mass with a laser or bipolar electrode is limited, preliminary reports regarding the efficacy of these therapeutic modalities is encouraging. See the chapter on *Laser Treatment in Gastrointestinal Disease*.

The opinions and assertions contained herein are the private ones of the authors and are not to be construed as official or reflecting the views of the Department of Defense, the U.S. Army Corps, or the Uniformed Services University of the Health Sciences.

LASER TREATMENT IN GASTROINTESTINAL DISEASE

DAVID E. FLEISCHER, M.D.

Laser treatment for gastrointestinal (GI) diseases is becoming more commonplace. In 1981, there were 12 GI units in the United States using lasers. Now there are more than 300. The growth has occurred for several reasons. Initial reports of the safety and efficacy have been encouraging. This information has persuaded the Food and Drug Administration to change its classification of laser, so that it is no longer considered an experimental device. Lasers are technically easy to use. Perhaps most importantly, the broad range of applications for treatment of GI and non-GI diseases has made them more affordable. The major gastrointestinal applications of lasers are GI bleeding and neoplastic diseases. It is likely, however, that the GI uses will expand with continuing technologic advances.

PHYSICAL PRINCIPLES

The word *laser* is an acronym for "light amplification by stimulated emission of radiation." This phenomenon occurs when a substance, whether gas, solid, or liquid, is excited (e.g., by heat) to a higher energy state and stimulated to emit light as it returns to a lower energy state. This process can be amplified when the photons produced interact between two mirrors. If one of the mirrors is only partially reflective, the laser beam can escape from the mirrored chamber. Laser light differs from other forms of light in that it is monochromatic and coherent. Because it is of one wavelength, it will have predictable, reproducible features. Because it is coherent, it can be sharply focused and large amounts of energy can be concentrated in a small area.

Three main types of lasers have been used therapeutically in medicine (Table 1). These are the argon, carbon dioxide, and neodymium: yttrium aluminum garnet (Nd:YAG) lasers. Each of these substances produces a different wavelength of light, and it is the wavelength that determines the unique properties of each laser (depth of penetration, visibility, and so on). Only the argon and the Nd:YAG lasers can be used with flexible waveguides; therefore, only these two have been used with flexible fiberoptic and video endoscopes. Technologic advances may allow use of the carbon dioxide laser with flexible instruments in the near future. Currently, more than 95 percent of all GI work is done with the Nd:YAG laser. It has the ability to penetrate more deeply than the argon laser, and because it is not absorbed in the red spectrum as is the argon beam, it can penetrate a clot which may overlie a bleeding point. Because of its greater versatility, it has become the preferred laser for treatment of GI diseases.

When the laser beam interacts with GI tissue, the effect, to a large extent, depends on the temperature that is generated in the tissue. With temperatures in the range of 60 °C, protein coagulates, and it is this coagulative effect that is sought when the laser is used to treat GI bleeding. At temperatures of 100 °C or greater, tissue water boils and vaporization occurs. This principle is applied when the laser is used to destroy neoplastic tissue.

APPLICATIONS

Gastrointestinal Bleeding

The first GI application in humans was for the treatment of upper GI bleeding. Lasers have now been used to treat both upper and lower GI bleeding, variceal and nonvariceal GI bleeding, and active bleeding and lesions that have recently bled but have stopped. How is it done? What are the results and how does it compare to alternative therapies?

Technique

Tissue effect will be determined by the power selected, the pulse duration, and the distance between the laser fiber and the tissue. Most effective coagulation with the Nd:YAG laser is achieved with powers in the range of 70 to 90 watts, short pulse durations (0.3 to 0.5 seconds), and distances of approximately 1 cm.

When treating actively bleeding varices, the beam is aimed at the bleeding site if it can be localized. A vasopressin bolus or intermittent balloon tamponade (e.g., with a Linton tube) may be used during the procedure to assist with visualization. There is a trend toward using chronic sclerotherapy following laser coagulation of varices to minimize rebleeding.

When treating an ulcer that is actively bleeding or a nonbleeding ulcer with a visible vessel, the laser beam should be aimed circumferentially around the bleeding

TABLE 1 Characteristics of Medical Lasers

Type	Wavelength (μm)	Penetration Depth	Visible	Use With Flexible Endoscope
Nd:YAG	1.06	Least superficial	No	Yes
Argon	0.5	Intermediate	Yes	Yes
Carbon Dioxide	10.6	Most superficial	No	No

point, then centrally. The purpose is to create edema which will staunch blood flow. There is divided opinion as to whether one should start at the rim of the ulcer or merely at the rim of the vessel before proceeding to treat the central vessel.

When treating nonbleeding angiodysplasia, technique varies according to the size of the lesion. If it is small (less than 3 mm), it can generally be treated with a single pulse aimed at the lesion. If it is larger, one attempts to coagulate it in parts, like slices of a pie, trying to burn the margin between the lesion and normal tissue. Laser-induced bleeding is very common, and if it occurs, energy should be directed to the center of the lesion. Colonic lesions are treated similarly but because the cecum is thin, the risk of perforation is greater. Attention must be given to reducing air insufflation so that the colonic wall is not further thinned by distention.

The coagulative techniques described here have evolved over a decade's experience with noncontact laser probes. Recently developed probe tips that attach to conventional fibers allow for contact therapy. In addition to giving the endoscopist the ability to tamponade the lesion prior to delivering the laser energy, heat distribution is different. Much lower energies are used.

Efficacy and Safety

Most endoscopists do not use the laser to treat variceal bleeding. The Nd:YAG laser, however, has been shown to be effective in an animal model of variceal bleeding, in large clinical series, and in a controlled trial.

For endoscopic control of nonvariceal bleeding, more published data exist about the laser than any other modality. In uncontrolled series, initial hemostasis is reported in more than 85 percent of cases using both the argon and Nd:YAG lasers. Reports from 11 randomized controlled studies are available, three with the argon laser and eight with the Nd:YAG. With both, laser results have been mixed. When patients with active ulcer bleeding or with visible vessels are evaluated separately, there is a trend showing that laser therapy is beneficial. A high quality study by Swain and colleagues from two London hospitals deserves emphasis. A total of 464 patients presenting with upper GI bleeding were seen. Of the 232 who had peptic ulcers, 147 had either active bleeding or stigmata of recent hemorrhage. Twenty-four patients were excluded. Of the remaining 123 patients, 62 were treated with the Nd:YAG laser and 61 served as controls. Cessation of bleeding was more common in the laser-treated group (p less than 0.02) and the mortality rate was less (p less than 0.05). It is extremely important to note that no perforations were reported in any of these 11 controlled studies. In uncontrolled series, perforation rates of 1 to 2 percent have been noted. Laser-induced bleeding is the most common complication.

Both argon and Nd:YAG lasers have been used to treat angiodysplasia of the upper and lower GI tract. It is generally held that successful obliteration of the lesions is possible. Clinical success depends upon whether or not the angiodysplastic lesions that are treated have been the cause of the bleeding and whether or not continued surveillance and treatment is carried out, since new lesions often develop. Treatment of angiodysplastic lesions is discussed in detail in the chapter on *Lower Gastrointestinal Bleeding*.

Alternative Endoscopic Therapy

For variceal bleeding, sclerotherapy is most commonly employed both for bleeding in the acute stage and for long-term control. Technically, endoscopic laser therapy and sclerotherapy are equally easy (or difficult) to perform, but repeated injection sclerotherapy is more apt to achieve the long-term goal. Therefore, even the endoscopists who prefer to use the laser to treat acute esophageal variceal bleeding embark on a course of sclerotherapy after laser treatment. See the chapter *Sclerotherapy of Esophageal Varices*.

Numerous endoscopic methods have been used to treat nonvariceal GI bleeding (Table 2). Unfortunately, there are few comparative data. The largest clinical experience in both controlled and uncontrolled series is with the laser. Of the nonlaser devices, the greatest interest currently is in the heater probe, the bipolar (multipolar) coagulator, and the injection devices. Early results with the multipolar coagulator (BICAP) and the heater probe have been encouraging and similar to those achieved with the laser. If these results hold up with increased use, the greater portability and reduced cost of these devices will weigh in their favor. Preliminary results using injection techniques for nonvariceal bleeding similar to those used to treat varices have been quite good. Either concentrated alcohol or variceal sclerosant solution is injected. The lack of comparative data makes it impossible to determine how these other modalities compare with endoscopic laser therapy (ELT).

TABLE 2 Endoscopic Treatment of Gastrointestinal Bleeding

Topical Therapy
  Tissue glues
  Clotting factors
  Collagen
  Ferromagnetic tamponade

Injection Therapy
  Variceal sclerosis
  Nonvariceal

Mechanical Therapy
  Balloons
  Hemoclips
  Sewing machine

Thermal Therapy
  Coagulation
    Monopolar
    Bipolar (multipolar)
  Heater probe
  Laser

Miscellaneous

Use of the laser for active variceal bleeding, focal nonvariceal bleeding, and angiodysplasia is well documented. There have also been other applications related to GI bleeding. In patients with nonbleeding esophageal varices, the laser has been used to obliterate the vessels in a fashion similar to sclerotherapy. When GI malignancies bleed, laser therapy is often beneficial. There are isolated reports of ELT for persistent bleeding from hemorrhagic gastritis, radiation colitis, and ulcerative proctitis. Finally, hemorrhoids have been treated with the laser.

Gastrointestinal Neoplasms

Lasers have been used to treat neoplasms throughout the GI tract. Tumors of the mouth, esophagus, stomach, duodenum, ampulla of Vater, colon, and rectum have been treated. The greatest experience is with esophageal and rectal disease. Because many GI cancers present at an advanced stage and because lasers have generally not been employed when more conventional approaches were available, in most instances treatment has been palliative. Laser therapy often can effectively relieve obstruction and has been useful in diminishing bleeding from GI neoplasms. It has not been effective for pain. In rare instances endoscopic laser therapy has been curative. It has been used when the neoplasm has been discovered early and the patient is not a candidate for surgery. It also has been employed to treat premalignant diseases in poor surgical risks when other approaches were not applicable (e.g., broad based villous adenoma) and to ablate polyps that develop in the rectal stump after colectomy in persons with familial polyposis syndromes.

Technique

Prior to ELT, one should obtain a barium radiograph and an imaging study (computed tomography or nuclear magnetic resonance). This information, added to that obtained during endoscopy, allows one to decide how treatment should best progress. The goal of therapy is generally to open an obstructed lumen to maximize intake of food or output of stool.

For esophageal cancer, the following technique is employed. It is best to be able to treat along the entire extent of tumor. If a standard endoscope will not pass to the distal margin, one may use a pediatric endoscope or pass a guide wire and dilate with Savary dilators. If one can begin treatment distally, it is possible to work back to the proximal margin. This allows for greater tumor destruction per session. When the laser beam is aimed at the tumor, the thermal burn causes edema prior to tissue necrosis, and by beginning distally one can withdraw and continue to treat. When treatment is begun proximally, tissue edema may prevent the endoscope from advancing distally, and this will limit the amount of tissue injury per session. The trade-off is that distal treatment is more difficult because it is carried out tangentially in most instances. For that reason, one may begin treatment at the proximal margin. If the lumen is severely narrowed, this often is the only option.

Most laser endoscopists use high power (90 to 100 watts) and long pulse durations (2.5 seconds or greater) to maximize thermal damage. Some investigators have used much lower energies trying to destroy the tumor by coagulation. These variables reflect the technique as it is practiced with noncontact fibers (preliminary work with contact probe tips which concentrate the energy using much lower power settings has been exciting). Maximal tissue necrosis occurs in 36 to 48 hours, so generally patients are treated every other day. At the beginning of each subsequent session necrotic tissue is removed either by repeat guide-wire dilation or excavation with endoscopic accessories. Treatments continue until maximal luminal patency is achieved.

Techniques are similar for colorectal cancer but there are some differences. Treatment of perianal tumors causes discomfort, and either local anesthesia or an epidural block is required. Often, a rigid proctoscope and a hand-held fiber offer technical advantages in the rectum. Treatment is begun, if possible, at the proximal margin.

Efficacy and Safety

The largest reported experience with ELT involves neoplasms of the esophagus and esophagogastric junction. Therapy is almost always palliative and usually for relief of obstruction. A number of institutions have treated more than 50 patients and results have been similar. Criteria have been defined which suggest that certain endoscopic factors influence the initial outcome. Exophytic, predominantly mucosal tumors are technically easier to treat and respond better than predominantly submucosal tumors. Neoplasms of the cervical esophagus are often difficult to treat when they abut the cricopharyngeus, and even when luminal patency is achieved dysphagia often may persist. If a sharp angulation exists at the esophagogastric junction, it is hard to maneuver the endoscope around the turn, and even if the lumen is opened, the rigid, horizontal, aperistaltic segment clogs easily. Short tumors, either primary or recurrent after esophagogastric anastomoses, respond very well. Extensive involvement is often associated with a large extraesophageal tumor load and overall prognosis is poor. Because laser therapy depends upon thermal destruction, it is not surprising that there is no difference in response for squamous cell or adenocarcinoma. Duration of benefit is hard to assess because often the patient has literally undergone every possible therapeutic alternative prior to ELT or is undergoing ancillary therapy. Studies are under way at some institutions to determine how laser treatment fits into the overall therapeutic armamentarium for esophageal cancer. The main complication has been perforation, which occurs at a rate of 5 to 10 percent.

In the United States, ELT for gastric cancer has been

used for tumors of the cardia, and the data are similar to those for esophageal cancer. Some patients with gastric outlet obstruction have been treated successfully. In Japan, there are several reports of large series of patients with early gastric cancers or borderline lesions cured by Nd:YAG laser therapy.

About 50 patients with neoplasms of the ampulla of Vater have been treated including both villous adenomas and carcinomas. Most patients were not candidates for surgery or had recurrences after surgery. Endoscopic laser therapy was indicated to relieve biliary obstruction or because of recurrent pancreatitis.

Lasers have been used in the large bowel to relieve obstruction caused by carcinoma, to treat villous adenomas in patients who were not candidates for surgery or in whom polypectomy could not be done, and to treat polyps recurring in rectal stumps of patients after colectomy with polyposis syndromes. Relief of malignant obstruction, particularly in the rectum, is generally feasible. Some series now include more than 100 patients with long-term follow-up.

FUTURE DEVELOPMENTS

Although the focus of this volume is on current therapy in gastroenterology and liver disease, it is impossible to put the topic of laser therapy in perspective without talking about the future. It must be remembered that laser application for gastrointestinal diseases is really in its infancy, the first patient having been treated little more than one decade ago.

At present, only a few wavelengths are available for use out of a light spectrum of hundreds. Conceivably, other wavelengths may have an element of specificity that would make their use safer and more effective. In the future, tunable (selectable) lasers will allow us to switch from one wavelength to another as we do with channels on the television set. Endoscopic ultrasounds will measure tumor size more precisely and computer adaptations should assist with more precise dosimetry. Tissue-sensitizing agents may render abnormal tissue more susceptible to laser destruction. The recent development of contact probe tips holds promise for a major breakthrough in the efficiency of energy delivery which may make smaller, portable, less costly lasers a reality.

It is particularly exciting to ponder potential new applications of laser therapy, all of which have either been performed in animal experiments or in a few patients. Endoscopic vagotomies have been performed. Attempts have been made to speed ulcer healing with low-dose laser energy. Experiments have been performed destroying malignant cells in tissue cultures with selective wavelengths. Lasers have been used to fragment gallstones in vitro. Percutaneously placed laser probes are being used to treat hepatomas and isolated hepatic metastases under ultrasound guidance. Benign and malignant biliary obstructions have been opened cholangioscopically. The future of lasers in the treatment of GI and hepatobiliary diseases is very bright.

DIFFUSE ESOPHAGEAL SPASM AND RELATED DISORDERS

ALAN G. SUNSHINE, M.D.
SIDNEY COHEN, M.D.

The precise cause of angina-like chest pain is sometimes difficult to determine. Approximately 10 to 30 percent of patients with anginal syndromes have normal coronary arteries or minimal atherosclerosis at cardiac catheterization. Patients without significant coronary disease are being referred for esophageal manometric studies in hopes of determining a cause for their symptoms. It is well established that the esophagus can cause serious chest pain, and it is suggested in the literature that patients with chest pain of esophageal origin will have either diffuse esophageal spasm or gastroesophageal reflux. In recent years, esophageal manometric laboratories have notably improved with the development of catheters and precise low compliant infusion systems. These systems have resulted in an increased incidence of the diagnosis of esophageal motility disorders but have also generated confusion as to the specific manometric patterns responsible for a patient's symptoms. The sensitivity of esophageal manometry in determining the cause of chest pain is unknown. More patients are found to have a nonspecific motor disorder of the esophagus instead of classic diffuse esophageal spasm, and only a minority of patients will have definitive manometric changes associated with their typical symptoms at the time of manometry. Because of the wide variability in the results of esophageal manometry, controlled trials designed to characterize the precise manometric abnormality and their specific therapies have been difficult. Therefore, most of the discussion in this chapter will outline the *empiric* treatments that are available to the clinician in the hope of conveying an organized approach to a difficult problem.

CLINICAL MANIFESTATIONS

The symptoms most frequently encountered in patients with esophageal motor disorders are those of dysphagia and chest pain. *Dysphagia* is seen in about 70 percent of patients, is provoked by eating either solids or liquids, and is nonprogressive. Occasionally, in the case of liquids, the patient is conscious of the fluid being forcefully ejected from the esophagus back into the nasopharynx, but frank regurgitation is uncommon.

Chest pain is one of the most characteristic manifestations, especially in younger patients. Chest pain is usually described as squeezing, is substernal in location, and radiates in the back, neck, jaw, or arms, making it sometimes indistinguishable from angina-like pain. The pain is usually associated with deglutition, especially foods that are of extreme temperatures. The pain, however, may also awaken a patient from sleep, be unrelated to meals, and be unprovoked in many cases. Weight loss is uncommon but occasionally a patient will avoid eating to prevent the occurrence of symptoms.

The incidence of esophageal dysfunction as a cause of chest pain is difficult to ascertain. In one prospective trial evaluating 200 patients, only 23 percent had abnormalities of the gastrointestinal tract, primarily of the esophagus. The classification of esophageal manometric abnormalities has evolved over the years in an arbitrary fashion. A wide range of manometric findings has been used to characterize patients with the diagnosis of *diffuse esophageal spasm* (DES). As can be seen in Table 1, there is overlap between the diagnosis of DES, the nutcracker esophagus, and other nonspecific motor disorders. This is in contrast to achalasia, in which total aperistalsis and a hypertensive nonrelaxing lower esophageal sphincter are definitive diagnostic criteria. The difficulty in diagnosis in patients with chest pain arises from the lack of specific presenting symptoms, manometric criteria, and the intermittent nature of the manometric changes at the time of patient evaluation. To overcome this ambiguity we have routinely utilized *provocative agents*, such as edrophonium chloride, to enhance the value of esophageal manometry. All patients with chest pain undergoing esophageal manometry who have had a negative cardiac evaluation are given 10 mg of intravenous edrophonium. In 120 patients evaluated with normal baseline manometry, provocative testing demonstrated significant manometric abnormalities and the development of typical symptoms in 34 percent. Seventeen percent of patients with negative baseline manometric results either developed typical chest pain or had manometric change but not both. As reported by others, approximately 50 percent of patients will have no significant change from baseline manometry despite the use of provocative agents. Ergonovine, another provocative agent, has been used to induce coronary spasm. We have evaluated those patients with negative coronary arteriograms and chest pain after ergonovine administration and found their symptoms to be esophageal in origin. The potential side effects and the lack of proven efficacy over edrophonium, however, has limited the use of ergonovine in our laboratory. Effective and accurate evaluation of patients with esophageal chest pain will occur if proper patient selection, provocative agents, and characterization of the esophageal motility disorders are utilized (Fig. 1).

TREATMENT

The treatment of esophageal motility disorders is quite variable, with no single agent being totally effective for any group of patients (Table 2). Because the symptoms are intermittent, it has been very difficult to define the correct agent for a specific symptom or even for any unique manometric abnormality. Secondary causes of esophageal spasm, such as gastroesophageal reflux, should be suspected in any patient with vague chest pain and a hypotensive lower esophageal sphincter (LES) pressure. Because the treatment for reflux disease is very effective, a Bernstein acid perfusion test should be administered in the hope of reproducing the patient's symptoms. This test, at the time of esophageal manometry, allows for the simultaneous documentation of any specific motor abnormality believed to be contributing to the patient's symptoms.

Anticholinergic Agents

Once secondary causes have been excluded, initial treatment involves the use of anticholinergics, such as *dicyclomine hydrochloride* (Bentyl) in doses up to 20 mg 4 times a day. The use of anticholinergics is based on the assumption that there may be supersensitivity to endogenous substances and neural transmitters, such as acetylcholine, leading to the development of esophageal spasm and symptoms. Because the symptoms are usually associated with eating, it is recommended that the patient take the medication 30 minutes before each meal.

Nitrates

If anticholinergic treatment is unsuccessful, oral or sublingual nitrates can be used. Because the basic pharmacologic action of nitrates is to relax smooth muscle,

TABLE 1 Manometric Criteria for Esophageal Motor Disorders

Diffuse Esophageal Spasm
  Simultaneous, nonperistaltic contractions (> 30% of swallows)
  Prolonged, repetitive contractions
  Spontaneous contractions
  High-amplitude contractions
  Periods of normal peristalsis
  Normal LES function in 70%, elevated LES pressure with or without impaired relaxation in 30% of patients

High Amplitude Esophageal Contractions (Nutcracker)
  High-amplitude contractions (mean > 120 mm Hg)
  Prolonged contractions
  Normal peristalsis

Nonspecific Motor Disorders
  Hypertensive (LES pressure > 35 mm Hg with normal relaxation)
  Combination of abnormal peristaltic sequences (< 30% of swallows)
    Simultaneous contractions
    Spontaneous contractions
    Low-amplitude contractions
    Repetitive contractions
    Prolonged contractions

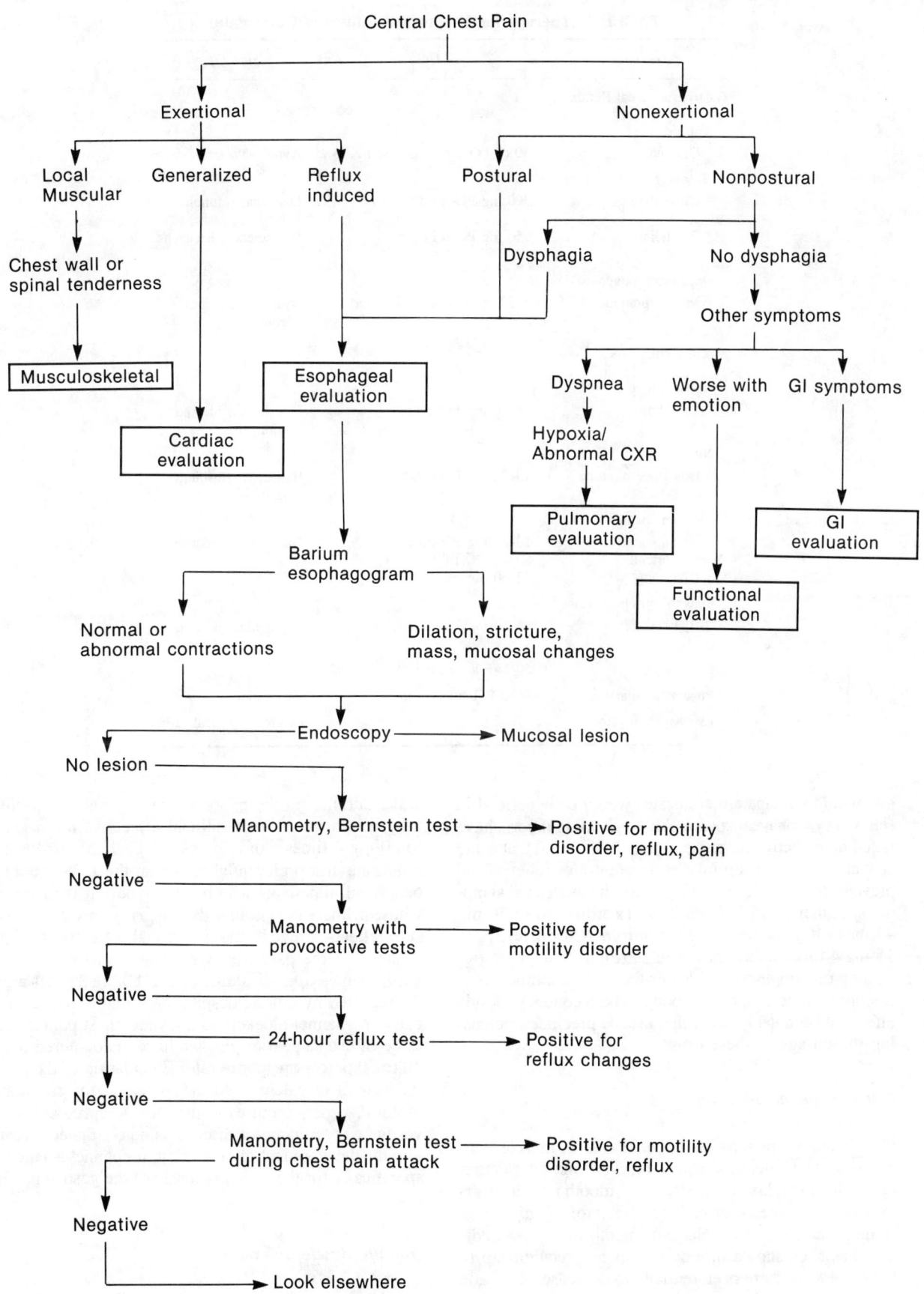

Figure 1 Evaluation of chest pain.

TABLE 2 Therapy for Esophageal Causes of Chest Pain

Treatment	Dose	Side Effects
Gastroesophageal Reflux		
Antacids		
Gaviscon	30 cc PO 1 hr p.c. and h.s.	Avoid with tetracyclines
H$_2$ Antagonists		
Cimetidine	300 mg PO q.i.d.	Diarrhea, somnolence, dizziness, rash
Ranitidine	150 mg PO b.i.d.	Somnolence, headache, rash
Dopamine Antagonists		
Metaclopramide	5–20 mg PO ½ hr a.c. and h.s.	Dystonic reactions, depression
Motility Disorders		
Anticholinergics		
Dicyclomine	10–20 mg PO q.i.d.	Dry mouth, blurred vision, dizziness
Nitrates		
Isosorbide dinitrate	10–30 mg PO q.i.d.	Headache, flushing, dizziness
Calcium-channel blockers		
Nifedipine	10–20 mg PO q.i.d.	Dizziness, headache
Verapramil	80 mg PO t.i.d.	
Diltiazem	30–60 mg PO q.i.d.	
Smooth muscle relaxant		
Hydralazine	25–50 mg PO t.i.d.	Lupus-like reaction, dizziness, edema
Bouginage	50–54F as needed	
Pneumatic dilatation	8–10 PSI for 20 sec	Perforation
Esophageal myotomy		Gastroesophageal reflux

one would anticipate that nitrates would be beneficial in relieving esophageal spasm. Although some reports have noted no objective response, others have found that acute as well as chronic administration of nitrates relieves and prevents the recurrence of chest pain and associated symptoms. Either *isosorbide dinitrate* (Isordil), 10 to 30 mg 4 times a day, or *erythrityl tetranitrate* (Cardilate), 10 to 15 mg 4 times a day, has been shown to reduce the frequency of symptoms and lower the high-amplitude contractions in the esophageal body. The frequency of side effects, most notably headache, usually precludes increasing the dosage of these drugs.

Calcium-channel Blockers

Calcium ions play an essential role in muscle contraction. The calcium-channel blockers inhibit calcium ionic flux and relax coronary artery smooth muscle. Various reports have described the effects of *nifedipine* on some parameters of esophageal smooth muscle. Nifedipine has been shown in a dose response relationship to lower LES pressure preferentially to decrease amplitude of esophageal high-amplitude contractions. In contrast, *verapamil* is noted to decrease contraction amplitude and wave duration in the baboon. Finally, another preliminary report notes the beneficial effects of *diltiazem* 30 to 60 mg 4 times a day, on esophageal spasm. Because nifedipine has preferential effects at the LES it is more beneficial in patients who have a hypertensive LES and whose primary symptom is dysphagia. In my experience, side effects prevent the beneficial effects at higher dosages. If the patient's symptoms are *primarily chest pain*, then *verapamil* is instituted at 80 mg 3 times a day. As reported by others, despite the initial enthusiasm for calcium-channel blockers to alleviate chest pain thought to be of esophageal origin, we have encountered only a 40 to 50 percent response rate. Elucidation of the potential benefit of calcium-channel blockers for esophageal motor disorders requires well-controlled protocols to investigate specific motor disorders and continued research into the development of new calcium-channel antagonists specifically for the smooth muscle of the gastrointestinal tract.

Smooth Muscle Relaxants

There is marked varibility in smooth muscle response to other pharmacologic agents. *Hydralazine* acts by direct relaxation of arteriolar smooth muscle, with minimal effect on other vessels. Because of its specific actions on smooth muscle, a single report of long-term administration of 25 mg 4 times a day suggested efficacy in preventing recurrent chest pain due to esophageal spasm upon bethanechol provocation. My experience with this drug has been of limited success because of fluid retention and postural hypotension-associated side effects.

Esophageal Dilatation

If the medical regimen described above fails to alleviate most of the patient's symptoms, repeated esophageal dilatation may be necessary. Again several studies have demonstrated conflicting results with bouginage. Most notably, there was no significant change in LES pressure or amplitude of contractions or significant reduction in major symptoms. There was, however, a sense of improvement once the study interval had ended, suggesting that a benefit may result due to the close physician-patient relationship. In general, patients who are refractory to medical therapy and who have normal LES pressures will be treated with *bouginage*. Patients who have failed to improve with medical therapy and are also found to have *hypertensive LES* pressure are candidates for *pneumatic dilatation*. I have seen dramatic results in relief of symptoms, most notably dysphagia, with dilatations.

Surgery

Only rarely will a patient be refractory to the regimen described above such that a *surgical* approach must be taken. When necessary, a long myotomy of the esophagus can be performed. A left thoracotomy provides excellent exposure for involvement of the distal two-thirds of the esophagus and the lower esophageal sphincter. When there is more extensive esophageal involvement, a right-sided approach to include the entire esophagus may be necessary. The length of the myotomy is determined by *preoperative manometric assessment*, and the incision should spare the normal lower esophageal sphincter. Lateral dissection of the muscle wall from the mucosa is essential to discourage subsequent healing of the myotomy.

Although symptomatic improvement is reported in 70 to 80 percent of patients, there is a definite risk of reflux esophagitis following extended myotomy. The lower esophageal sphincter should be involved in the myotomy if sphincter pressure is elevated or relaxation is impaired. If the myotomy includes the sphincter, a loose fundoplication is indicated.

Experience with long myotomy has not been good for several reasons: (1) persistent pain from spasm of the upper third of the nonmyotomized esophagus, (2) dysphagia secondary to myotomy or impaired sphincter function, and (3) post-thoracotomy chest wall pain. The best results have been achieved with a full myotomy of the entire esophagus, including the sphincter, together with a loose fundoplication.

ACHALASIA

DONALD O. CASTELL, M.D.

Achalasia is an esophageal motility disorder characterized clinically by slowly progressive dysphagia, often with associated regurgitation of ingested foods. There are two main functional defects in achalasia: (1) obstruction at the esophagogastric junction, and (2) abnormal esophageal peristalsis. Based on early x-ray studies, the obstruction was initially believed to be due to spasm of the cardia or lower esophageal sphincter (LES), hence the term "cardiospasm." Later, manometric studies showed absence of relaxation of the LES during swallowing, and this was called "achalasia." Currently available manometric techniques have shown that the motility abnormality is indeed dual. LES pressures are usually increased and display abnormal (incomplete) relaxation, producing a considerable functional obstruction. In addition, a total absence of peristalsis occurs in the lower two-thirds of the esophageal body. These functional abnormalities are the result of denervation of the distal esophagus and LES; histologic studies reveal degeneration of ganglion cells in the intermyenteric plexus. The specific etiology of this localized denervation is unknown.

The clinical presentation of achalasia may be quite variable. The majority of patients are between the ages of 20 and 40 years, although the disease does occur in children and in the elderly. The most common initial complaint is progressive dysphagia for both liquids and solids. Regurgitation of undigested food that has been eaten many hours previously is a common complaint, particularly at night, when it may result in aspiration and nocturnal coughing. Gastroesophageal reflux is unlikely because of the superprotective LES. However some patients describe a burning retrosternal pain similar to heartburn, probably secondary to the marked dilatation and stasis in the esophagus. Sometimes a more atypical form of chest pain may be a prominent early symptom in patients with achalasia.

DIAGNOSIS

As for most patients with dysphagia, barium esophagogram should be the initial diagnostic test. The characteristic findings include (1) smooth (beak-like) tapering at the distal end of the barium-filled esophagus, (2) an air-fluid level in the esophagus from retained secretions and food, and (3) esophageal dilatation, sometime showing the classic sigmoid appearance. The chest film may provide such clues as absence of the gastric air bubble or mediastinal widening. Such findings strongly suggest achalasia, but I prefer esophageal manometry as the method for establishing the diagnosis. Complete absence of peristalsis is a requirement and is usually accompanied by LES abnormalities of incomplete relaxation and elevated resting pressure (as already described). Occasionally the LES abnormalities are not clearly evident, and diagnosis is based on the manometric finding of total absence of peristalsis combined with typical roentgenographic defects. Delayed esophageal emptying of a radiolabeled meal of solid food should confirm the functional defect in these patients. Prior to accepting a diagnosis of idiopathic achalasia, all patients should undergo careful esophagoscopy to rule out a malignant lesion at the esophagogastric junction. These patients are more likely to be older (>50 years), to have a shorter history of dysphagia (<1 year), and to have a greater degree of weight loss (>15 pounds) than patients with idiopathic achalasia.

THERAPY

The optimal treatment for achalasia would restore esophageal peristalsis to normal and cause the LES to relax completely. Since neither of these goals is attainable, current therapies are directed at weakening the LES to allow gravity and any remaining contractile activity to move material into the stomach. This is usually attempted by either instrumental dilation or surgical esophagomyotomy of the LES muscle.

Pneumatic Dilation

The preferred method of instrumental dilation of the LES is pneumatic dilation. This has been a successful form of treatment for achalasia for over 30 years. Results of several large series reveal that excellent results can be expected in 75 to 85 percent of patients. If poor results are obtained with the first dilation, good results can be expected in many patients with a second procedure. Gastroesophageal reflux complicating pneumatic dilation is rare, less than 3 percent in most series. A more serious complication is perforation of the esophagus, which occurs in less than 5 percent of dilations.

The specific technique for pneumatic dilation varies considerably, with dilator bags of varying size and composition and with durations of actual inflation of the dilator within the LES ranging from only a few seconds to as long as 5 minutes. Since no information is available systematically comparing different techniques, the procedure used by most operators is more an art taught by those with greatest experience. The approach to pneumatic dilation used in our unit over the past 20 years is described in the next paragraphs.

Prior to all pneumatic dilations, the inflatable bag should be inspected to (1) observe the symmetry of the bag during inflation, (2) measure the circumference of the center and outer aspects of the bag and (3) submerge the bag under water to check for leaks.

The patient fasts overnight and is taken to the radiology suite where the entire procedure is performed. An Ewald tube is used to aspirate fluid from the dilated esophagus. Premedications include a Cetacaine spray to anesthetize the gag reflex and diazepam, given in 10-mg doses intravenously, as required to produce mild sedation and postprocedure amnesia. The pneumatic dilator is then advanced into the esophagus to a level at which half of the radiopaque strips surrounding the bag are above the diaphragmatic hiatus and the other half are in the stomach. As the bag is gradually inflated, the waist (LES) deformity surrounding the bag is noted on fluoroscopy, and should be maintained at the diaphragm. As the diameter of the bag increases, the bag may tend to move upward or downward. If this happens, the bag should be deflated and reinflated with a slight change in position to maintain the waist of the bag at the diaphragm. The bag is distended to its maximal degree as quickly as possible in an attempt to produce the most effective stretch of the LES. The degree to which the bag is distended depends on the maximal diameter of the bag. In the adult patient, a bag with a maximal diameter of 3.0 to 3.5 cm is used. Once the predetermined diameter of the bag is reached, the pressure (usually between 12 and 15 psi) is maintained for 60 seconds. The pressure is then completely released, and the bag is subsequently reinflated for an additional 60 seconds after a rest period of a few minutes. No more than two dilations are performed at a single session. If the dilation is successful, the patient experiences considerable pain while the balloon is inflated. This pain should resolve almost immediately following deflation. Persistent pain strongly suggests perforation.

After removal of the dilator, a small amount of barium (15 to 30 ml) is placed into the distal esophagus via nasogastric tube with the patient in the semiupright position. If a small perforation is noted extending beyond the lumen of the esophagus, the patient is restricted from eating or drinking and vital signs are closely observed. If the patient remains relatively asymptomatic, but shows a temperature spike to 100°F, antibiotics should be given immediately. Conservative treatment is usually sufficient in these patients. On the other hand, if barium is noted to flow freely into the mediastinum and left chest, immediate surgery is indicated. These patients usually exhibit symptoms of shock and develop severe pain in 1 or 2 hours. A positive Hammon's sign or subcutaneous emphysema indicates the presence of mediastinal air.

Esophagomyotomy

Surgical treatment of achalasia with distal esophagomyotomy (Heller procedure) has also been found to be quite effective. Excellent symptomatic improvement following this procedure has been described in 80 to 90 percent of patients. The most frequent complications are persistent dysphagia because of an inadequate myotomy and gastroesophageal reflux. Because of the latter, concomitant antireflux procedures have been advocated to reduce this complication. The necessity for this double procedure is controvesial.

Suggested indications for surgical therapy of achalasia are (1) several (more than two) unsuccessful attempts at pneumatic dilation, (2) esophageal rupture complicating pneumatic dilation, (3) difficulty in placing the pneumatic dilator because of extreme esophageal dilation, (4) inability to exclude esophageal neoplasm, and (5) achalasia in children under 12 years of age.

Dilation Versus Surgical Therapy

As already indicated, both the medical and the surgical treatment of achalasia are effective. Medical treatment is rarely associated with significant reflux; however, the risk of esophageal perforation is ever present. Improvement in dysphagia after dilation varies among studies, but is probably not so great as that occurring after myotomy. The time spent in the hospital is considerably less in patients who undergo pneumatic dilation. Best results with pneumatic dilation appear to be obtained in patients over age 45 who have had at least moderate esophageal dilatation and dysphagia for longer than 5 years.

An esophagomyotomy, on the other hand, may result in longer, more complete relief of dysphagia. Unfortunately, reflux is a major complication when an overzealous myotomy is performed. Present surgical mortality is very low; however, the morbidity and cost associated with major thoracic surgery are significant.

My personal recommendation, shared by many other experts, is to perform pneumatic dilation as the initial therapy and reserve myotomy for patients who fail to benefit from dilation. Other potential indications for myotomy are listed above.

Pharmacologic Approaches

Efforts to improve esophageal emptying in achalasia through pharmacologic means date back many years to observations in achalasia patients given amyl nitrite during barium swallow, in which case immediate relaxation of the cardia was noted. Recently *isosorbide dinitrate* has been shown to decrease LES pressure and increase radio-isotopic esophageal emptying. A clinical trial has suggested effective symptomatic improvement with long-term therapy, but many patients experienced headaches from this medication. Attempts to improve esophageal emptying with anticholinergics such as tincture of belladonna, atropine sulfate, and dicyclomine have been effective in isolated cases. An exciting new area of pharmacologic therapy may be developing with the calcium channel antagonists. *Nifedipine* (10 to 20 mg PO) has recently been found to significantly decrease the LES pressure in patients with mild-to-moderate achalasia and to greatly improve esophageal clearance of a radiolabeled solid meal. In addition, good-to-excellent symptomatic improvement for up to 18 months has been found in some patients when compared to patients receiving a placebo. It has been suggested that this calcium-channel blocker may be an effective medical therapy for mild-to-moderate achalasia. An apparently effective means of administration of nifedipine in these patients is sublingually just prior to meals. The patient can be advised to just chew the capsule until the medication is released into the mouth. Absorption is rapid, and maximal effects on esophageal pressures occur within 15 to 30 minutes.

Pharmacologic means for potentially improving patients with achalasia date back over 50 years, and although occasional agents are effective in maintaining patients on a long-term basis, few have withstood the test of time. My own personal suspicion is that successful long-term treatment for achalasia requires a procedure to alter the abnormal muscular obstructive component at the LES. This can be accomplished with either of the time-tested approaches: pneumatic dilation or a Heller myotomy. I remain skeptical whether pharmacologic therapy is likely to provide sustained benefit in these patients and await further clinical trials to resolve this question.

PHARYNGEAL DYSPHAGIA

WILLIAM J. RAVICH, M.D.

Pharyngeal dysphagia is not a disease but a symptom. In order to direct therapy, an accurate understanding of the nature and severity of swallowing impairment is essential. Neither the interest nor the skills of any single subspecialty, however, is comprehensive enough to analyze or treat the various causes of pharyngeal symptoms. It is difficult in many cases even to determine which subspecialty should be involved.

The Johns Hopkins Swallowing Center is a multidisciplinary center formed in recognition of the diverse skills required for the care of the dysphagic patient. Subspecialties involved include dentistry, gastroenterology, neurology, otolaryngology, radiology, and rehabilitation medicine.

Many patients referred to the center have symptoms suggesting a pharyngeal disorder. In this chapter I will describe some observations derived from the Swallowing Center experience with patients presenting with pharyngeal dysphagia, concentrating on the techniques available for the treatment of these patients.

BASIC PRINCIPLES

A number of basic principles govern the evaluation and treatment of patients with pharyngeal dysphagia, and attention to these principles is critical in directing therapeutic efforts.

First, the events of a pharyngeal swallow are too fast for either the eye to see (with fluoroscopy) or the hand to catch (on spot films). Significant structural, as well as motor, abnormalities can be missed when a routine barium swallow is used to assess the pharynx. A dynamic study (cine- or videoradiography) of swallowing by a radiologist experienced in the technique is essential in the evaluation of any patient suspected of having a pharyngeal disorder.

Second, patients who localize their dysphagia to the neck often have disorders of the oral cavity or the esophagus. Clinical and radiographic assessment should routinely include evaluation of the entire swallowing mechanism and not be limited to pharyngeal structure and function. The esophagus is a particularly frequent cause of pharyngeal symptoms.

Third, cough is an unreliable symptom of airway penetration. Many physicians and patients assume that if a patient does not cough, the airway is not in jeopardy. Unfortunately, a substantial proportion of patients with neurologic impairment of pharyngeal function also appear to have a deficient cough reflex. We frequently see patients who fail to cough even as barium is pouring down the trachea. Objective evaluation based on a dynamic contrast study is essential in assessing airway competence.

Fourth, a vigorous search for a structural obstruction should be part of the evaluation of every patient with dysphagia in whom the radiographic evaluation does not adequately explain symptoms. In practice, the onus is on the physician who withholds endoscopy as part of the evaluation.

Fifth, in patients with evidence of a neurogenic or myogenic cause of pharyngeal symptoms, treatable causes such as polymyositis, myasthenia gravis, hypothyroidism, hyperthyroidism, and Parkinson's disease must be excluded.

Sixth, an empiric approach is the best guide to therapy. For a variety of reasons, the precise influence of detected derangements in function and structure on the patient's symptoms is often unclear. In addition, the effect of specific interventions on swallowing cannot always be predicted. A step-by-step approach, relying on a combination of past experience and observation of effect based on a careful analysis of baseline and follow-up dynamic radiographic studies, is generally preferable.

Finally, the nutritional status of the patient is a critical, but often neglected, aspect of management. Whether the swallowing impairment is temporary or permanent, assurance of adequate caloric intake may require alternative means of feeding.

ANALYSIS OF DYSFUNCTION

The initial approach to management relies heavily on a careful analysis of clinical, radiographic, and endoscopic (pharyngoscopy and/or esophagoscopy) findings. Because the knowledge and skills required to evaluate all patients are not available within any one subspecialty, multiple consultations may be required to provide a complete assessment of the factors underlying symptoms and of the therapeutic options available. A joint discussion with all personnel who are or might become involved is often the best means of overcoming the intellectual distance between the subspecialties traditionally involved in the care of patients with pharyngeal dysphagia.

Clinical Examination

A clear description of symptoms is critical, as any physical, radiographic, or endoscopic findings must be put into context. Coughing or choking during swallowing strongly suggests the presence of an oral or pharyngeal disorder, while coughing after the meal or at night suggests esophageal disease.

Particular attention should be paid to the specific types of food which cause symptoms. Contrary to popular opinion, patients with neurogenic dysphagia often have the most trouble with liquids. These patients frequently do best with foods that have a gelatinous consistency and have enough intrinsic cohesiveness to pass an incompetent larynx without dripping into the airway.

Dysphagia with solids alone should be assumed due to a structural obstruction until proven otherwise. Because of its luminal diameter, the esophagus is likely to be responsible for solid food dysphagia. Patients often have modified their own diets prior to seeking medical attention. Such modifications should be specifically elicited. Occasionally patients presenting with pulmonary symptoms due to swallowing impairment deny difficulty swallowing because they have long before excluded solids from their diets.

Clinical examination should include an assessment of *oral cavity* structure and function. The condition of the teeth, including the adequacy of occlusion, is obviously important in the preparation of food for swallowing. A dry oral cavity should suggest xerostomia or the use of drugs with anticholinergic properties. Congenital or acquired (usually surgical) defects in maxilla, mandible, tongue, or hard and soft palate should be looked for.

The *tongue* should be evaluated for bulk and movement. Tongue enlargement can result from hypothyroidism, amyloidosis, or tumor. A serrated appearance on the margin of the tongue, representing the impression by the teeth, may be a subtle sign of enlargement. Wasting of the tongue or fasciculations suggests a neurologic disorder, though mild fasciculations present on extension only may be a normal, effort-related finding.

Additional signs of neurologic disease include buccal and tongue weakness, poor lip closure, an asymmetric palatine arch, or deviation of the uvula. The gag reflex should be assessed bilaterally. An absent gag reflex suggests the presence of a bulbar lesion which could involve the swallowing center, the neurologic area controlling swallowing which extends through much of the pons and medulla. The neurologic examination should include particular attention to cranial nerves V through XII, the nuclei of which are stretched out along the course of the swallowing center.

When abnormalities are noted, the appropriate subspecialty should be consulted for a more thorough assessment.

Radiographic Examination

A careful review of the findings on *cine-* or *videoradiography* is an essential part of the evaluation of any patient presenting with known or suspected pharyngeal dysfunction. This review is best done jointly by the clinicians and radiologist involved, and should assess not only the findings but also the adequacy of the study in answering pertinent clinical questions. Some patients have modified head position or bolus size to minimize symptoms. These self-imposed maneuvers should be noted. A conscious attempt by the radiologist to reproduce the situation that elicits symptoms may be required, including the use of a variety of barium-coated or barium-impregnated material.

The analysis of the dynamic study can be divided into oral, pharyngeal, and esophageal phases.

Oral Phase. The control of the bolus before, during, and after the initiation of swallowing should be assessed. Some patients have difficulty keeping material in the mouth during the oral preparation of food owing to impaired separation of oral cavity and pharynx. This can result in premature leakage into the pharynx. Others have an inadequate propulsion due to weak or uncoordinated movement of the tongue, causing oral retention often followed by post-swallow leakage into an unprotected larynx.

Pharyngeal Phase. The strength, symmetry, and completeness of the pharyngeal stripping wave; the adequacy of laryngeal closure, which involves both elevation of the larynx and tilt of the epiglottis; and the timing and extent of opening of the pharyngoesophageal segment should be assessed.

In addition to the presence of abnormal masses, pharyngeal pouches and webs involving the pharynx or pharyngoesophageal segment should be looked for. Though most gastroenterologists think of a Zenker's diverticulum whenever a pouch is mentioned, the majority of pharyngeal pouches are lateral and located in the valleculae. Most often these pouches represent an incidental finding and are not responsible for symptoms. If the pouch cannot be shown to retain material after the pharyngeal peristaltic wave has passed, its significance in the genesis of symptoms is dubious.

A worthwhile distinction can be made between direct penetration into the larynx during swallowing (*penetration*) and the inhalation of barium retained in the hypopharynx after pharyngeal swallowing is completed (*aspiration*). Direct penetration is most often due to neurologic or myogenic dysfunction. Though also frequently due to a neurologic or myogenic process, aspiration may result from a pouch, web, or an isolated disorder of upper esophageal function. In addition, review of radiographic studies done at the Swallowing Center indicates that pharyngeal dysfunction resulting in pharyngeal retention commonly occurs in association with esophageal dysmotility or structural disease. The possibility that esophageal disease may produce secondary dysfunction in the pharynx must be considered.

Esophageal Phase. Of patients presenting to the Swallowing Center with previously unexplained pharyngeal dysphagia, one-fourth have an isolated abnormality of esophageal function or structure on radiographic evaluation, while about one-third have combined disorders of the pharynx and esophagus in which either is capable of causing symptoms. Among the esophageal abnormalities demonstrated are esophageal stricture, Schatzki's ring, achalasia, and esophageal spasm. The treatment of these esophageal disorders usually results in symptomatic improvement of pharyngeal symptoms.

THERAPEUTIC APPROACHES

It is important for those caring for the dysphagic patient to have some understanding of how different subspecialties approach treatment. The following is intended as a brief overview of some of the therapeutic options and their indications.

Prosthodontics

The capacity to chew is obviously helpful in the ingestion of solid foods. In addition, the teeth are important in maintaining the proper alignment of the oral cavity. Though only occasionally implicated as the sole cause of swallowing difficulties in patients at the Swallowing Center, poor dentition or ill-fitting dentures may exaggerate the symptoms produced by disordered function or structure downstream.

In patients with congenital or acquired structural defects of the mandible, maxilla, tongue, or palates, a combination of oral reconstruction and prosthetic devices can produce dramatic improvement in swallowing. Obdurators are used to fill in the defects, preventing food from extruding into empty spaces where oral control and bolus preparation cannot occur. In patients with severe malocclusion, plates with specially designed ramps may be used to guide teeth into proper position for mastication. It is easier to secure these devices in an oral cavity in which at least some of the patient's own teeth remain.

Although not as successful for the neurologically impaired, similar devices can be tried in patients in whom loss of tongue mass or problems with alignment result from muscle wasting rather than structural abnormaliies.

Treatable Neurogenic and Myogenic Disease

The detection of pharyngeal paresis or inadequate elevation of the larynx suggests the presence of a neurologic or myogenic cause of dysphagia. Determining a specific diagnosis depends heavily on the detection of other physical findings and the judicious use of specific laboratory tests.

Disorders that require particular consideration are those susceptible to pharmacologic intervention. Polymyositis, myasthenia gravis, myopathies associated with hypo- and hyperthyroidism, and Parkinson's disease will respond to appropriate medical therapy.

Dysphagia associated with Huntington's disease can be ameliorated by phenothiazine compounds and haloperidol, drugs often used to decrease the severity of the choreiform movements that are the hallmark of this disease.

Chorea makes introduction of an appropriate-sized bolus into the mouth difficult. In addition, chorea of the tongue is often present, making control of the oral bolus difficult. Premature or delayed leakage into the pharynx is a common problem. Prolixin or haloperidol is useful in improving dysphagia.

What is remarkable in the few patients in whom the effects of this therapy on swallowing has been evaluated is the small, even subtherapeutic, doses of the medication to which they respond. In addition, as the dose is increased or as serum levels equilibrate, improvement can be followed by deterioration, possibly resulting from a sensitivity to the dyskinetic effects of the drugs which is not noted in normal individuals until much higher doses are used. Careful titration to obtain an optimal result in terms of swallowing is mandatory.

The Role of Pharyngeal Surgery

The frequency with which surgery is performed in patients with pharyngeal dysphagia varies considerably from institution to institution. Aside from the management of tumors, the otolaryngologist is most often asked to consider cricopharyngeal myotomy or resection of pharyngeal pouches.

Cricopharyngeal myotomy involves the incision of the cricopharyngeus—the main component of the upper esophageal sphincter—through a lateral neck incision. Its major indication is the presence of an isolated abnormality of upper esophageal sphincter function. This diagnosis is usually entertained on the basis of an incompletely opening pharyngoesophageal segment seen on barium swallow. Careful analysis of cineradiographic studies in patients referred to the Swallowing Center with a diagnosis of "cricopharyngeal achalasia" or "cricopharyngeal spasm" however, usually demonstrates profound abnormalities of pharyngeal function as well. Manometric confirmation that the upper esophageal sphincter is functioning improperly can only rarely be obtained. Cricopharyngeal myotomy in patients with diffuse impairment of pharyngeal function—as opposed to isolated upper esophageal sphincter dysfunction—is of questionable value, especially as additional damage to the peripheral nervous system and scarring at the pharyngoesophageal segment may actually make matters worse in an already impaired pharynx.

The role of *resection*, usually combined with *myotomy*, in Zenker's diverticulum is well established in otolaryngology. The myotomy is included because of manometric evidence of upper esophageal sphincter dysfunction and the clinical impression that diverticula are more likely to recur if myotomy is not performed. It is postulated that the pouch occurs through an area of relative weakness in the presence of increased pharyngeal pressure during swallowing resulting from sphincter dysfunction. Unfortunately, it is often impossible to intubate patients with large Zenker's diverticuli because the manometric catheter tends to preferentially pass directly into the pouch.

The surgical resection of lateral pharyngeal pouches is only rarely indicated. Most lateral pouches are incidental findings. Only pouches that remain filled after passage of the pharyngeal peristaltic wave should be considered potentially responsible for symptoms. In the Swallowing Center experience, these pouches are often associated with dysfunction elsewhere in the swallowing mechanism. In most cases, symptoms seem to correlate with these other abnormalities. A *double swallow rehabilitation* technique (see section on rehabilitation) is usually effective in diminishing symptoms from a pouch sufficiently to avoid surgery.

Gastroenterologic Considerations

As previously mentioned, patients often are inaccurate in localizing the level of obstruction. About one-third of individuals with obstructive lesions in the distal esophagus localize their symptoms to the neck. Conversely, about one-fourth of patients presenting to the Swallowing Center with pharyngeal dysphagia have a purely esophageal cause for their symptoms. This finding has two implications: first, that a careful examination of the esophagus is essential in patients presenting with pharyngeal dysphagia, and second, that esophageal disorders should be treated vigorously when they are found. The most common esophageal disorders causing pharyngeal dysphagia are esophageal stenosis (either due to Schatzki's ring or peptic stricture), gastroesophageal reflux without evidence of stricture formation, and idiopathic esophageal spasm. The treatment of these and other esophageal disorders is covered elsewhere in this book.

Rehabilitation Approach

The rehabilitation approach is aimed at the most efficient use of available resources. In terms of swallowing it concentrates on strengthening weak muscles where possible and consciously altering the way in which the patient swallows to *maximize pharyngeal clearance* and *minimize airway soiling*. The ultimate goals, as with other methods of treatment, include improved comfort, adequate nutrition, and airway safety. The rehabilitation approach, however, accepts that these goals often require substantial adjustments in the way the patient obtains his nutrition, adjustments that may be less than ideal from the patient's viewpoint.

The most obvious intervention is avoidance of foods that cause the greatest difficulty. Patients with problems in the oral preparation of foods or with a structural lesion obstructing the esophagus clearly recognize that foods that are chewy or stringy cause the greatest difficulty. Often patients have modified their diets to minimize symptoms. Depending on the alternatives available and the type of restriction required, modification of diet may be more or less acceptable.

For patients with impaired control of the oral phase of swallowing or incomplete laryngeal closure, thin liquids often cause particular difficulty, as they easily drip over the back of the tongue or into the incompletely protected larynx. Foods with a thicker consistency, such as thick liquids, puddings, jellos, and mashed potatoes, often are handled best. It appears that some degree of intrinsic cohesiveness prevents separation and diversion of a portion of the swallowed bolus. Some individuals who are unable to swallow either liquids or solids can be sustained entirely by means of a gelatinized diet.

As opposed to patients with masticatory or obstructive problems, neurologically impaired patients are less likely to have modified their diets appropriately. This failure may be due to the natural, but often inaccurate, impression that liquids are easiest to swallow, the relatively circumscribed role of foods with the necessary quality of cohesiveness in the average diet, and the influence of associated sensory and cognitive defects which limit the patient's ability to discriminate degrees of difficulty.

Beyond modification of diet, attempts to rehabilitate the neurologically impaired swallow involve the conscious alteration of a process that usually occurs without thought. Patients who leak before or after swallowing must learn to limit the quantity of material in the mouth at any one time and ensure that the mouth is cleared of material before the introduction of additional food. Chewing with the chin down may prevent leakage. Patients with a weak tongue may find that a coordinated extension of the head at the time of swallowing improves the efficiency with which food is introduced from mouth to pharynx.

In patients with *direct laryngeal penetration*, neck flexion decreases the distance that the larynx needs to elevate in order to protect the airway. This maneuver, in combination with the modification of the diet toward more cohesive foods, can often provide the margin of benefit required for adequate and safe hydration and nutrition.

In those with *pharyngeal retention*, the use of a *double swallow technique* is usually helpful. Because aspiration occurs during inspiration when substantial amounts of material remain in the pharynx at the end of a swallow, the goal is to minimize residual pharyngeal contents at the time of inspiration. Normally, swallowing occurs at any time during respiration and is associated with a temporary cessation of respiration. With the double swallow technique, the patient is instructed to consciously inhale just prior to swallowing. Post-swallow resumption of respiratory activity will begin with expiration, during which airway soiling is unlikely to occur. The patient is then instructed to swallow a second time before the next inspiration to clear the pharynx of as much residual material as possible.

SPECIAL PROBLEMS

Combined Dysfunction

Combined dysfunction of pharynx and esophagus is quite common in the Swallowing Center experience. In a series of 40 patients presenting with previously unexplained pharyngeal dysphagia, more than a third had combined disorders of pharynx and esophagus, either one of which could account for their symptoms (defined as the presence of a 50 percent decrease in luminal diameter or evidence of retention on barium study). In this situation, a decision must be made as to the most likely cause of the patient's symptoms. In many cases intensive treatment of the most treatable of the problems detected represents the best course, the response to therapy being used to confirm or deny its importance to the patient's clinical presentation.

Presumed Psychogenic Dysphagia

Many patients referred to the Swallowing Center have been previously diagnosed as having dysphagia of psychogenic origin. A careful investigation of these individuals reveals a cause for dysphagia in approximately three-fourths. In a series of 23 such patients, we were able to establish a cause in 16. Even in those in whom a cause is not found, it is not always clear that the problem is only emotional in origin. Only two patients were strongly suspected of having a purely psychogenic dysphagia on the basis of diffuse anxiety and unexplainable multisystem complaints. For the others, it is equally plausible that current technology does not permit proper assessment of the cause.

This is not to say that anxiety plays no role in dysphagia. Fear of cardiac disease, cancer, or sudden death from choking all represent legitimate reasons for anxiety. Often the anxiety produced by the symptoms has an important role in exaggerating the severity of symptoms beyond that expected from the degree of impairment detected. When the problem cannot be directly treated, and when reassurance fails to alleviate anxiety, *behavior modification* therapy may be useful.

Sedatives must be used with extreme caution in patients with impaired swallowing. These drugs are unlikely to help, except in doses at which mental acuity is severely impaired. In the presence of swallowing difficulties, the decreased attention to the act of oral preparation of food and the initiation of swallowing caused by sedatives may exacerbate the degree of disability. This is particularly dangerous in patients with symptoms suggesting airway soiling, such as coughing or choking during eating. Patients with both neurogenic and structural causes of dysphagia almost uniformly have more trouble when treated with tranquilizers than when these agents are withdrawn.

Alternative Means of Feeding

All too often patients are referred to the Swallowing Center in a severely malnourished condition. Consideration of tube feeding should not await severe weight loss. A starving patient is unlikely to be able to cooperate in a rehabilitation program. Often the patient compensates by taking an excessively long time to eat. For many, a major portion of the day is taken up in an often vain attempt to ingest an adequate number of calories. Such efforts are quite disruptive to normal activity. In addition, eating may be exhausting to those with swallowing difficulties, resulting in increasing difficulty as the meal goes on.

The reluctance of patients and physicians to implement tube feeding is unfortunate. Tube feeding is an excellent means of ensuring adequate caloric intake in patients in whom treatment is unlikely to bring rapid results. Because an already neurologically impaired pharynx may have increased trouble swallowing around a tube, an endoscopically or surgically placed feeding gastrostomy is generally preferable in anyone in whom tube feeding is likely to be required for an extended period of time. If oral feeding can be subsequently resumed, removal of the gastrostomy tube is followed by rapid closure of the surgical fistula. In patients who are able to eat food safely, but only in decreased amounts, tube feeding may be used to supplement oral feeding, taking pressure off the patient to eat unreasonable amounts of food.

The approaches to evaluation and management discussed here have evolved from the work of The Johns Hopkins Swallowing Center. They therefore represent the combined efforts of my colleagues in the Center, including Martin Donner, Bronwyn Jones, James Bosma, Susan Kramer, and Steven Rubesin (Radiology); Thomas Hendrix (Gastroenterology); Bernard Marsh and Haskins Kashima (Otolaryngology); David Buchholz (Neurology); Arthur Siebens, Patricia Linden, and Jeffrey Palmer (Rehabilitation Medicine); and Lowell Wiener (Dentistry).

FOREIGN BODY EXTRACTION FROM THE UPPER GASTROINTESTINAL TRACT

WILLIAM ALLEN WEBB, M.D.

In the United States as many as 1,500 people die annually as a result of foreign bodies entering the upper gastrointestinal (UGI) tract. Eighty percent of foreign body ingestion occurs in the pediatric age group. Most of these objects (80% to 90%) will pass spontaneously, but 10 to 20 percent will have to be removed endoscopically, and about 1 percent of patients will require surgery. Ninety percent of ingested foreign bodies will enter the GI tract and 10 percent will enter the tracheobronchial tree.

In 1937, Chevalier Jackson published a classic monograph on the management of foreign bodies of the upper airway and esophagus using the rigid endoscope. Until recent years very little progress in managing this problem had been made. The most significant advance in technique since Jackson's monograph is the use of the flexible endoscope to manage foreign bodies of the UGI tract. Use of this instrument has also resulted in placing the management of this problem primarily in the hands of the gastroenterologist. When both rigid and flexible endoscopy are available, I use rigid only to remove certain sharp foreign bodies from the esophagus in the pediatric age group. Overtubes may be used with the flexible endoscope in adults. In this chapter I will outline my procedures for managing coins, meat, sharp and pointed objects, and two special groups of foreign bodies (Table 1).

FOREIGN BODIES

Coins

Coins are the most common foreign bodies seen in the pediatric age group. One rarely encounters problems with the ingestion of a dime, for it is usually the larger coins that lodge at the level of the cricopharyngeus muscle or just below it. Anteroposterior (A-P) and lateral radiographs of the neck should be made to determine if the coin (or any radiopaque foreign body) is in the trachea or the esophagus. In the more anterior trachea, the A-P view will reveal the edge of the coin, while the flat surface will be seen on the lateral view. The reverse is true in the more posterior esophagus, with the flat surface being seen on the A-P view and the edge being seen on the lateral view (Figs. 1, 2).

In infants and children, radiographs from the base of the skull to the anus should be made to determine if more than one foreign body is present, or if one is located in the nasopharynx. The single most important thing to remember in managing coins (and other foreign bodies) is to *maintain an airway at all times*. Do not make matters worse or cause a catastrophe by dropping a for-

TABLE 1 Summary of Guidelines for Management of Ingested Foreign Bodies

I. History and physical examination.
  A. Odynophagia?
  B. Salivation?
    1. Esophageal obstruction indicated.
    2. Immediate endoscopy and removal should be done to prevent aspiration.
    3. Investigate reason for impaction.
  C. Swelling or crepitation in neck?
  D. Abdominal tenderness?
II. Radiographic examination.
  A. Radiopaque foreign body.
    1. A-P and lateral films of neck.
    2. Objects larger than 5 cm will probably not pass the pyloro-duodenal angle.
    3. Repeat x-rays should be made to note foreign body migration if more than a few hours have elapsed between last x-ray films and the time of endoscopy.
    4. A coin in the stomach requires an x-ray study no more frequently than once per week unless symptoms develop.
  B. Negative radiographs.
    1. Suspect radiolucent foreign body, e.g., fish bone.
      a. Thin barium studies may be helpful.
      b. Barium impregnated cotton not used.
    2. Asymptomatic patient with negative x-rays needs no further treatment.
    3. Endoscopy indicated if symptoms are present and persist for more than a few hours.
  C. Meat ingestion.
    1. No radiographs required.
    2. No barium studies required.
III. Anesthesia.
  A. Infants and children will usually require a general endotracheal anesthetic.
  B. Using flexible endoscopes, adults can be examined with intravenous diazepam (Valium) and meperidine (Demerol). They rarely require general anesthesia.
IV. Special considerations.
  A. Contemplation and practice with duplicate of foreign body is valuable.
  B. Children with impacted foreign bodies at the level of the cricopharyngeus muscle or cervical esophagus must have a controlled airway at the time of removal.
  C. Sharp and pointed objects.
    1. Can be removed with flexible or rigid endoscopes. (See text.)
    2. Overtube can be used to great advantage with flexible endoscope.
    3. IV antibiotics should be used.
V. Surgery is indicated for:
  A. Large or long objects not clearing the stomach in 3–5 days
  B. Perforation/bleeding.
  C. Obstruction.
VI. Choice of endoscopes.
  A. Rigid.
    1. General anesthesia used.
    2. Open laryngoscope used on pharynx.
    3. Used for foreign bodies in esophagus.
  B. Flexible.
    1. General anesthesia or IV sedation used.
    2. Used for all foreign bodies in esophagus, stomach, or duodenum.

Reprinted by permission from South Med J 1984; 77:1083–1086.

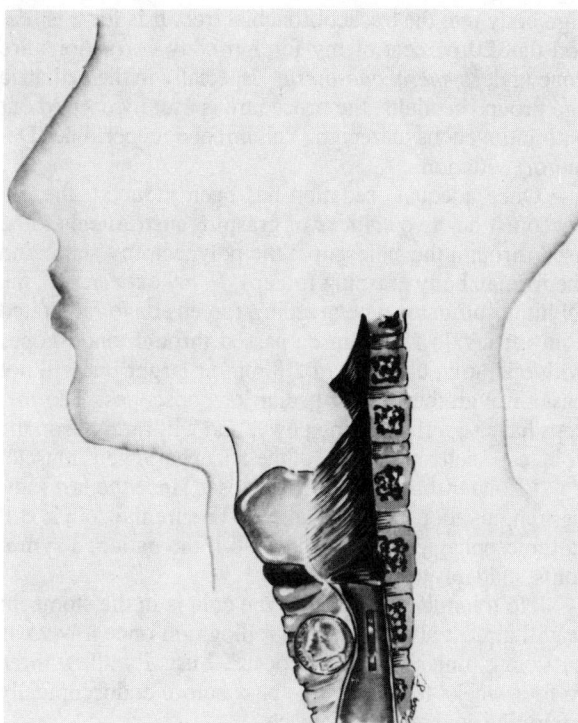

Figure 1 Artist's sketch showing the position of a coin in the trachea and the esophagus in the lateral view. Note how a coin in the trachea aligns itself with the slit in the vocal cords.

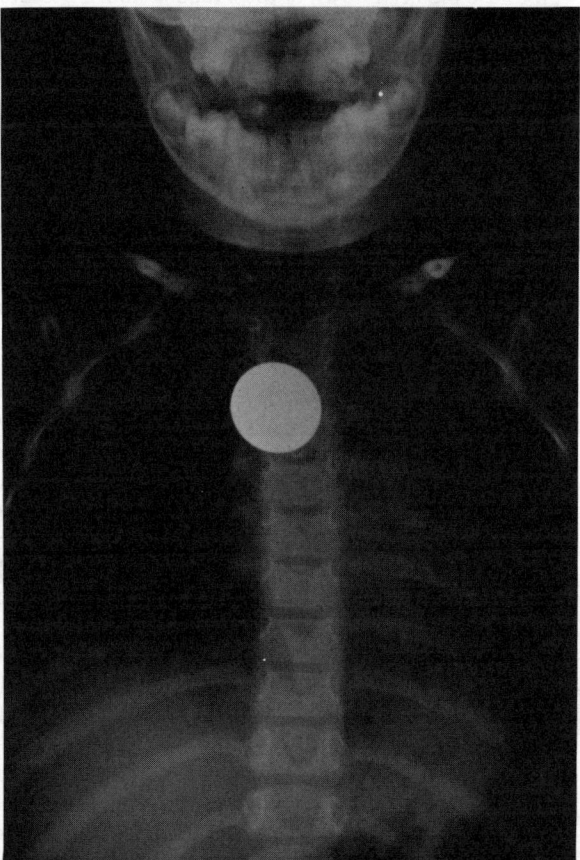

Figure 2 Anteroposterior radiograph demonstrating the position of a coin in the cervical esophagus.

eign body into the tracheobronchial tree. It is for this reason that 20 percent of my foreign body extractions are done under *general anesthesia*, especially in the pediatric age group. In adults, the procedure is usually carried out with intravenous diazepam (Valium) and meperidine (Demerol) sedation.

Once adequate sedation has been induced, the endoscopist has two choices of grasping instruments to be used through the endoscope: the polypectomy snare and the foreign body grasping forceps. In my experience, the Olympus alligator-type grasping forceps have facilitated coin retrieval. They can be passed through endoscopes with operating channels of 2.8 mm or larger but will not pass through the smaller pediatric endoscopes. The forceps have superb grasping power and will rarely drop the coin, especially at the level of the cricopharyngeus muscle.

If longer than an hour has elapsed since the last radiograph, another should be taken to be sure the coin is still in the esophagus. This is true also if the patient's symptoms suddenly disappear.

No treatment is needed if the coin is in the stomach; it will almost always pass. A radiograph once a week is sufficient, unless symptoms occur. I usually allow three to four weeks for the coin to pass before endoscopically removing it from the stomach.

I do not use magnets or balloon catheters to remove esophageal coins because one does not have adequate control of them. If endotracheal anesthesia is not used, it is well to use the head-down or the Trendelenburg position as the foreign body is being delivered into the hypopharynx.

Meat

Meat is the most common foreign body seen in the adult. A patient presenting with a history of meat impacted in the esophagus needs no radiographs or barium studies. The latter simply make the task of the endoscopist more difficult. If the patient is salivating and unable to handle his oral secretions, endoscopy should be done immediately to prevent aspiration. If the patient can handle his saliva, emergency endoscopy is not necessary. *Sedation* and *glucagon* (1 mg IV) will often relieve the obstruction if one is waiting overnight to perform endoscopy. Even if the meat bolus passes, the adult patient should undergo endoscopy because, in my experience, 97 percent of these patients have esophageal pathologic changes. (Cancer, however, is rarely the cause.) A child who has a coin hung in the esophagus and then passes it spontaneously does not need endoscopy if it is his first episode.

I do not use papain (meat tenderizer), since there have been reports in the literature of lethal complications. Aspiration of the papain from an obstructed esophagus, with resulting chemical pneumonitis, must also be considered.

If endoscopy is performed with flexible instruments soon after ingestion, the meat can be removed as a single unit, using a polypectomy snare. If the meat has started to fragment, however, it becomes more difficult to remove. In this situation, rigid instruments may be used to pull the fragments through the endoscope. Flexible instruments must be removed and reinserted repeatedly. I will sometimes use a foreign body overtube to facilitate reinsertion of the flexible endoscope. I prefer the Key Med overtube; and after lubricating it externally and internally, I put a No. 44 F Maloney rubber dilator through it and seat it proximal to the foreign body, just as if I were dilating the patient.

In recent years, I have often dealt with the fragmenting bolus of meat in a different manner. I first try to pass by the meat with a pediatric endoscope and assess the cause of the distal obstruction. If the stomach is entered, the endoscope is brought back proximal to the foreign body and is then used to push it *gently* into the stomach. If the endoscope cannot be passed beyond the meat, I will still try to push it into the stomach. In a patient with no prior history of dysphagia, this can usually be accomplished easily. To reemphasize, however, *gentle technique* and *good judgment* are essential.

After the meat has been removed from the esophagus, endoscopic assessment should be completed. If a peptic stricture is present and there is not too much reaction or edema from the foreign body, dilation should be performed immediately.

Sharp and Pointed Foreign Bodies

Sharp and pointed foreign bodies can be very challenging and difficult to manage, but fortunately they are not common. It is important to be extremely careful not to make the situation worse or to cause a complication, such as a perforated esophagus, that could be lethal. In this day of rapid transit, a patient can easily be moved to a center with an experienced endoscopist. It should not be considered a defeat to have to remove a foreign body surgically, for this is sometimes the safest means.

I believe that every gastroenterologist should have a good working relationship with an anesthesiologist and a rigid endoscopist. Nowhere in foreign body management is it more important than with these types of objects.

The open safety pin always represents a major problem. It is wise to remember Chevalier Jackson's axiom: "Advancing points puncture, trailing do not." If a safety pin is in the esophagus with the open end proximal, it is best managed with the flexible endoscope by pushing the pin into the stomach, turning it, and then grasping the hinged end and pulling it out first. An overtube or a rigid esophagoscope may be necessary with large open safety pins. Removal of multiple objects from the stomach is also made easier with an overtube.

The ingested razor blade is a traumatic experience for both the patient and the endoscopist. Fortunately, the single edge blade is usually seen today, rather than the older double edge blade. This can be managed with the rigid esophagoscope in both the child and the adult by pulling the blade into the instrument. In this type of foreign body removal, the foreign body, the forceps, and the endoscope often have to be removed as a unit. The razor blade can also be managed with the flexible endoscope and overtube, especially if it has reached the stomach.

In removing difficult foreign bodies, time spent in

forethought and planning will make extraction easier. If the foreign body can be duplicated and evaluated with a "dry run," the procedure will be easier and safer. These patients should be treated with *intravenous antibiotics* prior to the procedure.

I remove all sharp foreign bodies before they pass from the stomach because of the chances of perforation as they pass distally, usually in the area of the ileocecal valve. If this type of foreign body passes into the small bowel, *oral antibiotic bowel preparation*, as well as a *high-roughage diet*, is begun. Laxatives are not used. Daily radiographs are necessary in this situation, as opposed to the retained coin in the stomach. If the sharp foreign body fails to progress for three consecutive days, surgical intervention should be considered. If the patient becomes symptomatic, surgical intervention will also be necessary.

Other Specific Foreign Bodies

Elemental mercury that gets into the GI tract from a broken thermometer or the disrupted Miller-Abbott tube bag is not harmful, provided the gut is intact.

Toy batteries should be removed because of their potentially corrosive properties.

Plastic or cellophane packets of cocaine and heroin, when ingested to escape detection, can be a serious and possibly lethal problem. When located in the stomach or the colon, the bag(s) can be reached endoscopically without great difficulty. The bag must not be disrupted, however, because large quantities of the drug would then be absorbed. Often surgical removal is the safest means of managing this problem.

Foreign Bodies at the Level of the Pharynx and Cricopharyngeus

These foreign bodies, usually in the form of fish bones or the toy jackstone, require different management, in my experience. The gastroenterologist does not usually receive training with the indirect mirror technique for fish bones and if it becomes necessary to remove one, it is best done in the following manner. After sedation, the patient is placed in the supine position and the endoscopist stands at the head of the bed. An open rigid laryngoscope (anesthesiology type) is used, along with a surgical grasping clamp (Kelly) or McGill foreign body forceps. The patient can always identify the location of the foreign body, and it almost always will be anterior to the epiglottis in the base of the tongue or in the area of the tonsillar pillar. If removal is unsuccessful, the patient is placed in the left lateral position and flexible endoscopy is performed. The fish bone can often be felt initially with a gloved index finger.

The jackstone (Fig. 3) is difficult to remove because of its prongs. After general endotracheal anesthesia is administered, the endoscopist stands at the head of the table and elevates the epiglottis with the laryngoscope. The jackstone can usually be seen and can be grasped with

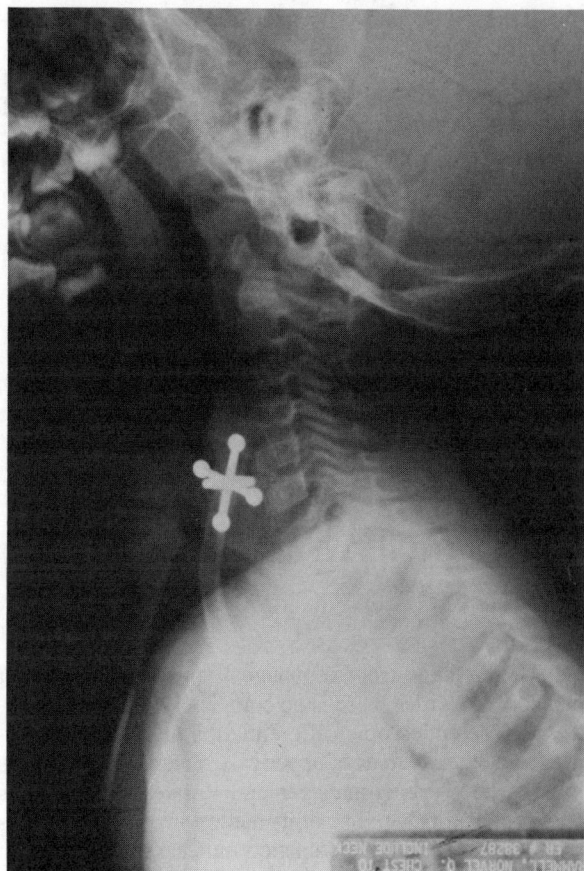

Figure 3 A child's jackstone with prongs caught behind the larynx above the thoracic inlet. See text for description of removal.

the Kelly clamp and removed in an everting or forceps delivery fashion. It is difficult to pull it out with a polypectomy snare if the sharp prongs are lodged posteriorly. Coins in this anatomic area, however, can still be managed as outlined previously.

The Radiolucent Foreign Body

Pieces of plastic, fish bones, glass, and pieces of wood can often be difficult to see on routine radiographs. If the patient has complained of swallowing a foreign body and it is not seen, thin barium is used to try to outline the object. Barium-impregnated cotton is not helpful, in my opinion. If the foreign body is identified radiographically in the hypopharynx or esophagus, endoscopy is performed. If no foreign body is seen radiographically, but the patient remains symptomatic, endoscopy is performed. If no foreign body is seen radiographically and the patient has become asymptomatic, no endoscopy is indicated.

POSTPROCEDURAL CONSIDERATIONS

Once foreign body extraction has been accomplished, one should always consider a *perforation* of the esophagus. If the extraction has been difficult, an immediate gastrograffin study should be done. In the follow-up period, one should diligently watch for signs and symptoms of perforation, such as fever, tachycardia, shortness of breath, chest pain, abdominal pain, and crepitation in the neck. The diagnosis is usually made with a chest film which shows mediastinal air. If the procedure is done on an outpatient basis, the family or parents must be counseled. This complication must be diagnosed early in order for the patient to survive.

SURGICAL INDICATIONS

Surgical indications for foreign body removal are fairly standard. Large objects not passing the pylorus in three to five days, and the complications of foreign bodies, such as bleeding, perforation, or obstruction, are the main indications. The toothpick is the foreign body that most frequently requires surgical removal in this country.

SCLEROTHERAPY OF ESOPHAGEAL VARICES

MICHAEL V. SIVAK Jr., M.D.

Hemorrhage from esophageal varices is a difficult problem for which there is no completely satisfactory solution. The endoscopic differentiation of variceal bleeding from other sources of upper gastrointestinal blood loss is essential to proper management. Variceal bleeding has a high mortality. Studies of its natural history in patients with compromised liver function indicate that more than 40 percent of patients will die within the first 6 weeks after onset and that the majority of deaths will be due to hemorrhage. If variceal hemorrhage is controlled initially but recurs during hospitalization, mortality is extremely high.

For those who survive a bleeding episode, variceal bleeding is likely to recur, and, long-term management of patients with prior variceal hemorrhage is difficult. Surgery may be an option for those with good liver function. The long-term use of pharmacologic agents such as propranolol has also been proposed, but data on the efficacy of this particular drug are conflicting. For those with poor liver function the therapeutic options are limited.

INDICATIONS FOR SCLEROTHERAPY

The immediate goals of endoscopic sclerotherapy of esophageal varices are control of active bleeding and prevention of recurrent bleeding. Since many deaths in patients with cirrhosis and esophageal varices are related to variceal hemorrhage, especially during the first 6 weeks after onset of bleeding, an attempt at reducing mortality may also be considered, although this is controversial.

Defining Acute Variceal Bleeding

Acute variceal bleeding is difficult to define. It is an intermittent process. Even when there is clinical evidence of hemorrhage, for example, hypotension and fresh blood in the stomach, it is unusual at endoscopy to find blood spurting from a rent in a varix. Adherent clot at the bleeding site is more common, but inability to localize the actual bleeding point is not unusual. In many cases the variceal bleeding is an inferred diagnosis because no other abnormalities are found.

Upper gastrointestinal bleeding in patients with known varices may originate from other lesions. Endoscopic diagnosis of variceal bleeding can be particularly difficult if a second potential source of blood loss is present in the upper gastrointestinal tract in association with varices, especially if bleeding is not active at the time of endoscopy and there are no stigmata of recent hemorrhage associated with either endoscopic finding. Despite the difficulties of endoscopic assessment, a reasonable degree of certainty with respect to the diagnosis of variceal bleeding is required before sclerotherapy can be considered. There are data to indicate that prophylactic sclerotherapy is beneficial in selected patients, but this has not been studied extensively, and with the exception of prospective trials, sclerotherapy should not be undertaken in patients who have not bled from varices.

There are numerous prospective trials of sclerotherapy that indicate that acute variceal bleeding is controlled in a high percentage of cases. In most series, however, *balloon tamponade* and/or *intravenous vasopressin* have been used in combination with sclerotherapy. Since variceal hemorrhage is intermittent, and since many patients will respond temporarily to these other measures, it is likely that sclerotherapy was actually performed to prevent recurrent bleeding in many reported series of patients. If there is adherence to a strict definition of acute variceal hemorrhage as endoscopically diagnosed active bleeding, it becomes more difficult to determine, by reference to published experience, whether spurting of blood from a varix can be stopped by endoscopic injection techniques. Despite this difficulty, there is a general consensus that active bleeding from a varix can be stopped by endoscopic injection.

The use of additional methods with sclerotherapy to control acute variceal bleeding does not diminish the value of published reports, but it does disguise some of the difficulties inherent in endoscopic control of active variceal bleeding. Emergency endoscopy for diagnosis alone during upper gastrointestinal bleeding has a complication rate significantly higher than that of routine diagnostic endoscopy. This is compounded by the technical problems inherent in all endoscopic hemostatic procedures, the foremost being the necessity of keeping the field clear of blood and clots. The latter can be difficult within the confines of the narrow tubular esophagus and can make precise placement of injections and control of the injection pattern extremely difficult or impossible.

Stabilization Period

Because of the difficulty of acute sclerotherapy, a valid argument can be made in favor of an attempt at stabilizing the patient by use of intravenous vasopressin and tamponade after it has been concluded by endoscopy that esophageal varices are the source of bleeding. The effectiveness of these methods has been established, but they can only be considered as temporary measures. Tamponade and intravenous vasopressin have potential complications, but these are minimized by recognizing the limitations of these measures and by careful attention to detail in their use. During the stabilization period the patient's intravascular volume deficit can be corrected, attention may be directed to any other medical conditions, and proper preparations can be made for the sclerotherapy procedure. It is difficult to document the value of controlled conditions when performing a technical procedure, but there is no doubt that greater success will be achieved at a lower cost in terms of complications if the procedure can be carried out in a calculated and precise fashion rather than hurriedly and with attention divided among multiple problems.

In some cases it may not be possible to stabilize a patient, and active bleeding may persist despite the use of intravenous vasopressin and tamponade. Given its intermittent nature, variceal bleeding may also resume as tamponade is discontinued. Furthermore, active bleeding may develop during and as a result of the sclerotherapy procedure. In any of these circumstances, the technical problems of endoscopic control of active bleeding may be unavoidable.

End Point of Sclerotherapy

Some reports suggest that sclerotherapy is less successful in the control of variceal bleeding in the short and intermediate term, and that a benefit results only after *variceal obliteration* is achieved. Most investigators believe that a series of procedures aimed at variceal obliteration is advantageous in the long-term control of recurrent variceal bleeding. In many patients it is possible to eliminate all endoscopic evidence of variceal channels, but this is not true in all patients. It may therefore be difficult to know when the maximum benefit from a series of injection procedures has been attained. Whether or not there are other acceptable end points remains problematic.

Surgery Versus Sclerotherapy

The majority of patients with cirrhosis and variceal bleeding are not surgical candidates with respect to the long-term prevention of recurrent bleeding because of poor liver function, ascites, and/or encephalopathy. In such cases therapeutic options are limited, although morbidity and mortality remain high.

There are no published data to guide the choice between surgical and endoscopic therapy in stable patients who have had documented variceal bleeding and who are good risks. Variceal hemorrhage may have ceased spontaneously or in response to measures such as balloon tamponade, and the patient's recent course may be stable, although the chance of recurrent bleeding remains high. During this time sclerotherapy may be proposed. If liver function is good, however, selective shunt surgery might also be considered. Whether surgery or sclerotherapy is superior with respect to morbidity, mortality, and efficacy in patients with prior variceal bleeding who are good risks is unknown. My view is that a selective shunt operation remains an option for such patients. Other factors, such as continued abuse of alcohol, may also influence this decision.

Extrahepatic Portal Hypertension

Although hepatic cirrhosis is the most common cause of portal hypertension, there are other causes. Many are vascular in nature, such as portal vein obstruction from a variety of causes. When this occurs in childhood it is frequently desirable to delay surgery, since further development of the collateral circulation may occur as the child approaches adolescence and a decrease in variceal hemorrhage may result. Sclerotherapy has been shown to control recurrent bleeding successfully in these patients.

Patient Selection for Sclerotherapy

My approach to the selection of patients for sclerotherapy is based on the following reasons.

Most patients who present with acute variceal hemorrhage documented by endoscopy are considered to be candidates for the procedure. An initial attempt is made to *stabilize* the patient when bleeding is acute and ongoing. This almost always includes the use of intravenous vasopressin and frequently of balloon tamponde in addition to the usual resuscitation measures to reverse hypotension and shock. If this is successful, sclerotherapy is usually begun in about 4 to 6 hours. When variceal hemorrhage persists despite these measures, sclerotherapy must be performed to stop bleeding. The technique of control of ongoing blood loss from a varix differs from that of the routine procedure.

If the patient has had documented variceal bleeding

but presents in stable condition, the decision for sclerotherapy is usually based on *liver function*. If this precludes surgery, sclerotherapy is begun. When hepatic function is adequate for surgery the decision to perform sclerotherapy is sometimes based on other factors, such as associated but unrelated medical conditions. In some cases liver function may be good, but surgical therapy is eliminated for technical reasons. Patients who have had prior unsuccessful surgery may undergo endoscopic therapy irrespective of their liver function status.

TECHNIQUE OF SCLEROTHERAPY

Virtually all aspects of endoscopic variceal sclerotherapy technique are empiric. For example, none of the sclerosing substances currently in use was developed specifically for esophageal variceal sclerotherapy. This multiplicity and heterogeneity of technique make comparison of results almost impossible. It is not known whether one method is more effective or has fewer complications than another. It is also possible that specific complications may be more closely associated with one method or sclerosing agent than with another. From a positive viewpoint, it appears that satisfactory results can be achieved with many of the varying techniques, and it is also possible that within broad limits there is no "correct" or optimal technique.

It is pointless to consider one aspect of technique apart from the other elements. For example, the selection of a sclerosing agent must be considered in relation to the number, pattern, and volume of injections as well as the concentration of the active agent and the schedule of procedures.

The variable elements in the technique of sclerotherapy are (1) selection of a sclerosing agent (or agents) and its concentration; (2) number, pattern, and volume of injections; (3) use or nonuse of various methods of compression; (4) intravariceal or paravariceal placement of injections; (5) schedule and number of procedures; and (6) the end point of therapy. Selection of a fiberoptic endoscope and injection device is also a matter of preference and there are numerous ones available for sclerotherapy.

Sclerosing Agent

At present, the substances and their concentrations in our sclerosant solution are sodium tetradecyl sulfate (0.75%) and hypertonic glucose (50%). Sodium tetradecyl sulfate is available in 1 and 3 percent solutions (Sotradecol, Elkins-Sinn, Cherry Hill, NJ). Our original solution consisted of 0.5 percent Sotradecol, 50 percent glucose and 3 to 4 units per milliliter of thrombin. The latter two substances were intended to promote thrombus formation within the vein, with the idea that this would enhance stasis and contact of the active sclerosing agent with the intima of the vein. Thrombin was eliminated because the amounts present in the solution were probably ineffective, the available preparation is a foreign protein, and because intravariceal thrombosis has been demonstrated with the use of a single sclerosing substance. Hypertonic glucose was included to increase the viscosity of the solution, which in turn might increase stasis within the varix and prolong contact of the more sclerosing tetradecyl sulfate molecule. It is likely, however, that the hypertonic glucose plays only a minor role.

Fifty milliliters of sclerosing solution are prepared before the procedure and divided into 10-milliliter syringes. A smaller syringe is easier for the assistant to control during injections.

Equipment

In addition to the sclerosant solution, the required items of equipment for the procedure are a twin-channel endoscope, a flexible unsheathed injector needle (American Endoscopy, Mentor, OH), a Sengstaken-Blakemore tube (for tamponade if hemorrhage is uncontrollable), and a standby vasopressin infusion. Intravenous diazepam and meperidine are used for sedation.

A double-channel fiberoptic endoscope is the preferred instrument; ideally this should have a larger diameter accessory channel for suction and one with a somewhat smaller diameter for insertion of the injection device. The main advantage of this instrument is that its large second channel is usually adequate for maintaining a clear field when there is active bleeding.

The injection device or injector was designed to our specifications. It consists of a single flexible tube, in contrast to other devices which have an inner and outer tube. With injectors of the latter design, the needle is attached to the inner tube and can be withdrawn into the outer tube. The needle itself in our injector is 25 gauge and 5 mm long and is fitted into a rounded metal collar attached to the end of the tubing. This injector has several advantages. It has a great degree of flexibility and responds and adapts readily to any motion that occurs in the esophagus during variceal puncture. The metal collar that houses the needle also prevents an excessive depth of variceal puncture, i.e., the depth of puncture is essentially predetermined by the length of the needle extending out from the metal collar. The injector can be forward loaded in the smaller diameter accessory channel of the endoscope. It will pass easily and safely through this channel as long as the distal tip of the instrument is not acutely deflected. The injector is placed in the accessory channel prior to passing the endoscope, and the point of the needle is positioned within the accessory channel about 1 cm back from the end of the insertion tube. It is also withdrawn into this position after each variceal puncture.

Injection

The placement of injections is controversial. It may be either *intravariceal* or *paravariceal*. It has been demonstrated that placement of injections is less accurate when varices are small, and it is therefore likely that some injections will be paravariceal even though intravariceal puncture is intended, and vice versa. The goal with paravariceal injection is to produce a fibrous reaction over the surface of the variceal vessels so that further bleeding is prevented. Intravariceal injections are thought to produce more immediate hemostasis by virtue of thrombus formation.

Sites of Injection. Intravariceal injections are performed beginning at the level of the esophagogastric mucosal junction. If varices are visible within the *cardia* these are also injected if possible. It is important to keep the needle about 2 cm from the end of the endoscope during injection to take advantge of the injector's flexibility. When working near the esophagogastric junction, this ideal relation may be difficult to maintain. When the injector has extended a shorter distance beyond the end of the insertion tube during variceal puncture, a sudden motion on the part of either the patient or the endoscopist may result in tearing of the varix.

After injecting all columns (there are usually four) at a given level, the fiberscope is withdrawn about 2 cm and injections are made in all columns at this new level.

Some variceal columns at a given level may be more difficult to target than others owing to the placement of the accessory channel within the endoscope insertion tube. The columns nearest the entry point of the needle into the endoscopic field align with the trajectory of the injector as it advances. Others may be more difficult to puncture because of their position. This can lead to overinjection of those that can be punctured without difficulty, and underinjection of those that are harder to reach. This is avoidable if *rotation* of the insertion tube is employed to allow for comfortable injection of all vessels at a given level.

Volume of Injection. The diameter of the varix and the change in its appearance during injection determine the injection volume, which ranges from a maximum of about 3.0 ml down to 0.5 ml. If a varix has a small diameter, a lesser volume usually produces rapid distention and blanching. There may be no observable change during injection of large diameter varices, in which case 2 to 3 ml may be injected. The maximum observable change in the appearance of a variceal vessel during injection appears to occur at a volume of about 3 ml, and greater amounts tend to result in increased back bleeding after withdrawal of the needle. A small amount of sclerosant should always be injected when a puncture is made, even if there is doubt that the needle is properly positioned in a varix. The average volume used during an initial procedure is about 30 ml. It is essential that a slow, steady injection pressure be maintained by the endoscopy assistant. Individual injections should be made over a period of 30 to 60 seconds, depending on the volume to be injected.

The endoscope should be advanced into the stomach after each set of injections at a given level. Estimation of the amount of blood in the gastric pool is the best way to assess the quantity of blood lost during the procedure. Air can also be removed to minimize the chance of an ill-timed eructation during subsequent injections.

All potential sites in the distal two-thirds of the esophagus should be injected during the first two sessions. Although variceal bleeding almost always occurs in the distal few centimeters of the esophagus, sclerotherapy will alter the pattern of blood flow within the varices. The intrinsic subepithelial variceal plexus seen at endoscopy is probably not the main esophageal collateral flow in portal hypertension. Rather, the extrinsic esophageal veins fulfill this function. These two systems are connected by perforating veins, and it is hypothesized that incompetence of the valves in these connecting vessels contributes to the formation of the endoscopically observable intrinsic variceal plexus. In this hypothesis, esophageal varices are actually a stagnant cul-de-sac for portal blood. Given this anastomosing plexus arrangement for variceal anatomy, it is illogical to think that treating a limited area of the esophagus, the distal few centimeters for example, will also eliminate flow and pressure in the more proximal vessels. If bleeding recurs, it may originate in these partially sclerosed proximal vessels.

Postinjection Bleeding. Bleeding is frequent after each injection. A slow ooze is permissible and usually stops in 1 to 2 minutes. If, however, a steady stream of blood issues from the puncture site and persists for longer than 30 seconds, the injection pattern for active hemorrhage as described below should be initiated.

Variceal Compression

Various methods of variceal compression may be employed during sclerotherapy in an effort to prolong contact of the sclerosant with the intima of the varix. The two basic approaches include use of an overtube sheath or placement of a balloon cuff over the insertion tube of the endoscope. Because of the plexus-type anatomy of the esophageal venous system and the interconnection of the luminal veins with the extrinsic esophageal veins via perforating veins, it is doubtful that injection of a varix with concomitant compression proximal to the point of puncture will enhance the effect of the sclerosant. It is more likely that the agent will disappear rapidly via the perforating and extrinsic veins. There is experimental evidence that supports this viewpoint. One potential advantage of compression devices, however, is that they provide another method for control of acute bleeding.

Schedule of Procedure

To control the patients' course during the early high-risk period of recurrent bleeding, two to three procedures including the initial one are performed during the first 10 days to 2 weeks. Sclerotherapy sessions are therefore performed at intervals of about 5 days. The aggressiveness of this schedule is offset by use of a relatively low concentration for the sclerosing agent. Nevertheless, one of the problems with performing procedures close together is that the maximum tissue effect of each procedure is realized only after a period of 5 to 7 days. The progressive chemical effect and delayed tissue response may add to the tissue damage that will occur with a subsequent procedure. When the interval between procedures is relatively short it may be difficult to estimate the overall and potentially incomplete effect of the previous procedure. The end result can be excessive damage to the esophagus if the endoscopist is not aware of this phenomenon.

A fourth sclerotherapy session is usually done 6 weeks after the first, and 2 months later a fifth procedure is performed. Additional procedures may be performed thereafter at intervals of 2 to 3 months depending upon the clinical and endoscopic response.

Rigid adherence to this schedule of procedures is *not* required nor necessarily desirable. After the first two sessions, the total number of procedures and intervals between them may be changed depending upon endoscopic assessment of the response to the initial injections. If, for example, variceal diameter was small at the outset, two sessions are often enough to control bleeding during the early course after the onset of hemorrhage. In some cases, numerous, severe, and/or extensive ulcerations may be encountered. Even if no untoward clinical events have resulted from this, it is usually prudent to delay further sclerotherapy until the inflammation subsides and the ulcer defects begin to heal.

Patients usually remain hospitalized between the first and second procedure. Conversion to outpatient status for subsequent procedures depends on a number of factors. Generally those patients with poor liver function remain hospitalized for other reasons, such as reduction of ascites and treatment of encephalopathy. Endoscopic assessment can also help in assessing the need for further hospitalization. If the varices are extensive at the outset, i.e., of large diameter and extension, and if there is little or no effect of the first sclerotherapy procedure apparent at the time of the second, then it is often best that the patient remain hospitalized until some results can be seen. Generally, the fourth (sometimes the third) session and those thereafter can be on an outpatient basis. Patients undergoing outpatient sclerotherapy must be reliable. They should also be required to remain geographically close to the hospital for at least 24 hours after a procedure, and they must be given specific instructions to follow in the event of a complication.

End Point of Therapy

The end point of a series of sclerotherapy procedures can be problematic. The aim of long-term therapy is complete obliteration of all variceal channels in the distal esophagus. Variceal obliteration is based on the subjective assessment of the endoscopic appearance of the esophagus after a series of sclerotherapy procedures. There may be no variceal channels apparent even to an experienced endoscopist. The mucosal surface is usually somewhat irregular and the normal esophageal vascular pattern is lost. This may be replaced by irregular small vessels that are probably remnants of the vasa vasorum of the varices. Small, short, faintly bluish vessels may frequently remain. Injection of these with a small volume of sclerosant solution (0.5 ml or less) usually results in rapid blanching and distention and the assistant may note that the resistance to the injection pressure is greater than usual. Small veins such as these are probably not likely to bleed. Repeated injections are also more likely to lead to ulceration or stricture formation. Whitish patches of mucosa may be present as well as small areas of ridge-like and pocket-like deformity that suggest mucosal scarring. Larger defects in the esophageal wall of one or more centimeters in diameter, sometimes with overhanging edges, or even bridges of mucosal tissue, are often present. These are residual defects of healed ulcers.

The number of sclerotherapy procedures required for endoscopic obliteration varies from patient to patient. It may depend on the diameter and extent of the varices at the outset, but assessment of these features at the outset does not reliably predict the number of sessions. The maximum number of procedures for a single patient in our series was 12. The average number is approximately 3.7. This is less than the number anticipated with our schedule because of early deaths from hemorrhage and hepatic failure. After obliteration, stable patients are followed endoscopically at intervals of 3 to 6 months for about 1 year, and thereafter at an interval of 6 months to 1 year.

Sclerotherapy for Active Variceal Hemorrhage

Sclerotherapy for active variceal bleeding is difficult and probably has a greater complication rate than that of procedures performed when there is no active bleeding. This cannot always be avoided even with the use of vasopressin and tamponade. The technique for control of acute bleeding differs in some aspects from that described above.

If possible, the *bleeding point* should be located. If this is impossible, then the standard injection sequence described above should be initiated beginning at the level of the esophagogastric junction or within the cardia. When the bleeding point is found, the first injection should be made about 1 or 2 cm proximal to this site on the same variceal column. Insertion of the injector needle directly into the bleeding point does not appear to have any advantage, and much of the sclerosant may be washed away. Although it is perhaps more logical to inject below the site of bleeding, it is usually not possible to obtain a clear field distal to this point. Furthermore, active variceal bleeding in a patient who has not had sclerotherapy is usually located near the esophagogastric junction, and injection distal to the bleeding point may be technically difficult or impossible. When any injection is made into a varix, the observable tissue blanching usually spreads upward and downward along the variceal column. Blood flow in esophageal varices has been shown to be bidirectional. Therefore, it is probably only necessary to place the first injection relatively close to the site of bleeding.

Active bleeding does not usually stop with one such injection. Additional injections must be placed to the left and right of the rent in the varix. Some of these will necessarily be paravariceal in position. An injection distal to the bleeding point may also be possible if and when flow subsides somewhat. In effect the bleeding point is bracketed by injections.

A repetition of this sequence of injections may be required when there is severe hemorrhage with a steady stream of blood coming from the rent in the varix. It is probable that this method of injection stops the bleeding by producing an acute inflammatory reaction with associated swelling and edema. This may require a few minutes to develop, and the delayed tissue response may lead to an excess of injections when the anxiety of an inexperienced endoscopist demands a more immediate response.

Active variceal bleeding often may stop momentarily even if it has been severe and persistent. A clot may then be seen protruding from a varix. In this case, injections should be carried out using the pattern for active hemorrhage as if active bleeding were present at the site of the clot. Such a clot is usually unstable, and it is frequently dislodged with the first or second injection. The endoscopist should nevertheless proceed calmly with the injection pattern for active hemorrhage.

RESULTS

The published results of a number of prospective trials of sclerotherapy indicate a favorable outcome with respect to transfusion requirements. In our series, comparison of the number of blood transfusions and episodes of bleeding prior to sclerotherapy with these same variables after initiation of sclerotherapy indicates a significant decrease in transfusion requirements. Approximately one-third of patients do not experience any further bleeding. About one-third have some episodes of bleeding while undergoing sclerotherapy, but these are generally less severe compared with prior episodes and their occurrence is probably related to the time and number of procedures required for variceal obliteration.

There are some published data that suggest that sclerotherapy results in a survival advantage for cirrhotic patients with variceal hemorrhage. When the outcome in patients in our series in whom obliteration was achieved is compared with that in patients without variceal obliteration, survival appears to be improved in the former group. Many deaths from hemorrhage occur in the period shortly after beginning sclerotherapy sessions. In most cases it is unlikely that varices will be obliterated after the first or second procedure. This suggested improvement in survival associated with sclerotherapy is a controversial issue that should be regarded as unresolved for the present.

Extrahepatic Portal Venous Obstruction

Patients who have responded especially well to sclerotherapy are those with extrahepatic portal venous obstruction. Although many patients with this type of disorder experience a decrease in variceal bleeding with increasing age and progressive development of other venous collaterals, most of the eight such patients in our series were adolescents or young adults (mean age, 21.8 years). Six had undergone prior operations to control variceal bleeding. On average they had sustained 7.6 episodes of bleeding and had a mean transfusion requirement of 23.5 units prior to sclerotherapy. After sclerotherapy (mean, 5.5 procedures) the mean transfusion requirement was 2.25 units and the mean number of bleeding episodes 0.9. at 24.4 months follow-up. Most of the bleeding was accounted for by one patient in whom obliteration was difficult to achieve.

COMPLICATIONS

A complication occurred in 12.3 percent of 171 patients who have undergone sclerotherapy using the above method (3.4% of 795 procedures). Most of the serious complications can be attributed to the initial sclerotherapy sessions in the series of procedures. Complications may be divided into minor, major, and relative ones. Among the minor complications are fever, minor chest x-ray abnormalities, transient chest pain, odynophagia, and abnormal motility patterns by esophageal manometry. None of these abnormalities is known to be clinically significant, although it is possible that they are manifestations of more serious but as yet unrecognized sequelae of sclerotherapy. The major complications include precipitation of bleeding, ulceration, perforation, and stricture formation. Esophageal ulceration may be considered as a relative complication.

Fever occurs after about 10 to 15 percent of procedures. It is generally low grade and persists for about 24 to 48 hours. Chest discomfort or pain occurs in about 25 percent of cases. Usually this is mild, is described as retrosternal burning or discomfort, and the complaint is elicited by questioning rather than offered spontaneously by the patient. More severe pain that requires medication for relief may also occur and may be due to esophageal spasm. It usually begins shortly after the procedure and persists for 6 to 10 hours. Transient localized chest x-ray abnormalities such as a small pleural effusion, have been noted occasionally.

A major complication occurs in about 2 to 3 percent of patients. These include esophageal necrosis with and without perforation, severe bleeding, and stricture formation. Severe bleeding has occurred immediately after and as a direct result of esophageal puncture. It has also occurred as a result of esophageal necrosis, and in these cases it may be arterial in nature or due to incomplete thrombosis of variceal vessels in the vicinity of an area of necrosis. Stricturing of the esophagus in our series occurs in only about 1 percent of patients. This contrasts with much higher incidences of this complication in other reported series of patients. The marked differences can probably be accounted for by differences in technique, since reports with the highest incidences include the use of paravariceal injection techniques. In most instances esophageal perforations have been "walled-off" and most have been surprisingly asymptomatic. Typically, perforations are discovered days or even weeks after a procedure and almost never present the catastrophic picture of a ruptured esophagus.

A characteristic tissue reaction to sclerosant injected into a varix is the formation of a yellowish plaque over the vessel. These are relatively flat but can be over 1 cm in diameter. They are usually multiple and evident by 4 or 5 days after a procedure. They persist for about 2 weeks and are frequently the forerunners of ulcers. On occasion the yellowish surface material may fall away to reveal a typical ulcer that usually has a black base. The plaques have been found in about 45 percent of cases; esophageal ulcers have been noted in about 30 percent of cases but the actual incidence may be somewhat higher.

Esophageal ulceration can be considered a "relative" complication because the majority of these heal, usually with scarring. The development and subsequent healing of an ulcer may even be desirable, since healing interrupts variceal blood flow. If yellow plaques or ulcers are encountered during later sclerotherapy sessions, injections should *not* be placed in their vicinity, since further tissue damage may lead to a larger ulcer and a complication. When these lesions are found to be extensive and numerous, it is advisable to postpone injection sessions. If they are relatively small and isolated, however, selective injections of distant and apparently non-treated vessels can be done safely.

Larger areas of ulceration and necrosis of the esophageal wall have also occurred. This type of lesion must be considered a complication, in contrast to the smaller plaques and ulcers—hence the designation of ulceration as a "relative" complication. Even large ulcers of 2 cm or more in diameter may still heal. Additional complications, however, such as perforation and bleeding, have developed in association with large areas of tissue destruction. Extensive necrosis is probably related to the quantity of sclerosant deposited and may occur as a result of an excessive number of injections in a small area, or a smaller number of injections of a concentrated sclerosant. The most serious examples of esophageal necrosis and ulceration in our experience have occurred after sclerotherapy for the control of active bleeding using the technique described above.

Other uncommon complications noted in our series include the development of colorectal varices with bleeding, respiratory failure with a clinical picture characteristic of adult respiratory distress syndrome, and mesenteric venous thrombosis.

CANCER OF THE ESOPHAGUS AND CARDIA: SURGICAL TREATMENT

MARK K. FERGUSON, M.D.
DAVID B. SKINNER, M.D.

Tumors of the esophagus and cardia are among the most challenging of problems confronted by the gastroenterologist and surgeon. The usual symptom at presentation is dysphagia, which is normally indicative of a large obstructing lesion and commonly produces a more severe degree of inanition than is initially seen with most other solid tumors. More than half of symptomatic patients have locally advanced or metastatic disease at presentation, resulting in an overall 5-year survival of less than 5 percent in previously published series. Standard surgical resection or radiation therapy increases survival to only 10 percent. Such results spur efforts toward earlier detection and more aggressive therapy. Cytologic screening via esophageal brushings obtained at regular intervals in high-risk patients is effective in detecting tumors at earlier stages, resulting in improved survival. A more radical therapeutic approach, involving a combination of aggressive surgical resection and adjuvant radiation therapy and chemotherapy, also shows promise in prolonging survival.

EVALUATION

Our staging work-up includes a barium swallow with axis views, esophagoscopy with biopsy, bone scan, and computed tomography (CT) of the chest and abdomen. In cases of adenocarcinoma a liver scan is indicated, as metastases to this organ may be isodense on CT scan and therefore undetectable. A gallium scan is useful in patients with squamous cell carcinoma. Bronchoscopy is done in those with tumors adjacent to the airways. On the basis of these studies we are able to predict with reasonable accuracy which patients are candidates for potentially curative treatment. The most frequent sites of tumor spread are regional lymph nodes and nodal drainage basins in the supraclavicular and celiac regions, followed by liver and bone. Involvement of contiguous mediastinal structures, including aorta, pericardium, and respiratory tract, is also common.

In one-third of patients, tumors are unresectable because of involvement of other mediastinal structures or distant metastatic disease. More than one-half of patients undergo surgical exploration, and nearly all have either a curative or palliative resection (Table 1). We do not advocate preoperative radiation therapy or chemotherapy for potentially curable cases, as there is no evidence that preoperative adjuvant therapy is more effective than

TABLE 1 Distribution of Treatment Modalities for Esophageal Carcinoma

Treatment	Patients (%)*
Resection	52
Bypass	8
Radiation and/or chemotherapy only	28
Intubation	4
None	8

* All stages of disease are considered.

postoperative therapy, or that preoperative therapy improves the length of survival. For those patients found to have stage I carcinoma (T1N0M0 or T2N0M0) by pathologic staging after resection, long-term survival rates are in the range of 80 percent, and in these patients preoperative adjuvant therapy is likely to be harmful.

SURGERY

Resection

Our initial treatment in favorable patients is resection. The choice of operation is based on the location, extent, and cell type of the tumor (Table 2). For potentially curable tumors we advocate en bloc removal of the esophagus and surrounding mediastinal structures, including the mesoesophagus and lymphatic drainage pathways. Contraindications to such resection include involvement of lymph nodes beyond limits of radical resection; an inability to obtain clear, deep margins at the limits of mediastinal dissection owing to involvement of the aorta or respiratory tree; or distant metastases. In such cases palliative (or standard) esophagectomy is performed whenever possible to prevent complications such as obstruction, hemorrhage, fistula, or abscess during subsequent irradiation or chemotherapy.

For patients in whom the proximal extent of tumor is 10 cm or more *below the aortic arch* at esophagoscopy, resection is performed through a left thoracotomy. This provides optimal exposure for a thorough dissection of the lower mediastinum and stomach and allows for reconstruction with an anastomosis below the level of the aortic arch or in the neck. If intraoperative staging confirms the preoperative clinical impression that the tumor does not extend outside the limits for resection, en bloc resection is indicated. For adenocarcinoma of the cardia extending into the stomach, a total gastrectomy with esophagectomy extending 10 cm above the proximal extent of the lesion is performed. For other carcinomas of the distal third of the esophagus, esophagectomy and partial gastrectomy are performed to include 10 cm of tissue on either side of the lesions. We routinely perform a pyloroplasty or pyloromyotomy in conjunction with esophagectomy to avoid problems with gastric emptying. For adenocarcinoma of the lower third of the esophagus, reconstruction of the esophagus is usually performed in-

trathoracically below the arch of the aorta. For squamous carcinoma a subtotal esophagectomy is done because of the incidence of multiple primary tumors.

Tumors of the *middle third of the esophagus* are approached through the right side of the chest. Mobilization of abdominal organs may be performed either through the diaphragmatic hiatus or through a separate midline laparotomy incision. The latter approach is necessary in the presence of obesity, previous intra-abdominal surgery, or inflammatory disease. In such cases we normally perform reconstructive anastomoses in the neck to avoid the difficulties of a high intrathoracic anastomosis. In case of an anastomotic leak, this approach also allows simple percutaneous drainage and avoids empyema.

Squamous carcinoma of the cervical esophagus usually involves the cricopharyngeal sphincter and is treated by total esophagectomy, bilateral modified radical neck dissections, and laryngectomy in conjunction with our head and neck surgical colleagues. In some cases it is necessary to perform a right thoracotomy to obtain adequate radical margins of resection, followed by removal of the remaining esophagus along its wall. In other instances, an esophagectomy without thoracotomy is performed through a combined cervical and abdominal approach (see below), followed by standard reconstruction.

For patients in whom radical resection is contraindicated owing to widespread disease or when operative risk is prohibitive because of poor physiologic status, standard esophagectomy can be performed. This eliminates symptoms of dysphagia and pain and prevents acute morbid complications. The operation is approached in a manner similar to that described above, based on tumor location. An alternative technique that is useful in some patients is blunt esophagectomy through a combined abdominal and cervical approach. Although we do not advocate this routinely, it is useful in those patients with carcinoma of the cardia, distal esophagus, or cervical esophagus, and in whom thoracotomy presents undue risk or a strictly palliative esophagectomy is planned. This technique has the disadvantage of providing incomplete staging, and complications from it sometimes necessitate urgent thoracotomy.

Reconstruction

Reconstruction is performed using either the stomach or colon following esophageal resection. Jejunum may be

TABLE 2 Distribution of Carcinoma of Esophagus and Cardia by Site and Histology

	Cardia and Lower Third	Middle Third	Cervical	Total
Squamous cell	9	25	15	49
Adenocarcinoma	39	6	1	46
Carcinosarcoma	2	2	1	5
Total	50	33	17	100

Note: All numbers are percentages.

employed in instances in which great length is not needed or in which adequate stomach or colon is not available, although microvascular anastomoses are usually necessary for long jejunal segments. The stomach may be used for an intrathoracic esophagogastrostomy following partial gastrectomy for lower third adenocarcinomas. Following total esophagectomy for squamous cell carcinoma a cervical esophagogastrostomy may be performed if no stomach has been resected. In other cases, particularly following total gastrectomy for lesions of the cardia, colon interposition is required. Although a more extensive procedure, colon interposition is preferred in patients who appear at operation to have highly favorable pathologic factors. This reduces the risk of reflux esophagitis, which occurs to a serious degree in about one-third of long-term survivors after esophagogastrostomy.

Postoperative Considerations

Radical dissection of the posterior mediastinal lymphatic tissues makes careful respiratory management essential immediately following operation. This frequently includes the use of positive pressure ventilation for several days postoperatively until significant diuresis indicates mobilization of sequestered fluid. Prophylactic antibiotics are given preoperatively and for 48 hours postoperatively. A barium swallow is obtained before a diet is commenced. Early postoperative complications may occur in up to 50 percent of patients (Table 3). Operative mortality in experienced hands is 10 percent or less, and is usually due to cardiovascular catastrophes, technical complications, or pneumonia.

Survival

With radical en bloc resection, the overall five-year survival in our consecutive series is 20 percent. Survival is independently and adversely affected by metastases to lymph nodes or full-thickness penetration of the esophageal wall. In the absence of lymph node metastases and the absence of full-thickness wall penetration, 2-year survival is 80 percent. In the presence of one but not both of these factors, 2-year survival free of disease is 50 percent. These results may be favorably modified through the use of adjuvant radiation therapy and/or chemotherapy.

Unresectable Tumors

Occasionally even palliative esophagectomy is not possible because of contiguous involvement of other mediastinal structures by the primary tumor, particularly the respiratory tree or the aorta. When obstruction is significant, or following the development of respiratory-esophageal fistula, attempts at palliation with gastrostomy and cervical esophagostomy usually fail to restore patient comfort and are often aesthetically unacceptable to family and friends. In such cases *esophageal exclusion*, performed by dividing both the esophagogastric junction and the cervical esophagus, and bypassing the segment with substernal colon or stomach, can provide significant palliation with only moderate operative morbidity. In poor-risk patients, restoration of alimentation can be achieved by a custom-made, extracorporeal, large-diameter esophageal prosthesis connecting a cervical stoma with a gastrostomy.

RADIATION THERAPY

Radiation therapy was the mainstay of treatment for esophageal tumors for many years. The overall five-year survival for patients undergoing curative radiation therapy is less than 10 percent, comparable to results of standard resection. The incidence of local recurrence following curative doses of radiation therapy is approximately 30 percent, however, and these patients are then at risk for local complications of obstruction, hemorrhage, and fistula formation. Such complications are only poorly remediable by conventional measures, and may require extra-anatomic bypass for palliation of symptoms. We use radiation therapy for patients who have tumors that are clearly unresectable, even for palliation, and who do not have such significant obstruction as to require bypass or abdominal feeding tubes. (See the chapter on *Cancer of the Esophagus: Radiation Treatment.*)

Intubation

Intubation of the esophagus has been popular in certain institutions for the palliation of esophageal tumors, especially those complicated by fistula or obstruction or which are unresectable. The ability to perform intubation is limited by an individual's esophageal anatomy and body habitus. It is not safe when significant angulation is present within or distal to the tumor or in the presence of severe kyphosis. Hospital mortality secondary to intubation is reported as 20 percent or higher. Intubation does not improve long-term survival and involves continued risk of local complications, including fatal tube erosion into vital mediastinal structures or aspiration with resultant pneumonia. We reserve this for patients with widespread disease in whom life expectancy is limited to weeks but who are miserable from continuous expectoration or night and day cough. Details of this type of technique are included in the chapter on *Esophageal Stricture.*

TABLE 3 Incidence of Early Nonfatal Postoperative Complications Following Esophagectomy

Complication	*Patients (%)*
Persistent pleural drainage or chylothorax	8
Pneumonia	6
Cardiac failure or arrhythmia	6
Bowel perforation or anastomotic leak	9
Wound infection	5

TABLE 4 Benign Esophageal Tumors

Intramural	Intraluminal
Leiomyomas	Fibrovascular polyps
Esophageal cysts	Papillomas
Fibromas	Adenomas
Giant cell tumors	Hemangiomas
Granular cell myoblastomas	

CHEMOTHERAPY

While chemotherapy has been used in the adjuvant treatment of carcinoma of the esophagus and cardia for many years, only recently has it been shown to have some effectiveness. The agents currently considered to be active against squamous cell tumors include cis-platinum and 5-fluorouracil (5-FU), while bleomycin, vindesine, and methotrexate may also be beneficial. In patients with adenocarcinoma, Adriamycin, mitomycin-C, and 5-FU have shown approximately a 30 percent frequency of response when used in combination. The concurrent administration of 5-FU and radiation therapy to locally advanced disease has been successful according to anecdotal reports. Long-term follow up of survival, recurrence, and complications is necessary before any of these adjuvant treatments becomes standard. Chemotherapy is also discussed in the chapter *Cancer of the Esophagus: Radiation Treatment*.

BENIGN TUMORS

Benign tumors of the esophagus (Table 4) are rare and normally asymptomatic. Intramural lesions include leiomyomas, cysts, fibromas, and a variety of less common tumors. Leiomyomas are by far the most common, infrequently causing dysphagia or chest pain. Diagnosis can be made confidently by an upper gastrointestinal series and esophagoscopy. *Endoscopic biopsy should be avoided* if leiomyoma is suspected. It causes adhesion between mucosa and tumor, complicating surgery, and is not likely to result in a histologic diagnosis. Enucleation should be considered if the tumor is large or symptomatic. Intraluminal lesions are even less common and include polyps, papillomas, adenomas, and hemangiomas. The latter should not be biopsied if recognized, as this may result in hemorrhage. None of the intraluminal tumors has proven malignant potential, and the indications for removal depend on the presence of symptoms or the need to establish a diagnosis.

CANCER OF THE ESOPHAGUS: RADIATION TREATMENT

EVA SARA ZINREICH, M.D.

Carcinoma of the esophagus accounts for 1.5 percent of all cancers and 7 percent of all gastrointestinal cancers in the United States. In spite of recent advances in surgery, radiotherapy, and chemotherapy, patient survival remains poor. The 5-year survival for esophageal carcinoma is 5 percent. A slightly better survival was reported from Japan and China; however, their populations are significantly different in that many of their patients have carcinoma in situ.

The form of therapy does not appear to alter survival. In spite of a significant decrease in operative mortality during the past 15 years, the 5-year survival for patients with surgically resectable esophageal carcinoma has not dramatically improved. Erlan reviewed 122 reports published between 1953 and 1978 covering 83,783 patients who had surgery for esophageal carcinoma. In this large series 58 percent of the patients were surgically explored, 39 percent had their tumors resected, 13 percent died in the hospital, and of the 26 percent who left the hospital only 4 percent survived 5 years. Of the 8,486 patients who were treated with radiation therapy 6 percent survived for 5 years. Radiation therapy has been used extensively in the management of patients with esophageal carcinoma. It has demonstrated an ability to cure a small percentage of patients. Cure is likely to be limited to patients who have lesions less than 5 cm in length and without lymph node involvement. Esophagectomy is likely to cure a similar percentage of patients, however, due to its attendant risks it has proven a less favored treatment modality than radiotherapy.

ANATOMY AND PATTERNS OF SPREAD OF ESOPHAGEAL CARCINOMA

The esophagus is a tubular structure 23 to 30 cm in length and is divided into three distinct parts: the cervical esophagus, the mid-third (T1–T8), and the distal esophagus. The cervical esophagus extends from the level of the cricoid cartilage to the thoracic inlet (C6–T1). It adjoins the larynx, trachea, vertebral column, laryngeal nerves, and the vascular supply of the head and neck.

The middle third of the esophagus extends from the thoracic inlet to 10 cm above the gastroesophageal junction (T1–T8). In this region the esophagus is closely apposed to the tracheobronchial tree, azygos vein, and aorta. Invasion of these adjacent structures may lead to a tracheoesophageal fistula and rapid exsanguination.

The distal esophagus extends from T8 to the gastroesophageal junction. It lies adjacent to the left atrial pericardium, descending aorta, inferior vena cava, and the left lower lobe of the lung.

The esophageal muscular layer is composed of external longitudinal and internal circular muscle fibers. This muscle layer is very thin and varies in thickness from 0.5 to 2.2 mm. The thin submucosa and muscularis layers of the esophagus provide little resistance to the direct invasion of tumor. In addition, serosa does not surround the esophagus, and therefore only loose connective tissue separates the esophagus from other mediastinal structures, facilitating tumor invasion into the adjacent organs.

More than 90 percent of esophageal carcinomas are of the squamous cell type. At the time of diagnosis, 70 percent of the patients already have metastasis to mediastinal and/or abdominal lymph nodes. The incidence of abdominal lymph node involvement is 35 percent for carcinomas of the lower esophagus and 15 percent for carcinomas of the upper esophagus. Supraclavicular lymph nodes are involved in 12 percent of all cases, with a higher incidence for lesions of the cervical esophagus. Lymph node metastasis carries a poor prognosis. Carcinoma of the esophagus can spread to any site within the body, and 30 percent of the patients have demonstrable distant metastasis on admission. The liver is the most frequent site of visceral involvement (30% to 50% in most autopsy series).

TREATMENT GUIDELINES

Treatment of esophageal carcinoma depends on the extent of involvement, stage (Table 1), and location of esophageal carcinoma. Prior to therapy the following work-up should be performed: (1) history and physical examination, (2) chest roentgenogram, (3) esophagogram, (4) bronchoscopy and esophagoscopy, (5) liver function tests and liver scan, (6) bone scan, (7) computed tomography scan of the chest and upper abdomen, and (8) electrocardiogram and pulmonary function tests. The information gained from the work-up will allow proper staging of the patients.

The aim of management of esophageal carcinoma is to provide a functional swallowing mechanism, acceptable cosmesis, and a good quality of life.

RADIATION TREATMENT FOR ESOPHAGEAL CARCINOMA

Radiation therapy can be used for curative or palliative intent. It can be used alone or in combination with surgery and/or chemotherapy. (There is a separate chapter on *Intraoperative Irradiation*.) Nearly all patients with squamous cell carcinoma of the esophagus are candidates for radiation therapy. Owing to the limited number of patients who benefit from esophagectomy, and owing to the substantial acute morbidity and mortality of this procedure, many investigators recommend radiotherapy rather than surgery for esophageal carcinoma.

TABLE 1 TNM Staging

Primary Tumor (T) (for all three segments of the esophagus)

T0	No demonstrable tumor in the esophagus
T1S	Carcinoma in situ
T1	A tumor that involves 5 cm or less of esophageal length, that produces no obstruction, and that has no circumferential involvement and no extraesophageal spread
T2	A tumor that involves more than 5 cm of esophageal length without extraesophageal spread or a tumor of any size which produces obstruction or involves the entire circumference, but without extraesophageal spread
T3	Any tumor with evidence of extraesophageal spread

Nodal Involvement (N)

Cervical esophagus: The regional lymph nodes in the cervical esophagus are the cervical and supraclavicular nodes

N0	No clinically palpable nodes
N1	Movable, unilateral, palpable nodes
N2	Movable, bilateral, palpable nodes
N3	Fixed nodes

Thoracic esophagus:
NX (clinical evaluation)
Regional lymph nodes for the upper, mid-thoracic, and lower thoracic esophagus that are not ordinarily accessible for clinical evaluation

N0	(Surgical evaluation) No positive nodes
N1	(Surgical evaluation) Positive nodes

Distant Metastasis (M)

MX	Not assessed
M0	No (known) distant metastasis
M1	Distant metastasis present, specify

Note: Details of the staging system are in the Manual for Staging of Cancer, by American Joint Committee for Cancer Staging and End Results Reporting.

Curative Radiotherapy

Curative radiation therapy is suitable for patients with lesions 5 to 10 cm long, with no evidence of metastatic disease or of tracheoesophageal fistula.

Cervical esophageal cancer has been managed with irradiation with a cure rate of 29 percent at 5 years.[1] Similar results were also reported by Newaishy (5-year survival).[2] While these results do not engender much optimism, they approximate the achievements of surgery in treating tumors of the cervical esophagus with substantially less acute morbidity and mortality.

Radiation therapy, when used alone for management of carcinoma of the thoracic esophagus, has a dismal result. The 29 percent 5-year survival reported by Pearson in 1969 has not been duplicated by other investigators. None of the 176 patients studied at the Princess Margaret Hospital survived 3 years.

Preoperative Radiotherapy

Preoperative radiotherapy is used to produce regression in tumor bulk, to sterilize microscopic disease in areas not resected, and to prevent metastasis and local recurrence of tumor resulting from the operation. The hope is that reduction in tumor size with preoperative radiotherapy will aid resectability and decrease operative mortality.

Nakayama instituted a three-stage treatment plan for esophageal carcinoma with a 37.5 percent 5-year survival in a limited number of patients.[3] He performed laparotomy with gastrostomy in the first week prior to preoperative radiotherapy. Then 2,000 to 2,500 rads were administered to the tumor using megavoltage equipment in four to five treatments. Three to 5 days later esophagectomy and cervical esophagostomy were performed. The esophagostomy was connected to the gastrostomy externally by means of an external tube. Reconstruction consisted of an anthethoracic cervical esophagogastrostomy during a third operation. Akakura, studying 110 patients with squamous cell carcinoma of the esophagus, revealed that preoperative radiotherapy doubled resectability and tripled the rate of cure.[4]

In contrast, a similar approach at Stanford University showed no improvement, using combined preoperative radiotherapy and surgical resection, over each modality used alone.

Postoperative Radiotherapy

Even though the Japanese report a limited impact of postop radiation in esophageal carcinoma, there is a place for this therapeutic modality in patients with positive resection margins, residual tumor in the mediastinum, and local recurrence after curative resection.

Palliative Radiotherapy

Since only 5 percent of the patients with esophageal carcinoma survive 5 years, 95 percent will need some type of palliative treatment. The aim of palliative therapy is to control dysphagia, chest pain, and malnutrition, and to provide an acceptable functional status.

Radiotherapy can provide good palliation, although the frequency and durability of relief of dysphagia vary. Of the 103 patients treated by Wara with irradiation, 66 percent had symptomatic improvement with a palliation of 6 months and a median duration of 3 months.[5] Often the palliation occurs near the end of irradiation. Patients with unresectable disease who lack evidence of metastasis or tracheoesophageal fistula are candidates for palliative radiotherapy or physiologic bypass surgery without removal of the primary tumor. Radiation therapy should be at full dose. One-third of patients treated with radiotherapy may have effective palliation of swallowing difficulties for the duration of their illness. Physiologic bypass will provide prolonged palliation when dysphagia recurs.

Technique

Treatment Volume

The treatment volume should include the primary tumor and adjacent lymphatics with a margin. The volume should be large enough to cover the known extent of tumor with at least a 5-cm margin, both proximally and distally. The width of the field should be 8 to 9 cm to cover the lymphatics in the mediastinum. Posteriorly, the treatment volume should cover the paravertebral fascia and the anterior half of the vertebral body. Anteriorly, it should cover the trachea with a margin. A computed tomography scan of the thorax is very important, since it provides the following information: the location of primary tumor, the extent of extraluminal spread, the special relationship of primary tumor to the spinal cord, and the volume of lung and heart in the irradiated field. This information is essential in formulating the optimum treatment plan. Since the radiotherapeutic dose that can be safely delivered to the spinal cord is less than the tumoricidal dose, opposing anterior and posterior treatment fields are not satisfactory. The radiotherapist has to select the treatment field to encompass the treatment volume with a high dose of radiation while avoiding excessive radiation to the adjacent normal tissues.

Dose and Method of Administration

Continuous Radiotherapy with Conventional Fractionation (180 to 200 rads per day). Experience gained with squamous cell carcinomas at other sites suggests that at least 4,500 to 5,000 rads are necessary to control microscopic disease and at least 6,000 to 7,000 rads are necessary to control gross disease. Doses beyond 7,000 rads are often associated with a high complication rate without improving the local control rate. The recommended treatment dose is as follows: 5,000 rads over 5 weeks delivered to the tumor volume described above, followed by 1,000 to 2,000 rads in 1 or 2 weeks delivered to a reduced volume tumor (with 1 cm margin). The total dose is 6,000 to 7,000 rads.

Split Course High Fractional Dose Therapy. This technique has been reported to give better relief of symptoms. The treatment is well tolerated and the patients spend less time in the hospital. The first course consists of 3,000 rads in ten fractions. Patients are treated only 4 days a week. After a treatment break of 2 weeks, a second course of treatment consists of 2,100 to 2,700 rads in seven to nine treatments. The total dose is 5,100 to 5,700 rads. The treatment volume is reduced after 4,500 rads (tumor and 1 cm margin).

Brachytherapy. Intracavitary irradiation can be delivered with a radium capsule or iridium seeds placed in a nasogastric tube which is then placed in the esophagus. Because of the rapid "fall" of the radiation dose from the source (capsule or seed), only superficial tumors can be treated electively with this modality. A larger tumor may be treated with this modality if, after an initial external administration of radiation, there is tumor shrinkage.

Preoperative Radiotherapy. Preoperatively, 4,500 to 5,000 rads are recommended with conventional fractionation (180 to 200 rads per day).

Postoperative Radiotherapy. Postoperatively, for residual tumor, continuous radiotherapy with conventional fractionation or split course high fractional dose therapy may be used.

Special Considerations: Involvement of Trachea or Bronchus. Tracheoesophageal fistula or bronchoesophageal fistula should not be treated because irradiation may exacerbate the problem, however, involvement of trachea or bronchus by tumor without fistula formation can sometimes be treated with radiotherapy. Care should be taken not to use a high fractional dose, which may cause rapid tumor necrosis and fistula formation. This may be avoided by using a daily dose and frequent treatment breaks to allow normal tissue healing. The following is a reasonable treatment schedule: 2,520 rads in 14 treatments with four treatments per week, followed by a 2-week break; then resume therapy with 2,520 rads in 14 treatments at four treatments per week, again followed by a 2-week treatment break; and finally an optional additional 1,080 to 1,620 rads in six to nine treatments to a cone down field. Patients should be informed about the risk of developing a fistula.

Side Effects of Radiotherapy

Excessive radiation to the spinal cord, lung, and heart can be avoided by careful treatment planning and the use of focus blocks to shield the normal tissue. With careful planning, radiation injury to these organs seldom occurs. Radiation-induced esophagitis usually occurs in the middle of the radiotherapy course, most often after a dose of 3,000 rads. If affected, patients will complain of mild to moderate substernal burning, difficulty in swallowing, and occasional chest pain radiating to the back. The symptoms can frequently be ameloriated with the use of analgesics (Tylenol with codeine elixir). Interruption of therapy for 1 to 2 weeks will allow these symptoms to subside, after which therapy will be reinstituted.

A later complication that may be encountered is esophageal stenosis due to increased fibrosis. These patients have increasing dysphagia, worse with solid foods. These symptoms are similar to those of recurrent esophageal carcinoma. Esophagoscopy will distinguish between the two. If the stenosis is mild, therapy is conservative with dilation and a semi-solid diet. If the stricture is advanced dilation becomes hazardous, necessitating a feeding tube or gastrostomy.

CHEMOTHERAPY

Agents with some documented activity against carcinoma of the esophagus include 5-fluorouracil (5-FU), mitomycin C, bleomycin, and cis-diaminochloroplatinum (cis-DDP). Patients with locally controlled disease who are suffering from distant metastases are good candidates for combination chemotherapy. Twenty percent of the patients respond to chemotherapy for a duration of 2 to 3 months.

The main role of chemotherapy in the management of carcinoma of the esophagus will probably be in adjuvant use combined with surgery or radiotherapy.

Preoperative bleomycin showed radiographic improvement in 11 of 18 patients with carcinoma of the esophagus (Wada).[6]

The use of chemotherapy with radiation can potentiate the cancericidal effect of the radiation therapy, thus increasing local control. Byfield reported excellent preliminary results with a combination of 5-FU and radiotherapy.[7] Four of six of his patients with unresectable lesions survived 6 to 21 months. The use of bleomycin with radiation in a series by Kolaric showed a 62 percent response rate.

At Wayne State University 54 patients treated with 5-FU, mitomycin C, and preopertive radiotherapy showed significant diminution of tumor size. Six patients showed no residual tumor in the resected specimens.

A recent report from the University of Pennsylvania described patients treated with combined radiotherapy and chemotherapy (5-FU and mitomycin). Thirteen patients with stage I or II disease received definitive treatment consisting of 6,000 rads for 6 to 7 weeks and 5-FU (1,000 mg per square meter per 24 hours) as a continuous intravenous infusion for 96 hours starting on days two and 28. Mitomycin (10 mg per square meter) was administered as a bolus injection on day two.

Palliative treatment of 5,000 rads (plus chemotherapy as described above) was delivered to six patients with stage III disease.

The treatment was well tolerated without significant hematologic problems. Four patients of 13 treated with definitive therapy relapsed, and ten of 13 patients are alive from four to 32 months after treatment. The use of Mitomycin C and 5-fluorouracil with radiation therapy provides increased local control. This approach is new, and its use may continue to show improvement in the survival data.

REFERENCES

1. Pearson JG. The value of radiation therapy in the management of esophageal carcinoma. J Thorac Cardiovasc Surg 1968; 103:291.
2. Newaishy GA, Read GA, Duncan W, et al. Results of radical radiotherapy of squamous cell carcinoma of the esophagus. Clin Radiol 1982; 33:347.
3. Nakayam K, Orihata H, Yamaguchi K. Surgical treatment combined with preoperative concentrated radiation for esophageal cancer. Cancer 1967; 29:778.
4. Akaura J, Nakamura Y, Kakegawa T, et al. Surgery of carcinoma of the esophagus with preoperative radiation. 1970; Chest 57:4.
5. Wara WM, Mauch PM, Thomas AN, et al. Palliation for carcinoma of the esophagus. 1976; Radiology 121:717.
6. Wada T, Matoumoto Y, Ama NOT. Chemotherapy of esophageal cancer with bleomycin. Prog Antimicrob Anticancer Chemother 1970; 2:696.
7. Byfield JE, Baron RE, Mendlesohn J, et al. Infusional 5-fluorouracil and x-ray therapy for non-resectable esophageal carcinoma. Cancer 1980; 45:703–708.

INFECTIOUS ESOPHAGITIS

PAUL A. KANTROWITZ, M.D.

Infectious esophagitis, resulting from depressed immunocompetence caused by disease and various therapeutic modalities, is increasingly common. Neoplastic disease and its treatment by chemotherapy, radiation therapy and bone marrow transplantation; organ transplants with attendant immunosuppressive therapy; diabetes and other debilitating diseases; and treatment with antibiotics and corticosteroids all predispose to infection by various organisms, including fungi, viruses, and bacteria. The most common agents causing infection of the esophagus are *Candida* and viruses of the herpes family: herpes simplex, varicella zoster, and, less commonly, cytomegalovirus. Other organisms, such as *Aspergillus* and *Lactobacillus acidophilus*, are even less frequently pathogenic.

CLINICAL SETTING

The clinical presentation of infectious esophagitis varies from incidental discovery at endoscopy in asymptomatic individuals to fulminant esophagitis with deep ulcerations and associated systemic dissemination. The intensity and duration of therapy selected will therefore depend on the clinical circumstances. The usual clinical setting for candidal or herpetic esophagitis is an immunocompromised host, such as a patient with hematologic or lymphoproliferative malignancy under treatment or with acquired immune deficiency syndrome (AIDS); following renal transplantation; or receiving corticosteroid therapy. Diabetics or patients receiving broad spectrum antibiotics, and occasionally normal (usually older) individuals, may also develop candidal esophagitis. Herpetic esophagitis can also occur in normal individuals.

DIAGNOSIS

The diagnosis of infectious esophagitis should be considered in patients with acute odynophagia. Swallowing may be painful enough to limit oral intake and result in weight loss and dehydration. Dysphagia and gastrointestinal bleeding may also occur, however, many patients with candidal or herpetic esophagitis do not experience any esophageal symptoms, and oral involvement may also be absent. The diagnosis can be suggested by careful single and double contrast barium esophagograms, although the sensitivity and specificity of radiographic studies are limited. The definitive diagnostic study is fiberoptic endoscopy with smear, culture, cytology and/or biopsy, though thrombocytopenia may preclude the latter. Yellowish-white plaques are typical of candidal infection. Demonstration of mycelial forms on smear or biopsy establishes that diagnosis. Serologic titers may occasionally be helpful. Herpetic infection is characterized grossly by vesicles; discrete, punched-out ulcerations; or diffuse esophagitis. At times, the appearance may be indistinguishable from that of candidal infection. The pathognomonic cytologic and histologic lesion of herpetic esophagitis is the Cowdry type A intranuclear inclusion body, usually seen in normal epithelial cells at the margins of ulcers. Less specific findings include multinucleated giant cells and ground glass nuclei. Multiple infections, such as those caused by combined *Candida* and herpes simplex virus, are being recognized with increasing frequency in immunocompromised hosts. Such polymicrobial infections can include highly invasive pathogens like aspergillus. Systemic infections may be difficult to detect, although careful physical examination, including skin and fundoscopic evaluation and blood and urine cultures, may permit such diagnoses.

THERAPY

The choice of therapy will depend on the severity of the esophagitis, the immune status and associated diseases of the patient, and the risk of systemic spread. The therapeutic benefit of the drug selected must be balanced against the danger posed by the disease in a given host, the risk of the drug itself, and the need for hospitalization when intravenous agents are employed. Effectiveness of therapy can be gauged by symptomatic improvement and, more definitively, by endoscopic examination. Periodic endoscopy is especially important in assessing candidal activity in patients with AIDS who are prone to chronic candidiasis but who may not have esophageal symptomatology. Therapeutic strategy in a more acute life-threatening situation, e.g., severe acute leukemia or treatment-induced neutropenia, where the risk of candidal dissemination is high, may entail use of a more toxic agent for a relatively short time, while in a patient with chronic immunosuppression such as AIDS, a longer course of a less toxic drug would be preferable. Therapy naturally will have to be modified if the patient fails to respond to a given agent. Whenever possible, antibiotics and corticosteroids should be omitted or decreased in dosage.

Candidal Esophagitis

Nystatin

In mild cases of candidal esophagitis, which are not severely immunocompromised and which do not have severe neutropenia, the drug of first choice is nystatin. This polyene antibiotic is both fungicidal and fungistatic. It binds to the sterol components of the fungal membrane, increasing membrane permeability and resulting in the loss of intracellular constituents. There is negligible absorption and the drug is extremely safe; it has been used extensively for many years. Its principal disadvantage is its somewhat unpleasant taste. In addition, large doses can produce transient diarrhea, nausea, and vomiting.

Although widely varying dosage schedules of nystatin have been employed, one reasonable plan is to start with 500,000 units of the oral suspension four times daily. If there is no appreciable improvement after several days, 200,000 units of the suspension can be given every 1 to 2 hours while the patient is awake; the increased frequency of administration may facilitate the antifungal effect. Additional benefit may be obtained by adding 0.5 percent methylcellulose, thus creating a more viscous suspension with presumably greater mucosal adherence. If at any time evidence of systemic candidiasis develops, amphotericin B should be employed.

Clotrimazole

Clotrimazole is a recently developed alternative therapeutic approach for mild candidal esophagitis. It is an imidazole antifungal agent that binds to membrane sterols and inhibits sterol synthesis, thus altering the permeability of the *Candida* membrane and causing injury or cell death. Uptake of nucleic acid precursors is also inhibited. The drug is given as a 10-mg troche—a large, slowly dissolving lozenge that is sucked until dissolved—four or five times daily. Larger doses may be given. The drug in troche form is absorbed by the mucous membranes of the oropharynx and sustained salivary drug levels are achieved. Protection against development of systemic candidiasis has also been observed with this agent. The troche is generally very well tolerated, though rare nausea and vomiting and occasional mild and generally unimportant serum transaminase elevations have been noted. Periodic assessment of liver function is advisable. Data on long-term administration are extremely limited. As with nystatin use, evidence of disseminated candidal infection should lead to prompt treatment with amphotericin B. Its use in tablet form is severely limited by gastrointestinal intolerance, the development of hematologic and biochemical abnormalities, and induction of the hepatic microsomal enzyme system that accelerates catabolism of the drug.

Ketoconazole

If a patient fails to respond to nystatin and/or clotrimazole therapy, but manifests no evidence of systemic candidal infection, another imidazole derivative, ketoconazole, can be employed. Ketoconazole can also be used as a primary treatment in patients who have moderately severe candidal esophagitis and who are also moderately immunocompromised. This drug acts in the same manner as clotrimazole. A single daily dose of 200 mg is given orally; a 400-mg dose is rarely employed. The advantages of ketoconazole include its ease and simplicity of administration, efficacy against *Candida* even in immunocompromised hosts, low incidence of side effects and toxicity, and low cost. Its effectiveness against *C. tropicalis* has been questioned. It may confer some protection against candidal dissemination and is the drug of choice in patients with chronic mucocutaneous candidiasis.

Ketoconazole requires an acid pH for its absorption. Bioavailability may be considerably diminished in patients with achlorhydria or undergoing treatment with drugs that markedly reduce gastric acidity. Antacids, H_2 blockers, and anticholinergics should therefore not be given until at least 2 hours after ketoconazole. Nausea, with or without vomiting, may occur early in a course of therapy; in such instances, dividing the daily dosage into two doses, or administering it with meals, may improve tolerance. Gynecomastia has also been observed, as have decreased serum testosterone, oligospermia, and loss of libido and potency. Rare anaphylactic reactions have been reported. The anticoagulant effect of warfarin can be potentiated.

Serum transaminase elevations occur in 5 to 15 percent of those given the drug, but these are usually transient, unassociated with symptoms, and reversible. Clinical hepatitis, usually with jaundice and with or without anorexia, nausea, vomiting, or malaise, is a rare complication. The biochemical abnormalities are most often consistent with hepatocellular injury, but at times suggest a cholestatic or mixed pattern. The mechanism of injury is considered to be a metabolic idiosyncrasy. The apparent incidence of symptomatic hepatic injury is one in 15,000. A few fatal cases have been reported; in some of these, ketoconozole administration was continued after clinical and laboratory evidence of hepatitis had been observed. Since this rare but most serious type of hepatotoxicity may be preventable by close monitoring of clinical and laboratory signs of liver dysfunction, patients should be instructed to report signs or symptoms suggestive of hepatitis, and periodic liver function tests should be obtained. Such testing could be performed at 2-week intervals for the first 2 months and then monthly. Detection of abnormal liver function tests should lead to closer monitoring; rising enzyme levels, even in the absence of symptoms, should lead the clinician to discontinue the drug or, at the very least, decrease the dosage and follow liver tests very closely. Clinical evidence of hepatitis, appearance of jaundice, or continuing rise in liver enzyme values should lead to immediate discontinuation of the drug.

Miconazole

Miconazole is also an imidazole derivative, with the same mode of antifungal action as clotrimazole and ketoconazole. Miconazole is administered intravenously. In the past it has been given as a 5 percent oral suspension but that preparation is no longer available. Six hundred miligrams of the drug in a glucose solution can be infused over 30 to 60 minutes. A number of important side effects have been reported, however: pruritus, which may be intense and persistent for weeks after the drug is discontinued; phlebitis; transient anemia and hyponatremia; thrombocytopenia; and hyperlipidemia. Moreoever, cases of cardiac arrest, respiratory arrest, and anaphylaxis have been described. In at least one instance, inadvertent rechallenge resulted in a second cardiac arrest. These substantial side effects have limited the overall usefulness of this agent in usual clinical circumstances, and considerable caution is advised in its administration. For example, the initial dose of 200 mg should be given with the physician in attendance. Miconazole does not cause nephrotoxicity and thus may be used in patients with impaired renal function.

Amphotericin B

The drug of choice in patients who have severe neutropenia, who are markedly immunocompromised, or who are suspected of having disseminated candidal infection is amphotericin B. Like nystatin, this is a polyene antibiotic which binds to the cytoplasmic membrane of the fungal cell, increasing its permeability. Unlike nystatin, it also affects membranes of host cells and can cause severe adverse effects. The drug is administered intravenously. It is not well absorbed by other routes. A test dose of 1 mg dissolved in 100 to 150 ml of 5 percent dextrose in water (D5W) should be infused over 1 to 2 hours and the patient's vital signs and general condition monitored. If the patient tolerates this well, then a therapeutic dose of 0.25 mg per kilogram of body weight dissolved in 500 mg of D5W can be infused over 6 hours on the following day. A daily dose of 0.3 to 0.5 mg per kilogram infused over 6 hours can then be given until esophageal symptoms have subsided or leukopenia has resolved; a less toxic drug may then be substituted. Amphotericin dosage can be increased more rapidly if clinical circumstances warrant it. Doses as low as 0.15 mg per kilogram per day have been utilized in an attempt to minimize toxicity. If lower dose therapy is unsuccessful, doses of up to 1 mg per kilogram per day can be given, but this increases toxicity.

The initial or first few infusions of amphotericin B frequently cause a febrile reaction, sometimes with chills, nausea, and vomiting. This can be minimized by administration of 50 mg diphenhydramine, 325 mg of acetaminophen, 50 mg of meperidine, and an antiemetic. Hydrocortisone, 25 to 50 mg, may be given intravenously or in the infusion bottle. Less frequently, severe reactions may occur with hypotension, bronchoconstriction, hypoxemia, and delirium. Anaphylaxis rarely develops. Hypokalemia may develop and require potassium supplementation. Anemia and thrombophlebitis are also common; the latter may be helped by alternate-day administration and the addition of a small amount of heparin to the infusion. Hepatocellular damage may also occur. A weekly hemogram and serum potassium and liver function tests should be performed.

The major toxic effect of amphotericin B is renal damage. This is dose-dependent and usually reversible if recognized early and treated by reduction in drug dosage and/or sodium loading. Renal function should be monitored once or twice weekly and dosage lowered or treatment stopped if serum creatinine rises above 3.0 mg per 100 ml. Late nephropathy is related to cumulative drug dosage and may be permanent. This potential for renal impairment has stimulated the development of alternative therapeutic approaches such as the imidazole compounds.

Flucytosine

The drug 5-flucytosine (5-fluorocytosine) is a synthetic, oral antifungal agent with a complex mode of action. It is transported into the fungal cell by cytosine permease, converted to 5-fluorouracil, and incorporated into fungal RNA. Intestinal absorption is very good and 90 percent of the drug is excreted in the urine. Its major advantages are that it can be given orally and it is better tolerated than amphotericin B. Side effects include bone marrow suppression (which may be fatal), reversible dose-related hepatoxicity in up to 10 percent of patients, and rash, nausea, vomiting, and severe diarrhea. Blood levels should be monitored, since flucytosine levels higher than 100 to 125 μg per milliliter are especially toxic. Twice weekly white blood cell and platelet counts should also be obtained. Flucytosine should be avoided or used with extreme caution in patients with impaired renal function or bone marrow depression. Its major disadvantage, which limits its use as a single antifungal agent, is the relatively high (10% to 15%) rate of resistant *C. albicans* strains.

Because of their synergism, flucytosine may be combined with reduced dosages of amphotericin B in patients with invasive or disseminated candidiasis. Even in combination therapy, however, the flucytosine dose of 50 to 150 mg per kilogram per day for 4 to 6 weeks must be reduced or the drug omitted in the presence of impaired renal function (which may in turn be caused by the amphotericin B) or bone marrow depression. As is the case with single drug usage, flucytosine blood levels must be monitored and twice weekly white cell and platelet counts obtained. The high incidence of severe adverse (or even fatal) effects of flucytosine has limited its usefulness in combination therapy, and such therapy should not be used for infections caused by flucytosine-resistant organisms. Therefore, candidal sensitivity to flucytosine should be demonstrated prior to its use; however, drug resistance can develop during its use.

Recommendation

For mild candidal esophagitis in patients without severe neutropenia, who are not markedly immunocompromised, or in whom there is no suspicion of systemic spread, nystatin or clotrimazole is the drug of choice (Fig. 1). If these agents are ineffective and there is still no suspicion of life-threatening systemic candidiasis, then ketoconazole can be employed. In patients with moderately severe infection or who are moderately immunocompromised, ketoconazole can be used as the initial drug. If there is severe neutropenia, concern about disseminated candidal infection, or if the patient is markedly immunocompromised, amphotericin B should be administered. When possible, concomitant antibiotic or corticosteroid medications should be reduced or omitted. Flucytosine may be given as an adjunctive agent to decrease the dose of amphotericin required, but only after candidal sensitivity has been shown. Initially, a 10- to 14-day course of therapy can be given. If there is per-

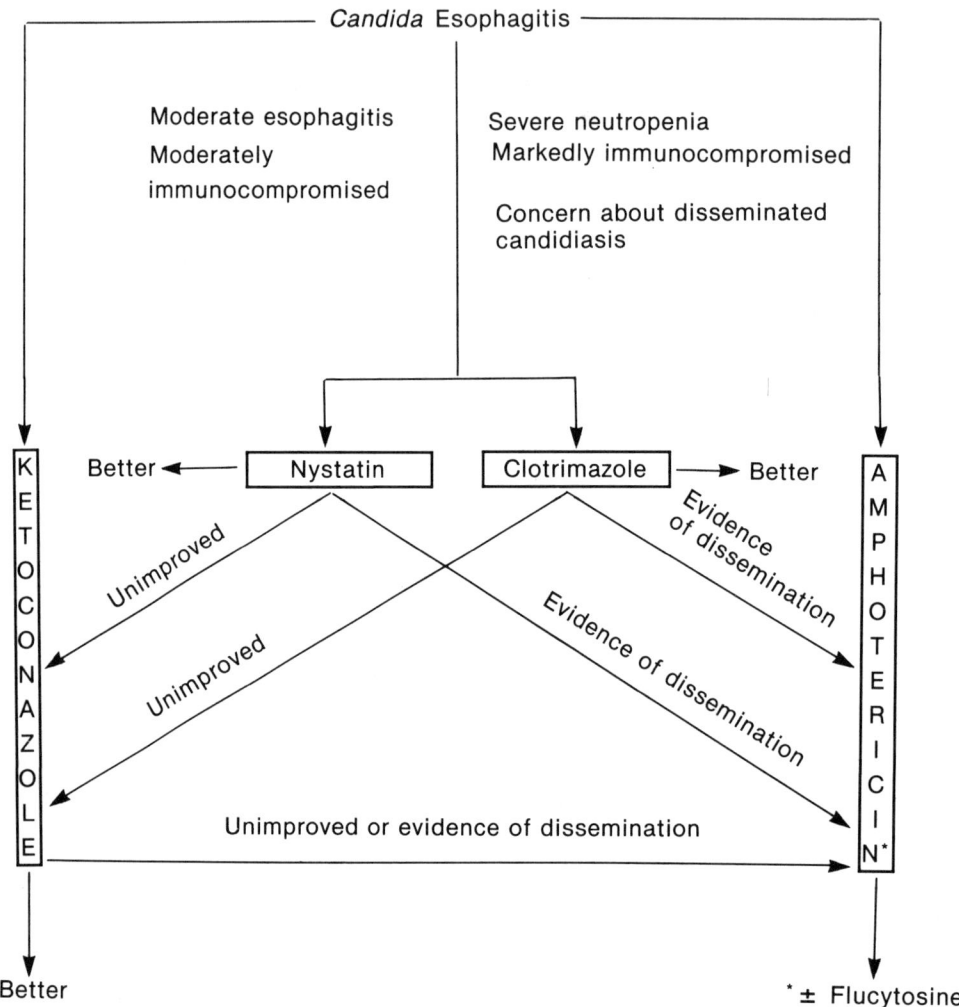

Figure 1 Selection of drug therapy in patients with *Candida* esophagitis.

sistence or recurrence of infection by clinical or—if necessary—endoscopic criteria, longer courses, and perhaps alternative drug selection, will be needed. Systemic infections will usually require 6 to 12 weeks of treatment. The role of long-term suppressive therapy or prophylaxis is not well defined, although there is increasing evidence for it.

Herpetic Esophagitis

Acyclovir

In the past few years, considerable knowledge has been acquired about acyclovir, an effective agent against herpes virus and varicella zoster virus. Acyclovir is selectively metabolized by virus-infected cells, interacting with virus-directed thymidine kinase which converts the drug to acyclovir monophosphate. This in turn is further metabolized to acyclovir triphosphate, which both inhibits viral DNA polymerase and is mistakenly but irreversibly incorporated into viral DNA during its synthesis. Because of the structure of acyclovir, its incorporation leads to termination of the DNA chain. By contrast, acyclovir interacts only minimally with uninfected human cells; this accounts for the drug's low toxicity.

Available experience suggests that acyclovir is effective against herpetic esophagitis. Antiviral treatment is generally unnecessary for acute herpetic esophagitis in immunocompetent individuals, but acyclovir treatment may be very helpful in extremely ill immunocompromised patients. The drug is given as an intravenous infusion of 5 to 6.2 mg per kilogram (200 to 250 mg per square meter) every 8 hours for 7 days. To avoid even transient crystal nephropathy, a dilute solution of the drug is given over an hour rather than as a bolus. Hydration should be well maintained, high urine output must be assured, and the use of other nephrotoxic drugs should be limited. Reduced doses should be used in patients with pre-existing renal disease. Since azotemia may occur even with these precautions, renal function should be monitored. Injection site thrombophlebitis is an infrequent occurrence and is probably due to the high pH of the acyclovir infusion. Infusion sites should be inspected frequently and changed every 72 hours or less. Rare and reversible central nervous system side effects have rendered patients lethargic, obtunded, and confused; tremors, hallucinations, agitation, seizures, and coma have also been noted. Acyclovir should be used with caution in patients with underlying neurologic abnormalities or with previous neurologic reactions to cytotoxic drugs.

STOMACH AND DUODENUM

DUODENAL ULCER

BASIL ISAAC HIRSCHOWITZ, B.Sc., M.B., B.Ch., M.D., F.A.C.P., F.R.C.P.E., F.R.C.P.

Duodenal ulcer (DU), which at some time affects one person in ten in our society, is in most cases a disease of long duration with multiple recurrences of a single ulcer crater in the duodenal bulb. Duodenal ulcers tend to heal spontaneously. About 20 percent of patients have only one or two attacks, and another 20 percent have, at some time, a major complication such as bleeding, pyloric obstruction, or perforation. Duodenal ulcer is not associated with later development of cancer. Several factors (e.g., smoking, anti-inflammatory drugs, and excessive acid secretion) may promote ulcer recurrence or delay healing.

DIAGNOSIS AND EVALUATION

Since the symptoms of duodenal ulcer may not always be typical or may be mimicked by other conditions (e.g., irritable bowel syndrome, biliary tract or pancreatic disease, hiatal hernia, or gastric ulcer), the first step in treatment requires that the dignosis of DU be firmly established. In many cases barium contrast studies may be diagnostic, but radiologic diagnosis (positive or negative) should be further supported by upper gastrointestinal endoscopy, which is the more definitive means of diagnosing a DU crater. Endoscopy provides additional information on the esophagus (e.g., esophagitis or hernia) and stomach (e.g., gastritis or gastric ulcer) which may further define the individual case. Every DU patient should have a fasting serum gastrin measured to rule out an underlying gastrinoma; if elevated, a gastric analysis should be performed to confirm gastric hypersecretion and to rule out the false hypergastrinemia of gastric atrophy. The diagnosis and treatment of gastrinoma (Zollinger-Ellison syndrome) is dealt with in a separate chapter in this volume.

Once the diagnosis of DU is established, the next step is to define the individual patient's disease profile and response to therapy over a period of time and to educate the patient in the symptoms, natural history, and complications of his or her disease, so that later relapses can be treated without full reinvestigation. It is perhaps self-evident that the best treatment of a chronic relapsing disease involves the physician and the patient in a mutually understood enterprise.

BASIS FOR TREATMENT

The factors predisposing to DU (DU disease) and the immediate or proximate causes of DU recurrence or complication are not well understood. What we know at present forms the basis for much of current therapy. In many, but not all, patients with DU there is a higher rate of basal and stimulated acid and pepsin secretion, more-so in males, so that the amount and concentration of both these digestive compounds entering the duodenal bulb per unit time in patients with DU is greater than in those without DU. Whether the pathophysiology can be equated with etiology is not clear, but reduction of secretion by a variety of medical or surgical means to levels in the normal range alleviates symptoms, promotes healing, and reduces the rate of relapse. The principal modes of therapy thus are directed toward reduction in acid (and pepsin) secretion. Conventional or traditional methods (e.g. diet, phenobarbital, and other psychotropic drugs) are not considered to be of value in current ulcer therapy. Coffee in any form may produce symptoms and should be proscribed. The patient should know that smoking, anti-inflammatory drugs, and strong family predisposition may make therapy less effective or may contribute to relapses. Women tend to have milder disease and fewer relapses than men.

TREATMENT STRATEGIES

Reduction of Acid. There are several ways in which we can reduce the acid/peptic load on the duodenal bulb: (1) postsecretory and surface coating agents, (2) alteration of neurohormonal controls, and (3) alterations of cellular mechanisms.

Postsecretory Therapy

Once acid is secreted, it can be neutralized in the stomach by food and by antacids. The average basal acid secretion in DU is about 6 mEq per hour compared to about 2 mEq per hour for normals, and with the stimulation by meals, the rate for perhaps half the day may be three or four times that amount. Thus, about 250 to 300 mEq per 24 hours require neutralization. Since food probably provides about one-fourth of this neutralization, at least 200 mEq of antacids are required per day for effective partial neutralization. Anatacids vary in potency from 0.3 to 4.2 mEq per milliliter (for potency and cost, see Table 1). If antacids are chosen, my preference is for a higher-potency (40 mEq/dose) liquid antacid, 1 and 3 hours after meals, continued for 4 to 6 weeks after the onset of a relapse. Antacids are also of value for occasional use for sporadic symptoms that may occur without an ulcer recurrence. Most patients learn to keep antacids handy for such use. Nowadays, however, the ease of use and effectiveness of other treatments, especially H_2 antagonists, have greatly reduced the role of anatacids as primary ulcer treatment.

Surface Coating Agents

As an alternative to antacid therapy, these agents act by combining with the slough in the ulcer base to form a protective coating, presumably allowing the ulcer to heal more readily. They include bismuth preparations, such as PeptoBismol or DeNol (DeNol is not available in the United States) and sucralfate (1 g four times a day for 6 weeks). Efficacy in promoting healing is similar to that of other drugs (Fig. 1). One possible advantage is a lack of systemic effects. Bismuth preparations cause black stools. Pepto Bismol contains salicylates and some authors caution against its use in peptic disease (see chapter on *Gastric Ulcer*).

Neurohormonal Alteration

The cause of basal hypersecretion in DU is believed to be due to the vagus, acting directly via acetylcholine as well as through the release of gastrin. This activity can be altered by medical (cholinergic muscarinic antagonists such as atropine and the synthetic anticholinergics or pirenzepine [not available in the United States]) or surgical means (vagotomy, preferably confined to the fundus). The vagus is highly sensitive to anticholinergics, and a dose of atropine, 0.4 to 0.6 mg sublingually 15 minutes

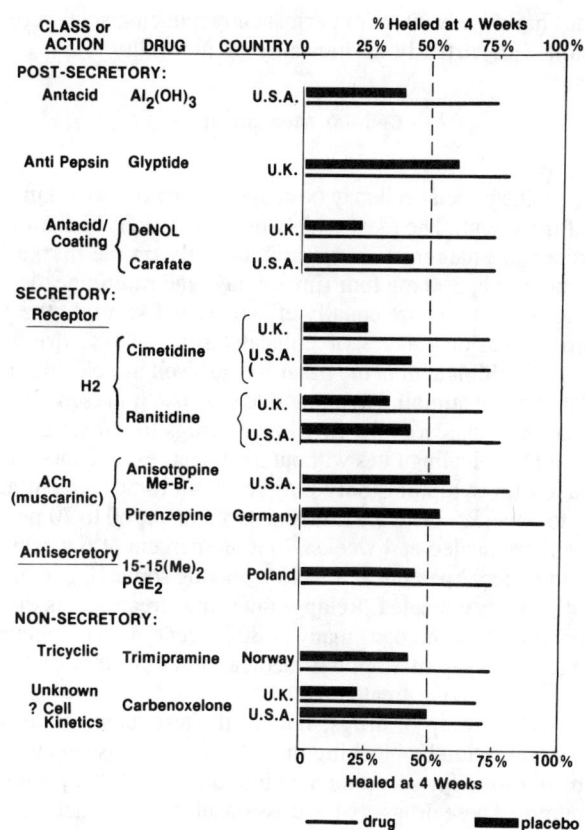

Figure 1 Duodenal ulcer healing with different classes of drugs. Relative percentage of patients healed with each class of drug (thin line), each compared to placebo treatment (thick line). *Note*: Most patients in the placebo group used antacids for relief of symptoms.

before meals and at bedtime or its equivalent, is adequate for modest control of acid. However, these medications tend to have side effects (e.g., dry mouth, urinary retention, delayed gastric emptying), which make them less desirable as first-line drugs for the treatment of DU. They may be useful as supplemental therapy, especially for hypersecretors, who are not fully responsive to H_2 antagonists.

For patients with ulcers that are difficult to treat or for patients with complications who qualify for surgical treatment (to be discussed), vagal denervation of the fun-

TABLE 1 Antacid Grouping According to Neutralizing Capacity and Cost

Approximate Dose for 40 mEq Antacid	Names of Antacids	Approximate Monthly Cost of 200–300 mEq/day ($)
10 ml	Titralac, Maalox TC, Delcid, Mylanta II	13–22
15 ml	Camalox, Gelusil II, Maalox Plus, Basaljel ES	17–35
20 ml	Gelusil, Riopan Plus	28
30 ml	Amphojel*	40
130 ml	Phosphajel*	175

* Contain only aluminum salts

dus has the advantage of permanently reducing acid secretion with virtually no mortality or morbidity.

Cellular Mechanisms

The parietal cell may be suppressed by different kinds of treatment. The most widely used are the H_2 histamine receptor antagonists. Two are currently on the market: cimetidine, 300 mg four times a day, and ranitidine, 150 mg twice a day are equally effective, and several others are in various stages of clinical testing. These drugs, which inhibit acid in the basal state as well as acid stimulated by all stimuli, have few side effects. At present they may be considered the first line of drugs for treating active DU. Healing rates without treatment, except antacids taken for symptoms only may reach 40 to 50 percent at 4 to 6 weeks. With H_2 antagonist treatment, 60 to 70 percent are healed at 4 weeks, 70 to 80 percent at 6 weeks, and 85 to 92 percent at 8 weeks, leaving some 10 percent of patients unhealed. Relapse rates after treatment is discontinued are high; as many as 80 percent of ulcers recur within a year of stopping medication regardless of the length of active treatment.

One group of drugs, now in the test stage, inhibits acid secretion by blocking the H^+-K^+-ATPase enzyme responsible for secreting acid into the lumen (the proton pump). These drugs are the class of substituted benzimidazoles. One of these, *Omeprazole*, has been tested clinically, and at a single daily dose of 40 to 60 mg, it completely inhibited acid secretion and produced 100 percent healing of DU in 2 weeks, thereby proving the underlying dictum of ulcer treatment: "No acid, no ulcer." However, the development of histologic gastric mucosal abnormalities resembling carcinoid tumors in female rats led to the temporary suspension of clinical testing for the present. Testing in the United States and abroad resumed in late 1985. The question raised is whether "no acid, no ulcer" carries some sort of price such as the problems of gastric tumors and possible susceptibility to orally ingested bacteria, as seen in patients with total anacidity due to pernicious anemia.

Another class of drugs being tested is the *prostaglandin E_2* series; several synthetic orally effective analogues have been tested with beneficial reduction in acid secretion (presumably acting on [adenosine 3':5' cyclic phosphate] cAMP-dependent pathways of acid stimulation) and on ulcer healing. Because these agents have widespread effects, the full range of side effects have not yet been evaluated. An additional benefit may accrue from an effect that has been described as "cytoprotective;" the exact nature of this phenomenon and particularly its specific effect, if any, on duodenal mucosa, including alkaline secretion, are not yet well enough understood for a thorough theoretic underpinning of the therapeutic potential of prostaglandins in DU.

Non-acid Active Drugs

Carbenoxelone (not available in the United States) and *trimipramine* (a tricyclic antidepressant) are at least two drugs that have been shown to lead to the healing of DU better than placebo (see Fig. 1). Mechanisms of action are unknown. With the availability of drugs of known action and effectiveness, they probably do not offer useful alternative treatment.

Overall, many treatments are equally effective in healing ulcers in the short term (see Fig. 1), but relapse is common after all of these. Medicines may heal duodenal ulcers, but do not cure the underlying disease.

SIDE EFFECTS OF TREATMENTS

Antacids. Diarrhea may be caused by Mg^{++}-containing antacids, constipation and phosphate depletion by aluminum hydroxide, and renal damage by sodium bicarbonate or calcium carbonate in excess.

Anticholinergics. These may cause dry mouth and urinary and gastric retention.

H_2 Antagonists. Cimetidine may produce mental changes, especially in sick or elderly patients, and antiandrogenic effects may cause gynecomastia and impotence in cases of prolonged maintenance therapy for hypersecretors. Ranitidine is much less likely to cause these effects and may be used safely in the place of cimetidine in such cases.

Carbenoxelone. Side effects are sodium retention and potassium depletion.

Trimipramine. This drug causes constipation and, at times, drowsiness. It may also cause excessive weight gain.

SPECIAL CASES

Renal failure. Doses of H_2 antagonists should be reduced by one-third for creatinine levels of 2.5 to 4 mg per deciliter and by one-half for creatinine levels over 4 mg per deciliter. Redosing after dialysis is needed. Antacids should be free of magnesium; aluminum toxicity may be a factor in both antacid and Carafate use.

Acutely Ill Patients. The evidence for prevention of DU activation due to physical stress is not very strong, and the routine use of H_2 antagonists intravenously in intensive care units and postoperatively is not justified by the evidence.

Patients with Rheumatoid Arthritis Receiving Continuous Steroid or Non-Steroidal Anti-inflammatory Therapy. If some of these patients develop DU, the dose of anti-inflammatory drug should be reduced or another drug should be substituted. H_2 antagonists should be given and, if effective, continued as long as other medications are needed. However, H_2 antagonists or antacids may not be effective in such cases.

Bleeding DU. There is no evidence that immediate intravenous administration of H_2 antagonists or other ulcer therapy is of benefit in controlling bleeding from a DU. Longer-term treatment to heal the ulcer should be considered on its own merits.

DU Relapses. Treating acute ulcer attacks with any one of a number of classes of drugs (see Fig. 1) leads

TABLE 2 Objectives of Treatment of Uncomplicated Active DU

Relief of symptoms
Healing the active crater
Prevention of relapse and of complications
Minimizing the socioeconomic consequences, preferably by keeping the patient ambulatory

to an improvement of 10 to 40 percent over placebo at 6 weeks, but relapse occurs after discontinuation of therapy. Since relapse is somewhat unpredictable in the individual case, Table 2 and the following schema provide a framework for management of DU.

SUGGESTED METHOD OF TREATMENT

The following steps are suggested for the treatment of duodenal ulcer:

1. For the acute attack (first encounter with patient), after confirming the presence of DU and measuring fasting gastrin, treat for 6 to 8 weeks with (a) H_2 antagonists or (b) antacids or (c) Carafate (a, b, c is my order of preference), expecting 75 to 90 percent healing rate. Watch compliance; symptoms usually disappear after 2 to 5 days and patients tend to stop taking medication when they feel better.
2. Stop treatment and await relapse. Retreat relapse as above and await relapse again. The type of therapy does not affect relapse. If relapse occurs rapidly when the patient is off treatment or if complications occur, place patient on partial or full long-term therapeutic maintenance with H_2 antagonists.
3. If the patient relapses on *maintenance* therapy or has complications, review compliance and possible deleterious habits or medication and re-evaluate the ulcer, including study of gastric secretion to rule out nongastrinemic hypersecretion. Increase dosage, change or add medication, and observe effects on gastric secretion and on the ulcer. Include follow-up endoscopy in the evaluation.
4. If, after obtaining the best possible medical result, the patient still has a nonhealing ulcer or has complications, fundic vagotomy should be recommended.

GASTRIC ULCER

DAVID Y. GRAHAM, M.D.

Chronic gastric ulcer is a recurrent disease of the human stomach generally confined to a nonacid-secreting mucosa of the antrum. In most cases gastric ulcer is primary, but in 20 to 30 percent of instances, it is associated with, or secondary to, duodenal ulcer. In many cases gastric ulcer occurs in patients with debilitating or chronic pulmonary, renal, hepatic, connective tissue, cardiovascular, or neoplastic disease. The treatment of these conditions may contribute to gastric ulcer, delay its healing, or impose other therapeutic considerations on the ulcer treatment. In a small number of patients, the gastric ulcer may represent a cancer, although few clinicians believe that a chronic gastric ulcer is a premalignant condition.

Macroscopic disruptions of the gastric mucosa can be either erosions or ulcers. An ulcer is a circumscribed break in the gastric mucosa that penetrates the muscularis mucosa. In contrast, a gastric erosion is a superficial mucosal disruption in which the damage remains superficial to the muscularis mucosa. There is scarring and fibrosis in the ulcer base of chronic gastric ulcers, whereas with acute ulcers there is no fibrosis. Acute ulcers can be thought of as large, deep erosions. The stomach has an amazing ability to repair acute injury, as exemplified by the rapid healing of surgical wounds. Gastric erosions and acute ulcers thus heal rapidly without specific therapy. With chronic gastric ulcers, in contrast, the normal reparative processes fail to heal an initial defect, suggesting an imbalance between destructive and reparative forces.

Endoscopically, it may be impossible to distinguish an acute ulcer from a chronic ulcer, particularly when the lesion is small (<1.0 cm). Large ulcers, which characteristically have intense scarring at the base, are easy to identify as such, both endoscopically and radiographically.

PATHOGENESIS

The pathogenesis of gastric ulcer disease remains unclear. It is generally best to think of the disease as an imbalance between factors acting to disrupt the mucosa (aggressive factors such as acid and pepsin) and protective factors (such as the presence of gastric mucus). Orally ingested nonsteroidal anti-inflammatory agents are aggressive factors important in the pathogenesis of gastric ulcer (but without a significant pathogenic role in duodenal ulcer). For example, the daily use of aspirin is associated with an increase in the risk of developing both acute and chronic gastric ulcers. This increase in risk is proportional to the number of tablets ingested per day; the relative risk becomes significantly greater in those who ingest more than 21 tablets of aspirin per week.

CLINICAL FEATURES

Patients with gastric ulcer usually seek help because of pain (dyspepsia), although the initial presentation may occasionally involve upper gastrointestinal bleeding, perforation, or gastric outlet obstruction. Clinically, the course of gastric ulcer is very similar to duodenal ulcer disease. John Fry, in his classic study of the natural history of ulcer disease, was unable to distinguish any major differences in the clinical pattern of the two diseases. The characteristic clinical course of gastric ulcer disease appeared in those patients with severe symptoms which gradually increased, finally peaking between seven and eight years after appearance, followed by the disease "burning out" as evidenced by progressively fewer patients complaining of symptoms.

The average patient with a gastric ulcer is older than the average patient with a duodenal ulcer, and the gastric acid secretory rate tends to be normal or low in patients with gastric ulcer, whereas secretion tends to be normal or high in patients with duodenal ulcer. There is a separate chapter on *Duodenal Ulcer*.

DIAGNOSIS

In many instances, an ulcer will first be identified by a barium contrast upper gastrointestinal series. The recommended approach to the patient with dyspepsia is currently changing, as it has become clear that endoscopy has a greater diagnostic yield compared with barium contrast x-ray studies in the initial evaluation of the dyspeptic patient.

In most large studies of drug therapy for gastric ulcers, between 2 and 5 percent of endoscopically and radiographically benign-appearing gastric ulcerations subsequently prove to be gastric carcinomas. The survival time in patients who undergo gastric resection of these early-diagnosed gastric cancers is superior to that in patients with advanced cancers. Therefore, it behooves the physician to distinguish these early cancerous diseases from ulcer disease so that appropriate therapy may be promptly instituted. If an ulcer is identified by roentgenogram, should the patient undergo endoscopy to obtain biopsy and cytology specimens to exclude malignancy? My answer is "yes," although there are certain exceptions, e.g., a young person with an obvious nonsteroidal anti-inflammatory drug–associated ulcer. A more important question is, "When should endoscopy be performed in the patient whose ulcer was diagnosed by an upper gastrointestinal series?" Radiologists claim 95 percent accuracy in distinguishing benign from malignant ulcers, but one must temper this reported high degree of accuracy with the fact that only 2 to 5 percent of radiographically identified ulcers will actually be malignant. Consequently, we review the results of the barium upper gastrointestinal (UGI) series with the radiologist. In my experience, a definite decision as to the benign nature of the process can be made in more than 60 percent of patients. If the ulcer is deemed radiographically benign, endoscopy can be performed at the first follow-up period (see below). This timing also allows the ulcer a chance to heal and provides further assurance that the ulcer is benign.

When endoscopy is performed, it is imperative that an adequate number of biopsies be taken. This generally translates into at least four biopsies with cytology or six to eight biopsies when cytology specimens are not taken.

THERAPY

The principles of therapy that are now considered standard for duodenal ulcers also apply to gastric ulcers, with some minor differences.

Healing the Ulcer

Effective ulcer therapies can be grouped into three types: (1) those that reduce or neutralize acid in the stomach; (2) those that coat the ulcer and protect it from aggressive factors; and (3) those that improve the mucosal resistance, enhance mucosal regeneration, or both. The simplest (and preferred) approach today is to reduce acid secretion.

Antacids. For years, the primary therapy was to use antacids to neutralize gastric acid; this therapy is effective in accelerating the healing of a gastric ulcer. The dose of antacid required to achieve healing is unknown, but recent studies have suggested that healing rates can be predicted, in part, by the degree of suppression of gastric acidity. Most commercially available liquid antacids are potent and low in sodium, so it makes little difference which one is chosen. For antacids to achieve healing rates similar to those seen with H_2 receptor antagonist therapy, seven doses per day (at least 60 mmole per dose) are probably required and, even then, the inhibitory effect on nocturnal acid secretion is less than with H_2 receptor antagonists. Side effects of antacid use includes phosphorus depletion, magnesium-aluminum toxicity (in patients with renal failure), and interference with the absorption (diminished bioavailability) of drugs such as digitalis, quinidine, isoniazid, barbiturates, and salicylates. Calcium carbonate may be associated with renal calcinosis and renal failure and thus should not be prescribed in large doses.

Histamine H_2 receptor Antagonists. Drugs that inhibit the secretion of acid by parietal cells include histamine H_2 receptor antagonists, cholinergic (muscarinic) receptor antagonists, prostaglandins, tricyclic antidepressants, and substituted benzimidazoles. H_2 receptor antagonists are effective in accelerating the healing of gastric ulcers. Two large clinical trials in the United States have shown that the healing rate is linear for up to eight weeks (by that time approximately 85% of ulcers originally ≤2.5 cm in diameter can be expected to have healed, in contrast to about 60% of placebo-treated ulcers) (Fig. 1). After 8 weeks, the percentage of patients undergoing healing for each additional week of therapy appears to lessen, possibly owing to a population of patients with more resistant disease.

The standard dosage recommended for *cimetidine* administration in the United States is 300 mg four times daily. *Ranitidine* is more potent than cimetidine, although

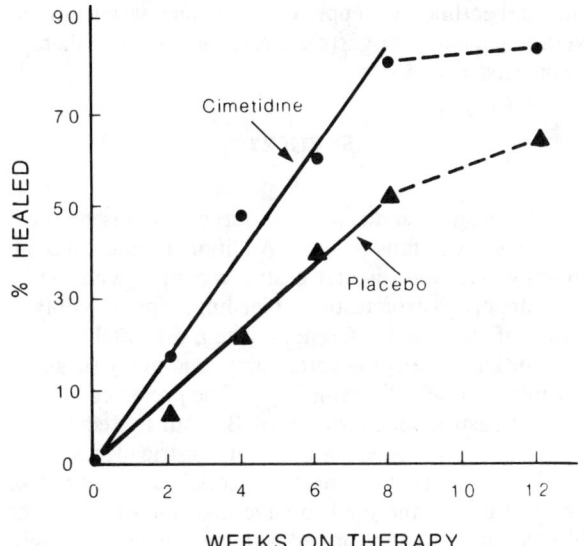

Figure 1 Comparison of placebo and cimetidine on healing rate in gastric ulcer. The solid line was constructed by the method of least squares. The dotted line is the actual healing rate from weeks 8 to 12. (Reprinted from Graham DY, et al. Healing of benign gastric ulcer. Ann Intern Med [in press].)

its half-life and pharmacokinetics appear to be very similar. Ranitidine can be given at a dosage of 150 mg twice daily and can achieve essentially the same effect on gastric acidity as obtained by cimetidine administered four times a day. Recent evidence has suggested that alternative regimens (cimetidine, 400 mg twice daily or 800 mg at bedtime, or ranitidine, 300 mg at bedtime) are as effective as the standard dosages in accelerating healing of duodenal ulcers; the effectiveness of these dosages in healing gastric ulcers is not yet known.

The main difference between cimetidine and ranitidine are side effects and cost. Both have proven to be remarkably safe. Cimetidine is metabolized in the liver by the cytochrome P450 pathway and may theoretically interfere with the metabolism of other drugs that are normally handled by the same processes.

Cholinergic (Muscarinic) Receptor Antagonists. Atropine analogues and synthetic anticholinergic drugs, e.g., Pro-Banthine, have been investigated in the treatment of ulcers; unfortunately, they are weak and nonselective in their ability to suppress gastric acidity. The frequent presence of side effects (delayed gastric emptying, reduced salivary secretion, pupil dilatation, and urinary retention) has prevented anticholinergics from being used as suppressors of acid secretion, they have fallen into disfavor and are not currently prescribed. Recently, a new agent, *pirenzepine*, which is a more specific muscarinic antagonist, has been promoted as an alternative antisecretory agent. It is still an experimental drug in the United States. Studies with gastric and duodenal ulcers have shown that the healing rate is proportional to the degree of acid suppression (directly related to the amount of drug administered). When dosages are used which achieve acid suppression equal to that achieved by H_2 receptor antagonists, typical anticholinergic side effects occur in about 20 percent of patients. Thus, it seems unlikely that these drugs will find a major place in treatment of gastric ulcer disease.

Synthetic *prostaglandins* of the PGE_2 series have been formulated for oral use, and, as with pirenzepine, a dose-response relationship has been demonstrated between the amount of drug administered, the reduction in acid secretion, and the ulcer healing rate. These findings suggest that reduction in acid secretion is the common denominator by which one can predict ulcer healing. Side effects (primarily diarrhea) become more common with the higher (and more effective) doses. The ultimate role of these agents in the treatment of gastric ulcer disease remains unknown.

Substituted benzimidazoles are new agents that inhibit the hydrogen-potassium adenosine triphosphatase enzyme that is responsible for the transfer of hydrogen ion from the parietal cell into the gastric lumen. Inhibition of this enzyme blocks acid secretion, regardless of the exciting stimulus. This type of drug is extremely potent and preliminary studies have shown excellent healing rates. Unfortunately, animal studies have revealed the development of carcinoid-like tumors in the stomachs of rats receiving high doses of drug for extended periods. The future of this drug, therefore, is uncertain.

Drugs That Coat the Ulcer

Two classes of drugs are used to coat the ulcer base by combining with the slough and mucus to provide a protective barrier: bismuth compounds (tripotassium-dicitrobismuthate) and sucralfate (an organic aluminum hydroxide sucrose octasulfide complex). Pepto Bismol (bismuth subsalicylate) would not be expected to form a protective barrier because it is hydrolyzed in the stomach to bismuth oxides and salicylic acid and is not recommended for ulcer disease. Pepto Bismol also has no antacid effect. Antiulcer bismuth preparations are not available in the United States, but clinical studies in Europe have shown them to be quite effective. Sucralfate has not yet been adequately studied in gastric ulcer disease, and currently I do not recommend it as primary therapy.

Drugs That Improve Mucosal Resistance

Carbonoxalone sodium was widely used in Europe, based on the premise that it improved mucosal resistance and enhanced mucosal regeneration. Side effects associated with the use of this drug were related to its aldosterone-like activity and limited its use. Once the H_2 receptor antagonists became available, the use of carbonoxalone sodium declined dramatically.

Theoretically, prostaglandin analogues should have a cytoprotective effect that might be useful in the treatment of ulcer disease, although recent studies have suggested that suppression of acid is more important. There is currently no evidence that cytoprotective effects alone have a role in the treatment of ulcer disease.

ASSESSMENT OF THERAPEUTIC RESPONSE

Symptoms are usually relieved within three or four days of beginning therapy, but the ulcer persists longer. We currently recommend that the first follow-up period be eight weeks after initiation of therapy, because the majority of ulcers would have healed by then. In most instances, the follow-up should be performed endoscopically to provide objective and specific information about the degree of healing and the state of the advancing healing edge. If there has been poor healing, malignancy should again be excluded by collecting cytology and biopsy specimens from the ulcer margins and base. If the ulcer has shown no signs of healing after eight weeks and there are no contributing factors, surgery is usually indicated. If the lesion is found to be benign, patient compliance should be evaluated and the patient scheduled for reevaluation after an additional eight weeks of treatment.

PREVENTION OF RECURRENCE

Recent studies have shown that nocturnal doses of H_2-receptor antagonists will reduce the recurrence rate of gastric ulcer. The recurrence rate in gastric ulcer can, in part, be predicted by the ease with which the ulcer heals. Ulcers that are difficult to heal (i.e., not completely healed by eight weeks) should be considered for maintenance therapy (400 mg of cimetidine or 150 mg of ranitidine at bedtime for approximately one year). In the average patient with gastric ulcer, maintenance therapy is not needed.

SURGERY

The primary indication for surgery in gastric ulcer is that the ulcer fails to heal. Additional indications include pyloric stenosis and gastric retention with extension, upper gastrointestinal bleeding, and possibly a history of multiple recurrences. The most suitable operation for gastric ulcer is antrectomy, and many surgeons now include a selective vagotomy. The preferred anastomosis is gastroduodenostomy or Billroth I. Recurrence rate after surgery for lesser curvature gastric ulcers is less than 1 percent. Pyloric channel ulcers behave more like duodenal ulcers and tend to have high recurrence rates unless vagotomy is performed with the antrectomy. Highly selective vagotomy without resection, while an excellent operation for duodenal ulcer disease, has not been shown to be the preferred operation for gastric ulcer or for pyloric channel ulcer.

GASTRITIS

Gastritis is difficult to diagnose because it does not cause characteristic symptoms, and the endoscopic impression of gastritis frequently is not confirmed by histologic studies. Therapy with antiulcer medications is not recommended for the treatment of gastritis. There is a separate chapter on *Stress Ulcer and Acute Erosive Gastritis*.

PEPTIC ULCER DISEASE: SURGICAL TREATMENT

JOHN L. SAWYERS, M.D.

Patients being considered for the surgical management of peptic ulcer disease should be diagnosed as having either duodenal or gastric ulcer. Patients with gastric ulcer should be classified as type I, II, or III gastric ulcer as defined by Johnson (Table 1).[1]

The incidence of duodenal ulcer has been decreasing in this country at a time when both medical and surgical treatment have been yielding improved results. The histamine$_2$ (H_2)-blockers, prostaglandin, and drugs under investigation, such as omeprazole, have reduced acid secretion to levels that permit healing of duodenal ulcers in most patients. Surgical procedures have been developed which have lower morbidity and mortality rates. Twenty years ago the indication for operation in one-half of patients undergoing surgical procedures was intractability. Now, fewer patients require operation for failure of medical treatment, but some patients still are resistant to medical treatment or have a recurring history of duodenal ulcer when medication is discontinued. These patients do benefit from operation for their duodenal ulcer.

OPERATIONS FOR CHRONIC DUODENAL ULCER

Proximal Gastric Vagotomy

Proximal gastric vagotomy (highly selective vagotomy, parietal cell vagotomy) without a drainage procedure is gaining increasing acceptance as the procedure of choice for patients who do not have gastric outlet obstruction. The operation was first performed in humans in Europe in 1969 and has become the preferred operation in the United Kingdom and Western Europe for patients with duodenal ulcer. Acceptance of the procedure has been slower in the United States, but it is increasingly used in medical centers as surgeons gain familiarity with it.

The operation is designed to denervate the parietal (acid-secreting) cells in the stomach while preserving va-

TABLE 1 Classification of Gastric Ulcer

Type I	Ulceration in the body of the stomach (antrocorpal junction)
Type II	Ulcer on the body of the stomach associated with duodenal ulcer
Type III	Distal prepyloric ulcer extending into the duodenal bulb (channel ulcer)

Adapted from Johnson HD. Gastric ulcer classification, blood group characteristics, secretion patterns, and pathogenesis. Ann Surg 1965; 162:996–1,004.

gal innervation to the antral-pyloric region so that near-normal gastric emptying of solid foods is maintained. Since the pylorus can be preserved as a sphincter, postgastrectomy disorders of dumping, alkaline reflux gastritis, postvagotomy diarrhea, and afferent or efferent loop problems are almost eliminated. Clinical evaluation of patients after proximal gastric vagotomy as compared with normal controls has shown no significant difference in terms of symptoms typical of postgastrectomy disorders (Fig. 1).

Proximal gastric vagotomy (PGV) cuts all the neuromuscular bundles between the anterior and posterior gastric nerves of Latarjet and the lesser curvature of the stomach cephalad to the "crow's foot" which is the terminus of the gastric nerves on the stomach near the incisura. The operation is extended 5 to 7 cm above the esophagogastric junction to sever any vagal fibers supplying the gastric fundus. The bare area on the lesser curvature is inverted with sutures to protect against lesser curve necrosis and vagal nerve sprouting. The hepatic, celiac, and antral vagus nerve branches are preserved. The technical aspects of the procedure are more difficult than truncal vagotomy and must be meticulously attended to ensure complete denervation of the parietal cell mass.

Recurrence Rate. Randomized studies in patients undergoing various ulcer operations show reduction in acid secretory responses after PGV to be equal to that following selective gastric vagotomy or truncal vagotomy and pyloroplasty. The ulcer recurrence rate after PGV ranges from 2 to 20 percent. As surgeons become more experienced in performing the procedure, the recurrence rate is less. There appears to be a learning curve in performance of PGV. The recurrence rate in series reported by experienced surgeons who have done 100 or more PGV operations ranges from 4 to 14 percent. If recurrent duodenal ulcer does develop after PGV, the ulcer will usually heal on therapy with H_2-blockers. Recurrent ulcers not responding to medical treatment may be managed by antrectomy with truncal vagotomy (Table 2). In the past, some of these latter patients may have had antral G-cell hyperplasia.

Morbidity and Mortality. Proximal gastric vagotomy has the lowest reported mortality of any operation ever used for duodenal ulcer. In a series of more than 5,000 patients the mortality rate was 0.26 percent. This procedure does not require an anastomosis or even opening of the gastrointestinal tract. Another major advantage of PGV is preservation of an intact innervated pyloroantral pump mechanism. While gastric emptying of liquids is slightly more rapid after PGV, emptying of solids into the duodenum is essentially normal. Patients do not require any dietary restrictions after operation. All other surgical procedures for peptic ulcer, such as antrectomy, pyloroplasty or gastrojejunostomy, destroy the integrity of the pyloric sphincter and may subject the patient to dumping syndrome and diarrhea. Dumping occurs to some degree in 20 percent of my patients undergoing pyloroplasty or antrectomy.

The safety and the minimal side effects of PGV offset the slightly higher ulcer recurrence rate. Follow-up results up to 14 years after PGV report ulcer recurrence rates similar to those after truncal vagotomy-pyloroplasty for duodenal ulcer. *For patients with duodenal ulcer without a tight outlet obstruction, proximal gastric vagotomy is the procedure of choice.*

Truncal Vagotomy

In 1943 Dragstedt reintroduced truncal vagotomy in the surgical treatment of duodenal ulcer.[2] Truncal vagotomy requires an ancillary procedure to drain the antrum. Gastrojejunostomy with truncal vagotomy has given way to pyloroplasty, except in patients with a large inflammatory mass around the pylorus which would render pyloroplasty dangerous. Truncal vagotomy-pyloroplasty (TV-P) and truncal vagotomy-antrectomy (TV-A) remain in common use for duodenal ulcer operations. Truncal vagotomy-pyloroplasty has a lower mortality rate but a higher ulcer recurrence rate than TV-A, but TV-A is the *best operation for controlling the ulcer diathesis* and consistently is reported to have an ulcer recurrence rate of

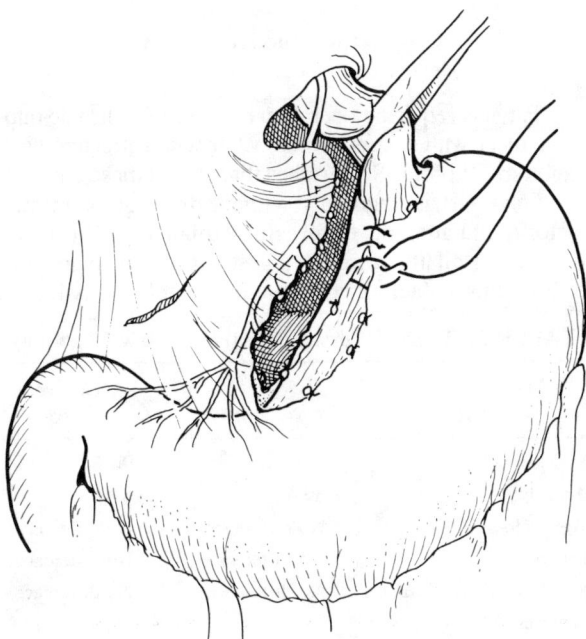

Figure 1 Proximal gastric vagotomy for duodenal ulcer. The vagus nerves are intact to the antrum and distal stomach. The parietal cell mass in the body and fundus is denervated. The bare area on the lesser curvature is being covered by serosa.

TABLE 2 Recurrent Ulceration After Proximal Gastric Vagotomy

Surgeon	Patients	Recurrence (%)
Amdrup	1,000	10
Barroso	728	4
Jenson	333	13
Johnson	433	9
Jordan	600	5
Kennedy	207	14
Sawyers	400	5
Van Heerden	240	6

1 percent or less. In more than 3,500 duodenal ulcer patients who underwent TV-A in the Vanderbilt University Medical Center, the ulcer recurrence rate is only 0.6 percent. The mortality rate was 1.6 percent. The mortality rate after TV-P is less than 1 percent, but the ulcer recurrence rate ranges from 5 to 15 percent.[3]

In a prospective randomized trial of TV-A versus TV-P (with all the operations done by the same surgeons)[4] the ulcer recurrence rate was 8.3 percent after TV-P and 1.1 percent after TV-A. There was no significant difference in the mortality rates, and the clinical results were judged to be the same. There is little reason then to subject good-risk patients to an operation (TV-P) with an increased risk of recurrent ulcer. By eliminating the hormonal (gastric) phase of gastric secretion, antrectomy provides additional protection against recurrent ulcer from incomplete vagotomy. *TV-A is preferred over TV-P except in poor-risk patients* in whom the lesser operative procedure of pyloroplasty may have an advantage over antrectomy, which requires distal gastrectomy and anastomosis.

In patients undergoing TV-A, gastrointestinal continuity may be re-established by Billroth I gastroduodenostomy, Billroth II gastrojejunostomy, or Roux-en-Y gastrojejunostomy. A *Billroth I anastomosis is preferred* unless the anastomosis appears difficult because of technical reasons which may increase the risk of an anastomotic leak. We no longer use the Billroth II because of the higher incidence of alkaline reflux gastritis and the possibility of afferent or efferent loop syndromes. Instead of a Billroth II, a Roux-en-Y gastrojejunostomy is preferred.[5]

Subtotal Gastric Resection

Adequate subtotal distal gastric resection without vagotomy was the standard operation for duodenal ulcer until Dragstedt's concept of vagotomy revolutionized the surgical treatment of duodenal ulcer. Vagotomy is now accepted as the basis for all operations to treat duodenal ulcer. The higher mortality and morbidity rate of subtotal gastric resection without any demonstrated superiority of the procedure has led surgeons to abandon this operation for duodenal ulcer. The operation is useful for *type I gastric ulcers*.

Selective Gastric Vagotomy

Selective gastric vagotomy (SGV) was proposed independently by Frankson and Jackson in 1948. The operation was designed to reduce acid secretion by vagally denervating the stomach but preserving parasympathetic innervation to the other abdominal organs. Results of our prospective randomized trial comparing truncal with selective gastric vagotomy are shown in Table 3. Selective gastric vagotomy is a more accurate method of achieving complete gastric vagotomy and preserves the inhibitory effect on gastric acid secretion that is mediated by way of the hepatic and celiac vagal branches which remain intact when SGV is done. Patients have a lower incidence of diarrhea following SGV than after TV.

A complementary procedure of *antrectomy* or a *drainage procedure* (pyloroplasty or gastrojejunostomy) *must* be done in association with SGV. The results of a randomized trial of SGV-A versus SGV-P differ from results of TV-A versus TV-P. The ulcer recurrence rate is less with SGV-P compared to TV-P. Postvagotomy diarrhea is less after SGV-A compared with TV-A. Selective gastric vagotomy lowers gastric acid secretion as much as TV.

The value of SGV has not been widely appreciated by surgeons. If antrectomy or pyloroplasty is indicated rather than PGV without drainage, then SGV should be done instead of TV, unless the procedure is an emergency or the patient such a poor risk that the additional operative time needed to perform SGV (about 45 minutes) is unwarranted.

Table 4 compares results of TV-P, SGV-P, and TV-A.

Obstructing Duodenal Ulcer

Patients requiring operation because of a chronic duodenal ulcer with obstruction do better with antrectomy and vagotomy. I prefer SGV rather than TV in these patients. Proximal gastric vagotomy without drainage is unsatisfactory, and attempts to forcefully dilate the obstruction with Hegar dilators through a gastrostomy have generally been unsatisfactory. Obstruction is defined as failure

TABLE 3 Truncal Versus Selective Gastric Vagotomy

Effect	Truncal Vagotomy	Selective Gastric Vagotomy
Visick I and II	93%	96%
Anacidity of aspirate	80%	84%
Weight loss	No difference	No difference
Dumping	No difference	No difference
Small bowel transit time	No difference	No difference
Diarrhea	15%	5%
Incomplete vagotomy (Hollander Test)	19%	2%

Table based on a prospective, randomized trial reported in Am J Surg 1968; 115-165. Sawyers JL, Scott HW Jr, Edwards WH et al. Comparative studies of the clinical effects of truncal and selective gastric vagotomy.

TABLE 4 Comparison of Surgical Results

	Mortality (%)	Ulcer Recurrence (%)	Visick (%)
Truncal vagotomy-pyloroplasty (TV-P)	0.5	10–15	65–75
Selective gastric vagotomy-pyloroplasty (SGV-P)	0.5	6–8	70–78
Truncal vagotomy-antrectomy (TV-A)	1–2	<1	66–75

to permit passage of a #40 F dilator through the lumen of the duodenal bulb after freeing periduodenal adhesions.

OPERATIONS FOR ACUTE DUODENAL ULCER

Perforated Duodenal Ulcer

The patient with an acute perforated duodenal ulcer is a surgical emergency. The traditional operation has been simple closure of the perforated ulcer with an omental patch as described by Graham. An increasing number of patients are being managed by definitive operation to control the ulcer diathesis. One-third of patients with a perforated duodenal ulcer treated only by simple closure will require a second operation for duodenal ulcer disease; one-third will require continuing medical treatment for duodenal ulcer; one-third will be asymptomatic. Proximal gastric vagotomy with patch of the perforated ulcer is our preferred operation because it provides control of gastric acid secretions to protect patients against ulcer symptoms but does not subject patients to symptoms of the postgastrectomy syndrome. The one-third of patients who do not need a definite ulcer operation are not harmed and the two-thirds who would have continuing ulcer symptoms are benefited.

Proximal gastric vagotomy with patch closure of the ulcer has been performed in more than 100 patients with no mortality and no severe postgastrectomy sequelae. The ulcer recurrence rate has been less than 2 percent. Good or excellent results (Visick I and II) have been achieved in more than 90 percent of patients. Truncal vagotomy-antrectomy and TV-P are alternative choices for definitive operations, but we have not used them in recent years. If there is severe contamination of the peritoneal cavity with peritonitis, then patch closure only is done. Patch closure alone should be elected in patients who are seriously ill with preexisting disease prior to onset of a perforated ulcer.

Bleeding Duodenal Ulcer

Patients with intermittent episodes of bleeding from duodenal ulcer may be managed by PGV if elective operation is done after bleeding has ceased. Patients requiring emergency operation for exsanguinating hemorrhage from a duodenal ulcer are usually elderly and frequently not good surgical risks. The treatment goal should be control of hemorrhage to save the patient's life. Truncal vagotomy-pyloroplasty with suture of the bleeding site is the operation of choice in most of these patients. The bleeding ulcer should be sutured with multiple nonabsorbable sutures placed above and below the bleeding site plus a U suture placed deep below the ulcer to ligate the underlying vessels.

In 18 selected good-risk patients requiring emergency operation for bleeding, we have suture ligated the bleeding vessel, closed the duodenostomy, and performed a PGV without drainage. Only one patient has had a minor rebleed which did not require reoperation. No recurrent ulcer or postgastrectomy problem has been encountered in these patients. Proximal gastric vagotomy with emergency suture of a bleeding duodenal ulcer should be limited to young, good-risk patients who have small posterior ulcers. Other aspects of this topic are discussed in the chapters *Duodenal Ulcer* and *Gastrointestinal Bleeding*.

Zollinger-Ellison Syndrome

Patients with Zollinger-Ellison syndrome are managed initially by H_2-blockers but should be considered for operation when ulcer control is achieved only by massive drug doses or when the possibility exists of excising the gastrinoma.

Total gastrectomy to remove the target organ has been the standard surgical treatment. For the past few years we have followed McClelland and his coworkers' suggestion of using PGV with excision of the gastrinoma if the tumor can be found.[6] All patients so managed have had reduction in acid secretion and resolution of their duodenal ulcer but required maintenance therapy with small doses of H_2-blockers. There is a separate chapter on *Gastrinoma*.

RECURRENT ULCERS

Recurrent ulcers are caused by failure of the first operation to control continued increased gastric acid secretion. The causes of recurrent ulcers are incomplete vagotomy, inadequate gastric resection, retained antrum on a duodenal stump, gastrinoma unrecognized at the first operation, or, rarely, G-cell hyperplasia. Surgical management depends on the cause. All patients should have serum gastrin levels measured, and, if elevated, a secretin test and a meal-stimulated gastrin test (for antral G-cell hyperplasia). Gastric analysis to include basal and stimulted acid secretion may help determine the completeness of vagotomy. We no longer use the insulin Hollander test. Others utilize sham feeding gastric analysis.

The management of patients with Zollinger-Ellison syndrome has been discussed. Patients with retained gastric antrum outside the acid stream need only to have the antral remnant excised. The rare patient with G-cell hyperplasia is treated by antrectomy. Most patients, however, have an incomplete vagotomy but all too often respond poorly to repeat vagotomy alone. Instead of doing a transthoracic vagotomy, we prefer doing a transabdominal truncal vagotomy with antrectomy. Patients with recurrent ulcer after PGV, SGV-P, or TV-P should have antrectomy and truncal vagotomy with a gastroduodenostomy (Billroth I). Those few patients with recurrent ulcer following SGV-A or TV-A and in whom serum gastrins are not elevated are best treated by a higher gastric resection and a repeat truncal vagotomy. Patients with Zollinger-Ellison syndrome with recurrent symptoms after lesser surgical procedures than a total gastrectomy require total gastrectomy. So far, our patients with Zollinger-Ellison syndrome managed by PGV have not developed a recurrent ulcer if maintained on cimetidine or ranitidine.

GASTRIC ULCERS

Although the incidence of duodenal ulcer disease is decreasing, the number of patient hospital admissions for gastric ulcer has not changed. The percentage of patients over 60 years of age with gastric ulcer increased from 40 to 48 percent between 1970 and 1978.

Surgical treatment of gastric ulcers is based on the type of ulcer (see Table 1). Approximately 60 percent of ulcers are type I, 25 percent type II, and 15 percent type III. All gastric ulcers may be managed by *distal subtotal gastric resection*, including the ulcer, with Billroth I gastroduodenostomy. If acid secretion is low, there is no duodenal ulcer, no ulcerogenic drug administration, and no alcoholism, this type of resection alone is sufficient. *Vagotomy* is added for all type II associated duodenal ulcers and type III (prepyloric) gastric ulcer patients and for type I gastric ulcer patients who are alcoholics or who need continued treatment with ulcerogenic medication, i.e., arthritics.

In addition to the usual indications for operation—*failure of medical treatment, perforation, hemorrhage, and obstruction*—the *possibility of malignancy* must be considered in patients with gastric ulcers. Endoscopy with multiple biopsies and brushing for cytologic study should be done in all patients with gastric ulcer. Upper gastrointestinal x-ray studies and gastric analysis are also performed. Only if all these diagnostic studies suggest that the gastric ulcer is benign should a trial of nonoperative treatment be undertaken. Patients are then reevaluated after 6 weeks of medical therapy to ascertain if the ulcer is healed and again at 12 weeks. If the ulcer has failed to heal completely by 12 weeks, operation is indicated.

Operation is also advocated for all patients with perforated gastric ulcer and for patients with bleeding gastric ulcers who require one or more blood transfusions. Patients with gastric ulcers are generally older and are more likely to continue to bleed or have early recurrent bleeding than patients with duodenal ulcers. Patients who develop a recurrent gastric ulcer should undergo operation without repeating the trial of medical therapy (Table 5).

TABLE 5 Criteria for Operation for Gastric Ulcer

Evaluation by roentgenography, gastroscopy with biopsy, and cytology—all benign or operate
Single test healing—reevaluate at 6 weeks for healing and 12 weeks for complete healing or operate
Single episode of hemorrhage requiring transfusion—operate
Recurrent ulcer—operate

Proximal gastric vagotomy for gastric ulcer has been reported from several surgical centers with controversial results. The recurrence rate following PGV for prepyloric ulcers (type III) ranges from 20 to 30 percent. Prepyloric or channel ulcers are best managed by selective gastric vagotomy and antrectomy (SGV-A). In a few surgical centers, type I gastric ulcers have been successfully treated by PGV alone. The gastric ulcer should be excised to rule out malignancy. Since the type I gastric ulcer characteristically occurs on the lesser curvature near the incisura, PGV may be technically difficult because the inflammatory reaction from the ulcer prevents identification and preservation of the gastric nerves of Latarjet. In my opinion, PGV for type I gastric ulcers needs further evaluation before it can be recommended for general use.

Truncal or selective gastric vagotomy with pyloroplasty for gastric ulcer has not been satisfactory in my experience because of an ulcer recurrence rate of 18 percent. The clinical results are not superior to those following antrectomy with ulcer excision, and the incidence of postgastrectomy sequelae is not diminished.

The high-lying gastric ulcer near the esophagogastric junction or fundus presents a technical challenge. Such ulcers must be biopsied or excised to rule out malignancy. To perform excision with antrectomy may necessitate total gastrectomy. Antrectomy leaving the ulcer in situ (after biopsy) is a satisfactory method and preferable to subtotal proximal gastric resection. In some patients the ulcer may be excised in continuity with the antrum and the remaining stomach "tubed" to permit anastomosis with the duodenum.

REFERENCES

1. Johnson HD. Gastric ulcer: classification, blood group characteristics, secretion patterns, and pathogenesis. Ann Surg 1965; 162:996-1004.
2. Dragstedt LR, Owens FM Jr. Supradiaphragmatic section of the vagus nerve in the treatment of duodenal ulcer. Proc Soc Exp Biol Med 1943; 53:152.
3. Herrington JL Jr, Sawyers JL, Scott HW Jr. A 25-year experience with vagotomy-antrectomy. Arch Surg 1973; 106:469.
4. Jordan PH Jr, Condon RE. A prospective evaluation of vagotomy-pyloroplasty and vagotomy-antrectomy for treatment of duodenal ulcer. Ann Surg 1970; 172:547.
5. Herrington JL Jr, Scott HW Jr, Sawyers JL. Experience with vagotomy-antrectomy and Roux-en-Y gastrojejunostomy in surgical treatment of duodenal, gastric and stomal ulcer. Ann Surg 1984; 199:590-597.
6. Richardson CT, Feldman M, McClelland RN, et al. Effect of vagotomy in Zollinger-Ellison syndrome. Gastroenterology 1979; 77:682-686.

GASTRINOMA

ROBERT T. JENSEN, M.D.
JERRY D. GARDNER, M.D.

Zollinger-Ellison syndrome (ZES) is characterized by hypersecretion of gastric acid due to hypergastrinemia secondary to a nonbeta islet cell tumor. Because these tumors contain and release large amounts of gastrin into the circulation, they are referred to as gastrinomas. A gastrinoma is found at surgery in 65 percent of patients, occurring in the pancreas in 42 percent, in the duodenum in 14 percent, and in other sites in 9 percent of cases—such as regional lymph nodes near the pancreas, or rarely, within the liver, ovary, or hilum of the spleen. Gastrinomas are malignant in 60 to 90 percent of cases, but they tend to grow slowly and are slow to metastasize. Currently 77 percent of patients with gastrinomas present with pain, usually due to a typical peptic ulcer. Up to 13 percent have esophageal symptoms, 50 percent have diarrhea, and in 18 percent diarrhea is the only symptom. Except for patients with far advanced metastatic disease, all symptoms in patients with gastrinomas are caused by excessive gastric acid secretion.

Approximately 25 percent of patients with gastronomas have evidence of multiple endocrine neoplasia type 1(MEN-1). MEN-1 is an autosomal dominant trait characterized by tumors or hyperplasia of multiple endocrine organs with hyperparathyroidism occurring in 98 percent, functional islet cell adenomas in 80 percent of patients and pituitary adenomas less commonly. Almost all patients with MEN-1 and ZES have multiple gastrinomas, and thus have a very low probability of surgical cure.

TREATMENT PHILOSOPHY

In patients with gastrinoma two therapeutic aims need to be considered. First, therapeutic decisions must be made to control gastric acid hypersecretion both short and long term. Second, because of the malignant potential of the gastrinoma, therapeutic decisions need to be made about the treatment of the gastrinoma itself. With the recent availability of potent antisecretory agents, hypersecretion of gastric acid can now be controlled medically in almost every patient, making routine total gastrectomy unnecessary. With the ability to control gastric hypersecretion, the natural history of the gastrinoma is becoming a more important determinant of long term prognosis.

CONTROL OF HYPERSECRETION OF GASTRIC ACID

Medical Treatment of Gastric Hypersecretion

The single most important determinant of successful medical management of hypersecretion of gastric acid is an adequate dosage of the antisecretory agent. Most studies show that relief of symptoms is not a good guide to ulcer healing or adequacy of therapy, although persistence of symptoms, especially diarrhea or epigastric pain, usually indicates the drug dosage is inadequate. *If gastric acid secretion is reduced to less than 10 mEq per hour for the last hour prior to the next dose of medication, peptic ulcers will heal and further peptic disease will be prevented.* In the small group of patients who have previously had a vagotomy and partial gastrectomy with a Billroth II gastroenterostomy, gastric acid secretion should be reduced to less than 5 mEq per hour. To assess the adequacy of antisecretory control a nasogastric tube should be passed into the antrum of the stomach, gastric secretion collected for 1 hour prior to the next dose of medication, a sample of the gastric secretion titrated to pH 7.0, and the acid secretory rate determined and expressed in milliequivalents per hour. The nasogastric tube can be properly placed without flouroscopy by passing the tube 50 to 55 cm and checking the recovery of instilled fluid by adding 50 cc of saline or water, of which 90 percent should be recovered. It cannot be overemphasized that *only by determining adequacy of suppression of gastric acid secretion can the adequacy of medical management be assessed.* In addition, long term medical management will be successful only in a compliant patient. The small number of patients who cannot or will not take medication regularly should not be considered for medical therapy with the antisecretory medications currently available, and should undergo total gastrectomy.

Intravenous Therapy

Most patients with ZES present with a long history of peptic ulcer disease, diarrhea, or esophageal symptoms, and treatment can be started with oral antisecretory medications. A few patients present with severe electrolyte or metabolic abnormalities and acute complications of their ulcer disease and cannot take oral medication. These patients should be treated with appropriate fluid and electrolyte replacement, nasogastric suction, and intravenous cimetidine or ranitidine. Ranitidine has been shown to be three to four times more potent than cimetidine, but either drug can be used and should be administered by continuous intravenous infusion after an intravenous bolus injection. Continuous intravenous infusion can be accomplished by adding intravenous cimetidine (or ranitidine) to 5 percent dextrose/water such that if the intravenous infusion rate is 75 ml per hour the patient will receive 3 mg per kilogram of body weight per hour of cimetidine (or 1 mg per kilogram per hour of ranitidine). If cimetidine is used, first administer a bolus injection of 150 mg, begin the intravenous cimetidine infusion at 1 mg per kilogram per hour (25 ml per hour), and after a few hours determine the gastric secretory rate for 1 hour. If gastric secretion is greater than 10 mEq per hour, give 2 mg per kilogram per hour of cimetidine (50 ml per hour), recheck the acid secretion, and continue increasing the cimetidine up to 6 mg per kilogram per hour until gastric secretion is controlled. If gastric acid secretion is still not less than 10 mEq per hour when giving 6 mg per kilogram per hour, an anticholinergic agent, such as Pro-Banthine, 15 mg IM every 6 hour, should be added.

Oral Therapy

For long term oral treatment, either cimetidine or ranitidine alone or with an anticholinergic agent should be used. Antacids are ineffective even in large amounts, probably because of the high acid secretion and rapid gastric emptying that occur in patients with gastrinoma. Ranitidine is preferable to cimetidine in men because high doses of cimetidine cause antiandrogen side effects (breast tenderness, gynecomastia, impotence). Ranitidine is also preferable in patients taking other medications that are metabolized by the hepatic mixed function oxidase system (Dilantin, Coumadin, theophylline, etc.) because cimetidine but not ranitidine, affects metabolism of drugs by the hepatic mixed function oxidase system. In women who are not taking medication that is metabolized by the hepatic mixed function oxidase system either cimetidine or ranitidine can be used, because equipotent doses of both drugs have the same duration of action. Even though ranitidine is three times more potent than cimetidine, ranitidine is three times more expensive.

If sufficient doses of cimetidine or ranitidine are used, gastric hypersecretion can be controlled in almost every patient with ZES. Patients should first be treated with cimetidine, 300 mg every 6 hours, or ranitidine, 150 mg. every 8 hours, and the gastric acid secretory rate determined the next day, 1 hour before the next dose of medication. If gastric acid secretion is greater than 10 mEq per hour in this hour, cimetidine should be increased to 600 mg every 6 hours or ranitidine to 150 mg every 6 hours and the secretory rate determined again. If the gastric acid secretory rate continues to be greater than 10 mEq per hour, cimetidine should be increased to 900 mg every 6 hours or ranitidine to 300 mg every 6 hours. If gastric hypersecretion is still not controlled, an oral *anticholinergic* agent such as isopropamide 5 mg every 6 hours can be added. Anticholinergic agents alone only inhibit gastric hypersecretion by 15 to 25 percent, but when combined with cimetidine or ranitidine can greatly increase the effectiveness of the histamine H_2 receptor antagonists. Anticholinergic agents should be continued for at least 3 days before the gastric secretory rate is redetermined. Side effects with anticholinergic agents, such as dry mouth, constipation, and visual changes, are usually dose related so that if the side effects become significant, the dose can be reduced. Anticholinergic agents should generally not be used in patients with prostatism, glaucoma, partial gastric outlet obstruction, or significant esophageal disease.

Dosage Requirements. To control gastric hypersecretion, most patients with gastrinoma require more than 1.2 g per day of cimetidine or 0.3 g per day of ranitidine, the doses used in treating routine duodenal ulcer. In recent large studies the median doses required were 3 to 5 g per day of cimetidine or 1 to 1.5 g per day of ranitidine. Patients with gastrinoma have been treated for more than one year with doses as high as 12 g per day of cimetidine or 6 g per day of ranitidine. High doses of either drug have been well tolerated without evidence of dose-related hepatic, renal, or central nervous system toxicity. The continued effectiveness of antisecretory control should be checked every 6 to 12 months even if the patient is asymptomatic or if at any time diarrhea, esophageal, or peptic symptoms develop and persist for more than one week.

Newer Drugs

Recently, several new drugs have been described which promise to facilitate medical management of patients with ZES but have not been approved for use by the Food and Drug Administration. More potent histamine receptor antagonists, such as famotidine, which is 40 times more potent than cimetidine, will probably soon be available. Other classes of drugs, such as omeprazole, a substituted benzimidazole which inhibits H^+-K^+-ATPase on the gastric parietal cell, also may soon by available. Famotidine has only a slightly longer duration of action than cimetidine or ranitidine, whereas omeprazole has a duration of action of at least 3 days. Recent studies suggest that hypersecretion of gastric acid will be controlled in most patients with omeprazole taken once a day.

Surgical Treatment of Gastric Hypersecretion

Parietal Cell Vagotomy

Most studies have shown that long-term medical management with cimetidine or ranitidine is effective, but many patients require more than 4.8 g per day of cimetidine or 1.5 g per day of ranitidine to control gastric acid hypersecretion. Furthermore, medication dose requirements slowly increase with time; thus, medication expense will become an increasingly important determinant of the feasibility of long-term medical management. Therefore, until more potent antisecretory agents such as omeprazole become available, in many patients with high antisecretory drug requirements, a parietal cell vagotomy should be considered. A recent study demonstrates that a parietal cell vagotomy will decrease basal acid secretion by 56 percent, decrease antisecretory drug requirement in more than 90 percent of patients, and allow control of acid secretion with less than 3.0 g per day of cimetidine. Although it is likely that drug requirements will increase with time as the gastrinoma progresses, in the patients followed for up to 24 months after a parietal cell vagotomy only one patient required an increased cimetidine dose to control gastric hypersecretion. If parietal cell vagotomy is considered, a surgeon who routinely performs this operation should be selected. The patient should realize that this operation reduces the drug requirement, but in no case will a patient be able to stop all antisecretory medication.

Parathyroidectomy

In patients with gastrinoma with the MEN-1 syndrome, medical control of gastric hypersecretion can be facilitated by correction of the hyperparathyroidism, which is almost invariably present by the time Zollinger-Ellison syndrome develops. Correction of the hyperparathyroidism may reduce the fasting gastrin concentration, increase responsiveness to a given dose of antisecretory medication, and decrease the basal acid output, all of which facilitate medical control of gastric hypersecretion. Correction of the hyperparathyroidism is recommended in those gastrinoma patients with MEN-1 in whom the hyperparathyroidism is symptomatic (for example, renal stones, and so on) or in those who have a high antisecretory drug requirement.

Total Gastrectomy

Total gastrectomy should now be reserved for patients who cannot or will not take antisecretory medication. In a recent review of all series published since 1978 involving 248 patients with gastrinoma undergoing total gastrectomy, the operative mortality was 5.6 percent overall and 2.4 percent for elective procedures. The true morbidity rate associated with total gastrectomy, however, is not apparent from most series. When total gastrectomy is performed, gastrinoma patients should be treated with oral calcium, vitamin D, iron, and monthly injections of vitamin B_{12}.

TREATMENT OF THE GASTRINOMA

All physicians agree that the ideal treatment of gastrinoma is total surgical excision. In long-term studies of patients with gastrinoma who survived total gastrectomy and subsequently died, at least 50 percent of the deaths were due to tumor progression. Aggressive surgery, however, is not warranted in most patients because the overall prognosis for most patients is good. In recent studies the 5-year survival for patients with metastatic or unresectable locally invasive gastrinoma was 14 to 70 percent, and for all patients with gastrinoma it was 42 to 80 percent. Recent studies provide a number of results that help identify which patients should be considered for exploratory surgery. Present studies report that preoperative imaging studies, such as CT scan, angiogram, and ultrasound, can identify more that 90 percent of patients with gastrinoma metastatic to the liver and 38 percent of primary gastrinomas. Almost every study demonstrates that the possibility of surgical cure is very low (<2%) in patients with MEN-1 and gastrinoma, probably because of the multiplicity of gastrinomas. In early studies up to 1981 involving 157 patients with gastrinoma, the surgical cure was only 5 percent, whereas in recent studies in patients with sporadic gastrinoma (i.e., without MEN-1) the cure rate was 20 percent overall and up to 50 percent in patients with an extrapancreatic gastrinoma. In most studies, in at least one-third of patients, no gastrinoma is found and, after long-term follow-up, none of these patients have died from tumor progression. Some studies suggest that excision of all gastrinoma visible at surgery will improve long-term prognosis. No studies have demonstrated that aggressive surgery in patients with advanced metastatic disease improves long-term survival.

Approach to Patients With Nonmetastatic Gastrinoma

The results outlined above suggest that, among patients in whom the gastrinoma has not metastasized to the liver, the gastrinoma is potentially resectable, and who do not have MEN-1, approximately 60 percent will have a tumor found at surgery. In 40 percent the resection will not be curative and in 20 percent the resection will be curative (in 40% no tumor will be found). If no tumor is found, present evidence suggests that it is very likely that tumor progression leading to death will not occur in the 10 years following surgery.

Therefore, at present it is recommended that all patients with sporadic gastrinoma, i.e., gastrinoma not associated with MEN-1, undergo preoperative imaging studies. First, a CT scan with intravenous contrast should be performed, which will identify more than 80 percent of patients with gastrinoma metastatic to the liver. If hepatic metastatic disease is not present and even if the CT scan demonstrates a probable primary gastrinoma, ultrasound and selective pancreatic and hepatic angiography should be performed. All patients without gastrinoma in the liver or gastrinoma that is judged unresectable should undergo surgical exploration. Even the 60 percent of patients with negative localization studies should undergo exploratory laparotomy, because recent studies suggest that small gastrinomas (≤ 1 cm) are frequently not identified preoperatively but may be found by an experienced surgeon. Preoperative transhepatic selective venous sampling for gastrin from portal venous tributaries has been claimed to be helpful by some workers but not by others, and until its value is proven further, it should not be performed routinely.

The single most important factor in achieving good surgical results is the expertise of the surgeon. Even many experienced pancreatic surgeons have little experience with islet cell tumors, with the difficulty in identifying extrahepatic gastrinomas, and with the technique of enucleating lesions within the pancreas. At surgery the entire pancreas shoud be examined, with a Kocher maneuver performed to examine the pancreatic head; and the duodenum, stomach, mesentery, liver, and splenic hilum should be examined carefully. Any suspicious lymph node or mass should be biopsied. Gastrinomas are occasionally multiple; therefore, even if one tumor is found, examination for others should be continued. If at laparotomy a gastrinoma is found in the pancreatic head and cannot be enucleated, a Whipple procedure is not recommended because at present no studies have demonstrated that this will enhance survival. In fact, given the morbidity and mortality associated with this procedure coupled with the slow growth of the tumor, a Whipple procedure may possibly decrease long-term survival. Gastrinoma in the pancreatic body and tail, as well as involved lymph nodes, should be resected when safe and possible. Solitary gastrinomas or a few isolated areas of gastrinoma in the liver should also be resected if safe and possible because some such tumors may represent multifocal primaries. If no tumor is found, a blind pancreatic resection should not be performed because this does not increase the cure rate. If cure is unlikely either because no tumor is found or because tumor is found but is not completely resectable, and if the preoperative antisecretory drug requirement is high, a parietal cell vagotomy should be performed.

Prior to surgery the dosage of intravenous cimetidine or ranitidine that reduces gastric acid secretion to less than 10 mEq per hour should be determined for each patient. This dose of antisecretory agent should be given by continuous intravenous administration throughout surgery and the postoperative period until the patient can resume oral medication. The antisecretory medication should not be stopped postoperatively until it is clear the patient has been cured. Because results of gastrin assays may take a number of days, a reasonable course is to treat the patient with the same antisecretory medication that was taken preoperatively and perform a fasting gastrin and secretin provocative test. If either of these two tests suggests incomplete resection, the patient should be maintained on oral medication and the minimum antisecretory dose to reduce gastric acid secretion to less than 10 mEq per hour should be determined. Patients with a normal fasting gastrin concentration and a normal secretin test postoperatively should be maintained on antisecretory medication for 3 months and then reassessed yearly with measurement of fasting gastrin concentration and a secretin provocative test.

Approach To Patients With Metastatic Gastrinoma

When gastric acid hypersecretion is adequately controlled almost all patients with metastatic gastrinoma remain asymptomatic until the gastrinoma becomes quite extensive. At what point chemotherapy should begin has still not been established. The response to chemotherapy is usually slow (months); and therefore, it should not be used as an attempt to control gastric acid hypersecretion. Streptozotocin and 5-fluorouracil, either alone or with Adriamycin, have been reported to reduce tumor mass. No cases of cure or even of complete disappearance of the gastrinoma have been reported with these chemotherapeutic agents. Approximately 60 percent of patients will show a decrease in tumor size, but the gastrinoma usually starts to grow again within 24 months of beginning chemotherapy even with continued treatment. Streptozotocin causes significant nausea and vomiting and can cause renal toxicity, requiring frequent monitoring of renal function. Of the two groups with considerable experience treating metastatic gastrinoma, one group recommends chemotherapy be used when there is objective evidence of metastatic tumor growth in the liver by CT scan or angiogram over a three to six month period. The other group does not use chemotherapy until the tumor becomes symptomatic (with local pain, anorexia, and so on).

LONG-TERM FOLLOW-UP

All patients with gastrinoma should be assessed for the adequacy of antisecretory therapy by determining the gastric acid secretion rate every 6 to 12 months or at any time that symptoms such as diarrhea, epigastric pain, or heartburn recur and persist. Possible tumor progression should be assessed at least every 2 years with a CT scan and ultrasound. All patients with gastrinoma with MEN-1 should be assessed at least every 2 years for hyperactivity of other endocrine glands. Hyperparathyroidism should be excluded by serial determinations of serum calcium and phosphate and a parathyroid hormone determination. Pituitary status should be assessed with serum prolactin determinations and pituitary sella size evaluated by CT scan. Adrenal status should be assessed by abdominal CT scan and an overnight dexamethasone suppression test.

ACUTE UPPER GASTROINTESTINAL BLEEDING

J. LOREN PITCHER, M.D., F.A.C.P.

There are few medical emergencies that provoke more urgency and anxiety for both the physician and the patient than acute upper gastrointestinal (UGI) bleeding. This common clinical problem accounts for an estimated 100 to 150 hospital admissions per year per 100,000 population in the United States and continues to be a therapeutic and economic challenge.

Despite major diagnostic and management advances, overall mortality from acute UGI hemorrhage has not decreased in the past 30 years. During this period, however, there has been a significant increase in the percentage of patients with UGI bleeding who are elderly, who often have serious underlying medical conditions, and in whom mortality may often be due to conditions other than the UGI bleeding. Thus, real improvements in reduced mortality, complications, transfusion requirements, and need for surgery in patients with certain bleeding lesions and in younger patients may be obscured by overall outcome data for all patients.

The cardinal rule that any amount of UGI bleeding is life-threatening until proven otherwise should prevail. A trickle of blood must always be considered as a harbinger of exsanguination even though 80 to 90 percent of patients will spontaneously cease bleeding.

In the past decade, seven prospective trials provided no evidence that a correct endoscopic diagnosis of the cause(s) of bleeding had any significant effect on either morbidity or mortality. Within these studies, however, were serious flaws in protocol design, inadequate stratification of patients, and often a lack of application of effective therapies for specific bleeding lesions, all of which make these studies of questionable value. Regardless, no one questions that endoscopy is the most safe, effective, and accurate method of diagnosing the cause(s) or site(s) of UGI bleeding in most patients. Recent advances in endoscopic techniques that (1) can effectively treat actively or recently bleeding lesions, (2) can identify lesions with a high probability of rebleeding or the need for surgical intervention, and (3) may preclude the use of unnecessary, ineffective, or potentially harmful therapies have opened a new era of optimism and realistic enthusiasm in the treatment of patients with UGI bleeding.

INITIAL PATIENT EVALUATION AND MANAGEMENT

Acute UGI bleeding may be massive, moderate, or mild and may be a single episode, intermittent episodes, or continuous. Fresh blood or "coffee grounds" in the emesis or in the gastric lavage return proves UGI bleeding if one can exclude paradoxic bleeding from the mouth, nasopharynx, or tracheobronchial tree and factitious bleeding (the swallowing of either human or animal blood). True melena is rarely found from a small bowel or proximal colonic source and hence its presence serves as a reasonable clue to UGI bleeding. Hematochezia, however, can occur in both UGI and lower GI bleeding. When bleeding is from the former rather than the latter source, the patient more often has signs and symptoms of significant blood volume loss.

A gastric lavage that is negative for gross or occult blood but is bile stained usually implies bleeding distal to the ligament of Treitz; however, a lack of duodenal-pyloric reflux of luminal contents, cessation of previous bleeding, or poor technique may yield a false-negative gastric lavage result.

The most common judgmental errors made in the initial evaluation and care of bleeding patients are to underestimate both the degree of blood loss (often due to a false reliance upon initial hematocrit values) and the potential gravity of the situation.

The patient's hemodynamic status must be rapidly and accurately assessed and monitored while resuscitative efforts are simultaneously initiated. Recumbent hypotension with or without clinical findings or hypovolemia and/or shock indicates a blood volume loss of 25 to 40 percent or more. For patients with recumbent normal blood pressures, a positive "tilt test" manifested by a rise in pulse rate of greater than 20 to 25 beats per minute and a diastolic pressure drop of greater than 10 to 15 mm Hg predicts a 10 to 20 percent loss of blood volume.

A relevant and expeditious history, physical examination, and review of available medical records should be accomplished while blood samples are drawn, large intravenous lines are established, and fluids, colloid, and blood replacement are initiated. In selected patients, a Swanz-Ganz catheter with thermodilution cardiac output capabilities and/or arterial monitoring lines may be indicated. Numerous studies have shown that the prediction of the actual bleeding site based upon history, physical examination, and prior known diagnoses is fraught with considerable error and cannot be relied upon.

Initial resuscitation always takes precedence over specific diagnostic and/or therapeutic measures; these can, however, usually be performed simultaneously.

Specific laboratory tests, always tailored to the patient's age, clinical history, symptoms, physical findings, and suspected or known underlying diseases should include complete blood count, urinalysis, prothrombin time, partial thromboplastin time, and careful review of the peripheral blood smear, with particular note taken of evidence of chronic anemia, hemolysis, vitamin B_{12} or folate deficiency, and platelet estimation. Blood chemistries should include, at minimum, blood glucose, creatinine, blood urea nitrogen, and liver function tests. Samples of blood may be obtained and stored and other tests run at a more expeditious time. In selected patients, serum and/or urinary amylase, electrolyte, and arterial blood gas measurements may be indicated. An electrocardiogram should be obtained in selected patients at admission and repeated in 24 to 48 hours or the patient monitored to uncover silent myocardial ischemia or infarction.

A portable chest roentgenogram, physical examination, and arterial blood gases provide reasonable assessment of pulmonary function status.

More detailed coagulation studies may be required when consumptive coagulopathy, liver disease, blood dyscrasias, drug ingestions, purpura, uremia, or other bleeding tendencies are suspected or apparent. Although it is often difficult to be certain when or if identified coagulation disorders are contributing to or causing the UGI bleeding, judicious replacement of appropriate clotting factors is usually indicated. Unless fresh whole blood less than one day old is available, this is usually best accomplished with fresh frozen plasma, platelets, or both. Specific clotting factor concentrates are rarely needed. Care must be exercised in using prothrombin complex concentrates, especially in patients with serious liver disease, because of the potential for inducing disseminated intravascular coagulation.

Critical vital signs and physiologic variables should be monitored and a flow sheet initiated to serially record all data and therapy. Patients with moderate and severe bleeding should have hourly measurement of urinary outputs obtained via an indwelling urinary catheter.

Deaths associated with UGI bleeding are often related to delayed resuscitation and/or insufficient volumes and rates of replacement therapy. Whole blood or packed red blood cells with isotonic fluids, colloid, or both are preferred when active bleeding and hypovolemia are present.

While one awaits blood products, Ringer's lactate (preferred if metabolic acidosis is present) or isotonic fluids should be infused at a rapid rate until the blood volume is minimally restored as indicated by improvement in blood pressure, pulse, clinical signs of hypovolemia, and other monitored, indicators of the patient's hemodynamic status.

Preference is given to maintaining a stable hematocrit above 30 to 34 percent with due precautions to avoid overexpansion of blood volume in patients at risk for congestive heart failure, variceal bleeding, or those with renal failure.

A team effort, to include *early surgical consultation* and *intensive care* provided by highly skilled nursing personnel, is important to optimal care and outcome.

Gastric lavage through a large-bore or a gastric tube is indicated when there is blood in the stomach. Although controlled studies are lacking to prove that iced or room temperature saline or water for gastric lavage either slows, halts, increases, or has no effect on active bleeding, clinical experience indicates that gastric lavage does slow or halt bleeding and is safe. Most importantly, lavage clears the stomach of blood to allow adequate endoscopic examination and/or therapy while precluding regurgitation and aspiration of blood during such procedures.

Gastric lavage should be accomplished using vigorous and forceful flushing and infusions of 100 to 250 ml of lavage solution with a 50-ml syringe, not a gravity flow system, so that organized clots can be broken up and blood flushed off the gastric mucosa. Return flow should be by either gravity or very gentle suction aspiration to avoid suction artifacts and damage to the gastric mucosa. Typically, the vigorous lavage will yield clear to pink return within 30 minutes. The lavage should not be discontinued until just before any diagnostic and/or therapeutic endoscopic procedures are performed.

Lavage solutions containing various vasoconstrictor agents are not commonly used or proven effective. One controlled, double-blind study comparing normal saline with an Aramine solution (300 mg per liter of normal saline) showed a benefit from the latter in reducing bleeding in a small number of patients.

SPECIFIC THERAPEUTIC ALTERNATIVES

Acid Neutralization or Secretory Inhibition

The use of antacids or histamine$_2$ (H$_2$) receptor antagonists has not been proved effective in stopping active bleeding from any lesion but may prevent rebleeding from ulcers; may be effective prophylaxis against bleeding in stress gastric erosions, as seen in patients on medical, surgical, trauma, and burn intensive care units; and may promote uncomplicated ulcer healing.

It is possible that the unproven or equivocal efficacy of these agents in some trials may be related to inadequate attention to proper doses to achieve near intragastric neutrality and to obviate the adverse effects on intragastric coagulation that may result from an intragastric pH of less than 6 to 7.

I prefer a combination of *cimetidine*, 300 to 400 mg IV every 4 to 6 hours by bolus injection or 50 to 65 mg per hour by constant infusion, plus a *potent antacid* (e.g., Mylanta II or Maalox T.C.) in doses of 15 to 45 ml every hour titrated to identify those amounts of both medications needed to maintain an intragastric pH of 6 to 7 for patients with peptic ulcer, reflux esophagitis with or without ulcer, and acute erosive gastritis/duodenitis secondary to drug, alcohol or gastric irritant ingestion.

I initially withhold H$_2$ receptor blockers in patients with gastric "stress" erosions or ulcers except those with central nervous system injuries or heptic coma. Reasonable but theoretical evidence suggests that, in other forms of gastric fundal "stress" bleeding, a secreting mucosa may be less vulnerable to erosions and ulceration than one blocked by an H$_2$ receptor antagonist.

Except in reflux esophagitis, with or without esophageal ulcer, and in patients with esophageal varices, antacids should be initiated via a nasogastric tube. After 48 to 72 hours of no significant bleeding and the necessary titration-calibration of the antacid/cimetidine therapy, comparable and then reduced oral doses may be utilized with due attention paid to the known side effects, contraindications, and drug interactions of these agents.

Angiotherapy

Selective and subselective catheterization of the mesenteric vasculature is now possible and allows the delivery of vasoconstrictor drugs and embolization therapy. I reserve this technique for very high-risk patients who fail to improve with more conventional and/or less hazardous and invasive procedures to control bleeding. No well-controlled studies are available, but control of bleeding has been reported in ulcer disease, diffuse mucosal erosions, Mallory-Weiss tears, and variceal bleeding when intravenous vasopressin fails.

Endoscopic Therapy

Thermal and Photocoagulation Methods. Of the endoscopic, hemostatic techniques evaluated to date, the most promising results, short of controlled studies, favor the application of techniques of coaptive electrocoagulation with either the available multipolar (BICAP) probe or the experimental heater probe. The combination of pressure and "slow" tissue heating from these instruments is felt to be more effective in controlling arterial bleeding. Neodymum: yttrium, aluminum, garnet (Nd:Yag) and argon lasers have proved effective in treating ulcer lesions to control bleeding and oozing and to prevent rebleeding. These have a greater erosive and perforation/penetration potential and are extremely costly, less portable, and less generally available than mono bipolar or multipolar electrocoagulation. The chapter *Laser Treatment in Gastrointestinal Disease* provides additional information.

Injection Therapy. Injection sclerotherapy of esophageal varices has been shown to be relatively safe and effective in the control of acute, actively bleeding varices, rebleeding from recently bleeding varices, and long-term control of variceal bleeding once obliteration of the varices is achieved. Control of bleeding has unfortunately not always and unequivocally been equated with increased short-, mid-, or long-term survival after an acute bleed but cost effectiveness has been demonstrated in one study. There is an excellent, well-referenced review of sclerotherapy by Conn and Grace.[1]

Of the sclerosing agents available in the United States, I prefer tetradecyl (Sotradecol) over sodium morrhuate or 95 percent ethanol. I specifically favor a mixed solution of equal volumes of 3 percent tetradecyl, 95 percent ethanol, and normal saline with methylene blue added as a marker (so-called TES solution). Such a mixture yields a solution of 1 percent tetradecyl, 32 percent ethanol, and 0.3 percent saline. This is an effective solution with a reasonable balance between efficacy and mucosal injury potential; it causes less fever, pleural effusions, chest pain, and other complications than fatty acid sclerosants such as sodium morrhuate. The use of single agents in full strengths yields too high an incidence of mucosal injury, ulcers, and other side effects. Perivariceal injections of these agents should be avoided when possible.

The technique is to inject 0.5 to 2.0 ml of TES solution at each site, with total volume not to exceed 26 ml per session. Varices should be injected in a circumferential fashion beginning at the esophageal gastric junction after the injection of the bleeding point of a recently bleeding or actively bleeding varix. I repeat injections in 48 hours in recently bleeding patients and then at 4- to 7-day intervals for three or four more sessions, followed by monthly injections until total obliteration of the varices has been achieved.

I consider reasonable indications for sclerotherapy to include active bleeding from esophageal varix at the time of diagnostic endoscopy; proven recent or recurrent variceal bleeding in Child's category B or C patients (especially those with severe clotting disorders); the absence of definitive therapy which would lead to a cure (i.e., splenic vein thrombosis); and proven, relatively recent variceal bleeding in a patient with large varices and a demonstrable cherry red spot, clot on a varix, submucosal hematoma around a varix, varix on a varix, black spot, red wale, or the so-called Mt. St. Helen's sign. (See the chapters on *Sclerotherapy of Esophageal Varices* and *Portal Hypertension*.)

Limited reports on the effectiveness of 95 percent ethanol injections to control ulcer and other arterial bleeding points and the use of endoscopic clipping and suturing techniques are too preliminary to recommend use of these techniques. Likewise, topical agents applied through the endoscope have no role in endoscopic therapy at this time.

Transhepatic Obliteration of Varices

Transhepatic obliteration of varices is of limited value because of the lack of controlled studies, the technical expertise required, the ease and accessibility of endoscopic sclerotherapy, and the theoretical disadvantage that this therapy may obliterate the paraesophageal veins which may act as a desirable portasystemic shunt.

Vasopressin

By its effect on splanchnic vasoconstriction and perhaps its reduction in intramural esophageal venous flow through its effect on smooth muscle action in the esophageal wall, both peripheral intravenous and mesenteric intra-arterial infusions of vasopressin may be equally effective in variceal bleeding. Because of its easy administration, the intravenous route is preferred at a rate of 0.2 to 0.9 units of vasopressin per minute. Close attention must be paid to the many adverse side effects of vasopressin, especially the unpredictable decrease in cardiac output, which may respond to appropriate doses of isoproterenol. A few patients who fail to respond to intravenous vasopressin may respond to mesenteric arterial infusions at doses of 0.1 to 0.4 units per minute. I prefer hemodynamic and cardiac output monitoring capabilities to be available during vasopressin infusion.

Vasopressin for the treatment of other sources of nonvariceal bleeding usually requires mesenteric intra-arterial infusion and often selective or subselective infusion into the vessel(s) directly supplying the bleeding site. Alcohol- or drug-induced gastritis may rapidly respond to vasopressin.

The use of sodium nitroprusside and propranolol for the control of acute bleeding, particularly variceal bleeding, cannot be recommended at this time.

Balloon Tamponade

Either the Sengstaken-Blakemore (S-B) tube with the Boyce modification or the Linton tube (the latter is preferred for gastric variceal bleeding only or Mallory-Weiss tear tamponade) can be safe and effective in the hands of experienced physicians. Permanent hemostasis utilizing this technique, however, occurs in only 40 to 50 percent of patients, and therefore it is generally relegated to the role of a procedure to halt acute variceal bleeding temporarily when vasopressin therapy and/or sclerotherapy fails. Details of a recommended safe and effective technique for the use of the S-B tube are available[2]. These instructions differ from those usually offered by the manufacturers of the various tamponade tubes.

Miscellaneous Medical Treatment

A number of therapeutic agents, including glucagon, anticholinergic drugs, somatostatin, prostaglandins, and

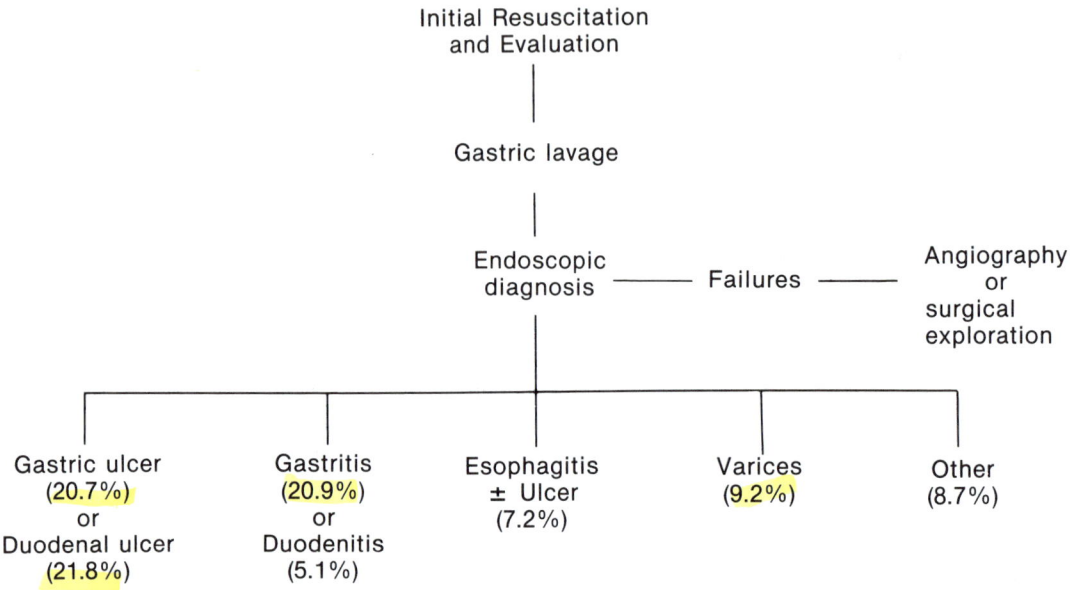

Figure 1 Initial management of acute upper gastrointestinal hemorrhage and approximate frequency of bleeding lesions.

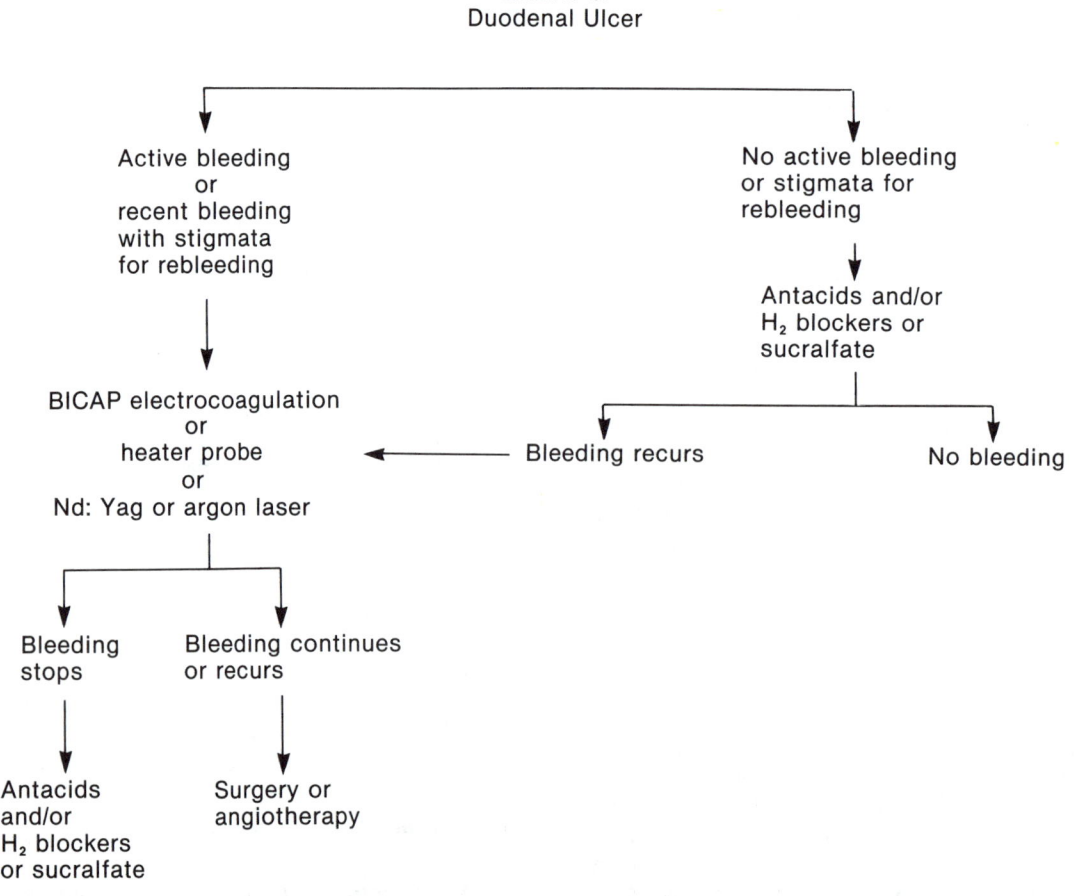

Figure 2 Management of acute hemorrhage from gastric or duodenal ulcer.

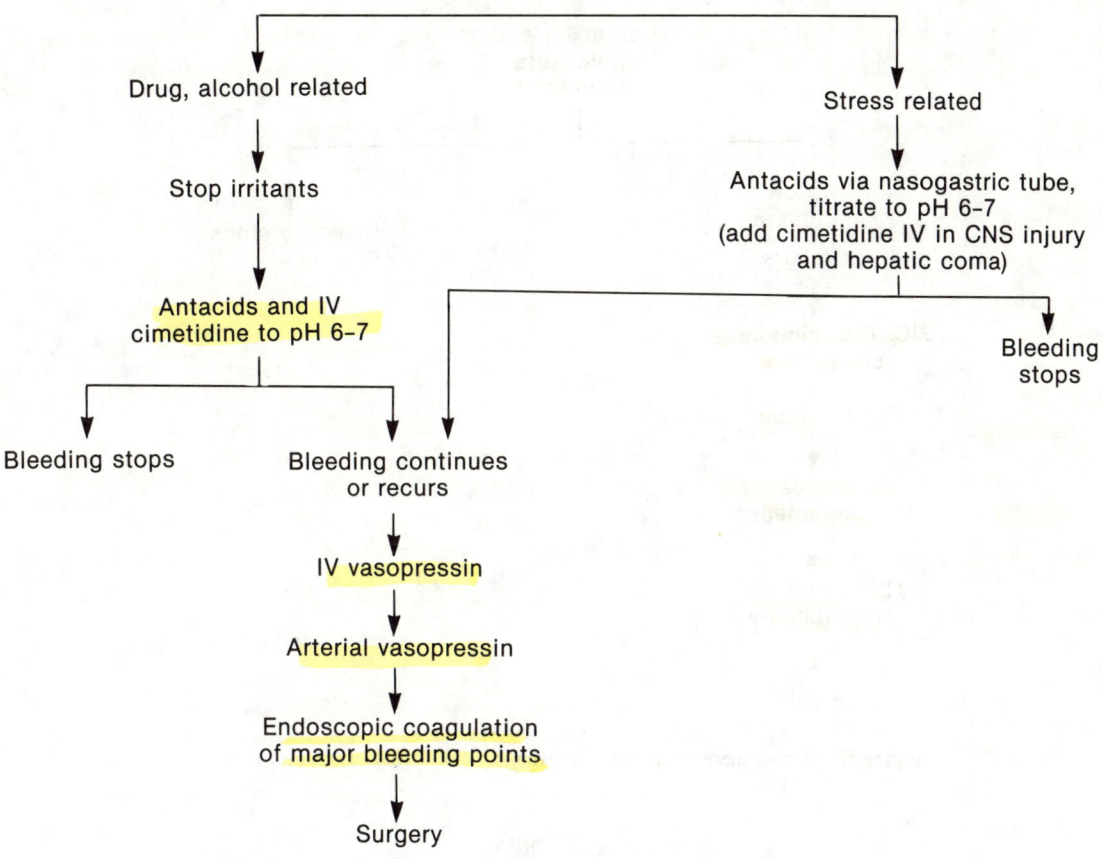

Figure 3 Management of acute hemorrhage from gastritis, duodenitis and erosions.

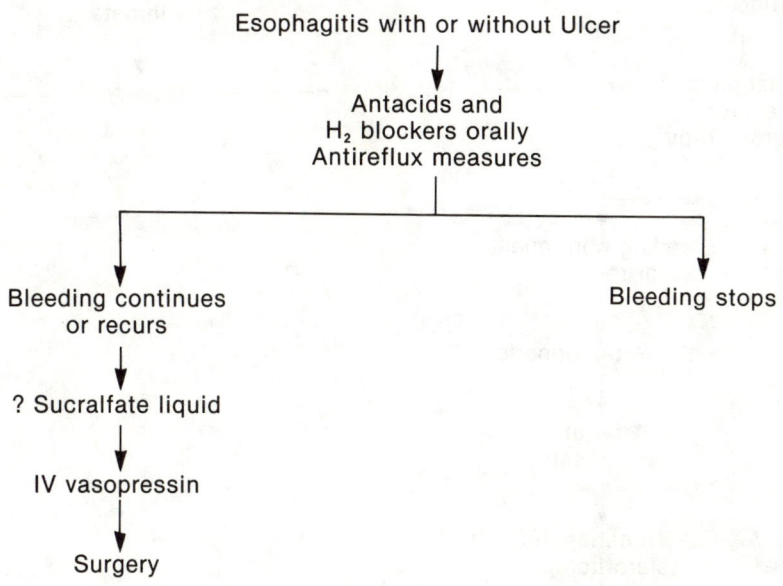

Figure 4 Management of acute hemorrhage from esophagitis, with or without ulcer.

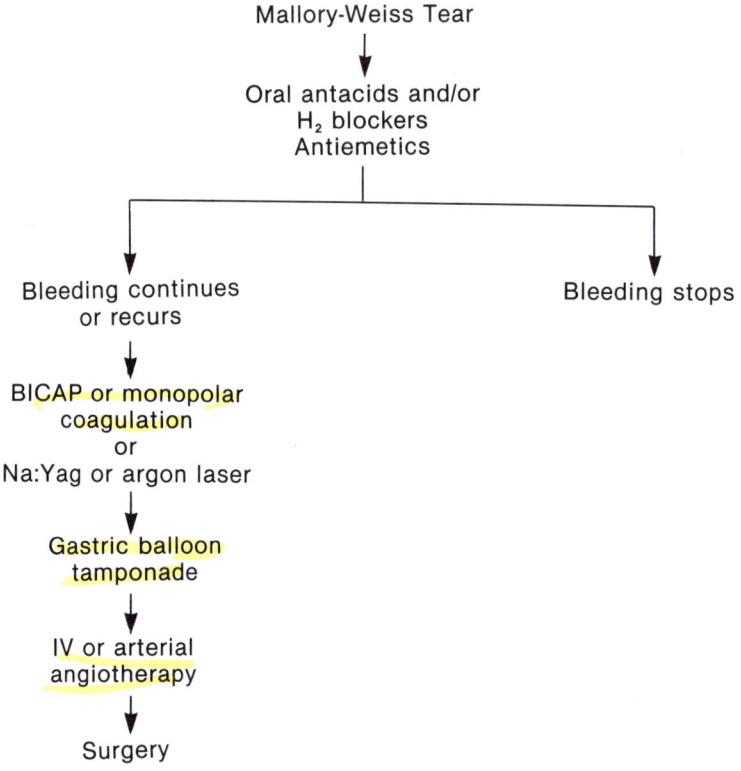

Figure 5 Management of acute hemorrhage from a Mallory-Weiss tear.

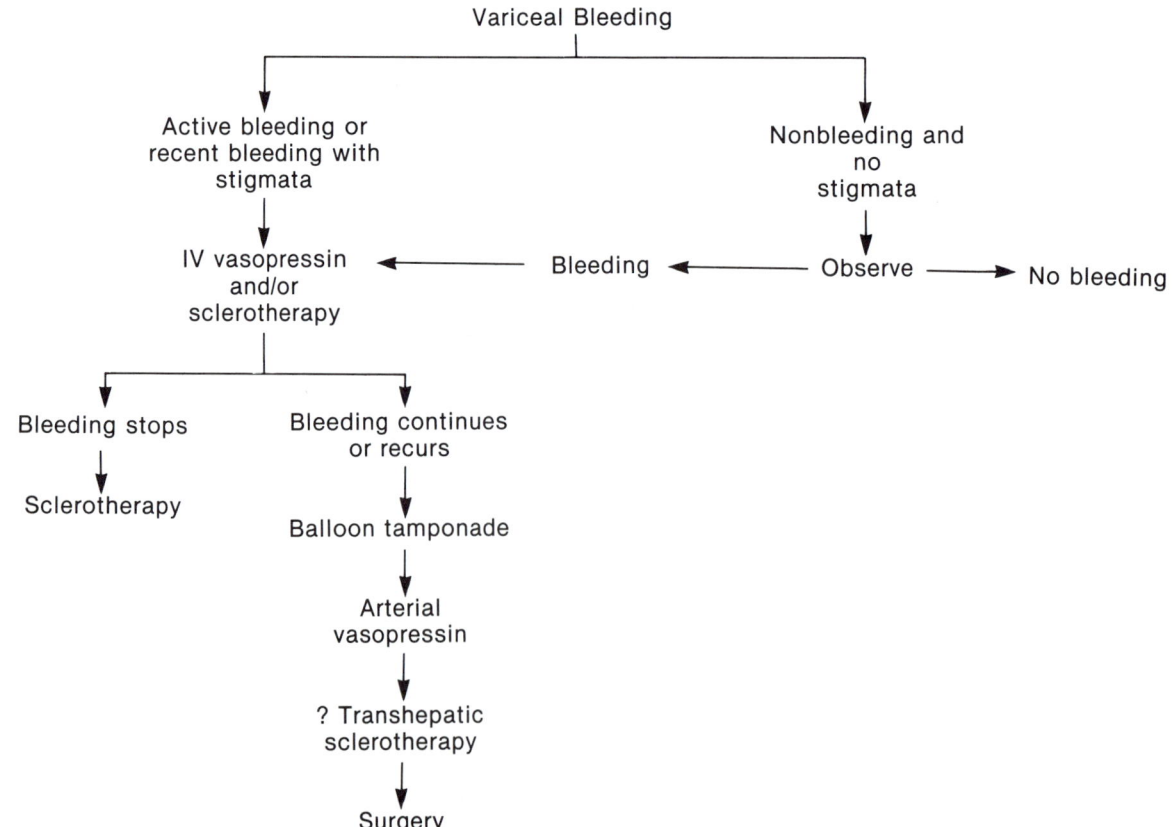

Figure 6 Management of acute hemorrhage from gastroesophageal varices.

sucralfate, are under investigation but none can be recommended at this time for routine use in the United States in actively bleeding patients. Seemingly, patients with diffuse erosive gastritis, may be the beneficiaries of some of these medications that have "cytoprotective" effects in the stomach.

Surgery

Surgical intervention to control bleeding is reserved for those who fail to stop bleeding spontaneously, have recurrent or continuous bleeding despite other modes of therapy, or who have specific lesions that are best treated and/or cured by surgery. Many factors, such as patient age, underlying medical conditions, the specific nature of the bleeding site, the amount, frequency, and rapidity of bleeding, the surgical expertise available, transfusion difficulties, patient's physiologic response and tolerance of the bleeding, and the availability of nonsurgical effective therapies, enter into the decision of when and on which patients surgery should be performed. No hard or fixed formulas can replace sound judgment and clinical experience in this arena. In some patients, surgical intervention may be the primary and most conservative approach to therapy. Discussions of preferred surgical procedures or techniques for various bleeding lesions are included in the chapters *Portal Hypertension, Peptic Ulcer Disease: Surgical Treatment* and *Sclerotherapy of Esophageal Varices*.

TREATMENT OF SPECIFIC CAUSES OF ACUTE UPPER GASTROINTESTINAL BLEEDING

A national, multicenter study involving 2,225 patients with 2,486 causes of UGI bleeding diagnosed by endoscopy identified eight common conditions which accounted for 93.9 percent of all final diagnoses. In order of frequency these causes were (1) duodenal ulcer (21.8%), (2) gastric erosions—gastritis (20.9%), (3) gastric and stomal ulcer (20.7%), (4) varices (9.2%), (5) esophagitis—esophageal ulcer (7.2%), (6) Mallory-Weiss tears (6.4%), (7) erosive duodenitis (5.1%), and (8) neoplasms (2.6%). It should be noted that several patients (11.7% of all patients) bled from or had more than one potential bleeding source identified in this study.

Figure 1 outlines the general and initial approach to most patients with acute UGI bleeding and displays the common specific causes and their approximate frequencies from a large multicenter study.

Figures 2 through 6 depict my current general preference for a stepwise approach to treating the major specific bleeding lesions. For specific details on each therapeutic alternative in the schematic diagrams, reference should be made to that section on specific therapeutic alternatives in this chapter. Fixed rules must be avoided, however, and each patient's care must be individualized based upon a multitude of clinical factors present. There can be no substitute for sound clinical judgment and extensive clinical experience in treating these patients with acute upper GI bleeding.

In selected patients with torrential bleeding, endoscopy and/or other forms of medical therapy are impossible or futile and surgical intervention is mandated.

Regardless of the immediate therapy being rendered or the status of the patient's bleeding, physicians should always be contemplating the next logical therapeutic step to be taken should the current therapy fail or complications of therapy develop.

Some recommended treatments in Figures 2 through 6 may not have been proved to be safe and effective in well-controlled studies. A combination of factors, however, such as relative safety of a treatment, the cumulative weight of uncontrolled clinical trials, current concepts of pathophysiologic mechanisms, and experimental/theoretical considerations have been incorporated in the recommendations. Occasionally, when the stakes are high, when the remaining therapeutic options are limited or carry a known high mortality rate for a specific patient's overall condition; and when a relatively simple, safe, clinically effective albeit unproven therapy is available, one may elect to "have a shot at it" after obtaining informed consent.

Other Bleeding Lesions

Bleeding arteriovenous malformations and angiodysplasia may be treated by BICAP electrocoagulation, Nd:Yag or argon laser, or monopolar electrocoagulation in that order of preference. Bleeding neoplasia may be treated by the same modalities above plus surgical resection or snare coagulation (when the lesion is polypoid). Bleeding aortoenteric fistula requires surgical intervention. The chapter *Laser Treatment in Gastrointestinal Disease* has numerous helpful details.

REFERENCES

1. Conn HD, Grace ND. Portal hypertension and sclerotherapy of esophageal varices; a point of view. Endoscopy Review 1985; May/June:39–53.
2. Pitcher JL. Safety and effectiveness of the modified Sengstaken-Blakemore tube: a prospective study. Gastroenterology 1971; 61:291.

GASTROINTESTINAL BLEEDING IN CHILDREN

JEFFREY S. HYAMS, M.D.

The management of the infant or child with gastrointestinal bleeding involves three sequential steps. First, if intravascular volume has been significantly compromised *fluid resuscitation* should be vigorous and precede diagnostic studies. Second, the exact *site* of the hemorrhage is identified. Third, *specific therapy* based on the age of the patient and diagnosis is instituted.

General Measures

The presence of tachycardia and orthostatic hypotension in a child reflects the need for immediate intravascular volume replacement. A large-gauge venous catheter should be immediately inserted and normal saline or lactated Ringer's solution infused rapidly until the blood pressure rises and peripheral circulation is restored. In general, 10 to 20 ml per kilogram of crystalloid may be infused as a bolus without fear of overexpanding the intravascular volume. With massive bleeding, whole (preferably fresh) blood should be given to maintain volume as well as to replace red blood cells. After the bleeding has stopped, packed cells can be given, generally with a 10 ml per kilogram transfusion of packed cells (maximum 250 ml) given over 2 to 3 hours, depending on the degree of anemia. Underlying coagulopathies are treated with vitamin K (1 mg per year of age, maximum 10 mg, given intramuscularly), platelets, and fresh frozen plasma as necessary. In the patient who has bled from esophageal varices, care must be taken not to overexpand the intravascular volume, as bleeding may be exacerbated. Central venous pressure monitoring may be required.

Gastric lavage with saline is effective in children to clear blood in the stomach to permit endoscopy. Care must be taken, however, not to produce hypothermia in young children with iced lavage fluid. Further therapy then depends on the specific diagnosis.

Upper Gastrointestinal Bleeding

In general, upper gastrointestinal bleeding in a child falls in one of two categories. The first includes those disorders in which mucosal erosion or ulceration is important (esophagitis, Mallory-Weiss tear, gastritis, duodenitis, gastric ulcer, duodenal ulcer) and in which the aim of therapy is either to neutralize or prevent the release of gastric acid. The second category is variceal hemorrhage, for which a number of therapeutic alternatives are available in children.

Peptic Diseases

Antacids

In the case of an acute, severe mucosal hemorrhage, 0.5 ml per kilogram (maximum 30 ml per dose) of a high-potency liquid antacid should be given every 1 to 2 hours to maintain gastric pH at ≥ 5. If a nasogastric tube is in place, hourly measurement of gastric pH can be performed and therapy adjusted accordingly. Thereafter, the same dose can be given 1 and 3 hours after meals and at bedtime to complete a 4 to 6 week course. Serious drawbacks associated with antacid use in children include poor patient acceptance because of unpalatability, inconvenience of frequent administration, diarrhea or constipation, and potentially high sodium load. Both magnesium and aluminum contained in some antacids may be absorbed and cause toxicity, particularly if there is impaired renal function. These problems are particularly important in infants. Rarely, aluminum-containing acids cause hypophosphatemia.

Histamine$_2$-receptor Antagonists

Cimetidine has an anecdotally established place in the treatment of peptic disease in children. Unfortunately, there are no controlled studies to allow us to determine its efficacy or exact dosage requirements. I use 7.5 to 10 mg per kilogram doses given every 6 hours in the acutely ill patient, and subsequently before meals and at bedtime in the convalescent patient. The liquid form of this medication (300 mg per 5 ml) can be given to children who cannot swallow tablets. Patients with peptic ulcer are generally treated for 6 weeks. In patients with recurrent peptic ulcer disease I have had success with a single nocturnal dose of 10 mg per kilogram given prophylactically for 6 to 12 months following the usual 6-week treatment course. Cimetidine is usually well tolerated, although some children will develop diarrhea. Since cimetidine may inhibit microsomal drug metabolism, care must be taken in the concomitant administration of phenytoin, diazepam, and theophylline. Theophylline in particular is commonly used in the intensive care nursery, where gastrointestinal bleeding is common, and careful monitoring of theophylline levels is necessary if cimetidine is administered in this setting.

I have used ranitidine more and more often in older patients and have found it to be as effective as cimetidine. I use 2 mg per kilogram doses (maximum 150 mg) given orally twice daily, or 1 mg per kilogram doses (maximum 50 mg) given intravenously every 8 hours.

Histamine$_2$ receptor antagonists are not the agents of choice in the prophylaxis of gastrointestinal tract bleeding in severely ill children. I recommend the frequent administration of antacids to maintain gastric pH at ≥ 5.

Anticholinergic Drugs

Anticholinergics have little use in the management

of peptic disease in children. Their effectiveness is unknown and the incidence of side effects quite high.

Sucralfate

Theoretically, sucralfate would appear to be an ideal agent to treat peptic ulcer disease in children. Its effects are purely local and there is no significant systemic absorption. Unfortunately, it is only available as a large tablet, making it impossible to administer to most children. In my limited experience with this drug in adolescents it has worked as well as antacids or H_2 receptor antagonists.

Additional Therapy

In the child with uncontrolled gastric or duodenal mucoscal hemorrhage both angiographic and surgical intervention can be considered. Selective arterial infusion of vasopressin (0.0050 units per kg per minute, maximum 0.40 units per minute) has proven effective in the treatment of severe gastritis in some children. Arteriographic embolization may also be attempted if a specific vessel can be shown to be causing the hemorrhage. These more aggressive interventional techniques are rarely required but are preferable to gastric surgery if *experienced* vascular radiologists are available. Intractable bleeding requires definitive surgery.

Diet

Dietary manipulations are generally not of significant value in the treatment of peptic disease in children. I do, however, proscribe the intake of caffeine-containing foods based on their ability to increase gastric acid secretion. Bland diets and the frequent administration of milk are of no use, and probably will not be followed. Adolescents are advised to refrain from drinking alcoholic beverages and smoking.

Esophageal Varices

The most common cause of portal hypertension in children is extrahepatic portal vein obstruction. Since in this entity liver function is normal, bleeding episodes are generally better tolerated than in patients with underlying cirrhosis. In the absence of abnormal coagulation studies, hemorrhage is often self-limited, as the bleeding itself decompresses the portal system. Judicious sedation with morphine or meperidine is very helpful in allaying fears and sedating the child with hematemesis secondary to portal vein obstruction. Clearly, sedation must be used with great care if at all in the child with intrinsic liver disease. The therapeutic alternatives for children with continued variceal hemorrhage, whatever the underlying cause, are similar to those in adults and include the use of vasopressin, a Sengstaken-Blakemore tube, variceal sclerosis, and shunt surgery. Since aspirin intake often may precipitate variceal hemorrhage, its use is absolutely contraindicated.

Vasopressin

In children vasopressin may be administered as an intravenous bolus or by continuous infusion. The bolus dose is 0.3 U per kilogram (maximum 20U) diluted in 2 ml per kilogram of 5 percent dextrose in water, given over 20 minutes. This may be followed by continuous infusion of 0.2 to 0.4 units per 1.73 square meters per minute, if necessary. Administration through a peripheral vein is effective and catheterization of the superior mesenteric artery is not required. If the bleeding ceases, the infusion is maintained at the effective dose for 12 hours and then gradually tapered over the next 24 to 36 hours. Although generally well tolerated in children, the use of vasopressin may be associted with hypertension, reduced cardiac output, peripheral ischemia, abdominal cramping, and hyponatremia. No experience with the less toxic vasopressin analogue, glypressin (triglycyl-lysine vasopressin), has been reported in children, but, its apparent efficacy, safety, and ease of administration suggest a potential use in pediatric patients.

Balloon Tamponade

Although a Sengstaken-Blakemore tube may be fashioned for the pediatric patient, its use is associated with the same serious complications as seen in adults, including esophageal rupture, pulmonary aspiration, and airway obstruction. It is rare to have to use this device in children with variceal bleeding.

Variceal Sclerosis

This technique may well represent a great advance in the treatment of portal hypertension in children. Since variceal bleeding secondary to extrahepatic portal vein obstruction often diminishes following early adolescence, a palliative procedure such as sclerosis is much preferred to portosystemic shunt surgery. Additionally, since shunt surgery may be technically difficult in very young children, variceal sclerosis may sustain a child until he is a better candidate for surgery.

Although initial attempts at variceal sclerosis in children employed rigid endoscopy, I favor the use of the newer flexible instruments. Unless it is contraindicated by the patient's overall condition, most young children are better treated under general anesthesia than under sedation. Protecting an infant's or young child's airway with an endotracheal tube decreases the risk of the procedure and allows the endoscopist to proceed at a more relaxed pace. Once the varices are inspected and their size and location noted, injections are begun at the cardia with the needle inserted either directly into or alongside each varix. I currently use 5 percent sodium morrhuate and will inject 0.5 to 1.0 ml of sclerosant into each of the multiple sites to a maximum of 7 to 10 ml per session. The patient is maintained in a semi upright position during the procedure to provide drainage of blood into the stomach. Clear liquids are allowed 6 to 8 hours following each sclerosis session if the patient's overall condition permits, and solid food is given starting the following day. The variceal sclerosis sessions are performed weekly until all the varices have been obliterated. Three to five sessions are usually required. Follow-up endoscopy is performed at 3 to 6 month intervals and repeat sclerosis performed for the emergence of new varices. Complications of variceal sclerosis in children are similar to those seen in adults and include bleeding, esophageal ulceration, and stricture formation. There is a separate chapter in this volume on *Sclerotherapy of Esophageal Varices.*

Portosystemic Shunts

I feel that portosystemic shunt procedures should be undertaken only as a last resort in most children with portal hypertension. Shunt surgery may make later attempts at hepatic transplantation in children with intrinsic liver disease more difficult by disrupting normal portal anatomy. In children with portal vein thrombosis, attempts at variceal sclerosis should precede consideration of shunt surgery.

In children with cirrhosis, shunt procedures are similar to those in adults, although the distal splenorenal shunt is generally preferred. In children with portal vein thrombosis, central splenorenal shunts and mesocaval shunts are usually performed. Recent work has suggested that jugular vein interposition between the superior mesenteric vein and the inferior vena cava may be an effective procedure, even in very young children. Other surgical procedures, such as splenectomy alone and variceal ligation, are of no use in treating portal hypertension in children, since they are associated with a high incidence of rebleeding. The chapter on *Portal Hypertension* provides additional details.

Propranolol

No controlled trials using propranolol to prevent bleeding from esophageal varices have been performed in children. One report has documented a significant reduction in splenic pulp pressure in children with portal hypertension following propranolol administration at a dosage sufficient to decrease the resting pulse by 25 percent. Doses ranged from 2 to 8 mg per kilogram per day. I would urge caution in using this drug in young children before more published experience is available.

LOWER GASTROINTESTINAL HEMORRHAGE

Many disorders, with each having a predilection for a particular childhood age group, may be responsible for rectal bleeding in the pediatric population.

Infants

Anal fissures account for the overwhelming majority of episodes of bleeding in infants. Reassuring parents of the benign nature of the problem is the most important therapeutic step. In the presence of constipation a stool softener (Colace, ½ to 2 teaspoons per day) should be given. Scrupulous local care is important, and occasionally the application of hydrocortisone cream in an anesthetic base (Anusol-HC) may be helpful. *Protein-sensitive enterocolitis* can be seen following the administration of cows milk, soy milk, and even breast milk. Use of a protein-hydrolysate formula (Pregestimil) is usually sufficient and may need to continue for several months. If the initial illness was severe, I withhold the offending protein until at least 1 year of age. Rectal bleeding in the presence of fever and loose stools suggests *infection*, particularly with *Salmonella*. The incidence of bacteremia in children under 1 year of age with *Salmonella* gastroenteritis is more than 25 percent, and empiric antimicrobial therapy (ampicillin or chloramphenicol) should be started parenterally in the sick infant pending the results of blood cultures. If no bacteremia is present the antibiotics can be safely discontinued. Enterocolitis associated with *Hirschsprung's disease* must be treated with colonic decompression with a rectal tube, broad-spectrum antibiotic therapy (ampicillin, gentamicin, clindamycin), and a temporary colostomy or ileostomy. *Intussusception* generally occurs between the ages of 6 months and 2 years. Attempts at hydrostatic reduction with a barium enema can be attempted if there is no evidence of peritonitis or free gas in the abdomen. Sedation should be routinely used (meperidine, 1 to 2 mg per kilogram IV) prior to the procedure. Glucagon has no proven value in this setting. If the intussusception does not readily reduce, laparotomy is indicated. *Duplications* and *midget volvulus*, uncommon causes of bleeding, are treated surgically.

Toddlers

Many of the disorders discussed previously may also be seen in toddlers. *Meckel's diverticulum* is seen in both infants and toddlers and is treated surgically. *Juvenile polyps* frequently spontaneously slough and require no therapy. Persistent bleeding is often troublesome to patients and parents, however, and I will remove persistent polyps at colonoscopy. In 25 percent of cases more than one polyp is present. *Henoch-Schönlein* purpura is usually seen in toddlers and generally does not require therapy. In patients with severe cramping and rectal bleeding, intravenous methylprednisolone (2 mg per kilogram per day divided into two doses) can be helpful. It is continued for several days and then tapered over 2 weeks. Recurrence of symptoms is not uncommon. The *hemolytic-uremic syndrome* is an important cause of bloody diarrhea and is often initially confused with an infectious enteritis or idiopathic bowel disease. Intensive supportive care and early dialysis are crucial to facilitating recovery. Bowel perforation is common, requiring surgical intervention.

School-Age Children

Diagnostic overlap with the two younger groups is also seen in school-age children. The treatment of *inflammatory bowel disese,* a common cause of persistent rectal bleeding in this age group, is discussed elsewhere in this text. *Hemorrhoids* are rare in children and are always external. If present, constipation should be treated with either bulking agents or stool softeners. Local care with an anesthetic-hydrocortisone cream is often helpful. The clinician should also be alerted to the presence of occult portal hypertension in the child with hemorrhoids. *Intussusception* in this age group requires a careful search for a lead point such as a polyp, lymphoma, foreign body, and rarely, a Meckel's diverticulum.

STRESS ULCER AND ACUTE EROSIVE GASTRITIS

MICHAEL J. ZINNER, M.D., F.A.C.S.

Stress ulcerations are acute superficial lesions that occur in the gastric mucosa in patients subjected to overwhelming physiologic stress. The lesions occur early and have been endoscopically verified to exist within hours of the injury. Early they appear as interspersed areas of hyperemia and pallor which quickly give rise to submucosal microvascular congestion and accumulation of polymorphonuclear cells. By 24 and 48 hours, these lesions can lead to true ulcerations and loss of mucosal integrity.

The incidence in surgical intensive care units varies depending upon the setting and the scrutiny with which the patients are investigated. The accepted range is between 10 and 100 percent of all intensive care unit patients. A number of risk factors have been identified which contribute to the incidence of these lesions, including sepsis, peritonitis, respiratory failure, jaundice, renal failure, and hypotension. In the burn patient, the incidence ranges from approximately 25 to 33 percent. Eighty percent of patients with greater than 30 percent body surface burn will manifest some form of stress ulceration in the untreated state. Approximately 20 percent of these will manifest signs of true upper gastrointestinal bleeding.

The pathophysiology of stress ulcers is not entirely clear; however, the role of acid appears to be key. In an attempt to identify this role in one prospective study, 50 severely injured casualties were evaluated. Nine of these patients developed post-traumatic stress ulcer bleeding confirmed at either surgery or autopsy. In the first three to four days following injury, none of these patients had hypersecretion of acid as measured by nasogastric aspirate. The only group that did manifest hypersecretion of hydrochloric acid were those patients with neurosurgical trauma. The amount of acid withdrawn from the nasogastric tubes of patients sustaining trauma to the trunk or extremities was normal or less than normal. The explanation for this normal or low-normal acid secretion has little to do with the ability of the stomach to secrete acid, but appears to be related to the ability of the gastric mucosa to prevent the back diffusion of acid from the lumen into the mucosal cells. Normally, the parietal cells secrete hydrogen and chloride against an electrochemical gradient into the lumen of the stomach. The high concentration of acid remains in the lumen and the gastric mucosal barrier prevents the hydrogen from reentering the parietal cells. In the process the parietal cells eliminate HCO_3^-, which acts as a local buffer. The high HCl concentration in the lumen and high HCO_3^- in the cell maintains integrity. A number of experimental studies have demonstrated that agents such as aspirin, urea, and bile salts disrupt this normal gastric mucosal barrier and allow significant concentrations of H^+ to leave the lumen of the stomach and enter the surface cells. It appears that this increased H^+ ion back diffusion is the contributing agent to the development of stress ulcerations.

In the mid-1980s, endoscopy is the best way to confirm the diagnosis of acute hemorrhagic gastritis or stress-induced gastric ulcers. Angiography plays a role in the diagnosis but is more important in the treatment.

MEDICAL TREATMENT

The medical treatment of upper gastrointestinal bleeding from stress ulcer sources begins with lavage. Although iced saline lavage may be useful in keeping ancillary and medical personnel close to the critically ill patients, there is still controversy as to the use of ice or saline. Extremely cold temperatures are known to contribute to clotting disorders in both experimental settings and in humans. In addition, saline is isotonic and does not tend to remove red cells as effectively as water. I no longer recommend either iced saline or ice water, but would use water lavage to clear the upper gastrointestinal tract for endoscopy and then switch to saline to prevent the electrolyte complications of water irrigation. If irrigation is unsuccessful in stopping the bleeding, two additional procedures can be used. First is the addition of antacids to the irrigation fluid. This has been shown to be effective when the pH is raised to 7.0 but this was in uncontrolled trials. The second procedure is the addition of topical vasoconstrictor agents such as Levophed. Levophed is used by adding two ampules (8 mg) to 100 ml of saline irrigant; this solution is left in the stomach for approximately 15 minutes and then gently irrigated. This technique is useful when patients are bleeding from superficial erosions but is ineffective in any other form of bleeding.

In patients who continue to bleed from acute superficial ulcerations, angiographic localization of the bleeding site and infusion of vasopressin into the celiac artery or left gastric artery has proven to be effective. Unlike patients with portal hypertension, the direct arterial infusion of vasopressin is more effective than intravenous infusion. The doses used are the same as those for patients with portal hypertension, i.e., 0.2 U per min. Several of the contraindications include water intoxication, congestive heart failure, and angina. This technique should be effective in 80 percent of patients who are bleeding from acute hemorrhagic gastritis.

SURGICAL TREATMENT

Medical management to control bleeding should be effective in more than 75 percent of patients. For those patients who continue to bleed, the surgical alternatives available include all the standard techniques for treatment of peptic ulcer disease. There are no large prospective control trials that favor one form of therapy over another. By combining data from numerous trials, however, certain trends become obvious. Vagotomy and pyloroplasty in the patient who does not stop bleeding after conventional techniques has an estimated mortality of 33 percent with a rebleeding rate of 40 percent. Resection alone can be expected to result in a mortality of approximately 48 percent with a rebleeding rate of 55 percent. The estimated mortality from vagotomy and antrectomy is 40 percent with a rebleeding rate of 17 percent. This information leads me to recommend vagotomy and resection for patients who will tolerate such a procedure. Recently, a prospective trial compared gastric devascularization with vagotomy and pyloroplasty or vagotomy and antrectomy. Gastric devascularization is a rapid and simple procedure and resulted in a mortality of 33 percent and a rebleeding rate of 9 percent as compared with vagotomy and pyloroplasty, with a mortality of 55 percent and rebleeding rate of 61 percent. The operation of gastric devascularization should be considered as a potential salvage procedure in critically ill patients who may not be able to survive a major gastric resection. In general I do not favor total gastrectomy for this disease because of the high mortality associated with it.

PROPHYLAXIS

It should be clear that once bleeding occurs it is a serious complication in an already compromised host. The best treatment is prophylaxis. Numerous clinical studies have reported use of either antacids, cimetidine, or nutrition to prevent stress ulcerations. We have recently reported on a large series of patients in a randomized prospective controlled clinical trial comparing cimetidine, antacid titration, and placebo for the prevention of stress-induced gastric ulcers in an intensive care unit. The trial was conducted over a 2-year period and 300 patients were entered. They were randomized to one of three treatment groups with 100 patients in each group. Group 1 consisted of patients treated with cimetidine, 300 mg every 6 hours. Group 2 consisted of patients treated with antacid titration using Maalox TC to titrate the pH greater than 4.0 on an approximately 2-hour dosage schedule. Group 3 was a control group and they received placebo. All patients were admitted to the surgical intensive care unit with an anticipated stay of greater than 48 hours or they were excluded from the study. The end point of this study was bright red bleeding from the nasogastric tube or persistent guaiac positive nasogastric aspirate over at least two nursing shifts (16 hours). The average length of stay, mortality, and severity of illness were the same for all three groups of patients. Most patients were general surgical or cardiac surgical patients following operation.

The incidence of upper gastrointestinal bleeding in the control group was 20 percent. In the cimetidine treated group it was 14 percent. There was no difference between these two groups. The incidence of upper gastrointestinal bleeding in the antacid treated group was 5 percent. This was a statistically significant improvement over the no treatment group. The incidence of upper gastrointestinal bleeding that required transfusion was 7 percent in the no treatment group, 5 percent in the cimetidine treated group, and 1 percent in the antacid treated group.

In the group of patients we investigated, 75 percent in the no treatment group had a gastric pH less than 4.0 for a minimum of 8 hours. In the cimetidine treated group, with a fixed dose of cimetidine every 6 hours, one-third of the patients had a gastric pH less than 4.0 for at least 8 hours, indicating the presence of acid in the stomach. Among the patients with antacid titration none had significant amounts of gastric acid because of our titration regimen. In 88 percent of the patients on the antacid titration regimen, 20 ml of Maalox TC (approximately every 2 hours) was sufficient to keep their gastric pH over 4.0

We attempted to identify any complications of either drug regimen and could not. There was a higher incidence of regurgitation and diarrhea in the patients receiving antacid but this was not statistically significant.

Alternate Agents

Although antacid titration is extremely effective in preventing bleeding in the intensive care unit setting, it is not universally employed. No other form of prophylaxis is as effective, but no other form of prophylaxis is as labor intensive. The technique requires moderate work and attention to detail. For this reason other forms of therapy are now under investigation. Sucralfate has been shown in small studies to be as effective as antacids with virtually no side effects. It has the advantage of being simple to administer with no systemic actions. We will await further trials before we can recommend this agent.

The new H_2 blocker, ranitidine, has been very successful in the treatement of chronic peptic ulcer disease, but it will probably be no more effective than cimetidine in stress prophylaxis—that is, not effective.

One of the most interesting new areas of clinical investigation in this area is the use of prostaglandins for prophylaxis. There are a number of multicenter clinical trials currently underway to evaluate at least two different prostaglandin analogues. Although it is too early to comment on these trials, these agents have the theoretical advantage of being both antisecretory and cytoprotective to the gastric mucosa.

ALKALINE REFLUX GASTRITIS

THOMAS R. GADACZ, M.D., F.A.C.S.

Reflux of alkaline material into the stomach and esophagus may produce inflammation, which can produce symptoms, signs, and complications. Alkaline reflux gastritis has also been termed bile reflux and reflux gastritis. These nonspecific terms are the result of our lack of knowledge concerning the pathogenesis and treatment of this inflammatory process. Correlations among symptoms, findings, and the severity of inflammation are often lacking. In most affected patients the causative factors are poorly understood and may be multiple. At one time reflux esophagitis and gastritis were thought to occur only in postoperative patients, usually following an ulcer operation. It has now been well established that reflux esophagitis and gastritis can occur in a patient who has not undergone an operation.

ALKALINE REFLUX ESOPHAGITIS

Alkaline reflux esophagitis is probably uncommon although the frequent use of esophageal pH monitoring has made it evident that an increase in pH of five to seven has been associated with symptoms of reflux alkaline esophagitis. A patient with alkaline reflux esophagitis usually presents with symptoms of dysphagia, substernal burning, and regurgitation. Occasionally the patient may describe a bitter taste, which is usually associated with bile, as opposed to a sour taste, which is associated with acid. The diagnosis of alkaline reflux esophagitis is confirmed by inflammatory changes and/or ulceration at endoscopy and confirmed by biopsy. Alkaline reflux esophagitis is usually associated with alkaline reflux gastritis, and treatment of the gastritis generally results in resolution of the esophagitis. An exception to this relationship is the reflux esophagitis following a total gastrectomy with reconstruction with a loop of jejunum. Alkaline reflux esophagitis can be alleviated by converting the loop to a Roux-en-Y or by a large side-to-side jejunojejunostomy 45 cm from the esophagojejunostomy.

REFLUX GASTRITIS

Since alkaline reflux gastritis is a more common disease than alkaline reflux esophagitis, it is the main focus of this chapter. The most common symptom of gastritis is epigastric pain. Nausea and vomiting may occur and in severe cases anorexia and weight loss may also be present. Weakness associated with chronic blood loss and anemia occurs in a small percentage of patients. Physical examination is usually normal, although mild epigastric tenderness may be present. Agents that have been associated with gastritis include acid, pepsin, drugs, alcohol, and viruses. Acid injury is usually confirmed by low pH and the Histalog test confirms the presence of a significant amount of acid. Although the clinical symptoms are similar, these other forms of gastritis should be differentiated from alkaline reflux gastritis. Some of the endogenous substances that have been implicated in the development of alkaline gastritis include bile salts, lysolecithin, and trypsin. Trypsin can cause damage in an alkaline environment but the enzyme is inactivated in an acid environment. Bile salts have received extensive evaluation and have been shown to damage the gastric mucosa. Damage depends not only on the concentration of the bile salts but also on the type of bile salt. Factors such as pH, conjugation of the bile salts, and prior injury to the gastric mucosa are all factors that influence bile salt damage. The correlation between damage to the stomach and symptoms is usual but not universal. It is not unusual to see significant bile pooling in the stomach with minimal visual and biopsy evidence of gastritis. Other patients may have minimal changes in the stomach yet quite severe symptoms. These patients should be evaluated for other causes of abdominal pain, especially chronic pancreatitis.

Another concept that has been disproven is the association between gastritis and ulcer operations. In one study on alkaline reflux gastritis, about half of the patients had had a cholecystectomy, a fourth an ulcer operation, and 15 percent had had no previous operation. It appears that cholecystectomy has a permissive influence on the development of reflux gastritis. Many patients have no symptoms of reflux gastritis after an ulcer operation but at a later date when a subsequent cholecystectomy is performed, about 20 percent develop bile gastritis.

Diagnosis

The diagnosis of reflux gastritis may be difficult to establish. Frequently other diseases must be ruled out. The work-up of a patient with significant symptoms of epigastric discomfort should include endoscopy with biopsy. Bile gastritis may be suspected if there is pooling of bilious material in the stomach and gross and microscopic evidence of gastritis. A sample of bile should be taken at this time to determine the pH and bile salt concentration. An upper gastrointestinal and gallbladder series or sonogram may help rule out other problems, such as abnormal gastric emptying and gallstones. Serum amylase and liver function tests should be obtained to rule out pancreatitis and hepatitis. If the pH of the gastric aspirate is low, then acid is the most likely cause of inflammation and the patient does not have alkaline reflux gastritis. The bile salt concentration in patients with alkaline reflux gastritis usually exceeds 2.5 mM. These patients may have an increase in the secondary bile salt (deoxycholate). The basal acid output is usually negligible and the maximal acid output is usually low (less than 0.5 mEq of hydrogen ion per hour). Once other diseases, such as gastric and duodenal ulcer, marginal ulcer, alcohol-drug-induced gastritis, cholelithiasis, hepatitis, and pancreatitis, have been ruled out, the diagnosis of alkaline reflux gastritis cn be made with some assurance. The combination of bile pooling in the stomach, a high gastric pH, and gross and histologic evidence of gastritis strongly supports such a diagnosis. Reproduction of the patient's pain with gastric instillation of his own stomach juice or an alkaline solution but not with saline or acid was suggested by Warshaw as a relatively reliable predictor of favorable response to operative bile diversion.[1] A completely negative test was rarely followed by a favorable operative result.

Medical Treatment

Most of these patients can be managed without operation. Antacids can be very successful provided the antacid has the capacity to adsorb bile salts. Since gastric acid generally is not a problem in these patients, acid neutralization is not a major requirement for the antacid. Antacid is usually given as the initial treatment (30 ml between meals and 60 ml at bedtime). Since considerable reflux and pooling occur in a recumbent position, these patients should avoid large meals before bedtime and either elevate the head of the bed on blocks or insert a large foam wedge under the sheets to prevent reflux and to facilitate gravity drainage of the stomach. *Magaldrate* is a very effective antacid which binds bile salts. If magaldrate does not provide adequate relief, *cholestyramine* is prescribed and given at the same times (one packet between meals and at bedtime). Cholestyramine is not very palatable and patient compliance is frequently a problem. Hyperchloremic acidosis is a complication of cholestyramine. It occurs because the resin adsorbs bile salts and releases chloride. Complaints of muscle cramps and weakness should suggest this metabolic problem. Serum electrolytes should be determined to detect this complication and cessation of cholestyramine usually resolves the problem. *Metoclopramide* (5 to 10 mg orally before meals and at bedtime) may also be helpful by improving gastric emptying. Poor gastric motility occasionally contributes to pooling of bile in the stomach. Antacids, cholestyramine, and metoclopramide should not be given simultaneously, since there will be decreased bioavailability of these agents. The recommeded approach is to begin treatment with antacids alone. If this is unsuccessful, then prescribe cholestyramine. If this does not prove to be successful a combination of antacids and metoclopramide should then be tried. Once the patient starts improving the treatment is gradually stopped. If symptoms recur, antacids, cholestyramine, or metoclopramide are again tried. Various combinations may be needed until successful managment is achieved. I have tried cimetidine in several patients and have not had much success, although one study demonstrated a 60 to 70 percent improvement. Other agents, such as *sucralfate* and *prostaglandin analogs*, have some theoretical basis for the treatment of reflux gastritis but their value has not yet been confirmed by clinical trials. Future studies of these agents may demonstrate their usefulness.

Operative Treatment

Occasionally symptoms or complications become so severe that the patient should be considered for operation. The indications for operation generally include weight loss, anemia associated with chronic bleeding, and severe pain. Generally I try to avoid operating on these patients if pain is the only problem. Some of these patients may have chronic pancreatitis as their major problem and this diagnosis may be difficult to establish and distinguish from alkaline reflux gastritis. When operative treatment is indicated, the object of the operation is to divert duodenal contents from the stomach. Before such an operation is contemplated it is imperative to assess the acid secretory capacity of the stomach. A standard Histalog test should be done and if the maximal acid output is greater than 3 or 4 mEq per hour, the diagnosis of reflux gastritis should be doubted. If there is significant acid secretion, it is usually not advisable to proceed with an operation that diverts duodenal material from a gastroenteric area, since a more severe complication, such as marginal ulcer, may result from the unbuffered effects of acid on the jejunum. The preferred operation for reflux gastritis is a 45-cm Roux-en-Y jejunal loop. This is usually accompanied by a vagotomy and Billroth II. About 85 percent of the patients requiring operative treatment will obtain a good result. A gastric perfusion test, described earlier in this chapter, has been used as a possible predictor of operative results. It is usually not very reliable. An ileal loop has also been used as treatment but is much less effective than a Roux-en-Y. It consists of a 20-cm segment of jejunum interposed between the stomach and duodenum. Fewer than 5 percent of patients with alkaline reflux gastritis require operative treatment.

REFERENCE

1. Warshaw AL, Schapiro RH. Alkaline reflux gastritis. In: Bayless TM, ed. Current therapy in gastroenterology and liver disease 1984–1985. Toronto: BC Decker, 1984:90.

DISORDERS OF GASTRIC EMPTYING

ROBERT S. FISHER, M.D.

The functions of the stomach are fourfold: (1) to act as a storage receptacle for ingested food; (2) to triturate the solid components of a meal to particles less than 1 mm in size, which are then emptied into the duodenum in the same way as are liquids; (3) to initiate the early stages of digestion; and (4) to deliver nutrients into the duodenum and small intestine at a rate that will maximize digestion and absorption.

PHYSIOLOGY

To diagnose and treat gastric motility disorders effectively, an understanding of normal stomach physiology is essential. Although a comprehensive discussion of gastric physiology would be inappropriate for this chapter, some highlights will be reviewed. Both the secretory and motor functions of the stomach are highly specialized activities related to different regions of the stomach. For example, the fundus and body are rich in parietal and chief cells, which secrete acid and pepsinogen, respectively. The pyloric gland cells and perhaps those of the cardia secrete much mucus. Similarly, the emptying of liquids from the stomach is controlled mostly by motor activity in the fundus and proximal body of the stomach, whereas the emptying of solids is related predominantly to antral and pyloric motility.

PATHOPHYSIOLOGY

A number of factors may influence gastric motility, such as the volume of the meal, which may stimulate mechanoreceptors by distending the wall of the stomach, and the chemical and physical composition of meals, which may interact with osmoreceptors, stimulate the release of active peptides from the small bowel mucosa, or stimulate a number of enterogastric neural reflexes. Abnormal gastric motility may be associated with either rapid or delayed stomach emptying. Rapid stomach emptying may produce a number of symptoms, including lightheadedness, abdominal pain, diaphoresis, tachycardia, and even diarrhea. This constellation of symptoms has been referred to as the *dumping symdrome*. Potential causes of the dumping syndrome include duodenal or jejunal overdistention, rapid intestinal transit, maldigestion, reactive hypoglycemia, and increased gas production. Symptoms may be mediated by the release of active agents such as serotonin, prostaglandins, vasoactive intestinal polypeptide, insulin, and others. Rapid stomach emptying may occur in hyperthyroidism and gastrinoma, but is usually the result of gastroduodenal surgery.

Delayed stomach emptying is much more common and can be subdivided into two major categories: delayed emptying due to increased gastroduodenal junction resistance, often referred to as mechanical obstruction; and delayed emptying due to failure of the stomach to generate an effective propulsive force, i.e., functional obstruction or gastroparesis. A variety of nonspecific symptoms may suggest that stomach emptying is prolonged, including early satiety, postprandial abdominal distention or bloating, epigastric pain, nausea, vomiting, and weight loss. Vomiting of undigested food may occur immediately or hours after food has been ingested. An audible succussion splash over the abdomen may provide a clue to delayed emptying of the stomach.

A number of disorders may produce mechanical obstruction of the stomach. *Duodenal* and *pyloric channel ulcers, pyloric strictures, benign hypertrophic pyloric stenosis*, and *tumors of the stomach* may all decrease the size of the lumen at the gastric outlet, thereby impeding gastric emptying. Both *incomplete relaxation of the pylorus* and *gastroduodenopyloric dyskinesia* are hypothetical disorders which to date have not been clearly demonstrated. Incomplete relaxation of the pylorus might create a condition analogous to achalasia with its incomplete relaxation of the lower esophageal sphincter. Gastroduodenopyloric dyskinesia might be associated with an ineffective gastroduodenal pressure gradient and/or poor timing between gastroduodenal contractions and pyloric relaxation. Clinical demonstration of these disorders will require improvement in the techniques available for evaluating gastroduodenal motility.

There are many causes of gastroparesis, or functional gastric outlet obstruction (Table 1). The subdivision is somewhat artificial, and there is certainly a great overlap among the groups. A comprehensive discussion of each of these disorders is clearly beyond the scope of this chapter; nevertheless, the protean causes of gastroparesis must be considered in order to treat the problem effectively. A number of pharmacologic agents may alter the electromechanical events associated with normal gastric motility. In most cases these effects can be rapidly reversed when the agents are discontinued. Similarly, an imbalance of electrolytes may change gastric motility. Certain metabolic disorders may create electrolyte or abnormal neuromuscular reactivity by virtue of excessive or deficient release of hormones. Elevated blood glucose levels have been demonstrated in some cases to slow stomach emptying. Whether infiltrative gastropathies impede gastric emptying by interfering with neural conduction or muscle contractility has not been determined. Certain systemic diseases have been associated with delayed stomach emptying. Scleroderma and dermatomyositis may affect nerves or muscles directly or may disrupt gastric emptying by virtue of concomitant vasculitis. The mechanism by which Crohn's disease slows gastric emptying has not been elucidated. Certain infections have been identified as occasional causes of gastroparesis. These episodes usually are self-limiting and reversible over time. Recently, attention has been drawn to the occurrence of gastroparesis in certain psychiatric disorders, such as anorexia nervosa, bulimia, and psychogenic vomiting. Positive responses to treatment with gastrokinetic agents have been reported.

TABLE 1 Functional Obstruction of the Stomach (Gastroparesis)

Drugs
  Anticholinergic agents
  Beta-adrenergic agonists
  Calcium channel blockers
  Cytostatic drugs
  Dopamine agonists
Electrolyte Imbalance
  Hypokalemia
  Hypocalcemia
  Hypomagnesemia
Metabolic Disorder
  Diabetes mellitus
  Hypothyroidism
  Hypoparathyroidism
  Pregnancy
Vagotomy
Infiltrative
  Amyloidosis
  Pernicious anemia
  Malignancy
Systemic Diseases
  Scleroderma
  Dermatomyositis
  Infections
    Nonbacterial (viral) gastroenteritis
    Guillaine-Barré syndrome
    Botulism
  Crohn's disease
Psychiatric Disorder
  Anorexia nervosa
  Psychogenic vomiting
  Bulimia
Neuromuscular Disorders
  Myotonic dystrophy
  Diabetes mellitus (autonomic neuropathy)
  Chronic idiopathic intestinal pseudoobstruction
  Aberrant gastric pacemaker (tachygastria)
  Familial megaduodenum syndrome
Idiopathic

Abnormal stomach emptying has been reported in a host of neuromuscular diseases. It could be argued that many of the causes of gastroparesis listed in Table 1 also represent neuromuscular dysfunction, which serves to emphasize the difficulty with any classification of these disorders. Diabetic gastropathy has received the most attention and is probably a manifestation of the autonomic neuropathy often seen as a complication of longstanding diabetes mellitus. Chronic idiopathic intestinal pseudoobstruction is a neuromuscular disorder that may involve any or all portions of the gastrointestinal tract. Abnormalities of the myenteric plexus have recently been seen in a number of patients. Several cases of an aberrant distal antral pacemaker, referred to as *tachygastria*, have been reported. Finally, in our center we are seeing an increasing number of patients with unexplained upper gastrointestinal tract symptoms due to gastroparesis, but this experience is not unique to our center. One wonders whether gastroparesis may explain the symptoms in some patients previously labeled as having functional or nonulcer dyspepsia.

DIAGNOSIS AND ACUTE MANAGEMENT OF GASTRIC OUTLET OBSTRUCTION

Let us now turn to diagnosis and treatment. The first step in the treatment of delayed gastric emptying is to diagnose it. Symptoms such as nausea, vomiting, postprandial abdominal pain, bloating or abdominal distention, and early satiety should suggest the possibility of an abnormality in emptying of the stomach contents. The presence of a succussion splash on physical examination would corroborate this impression. A careful history and physical examination may provide important clues to the cause of gastric obstruction. A past history of peptic ulcer disease, pyloric stenosis of the newborn, pernicious anemia, scleroderma, thyroid disease, abdominal surgery, or psychiatric illness might be helpful. Similarly, findings of neuropathy or autonomic dysfunction might suggest certain etiologic agents. A common mistake in the evaluation of a patient for abnormal stomach emptying is to perform an upper gastrointestinal tract barium roentgenogram followed by upper endoscopy as soon as the diagnosis is suspected. Usually when these procedures are performed early, they do not succeed in including or excluding mechanical obstruction because of the presence of marked gastric dilatation and copious amounts of food in the stomach.

An acute emergency should be excluded by performing a number of laboratory tests, and obtaining a roentgenographic obstructive series with erect and decubitus views plus an ultrasonogram to examine the gallbladder, biliary tract, and pancreas. An attempt should be made to remove retained food from the stomach using a large-bore tube. Next, an *indwelling nasogastric tube* should be placed in the distal stomach and connected to intermittent suction to *decompress* the dilated stomach. Whether a patient has mechanical or functional gastric outlet obstruction, gastric decompression is an important early therapeutic step for restoring muscle tone to the walls of the stomach. For mechanical obstruction, the older literature would suggest that decompression accompanied by intravenous fluid maintenance should be limited to 48 to 72 hours. Remember, however, that most of these reports were written before peripheral or parenteral alimentation was available to maintain or improve nutrition over extended periods. If there is a suspicion of peptic ulcer disease, intravenous H_2 receptor blockers should be administered empirically. I do not feel pressured to remove the nasogastric tube. Following several days of gastric decompression and nutritional support, *endoscopic* examination should be performed to detect benign or malignant lesions of the stomach and duodenum or a stricture of the gastric outlet. If endoscopy does not provide an answer, barium roentgenography should be considered. In most cases mechanical gastric outlet obstruction is treated surgically.

If the endoscope passes easily through the gastroduodenal junction and no lesion is detected, this suggests that functional obstruction or gastroparesis may be the cause of the symptoms. This impression can be documented by *measuring gastric emptying* using a test meal labeled with gamma-emitting radionuclide. There are a number of patients with symptomatic gastroparesis in whom liquids empty normally from the stomach but solids are delayed. Therefore, a labeled solid test meal should be employed; however, administration of a solid test meal to a patient with mechanical gastric outlet obstruction would be a mistake. In those few cases in which functional and mechanical obstruction cannot be differentiated using endoscopic and roentgenographic techniques, a radionuclide solid test meal should be withheld until normal emptying of liquid is demonstrated by performing a saline load test, measuring the residual gastric volume after clamping the nasogastric tube overnight, or both.

Measurement of Gastric Emptying

Over the years, a number of techniques have been utilized to measure gastric emptying. Barium roentgenographic studies are limited because they are quantitative and associated with high radiation burdens. Intubation techniques are inconvenient, uncomfortable and provide data only on emptying of liquids from the stomach. In 1966, Griffith and his colleagues introduced chromium-51-labeled porridge as a gamma-emitting radionuclide labeled meal to quantitate gastric emptying.[1] Over the years gamma-counting probes were replaced by rectilinear scanners, which have been supplanted by sophisticated gamma cameras on line to dedicated computers. *Radionuclide scintigraphy* using *solids alone* or *combined solid-liquid* test meals is the test of choice for making a diagnosis of gastroparesis. Gastric emptying can be observed by reviewing serial scintigrams obtained for either the solid or liquid compomentor of a test meal (Fig. 1), and using computerized data analysis. Emptying curves can be established for both components of the test meal (Fig. 2).

Causes of Gastroparesis

Once a diagnosis of functional gastric outlet obstruction, or gastroparesis, has been documented (Table 2), an effort should be made to rule out correctable causes. For example, certain pharmacologic agents may be responsible, and certain reversible psychiatric or medical diseases may play a role. A comprehensive neurologic examination, including computed tomography of the head and evaluation of cranial and peripheral nerve function, is essential. Medical disorders with specific treatments, such as hypothyroidism, hypoparathyroidism, and Crohn's disease, should be excluded. Esophageal and anal tonometry may provide clues to underlying systemic diseases.

THERAPY FOR GASTROPARESIS

Having made a diagnosis of gastroparesis, one must now proceed to specific therapy whenever possible and, if not, to nonspecific therapy (Table 3).

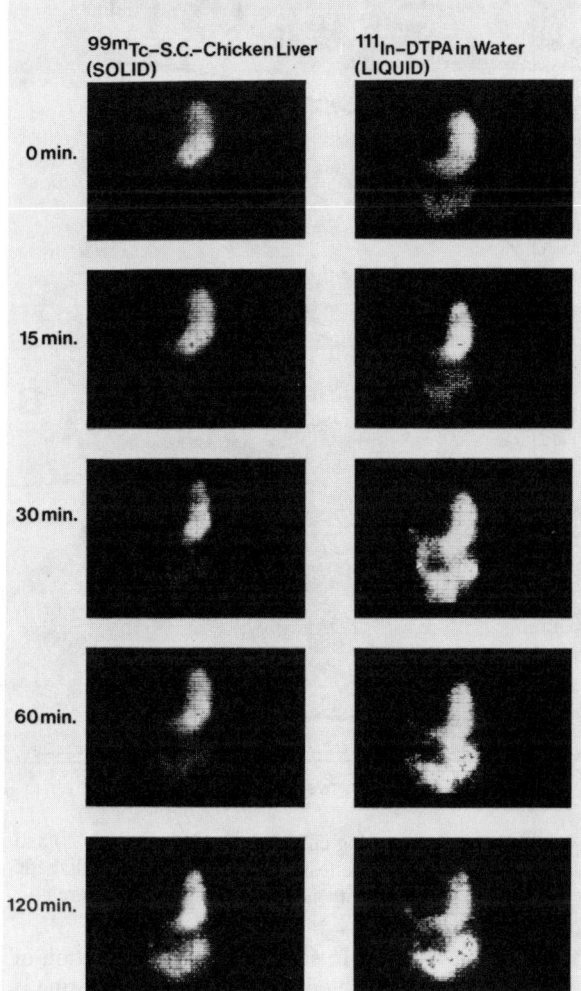

Figure 1 Serial scintigrams in a patient with diabetic gastroparesis immediately and at 15, 30, 60, and 120 minutes after ingestion of a test meal. Emptying of both the solid component (technetium-99-m-chicken liver) and the liquid component (inilium 111-water) is shown.

Dietary Manipulation

The efficacy of dietary manipulation in the treatment of patients with gastroparesis has not been tested. An empiric trial of several dietary manipulations may be worthwhile. After a period of gastric decompression using a nasogastric tube, it may be beneficial to feed a patient with frequent small, low-volume liquid feedings. A number of patients tolerate liquids before the ability to handle solid food returns. It is probably best to limit lactose and fat content during the initial stages of realimentation. In some patients it may be necessary to bypass the stomach for a while by instilling liquid supplements directly into the small intestine distal to the ligament of Treitz. This can be done with a nasointestinal feeding tube or by creating

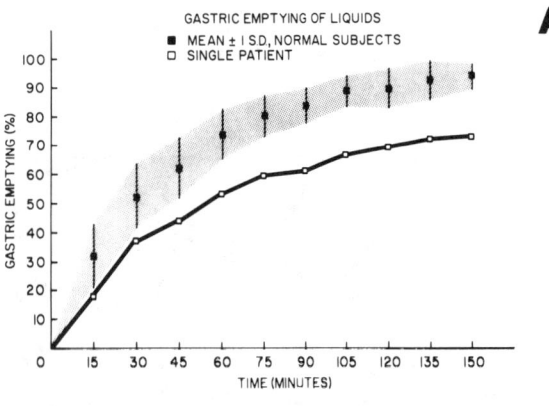

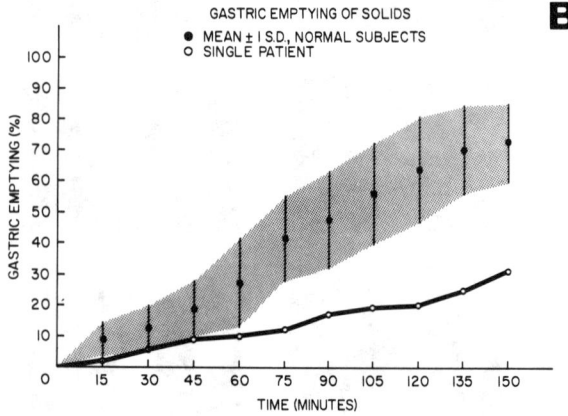

Figure 2 Gastric emptying curves for both the liquid (A) and solid (B) components of the test meal in a patient with diabetic gastroparesis compared with normal values (stippled areas).

a feeding jejunostomy. In some patients introduction of food into the stomach, duodenum, and small intestine is not tolerated. These patients may require home parenteral alimentation. In many cases the ability to tolerate oral feedings of relatively normal meals will return after a time using these measures.

TABLE 2 Diagnosis of Gastroparesis

Suspicion
   History and physical examination
Exclude acute process
   Complete blood count, amylase
   Obstructive series, i.e., flat plate of abdomen
Gastric lavage (Ewald tube) followed by nasogastric suction
   Peripheral or parenteral alimentation
Upper gastrointestinal endoscopy
Upper gastrointestinal roentgenography
Radionuclide gastric scintigraphy
Measurement of gastric emptying
   Intubation techniques
      Saline load test
      Residual volume measurement
      Nonabsorbable dyes
   Radionuclide gastric scintigraphy*

* Method of choice

TABLE 3 Treatment of Gastroparesis

Treat underlying medical illness
Eliminate causative drugs
Correct electrolyte imbalance
Dietary manipulation
   Small, frequent liquid meals
   Decrease lactose and/or fat in diet
   Enteral alimentation
   Home parenteral alimentation
Antiemetic Agents
   Phenothiazines
   Antihistamines
   Anticholinergics (?)
Gastrokinetic Agents
   Bethanechol
   (Cisapride)
   Metoclopramide
   Domperidone
Behavior modification
Psychotherapy
Surgery

Antiemetic Agents

For years the approach to pharmacologic treatment of gastroparesis has been limited to treating its associated symptoms, nausea and vomiting. The phenothiazines, especially the halogenated forms such as prochlorperazine and thiethylperazine, are potent antiemetics by virtue of their action as dopamine receptor blockers at the chemoreceptor trigger zone. These agents are not usually effective against central types of vomiting and may be associated with side effects such as sedation, hypotension, and extrapyramidal manifestations. On occasion, conventional antihistaminic agents (H_1 blockers) and antimuscarinic agents (anticholinergics) may be useful to treat or prevent vestibular-induced nausea and vomiting. These same agents, however, may aggravate or exacerbate gastroparesis from other causes. Recently marijuana (tetrahydrocannabinol) has been shown to be effective in treating severe nausea and vomiting in some patients. A role for marijuana in treating symptomatic gastroparesis has not been established.

Gastrokinetic Agents

The most effective agents that have been used to treat gastroparesis have been termed prokinetic agents or more specifically, gastrokinetic agents. The prototypical gastrokinetic agents are the cholinomimetic agent *bethanechol*, the central and peripheral dopamine antagonist *metoclopramide*, and the peripheral dopamine antagonist, *domperidone*. As shown in Figure 3, each of these agents has a distinctive structure.

Cholinomimetic agents are those that reproduce totally or in part the effects of acetylcholine. They may be structural analogues, like bethanechol; they may inhibit acetylcholinesterase, like edrophonium, or they may release acetylcholine from nerve endings, like the new

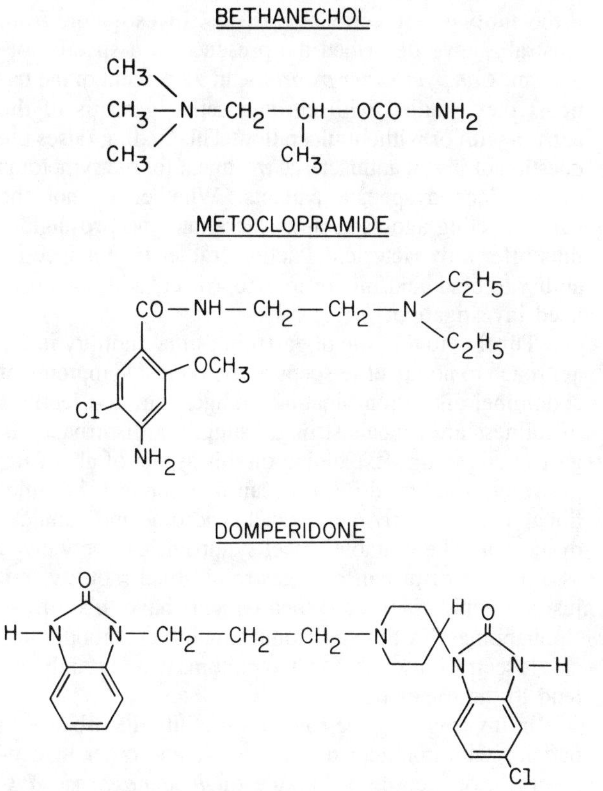

Figure 3 Chemical structure of three prototypical gastrokinetic agents.

agent, cisapride. To date bethanechol has received the most attention. It has a selective muscarinic action with predominant effects not only on the bladder but also on the gastrointestinal tract, manifested by increased amplitudes of esophageal, gastric, small intestine, colonic, and gallbladder contractions as well as elevated resting lower esophageal sphincter pressure. These effects would suggest that bethanechol might be useful to treat patients with delayed esophageal transit, gastroesophageal reflux disease, gastroparesis, small intestinal motility disturbances, and gallbladder stones. Despite bethanechol's varied potential clinical uses, there is little evidence for clinical efficacy in these conditions. Perhaps this is due in part to its potential side effects, which include excessive salivation, blurred vision, headaches, abdominal cramps, nausea and vomiting, bladder spasm, flushing, and sweating. To date, there are only limited published data on cisapride.

The other major category of gastrokinetic agents includes the dopamine antagonists. Metoclopramide is a drug chemically related to procainamide which exhibits dopamine receptor antagonism at both central and peripheral sites. Metoclopramide has a threefold mode of action: It may increase acetylcholine release from postganglionic cholinergic nerve terminals; it may sensitize muscarinic receptors to acetylcholine; and, most importantly, it antagonizes dopamine receptors. In addition to its prokinetic effects, metoclopramide has central antiemetic effects as well. Dopamine receptors are found throughout the body, not only in the gastrointestinal tract but also in the central nervous system, the nigrostriatum, the emesis center, the chemoreceptor trigger zone, the medulla oblongata, the urinary bladder, the ureters, and in selected blood vessels. Blockade of dopamine receptors with metoclopramide has been reported to increase the amplitudes of esophageal, stomach, and small intestinal contractions. It may increase resting lower esophageal sphincter and pyloric pressures, and it may improve the coordination between antral and duodenal contraction and pyloric relaxation. Some published data suggests that, because of these effects, metoclopramide may be useful to treat patients with gastroparesis due to diabetes mellitus, vagotomy, gastroesophageal reflux disease, anorexia nervosa, pregnancy, and unexplained causes. In addition, metoclopramide has been employed to empty the stomach before emergency anesthetization, endoscopy, or surgery. Metoclopramide has been prescribed at doses ranging from 5 mg to 20 mg, 30 minutes before meals and at bedtime. An unfortunate aspect of metoclopramide use is the relatively high incidence—20 to 30 percent—of side effects, including agitation, irritability, drowsiness, akathisia, increased prolactin secretion, and extrapyramidal effects. Metoclopramide is available for both oral and intravenous use.

A new prokinetic agent, under vigorous investigation in the United States but approved in many other countries, is domperidone. Like metoclopramide, domperidone blocks dopamine receptors, but unlike metoclopramide, domperidone is predominantly a peripheral dopamine antagonist. Therefore, it has fewer side effects. Domperidone is being tested orally in doses ranging from 10 to 30 mg, administered 30 minutes before meals and at bedtime.

Other therapeutic modalities available to treat these patients include *behavior modification* in selected patients who can undergo a program of operant conditioning for ingested food. *Psychotherapy* may be helpful in patients with obvious psychiatric disorders such as anorexia nervosa or psychogenic vomiting. Finally, *surgical* therapy may be employed in selected cases, but only after every effort is expended to ensure normal esophageal, small intestinal, and colonic motility.

REFERENCE

1. Griffith GH, Owen GM, Kirkman S, et al. Measurement of rate of gastric emptying using Chromium-51. Lancet 1966; 1:1244.

FUNCTIONAL DISORDERS OF THE UPPER GASTROINTESTINAL TRACT

GARY A. NEWMAN, M.D.
RICHARD W. McCALLUM, M.D., F.A.C.P.,
F.R.A.C.P.(Austral), F.A.C.G.

NONULCER DYSPEPSIA

Dyspepsia, or more appropriately nonulcer dyspepsia, refers to a symptom complex which includes heartburn, indigestion, abdominal/epigastric pain or burning, postprandial bloating and early satiety sensations, and even nausea and vomiting. The syndrome, which can account for up to 40 to 60 percent of all patients referred to gastroenterologists, includes various functional problems such as nervous dyspepsia, abdominal pains for which no organic cause can be found, and the visceral or somatic manifestations of psychiatric disease.

In dealing with nonulcer dyspepsia, a brief understanding of its presumed pathogenesis is necessary. First of all, the existence of gstroesophageal reflux, complicated esophageal disease (i.e., strictures, achalasia), peptic ulcer disease, pancreatic disease, small bowel mucosal disease, or biliary tract disease must be ruled out. Once this is accomplished endoscopically or otherwise, the treatment of nonulcer dyspepsia can be directed toward the suppression or neutralization of gastric acid, the enhancement of gastrointestinal motility, or the psychologic and emotional aspects of the disease.

Recent reports have suggested that patients with nonulcer dyspepsia have histologic increases in the gastroduodenal mucosal neutrophil count, possibly indicative of ongoing low-grade inflammation that is not yet endoscopically visible. This patient group, however, has never been shown to be hypersecretors and significant bile reflux has never been documented. Further, while patients have reported significant improvement of their symptoms with antacid ingestion, acid neutralizing compounds have not been consistently shown to be significantly more effective than placebo. Along these lines, H_2 antagonists, most notably cimetidine, have not been shown to be significantly better than placebo in controlling the long-term or recurrent symptoms of nonulcer dyspepsia.

Anticholinergic agents have also been used, but again there is little controlled evidence of a significant advantage over placebo. Nonetheless, *pirenzepine*, a new anticholinergic, acid-suppressing drug with selective antimuscarinic (MI) activity (thus avoiding antimotility side effects), has shown promise. Preliminary reports in peptic ulcer disease indicate that, used alone, its acid-suppressing properties are not impressive. Its most useful role may be to augment the acid inhibition induced by other agents. It may also be of some use if nocturnally administered.

Another new component in the increasing spectrum of nonulcer dyspepsia and gastroduodenal inflammation is the entity of "infectious" gastritis. Investigators from Australia have described the presence of a specific organism, *Campylobacter pyloridis*, in 95 percent of the patients they studied with chronic active gastritis of the antrum with or without ulceration. This finding raises the question of in situ antibacterial treatment for the symptoms of nonulcer dyspepsia patients. Whether or not the surface-acting agents such as sucralfate and prostaglandins offer any bactericidal action, rather than a specific ability to bind acid/bile or to cytoprotect, will obviously need investigation.

Turning to the role of gastrointestinal motility in the approach to nonulcer dyspepsia, the typical symptoms of abdominal distention/bloating, indigestion, and feelings of fullness after meals strongly suggest a disturbance in gastric emptying. Expanding on this aspect of abnormal gastrointestinal motility, one can interconnect the functional diseases of irritable bowel syndrome and nonulcer dyspepsia. The irritable bowel syndrome can be viewed as a diffuse disturbance of gastrointestinal motility, not just a colonic disorder. When patients have this diffuse "unhappiness" of the gastrointestinal tract smooth muscle, it seems reasonable that symptoms can certainly extend to the upper tract.

In investigating the role of a motility disturbance in patients with nonulcer dyspepsia, we and other investigators have identified the role of *duodenogastric dyssynchrony*. Normally there is a coordination of aborally conducted contractions that begin in the proximal stomach, extend into the antrum, and then progress through the duodenum and small bowel. Observations in patients with duodenogastric dysfunction show that multiple and often high-amplitude contractions of the duodenum can be observed without any indication that they initiated in the antrum. Moreover, these contractions seemed to be conducted toward the antrum rather than aborally toward the small intestine. This creates a relative duodenal block and presumably contributes to abdominal pain, duodenogastric reflux, bile reflux gastritis, nausea, and even vomiting.

In accordance with the above, manometric abnormalities have been recently documented in patients with functional upper gut symptoms. Measurements in the stomach revealed decreased antral phasic pressure activity after a solid meal, while probes in the small intestine showed unpropagated bursts of phasic and tonic activity.[1]

Another interesting aspect of gastric motility and its relationship to nonulcer dyspepsia is the concept of *electrical dysrhythmias* of the stomach and small bowel. At this point, longer and better studies in normal subjects are a prerequisite before one goes beyond the stage of postulating that some groups of patients with symptoms consistent with nonulcer dyspepsia may have dysrhythmias of the wavelike electrical rhythms of the stomach and small intestine. These abnormalities could vary from tachy- to bradyarrhythmias using the cardiology blueprint. The accompanying impairments in motility and/or gastric emptying could explain the patient's symptoms.

With the lack of specific gastrointestinal antiarrhythmic agents, treatment of these profound postprandial symptoms is currently aimed at reorchestrating a normal aboral propagation of motility. This is best accomplished by the prokinetic agents metoclopramide (note its similarity to procainamide, Fig. 1) and domperidone (still experimental in the United States, Fig. 2), which are the most promising drugs at this time.

Metoclopramide is a dopamine antagonist and partial cholinergic agonist that stimultes motility of the upper gastrointestinal tract without stimulating gastric, biliary, or pancreatic secretions. It increases the resting tone of the lower esophageal sphincter and increases and coordinates the tone and amplitude of gastric (primarily antral) contractions while relaxing the pyloric sphincter and duodenal bulb. It also increases aboral peristalsis in the duodenum and jejunum. *Domperidone* is similar to metoclopramide in that it is a dopamine antagonist and prolactin releasing agent, but it does not cross the blood-brain barrier and does not enter the central nervous system, resulting in no extrapyramidal side effects. In addition, domperidone neither augments acetylcholine release nor sensitizes muscarinic receptors as metoclopramide does. Therefore, it is not antagonized by either atropine or other anticholinergic agents.

Both domperidone and metoclopramide have been evaluated in patients with postprandial upper gastrointestinal distress or chronic postprandial dyspepsia. In placebo controlled trials, both metoclopramide (Reglan in the United States and Maxalon in England), given in a dose ranging from 5 to 15 mg orally one-half hour before meals, and domperidone (to be marketed as Motilium), given in a dose ranging from 10 to 30 mg orally prior to eating, have shown significant benefit over placebo.

Finally, the psychologic stresses and emotional tensions that are known to affect bowel function may be playing a role in some patients with classic nonulcer dyspepsia. In reviews of the Scandinavian experience with nonulcer dyspepsia, a majority of the patients showed signs and symptoms of inner tension, autonomic disturbances, and complaints of fatigability, irritability, and hostile feelings. The patients were also found to have an increased incidence of phobias, sleep disturbances, and obsessive-compulsive symptoms. Further, recent reports in the United States indicated that many patients with functional upper tract symptoms and normal manometry of the stomach and proximal small bowel had some level of psychiatric problems.

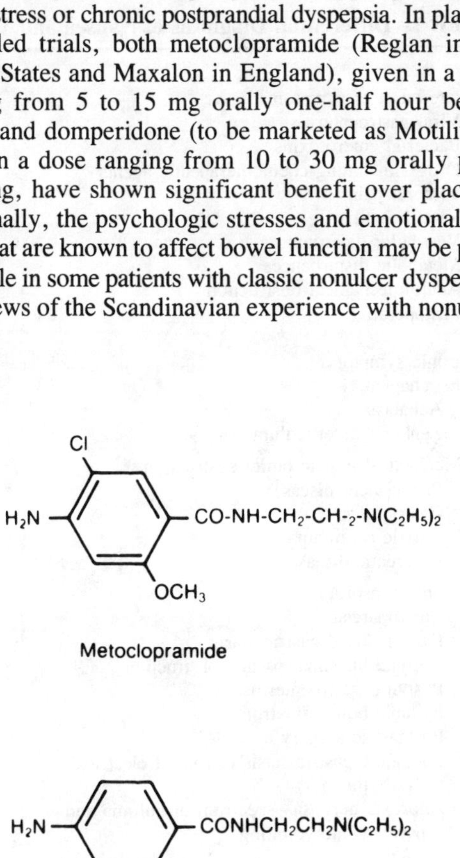

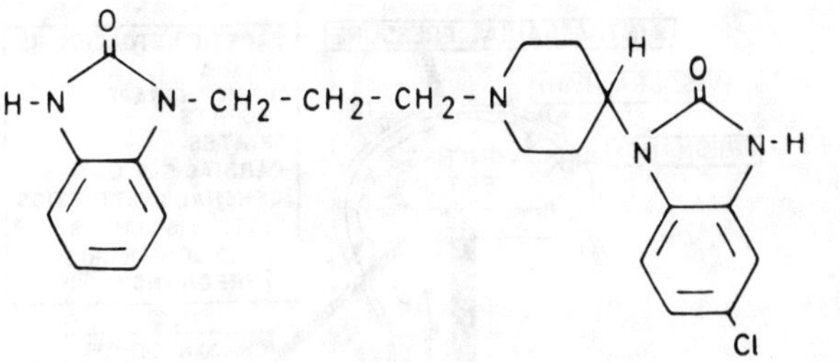

Figure 2 Chemical structure of domperidone.

The experience with the treatment of irritable bowel syndrome (IBS) is clearly an appropriate area for comparison. Patients with classic IBS are often sensitive, anxious, depressed, and may have abnormalities in learned illness behavior. Medical therapy in association with intensive psychotherapy has been shown to be more efficacious in IBS than medical therapy alone. This "holistic" approach in the absence of response to the standard medical therapies noted above may be necessary in selected patients with refractory, chronic, and relapsing dyspeptic symptoms. The chapter *Functional Illness* provides additional suggestions. Further information on nonulcer dyspepsia can be found in articles by Lagarde and Spiro[2] and Petersen[3].

NAUSEA AND VOMITING

The characterization and treatment of nausea along with unexplained vomiting is a difficult diagnostic challenge. While a precise description of the sensation of nausea is elusive, vomiting is a more physical and objective complaint and involves a complex interaction between the gut and central nervous system (Fig. 3).

The differential diagnosis of nausea and vomiting is wide-ranging (Table 1). Because of the multiple etiologic factors involved, extensive investigations are often necessary to pinpoint the cause and direct therapy at the appropriate source.

First of all, the usual history and physical examination, standard laboratory tests, and plain abdominal films are obtained. The determination of acute versus chronic/recurrent symptoms, the temporal relationship of vomiting to meals, and the association of other systemic complaints are the most significant points. In this initial part of the investigation, it is important to keep in mind

Figure 1 Structural formula of metoclopramide and procainamide.

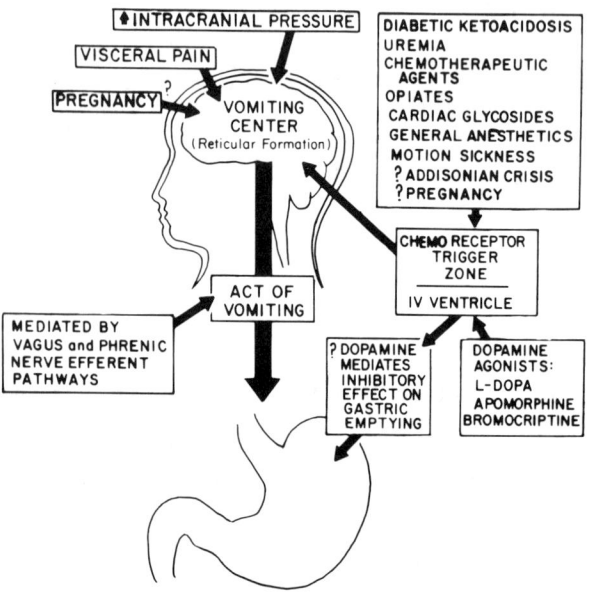

Figure 3 The central control of vomiting.

that vomiting can occur in healthy people as part of a strong emotional response, or in neurotic patients as a manifestation of underlying pathologic factors. Psychogenic vomiting can be recognized early by its classic pattern. The patient often has a long personal or family history of vomiting. Although the vomiting can often be suppressed, delayed vomiting is less common than vomiting directly after a meal. Stressful situations are often a precipitating factor in the reflex. Concealed vomiting and cyclic vomiting usually also fall into this psychogenic category. Bulimia is discussed in the chapter *Anorexia Nervosa and Bulimia*.

In the further investigation of unexplained vomiting, a standard saline load test may be useful in ruling out gastric outlet obstruction or gastric atony, but the key to revealing true mechanical obstruction or mucosal disease involves the use of upper endoscopy and/or barium studies. Peptic ulcer disease, pancreatic disease, or an upper tract malignancy can usually be defined and appropriately treated.

If mechanical obstruction is not present, more general disease states must be considered, and endocrine, neurologic (both central and peripheral), and more intensive psychiatric assessments are reasonable. At this point, therapeutic trials can be attempted, but if the patient's symptoms remain refractory, a thorough search for motility disorders is necessary.

Gastroparesis can be idiopathic or can occur secondary to drugs (anticholinergics, beta-adrenergic agents, opiates, tricyclic antidepressants). It is also seen after gastric surgery (e.g., after gastrectomy or vagotomy), in the diabetic patient, in metabolic disorders (e.g., acidosis, hypothyroidism), in connective tissue disease (primarily scleroderma), and in achlorhydric states, such as pernicious anemia. Disorders of gastric electrophysiology (dysrhythmias) have been reported in patients with unexplained nausea and vomiting, and upper tract symptoms can be seen in patients with classic irritable bowel syndrome.

While gastric manometry and electrophysiology studies can be obtained in some centers, radioisotope scanning is currently the most useful and available method for measuring both solid and liquid gastric emptying and is the test primarily relied upon to document emptying dysfunction.

Drug therapy for nausea and vomiting should always be aimed at the cause, if it can be delineated. Patients with symptomatic gastrointestinal upset from a labyrinthine source, i.e., motion sickness, can best be treated with *meclizine hydrochloride, diphenhydramine* preparations, *promethazine hydrochloride*, or *scopolamine* patches. Patients with immediate postoperative gastrointestinal distress often respond to *benzquinamide hydrochloride, prochlorperazine, trimethobenzamide hydrochloride, haloperidol* preparations, or to *phenothiazines*.

Patients receiving cancer chemotherapy develop severe nausea and vomiting both as a learned response prior to the actual administration of the drugs and, of course, secondary to the actual instillation of the noxious agents. The control of emesis in this case depends on the suppression of the peripheral and central pathways of emeto-

TABLE 1 Differential Diagnosis of Nausea and Vomiting

Acute onset of symptoms
   Viral gastroenteritis
   Bacterial enterotoxins
   Drugs, including chemotherapeutic agents
   Visceral pain
   Viral hepatitis
   Vestibular disorders
   Metabolic disturbances
   Acute mechanical obstruction
   Postoperative

Chronic symptoms
   Esophageal
     Achalasia
     Zenker's diverticulum
   Mechanical gastric outlet obstruction
     Peptic ulcer disease
     Gastric ulcer
     Gastric carcinoma
     Pancreatic disease
   Motility disorders
     Gastroparesis
     Drug-induced gastric stasis
     Chronic intestinal pseudo-obstruction
     Postviral gastroenteritis
     Irritable bowel syndrome
     Postgastric surgery
     Idiopathic gastric stasis (? role of electrical dysrhythmias)
     Anorexia nervosa—spectrum of bulimia and psychogenic vomiting
   Miscellaneous
     Pregnancy
     Increased intracranial pressure
   Psychogenic vomiting
     Self-induced
     Rumination

genesis and the chemoreceptor trigger zone. While prochlorperazine has been of little consistent use, particularly when the intensely emetogenic agent cisplatin is used, high-dose intravenous *metoclopramide* is useful in increasing the number of patients without vomiting at all. Further, intravenous *dexamethasone* has been found useful in controlling nausea and vomiting in these chemotherapy patients, and *tetrahydrocannabinol*, acting centrally, has been used with varying success.

In the postgastrectomy, postvagotomy patient with nausea and vomiting, the symptom complex may be due to either the disruption of motility or to bile reflux gastritis causing delayed emptying. Therapy with either prokinetic agents (discussed below) or with drugs such as cholestyramine, aluminum containing antacids, or sucralfate is reasonable. Bile reflux gastritis is discussed in a separate chapter.

The treatment of delayed gastric emptying without true mechanical obstruction deserves an additional note as the newer prokinetic agents are becoming more widely used. Metoclopramide, whose pharmacology has already been described, acts centrally as an antiemetic agent and peripherally to accelerate gastric emptying by increasing gastric tone and amplitude of the antral contractions. The drug also decreases relaxation of the proximal stomach, relaxes the pylorus and duodenal bulb, increases peristalsis in the duodenum and jejunum, and accelerates intestinal transit time from the duodenum to the ileocecal valve.

Domperidone is a benzimidazole derivative that is a specific dopamine antagonist. It stimulates the gastrointestinal tract and has antiemetic properties but does not readily cross the blood-brain barrier and rarely, if ever, causes extrapyramidal side effects. The usual dose of domperidone in various studies has ranged from 40 to 120 mg orally every day usually in four divided doses. While the oral form may be available soon in the United States, an intravenous preparation will not be pursued. The drug does have a potent effect on prolactin secretion, with other reported side effects including dry mouth, headache, and nervousness. While domperidone appears to be no better than metoclopramide as a prokinetic agent, its minimal side effects make it an attractive agent for long-term use, which can often be necessry in patients with diabetic gastroparesis or idiopathic gastric stasis. The drug may also be particularly useful in the treatment of the nausea and vomiting accompanying levodopa therapy for patients with Parkinson's disease, as it will not deplete central dopamine stores.

A mention of *naloxone* in the treatment of delayed gastric emptying should be made. The opiate peptides have been identified in the entire gastrointestinal tract, and it is well known that morphine has an inhibitory effect on gastric emptying which can be demonstrated by the systemic or intracerebroventricular administration of the gent. Naloxone is a potent opiate (mu) receptor antagonist and may be able to accelerate gastric emptying by antagonizing endogenous inhibitory peptides or by a direct effect on smooth muscle. While small isolated doses (2 mg via intravenous bolus) of naloxone may inhibit gastric emptying, sustained doses (1.6 mg subcutaneously daily) have been shown to markedly accelerate both solid emptying and small intestinal transit in a group of patients with intestinal pseudo-obstruction. Further studies on naloxone and its oral equivalent *naltrexene* are necessary.

A summary of the effective antinauseants/antiemetics currently available in the United States is presented in Table 2.

It is also important to note that there are multiple *behavioral strategies* for reducing nausea and vomiting. Hypnosis with guided imagery for relaxation, progressive muscle-relaxant training, multiple muscle-site electromyographic biofeedback, and system desensitization have all been used with some success. While these techniques have been primarily used in the anticipatory nausea seen in chemotherapy patients, their application, along with psychotherapy and counseling, may be extended to patients with functional nausea and vomiting.

If all attempts at symptomatic control fail, a trial of therapy with parenteral feeding may become necessary. Finally, the consideration of surgery involving a gastric bypass or drainage procedure is a difficult decision and lies beyond the scope of this chapter. There is a review of nausea and vomiting by Hanson and McCallum[4] and a discussion of unexplained vomiting by Malagelada and Canillieri[5].

HICCUPS

Hiccups, defined as the brief involuntary inspirations cut short by glottic closure, can be precipitated by many stimuli. While peripheral causes of persistent hiccups include gastric distention, intra-abdominal/diaphragmatic inflammation, and even tympanic membrane irritation, central causes encompass any central nervous system insult from infection to tumor. To complete the list, one should remember that intractable hiccups also occur in the setting of uremia and hyponatremia and also secondary to various drugs (e.g., Aldomet, diazepam, and sodium pentothal).

The management of hiccups is usually aimed at inhibiting or interrupting the irritated reflex arc. The traditional home remedies of gagging, breathing into a paper bag, ingesting granulated sugar, or drinking a glass of water while bending over head down are all worth a try. More complicated approaches include nasogastric intubation with gastric decompression, pharyngeal intubation, or high pressure O_2 inhalation.

Drug treatment with chlorpromazine (25 to 50 mg PO or IV) and metoclopramide (10 mg PO or IV) may be effective. Quinidine, atropine, amphetamines, and ephedrine have also been used. Hiccups are reviewed by Kaufman[6].

Eructation/Bloating

Excess upper gastrointestinal tract gas can result in repetitive and excessive eructation or complaints of up-

TABLE 2 Effective Antinauseant and Antiemetic Agents Available in United States

Phenothiazines (Prochlorperazine, Trifluoperazine)
  Mechanism: Acts primarily through the chemoreceptor trigger zone and on the vomiting center itself
  Adverse Effects: Extrapyramidal reactions, drowsiness, dizziness, hypotension, hypersensitivity reactions, blood dyscrasias, gynecomastia, cholestatic jaundice
  Dosage: Trifluoperazine (Stelazine)
    1–2 mg PO b.i.d./t.i.d.
    1–2 mg IM b.i.d./t.i.d.
    Prochlorperazine (Compazine)
    5–10 mg PO t.i.d./q.i.d.
    1–2 mg IM t.i.d./q.i.d.
    25 mg PO t.i.d./q.i.d. (as a suppository)

Butyrophenone (Haloperidol)
  Mechanism: Acts as a dopamine antagonist and antagonizes the chemoreceptor trigger zone
  Adverse Effects: Marked extrapyramidal effects, insomnia, confusion, lethargy, decreased seizure threshold
  Dosage: Haloperidol (Haldol)
    1–5 mg PO b.i.d./t.i.d.
    2.5–5.0 mg IM with dose titrated for symptoms

Metoclopramide Hydrochloride
  Mechanism: Dopaminergic antagonist and partial anticholinergic agent with both peripheral and central effects; increases antral contractions, increases jejunal and duodenal peristalsis, increases lower esophageal sphincter pressure
  Adverse Effects: Extrapyramidal reactions, sedation, restlessness, prolactin elevation, galactorrhea
  Dosage: Metoclopramide hydrochloride (Reglan)
    10–20 mg PO ½ hr p.c. and q.h.s.
    1–2 mg/kg IV ½ hr prior to treatment and then 22 hr × 3 (for cancer chemotherapy-induced emesis)

Trimethobenzamide Hydrochloride
  Mechanism: Acts on chemoreceptor trigger zone; useful for postanaesthetic and postsurgical nausea/vomiting
  Adverse Effects: Extrapyramidal symptoms, hypersensitivity reactions
  Dosage: Trimethobenzamide hydrochloride (Tigan)
    250 mg PO t.i.d./q.i.d.
    200 mg IM t.i.d./q.i.d.
    200 mg PO t.i.d./q.i.d. (as a suppository)

Benzquinamide Hydrochloride
  Mechanism: Nonphenothiazine with antiemetic, antihistamine, and mild anticholinergic actions; primarily used for postsurgical nausea/vomiting
  Adverse Effects: Drowsiness, dry mouth, tremors, fatigue, blurred vision, sedation
  Dosage: Benzquinamide hydrochloride (Emete-Con)
    50 mg IM × 1, then q1h × 1, then q3–4h p.r.n.

Promethazine Hydrochloride
  Mechanism: Phenothiazine derivative with additional antihistamine activity
  Adverse Effects: Dry mouth, blurring of vision, dizziness
  Dosage: Promethazine hydrochloride (Phenergan)
    12.5–25.0 mg PO/IM presurgery

Dimenhydrinate
  Mechanism: Depresses hyperstimulated labyrinthine function; useful in motion sickness
  Adverse Effects: Drowsiness, dizziness, dry mouth
  Dosage: Dimenhydrinate (Dramamine)
    50–100 mg PO q4h

Scopolamine
  Mechanism: Belladonna alkaloid with anticholinergic effects; probably acts to prevent motion sickness nausea by inhibiting the vestibular input of the chemoreceptor trigger zone
  Adverse Effects: Dry mouth, difficulty urinating, acute narrow-angle glaucoma, disorientation, memory disturbances
  Dosage: Scopolamine (Transderm Scop)
    One disk applied cutaneously (4 hr prior to expected insult) then q3 days p.r.n.

per abdominal bloating and pain. The gases involved include O_2, N_2, H_2, CO_2, and CH_4, with their primary sources being swallowed air, gut production via chemical reactions or bacterial metabolism, or diffusion from the blood into the gut lumen.

Swallowed gas, primarily O_2 and N_2, can arise from gases trapped in foods, during ingestion of liquids or solids (particularly in the supine position), and via the nervous habit of swallowing or aspirating air (aerophagia). The latter can occur at any time but may be worse during times of stress. It may result from the actual gulping of air, but much of the problem in patients who complain of "belching" rests with the unconscious inhalation of air. It is thought to be an unconscious "sucking in" or actual "aspiration" of air at points during the day associated with an automatic and unconscious relaxation of the upper esophageal sphincter. This then causes esophageal distention and the resultant rejection of the air based on an esophageal burping mechanism; the net result is eructation. Studies have shown that such air does not actually end up in the stomach, but is expelled efficiently by the esophagus after it reaches different levels, probably quite proximal within the esophagus. This cycle falls into the realm of an unconscious nervous tendency and may be very difficult to treat.

Gas can be produced in the gut when gastric acids or fatty acids produced from lipid metabolism react with endogenously produced bicarbonate to produce CO_2. Further, intestinal bacteria can produce large amounts of H_2 from nonabsorbable carbohydrates, and gut anaerobes can produce significant quantities of CH_4. Gases can be removed from the gut via eructation, passage of flatus, metabolism by intestinal bacteria, or via diffusion back into the blood. Eructation, the primary focus of this discussion, may occur when the basal pressure of the lower esophageal sphincter (LES) is low, when a transient increase in intragastric pressure occurs, or during transient but complete LES relaxation associated with swallowing. Further, some transient relaxations may be nonswallow-related and can be precipitated by esophageal or gastric distention.

Most of the patients who complain of repetitive belching are simply expelling swallowed air that has lodged in the esophagus. Cycles of purposeful air swallowing to precipitate belching may occur in an effort to relieve any discomfort but only exacerbate the problem. The patient rarely recognizes this and instead views his problem as increased gas production from some digestive abnormality.

Nonetheless, ruling out true organic abdominal or thoracic disease is necessary in many cases. Gastric outlet obstruction of any origin can result in trapped air and belching. Foul-smelling belching may be seen in patients with gastric bezoars. Milk/carbohydrate intolerance will usually not result in excessive upper tract gas but may be useful to investigate. Finally, we have seen severe eructation in diabetics with gastric stasis and have also seen complaints of abdominal bloating and belching in patients with small bowel overgrowth and in achlorhydric patients. Beyond the use of prokinetic agents, the use of ingested acids to minimize bacterial colonization has proved useful.

If true disease is not found, treatment is often difficult. For the patient with excessive eructation, the ingestion of hot water is a home remedy with variable results. The beneficial effect of simethicone, 40 to 80 mg orally four times a day, is also poorly documented. Acting as a surfactant, this agent may break up air bubbles but probably does little to the resulting gas released. Charcoal has been widely presented as an absorber of gas, but again, controlled studies on proven gastric gas diminution or a significant clinical effect on eructation are lacking. Metoclopramide and the newer prokinetic agents may be of some use in patients with complaints of bloating where there is really no evidence that they actually have excessive intestinal gas, but there is evidence that they tolerate the gas present poorly and/or could have slow gastric emptying. The patient should also be alerted to the fact that his complaints may be related to excessive air swallowing and, although bothersome, are benign. The patient should avoid reclining after meals and may benefit from a low-fat, low-nonabsorbable carbohydrate, low-lactose diet. Behavioral training is evidently of some help in patients with minimal symptoms but rarely helps those with severe complaints. (For additional information, see chapter, *Intestinal Gas*.)

RUMINATION

Rumination is a process whereby food is transferred from the stomach to the mouth, usually within 15 to 20 minutes after ingestion. Some of the food is chewed and reswallowed while some is ejected from the mouth. The act itself can either be involuntary, or voluntary with some patients actually putting their fingers down their throats or contracting their abdominal muscles to bring the food into their mouths.

Ruminators tend to be young patients, some younger than 17, with the onset of symptoms often becoming apparent by age 10 or younger. The patients usually seek medical evaluation on the advice of concerned family members who are either repelled by the habit or fear a more severe, more widespread problem. While the young ruminators tend to downplay the disorder and appear quite cheerful, the adult ruminators can often be depressed and anxious.

The possible association of significant regurgitation and vomiting in infants and rumination later on in the young adult is an interesting but totally unproven one. It is felt that gastroesophageal reflux in infancy is transient between the ages of 6 months and 2 to 3 years and that a resolution usually occurs over time. Infants with severe problems can present with either failure to thrive or pulmonary complications, and we have reported a delay in gastric emptying of liquid formula in this group which apparently improves with time.

We have been intrigued by the possibility of anatomic defects being present in the population of young adult and adult patients with rumination. While LES pressure measurements have been normal in this group, it is possible that some impairment of the angle of His or in the gastric sling fibers could lead to a failed valve mechanism and free reflux. These patients often present to the gstroenterologist for the evaluation of reflux disease, but true complaints of heartburn are rare. Further, despite the long duration of presumed rumination, complicating problems of weight loss, aspiration, coughing, or nocturnal regurgitation are usually absent. While pH studies of the esophagus can show an acid milieu during the events of reflux, motility studies and endoscopy are usually normal and gastric emptying studies have shown normal or even rapid emptying rather than delayed rates. We have actually recommended fundoplication of the gastroesophageal junction in one patient in whom the volume and social embarrassment of the problem were not acceptable. The outcome was successful, and this should be kept in mind as a last resort.

Other approaches include psychotherapy and mechanical restraints, including a device known as a "ruminator cap" which keeps the patient's jaws shut when placed postprandially, plugging the nostrils, or restraining the arms so that self-gagging cannot be carried out. The passage of time and reassurance of patient and family that a disease process is not being missed and that severe complications do not occur play an important role.

ABDOMINAL EPILEPSY

Abdominal epilepsy is a rare cause of abdominal pain in children and young adults. The criteria for diagnosis include intermittent abdominal pain of unknown cause associated with occasional alterations of mental status during the attacks, an abnormal EEG, and a response to anticonvulsant therapy.

The pains are often periumbilical, are described as sudden in onset, and can last from minutes to hours. The patients can complain of nausea and vomiting during the attacks and there are reports of altered consciousness and postattack fatigue.

While the EEG abnormalities seen in these patients are somewhat nonspecific, generalized slow wave dysrhythmia and paroxysmal 6 and 14 per second positive spikes seem the most prominent findings. Sleep studies may be necessary for case detection.

Whether anticonvulsants such as phenytoin (Dilantin, 300 mg orally daily) or phenobarbitol (90 mg orally daily) control the reported pain centrally or peripherally is unknown. there have been no studies evaluating the effect of Dilantin on either gastrointestinal motility or disorders in which an abnormal gastrointestinal electrical rhythm is suspected. The one study of Dilantin in irritable bowel syndrome showed it to be more effective than placebo. Occasionally a teenager with unrecognized lactose intolerance may present with recurrent abdominal pain, as discussed in the chapter *Recurrent Abdominal Pain in Childhood and Adolescence*. Zarling has published a review of abdominal epilepsy[7].

REFERENCES

1. Malagelada J-R, Stanghellini V. Manometric evaluation of functional upper gut symptoms. Gastroenterology 1985; 88:1223.
2. Lagarde SP, Spiro HM. Non-ulcer dyspepsia. Clin Gastro 1984; 13:347.
3. Petersen H. Further investigations and treatment of non-ulcer dyspepsia. Scand J Gastro 1982; 17 (Suppl 72):130.
4. Hanson JS, McCallum RW. The diagnosis and management of nausea and vomiting: a review. Am J Gastro 1985; 80:210.
5. Malagelada J-R, Canillieri M. Unexplained vomiting: a diagnostic challenge. Ann Int Med 1984; 101:211.
6. Kaufman HJ. Hiccups: causes, mechanisms, and treatment. Pract Gastro 1985; 9:12.
7. Zarling EJ. Abdominal epilepsy: an unusual cause of recurrent abdominal pain. Am J Gastro 1984; 79:681.

OBESITY

THOMAS POZEFSKY, M.D.

The physician is justifiably concerned with the overweight patient when the degree of obesity is sufficient of itself to constitute a physical health hazard, or when a coexisting medical condition, such as diabetes or hypertension, is exacerbated by the increased weight. While such physical health considerations should and frequently do motivate the obese patient to attempt weight reduction, this is not always the case. Very commonly patients are motivated simply by unhappiness with their appearance. To them their weight constitutes a "mental health" hazard; and, of course, the patient's psychological well-being is also the physician's legitimate concern. Achieving and maintaining weight loss is a difficult and lifelong undertaking. To facilitate this process it is important for the physician to provide or reinforce motivation by clearly defining the physical health benefits to be derived from weight reduction, by understanding the patient's objectives (even when cosmetic), by helping to define realistic weight goals, by providing a specific diet plan, and by empathizing with the patient's ongoing struggle to deny himself food.

INITIAL EVALUATION

The primary purposes of the initial history, physical examination, and laboratory evaluation are self-evident. Onset and progression of the weight problem are characterized, the degree of obesity is quantified, the presence of underlying genetic or endocrine-metabolic disease of etiologic significance is sought, and symptoms or disease processes complicating the obesity and potentially ameliorated by weight reduction are identified (Table 1). Details of the initial physical examination should not be compromised. Obese patients frequently view themselves as metabolically abnormal, capable of gaining weight while consuming no more, and often fewer, calories than those around them. Consequently, confidence in the physician and the therapeutic program can be jeopardized if the clinical evaluation is viewed as too superficial to detect underlying metabolic disease. In this context it is useful to ask the question: "Why do you think you are overweight?" Some will frankly assume responsibility by acknowledging overeating (even binging), or lack of exercise. Others will respond in metabolic terms, and it is these patients who must come away from the initial examination feeling that their "metabolism" has been adequately evaluated. It is likely that patients with the "metabolic mentality" are more inclined to seek therapy from an internist, endocrinologist, or related subspecialist, while those who frankly acknowledge overeating gravitate toward more psychiatrically oriented programs.

Just as obesity can be caused by and/or lead to abnormalities in the patient's physical health, so it can be caused by and result in psychiatric disturbance. In such patients overeating is often stimulated by anxiety, depression, boredom, fatigue, and cravings rather than by hunger. It is estimated that binging (complete loss of control over food intake) occurs in one-half to two-thirds of overweight patients. Desperate attempts to prevent weight gain include the induction of vomiting and the abuse of diuretics and laxatives. Not only depressed by their weight, such patients are mortified by their inability to control such a fundamental biologic activity as food intake. The whole problem takes on the character of a substance abuse, and as such, it is obvious that there must be a psychologically oriented component to the evaluation and management of these patients. The evaluation outlined in Table 1 does not adequately define the psychological dimension. Most internists (and gastroenterologists) are not comfortable doing a detailed psychologic assessment. Yet sensitivity to this aspect of the problem is important in establishing rapport with the patient. As outlined later in this discussion, it may be wise at some point in the therapeutic program to collaborate with a behavioral psychologist in undertaking a formal analysis of eating behavior. One explanation for the poor overall results of nutrition-metabolism oriented programs on one hand and behavior oriented programs on the other is that both disciplines are required for the proper management of practically all patients.

TABLE 1 Initial Evaluation of the Obese Patient

Onset and Progression	Etiology	Complications
History:		
Age at onset and first diet	Symptoms of:	Symptoms of:
Weight at high school graduation, college graduation, marriage, discharge from service, after deliveries, menopause, one year ago	Hypothyroidism	Diabetes
	Hypogonadism	Hypertension
	Polycystic ovary	Congestive heart failure
	Hypoglycemia	Pickwickian syndrome
	Intracranial mass	Sleep-apnea
	Depression	Degenerative joint disease
Success of previous efforts (diet clubs, physician supervised diets, personal diets, use of diet pills): amount of weight lost, how long sustained	Anxiety	Gout
	Family history of obesity	Gallstones
	Use of antidepressants	Esophageal reflux
	Exercise level	Menstrual irregularity
Lowest, highest adult weight and "typical" weight last 5–10 years		
Physical Examination:		
Height	Slow reflexes, goiter	Hypertension
Weight	Striae, buffalo hump, central fat distribution	Right upper quadrant tenderness
Wrist circumference*		Varicose veins, phlebitis
	Hirsutism	Asterixis, facial rubor, somnolence
	Small testes	
	Papilledema	Intertrigo
	Retinitis pigmentosa, polydactyly (Bardet-Biedl syndrome)	Joint tenderness or deformity
	Hypotonia, mental retardation (Prader-Willi syndrome)	
Laboratory Tests†:		
	Thyroxine, TSH	HDL and LDL cholesterol
	24-hr urine free cortisol	Triglyceride
	Testosterone, FSH and LH	Blood sugar, GTT
		Blood gases, spirogram
	Androstenedione	Roentgenograms of back, knees, hips
	CT scan of head	Uric acid
		Gallbladder sonogram

* Used to calculate body frame size (see text and Table 2).
† A minimum laboratory evaluation includes a CBC, urinalysis, spirogram, EKG, chest film, serum thyroxine, multichannel blood analysis (glucose, creatinine, electrolytes, uric acid, liver function studies), triglycerides, and HDL and total cholesterol.

FIRST RETURN VISIT

Discussion of Results

The purpose of the first return visit is to review the findings of the initial evaluation and present the specifics of the diet program to the patient. In most instances the obesity is found not to be secondary to an identifiable underlying disease process. Consequently, it should be made clear that the principal component of the weight control program will be restriction of food intake. One need not directly contradict those patients who perceive themselves to be metabolically abnormal. It is fair to tell them that medical researchers have identified several metabolic and hormonal differences between obese and thin people. However, as these differences disappear when the obese patient loses weight, they are the result rather than the cause of obesity. The patient's perception of a primary metabolic error may be correct, but since the error has thus far escaped detection, control of food intake must be the basic therapeutic approach. An increase in fat cell number is associated with early onset obesity and persists despite weight reduction. The significance of this finding in terms of ability to lose weight and maintain weight loss is speculative, although long-term success is poorest in those with obesity of adolescent or preadolescent onset.

Coexistent risk factors identified in the patient and known to be responsive to weight reduction (hyperglycemia, hypertriglyceridemia, increased low-density lipoprotein, cholesterol, decreased high-density lipoprotein cholesterol, and hypertension) should be discussed. Physical conditions complicating obesity and their potential response to weight reduction require elaboration. All this serves to reinforce whatever motivation the patient brings to the process.

Set Weight Goals

At this point weight goals should be discussed. Body frame size is estimated from the ratio of height to wrist circumference (Table 2). Ideal body weight is determined from the Metropolitan Life Insurance Company table (Table 3) as the midpoint of the ideal weight range for a given height and frame size. Percent overweight is the ratio of the patient's actual weight to his ideal weight. A weight greater than 120 percent of ideal shortens life expectancy even in the absence of coexistent risk factors. Such patients are considered obese. Patients 110 to 120 percent of ideal are considered overweight.

The initial objective should be to decrease weight to 120 percent of ideal. When this is achieved, risk factors and residual physical symptoms can be reassessed as a guide to further weight reduction. In the patient without risk factors or physical symptoms who is within 120 percent of ideal, the need for weight reduction lies in the psychological sphere. Cosmetic considerations are usually paramount, and the patient must suggest the weight goal. The role of the physician is to be sure the desired weight is not inappropriately low as gauged both by the patient's weight history and the ideal weight range indicated in Table 3.

General Principles of the Diet

The patient must now be told what to eat. The only imperative in the design of a diet is that it be hypocaloric. The balanced low calorie diet recommended by most nutritionists and diet clubs, and typified by the American Diabetes Association exchange list diet, is widely used. Its attractiveness follows from its nutritional adequacy (except for calories), and from the flexibility it gives patients in food selection. Theoretically, it can be followed indefinitely, with minor upward adjustments in calorie intake when the patient achieves his weight goal.

TABLE 2 Estimation of Frame Size from the Ratio of Height to Wrist Circumference*

Frame Size	Male	Female
Small	> 10.4	> 11.0
Medium	9.6–10.4	10.1–11.0
Large	< 9.6	< 10.1

* Height (inches); wrist circumference (inches)

TABLE 3 Ideal Body Weight According to Sex and Height*

Height Feet	Height Inches	Small Frame	Medium Frame	Large Frame
Men				
5	2	128–134	131–141	138–150
5	3	130–136	133–143	140–153
5	4	132–138	135–145	142–156
5	5	134–140	137–148	144–160
5	6	136–142	139–151	146–164
5	7	138–145	142–154	149–168
5	8	140–148	145–157	152–172
5	9	142–151	148–160	155–176
5	10	144–154	151–163	158–180
5	11	146–157	154–166	161–184
6	0	149–160	157–170	164–188
6	1	152–164	160–174	168–192
6	2	155–168	164–178	172–197
6	3	158–172	167–182	176–202
6	4	162–176	171–187	181–207
Women				
4	10	102–111	109–121	118–131
4	11	103–113	111–123	120–134
5	0	104–115	113–126	122–137
5	1	106–118	115–129	125–140
5	2	108–121	118–132	128–143
5	3	111–124	121–135	131–147
5	4	114–127	124–138	134–151
5	5	117–130	127–141	137–155
5	6	120–133	130–144	140–159
5	7	123–136	133–147	143–163
5	8	126–139	136–150	146–167
5	9	129–142	139–153	149–170
5	10	132–145	142–156	152–173
5	11	135–148	145–158	155–176
6	0	138–151	148–162	158–179

* Weights at ages 25 to 59 based on lowest mortality. Weights are in pounds, in indoor clothing weighing 5 pounds in men and 3 pounds in women, and shoes with 1 inch heels. Metropolitan Life Insurance Company, 1983. (Source of basic data, 1979 Build Study Society of Actuaries and Association of Life Insurance Medical Directors of America, 1980.)

Unfortunately, fewer than 30 percent of patients following a balanced low calorie diet lose more than 20 pounds; fewer than 5 percent lose more than 40 pounds. Hence, this diet rarely has a significant impact on the more obese patient who is of greatest medical concern. It is precisely the diet's variety that appears to be at fault. The overweight patient needs rigidity rather than flexibility—the fewer choices the better. He has already demonstrated an inability to make appropriate food selections, and prefers explicit guidance by the physician. Beyond this, poor control over the intake of certain specific foods appears to be characteristic of many very obese patients. These foods are generally rich in carbohydrate and sweet (chocolate, ice cream, Coca-Cola, cookies, cake), "starchy" but not sweet (bread, pasta, crackers, pizza), or salty and crunchy (chips, pretzels). The small amounts of such foods permitted on the balanced low calorie diet stimulate overeating just as small quantities of alcohol in the diet of the alcoholic lead to its overindulgence. Consequently, although the low calorie diet makes sense nutritionally, it may not behaviorally.

One reason for surprisingly good initial adherence to the protein-supplemented modified fast by very obese patients and accompanying large weight losses is the removal of all food choices, including binge stimulators. The central problem with the protein-supplemented modified fast is that patients living exclusively on this synthetic diet do not learn how to control the intake of real food during the period of weight loss. When appetizing foods are finally reintroduced (as eventually they must), control is lost and weight regained. On theoretical grounds a diet that is very restrictive intially, giving the patient few choices and eliminating potential binge stimulators (particularly carbohydrate), would seem best. As weight is lost and the patient gains confidence in his control over food intake, flexibility in the form of food choices can be introduced, variety increased, and the diet balanced nutritionally. Aggressive dieting is particularly well suited to the very overweight patient who, while losing some weight with previous dieting efforts, may never have reached an acceptable weight goal. Rapid weight loss strongly reinforces the patient's dieting effort. He can, perhaps for the first time, anticipate success in realizing goal weight in months rather than years.

In behaviorally oriented weight control programs rigid diet is usually scrupulously avoided. A limit on total caloric intake may be the only nutritional recommendation (e.g., 1,200 kcal for women, 1,500 kcal for men). The emphasis instead is on eating behavior. The therapist's presumption is that the more rigid the diet, the more likely is deviation to occur along with the attendant risk that the first "cheat" will beget a second, and ultimately a binge ("I've already blown it so what's the difference what I eat?"). This concern is real, but has to be balanced against the fact that the dieter initially is well motivated and often can follow a rigid diet for relatively long periods of time as experience with large resultant weight losses as experienced with the protein-supplemented modified fast has shown. Failure to capitalize on this opportunity may jeopardize the obese patient's chance to lose enough weight to make a difference physically and psychologically, and thereby to provide the motivation necessary to maintain weight loss. Weight reduction has amounted to only 10 to 15 pounds on average in programs that are exclusively behaviorally oriented. Obviously, when a rigid diet of the type described below is prescribed, the physician must be alert to the potential for binges induced by excessive rigidity, and be prepared to respond to transgressions by increasing flexibility.

Semistarvation

Diets are outlined in Tables 4 through 6 that meet the needs of virtually all adult patients. (The nutritional composition of each diet is given in Table 7). The highly motivated individual who is grossly overweight (for example, a man with more than 65 pounds to lose or a woman with more than 45 pounds to lose) can be started on a semistarvation regimen of calorie-free fluids and vegetable salads for a week (see Table 4). Since carbohydrate intake is substantially below 100 g per day, ketosis develops; ketosis suppresses the appetite in many patients. Urine ketones are monitored by the physician as a check on compliance. The patient can also monitor urinary ketones and, having been told that this is an index of massive fat breakdown and utilization, is reinforced in the dieting effort. After initiation of the diet, brief office visits are set up weekly. Foods of low carbohydrate content are added on a weekly or biweekly basis as indicated in Table 4 and discussed below in the section Follow-Up Visits. Carbohydrate-containing foods are cautiously added as goal weight is approached. Within a few pounds of weight goal greater flexibility is introduced by the addition of a fixed number of calories daily (e.g., 150 kcal for women, 200 kcal for men). The specific food choices are left to the dieter with instructions to avoid foods traditionally poorly controlled. The anticipated rate of weight loss is greater the higher the initial weight, and is greater in men than women of the same weight. Males over 250 pounds can expect to lose 45 pounds or more in the first ten weeks. For females over 200 pounds the anticipated weight loss in the same time frame is 25 pounds or more.

Despite the aggressiveness of this approach, side effects are few and easily managed. Postural lightheadedness due to salt and water loss is the most common complaint and can be controlled by salt supplementation. Insomnia responds to a mild hypnotic, headache to over-the-counter analgesics. Hyperuricemia routinely occurs because of competition between uric acid and ketones for excretion by the renal tubules. Gouty arthritis is infrequent, mild, and responds to Indocin or colchicine. If there is a prior history of uric acid elevation, gout, or uric acid stones, a 24-hour urine collection to measure uric acid excretion should be obtained before and after the first week of dieting. Hyperuricosuria which increases as a result of the diet mandates a different dietary approach. Ketogenic diets are contraindicated during pregnancy because of potential harm to the developing fetal central nervous system.

Low Calorie Ketogenic Diet

When lesser amounts of weight are to be lost (25 to 65 pounds for men, 20 to 45 pounds for women), or for the larger patient who rejects the semistarvation approach as "too radical," a ketogenic diet as outlined in Table 5 may be used. Food intake initially is equivalent to that reached after about 8 weeks of dieting by the semistarvation method described above. Because carbohydrate intake is very limited ketosis will develop, but ketonemia and ketonuria are less intense, as is the attendant dehydration. Patients are seen every 10 to 14 days, and noncarbohyrate-containing foods are added as shown in Table 5 (and further elaborated in the section Follow-Up Visits). Ultimately, as goal weight is approached, specific carbohydrate-containing foods are cautiously added, followed by the introduction of greater flexibility in food selection by the addition of a fixed number of calories daily. The specific food choices to be left to the dieter. Weight loss in the first 10 weeks is about 30 pounds for men, 15 to 20 pounds for women. Side effects are insignificant, although hyperuricemia and hyperuricosuria are potential problems.

TABLE 4 Semistarvation Diet*

Week 1: Unlimited fluids include coffee, tea, club soda (or Perrier), and water. Minimum of 48 oz water required. Six oz skim milk to "lighten" coffee or tea. Unlimited unsweetened lime or lemon juice (to make lime- or lemonade). Artificial sweetener (saccharin, aspartame). Three 8-oz cups of salad (four cups for men) using lettuce, tomato, celery, cucumber, radish, green pepper, mushroom, onion, and carrot. Unlimited diet dressing (up to 25 kcal/tbsp) or vinegar and lemon. Seasonings (including salt), herbs, and spices. Supplemental multivitamin (Theragran-M), potassium (50 mEq as Kaylite), calcium (400 mg as two Tums), and if postural lightheadedness develops, 3–5 g salt (Thermogram).

Week 2: Boiled or steamed vegetables, such as string beans, asparagus, broccoli, cauliflower, brussels sprouts, zucchini, spinach, eggplant, cabbage, may be substituted for salads.† Add unlimited diet sodas.

Week 3: Add 3½ oz can of water packed tuna fish (7 oz can for men). Add 2 cups bouillon (Lipton Trim).

Week 4: May substitute 3½ oz cooked weight (7 oz for men) of poultry, fish, or shellfish for tuna fish if desired.

Week 5: Add an egg (2 eggs for men). If scrambled or fried use Pam or Teflon pan.

Week 6: Add 1 tbsp diet mayonnaise or margarine.

Week 7: Add 6 oz 1% fat cottage cheese (8 oz for men). The carbohydrate in cottage cheese will reduce the degree of ketosis.

Week 8: Increase chicken, fish, or shellfish allotment to 6 oz (9 oz for men). Veal or liver may also be included.

Week 9: Add 1 oz hard cheese (cheddar, Swiss, American, etc.) or 2 oz low-fat hard cheese (Lite-Line).

Week 10: May substitute beef, lamb, or pork for poultry, fish, shellfish, veal, or liver, but only twice a week (3 times a week for men).

Weeks 11 and thereafter: No additions until the patient is 20 pounds from goal weight (25 pounds for men), or until weight begins to plateau. Then add 1 fruit selection (2 for men) from fruit list below.‡ This probably will terminate ketosis.

10 Pounds from Goal Weight (15 pounds for men): Add either a small baked potato, ½ cup (boiled and drained) rice, beans, or corn, or 2 thin slices bread (e.g., Hollywood bread).

5 Pounds from Goal Weight (8 pounds for men): Add a fixed number of calories of the patient's choice, avoiding binge triggering foods. The number of calories added depends on the concurrent rate of weight loss but might be 150 kcal per day (200 kcal per day for men). If weight loss is rapid, a greater number of calories may be added.

* The schedule of food additions, in terms of amount and timing, can be viewed as flexible. Physician initiated alterations in the precise amount of food added and the timing of additions should conform to the overall strategy of adding as little as possible consistent with the patient's capacity to comply, and avoiding carbohydrate containing foods (particularly potential binge stimulators) until goal weight is approached. Daily rations are shown unless otherwise stated.

† Other vegetables (cooked or raw) that may be included are bean sprouts, beet greens, chard, chicory, collard greens, dill pickles, dandelion greens, escarole, kale, mustard greens, okra, sauerkraut, summer squash, watercress, and wax beans.

‡ Fruit list (unsweetened if canned, or fresh):

Apple (2-in diameter)	1	Figs (dried)	1 small	Papaya	⅓ medium
Applesauce	½ cup	Fruit cocktail	½ cup	Peach	1 medium
Apricots (fresh)	2 medium	Grapefruit	½ small	Pear	1 small
Apricots (dried)	4 halves	Grapefruit juice	½ cup	Pineapple	½ cup
Blackberries, raspberries, strawberries	1 cup	Grapes	12	Pineapple juice	⅓ cup
Blueberries	⅔ cup	Grape juice	¼ cup	Plums	2 medium
Cantaloupe (6-in diameter)	½	Guava	1 small	Prunes	2
Cherries	10 large	Honeydew (7-in diameter)	¼	Raisins	2 tbsp
Cider	⅓ cup	Mango	½ small	Relish	2 tbsp
Dates	2	Nectarine	1 medium	Tangerine	1 large
Figs (fresh)	2 large	Orange	1 small	Watermelon	3×1×½-in slice
		Orange juice	½ cup		

Balanced Low Calorie Diet

A balanced diet of 1,200 kcal and 150 g of carbohydrate daily is shown in Table 6. It can be used for women with less than 20 pounds of weight to lose and, in slightly liberalized form, (1,500 kcal and 170 g of carbohydrate daily) for men with less than 25 pounds to lose. While carbohydrate is present in the form of fruit, some starchy vegetables, and bread, the patient's choices are still limited and most of the binge provoking foods mentioned previously are excluded. Because carbohydrate intake exceeds 100 g per day, ketosis does not develop. Patients are seen every 10 to 14 days initially for the addition of specific foods, then for the introduction of greater flexibility in food selection by the addition of a fixed number of calories daily.

Body Measurements

Although the patient's total caloric intake may vary only slightly from week to week, the rate of weight loss will not be constant. This is explained largely by variations in the state of hydration. For example, fluid retention may follow for a day after a meal of high sodium content; and in women it may occur simply on a cyclic basis. Concomitant fat loss can thereby be obscured. Nothing is more frustrating to the dieter than a week of no weight loss or even weight gain despite diligent dieting. In this setting patients often comment on an apparent loosening of their clothes despite the absence of weight loss. This is because fat loss leads to a reduction in certain body dimensions which are unaffected by the retention of fluid. Reductions in body dimensions can be quantified and knowledge of them will help sustain motivation. The following body dimensions should be measured by the patient (undressed) at the start of the diet, and before each subsequent visit: bust (or chest), waist, hips, thigh (at the level of the pubic symphysis), and upper arm (largest circumference). From the behavioral viewpoint, the initial prediet data may so mortify the patient as to underscore the need to lose weight. As time goes on, careful measurements keep the patient in better touch with bodily change than weight which is, after all, only an ab-

TABLE 5 Low Calorie Ketogenic Diet

Initial Diet:*

- Breakfast: Cup of bouillon (Lipton Trim).
  One egg (two for men). If scrambled or fried use Pam or Teflon pan.
- Lunch: One 8-oz cup of vegetable salad (two for men). Use lettuce, tomato, celery, cucumber, radish, green pepper, mushroom, onion, and carrot. Unlimited diet dressing (up to 25 kcal/tbsp) or vinegar and lemon.
  6 oz 1% fat cottage cheese (8 oz for men).
- Supper: One Lipton Cup of Soup.
  5 oz cooked weight (8 oz for men) poultry, fish, or shellfish (boiled, baked, broiled, or steamed).
  One 8-oz cup of vegetable salad with dressing (two for men), see lunch above; or one 8-oz cup (two for men) of boiled or steamed vegetables such as string beans, asparagus, broccoli, cauliflower, brussel sprouts, eggplant, zucchini, spinach, and cabbage.†
- Bedtime: One 8-oz cup of vegetable salad with dressing or cooked vegetables (two for men) as described above.
- Fluids: Unlimited fluids include water, black coffee, tea (with or without lemon), club soda, diet sodas, and unsweetened lime and lemon juice (to make lime- or lemonade). Six oz skim milk to "lighten" coffee or tea.
- Other: Seasonings, spices, herbs, and artificial sweetener. 1 tbsp diet mayonnaise or margarine. Supplemental multivitamin (Theragran-M), potassium (50 mEq as Kaylite), calcium (400 mg as 2 Tums), and if postural lightheadedness develops, 3-5 g salt (Thermogram).

Changes at 10 to 14 Day Intervals:

Increase poultry, fish, and shellfish allotment to 7 oz (10 oz for men).
Substitute beef, lamb, pork, veal, or liver for poultry, fish, or shellfish twice a week (3 times a week for men).
Add 1 light beer, 6 oz dry wine, or 1½ oz liquor.
Add 1 oz hard cheese (cheddar, Swiss, American, etc.) or 2 oz low-fat hard cheese (Lite-Line). For men, 2 oz of any hard cheese may be added.

10 Pounds from Goal (15 for Men):

Add 1 fruit from the fruit list (see Table 4, third footnote). For men add 2 fruits.

5 Pounds from Goal (8 for Men):

Add either a small baked potato, ½ cup (boiled and drained) rice, beans, or corn, or 2 thin slices bread (e.g., Hollywood bread).

Within a Few Pounds of Goal:

Add a fixed number of calories of the patient's choice, avoiding binge triggering foods. The number of calories added depends on the concurrent rate of weight loss but might be 150 kcal per day (200 kcal per day for men). If weight loss is rapid, more calories may be added.

* Although the specific foods are divided into three meals and a bedtime snack, this is for convenience only. The patient may change the timing and sequence of foods to accommodate his life style.
† Other vegetables (cooked or raw) that may be included are listed in Table 4, second footnote.

straction. Other factors which contribute to variations in weekly weight loss include the drop in basal metabolic rate which occurs within the first two weeks of dieting, variations in exercise, and differences in the weight of clothing and of bladder, bowel, and stomach contents at the time of weigh-ins.

FOLLOW-UP VISITS

Brief follow-up visits should be scheduled weekly for patients dieting most aggressively (semistarvation), and at intervals of 10 to 14 days for the remainder. These continue until goal weight is achieved. The interval between visits is then lengthened to 3 weeks or longer if weight is well maintained. The ultimate objective is to have the patient managing independently. The entire process often extends beyond a year. The purposes of these follow-up visits are to measure weight change, to determine urine ketones semiquantitatively (when a ketogenic diet has been recommended), to record changes in body dimensions, to make food additions as shown in Tables 4 through 6, to treat physical complaints to introduce other important behavioral components such as diet diary keeping and exercise, and to respond sympathetically to the emotional stresses incident to giving up food and losing weight. The physician is viewed as an authority figure and his or her personal approval is important to the dieter. Success should be commended. The patient who is doing poorly will be depressed and guilt-ridden and sees the physician as impatient, critical, and disapproving. Inevitably these projections are partly true. Nevertheless, encouragement is the appropriate response to the dieter who slips! An unkind word from a frustrated physician can make follow-up visits more painful for the patient and lead to his dropping out of the weight control program.

The Diet Diary

The diet diary is a powerful behavioral tool for helping patients regain control over food intake. At the second or third follow-up visit the dieter is asked to record the foods eaten and their estimated caloric content immediately after each meal. He then calculates total daily calorie intake. At subsequent follow-up visits the calorie total for each day is reported to the physician, who notes high values indicating loss of control. The foods eaten and the specific reasons for overeating on these days should be discussed briefly. In this way the physician can develop a feeling for the circumstances surrounding overeating. The average daily calorie intake for the 1- to 2-week period between visits is then calculated and recorded. Diary keeping may be further refined by having the patient record carbohydrate intake as well to scrutinize the intake of foods over which control may be poor. Behavioral psychologists ask for a detailed description of the setting in which food is consumed and the feeling states surrounding food ingestion. Discussions of this material are time consuming and generally beyond the scope of the internist or gastroenterologist and are best left to those specifically trained in this area.

Beyond helping the patient and physician to understand the causes of overeating, the diet diary is of value

TABLE 6 Balanced Low Calorie Diet

Initial Diet*:	
Breakfast (select 1 or 2)	
Breakfast 1	
One fruit (see Table 4, third footnote).	
One cup cereal (bran or corn flakes, puffed rice or wheat, oatmeal or farina).	
8 oz skim milk	
Breakfast 2	
One fruit.	
One egg (two for men). If scrambled or fried use Pam or Teflon pan.	
One thin slice bread (two for men), e.g., Hollywood bread.	
One tsp butter or margarine or 1 tbsp cream cheese or Neufchatel cheese.	
Lunch:	One fruit
	One 8-oz cup of vegetable salad (two for men). Use lettuce, tomato, celery, cucumber, radish, green pepper, mushroom, onion, and carrot. Unlimited diet dressing (up to 25 kcal/tbsp) or vinegar and lemon.
	Select either A, B, or C
	A. 6 oz 1% fat cottage cheese (8 oz for men) *or* 3 oz farmer cheese (4 oz for men) *or* 1½ oz mozzarella, ricotta, feta, parmesan, or Lite-Line cheese (2 oz for men)
	B. 2 eggs, if scrambled or fried use Pam or a Teflon pan
	C. 3½ oz shellfish, or water packed tuna fish.
Supper:	One fruit.
	One Lipton Cup of Soup
	5 oz cooked weight of poultry, fish, veal, or liver (8 oz for men), or 7 oz shellfish (9 oz for men).
	A starchy vegetable or bread (select 1): Either a small baked potato, a small ear of corn, ½ cup of rice or beans, 2 thin slices bread, 4 melba toast, or 6 saltines.
	One 8-oz cup of salad (two for men) as described for lunch, or an equivalent amount of boiled or steamed vegetables. Use string beans, broccoli, asparagus, cauliflower, brussel sprouts, eggplant, zucchini, spinach, or cabbage.†
	2 tbsp of sour cream, or 1 tsp of butter, margarine, or mayonnaise.
Fluids:	Unlimited fluids include water, black coffee, tea (with or without lemon), club soda, diet sodas, bouillon (Lipton Trim), and unsweetened lime and lemon juice (to make lime- or lemonade). Six oz skim milk to "lighten" coffee or tea. 6 oz of tomato or V8 juice.
Other:	Seasonings, spices, herbs, and artificial sweetener. Supplemental mulivitamin (Theragran-M).
Changes at 10 to 14 Day Intervals:	
	Substitute 5 oz beef, lamb, or pork (8 oz for men) for poultry, fish, shellfish, veal, or liver twice a week (3 times a week for men).
	Add 1 light beer, 6 oz dry wine, or 1½ oz liquor.
	Add a second starchy vegetable selection from the supper list.
	Add a fixed number of calories of the patient's choice when the dieter is within 5 pounds of goal weight. Avoid binge triggering foods. The number of calories added depends on the rate of weight loss but might be 150 kcal per day (200 kcal per day for men). If weight loss is rapid more calories may be added.

* Although the specific foods are divided into three meals and a bedtime snack, this is for convenience only. The patient may change the timing and sequence of foods to accommodate his life style.
† Other vegetables (cooked or raw) that may be included are listed in Table 4, second footnote.

in other important respects. First, the recording of food intake is a "consciousness raising" experience that serves to discourage deviations from the diet. The principle that the act of observation itself alters behavior appears to apply in the behavioral sphere as it does in the physical sciences. The patient is embarrassed to present a diary replete with "cheats" to the physician. Far more important, the dieter is uncomfortable confronting his own lack of control. While some will fabricate information, most see this as pointless, particularly if the physician takes the information seriously and uses it as a basis for discussion at follow-up visits. Rather, resistance takes the form of not having the data, along with attendant excuses (e.g., "It was too time-consuming." "I simply forgot." "It was lost." "I ate out frequently and didn't know how the foods were prepared."). Second, the patient acquires valuable nutritional information. Many are surprised at the high caloric content of the foods they had not considered "fattening." A patient's frustrating and self-defeating perception of an intrinsic metabolic defect as the explanation for his obesity may thus be altered. Third, an estimate of the patient's actual caloric requirement can be made from the weekly averages of caloric intake and the rate of weight loss. The central assumptions are that a pound of fat is lost for every 3,500 kcal of negative caloric balance, and that all of the patient's weight loss is fat. These assumptions are approximately true if the degree of ketosis is about the same on the starting and termination dates used for the calculation (to minimize errors due to changes in state of hydration incident to varying degrees of ketosis). The period of observation should be long enough (perhaps 8 to 12 weeks) and the amount of weight lost large enough to minimize the impact of small errors in estimates of caloric intake and in the actual measurement of weight change. In the final analysis, for the dieter to maintain weight loss he must have some concept of the caloric content of the foods he eats and of his daily caloric requirement. This information is best derived from diary keeping.

Exercise

Exercise is the only practical and effective way to enhance the disposal of ingested calories. Dieters frequently abuse diuretics and laxatives for this purpose with resultant dehydration rather than calorie loss. Some at-

TABLE 7 Daily Caloric and Nutrient Intake

	Women				Men			
	Kcal	Protein	Fat	Carbohydrate	Kcal	Protein	Fat	Carbohydrate
		(g per day)				(g per day)		
Semistarvation Diet								
Week 1	301	16	7	52	369	19	9	65
2	307	21	7	51	377	25	10	63
3	445	47	10	53	634	75	16	65
4	456	46	11	54	656	72	16	66
5	545	52	18	54	832	86	30	67
6	595	52	23	55	882	86	35	68
7	715	73	25	61	1,042	114	37	76
8	841	92	29	63	1,167	130	42	79
9	943	102	36	64	1,375	143	59	80
10	1,063	102	50	64	1,645	142	90	78
11+[1]	1,103	102	50	73	1,725	144	91	98
12+[2]	1,193	105	50	92	1,815	146	91	117
Low Calorie Ketogenic Diet								
Basic Diet	863	84	29	76	1,316	125	47	112
Change 1	937	96	31	76	1,390	138	49	112
2	1,116	98	50	78	1,747	141	88	113
3	1,234	98	62[3]	81	1,865	141	100[3]	116
4	1,336	109	68	82	2,073	154	116	117
5[4]	1,376	109	68	92	2,153	155	117	136
6[5]	1,466	112	69	111	2,243	158	118	155
Balanced Low Calorie Diet								
Breakfast 1								
Basic Diet	1,221	94	27	158	1,508	120	38	183
Change 1	1,318	93	39	157	1,749	119	66	182
2	1,436	93	51[3]	160	1,867	119	78[3]	185
3	1,526	96	51	179	1,957	122	78	204
Breakfast 2								
Basic Diet	1,171	88	39	127	1,585	122	56	160
Change 1	1,268	87	50	126	1,826	122	84	159
2	1,386	87	62[3]	129	1,944	122	96[3]	162
3	1,478	90	63	148	2,034	124	96	181

[1] 20 pounds from goal weight in women, 25 pounds in men.
[2] 10 pounds from goal weight in women, 15 pounds in men.
[3] Alcohol is considered a fat for purposes of this table.
[4] 10 pounds from goal weight in women, 15 pounds in men.
[5] 5 pounds from goal weight in women, 8 pounds in men.

tempt to induce vomiting; this is both dangerous and abhorrent to the patient. Effecting a life-style change that includes regular exercise is difficult. Lack of time is a commonly cited and often real obstacle. Important, too, but less often verbalized, is self-consciousness about appearance while exercising. Sometimes the problem is simply ignorance of how to go about exercising and what kind of exercise to do. Exercise diary keeping helps to establish a regular pattern of exercise. Once the patient has begun to keep his diet diary consistently, he is asked to begin monitoring exercise. The number of calories burned for each planned exercise period is calculated and recorded by the patient using Table 8. Although the dieter need not exercise every day, a reasonable initial goal would be to average 700 kcal per week (equivalent to about 1 mile of walking daily at a comfortable pace). This combusts about 10 pounds of fat yearly, a value that may seem trivial from the point of view of weight loss, but is significant for weight maintenance. The patient is often surprised by the relatively small caloric dividends of exercise, but it is important that he recognize the substantial amount of physical effort required to burn "harmless" snacks. This reinforces adherence to the diet. Beyond increased caloric expenditure, an anticipated improvement in cardiovascular conditioning should be stressed. Patients will find that, with time, they can do more with less effort. It should be pointed out that exercise can help compensate for the drop in basal metabolic rate incident to dieting. Exercise is often associated with an improvement in mood. It influences the changes in body composition occurring with dieting in a salutary way by reducing loss of lean muscle mass. Its effect on appetite is debated; studies show both stimulation and inhibition. In either event the effect is small. Excessive exercise is time consuming, painful, and hazardous, and should be discouraged.

TABLE 8 Calories Used for Each Minute of Continuous Exercise*

Activity	Weight in pounds					
	120	150	170	200	220	250
	kcal/min					
Volleyball, moderate	2.7	3.4	3.9	4.6	5.0	5.7
Walking, 3 mph	3.2	4.0	4.6	5.4	5.9	6.8
Table tennis	3.2	4.0	4.6	5.4	5.9	6.8
Bicycling, 5.5 mph	3.8	4.7	5.3	6.3	6.9	7.9
Calisthenics	3.9	4.9	5.6	6.6	7.2	8.2
Golf	4.3	5.4	6.1	7.2	7.9	9.0
Skating, moderate	4.3	5.4	6.1	7.2	7.9	9.0
Walking, 4 mph	4.6	5.8	6.6	7.8	8.5	9.7
Aerobics	4.6	5.8	6.6	7.8	8.5	9.7
Tennis, doubles	4.8	6.0	6.9	8.1	8.9	10.1
Badminton	5.2	6.5	7.4	8.7	9.6	10.9
Canoeing, 4 mph	5.6	7.0	7.9	9.3	10.2	11.6
Swimming, breaststroke	5.7	7.2	8.1	9.6	10.5	12.0
Tennis, singles	6.0	7.5	8.5	10.0	10.9	12.5
Bicycling, 10 mph	6.5	8.1	9.2	10.8	11.9	13.6
Swimming, crawl	6.9	8.7	9.8	11.6	12.7	14.5
Jogging, 11 min mile	7.3	9.1	10.4	12.2	13.4	15.3
Skiing, downhill	7.6	9.5	10.7	12.7	13.9	15.8
Racquetball	7.6	9.4	10.7	12.7	13.9	15.8
Handball	7.6	9.5	10.7	12.7	13.9	15.8
Mountain climbing	8.0	10.0	11.3	13.3	14.6	16.6
Squash	8.1	10.2	11.5	13.6	14.9	17.0
Skiing, cross-country	8.7	10.8	12.3	14.5	15.9	18.0
Running, 8 min mile	11.3	14.1	16.0	18.8	20.7	23.5
Running, 5 min mile	15.7	19.7	22.3	26.3	28.9	32.8

* The figures were developed under standardized conditions at the Human Performance Research Center at Brigham Young University, Provo, Utah. Factors such as ambient temperature and clothing can affect values.

ADDITIONAL SUPPORTIVE MEASURES

Most dieters starting the program described above do well initially. Rigid adherence to the diet and rapid weight loss may continue for 6 months or more in the very obese. For all patients weight loss eventually decelerates and ultimately stops. Some will reach goal weight, but the majority will not. One strategy for the patient whose weight loss has stopped near goal weight and in whom risk factors have been normalized is simply to revise the goal upward. In this instance the reason for additional weight loss is aesthetic, and the selected goal not an absolute. In patients far from goal weight additional supportive measures are necessary.

Formal Psychologically Oriented Therapy

Reasons for the deceleration of weight loss include the decline in basal metabolic rate with dieting, the lowered caloric requirement incident to the patient's becoming smaller, and the gradually increasing caloric intake called for by the diet. Unquestionably most important, however, is deviation from the diet. The reasons for deviation are multiple; almost invariably they are fundamental to the cause of obesity in the first place. The patient may now know them, or knowing them feel powerless to affect them. Frustration over the slowing rate of weight loss is frequently mentioned, as is boredom with the limited food selections. These can be dealt with respectively by removing some of the foods previously added or by adding new ones, perhaps some suggested by the patient. This occasionally is effective, but in most instances the problem lies not with the diet. The most important reasons are the most difficult to reverse, and sometimes even to identify. This is not surprising in view of the well-known refractoriness of obesity to all forms of therapy.

Common underlying reasons for deviations from the diet include eating to satisfy emotional needs rather than hunger (depression, anxiety, boredom, fatigue), specific food cravings, and premenstrual (and possibly hormonally mediated) food cravings. Dieting, rapid weight loss, and thinness attract attention to the dieter who is often shy, unaccustomed to such attention, and uncomfortable with it. There is an abiding fear about what others who have been so supportive during the dieting process will think but not say if and when weight is regained. Also, there may be disappointment when long held fantasies about life as a thinner person prove unrealistic. Surprisingly, hunger is rarely offered as an explanation. Dieters sometimes refer to "poor eating habits" as the cause of deviation, implying a somewhat more benign underlying psychologic process. Even if a significant emotional disturbance does not appear to motivate eating in such patients, it may follow dieting simply because of interference with familiar and comfortable patterns of food intake.

It is thus obvious that in some patients, and probably in most, a psychologically oriented component to the weight reduction program should be introduced. This may take the form of counseling by a therapist interested in the problem of substance abuse as it applies to overeating. The patient's spouse and other family members can be included. Lay support groups such as Overeaters Anonymous are helpful, particularly when they include role models who have dieted successfully. For many, a formal behavior modification program is best. The patient should be an important guide as to which form of psychologically oriented therapy might be best. Some will reject a group format, others will already have had negative experiences with individual counseling.

It is beyond the scope of this chapter to describe behavior modification techniques in detail. Patients must be referred to an existing program which may be found in a university setting, at a local psychiatric hospital (or the psychiatry department of a general hospital), or pehaps in the private sphere. Generally, it is done in a group setting, on a weekly basis, and with an experienced therapist. Diet diary keeping is central and the information recorded includes the foods eaten, their caloric content, the reasons for eating, the location of and activities surrounding eating, and associated feeling states. An attempt is then made to identify internal cues (e.g., anxiety) and external cues (e.g., passing a bakery, seeing food advertisements on television) for eating. Alternative outlets for internal cues, such as calling a friend or exercising, are sought. External cues are either removed or minimized. The location and circumstances of eating are restricted. A system is developed to reward the attainment of short-term goals either through group recognition or by self-administered rewards, e.g., the purchase of new clothes in a smaller size. Flexibility is important at this point in the dieting process. Minor deviations should not be viewed as tantamount to failure, a perception that justifies further discouragement, deviation, and even binging. A group setting is particularly useful because it helps the patient realize that he is not alone in the difficult struggle to control food intake. The transition from a metabolically oriented program supervised by the internist or gastroenterologist to one that has a behavioral focus primarily is difficult to orchestrate in the private practice of medicine. This accounts in significant measure for poor long-term results.

Appetite Suppressants

A wide variety of drugs (digitalis, thyroid hormone, chorionic gonadotropin, "starch blockers") have been used to facilitate weight reduction, but only appetite suppressants have established efficacy. Appetite suppressants are structurally related to the naturally occurring sympathomimetic amines. They are presumed to act by releasing norepinephrine or dopamine from adrenergic nuclei in the central nervous system. In addition to appetite suppression they produce psychomotor stimulation. With respect to enhancement of weight reduction they all seem to be equally effective. The established duration of efficacy is limited to 20 weeks because high dropout rates in longer term studies preclude firm conclusions. Tachyphylaxis is common and side effects can be significant, particularly insomnia and blood pressure elevation.

Although not to be recommended for all dieters, appetite suppressants can be a useful adjunct when compliance falters with episodic loss of control. Schedule II drugs like dextroamphetamine (Dexedrine), methamphetamine (Desoxyn), and phenmetrazine (Preludin) should be avoided because of their high potential for abuse. Phendimetrazine, a Schedule III drug, can be administered either one hour before meals (17½ to 70 mg in short-acting form, supplied generically as 35-mg tablets) or as a single dose before 3 PM (long-acting form, supplied in 105-mg capsules as Prelu-2). Fenfluramine (Pondimin) produces drowsiness rather than central nervous system stimulation, and can be useful before the evening meal in patients who snack throughout the evening (20 to 40 mg one hour before supper, supplied as short-acting 20-mg tablets). The nonprescription sympathomimetic agent phenylpropanolamine is promoted directly to the public for weight reduction. Studies lasting 2 to 4 weeks show it to have significant, though minimal, appetite suppressing effect. No more than a 2-week supply of an appetite suppressant should be prescribed at one time. Effectiveness, either as continued weight loss or weight maintenance, should be closely monitored. It may be well to recommend that regular daily use be avoided; rather, the medication can be used "as a crutch" only when an impending loss of control is anticipated. Intermittent use may minimize the development of tachyphylaxis and the potential for dependence.

WEIGHT MAINTENANCE

Obese patients who have lost weight previously recognize that weight maintenance is at least as difficult as weight reduction, having already succeeded at losing weight and failed at maintaining the loss. It is clear to them that a long-term perspective is necessary. Those who are dieting for the first time must be educated early to the fact that dieting, i.e., the conscious exercise of restraint over food intake, does not end with the attainment of goal weight. Failure to accept this harsh reality will inevitably lead to weight gain. Theoretically, the process ends only when the patient is able to maintain optimal weight comfortably and independently through control of food intake and regular exercise. This ideal is rarely, if ever, totally accomplished.

Operationally, the process of weight reduction should blend imperceptibly into that of weight maintenance. This will follow from the previously outlined strategy of gradually increasing caloric intake so that the patient approaches goal weight asymptomatically rather than abruptly. At goal weight the diet must come close to meeting the patient's need for nutritional balance and variety, with subsequent minor adjustments being made early in the period of weight maintenance. Office visits are spaced farther apart but the self-monitoring of calorie (and carbohydrate) intake and of exercise continues. If the patient falters, the time interval between office visits can be shortened. Patients have a need to "internalize" control of food intake, i.e., to function independent of the physician. They may wish to discontinue visits prematurely, and great care must be taken to endorse the cessation of visits only when control seems good. The patient who has lost substantial weight but nevertheless has stabilized above goal may suggest discontinuation of visits, stating: "I don't see that progress is being made." Either he has failed to learn that stabilization at a lower weight is a significant accomplishment; or, he perceives that the physician is disappointed with his failure to lose more weight. These misconceptions must be clarified. Particularly at risk for weight gain is the dieter whose weight, after a period of stabilization, begins to fluctuate wildly from week to week, with the general trend being slowly upward. Clearly, such patients are losing control, alternating fasting with feasting, and need more rather than less reinforcement. Long-term follow-up studies show that continued contact with the therapeutic program and regular exercise characterize successful patients.

Patients who discontinue treatment and return to diet

again after regaining weight merit comment. For them very rigid dieting seems to work poorly. Excessive dietery restriction must lead first to minor deviations, then binges followed by fasts. In such patients it is probably best to prescribe a flexible regimen consisting of a fixed total daily calorie and carbohydrate intake (e.g., 1,000 kcal and 100 g of carbohydrate for women, and 1,500 kcal and 150 g of carbohydrate for men) without reference to specific foods, along with regular follow-up visits and the other self-monitoring techniques described above.

SURGERY

Surgical intervention to alter nutrient ingestion or absorption may be considered for the morbidly obese patient (more than 100 pounds or 100 percent above ideal weight) who cannot control his weight by dieting. The risk:benefit ratio has proved most favorable in patients aged 20 to 50 years. Jejunoileal bypass was introduced for this purpose first, and results in dramatic weight loss through a combination of malabsorption and decreased appetite. Though it is generally effective, initial enthusiasm has waned because of side effects. Diarrhea may be intractable, leading to very uncomfortable proctitis and hemorrhoids. Patients are afraid to eat because of the almost immediate need to defecate. Fatal cirrhosis has been reported, along with serious nutritional deficiencies resulting from malabsorption and the blind loop syndrome. Polyarthralgias and renal stones also occur. For these reasons gastric bypass, and more recently gastroplasty, have become more popular. The latter procedure involves partitioning the stomach, creating a small (35 to 50 ml) upper reservoir emptying into the larger distal portion of the stomach through a narrow channel (9 to 12 mm in diameter). Early satiety is then experienced. Overeating leads to nausea and vomiting. The incidence of long-term complications of gastroplasty is not known as yet, but the problems reported thus far appear to be less serious than with jejunoileal bypass. Gallstones frequently develop. Deficiencies in water-soluble vitamins, loss of bone mineral, and hepatic damage resembling alcoholic hepatitis have also been reported. Although patients lose only 50 percent of excess weight on average, they usually are gratified by the results. Unfortunately, some weight gain after the first year is common owing to dilatation of the upper gastric reservoir and/or the channel between the upper and lower segments of the stomach. A conscious effort by the patient to curtail binging is necessary to prevent dilatation of the upper reservoir. External banding of the channel has recently been introduced to prevent its dilatation. Surgical revision may prove necessary in a significant number of patients as weight is regained. Gastroplasty can also be defeated by the continuous sipping of calorie-dense liquids.

For patients who lose large amounts of weight either by dieting or surgical intervention, cosmetic surgery may be desirable to remove unsightly skin folds about the abdomen, thighs, and upper arms. This surgery should be delayed until weight loss has been successfully maintained for at least 6 months. Suction lipectomy is an effective procedure to remove localized accumulations of fat no more than 8 inches in diameter.

ANOREXIA NERVOSA AND BULIMIA

PAUL E. GARFINKEL, M.D., M.Sc., F.R.C.P.(C)

Anorexia nervosa is characterized by self-imposed starvation due to a relentless pursuit of thinness and fear of fatness. Bulimia is characterized by episodic patterns of binge eating with a sense of loss of control and depressive moods. Bulimia can occur as a symptom in many illnesses, including anorexia nervosa, and as a separate syndrome with little weight loss. The hallmark of these eating disorders is the distorted drive for thinness and subsequent dieting. The person states that she feels her body to be too large no matter what she weighs, and she offers no explanation for this—merely that she feels better the thinner she is.

Anorexia nervosa occurs in about 1 percent of young women and bulimia occurs in 2 to 3 percent of women. More mild variants of these disorders occur in about 5 percent. About 95 percent of cases are female (hence the use of the feminine form to refer to patients throughout this chapter). These eating disorders remain serious problems, causing significant mortality (about 5%) and morbidity (about 25% of patients develop a chronic form).

Because there is a denial of illness, there may be a variety of presentations. Because of increasing awareness of these disorders, some cases are discovered by a schoolteacher, parent, or friend. Other patients see a physician for amenorrhea or because of emotional sequelae such as depressed mood and social withdrawal. It is also common to have such gastrointestinal symptoms as bloating and early satiety due to reduced gastric emptying; or alternating diarrhea and constipation due to surreptitious laxative misuse; or hypokalemia and parotitis due to vomiting. Because of the acidic nature of vomitus some patients present to dentists with erosion of dental enamel.

There are a number of cultural, familial, and individual risk factors for these disorders. The cultural component involves the pervasive emphasis on thinness in young women. This is responsible for the increased prevalence of these diseases in certain professions, such as dancing and modeling. Pressures on women to perform to please others are also important here. Depressive illness, alcoholism, and eating disorders are all more common in the families of bulimics and anorexics than in the general population. Family patterns in which independence is discouraged may be another contributor. Family stresses, including separation and losses, often precede the onset. Factors within the individual include fears of the demands of maturation and the increased independence this requires. These in turn are related to an underlying sense of personal helplessness and fear of losing control. People with eating disorders have a lowered sense of self-worth which is bound to external criteria, such as parental approval, high grades, and a look or an image that is culturally sanctioned. Many people with anorexia nervosa also have a disturbance in self-perception; they either do not recognize the extent of their weight loss or they continue to feel a particular part of the body is too fat no matter what they weigh.

People with bulimia share many of the features of the anorexic but also display some differences. In particular, they tend to have been heavier before the onset of the disease and they come from heavier families. They are also much more impulsive, and this is manifested by their difficulties with control of alcohol and street drugs and stealing.

DIAGNOSIS

Young adults lose weight for various reasons, including (1) chronic wasting illnesses (e.g., Crohn's disease); (2) endocrine diseases (hyperthyroidism, hypopituitarism, Addison's disease, diabetes mellitus); and (3) functional disorders (schizophrenia, depression, and conversion disorders with psychogenic vomiting).

The diagnosis of anorexia nervosa or bulimia is based on a good clinical interview. Here the important features include the drive for thinness, fears of weight gain, and fears of losing control of eating. There is generally a normal appetite, as is not the case in depression when a true "anorexia" occurs. It is rare that laboratory investigations are necessary to arrive at a diagnosis. However, if a metabolic disorder is being considered, tests of pituitary function (luteinizing hormone, follicle-stimulating hormone, growth hormone) or end-organ function (cortisol) can be of use.

While investigations are generally not needed for diagnostic reasons they are helpful to determine the metabolic sequelae. Important laboratory investigations include complete blood count, electrocardiogram, electrolytes, tests of liver, kidney, and thyroid function, serum amylase and creatine phosphokinase (some bulimics misuse ipecac to induce vomiting; ipecac contains emetine which is a muscle poison and can lead to a progressive peripheral and cardiomyopathy). More specialized investigations such as a computed tomography (CT) scan and upper and lower gastrointestinal series are not routinely ordered but should be if indications warrant.

TREATMENT

Attitude of the Physician

People with serious eating disorders are often mistrustful of physicians whom they think are interested only in refeeding them or in making them lose their will and become fat. The physician must encourage normal eating habits and weight without making this a battleground or the only focus of treatment. Anorexics are also often worried about being deserted. The physician must emphasize that he or she will continue to treat the patient over a long period of time and may focus on many different issues as necessary. The goal of treatment is not control of the anorexic but rather relief of suffering. It is helpful to have a firm, nonjudgmental attitude and to reinterpret the individual's low body weight not as a sign of self-control but as something to which the patient has become a slave. For the patient to become motivated to receive help, it is important to focus on symptoms that she herself views as being problems.

There is great value in education. Patients benefit from learning about body size and body weight regulation, and the effects of starvation on the body, including its effects on thinking, feelings, and behavior; and dietary misconceptions can be clarified. The effects of vomiting and laxatives on bodily functions should be discussed. It is equally important to have a frank discussion with the patient about cultural attitudes regarding women's body sizes and how easily individuals can be manipulated by cultural phenomena. It is also important to discuss issues of self-esteem and how in this circumstance the individual is relating her self-worth entirely to a body size or weight, to her disadvantage.

Indications for Admission to Hospital

Most patients with anorexia nervosa and bulimia can be treated entirely as outpatients. However, a significant subgroup requires hospitalization, depending on the following: (1) the severity and rate of weight loss—for example, when patients have lost about 30 percent of their body weight or when the weight loss has been rapid; (2) an unending cycle of bulimia and vomiting which cannot be interrupted for even one day often requires the external control of a hospital environment; (3) failure of outpatient treatment; or (4) treatment of a variety of complications, including persistent hypokalemic alkalosis, depression, suicide attempts, and so on.

IN-HOSPITAL TREATMENT PROGRAM

Important components of in-hospital management include the following:

1. A weight range should be set as a goal. This usually is about 90 percent of average for the person's age and height. Rather than a single weight, a range of 3 to 4 pounds should be chosen so that the person recognizes that there can be normal fluctuations in weight. Most patients can tolerate gains of 1 to 2 kg per week.
2. Methods of weight restoration. A safe and effective technique involves a program of bedrest and close nursing observation during and after meals, together with nutritional education and emotional support. Bedrest allows the medical staff to assume control over the situation. It also tends to erode the patient's denial by emphasizing that she is ill, and the restriction of activities may be used as part of a reward system to encourage weight gain. I tend to allow the patient out of bed for increasing periods of time as weight is being restored. However, some physicians recommend that the patient remain in bed until she has reached her target weight. Both methods are effective. More detailed reward systems in which patients are allowed increasing privileges, such as off ward activities, visitors, phone calls, and so on, are effective but are often not required and have the undesirable effect of becoming the focus of treatment, with the patient negotiating endlessly with staff for various privileges.

   In very rare instances nasogastric feedings or total parenteral nutrition may be required, but these should be used only in life-threatening circumstances when all else has failed; fewer than 1 percent of patients require these. There are some instances in which severe anxiety interferes with the patient's beginning to eat. Emotional support from the staff and relaxation exercises are helpful here. Occasionally drugs such as a relatively short-acting benzodiazepine (lorazepam, 0.5 mg) or a sedating neuroleptic (chlorpromazine, 25 mg) may be used before meals for a few weeks.
3. The patient should be weighed three times weekly at a standard time (in the morning before breakfast and after voiding) and in standard clothing and the patient is told the readings on the scales. Staff should be alert to the patient's possible attempts to increase weight artificially (e.g., drinking large volumes of water); these should be dealt with firmly but not with punishment.
4. Dietary re-education must be provided to dispel myths or strange beliefs about food. To prevent gastric dilatation the patient should initially receive about 1,500 calories per day. This may be increased to 2,500 to 3,500 calories over 2 weeks. For some people who are unable to consume this in meals, high-calorie liquid drinks (Ensure) may be used as supplements. Patients are given the same opportunity to select foods as are other patients, but they are not permitted food idiosyncracies, e.g., complete avoidance of carbohydrates, fats, or high-calorie foods.
5. Patients should not be allowed to have access to foods on their own or to the hospital kitchen or vending machines. This is especially important for patients who have been bulimic or engaged in self-induced purging. Similarly, patients who vomit or misuse laxatives must be accompanied to the bathroom.
6. Hospitalization or a day care program should continue for about 2 weeks after the patient's weight has been restored to above 90 percent of average to demonstrate to her that control can be maintained in this range. During this phase she should be allowed more control over the choice of diet.

THE ROLE OF MEDICATION

It was previously noted that small doses of neuroleptics may be useful to reduce anxiety over gaining weight, and for this purpose the neuroleptics have a limited value. Side effects such as hypotension and a reduced convulsive threshold restrict their use. Also, as noted, a short-acting benzodiazepine may be used for the same purpose. However, the bulimic group who have a high propensity for addictions should not receive minor tranquilizers. The anticonvulsants, carbamazepine and phenytoin, have been found to be useful in a minority of patients with bulimia, but further study is needed before these drugs are more widely used.

The antidepressant medications, the tricyclics and monoamineoxidase inhibitors (MAOIs), have not been shown to have much value in the restricting group of anorexics. There are at least four controlled studies, however, which have demonstrated the efficacy of antidepressants in treating bulimia. I limit their use to those patients who have depressive features that do not remit after weight restoration. Generally these patients should be treated with a nonsedating tricyclic with the least antihistaminic and anticholinergic properties. *Desipramine* is useful because of its low incidence of these side effects. Given the dietary interactions of the MAOIs and the bulimics' impulsive tendencies to overeat, caution should be exerted in their use.

Because of the effects of starvation, delayed gastric emptying can occur and may produce symptoms of bloating and gastrointestinal discomfort which may persist for several months after weight is restored. While metoclopramide has been used for this problem, its tendency to cause depression restricts its value in this population. I prefer to use *domperidone* under these circumstances.

Certain medications must be avoided. Frequently, anorexics and bulimics are given thyroxine because their laboratory values are in the low-normal range. The thyroid response to starvation is one of conservation-adaptation and this does not require treatment. Moreover, a large proportion misuse the thyroxine by doubling up the medication to lose more weight. Insulin was once widely prescribed to stimulate the patient's hunger and because of its anabolic properties. Given the fact that these patients are very hungry but are frightened of giving in to the impulse to eat, and given their increased sensitivity to insulin, using insulin must be considered dangerous. Some patients present to physicians complaining of feeling bloated and stuffed as a description of their dissatisfaction with their body size. At times they may be given a diagnosis of idiopathic cyclic edema and be placed on a diuretic. Again they have a tendency to misuse this medication to reduce the readings on the scale.

OUTPATIENT TREATMENT PROGRAM

Many patients do not require management in hospital, and all of those who are treated in hospital require outpatient follow up. The outpatient program involves (1) monitoring eating and weight; (2) monitoring appropriate biochemical indices (patients may require monitoring of potassium if hypokalemia has been a problem; for some, potassium supplements are necessary); and (3) ongoing psychotherapy, both for the individual and often for family members.

Eating and weight can be dealt with in the following way:

1. Patients should be encouraged to throw out their scales and be weighed weekly by their doctor.
2. When encouraging weight gains modest increases of 0.5 kg per week are reasonable.
3. The patient must continue eating three meals per day of moderate caloric intake, even if she is binge eating. Binge eating on 1 day should not be followed by a restriction of intake, as this perpetuates the pattern.
4. Patients often benefit from record keeping of dietary intake. This includes the patient recording what she has eaten, the time and the place when binge eating occurs, and the feelings and events associated with this.
5. Exercise should be limited (30 minutes per day); if it becomes compulsive the patient should not be permitted any exercise at all.
6. The patient should know that if her weight falls below her goal range, the treatment will alter (this may involve more focus on nutrition in the treatment, addition of liquid suplements, and restricting activities).

The psychological treatment has a number of components:

1. An educative role as described earlier.
2. Correcting faulty thinking patterns. These patients have a variety of distortions in their thinking, most notably, an all-or-nothing pattern that does not allow them to see in-betweens in their lives. Repeated emphasis on correcting this is useful.
3. Reinterpretation of their distortions regarding their body. This involves having the individual learn to trust how others see her and to feel her body as a source of comfort and pleasure.

TABLE 1 Complications of Anorexia and Bulimia

	Frequency	Course	Treatment
Cardiovascular System			
Bradycardia	Common	Starvation	Responds to weight restoration
Hypotension	Common	Starvation, fluid depletion	Responds to weight restoration
Arrhythmias	Infrequent	Usually provided by exercise in starvation; may be due to hypokalemia	Responds to weight restoration or potassium supplements
Cardiomyopathy	Rare	Emetine toxicity from ipecac	Stop the ipecac
Electrolytes			
Hypokalemia	Common	Loss of potassium from multiple routes (vomiting, diarrhea, and diuretics)	Prevent purging; may need a potassium supplement
Hyponatremia	Rare	Salt restriction and water intoxication (to meet weight goals)	Well-balanced diet with appropriate amounts of fluids
Edema	Common	Not clearly understood	Elevate feet for 1 hr t.i.d.; avoid salt; do not use diuretics
Gastrointestinal System			
Parotitis	Common	Mechanical trauma; starvation	No specific treatment; stop binges and vomiting
Early satiety	Common	Delayed gastric emptying	Domperidone 10 mg t.i.d.
Gastric dilatation	Rare	Rapid refeeding	Avoid oral feeding; use IV feeding
Constipation	Common	Starvation; reliance on laxative	Use diet—emphasis on dietary bulk, fruits, vegetables and try to avoid laxatives
Dental caries	Common	Acidic nature of vomitus	Dental consult
Persistent Amenorrhea	Infrequent	Low weight; emotional stress	Restore weight to >90% of average
Hematologic Changes			
Anemia	Infrequent	Bone marrow hypoplasia; due to starvation	Weight restoration; may need iron
Thrombocytopenia	Rare	Starvation	Weight restoration
Hypercholesterolemia	Common	Unknown	Balanced diet
Hypercarotenemia	Infrequent	Ingestion of high carotene foods	Balanced diet

4. Affective expression. The psychotherapy must help the person learn to recognize different feeling states and to respond appropriately to these. Especially important is recognizing feeling states which trigger binge eating. Anxiety, depression, and boredom are common initiators of a binge. Patients can learn that this may be prevented by more appropriate behaviour, e.g., relaxation exercises, meeting a friend, etc.
5. Self-esteem has been tied to weight and to a look. The person should gradually recognize that self-esteem can be built up by factors outside of this.
6. Structuring time is very important. These patients are most vulnerable to difficulties when alone in the evenings, especially after a difficult day of work or school. Having other people present can be useful; or a structured activity can prevent binge eating.
7. Family therapy is important; the family should not be blamed for the disorder. They require advice regarding what the illness involves. At times they need advice about effective parenting and must allow the individual to separate emotionally and physically from the family.
8. For many, group therapy and support groups help, as an adjunct to the ongoing treatment program.

COMPLICATIONS

The complications of anorexia nervosa and bulimia may be due to the starvation process itself, to artificial attempts to control weight (by vomiting, laxative, or diuretic misuse), to the weight-restoring treatments, or to the psychological sequelae. Some of the complications are described in the accompanying table.

GASTRIC CARCINOMA

JOHN R. STROEHLEIN, M.D.
JAFFER A. AJANI, M.D.

Gastric cancer claims more than 14,000 lives annually and accounts for almost 3 percent of all newly diagnosed cancers in the United States. The importance of gastric cancer is partially obscured by its declining incidence. In 1930, gastric cancer was the most frequent cause of death from cancer. The age-adjusted death rate has fallen from 37.5 per 100,000 population for males and 27.5 per 100,000 for females in that year to an estimated 8.6 per 100,000 for males and 4.3 per 100,000 for females in 1980 (Tables 1, 2).

It appears that dietary habits may affect the development of gastric cancer. This, in part, has led to recommendations to decrease ingestion of smoked, salted, or nitrate-preserved foods, and to maintain a diet high in fiber, low in fat, and one that contains ample quantities of fresh fruits and vegetables. The role of specific dietary products, such as vitamins or antioxidants, has not been established, and it is unlikely that this will be subjected to prospective studies regarding gastric cancer. Pending some primary preventive measures, endoscopic polypectomy, a secondary preventive measure, remains the only "established" method for preventing gastric cancer in the small percentage of patients affected by gastric adenomas. Clinical emphasis must currently focus on early diagnosis and optimal treatment of established disease.

DIAGNOSTIC CONSIDERATIONS

It is no challenge to diagnose advanced gastric cancer heralded by weight loss, pain, anemia, and a palpable mass or large ulcerated malignancy. What is of greater importance is to (1) know who is more likely to have gastric cancer and (2) appreciate more subtle manifestations of this disease so that diagnosis can more often be established at an earlier stage. The potential for early diagnosis has been well established and its importance underscored by dramatic differences in survival.

Our approach is to assess the relative possibility of gastric cancer and be alert for early endoscopic and roentgenographic signs of disease. Unless one is aware of these diagnostic subtleties they will not be recognized. Diligence is essential to increase the proportion of gastric cancers diagnosed at an early stage. Roentgenographically, this requires *air-contrast techniques* to identify subtle mucosal abnormalities, including flattening or depression of the mucosa, which is one of the more common types of early gastric cancer. It takes considerable experience to appreciate these changes *endoscopically*. Recognition of these patterns is of more than academic interest and is reflected by a two- to fourfold increase in the percentage of cancers that have been diagnosed early since the development of air-contrast techniques, endoscopy, and biopsy.

It is important to inspect carefully the gastric mucosa in its entirety and perform *six or more biopsies* of any *mass* lesion, *ulceration*, area of *discoloration*, unexplained *mucosal depression*, or *prominent folds*. Polyps suitable

TABLE 1 Changing Death Rate* from Gastric Cancer

	Average/100,000 Population	
Decade	Male	Female
1940	32.5	19.9
1960	16.9	8.1
1980	8.6	4.3

* Primarily due to fewer "intestinal-type" gastric cancers

TABLE 2 Gender-specific Mortality from Gastric Carcinoma

	Mortality/100,000 Population	
Country	Male	Female
Japan	66.1	31.2
Portugal	40.6	20.9
Finland	30.7	15.0
Canada	14.4	6.7

for endoscopic polypectomy should be removed completely because of 1) variation between individual biopsy specimens and histologic inspection of a lesion macroscopically removed, and 2) removal of adenomas prevents future malignant deterioration. Other members of the family may require surveillance when gastric cancer or adenomatous polyps are diagnosed in relatives.

PREOPERATIVE MANAGEMENT

Preoperative evaluation should include gastroscopy with biopsy. This may yield a great deal of information about the submucosal extension of cancer or presence of multifocal disease. The former may be manifested by nodule formation a few centimeters removed from the apparent confines of cancer, and the latter has been variously reported to occur in 2 to 20 percent of cases.

Standard preoperative evaluation, as required for any major surgical procedure, is indicated. Cross-sectional imaging may be useful in identifying gastric wall thickening or mass effect, intra-abdominal tumor extension, or metastatic disease. Its use has been advocated to stage patients preoperatively, based in part on thickness of the gastric wall, and to select for surgery those who are more likely to have curative resection. We do not rely heavily on the preoperative computed tomographic appearance in deciding whether or not to recommend surgery unless there is widespread metastasis, the patient is a poor risk for surgery, the primary cancer is clearly unresectable, or a lesion would require total gastrectomy with only palliative intent. Resection offers the only effective surgical palliation and, in cases of lesions involving the body or antrum should not be precluded in the symptomatic patient who has minor roentgenographic signs of advanced disease.

Mechanical and antibiotic bowel preparation should be given in view of the involvement of the transverse mesocolon in some cases, which may result in inadvertent intraoperative injury or need to resect the transverse colon. Malnourished patients should be nutritionally replenished in view of the required anastomosis. Preoperative radiation and neoadjuvant chemotherapy have no established role.

SURGERY

Retrospective evaluation of data from several centers has demonstrated that *radical subtotal gastrectomy* is the procedure of choice for lesions of the body or antrum. This procedure involves removing the cancer en bloc with about 75 percent of the stomach and draining lymph nodes. Multiple frozen sections help establish adequacy of resection prior to anastomosis; however, cancer cells may be sparsely distributed and difficult to identify on frozen section alone. Consequently, if there is any question, the margin of resection should be extended so the anastomosis is free of cancer cells. The first portion of the duodenum, gastrohepatic ligament, entire omentum, and celiac and other regional nodes are also removed, and some surgeons advocate *bilateral oophorectomy* because the ovaries are frequently involved with metastasis.

For lesions that approach the gastroesophageal junction, an *extended total gastrectomy* is necessary. This usually requires splenectomy in addition to removal of structures described above.

Patients do remarkably well following *Roux-en-Y esophagojejunostomy* or *loop jejunostomy*. A sleeve resection with pull-through anastomosis is not advised. Reconstruction following subtotal gastrectomy usually requires a *Billroth II* or *Roux-en-Y type anastomosis*. Placement of a small-caliber feeding jejunostomy can facilitate postoperative enteral nutritional support.

Although survival primarily depends on stage at diagnosis, direct extension of tumor to contiguous structures should *not* preclude resection for cure in a good risk patient with no evidence of distant metastasis (Table 3). This may require distal pancreatectomy, transverse colectomy, or partial left-sided hepatectomy. We have followed patients who have enjoyed years of disease-free survival after resection of gastric cancer locally extending into adjacent structures (Table 4).

Palliative resection (not including extensive lymphadenectomy, omentectomy, or removal of adjacent structures) is indicated for relief of symptoms provided

TABLE 3 Five-Year Survival After Curative Resection of Gastric Cancer

Involvement	Survival (%)
Limited to mucosa	90–95
Limited to submucosa	85–90
Invasive, nodes negative	45–50
Invasive, nodes positive	10–15

TABLE 4 Other Factors Reported to Affect Survival in Gastric Cancer

Factor	Adverse Effect
Cancer type	Scirrhous or infiltrating type
Involvement	Lymphatic or vascular invasion
Differentiation	Poorly differentiated
Sex	Males worse with advancing age
Node morphology	Sinus fibrosis

the procedure does not require total gastrectomy, transection of gross tumor, or unacceptable risk to the patient. Resection is the only effective surgical palliation. Bypass gastrojejunostomy, gastrostomy, or jejunostomy is usually ineffective for palliation and rarely alleviates symptoms or prolongs survival. When conditions preclude resection, the abdomen should be closed without further surgery.

ADJUVANT THERAPY

Radiation

There is no established adjuvant therapy for gastric cancer. If permanent sections reveal cancer cells at the anastomosis, restricted field radiation therapy, alone or with 5-fluorouracil (5-FU), should be given. Otherwise, we generally do not recommend radiation therapy except for palliation of recurrent disease. Newer techniques and intraoperative radiation therapy are under investigation and theoretically have merit, because the pattern of failure of gastric cancer are primarily local, regional, or both as illustrated in Table 5. (See also the chapter *Intraoperative Irradiation.*)

Chemotherapy

More than 23 studies conducted in this country have been published describing the use of combination chemotherapy following curative resection of gastric cancer. Many of these involved small numbers of patients or were uncontrolled. On balance, there is no established advantage to postoperative chemotherapy alone or in combination with radiation or immunotherapy. Consequently, patients should be considered for adjuvant therapy under protocol. In lieu of this, 5-FU, doxorubicin, and mitomycin may be given to patients at high risk of recurrence, using standard dosages described in the section on treatment for advanced disease. Adjuvant therapy does not appear to be indicated for patients with early gastric cancer (confined to mucosa and/or submucosa) even if nodes are positive.

POSTOPERTIVE AND SUPPORTIVE CARE

Following gastric resection, we begin giving all patients vitamin B_{12} injections so this will not subsequently be overlooked. Iron supplementation is often necessary.

TABLE 5 Initial Patterns of Failure*

Local-Regional (65%)	(%)	Distant (35%)	(%)
Gastric bed	55	Liver	50
Lymph nodes	40	Lung	25
Peritoneal cavity	40	Bone	15
Anastomosis	25	Other	10

* Subheadings not mutually exclusive

TABLE 6 Follow-up of Patients with Postoperative Years 1 and 2

Interval (mo)	Evaluation
3–6	History, physical examination, complete blood count, chemistries, CEA*
6–12	Above (3–6 mo) components, gastroscopy with biopsy, CT scan and chest roentgenogram
As needed	Determined by clinical symptoms, signs, or laboratory abnormalities

* CEA is of limited value for surveillance of gastric cancer.

Steatorrhea typically accompanies gastrectomy, and we usually advise reducing fat caloric intake to about 30 percent of total calories. Restricting fluids with meals and intake of rich hyperosmolar foods, in our experience, almost always controls symptoms of dumping. If a patient has unexplained diarrhea, increased steatorrhea, or nutritional deficiencies, consider the possibility of celiac-sprue unmasked by gastric surgery. Frequent (4 or 5) nutritionally sound feedings per day should be provided.

Nausea associated with impaired gastric emptying frequently accompanies *retroperitoneal extension* of cancer. Prospective studies and personal experience demonstrate efficacy of metoclopramide, 10 to 20 mg orally three times a day, before meals. *Pain* secondary to cancer involving the upper abdomen or retroperitoneum may be partially alleviated by a celiac block. This applies to gastric as well as pancreatic or other retroperitoneal cancers. When analgesics are required for chronic pain they should be given on a scheduled basis using drugs that have intermediate or long duration of action and are well absorbed. If analgesics cannot be taken orally or need to be supplemented, rectal suppositories may be used, obviating the need for injections.

Approximately 85 percent of patients who develop recurrent disease do so within 2 years following surgery. This is the interval when surveillance is most important. Patients who develop solitary metastasis or anastomotic and/or stump recurrence should be considered for repeat resection or metastasectomy if, on careful examination, there is no evidence of metastatic disease elsewhere and provided the surgical risks are acceptable. There is a trend toward combining frequent, limited, noninvasive clinical and laboratory assessment with less frequent, more extensive examination. There are no hard

TABLE 7 Single Agent Chemotherapy for Gastric Cancer*

Drug	Approximate Response Rate (%)	Range (%)
Doxorubicin	26	25–36
Mitomycin	30	27–32
Cisplatin	20	18–26
5-Fluorouracil	22	21–23
Nitrosoureas	12	8–18

* Response varies with prior therapy, performance status and other factors.

TABLE 8 FAM Chemotherapy for Gastric Cancer (8-Week Cycle)

Drugs	Dosage (mg/M² IV)*	Day Therapy Given
5-Fluorouracil	600	1, 8, 29, 36
Doxorubicin	30	1, 29
Mitomycin	10	1

* Must be adjusted for toxicity and anticipated tolerance

TABLE 9 FAP Chemotherapy for Gastric Cancer (4-Week Cycle)

Drugs	Dosage (mg/M² IV)*	Day Therapy Given
5-Fluorouracil	600	1, 8, 29, 36
Doxorubicin	30	1, 29
Cisplatin	100	1, 29

* Must be adjusted for toxicity and anticipated tolerance; requires hydration/diuresis

TABLE 10 Alternate Dosage Schedule of FAP Chemotherapy for Gastric Cancer (3- or 4-Week Cycle)

Drugs	Dosage (mg/M² IV)*	Day Therapy Given
5-Fluorouracil	500–600	1, 2, 3, 4, 5
Doxorubicin	30–40	1
Cisplatin	20	1, 2, 3, 4, 5

* Must be adjusted for toxicity and anticipated tolerance

data as to optimal studies or interval of follow up. Postoperative surveillance provides an opportunity to look for complications of therapy as well as recurrent disease (Table 6).

TREATMENT FOR ADVANCED DISEASE

Radiation

Radiation therapy for advanced disease should generally be reserved for specific palliative problems, such as obstruction at the esophagogastric junction, bleeding, or pain due to tumor extension or skeletal metastasis. Symptoms can usually be effectively palliated using a minimum of 3,000 rads given in ten fractions over 2 weeks. Smaller fraction, 200 rads per day, (5,000 rads total dose) therapy may be preferable for malignant obstruction involving the upper gastrointestinal tract. High-dose short-term therapy should be used for patients with widespread disease and limited duration of survival. Smaller fraction, high total dose therapy for locally recurrent disease may be given with 5-FU chemotherapy.

Chemotherapy

More than 30 single agents have been studied for their activity against gastric cancer. No survival benefit has been established. Of these, 5-FU, doxorubicin, mitomycin C, the nitrosoureas, and cisplatin enjoy the highest response rate (Table 7). 5-Flourouracil can be given to patients who do not qualify for more aggressive combination chemotherapy.

Combination chemotherapy, usually involving some combination of the drugs mentioned above, has been the subject of more than 60 reports since Reitemeier and Moertel's publications in the early 1970s. The recent trend is to combine 5-FU, doxorubicin (adriamycin), and mitomycin (FAM) in the dosage schedule outlined in Table 8.

In comparative trials, the FAM regimen and 5-FU-doxorubicin-Methyl CCNU achieved higher response rates (25% and 30%) than other combinations, including addition of investigational agents. Adding a nitrosourea to FAM does not enhance its activity.

Bone marrow toxicity is often the dose-limiting factor for FAM chemotherapy and may require substituting cisplatin for mitomycin (Table 9). This likewise results in serious marrow toxicity after multiple courses of therapy.

Another dosage schedule of these agents can be more easily and safely administered on an outpatient basis and is under investigation at two comprehensive cancer centers (Table 10).

Although far from ideal, FAM appears to be as effective as any form of combination therapy, with reported response rates ranging from 16 to 45 percent and averaging 32 percent when the results of nine studies involving more than 300 patients are combined. Although it is gratifying to note that some patients with advanced disease respond well to therapy, new therapeutic approaches are necessary to increase survival for the majority of patients to survive.

Laser Palliation

Interventional endoscopy has provided the opportunity to palliate some patients with symptomatic advanced disease. If obstructive symptoms are refractory to radiation with or without chemotherapy, laser therapy combined with balloon dilation should be tried if the patient's survival time is anticipated to exceed 6 to 8 weeks. This therapy should be started while the gastric lumen can be easily identified so the laser beam can be directed with maximum safety. Laser uses in gastroenterology are discussed in the chapter *Laser Treatment in Gastrointestinal Disease*.

PREMALIGNANT CONDITIONS OF THE STOMACH

ROBERT G. STRICKLAND, M.D., F.R.A.C.P., F.A.C.P.

GASTRIC CANCER IN PERSPECTIVE

The incidence of gastric cancer in the United States population (currently 9 per 100,000) has declined steadily since the 1930s when it was the most common form of cancer. Over the past 15 years, a similar trend toward decreasing gastric cancer rates has become evident worldwide, including such high incidence regions as Japan. In the United States, gastric cancer is now the third most common digestive malignancy, having fallen slightly below pancreatic cancer in overall frequency. The leading digestive organ malignancy in this country, colorectal cancer, is approximately five times as prevalent as gastric cancer. In spite of these trends, an estimated 25,000 new cases of gastric cancer occurred in the United States in 1984. In addition, regional differences, apparently based on ethnicity, continue to be evident. Thus, in the southwestern United States, gastric cancer rates among Hispanic and Native American populations have been observed to be two to three times those among white populations in the same region.

The prognosis for gastric cancer in the United States population continues to be grim. Relative 5-year survival has shown no significant improvement, remaining at 10 to 15 percent over the past 15 years. It is clear from the observations of workers in Japan, and some selected centers in the West, that detection of gastric cancer at an early stage can dramatically improve survival. In Japan, the detection of early gastric cancer has largely resulted from mass screening of the population by roentgenography and/or endoscopy. Such an approach would be impractical in the United States, where the relative frequency of gastric cancer is approximately eight times lower than in Japan.

Premalignant conditions and lesions of the gastric mucosa have been identified as risk factors for either the coexistence or later development of some forms of gastric cancer. Detailed upper gastrointestinal evaluation of symptomatic patients with these conditions, together with periodic screening of selected asymptomatic subjects in these risk groups, offers the best chance of improving the outcome of gastric cancer in Western populations.

CLASSIFICATIONS AND ETIOLOGY

Adenocarcinoma accounts for more than 90 percent of gastric malignancies, and the histopathologic (Lauren) classification into intestinal and diffuse types is used for both advanced and early carcinomas. The intestinal type is a well-differentiated tumor, occurs in older patients, and is consistently associated with marked atrophic gastritis in the remainder of the stomach. Diffuse gastric cancer is poorly differentiated, affects younger age groups, and an associated atrophic gastritis is less consistently observed. There is good evidence that the temporal change in the incidence of gastric cancer has been largely due to a decrease in the incidence of the intestinal type, and the relative frequency of diffuse tumors is now greater than in the past.

Both familial and environmental factors are believed to influence the development of gastric carcinoma. Genetic influences are significant in diffuse gastric cancer but are less evident in the intestinal type. On the other hand, environmental factors are believed to be particularly relevant to the development of the intestinal type of gastric cancer. A popular hypothesis relates the initiation of this type of gastric cancer to the in vivo formation of nitrosamines which results from gastric hypo- or achlorhydria and bacterial reduction of dietary nitrates to nitrites. Patients with achlorhydria have been shown to have increased concentrations of nitrite and nitrosamines in gastric juice, but there is no direct evidence that these alterations are responsible for the initiation of gastric carcinogenesis. Furthermore, suggestions that chemoprevention (inhibition of intragastric nitrosamine formation) by ascorbate may be possible are also unproven at this time.

PREMALIGNANT CONDITIONS AND PREMALIGNANT LESIONS OF THE STOMACH

Morson has emphasized the importance of distinguishing precancerous conditions and precancerous lesions (Table 1). The former refers to a clinical state associated with an increased risk of cancer. A precancerous lesion, on the other hand, is a histopathologic abnormality in which cancer is more likely to arise than in its apparently normal counterpart. A number of clinical disorders are considered to be associated with an increased risk of gastric cancer, including pernicious anemia, chronic atrophic gasritis, gastric polyps, gastric stumps (postgastrectomy), gastric ulcer, Menetrier's disease, and certain immunodeficiency syndromes. The histopathologic abnormality of the gastric mucosa which occurs in a majority of these conditions, and has in the past been most closely linked to gastric carcinoma, is intestinal metaplasia of the epithelium. It is important to note, however, that neither the premalignant conditions nor the precancerous change of intestinal metaplasia imply inevitability of malignant transformation of the mucosa. They are simply markers of an increased probability of such change.

Most recently, the concept of epithelial dysplasia in the gastric mucosa has emerged. This histopathologic change has been most commonly (but not exclusively) observed in association with intestinal metaplasia and with the intestinal type of gastric cancer. The histologic features that define gastric mucosal dysplasia were developed by a World Health Organization expert Committee on Precancerous Conditions of the Stomach. They include epithelial cellular atypia, abnormal differentiation, and disorganized mucosal architecture. The degree of epithelial dysplasia is classified into three grades—mild,

TABLE 1 Precursors of Gastric Cancer

Premalignant Conditions

Pernicious anemia
Chronic atrophic gastritis
   Type A, Type B
Gastric polyps (sporadic); polyposis syndromes
   Adenomatous
   Hyperplastic (rarely)
   Carcinoids
Gastric stumps
Chronic gastric ulcer (?)
Menetrier's disease
Immunodeficiency syndromes
   Common variable immunodeficiency
   Ataxia-telangiectasia

Premalignant Lesions

Intestinal metaplasia (incompletely differentiated type)
Epithelial dysplasia

---

moderate, and severe—according to the severity of the changes. The basis for this classification remains a subjective one. Thus, the distinctions between mild dysplasia and inflammation-associated regenerative change, and between severe dysplasia and intramucosal carcinoma, remain problematic. The natural history of gastric epithelial dysplasia and its usefulness as a more specific marker of gastric cancer risk are areas of current research interest.

Methods of Clinical Evaluation

The primary goal in the evaluation of premalignant conditions of the stomach is the detection of gastric cancer at an early and potentially curable stage. Double-contrast radiography can detect larger focal gastric lesions such as ulcers and polyps. It lacks sufficient sensitivity, however, in the identification of more subtle focal surface abnormalities which may be the site of early gastric cancer. It is therefore of very little use in selecting those patients in need of endoscopic examination. The most direct method of identifying early gastric cancer is through the use of endoscopic examination of the stomach with targeted biopsy or endoscopic excision (polypectomy, "large particle biopsy") of any visible mucosal abnormality. Multiple stepwise biopsies, cytologic studies of a flat mucosa lacking focal surface abnormalities, or both may also be used, though the yield of such sampling is far smaller than that using directed biopsy of visible lesions.

An ingenious approach to the identification of focal mucosal abnormalities, which could be the site of early gastric cancer, is the technique of chromoendoscopy. This method, developed by Japanese workers, involves endoscopic dyeing of the mucosa with methylene blue and congo red. The lesions of early gastric cancer appear as bleached areas in contrast to the surrounding red-colored mucosa. There are no reports of the use of chromoendoscopy in Western populations at risk for gastric cancer, but it appears to be a technique worthy of study.

A second goal of upper endoscopy in the evaluation of patients with premalignant conditions of the stomach may be the identification of epithelial dysplasia. The full significance of gastric mucosal dysplasia is not yet established. Potentially, its presence may provide an additional and more sensitive marker of cancer risk so that subsets of patients with a given premalignant condition may be identified for intensive surveillance.

SPECIFIC PREMALIGNANT CONDITIONS AND THEIR MANAGEMENT

Pernicious Anemia and Chronic Atrophic Gastritis

Severe atrophic gastritis or gastric atrophy affecting the body and fundus of the stomach, and in general sparing the antral mucosa, is the central pathologic lesion leading to pernicious anemia. The prepernicious anemia state can also be recognized and has been termed type A gastritis. This condition causes identical morphologic and functional changes of the gastric mucosa and similar immunologic aberrations to those present in established pernicious anemia. The risk of gastric cancer is increased in pernicious anemia and probably also in type A gastritis. The reported magnitude of risk has been variable but approaches a three- to fourfold increase compared with that in the general population. The contribution of these precursors to the overall occurrence of gastric cancer in a given population, however, is small ($<10\%$). This observation appears to contradict the finding that most patients with the intestinal type of gastric cancer display extensive chronic atrophic gastritis. The gastritis that accompanies a majority of intestinal type gastric cancers, however, is type B in distribution, i.e., antral-predominant with variable involvement of the body and fundic mucosa. This form of atrophic gastritis, in contrast to that present in pernicious anemia and the prepernicious anemia state (type A), is rarely accompanied by gastric autoantibodies and is an extremely common finding in otherwise healthy aging subjects.

Two distinct management decisions arise in patients with pernicious anemia or atrophic gastritis (type A or B). First, in patients with symptoms or signs that could indicate the presence of gastric malignancy (upper gastrointestinal symptoms, unexplained weight loss, anemia, occult gastrointestinal bleeding), complete investigation as outlined in the previous section is clearly indicated.

The second management decision is whether asymptomatic patients with these conditions should undergo endoscopic surveillance. Repeated endoscopy in this mostly elderly population is not without risk and is costly, and the overall yield of detecting early and curable cancer is very low in relation to the size of the populations at risk. Thus, with the possible exception of younger patients or those with a family history of gastric cancer, routine surveillance of patients with pernicious anemia or atrophic gastritis cannot be recommended. Perhaps initial screening with the purpose of identifying those patients showing polyps (see following section) and/or epithelial dysplasia followed by selective surveillance of these subpopulations may lead to a higher yield at lower overall cost and risk. An initial study of this approach in pernicious anemia revealed that 33 of 80 patients had dysplasia and 18 of 80 had polyps. In seven of the nine patients showing moderate or severe dysplasia, the biopsy specimens were obtained from mucosal areas with visible surface abnormalities. Until the evolution of these lesions is more fully defined, this approach to selective surveillance cannot be firmly recommended.

An additional investigative approach to identifying high-risk patients from among those with pernicious anemia or atrophic gastritis has involved the staining of endoscopic biopsies for sulfomucins, a marker of incompletely differentiated intestinal metaplasia. One study has suggested that strongly positive staining for sulfomucins indicated high specificity (94%) for the presence of carcinoma. Sensitivity of this finding was, however, low (34%). Other histochemical markers of incomplete intestinal metaplasia and increased risk of cancer identified by Japanese workers are reduced aminopeptidase and absent alkaline phosphatase staining. Further study of the application of special staining techniques to endoscopic biopsies is needed before this approach is used in clinical practice.

Gastric Polyps

Gastric polyps are discovered in approximately 2 percent of upper endoscopic examinations. A majority of the polyps (80%) are epithelial. Epithelial polyps of the gastric mucosa include hyperplastic (regenerative) polyps and neoplastic (adenomatous) polyps. The essential histopathologic difference between hyperplastic and adenomatous polyps is that the epithelium is normal in the former and dysplastic in the latter. The relative frequency of the different types of gastric epithelial polyps is well established. A majority (75% to 90%) are hyperplastic. Hyperplastic polyps are smooth surfaced, usually sessile, and may be single (50%) or multiple (50%); most (85%) are small (<1 cm) and they carry a very low (1%) risk of malignant change. Adenomatous polyps, on the other hand, are usually single, larger in diameter (>1 cm), and display a lobulated surface; they carry a substantial risk of malignant transformation (average, 40%). It should be noted, however, that in spite of these differences in risk of malignant change in hyperplastic and adenomatous polyps, carcinoma may still develop elsewhere in the stomach of patients with either type of polyp. This is because both types of polyp are significantly associated with atrophic gastritis and intestinal metaplasia of the nonpolyp-bearing mucosa. It is important to establish this association even though its extent may have been overestimated in the past (small single or relatively few hyperplastic polyps more commonly arise in normal gastric mucosa).

In addition to the association with atrophic gastritis, hyperplastic and adenomatous polyps are seen in association with the polyposis syndromes—in particular, with polyposis coli where there is a significant risk of malignant transformation. Multiple hyperplastic polyps are also seen in the Cronkhite-Canada syndrome and Cowden's disease, but in these disorders there is no increased risk of malignant change. In the Peutz-Jeghers syndrome, gastric hamartomatous polyps occur in 25 percent of patients and there appears to be a significant risk of gastric carcinoma in this rare condition.

Gastric carcinoids present as single or multiple sessile polyps with a yellowish-pink color. They represent approximately 1 percent of all gastric polyps and may become locally invasive or, rarely, metastatic. The carcinoid syndrome is unusual. Recent studies have indicated a substantial association of gastric carcinoids with pernicious anemia and type A atrophic gastritis.

In a majority of instances, gastric polyps are asymptomatic or associated with vague upper abdominal complaints. Less than 10 percent of gastric polyps bleed significantly and intermittent gastric outlet obstruction is rare.

The management of patients with gastric polyps thus involves several considerations, including whether polyps are symptomatic or asymptomatic, whether there are single or multiple polyps, their size, the presence of associated conditions such as atrophic gastritis, and, most important, the histologic nature of the polyp(s). While forceps biopsy sampling of gastric polyps is not entirely satisfactory in ruling out neoplastic foci, it remains preferable to endoscopic polypectomy as the first step in evaluation. This approach is predicated on the relatively low frequency of adenomatous polyps in the stomach and the observation that hemorrhage is more frequent (4%) with gastric than with colonic polypectomy.

The following strategy in approaching the patient with gastric polyp(s) is suggested (Fig. 1). The polyp(s) should be biopsied, and stepwise biopsy specimens of nonpolyp-bearing mucosa of the gastric antrum and body should also be taken. If the polyp is hyperplastic and small (<1 cm), and the nonpolyp-bearing mucosa is normal, the patient may be followed up expectantly with repeated endoscopy only if clinically indicated. If the hyperplastic polyp occurs against a background of atrophic gastritis or a polyposis syndrome, endoscopic surveillance every two years may be advisable; however, as indicated in the previous section, the value of this approach remains to be established by prospective studies. Symptomatic hyperplastic polyps, most of which will be larger than 1 cm, can be removed by endoscopic polypectomy or surgery, the choice being determined largely by the size and location of the polyp and local experience with these two therapeutic modalities. In practice the decision to proceed with removal of hyperplastic polyps is often influenced by other factors, such as age and associated disease. High-risk patients in whom symptoms are not life-threatening may be better served by continued observation.

If the polyp is adenomatous on biopsy (most will be single polyps) polypectomy is more clearly indicated irrespective of its size or whether it is symptomatic. Furthermore, periodic endoscopic surveillance (2-year inter-

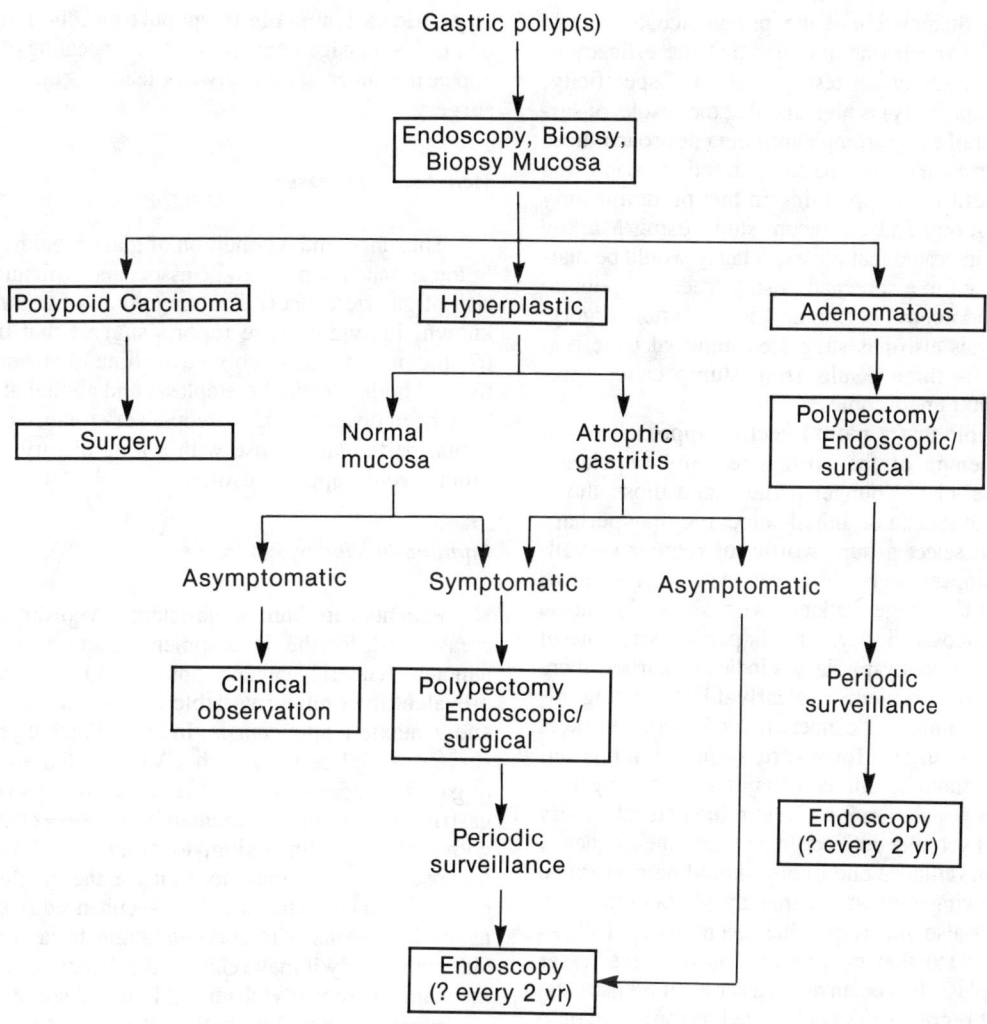

Figure 1 A suggested approach to management and surveillance of gastric polyps.

vals) after polypectomy is desirable in such patients with or without associated atrophic gastritis. In some high-risk patients with an adenomatous polyp, however, periodic observation of the patient and the polyp may be the preferred course.

Gastric Stumps

A majority of studies (but not all) involving the long-term follow-up of patients who have undergone partial gastrectomy for benign peptic ulcer disease reveal an increased incidence of carcinoma of the gastric remnant beginning 15 years after operation. Those with Billroth II anastomosis appear most susceptible and the risk extends to patients operated on for either gastric or duodenal ulcers. The magnitude of risk for the development of stump carcinoma was probably overestimated in earlier studies and is probably in the 3 to 6 percent range, representing a two to threefold increase over that expected. A majority of stump carcinomas originate in the region of the stoma. Once these tumors become symptomatic, resectability rates and survival (5% at 5 years) are very low. The histogenesis of stump carcinoma is believed to be similar to that of gastric cancer developing against a background of atrophic gastritis or pernicious anemia. Atrophic gastritis of the remnant following partial resection is almost universal, and changes of intestinal metaplasia and epithelial dysplasia have been observed with varying frequency in this setting. In contrast to atrophic gastritis in the nonoperated stomach, visible lesions do not correlate well with either dysplasia or early cancer in the gastric stump. Multiple biopsies (up to 20) of the remnant are therefore needed to provide histologic documentation of these lesions in the operated stomach.

As previously discussed in relation to atrophic gastritis and pernicious anemia, symptomatic postgastrectomy patients must undergo full upper gastrointestinal evaluation. Asymptomatic patients would also appear to represent a group worthy of surveillance for detection of early gastric cancer. The prevailing view, however, does not favor such an approach, at least in populations (such as the United States) where the prevalence of gastric cancer is low. Even if one assumes that the efficacy of endoscopy as a screening test (sensitivity, specificity, reliability, acceptability) is high and that the results of surgical treatment of early stump carcinoma approach those for early gastric cancer in the unoperated stomach, the estimated benefit is disappointing in this predominantly elderly population. Thus, a recent study using Markov chain analysis indicated that life expectancy would be marginally improved in a screened postgastrectomy population (annual endoscopy) beginning 15 years after surgery. Another analysis also has suggested minimal benefit at significant cost—three deaths from stump cancer prevented by 1,000 endoscopies.

It is possible that a more selective approach to endoscopic screening of the postgastrectomy population would be beneficial. Younger patients and those showing epithelial dysplasia on initial screening may perhaps represent such select groups worthy of regular surveillance. There appears to be, however, no clear consensus yet on how to manage patients who show dysplastic changes on mucosal biopsy. This is particularly true of those showing severe dysplasia. As indicated earlier, there may be diagnostic problems in clearly differentiating this lesion from intramucosal cancer. Indeed, some workers advocate gastric surgery for severe dysplasia in this setting. Clearly, though, this is a major undertaking in a mostly elderly population for a lesion, the natural history of which is not yet fully defined. In addition, the frequency with which surveillance endoscopy should be performed in patients showing mild or moderate dysplasia of the remnant mucosa is also uncertain. One recent 3-year follow-up study indicated that no progression of these lesser grades of dysplasia had occurred in a series of 58 patients. In fact, actual regression was observed in some patients. The authors suggested that reexaminations might therefore be carried out every 3 to 5 years. In view of all these uncertainties it is clear that additional prospective studies of selective surveillance will be needed before any firm recommendations can be made for patients with gastric stumps.

Gastric Ulcers

The existence of so-called ulcer cancer, that is, the development of carcinoma in a preexisting peptic ulcer, has been debated for many years. If this sequence occurs at all (and it is almost impossible to establish proof of such a transition) it is rare. A small proportion (<5%) of apparently benign gastric ulcers (defined by endoscopic visualization, multiple target biopsies, and brush cytology) will later prove to be malignant, either at follow-up endoscopy or following surgical resection for incomplete healing. In a majority of such situations it is most likely that the ulcer was malignant from the outset and evaded discovery despite optimal diagnostic methods. While it is uncommon, this type of occurrence emphasizes the importance of following benign gastric ulcers to complete endoscopic healing. The higher the background incidence of gastric carcinoma in the population, the more important is this management approach. Nonhealing of a benign-appearing ulcer should always lead to consideration of surgery.

Menetrier's Disease

This uncommon condition of giant rugal hypertrophy of the stomach appears to be associated with an increased risk of gastric cancer. The magnitude of this risk is not known. Individual case reports suggest that the hypertrophic process may evolve over time to atrophic gastritis, and both intestinal metaplasia and epithelial dysplasia have been observed. Endoscopic surveillance of such patients, particularly those with a long history of the disorder, would appear justified.

Immunodeficiency Syndromes

Patients with immunodeficiency syndromes are at increased risk for the development of a number of malignancies. Gastric cancer appears to be particularly prevalent in common variable immunodeficiency (CVI) and in ataxia-telangiectasia. Indeed, a recent prospective survey of 220 patients with CVI revealed an incidence of gastric cancer 47 times that expected. Severe atrophic gastritis occurs in approximately 50 percent of patients with CVI, and this lesion, together with impaired immunosurveillance, may account for the heightened risk of gastric cancer. The basis for the enhanced risk of malignancy in patients with ataxia-telangiectasia is unknown, although clearly it may relate to the defective DNA repair mechanisms recently observed in this disorder. There is no reported experience with endoscopic surveillance in these patients, but in view of the above observations this approach should be considered, particularly in those with CVI and associated atrophic gastritis.

CONCLUSIONS

There are a number of premalignant conditions that appear to place the stomach at higher risk for the develop-

TABLE 2 Current Limitations of Routine Surveillance Endoscopy in Asymptomatic Patients with Pernicious Anemia, Atrophic Gastritis, or Gastric Stumps

Target populations mostly elderly, with associated diseases that may increase risk of repeated endoscopy and surgery

Acceptability of repeated endoscopy in absence of symptoms is low

Yield of detecting early cancer low in relation to size of population at risk (especially true in U.S. where prevalence of gastric cancer is low)

Cost: benefit ratio unacceptable

New methods directed toward selective surveillance (dysplasia, incompletely differentiated metaplasia) not yet applicable to practice setting (see text)

ment of carcinoma. The statistical risk in any of these conditions is not fully defined and may be declining in parallel with a worldwide decrease in the incidence of this tumor. The magnitude of risk in each of these conditions is in any case small. Nevertheless, patients with these premalignant conditions who develop upper gastrointestinal symptoms should undergo full evaluation, including endoscopy and sampling of any visible mucosal abnormalities. The management of these premalignant conditions has been reviewed, particularly from the perspective of endoscopic surveillance of asymptomatic individuals so that cancer can be detected at an early and potentially curable stage. There are significant problems with this approach at the present time (Table 2), and there is a great need to develop new methods to identify patients with a more substantial risk of the development of gastric cancer.

The detection of gastric epithelial dysplasia shows promise in this regard, and the results of prospective studies of patients with this lesion are awaited with interest.

Even if this approach is successful, its impact on the detection of most gastric cancers at an early and potentially curable stage remains uncertain. As indicated in this review, the incidence of the intestinal type of gastric cancer is decreasing. This form of gastric cancer is the one most likely to be favorably influenced by surveillance of known premalignant conditions. By contrast, diffuse gastric cancer is becoming relatively more common but the precursors of this tumor are currently not well defined. Until the factors involved in its development are better understood, present methods of surveillance may have little impact on the outcome of this increasingly important form of gastric cancer.

INTRAOPERATIVE IRRADIATION

LEONARD L. GUNDERSON, M.D., M.S.

Although useful palliation can be achieved in many patients when conventional modalities (external beam irradiation and chemotherapy with or without resection) are used in the treatment of locally advanced gastrointestinal malignancies, local control and long-term survival are rare owing to the limited radiation tolerance of the surrounding organs and tissues. For unresected lesions or lesions with subtotal resection and residual disease, local control and cure occur in 5 to 30 percent of patients,[1] but external beam radiation doses required to accomplish such results are 6,000 to 7,000 rad or more. Such doses exceed the radiation tolerance of some organs and structures in the abdomen and pelvis. The tolerance of the stomach, small intestine, and spinal cord is 4,500 to 5,000 rad over five to five and a half weeks; of the entire liver, 2,500 to 3,000 rad over three to four weeks; and of both kidneys, 2,000 to 2,500 rad over two to three weeks. Portions of the large bowel and bladder can safely receive 6,000 to 7,000 rad, but at the upper dose level the volume of organ must be small or the risk of complications will be excessive.

In view of the dose limitations of external beam techniques, intraoperative radiation (IORT) has been used in the United States and Japan in the last two decades in an attempt to improve the therapeutic ratio of local control versus complications.[2-8] These objectives are achieved by (1) decreasing the volume of the irradiation "boost field" by direct tumor visualization and appositional treatment, (2) excluding all or part of dose-limiting sensitive structures by operative mobilization or shielding and/or the use of appropriate electron beam energies, and (3) increasing the "effective" dose to the tumor volume due to (1) and (2).

Although early investigators in Japan[2] and the United States (Howard University[3-6]) generally delivered intraoperative radiation to the site of interest with a single dose of 2,000 to 4,000 rad with electron beams and rarely used any supplemental external beam irradiation, those at Massachusetts General Hospital (MGH)[5,6] and the Mayo Clinic[6,7] preferred to use intraoperative electrons as a "boost" dose in conjunction with conventional fractionated external beam radiation and resection whenever feasible. This approach is similar to that employed in patients with malignancies such as head and neck, breast, and gynecologic tumors in whom combined external beam and "boost" techniques are commonly employed. The only difference is the method of delivering the boost dose (i.e., for head and neck and breast tumors interstitial implants are used; for gynecologic tumors, intracavitary insertions; and for intra-abdominal, pelvic, or thoracic tumors, intraoperative electrons).

There are several potential advantages of a combined external beam-intraoperative approach over intraoperative irradiation alone: improvement in local-regional control because of a decreased risk of marginal recurrence (areas at risk are included in the external beam field) and the radiobiologic advantages of fractionated irradiation, and less risk of normal tissue necrosis. The excellent long-term results achieved with head and neck, breast, and gynecologic malignancies support the concept of combining external beam and boost dose irradiation techniques, since good local control has been achieved with relatively little morbidity to dose-limiting normal tissues.

In pilot studies from MGH and the Mayo Clinic an IORT dose of 1,000 to 2,000 rad has been combined with fractionated external beam doses of 4,500 to 5,000 rad (25 to 28 fractions of 180 rad in five to five and a half weeks) and, when safely feasible, subtotal or gross total resection of disease (resections done with gastric and colorectal lesions but not with initially unresectable pancreatic or biliary duct tumors). The biologic effectiveness of single-dose irradiation is considered equivalent to two to three times the efficacy of that quantity of fractionated external beam treatment.[9] In view of that, the effective dose in the IORT boost field, when added to the 4,500 to 5,000 rad delivered in 25 to 28 fractions with external beam techniques, is 6,500 to 8,000 rad for an IORT dose of 1,000 rad, 7,500 to 9,500 rad with a 1,500-rad boost, and 8,500 to 11,000 rad with a 2,000-rad IORT dose.

Given the advent of the aggressive treatment approaches described in this chapter, a recommendation of therapeutic nihilism for locally advanced gastrointestinal malignancies is now inappropriate, as tools exist for greater long-term local control with or without cure. Patient symptoms and diagnostic roentgenographic changes due to irradiation fibrosis, however, can mimic tumor persistence or regrowth, and the radiation oncologist needs to be an active member of the follow-up team. Often only time and serial radiographs over a 6- to 12-month period will resolve the issue. Randomized trials by site are needed to determine if the observed differences seen in prospective nonrandomized trials are real or are due to differences in case selection.

The intent of this chapter is to discuss, by site, the indications for and potential of aggressive combined techniques that include IORT. Previous results obtained with only external beam techniques with or without resection will be provided to demonstrate the need for higher doses of irradiation. Technical considerations of and results with IORT in the MGH and Mayo pilot studies will be presented, and the potential for the future will be discussed.

UPPER GASTROINTESTINAL MALIGNANCIES

Gastric Cancer

Treatment Alternatives

External beam irradiation has been shown to have good palliative and occasional curative potential in patients with residual disease after resection or in those with unresectable lesions, but its greatest benefit has been when used in combination with chemotherapy. In a randomized series from the Mayo Clinic,[10] 5-fluorouracil (5-FU) was utilized during the first three days of irradiation in half the group: For the combined treatment group, mean and overall survival were improved (13 versus 5.9 months and 3 of 25 patients, or 12%, versus 0 of 23 patients surviving five years). In a recent randomized study by the Gastrointestinal Tumor Study Group,[11] a combination of irradiation and 5-FU followed by maintenance 5-FU-MECCNU was statistically superior to 5-FU-MECCNU alone for long-term survival, with a plateau of 20 percent between the second and third years of follow-up (p <0.05).

Intraoperative radiation has been used in the management of gastric cancer primarily in Japan.[2] Abe and colleagues use pentagonal cones to deliver single doses of 2,800 to 4,000 rad to the tumor bed and major nodal sites after gastrectomy. Although a formal randomization procedure was not performed, patients were selected for IORT on the basis of the day they were admitted to the hospital. In a prospective study, 110 patients were treated by surgery alone and 84 patients by surgery plus IORT with results as shown in Table 1. The five-year survival is very similar in patients with stage I disease, but there is a suggestion of a survival advantage for the IORT group in both stage II (77.6% versus 54.5%) and stage III (44.6% versus 36.8%) disease. The most impressive difference, however, is for stage IV patients who had residual disease without distant metastases. In this subset, no survivors were seen among 18 patients treated with operation alone compared with a 19.5 percent five-year survival rate in 27 patients treated with surgery plus IORT. Unfortunately, these data do not answer the question of whether IORT would be more effective than conventional external beam irradiation plus chemotherapy or whether the combined use of both irradiation modalities would be even more effective, and randomized trials are needed.

Failure Patterns

Patterns of tumor progression were not analyzed in detail in any of these trials to determine whether local persistence or progression was a major factor with regard to either quality or duration of life. The long-term survival figure of 20 percent seen with external beam irradiation and chemotherapy in the Gastrointestinal Tumor Study Group trial and with IORT in the Japanese experience closely parallels the incidence of patients with gastric disease undergoing curative resection who failed only in the local regional area in the University of Minnesota reoperative series (29% of failure group and 23% of total group at risk[12]). The remainder of patients who fail after curative resection and a large percentage of patients treated for unresected or residual disease have a component of failure in the liver or peritoneal cavity in spite of attempts at prevention of such with combined drug chemotherapy.

TABLE 1 Gastric Cancer: Five-Year Survival Versus Treatment Method in the Japanese Trials

	Surgery		Surgery + IORT	
	No. at Risk	% SR	No. at Risk	% SR
Stage I	43	93	20	88
Stage II	11	55	18	78
Stage III	38	37	19	45
Stage IV (no distant metastases)	18	0	27	20

IORT = intraoperative radiation; SR = survival rate

TABLE 2 Pancreatic Cancer: Comparison of Results

Series	No. of Pt	Median Survival (mo)			Local Failure*	
		Total Group	RT	RT + CT	No.	%
Radical operation, MGH (26 postoperative survivors)	31	10.5	——	——	13/26	(50)
Regional, Unresectable						
Mayo Clinic, external beam RT						
Untreated	67	6.0	——	——	——	——
3,500 rad/4 wk ± 5-FU	64	——	6.3	10.4	——	——
GITSG						
4,000 rad/6 wk + 5-FU	79	——	——	6.9	——	——
6,000 rad/10 wk ± 5-FU (XRT, 25 pt; XRT + CT, 75 pts)	100	——	5.1	8.7	——	——
Duke Curative Group						
6,000 rad/10 wk ± chemotherapy (RT, 9 pt; RT + CT, 11 pt)	20	——	8	10	——	——
Thomas Jefferson University Hospital						
6,300–6,700/7–9 wk external RT ± CT	46	——	7.3	12.4	36/46	(78)
External + I[125] implant ± CT†	26	——	5.5 (7.3)	11.3 (12.5)	5/26	(19)
Massachusetts General Hospital						
I[125] + external beam (4,000–4,500 rad/4.5–5 wk)	12	12	——	——	4/12	(33)
External + IORT (4,500–5,000 rad ± CT)	29	16.5	——	——	10/29	(34)
Mayo, external + IORT						
5,000 rad/180 rad per fraction plus 2,000 rad IORT	44	12.2	——	——	3/42	(7)
Japanese						
IORT alone		6	——	——	——	——
IORT + 4,000 rad external		10	——	——	——	——

* In evaluable patients
† Median survival external + implant: open figures = early postoperative deaths included; ( ) = excluded
RT = radiation, CT = chemotherapy, IORT = intraoperative radiation, XRT = external irradiation, I[125] = Iodine[125], MGH = Massachusetts General Hospital, GITSG = Gastrointestinal Tumor Study Group.

Pancreatic Cancer

Treatment Alternatives

For unresectable lesions, definite palliation and occasional cure can be obtained using external beam irradiation[13-16]. The duration of palliation appears to increase as the dose of irradiation is increased from 4,000 rad in four to six weeks[13] to 6,000 to 6,500 rad in seven to ten weeks,[14-16] and a combination of radiation and chemotherapy increases survival when compared with radiation alone (Table 2). Even in the high-dose series from Thomas Jefferson University, however, local failure was documented in at least two-thirds of patients[16].

In an attempt to improve local tumor control without increasing normal tissue morbidity, specialized radiation therapy techniques have been used to increase the irradiation dose to tumor volume. These have included IORT alone[2-4] or the use of iodine 125 implants[16-17] or intraoperative electrons as a boost dose in combination with external beam irradiation.[5-7,18] With IORT alone, results parallel those of the Mayo Clinic results with only surgical bypass or low-dose external irradiation. The Japanese now use external beam irradiation in combination with IORT. This combination has resulted in a lower incidence of local failure in most United States series, and improved median survival in some, when compared with conventional external beam irradiation, but it is uncertain whether this is due to superior treatment or case selection (see Table 2). While the combination methods deliver a much higher effective dose of irradiation than external beam alone, prospective randomized trials are needed to determine if a therapeutic gain will result from the more aggressive techniques.

Failure Patterns

While slight gains in median survival may be achieved by improving local tumor control, a serious distant failure problem may prevent significant improvements in long-term survival. In a Mayo Clinic pilot trial combining external beam and IORT, local progression has not been a major problem (Tables 2, 3), but median survival has shifted only slightly to 12.2 months.[7] A majority of patients with disease progression have demonstrated liver metastases, peritoneal seeding, or both. In the latest analysis of the MGH data, distant failure has also been a significant problem, occurring in 12 of 29 patients at risk.[18]

Biliary Duct

Treatment Alternatives

Significant palliation and occasional cure can be obtained with external beam irradiation to doses of 4,000 to 6,000 rad in four to seven weeks, but long-term local control is rare.[1] In a series by Kopelson, one-year survival was improved when 5-FU was added to external beam irradiation for treatment of advanced primary lesions.[19]

An alternative palliative approach used in some institutions is the placement of percutaneous transhepatic catheters or intraoperative U tubes through areas of obstruction to allow immediate decompression. This does nothing to treat the tumor, however, and is best used in combination with irradiation.

The use of intraoperative electrons as the sole treatment modality has been reported for unresectable lesions by several Japanese groups.[2] Although early bile duct recanalization was observed, four of five patients in the series by Todoroki et al experienced regional recurrence and the longest survival was 18 months.[20] This suggests that tumor had extended beyond the small volume encompassed by the IORT cones (no external beam irradiation was used).

The temporary insertion of sealed radioactive sources via transhepatic catheters can deliver localized high-dose irradiation and is especially attractive in view of its potential wide applicability. Published series have shown decent short-term results, but local failures are excessive if only transcatheter irradiation is used.

Both of the specialized methods have limitations if used as the sole method of treatment. We prefer to delivery 4,500 to 5,000 rad in 25 to 28 fractions over five to five and a half weeks to the primary lesion plus nodal areas with electrons or transcatheter sources as a boost dose: 1,500 to 2,000 rad with intraoperative electrons; 2,000 to 3,000 rad at a 0.7 to 1.0 cm radius with transcatheter sources.[21] An intraoperative electron boost is used when feasible, as stomach and duodenum can be displaced out of the boost field. For a 12- to 18-month period from initiation of treatment, it is difficult to distinguish problems related to the indwelling tubes, possible persistence of tumor, or radiation fibrosis. Patients deserve aggressive support, and the radiation oncologist needs to be an active member of the follow-up team. While early results with the combined techniques are encouraging (Tables 3, 4), patient numbers are small.

Failure Patterns

Extrahepatic bile duct lesions represent the best disease model in upper gastrointestinal sites for the translation of local control into improved survival. A majority of proximal lesions are either unresectable or have gross or microscopic residual disease remaining after attempts at resection, owing to the anatomic location and operative limitations. At the time of initial presentation, peritoneal seeding is present in only 5 to 10 percent of those with ductal primary tumors, and local regional failures are a common cause of death. In contrast, peritoneal seeding is present initially in at least 20 per-

TABLE 3 Incidence and Patterns of Failure of Gastrointestinal Intraoperative Radiation at the Mayo Clinic

Site	Failure		Patterns of Disease Progression (any component)*										
			CF			LF			DM			PS		
	No.	%	No.	%	(%)	No.	%	(%)	No.	%	(%)	No.	%	(%)
Pancreas	30/42	(71)	2	7	(5)	3	10	(7)	21	70	(50)	12	40	(29)
Biliary	0/8		—	—	—	—	—	—	—	—	—	—	—	—
Colorectum	13/35	(37)	1	8	(3)	4	31	(11)	11	85	(31)	2	15	(6)
Resected, residual†	11/27	(40)	1			2			9			2		
Unresectable, resected after external RT‡	2/6	(33)	0			1			2			0		
Recurrent, unresectable after external RT	0/2		0			0			0			0		

Note: This analysis was done in March 1985

* Open percentages are percentages of patients who failed and closed percentages are percentages of the total at risk
† Primary 3/9; recurrent 8/18
‡ Primary 0/2; recurrent 2/4

CF = central failure in intraoperative irradiation field; LF = local failure in external beam field; DM = distant metastases; PS = peritoneal seeding, RT = radiation

TABLE 4 Biliary Duct Cancer: Survival and Status by Treatment Method at the Mayo Clinic

Status	No. of Pt	Survival Incidence and Duration in Months ( ) by Method*			
		XRT	XRT + 5-FU	XRT + Ir[192]	XRT + IORT
Alive, NED	6	----	----	1(41)	5 (1,7,9,15,22)
Uncertain	1	----	----	1(18)	----
With disease	1	1(29*)	----	----	----
Dead, NED	2	----	----	----	2,(4,37)
Uncertain	1	----	----	----	1(6)
With disease	11	5 (6,8,14,16,39*)	3 (10*,11*,16)	3 (10,12,18*)	----
Totals	22	6	3	5	8

Note: This analysis was done in March 1985
* Subtotal resection before XRT in 4 patients and total resection with right lobectomy in a fifth (dead at 39 mo); remainder of patients were unresected
NED = no evidence of disease; XRT = external irradiation; 5-FU = 5-fluorouracil; Ir[192] = Iridium[192]; IORT = intraoperative radiation

cent of patients with gallbladder primaries. If the bile duct is surgically violated to obtain tissue diagnosis for bile duct primaries, the incidence of peritoneal seeding may rise to 40 percent, and aggressive local treatment techniques become less appropriate. Therefore, thin needle percutaneous biopsy may be a preferable method to achieve a tissue diagnosis.

Colorectal Cancer

Local Failure After Conventional Treatment

External beam irradiation has been combined with surgical resection, chemotherapy, and/or immunotherapy for locally advanced disease. When radiation is combined with surgery for residual disease after resection or for initially unresectable disease, although local control and survival can be achieved in some patients, the risk of local recurrence is too high at 30 to 50 percent.[1] In a recent Mayo Clinic series, 44 patients with locally advanced rectal cancer received 5,000-rad split-course irradiation with or without immunotherapy.[22] Among the patients in whom site of initial tumor progression could be evaluated, 28 of 31 experienced local progression, and in 17 (55%) it was their only site of failure.

Intraoperative Radiation plus External Irradiation

In an attempt to decrease local recurrence and improve survival, both MGH and the Mayo Clinic have initiated pilot studies which add an intraoperative electron boost to the fractionated external beam doses of 4,500 to 5,000 rad in 180-rad fractions with or without resection. The IORT dose varies from 1,000 to 2,000 rad depending on the amount of disease remaining after attempted resection: microscopic residual, 1,000 rad; gross residual <2 cm, 1,500 rad; gross residual ≥2 cm or unresectable, 1,750 to 2,000 rad.

In the published MGH trial of 32 patients, local control was improved in patients with residual disease and in those whose tumors were initially unresectable, and survival was better in the latter group when compared with historical controls treated only with preoperative irradiation and resection.[23] In their ongoing trials, survival in the patients with recurrence is stable at nearly 40 percent between three and four years, in contrast to an expected long-term survival of 5 to 10 percent after treatment with standard techniques.[6] The incidence of moderate or severe complications has not appeared to increase as a result of the aggressive combinations.[24]

In a series of 35 patients treated at the Mayo Clinic, results parallelled those achieved at MGH, but the follow-up was not as long (see Table 3). Disease progression occurred in only two of eight patients (25%) when resection was preceded by the external beam component of irradiation (5,000 rad in 28 fractions) compared with 11 of 27 patients (40%) when resection was performed before external irradiation. Similar improvements in disease control were found in the MGH series when irradiation preceded the resection.

REFERENCES

1. Gunderson LL, Tepper JE, Dosoretz DE, Kopelson G, Hoskins RB, Rich TA, Russell AH. Patterns of failure after treatment of gastrointestinal cancer. Cancer Treatment Symposia 1983; 2:181–197.
2. Abe M, Takahashi M. Intraoperative radiotherapy: the Japanese experience. Int J Rad Oncol Biol Phys 1981; 7:863–868.
3. Goldson A. Preliminary clinical experience with intraoperative radiotherapy. J Nat Med Assoc 1978; 79:493–495.
4. Goldson AL. Past, present and future prospects of intraoperative radiotherapy (IOR). Seminars in Oncology 1981; 8:59–65.
5. Gunderson LL, Shipley WU, Suit HD, et al. Intraoperative irradiation: a pilot study combining external beam photons with "boost" dose intraoperative electrons. Cancer 1981; 49:2259–2266.
6. Gunderson LL, Tepper JE, Biggs PJ, Goldson A, Martin JK, McCullough EC, Rich TA, Shipley WU, Sindelar WF, Wood WC. Intraoperative ± external beam irradiation. Current Problems Cancer 1983; 7(11):1–69.
7. Gunderson LL, Martin JK, Earle JB, Byer D, Voss M, Fieck J,

Kvols L, Rorie D, Martinez A, Nagorney DM, O'Connell MJ, Weber F. Intraoperative and external beam irradiation ± resection: Mayo pilot experience. Mayo Clin Proc 1984; 59:691–699.
8. Sindelar ST, Kinsella T, Tepper J, Travis EL, Rosenberg SA, Glatstein E. Experimental and clinical studies with intraoperative radiotherapy. Surg Gyn Obstet 1983; 157:205–219.
9. Suit HD. Radiation biology: a basis for radiotherapy. In: Fletcher GH ed. Textbook of radiotherapy. 2nd ed. Philadelphia: Lea and Febiger 1973; 75.
10. Holbrook MA. Radiation therapy. Current concepts in cancer, Chapter 44 - gastric cancer: treatment principles. JAMA 1974; 228:1289–1290.
11. Schein PS, Novak J for GITSG. Combined modality therapy (XRT-chemo) versus chemotherapy alone for locally unresectable gastric cancer. Cancer 1982; 49:1771-1777.
12. Gunderson LL, Sosin H. Adenocarcinoma of the stomach: areas of failure in a reoperation series (second or symptomatic looks): clinicopathologic correlation and implications for adjuvant therapy. Int J Radiat Oncol Biol Phys 1982; 8:1–11.
13. Moertel CG, Childs DS Jr., Reitemeier RJ, Colby MY Jr, Holbrook MA. Combined 5-fluorouracil and supervoltage radiation therapy of locally unresectable gastrointestinal cancer. Lancet 1969; 2:865–867.
14. Haslam JB, Cavanaugh PJ, Stroup SL. Radiation therapy in the treatment of irresectible adenocarcinoma of the pancreas. Cancer 1973; 32:1341–1345.
15. Gastrointestinal Tumor Study Group. Comparative therapeutic trial of radiation with or without chemotherapy in pancreatic carcinoma. Int J Radiat Oncol Biol Phys 1979; 5:1643–1647.
16. Whittington R, Mohiuddin M, Cantor RI, Rosato FE, Biermann WA, Weiss SA, Solin L, Pajak TF. Multimodality therapy of localized unresectable pancreatic adenocarcinoma. Cancer (in press).
17. Shipley WU, Nardi GL, Cohen AM. Iodine-125 implant and external beam irradiation in patients with localized pancreatic carcinoma: a comparative study to surgical resection. Cancer 1980; 45:709–714.
18. Shipley WU, Wood WC, Tepper JE, Warshaw WL, Orlow EL, Kaufman D, Battit GE, Nardi GL. Intraoperative electron beam irradiation for patients with unresectable pancreatic carcinoma. Ann Surg 1984; 200:289–296.
19. Kopelson G, Harisiadis L, Tretter P, Chang LH. The role of radiation therapy in cancer of the extrahepatic biliary system: an analysis of thirteen patients and a review of the literature of the effectiveness of surgery, chemotherapy and radiotherapy. Int J Radiat Oncol Biol Phys 1977; 2:883–894.
20. Todorki T, Iwasaki Y, Okamura T, et al. Intraoperative radiotherapy for advanced carcinoma of the biliary system. Cancer 1980; 46:2179–2184.
21. Buskirk SJ, Gunderson LL, Adson MA, Martinez A, May GR, McIlrath DC, Nagorney DM, Edmundson GK, Bender CE, Martin JK. Analysis of failure following curative irradiation of gallbladder and extrahepatic bile duct carcinoma. Int J Radiat Oncol Biol Phys 1984; 10:2013-2023.
22. O'Connell MJ, Childs DS, Moertel CG, et al. A prospective controlled evaluation of combined pelvic radiotherapy and methanol extraction residue of BCG (MER) for locally unresectable or recurrent rectal carcinoma. Int J Radiat Oncol Biol Phys 1982; 8:1115–1119.
23. Gunderson LL, Cohen AM, Dosoretz DE, Shipely WU, Hedberg SE, Wood WC, Rodkey CV, Suit HD. Residual, unresectable, or recurrent colorectal cancer: external beam irradiation and intraoperative electron beam boost ± resection. Int J Radiat Oncol Biol Phys 1983; 9:1597–1606.
24. Tepper JE, Gunderson LL, Orlow E, Cohen AM, Hedberg SE, Shipley WU, Blitzer PH, Rich T. Complications of intraoperative radiation therapy. Int J Radiat Oncol Biol Phys 1984; 10:1831–1839.

HYPOCHONDRIASIS, HYSTERIA, AND DEPRESSION

MARK L. TEITELBAUM, M.D.

HYPOCHONDRIASIS

The hypochondriacal patient is preoccupied with the anxious and fearful worry that he is physically ill despite medical evidence to the contrary. He is preoccupied with worries about health, often to the point of interference with social and occupational function. He is also particularly resistant to reassurance by a physician and has great difficulty in trusting the doctor. The worry about disease is generally phasic with a waxing and waning, often in response to life circumstances. The hypochondriacal patient is often a sensitive and self-centered person who responds to loss, rejection, or rebuff with nonspecific symptoms such as pain, fatigue, and weakness, which become the focus of his worry. He usually craves a relationship with a powerful and protective "parent figure" in order to feel whole and well, yet at the same time is fearful of this closeness because of his vulnerability to being hurt.

For this patient the doctor-patient relationship itself is the treatment. Technologic medicine has virtually nothing to offer this patient and furthermore is often potentially dangerous. The establishment of a stable, long-term, and trusting doctor-patient relationship is the goal in management of the hypochondriacal patient in the medical setting. To do this is no easy task. For the physician to take on such a patient, he or she must be willing to risk failing and become one of a series of devalued physicians whom the patient has discarded as seemingly useless to him, as he proceeds on his way to more "doctor shopping." The task for the physician in his attempt to establish a stable and trusting long-term relationship with a hypochondriacal patient requires that he be sufficiently able to provide engagement, intimacy, and concern with a minimum of anxiety on his part, while at the same time being able to retain his freedom to set limits on inappropriate demands for time, diagnostic tests, and treatments without feeling excessively guilty. The physician must be prepared to make errors on both sides of this equation and be flexible enough to adjust his behavior when he recognizes his mistake.

On the one hand, the physician may find himself having difficulty setting limits on unreasonable demands, feeling controlled by the patient, and being manipulated to act in ways against his better judgment. Eventually the physician begins to feel resentful and angry toward the patient in this situation. The recognition of his own anger toward the patient under these circumstances can be used as a signal to alter his behavior by firmly, yet kindly, beginning to set limits. By doing so, the physician prevents his own anger from becoming excessive and eventually leading him to become either subtly or overtly rejecting of the patient and thereby driving him out of treatment. On the other hand, he may find himself having difficulty engaging the patient in a meaningful way, setting limits excessively, and trying to avoid the patient. The physician may become aware of anxious feelings about involvement with the patient and guilty feelings about his avoidance. Efforts to modify his approach by relaxing some of his limit-setting are needed at this point to maintain a relationship with the patient and prevent his emotional withdrawal from driving the patient out of treatment. Fluctuations in the physician's feelings and behavior between these two extremes are to be expected in the course of establishing a relationship with the hypochondriacal patient. With experience, a middle course between the two extremes that is satisfactory to the physician and therapeutic for the patient can be navigated.

It is important to keep in mind that the setting of limits on excessive demands for time and attention should be based upon the realities and limits of any interpersonal relationship. The physician is a human being and realistically can provide just so much time, attention, energy, and support. The setting of limits on unreasonable demands for potentially harmful and unnecessary diagnostic tests and treatments should be based upon the reality of the hazards to the patient compared with their potential helpfulness.

The provision of regular appointments "to discuss the patient's difficulties" is a useful and simple way to structure the treatment. Some patients initially require weekly contact. For many—those whom the physician is able to engage and who begin to trust the physician to some degree—less frequent contact can be arranged. Frequency of contact, however, is not so important as quality of contact. For quality contact, time must be allowed to permit open discussion and the unfolding of a relationship. Less frequent contacts of 20 or 30 minutes are more valuable than frequent contacts of 10 or 15 minutes that are pressured and rushed. As a relationship unfolds, the physician can gradually suggest to the patient that a discussion of personal matters might be helpful. For some hypochondriacal patients, it may be possible, over time, to illuminate the connection between his symptomatic complaining and troublesome life events that have provoked disappointment and dissatisfaction. For many hypochondriacal patients, this degree of illumination is impossible, and a more modest goal should be sought: a stable doctor-patient relationship, the development of trust in the doctor, and a diminution of "doctor shopping."

The use of psychotropic medications in the management of the hypochondriacal patient may be considered when significant symtoms of anxiety or depression are associated with hypochondriacal concerns. For the hypochondriacal patient with associated symptoms of anxiety, small doses of a minor tranquilizer such as diazepam, used intermittently during exacerbations of anxiety, can be helpful. In such instances, alprozolam can be given in doses of 0.25 to 0.5 mg, two to four times a day. For patients with associated insomnia, the bulk of the daily diazepman dose can be given at bedtime. Significant anxiety in the hypochondriacal patient usually is phasic, and minor tranquilizers are best used intermittently when severe symptoms of anxiety are present. The chronic use of minor tranquilizers should be avoided. For the hypochondriacal patient with symptoms of depression, the use of a tricyclic antidepressant may be warranted. The use of antidepressants will be discussed in further detail in the discussion on the management of the depressed patient.

Consultation with a psychiatrist should be considered in patients with hypochondriacal complaints. Such consultation can be of help when questions of diagnosis remain, for the particularly troubled hypochondriacal patient with marked difficulties in interpersonal relating, and for the hypochondriacal patient with significant associated symptoms of anxiety, depression, or other serious psychiatric symptomatology. For some hypochondriacal patients, collaborative treatment by both internist and psychiatrist may be the best plan of management.

HYSTERIA

The hysterical patient is a polysymptomatic complainer, usually of life-long duration, whose complaints occur in the absence of evidence of significant bodily diseae. The patient with hysterical symptoms may also be hypochondriacally fearful and worried, but sometimes may appear paradoxically indifferent or unconcerned. Among his multiple symptoms he may have classic conversion symptoms, i.e, alterations or losses of specific neurologic function, such as paralysis, sensory loss, or blindness. Irritable bowel syndrome is sometimes found in patients with multiple hysterical complaints. The hysterical patient is best conceptualized as communicating to the physician dysphoria and dissatisfaction about his life through his bodily complaints. Often he is found to be a troubled individual whose life may be quite disorganized. Like the hypochondriacal patient, he may be having difficulty in a number of areas of his life, particularly in his interpersonal relationships. The hysterical patient often presents to the physician with an exacerbation of symptomatic complaints during a period of difficulty in an important interpersonal relationship in his life, such as that with his spouse, lover, parent, or another physician. Such interpersonal difficulty has often led to either actual or perceived abandonment or rejection by the "significant other." Feelings of disappointment, anxiety, anger, and depression sometimes accompany the symptomatic complaints that are arising in such a setting. The hysterical patient often gives the impression that he is seeking "a safe haven" in the form of the doctor-patient relationship.

As with the hypochondriacal patient, the establishment of a stable, trusting doctor-patient relationship is the basis for treatment, and the problem facing the physician again is the balancing of engagement, empathy, and support with kind but firm limit-setting on unreasonable demands for time, attention, and dangerous demands for unneeded diagnostic tests and therapeutic procedures. As with the hypochondriacal patient, the illumination of the connection between symptomatic complaining and life events may sometimes be possible, but for the majority of hysterical patients, the establishment of a stable and trusting doctor-patient relationship, which affords protection of the patient from excessive "doctor shopping" and exposure to unneeded diagnostic procedures and treatments, are more realistic goals.

Dealing with the hysterical patient who is markedly angry often poses a special problem for the physician. As with all emotionally distraught patients, the degree to which the physician can remain calm and supportive in the face of this emotional storm will determine whether he or she can be helpful to the patient. Most emotional storms subside in the face of a calm and nonrejecting physician. The patient's anger can be best looked upon as a response to those same events in his life that have brought him to the physician in the first place. The problem for the physician is often that this anger is displaced onto him, and he is faced with an angry patient who is critical and devaluing of his attempts to help. In dealing with such a situation, a helpful approach is a kind but firm confrontation of the patient with the fact that angry devaluation of the physician is basically self-defeating and calculated to disrupt a relationship that the patient clearly needs. Such confrontation should only be attempted when the physician is in control of his own anger. If the physician is excessively angry at the patient because of the patient's attack on him, the confrontation will be experienced by the patient as a counter-attack and will drive the patient out of treatment. The angry devaluing of the physician's attempt to establish a relationship with the patient can often be experienced by the physician as an attack on his ability to be therapeutic. Such an attack often stimulates doubts within the physician that the doctor-patient relationship will be enough, which in turn may stimulate a tendency in the physician to want to "do something." As with the hypochondriacal patient, the "doing" for the hysterical patient is simply the attempt to establish and maintain a stable and trusting relationship with the patient. Attempts to quickly alleviate the patient's suffering and the physician's own feelings of helplessness when being devalued by the patient can lead to a repetition of unneeded diagnostic tests and dangerous therapeutic maneuvers that the patient generally has been through many times before.

The judicious use of minor tranquilizers or tricyclic antidepressants in selected hysterical patients with significant symptoms of anxiety or depression is sometimes warranted. Details of the use of minor tranquilizers can be found in the section on the management of the hypochondriacal patient. A discussion of the use of tricyclic antidepressants will follow in the section on the management of the depressed patient.

Psychiatric consultation should be considered for the hysterical patient when diagnosis is uncertain, in the presence of significant associated symptoms of depression, anxiety, or other psychiatric symptomatology, and for help in the management of a particularly difficult patient whose personality makes the establishment of a relationship problematic. For selected hysterical patients, collaborative treatment by both psychiatrist and internist may be warranted.

DEPRESSION

Depressed patients are seen commonly in the medical setting. Depressed mood, loss of interest and energy, low confidence, and vegetative disturbances such as insomnia, poor appetite, and constipation identify the typical depressed patient. The distinction between a patient with a grief response who is reacting to life circumstances and a patient with a major depressive illness is important.

Patients suffering from major depressive illness often become depressed "out of the blue," often have family histories of depression and/or suicide, and histories themselves of past episodes of depression and/or mania. Their mood state is relatively unresponsive to outside influence. Feelings of guilt and self-reproach, severe vegetative symptoms, and psychomotor retardation are often prominent. The grief-stricken patient, on the other hand, displays a mood disturbance that is responsive to the environment. Painful feelings of sadness seem to appear and disappear as waves of distress that come and go. Guilty feelings and vegetative disturbances are much less prominent.

A grieving patient whose sad mood is in response to environmental events generally has had the experience of some recent loss. Loss of an important person through death or abandonment, loss of a job, home, or money—all can precipitate a depressive response. More subtle events, such as losses of health, independence, attractiveness, or the sense of mastery and control can also precipitate a grief reaction. The losses experienced may precipitate feelings of shock, anger, and sadness, which may appear and disappear in alternating fashion. Self-esteem is generally preserved. In a patient with physical illness, a grief reaction may be related to the meaning that the particular illness has for him; for example, a perfectionistic person, who needs a sense of being in total control, might experience a grief reaction when ill with a diarrheal disorder.

The management of the depressed patient involves the following:

Assessment of the Patient's Suicide Potential

Previous suicide attempts, concrete and definite plans, features in the patient's presentation suggestive of true depressive illness, the lack of a social support system, and the presence of serious physical disease can all be considered risk factors. A seriously depressed patient with high suicide potential should be treated as an inpatient in a psychiatric hospital.

Provision of Psychologic Support

The physician's task in providing psychologic support for the depressed patient involves his attempt to reverse the lowered self-esteem, pessimism, and guilt that the patient is experiencing. Scheduling of appointments and demonstrating a willingness to listen serve to mobilize powerful forces against lowered self-esteem and pessimism. By offering himself, his time, and his empathy to the depressed patient, the physician in essence is communicating to the patient not only that he feels that the patient is worth his time and effort, but also that he believes that there will be a future for the patient! Clear statements to the patient that depression is treatable and invariably gets better is also helpful in combating hopelessness about the future. Explanations that vegetative symptoms, such as poor sleep, are symptoms of depression and will improve as depression improves also encourage optimism. The depressed patient often feels himself a burden on his family, friends, and physicians. Comments emphasizing that love and dependent care are well deserved by the patient can be soothing. Statements to the effect that, in the physician's opinion, the patient has "suffered enough" can also be helpful in alleviating painful feelings of guilt.

Use of Antidepressant Medication

A patient with symptoms of major depressive illness usually require pharmacologic intervention along with psychologic support. The tricyclic antidepressants are the drugs of choice for treatment of such a patient. Treatment with amytriptyline can be instituted with doses of 50 to 75 mg a day. The dose is then titrated upward, usually to the range of 100 to 200 mg a day. Elderly patients should be treated with lower doses, starting with 25 to 50 mg a day. Often a maximum dose of 75 to 100 mg a day is sufficient.

Side effects are usually related to the sedative and anticholinergic properties of the drug, with drowsiness and dryness of mouth being two frequently encountered symptoms. Drowsiness is often transient and improves as treatment progresses. Dry mouth can be combatted by the use of chewing gum or hard candy. A patient with prostatic hypertrophy or glaucoma may have problems with urinary retention or an increase in intraocular pressure. Orthostatic hypotension can also be a problem, particularly in the elderly. With an elderly depressed patient, the monitoring of blood pressure prior to dosage increase is strongly recommended. When oversedation and drowsiness become problematic, less-sedating tricyclic antidepressants, such as imipramine (100 to 200 mg per day) can be substituted. When orthostatic hypotension is a problem, nortriptyline in doses of 75 to 125 mg (25 to 75 mg for the elderly) may be tried. When anticholinergic side effects are troublesome, a drug such as desipramine (100 to 200 mg per day) may be substituted.

All the tricyclic antidepressants can be given in one dose at bedtime. This is often most convenient for the patient, maximizes what sedative potential the drugs have as an aid to sleep, and minimizes some of the side-effects that occur during the day. In elderly patients, if the drugs are given in this way, particular attention must be paid to the possibility of orthostatic hypotension upon getting out of bed in the morning. With all the tricyclic antidepressants there is a lag before symptomatic improvement occurs, the patient requiring treatment with the drug at a therapeutic dose for 2 to 3 weeks to get the maximum effect.

Consultation with a psychiatrist should always be considered for a patient with symptoms suggestive of major depressive illness or in whom suicide risk is believed to be great. The majority of patients with major depressive illness require ongoing consultation with, or treatment by, a psychiatrist. However, many depressed patients who are suffering from grief responses can be managed by the primary care physician alone.

FUNCTIONAL ILLNESS

PHILIP A. TUMULTY, M.D.

A very large proportion of the patients seen by a clinician have illnesses that are entirely or in part due to emotional factors. One of our most brilliant internists, Dr. Louis Hamman, once reported that one-third of the patients he saw in consultation had illnesses that were entirely functional, and in another one-third, psychophysiologic factors played an important role. Experiences in my own practice echo his.

Physician Attitude

I smile when I hear young clinicians say, "I wish I were a consultant like you—you must get only interesting organic problems referred to you." They don't realize that the more one becomes recognized as a consultant, the more functional illness one must deal with because very often referring physicians are not sure whether a patient has a functional disorder or some obscure organic disease; they may be anxious, for a variety of reasons, to pass on to a consultant a difficult functional problem they do not want to handle themselves. Make no mistake:

The proper management of a major functional illness requires the very best efforts of a skilled clinician, certainly no less than does a complicated organic problem.

It has been my impression through the years that many patients with functional illnesses are not well managed, for a variety of reasons. In many instances, the functional aspects of a patient's health problem are quickly passed over or even completely ignored, and the patient is treated for some inconsequential or even nonexistent organic disorder, such as a hiatus hernia, hypoglycemia and so forth. The result is that the patient's symptoms become more and more deeply embedded, and finally immutable, as each new physician whom the patient sees fails to make clear the real nature of the illness, and what must be done to manage it effectively. The physician's failure may be compounded, because in a sense, functional illness is an "infectious" disease which is often contracted by other members of the family; children and spouse eventually may be affected by it.

Why are many patients who have functional disorders so frequently managed so poorly? There are a variety of reasons.

Many physicians are "turned off" by functional illness. One hears it said by young physicians that "I got into this specialty to get away from those kinds of patients. They are a nuisance, they take up a lot of your time, and they keep coming back with the same old complaints, or new ones that are even worse. You simply cannot get them well. They just don't want to become well. They enjoy being sick!"

During their clinical education, many young physicians feel an intense pressure to learn about a welter of technical matters concerning organic disorders, and they may regard the functional aspects of their patient's health problems as secondary matters for which they have neither the time nor the interest. Alas, their instructors or clinical models may likewise have little of either. Current clinical education of our young physicians stresses the disease state and its recognition and treatment through the employment of a variety of special techniques and not the management of the *total* factors—functional as well as organic—which actually comprise the patient's illness. It is only through meaningful dialogue with the patient that all of these factors can be disclosed and effectively altered. While the modern clinician is, indeed, a doer, he or she is often unfortunately not a conversationalist, and the ability to carry on meaningful dialogue with patients may not be a technique that has been taught or acquired. To have a meaningful dialogue with sick persons means that one must understand something about human nature and its reactions to various stimuli and circumstances, which differ from patient to patient, depending upon such factors as intellectual capacity, ethnic, social, and economic background; experience; and so forth.

Clearly, these matters are not taught in medical school, and probably they cannot be. Perhaps only through working closely with many people can they be learned, and this to a large degree depends upon the individual physician's interest and sensitivity. Unfortunately, both these requisites are sometimes lacking, and the ability to have a positive impact upon a patient through conversation is never acquired. The result is that the physician becomes a technician—one who does things to the patient, some of them scientifically quite remarkable, but who cannot sensitively discern the human issues and reactions and who cannot positively affect these through the strength of his or her own spirit expressed through conversation.

A practical and most important corollary to the failure of some physicians to conduct effective dialogue with their patients is the fact that to accomplish this takes time, a very great deal of time, which is very costly for both the physician and the patient. In the time required for a follow-up visit with one of my patients who has an emotional problem, for example, a colleague in some specialty area can perform some type of technical procedure upon a patient and realize a much larger fee. Most unfortunately, insurance companies and other agencies fail to adequately reimburse a clinician merely for *talking* with patients—one must *do* something to them to really earn one's keep! And yet, truthfully, isn't effective conversation with a patient the most valuable diagnostic and therapeutic "technique" of all?

Inappropriate Psychiatric Referral

Poor management of functional illness also results when the physician tells the patient that all of the diagnostic studies are normal, the patient's symptoms are emotional in origin, and that therefore the patient should see a psychiatrist in consultation.

I realize that I am broaching delicate issues at this point in my discussion, but frankly, I am of the opinion that most patients with functional illness do not need formal psychotherapy, and furthermore it is much wiser *not* to urge them to seek psychiatric help, at least not initially, although it may become appropriate later.

I believe this for two main reasons, first, despite the sophistication of this era, to many patients, being advised that they need to see a psychiatrist is a serious indication that they are losing control of themselves emotionally; that they are no longer able to call their own shots; and that there is something lacking or unsound or weak or different about them. Therefore, at a time when the patient needs so badly to maintain and, if possible, increase his self-esteem, the advice that he must see a psychiatrist may undermine what little self-confidence remains and even cause panic.

I believe that the key concept that must be presented to the patient at the outset of the management of a functional illness is that, while it is evident that here and now the patient is going through a very stormy period, and the storm is a severe and distressing and frightening one, the patient is still very much in control of the situation. He has a strong arm at the helm and can ride out the storm. The premature insistence that the patient must see a psychiatrist will, in some instances, destroy this feeling of still being in control of self.

Secondly, I am convinced that many patients with functional illness do not get sufficient practical help from the type of therapy they are given by some psychiatrists. Specifically, I refer to the type of psychotherapeutic approach which seeks to explain and to reveal to the patient through detailed analysis of self and past *why* he reacts as he does. The patient is not primarily concerned with the question, "*Why* do I react as I do?" nearly so much as with the question, "Reacting as I do, what in a practical way can I do about it? I am what I am—I am not seeking a theoretical explanation of why I am this way, but being what I am, in practical terms, what can I do to control and to modify and to manage myself in these particular situations more effectively, so that I am no longer made sick by them?"

Common Sense Support

Patients want positive direct, uncomplicated, straightforward, sensible, realistic help with the problems of everyday living as they exist within themselves, and not a detailed unearthing and analysis of how the problems got there in the first place. They want practical help and not explanations, in useful terms, not theoretical ones, not magical in scope, but realistically forward-moving and positive.

Another reason some physicians are highly reluctant to become involved in their patient's emotional problems, is that they simply do not fully understand what their role should be, and they are fearful of their inability to play it adequately. Thus, they are concerned that the patient will expect them to have quick, smart, satisfying answers and solutions to their sometimes very involved problems. The physician is afraid that he or she will be expected to create something for the patient that cannot possibly be produced and to achieve results that simply cannot be had. Actually, all such patients really want is understanding, a chance to tell their story fully and reassuring common sense support and sound direction which has practical meaning.

Since most of the problems patients have usually involve matters that are common to so many of us, a clinician of any experience and sophistication should be able to give needed support, understanding, and practical advice.

PATIENT MANAGMENT STEPS

What should be the general approach of a clinician to the management of the patient with functional illness? For the sake of conciseness, let us consider this question in a series of steps.

Diagnostic Evaluation

In the first step, the clinician must reasonably exclude the possibility of latent organic disease by carrying out appropriate studies and consultations. Without such a survey, it is impossible to exclude organic factors. It is the experience of all of us that some exceedingly important organic disorders may exactly duplicate the manifestations of classic functional illness and, the experienced clinician has learned the hard way that the early stages of serious organic disease may masquerade as a functional illness. Furthermore, in this day of "scientific medicine," many patients will simply not accept the fact that they have a functional disorder until organic possibilities have been reasonably excluded by appropriate investigation. This does not mean that the clinician "shoots the works" diagnostically just to please the whim of a patient. What it does mean is that at the conclusion of the initial conference with the patient, following completion of the history and physical examination, the physician explains in terms the patient understands that his particular symptoms could be due either to an organic disorder or to the stresses of circumstances and interpersonal relationships, and that the role of the physician is to evaluate meticulously all of the clinical evidence until the true cause of the illness is fully understood. In coming to a final diagnosis, the physician will, of course, look carefully at both sides of the street. If the physician has carried out a very thorough history and physical examination, he or she will at this point already have won the patient's confidence and set the stage for a satisfying relationship.

Review of Study Results

When the diagnostic evaluation has been completed, the clinician takes the second step at the next meeting by reviewing with the patient the results of the studies, explaining the scope and significance of each test in meaningful terms so that the patient appreciates that the cause of his symptoms has been pursued in a very careful and organized way. The physician concludes this step by stating that a careful and logical synthesis of the total evidence gathered indicates that the symptoms are not due to any significant organic disorder, but rather to psychophysiologic or functional factors.

Explanation of Functional Illness

The third step is to explain to the patient, in easily understood terms, what is meant by functional illness, and then, just as important, what is *not* meant by functional illness. Often, at this stage of the interchange, the patient will be resentful and conclude that the doctor is telling him that his symptoms are imaginary or put on, or that he is "crazy" or losing control of himself, or that he is peculiar or different or odd.

Therefore, it is critically important at this point to make it crystal clear to the patient that his symptoms are exceedingly real and very valid, but that they are not the product of structural abnormalities but rather the result of the physiologic response to stress. Several examples of this interrelationship between stress and body function should be presented to the patient in keeping with the patient's intellectual capacities. For example, when we are embarassed, we flush, when we are frightened, we sweat and our hearts beat faster, when we are under pressure our bowels may stop functioning or overfunction; and so forth. We are all familiar with the expression, "What a headache he is!"

Patient's Reactions. The patient's reaction at this juncture is often one of disbelief, anger, resentment, or insincere acceptance at a very superficial level. The physician must be prepared to accept this unhappy and negative response and not be perturbed or discouraged and above all, the physician must not be forced into backing off and suggesting that possibly some minor organic factors might be playing some role. Unequivocal recognition and understanding by the patient of what is truly causing the illness, and the significance of what the physician is saying, are of the greatest importance at this juncture if the patient is to be cured.

It is at this stage, unfortunately, that many physicians fumble the ball, and the patient grabs it and runs away with it. When the patient demurs, the physician must be understanding but persistent in firmly restating his or her conclusions. Unfortunately, the fear of legal suits which haunts many physicians and sometimes directs their philosophy of patient care, holds them back from dealing with patients who have these sorts of problems in this straightforward, positive, definite approach that is so essential. So they hedge, and they back and fill, as they become self-protective. The patient limps on with his chronic functional illness, no better and probably worse because his convictions of hidden organic disease have become deeper and deeper as a result of his encounter with a physician who practices what might be called "self-defensive medicine."

Discussion of Interpersonal Factors

The fourth step is to discuss with the patient the kind of factors in his life which are most commonly responsible for the development of a functional illness. I have given much thought to this issue, and while the specific causes of functional illness are as varied as the human personality, I think one can make certain basic generalizations. First, the factors are always interpersonal. Second, they are always items that affect us in our most sensitive areas. They are most often little items, but ones that have very special and major significance for us, sometimes for reasons that are quite unclear to us.

At this stage of our conversation, I find it helpful to tell my patient that if he and I were playing a game in which I would list on a piece of paper all the various things that affect me in my areas of deepest reactivity and sensitivity, and he would do likewise, and if we then exchanged our lists and compared them, he would say, after looking over my list, "Doctor, you don't mean to tell me that this or that item could possibly be important and significant to you!" And I'm certain I would say the same thing about his list. Some of these items I am sure are the products of our genes, and still others the result of little things and big things that have happened to us since our very earliest days. Like a computer, little circuits have been turned on within us, through the years, to which we continue to react.

As I perceive it, there are two major mechanisms most often responsible for functional illness in the area of interpersonal relationships: First, *frustration*—something is keeping me from achieving some need which means a great deal to me; secondly, *ambivalence*,—for one set of reasons which mean a great deal to me, I want to walk sharply to the right, and for another set of reasons, meaning an equal amount to me, I want to walk sharply to the left, and so I find myself pulled apart and torn in the middle.

Self-Treatment Measures

Lastly, the patient is advised that there are a series of steps which he must take to recover from this functional illness, which he can do completely, though it may take considerable time, much self-discipline, and a great deal of patience. There will be periods of success, followed by some perids of discouragement, but ultimately the regaining of peace and well-being will be the reward.

The first of these curative steps the patient has already accomplished, namely, the completion of a very meticulous *evaluation* of his symptoms to determine the role and proper management of any organic factors.

The second step is to develop an *understanding* of the real nature of functional illness, and how it differs from organic illness, and especially how it differs from imaginary illness, or wanting to be sick, or putting on, or hysteria, or losing control of one's self, or being emotionally unstable, and so forth.

The third step to *comprehend* fully that functional illness is as natural as human nature itself, and just as common, and that there is no one who goes through life who does not sooner or later suffer the consequences of functional illness to a greater or a lesser degree, and frequently over and over again.

Finally, the patient must *appreciate* that functional illness is particularly likely to occur in individuals who are perceptive and sensitive and thoughtful and imaginative and reactive, and those who are somewhat perfectionistic and obsessive, for these are the kind of persons who feel deeply and who respond keenly to people and to life's encounters. So, having a functional illness is nothing to be ashamed of or to fear. It is simply something that must be overcome, and this the patient can do with your help.

In attempting to understand the nature of functional illness—what it is and also what it isn't—the patient should ask himself the difficult question, "What are the factors in my life which might be responsible for this illness? What items might be causing frustration? What items might be causing ambivalence?" All of these various factors must be ferreted out and examined, recognized and accepted as real, and be understood for what they are and for the negative effects they are producing.

Having recognized the factors, the patient must then ask the hardest question of all: "What can I do about them?"

In attempting to answer this question, it is well to think in terms of *modification* rather than in terms of *change*. Once in adult life, how many of us can realistically think in terms of producing major changes either within ourselves or without? How many of us can completely rid our lives of the factors that are causing frustration and ambivalence? No, modification is surely the word, and not change, and many times, although we surely wish it could be otherwise, it is modification not of the situation, but of our reaction to it.

Practical Measures

Another key word to add to the concept of modification is the word practical, for our decisions and our resolutions and our actions must have practical meaning and be within the reach of attainment. Thus, recovering from a functional illness usually has to be thought of in terms of achieving practical modifications in those features of one's life which self-questioning has indicated are causing illness.

What are the courses of action a wise man adopts when he cannot rid himself of something that is noxious to him? They are few, they are practical, and they are simple: (1) he attempts to avoid it as best he can; (2) he tries to substitute something for it; (3) he endeavors to alter it or to modify his own reaction to it; and (4) he learns to adapt to it, and to put up with it. A wise man does not continue to chew on the same old bone.

These are the alternatives open to the patient in meeting his problems. There is no mystic formula, there is no magic wand, there are no easy solutions. Complete bliss and happiness and self-satisfaction are not the goals, for who on earth has them? The goal is simply not to be made chronically sick by factors from which we cannot escape, and this can be brought about only through persistent effort based on self-discipline and maturity.

Some practical aids are the development of interests and hobbies, and the practical organization of one's work and responsibilities so that they create less unremitting stress. Most important of all is the advice that the patient learn to heal himself in the wounds of others by devoting a significant portion of time and energies to activities that deal with the problems and miseries of persons even more ill and unfortunate than himself.

What must be done is clear. The goal is a middle ground of a reasonable degree of satisfaction and peace, which comes only to those who, with wisdom and maturity and self-discipline, walk through the steps I have outlined. It should be made clear to the patient that either he can make these necessary adjustments, or his sick way of living will undoubtedly continue. There is no alternative route. The choice is his, but the physician will be helping and advising the patient during the long journey.

Finally, which patients with functional illness should be referred to psychiatrists? Certainly patients who have major emotional and personality disturbances should seek psychiatric help, but also those patients who simply cannot accept the fact that their illness is a functional one, or who despite your best efforts, cannot comprehend the nature of functional illness or cannot discern for themselves the factors in their lives which are responsible for their illness. Finally, patients who are thoroughly incapable of altering or affecting in any significant way the things in their lives that are making them sick should be referred to a psychiatrist.

This then, is one physician's approach to the management of functional illness. Does it work? My impression is that it is reasonably successful, for it is based upon telling the patient the truth about himself and his problems in a kind and gentle way. It is based upon interest and understanding. The nature of man is such that his intellect cannot reject the truth when it is presented clearly, and his spirit will always respond to genuine interest and caring.

CHRONIC ABDOMINAL PAIN: A COGNITIVE BEHAVIORAL TREATMENT APPROACH

HARRY S. SHABSIN, Ph.D.

Chronic abdominal pain is pain of noncarcinogenic origin which continues for 6 months or longer and fails to respond to various forms of medical management. Often individuals with such pain have a lengthy diagnostic history and may have been to a number of specialists in an attempt to find a cure for their symptoms. Often these individuals have taken, or are taking, a variety of drugs, including antidepressants, anxiolytics, and narcotic-analgesic medications. Such patients may also have undergone one or more operations in an effort to rid themselves of their symptoms. Continued failure to relieve chronic pain can lead to frustration on both the physician's and the patient's part; the physician may begin to feel that the patient is malingering, while the patient may begin to lose faith in the medical community and its therapeutic abilities.

In providing treatment to the patient with chronic abdominal symptoms, it is important to consider the personality characteristics of many of these patients. Studies investigating individuals with chronic abdominal pain, such as that often associated with the irritable bowel syndrome, show them to be more anxious or hysterical than normal controls. Depression is also cited as a major factor in chronic pain syndromes, although its occurrence does not appear to be any more prevalent than other psychological characteristics. Depression associated with chronic pain is often reactive in nature and may be more representative of difficulties in coping with a chronic condition than a contributing cause of pain. Using the Minnesota Multiphasic Personality Inventory (MMPI) comparisons of patients with organic disorders, such as peptic ulcer, to those with psychosomatic disorders, such as mucous colitis or tension headache, have found persons with psychosomatic complaints to score higher on scales indicative of hypochondriasis, hysteria, and depression. Elevation of these MMPI scales is typical of individuals likely to react to stress or to avoid difficult situations by somatizing or developing complaints of physical distress. Such individuals are especially prone to developing abdominal symptoms, but similar MMPI profiles are obtained for a variety of chronic pain symptoms, including low back pain, migraine, and pain of musculoskeletal origin.

Once it becomes clear that a patient is not responding to medical management, and more importantly, is unlikely to respond in the future, an understanding of the psychological profile of the chronic pain patient becomes an important factor in continuing to provide treatment. The patient who keeps returning with complaints of chronic pain more than likely has an increased level of anxiety, tends to overreact to a variety of situations, especially illness, and may be experiencing a good deal of stress and fear as a result of his symptoms, without really understanding the nature of these symptoms or why they are occurring. Because of this lack of insight, patients may come to the physician with physical complaints' but actually be seeking help for difficulties that might be more appropriate for the psychologist, social worker, or psychiatrist. If the primary health care provider is to continue to help the patient at this point, he or she needs to look at the presenting complaint and the patient in the broader perspective of the psychological and social situations in a person's life which may be contributing to that person's symptoms.

Interacting With The Patient In Chronic Pain

An important first step in helping the patient with chronic pain is the establishment of an understanding and supportive rapport. Patients who feel they are not taken seriously or who are told the pain is "in your head" will very often become resentful or fail to respond to therapy. This in turn may cause them to abandon treatment or to become more entrenched in the belief that difficulties arising from their symptoms are all physical in nature. Several suggestions are offered below which may be helpful in initially dealing with the patient with chronic abdominal pain.

First, *accept the patient's symptoms*. No matter how negative the physical findings are or how obscure the description of the symptoms, the most useful strategy for establishing a therapeutic relationship with the patient is to accept the physical complaint as real. Patients who come to the doctor because of a physical problem will often feel rejected and lose confidence and trust in the physician if their physical symptoms are denied. Accepting the patient's symptoms as real will help in overcoming patient resistance to exploring nonphysical factors related to chronic pain symptoms.

Second, *allow enough time to talk to and listen to the patient*. In patients with chronic pain, the quality of the time spent during a visit is often as important as the medical assistance received. Enough time should be set aside to talk about and become familiar with the patient's problem. Often patients show improvement in chronic symptoms if they are just allowed to talk without interruption about their difficulties. At times, however, it may be necessary to draw the patient out in order to establish a helpful therapeutic relationship.

Third, *dispel misconceptions and fear about chronic abdominal (or other) symptoms*. Many patients with chronic abdominal symptoms have exaggerated fears or irrational beliefs about their symptoms. This may lead them to feel their symptoms are becoming worse, even when faced with evidence to the contrary. This fear can also lead to increased anxiety which may exacerbate their pain or cause more requests for medical appointments or emergency room visits.

Misconceptions about chronic pain symptoms can also lead to decreased social, family, recreational, and work activities, which in turn can lead to feelings of isolation, helplessness, or depression. A fear of death and dying often underlies these psychological reactions to a chronic condition. Patients with chronic pain often feel they have a degenerative or progressive disease for which the correct diagnosis has been missed, in spite of repeated tests and reassurances to the contrary. Many times a fear of cancer is at the base of this type of concern.

Finally, *provide information and encouragement*. One of the best ways to dispel misconceptions and fears about a chronic condition is to go over the nature of the symptoms with the patient, explaining some of the realistic expectations patients should have and examining unrealistic expectations they may have. Finding out what the patient thinks his symptoms mean is also useful in this regard. Patients should be encouraged to be as active as possible, and to return to work or continue to work whenever feasible. Any misperceptions about not being able to engage in a normal and active life to the fullest extent possible should be discouraged. Many times, a fear of exacerbating symptoms or making a chronic condition worse, rather than the actual symptoms themselves, is the reason a person begins restricting social and professional activities. Giving reassurance and guidance can be quite helpful to the patient, but this requires patience and persistence, as it often needs to be repeated on many occasions.

While the procedures outlined above are useful, at times they may not be enough. The patient with chronic pain may continue to find his life disrupted, to make unreasonable demands on physician and family, or be unable to deal with a chronic medical condition. If such is the case, a more direct approach may be needed.

COGNITIVE-BEHAVIORAL PAIN MANAGEMENT

One successful strategy for treating the patient with chronic abdominal pain is based on a combination of cognitive and behavioral psychotherapeutic principles. This form of pain management involves identifying and modifying those factors in a person's life which contribute to or reinforce pain perceptions and behaviors. Often such reinforcers may include the behavior of others, such as family members and friends, as well as that of the individual to be treated. Three general components of a cognitive-behavioral program which can be used to help the patient with chronic pain involve *family therapy, cognitive psychotherapy,* and *self-control strategies,* such as biofeedback and relaxation training.

Family Therapy

It is almost impossible for an individual to experience chronic pain without family and friends becoming involved. Those close to the person in pain almost always want to help, but often feel frustrated or helpless. Family therapy for the patient with chronic pain involves informing family members about ways they can help the patient decrease his symptoms. It also provides a means for the therapist to direct the behavior of family and friends toward reinforcing nonpain behavior while extinguishing illness behavior.

Out of concern and love for the person in pain, family members or close friends may begin to treat the person with chronic pain differently, as if he were sick. While this type of behavior may be appropriate for acute pain, it can serve to increase pain in the person with chronic symptoms by eliciting the pain as a conditioned response. Chronic pain can become conditioned in such a fashion through reinforcement, or secondary gain, occurring from alterations in attention received by the person in pain, the provision of small favors, or by changes in responsibilities as a result of the pain symptoms. In addition, solicitous inquiries into how a person is feeling only serve as reminders of pain and focus the attention of the individual on his symptoms. Instead, those who interact with the person with chronic pain should be instructed to allow that person to fend for himself as much as possible, to encourage increases in activities, and, perhaps most importantly, to give attention to the person with chronic pain when he is behaving as if his pain symptoms were better rather than when his pain appears to be increased. Discussion should center around topics other than the symptoms related to the pain, and inquiries about the affected person's health should be greatly reduced, if not eliminated. This type of family therapy will not only help the patient by reducing reminders and reinforcers of pain symptoms, but will also help the family adjust by providing guidance on how they can help the individual with chronic pain feel better.

One caveat is in order at this point. Often complicated family interactions have already been established surrounding the individual with chronic pain, and family members and friends may find it difficult to decrease the attention paid to the "sick" person. It is sometimes more productive to discuss the reduction of illness behavior in terms of distraction. This can be accomplished by telling family and friends that they will be helping the patient by not continually reminding him he is in pain, by not discussing symptoms, and by treating him as if he were well. This approach is often useful; however, it is sometimes the case that secondary gain has accrued to other family members as a result of a chronic pain syndrome. If such is the case, different strategies than those discussed above need to be employed in the effective use of family therapy.

Cognitive Psychotherapy

Cognitive psychotherapy addresses the cognitions or internal dialogue a person has related to his symptoms. Individuals' thoughts about their symptoms usually affect how they will respond when experiencing pain. Misconceptions or negative statements about themselves often lead to increased pain perception and disability in patients with chronic pain. Cognitive psychotherapy is aimed at providing alternative preceptions about chronic pain so that symptoms are viewed in a more positive and productive context. Cognitive psychotherapeutic strategies provide a framework for change and increase the likelihood for successful therapeutic outcomes.

Although the concept of cognitive psychotherapy for managing pain is fairly straightforward on a theoretical level, its implementation can be as varied as are the patients who present with chronic pain. Because of this, an important step in this form of pain management is to have the patient keep a daily record of cognitions about pain symptoms. Along with this information, it is also useful to have patients record the amount of pain they are experiencing as well as the events surrounding their pain episodes. This type of daily record is not only useful for the therapist, but is often helpful in allowing patients to become more aware of the relationship between stressful events in their lives, their cognitions, and their symptoms. In addition, patients who state that they are in constant pain often find that their pain actually fluctuates throughout the day, and that they are not in as much pain as they had imagined. Data should be written down by the patient as often as necessary to provide a clear picture of the pain complaint and events surrounding it.

Once data collection has begun, the therapist can begin to assess the patient's attitude about his pain and help reorient this attitude as needed. For instance, the patient who experiences a moderate amount of pain at work but whose cognitions are, "What if my pain gets worse?", "I'd better go home now in case my pain gets worse", "I know my doctor missed somthing, I'd better go to the emergency room", will likely find himself increasingly incapacitated by his symptoms, becoming more disabled as time goes by. In contrast, the patient who, under the same conditions, says "This will go away in a little while", "I'm going to ignore this", "I know there is nothing seriously wrong with me'', will be much better able to cope with chronic pain and will be much less likely to experience psychological complications as a result of his symptoms. In addition, by learning to change congitions about symptoms, individuals successfully using these strategies will often report decreased levels of pain as the stress and anxiety resulting from their symptoms decrease.

Self-Control Strategies

Patients with chronic abdominal pain often report their symptoms becoming worse when under stress or tension. Problem solving, a form of stress management, offers a technique for reducing stress by helping the patient develop coping skills. Problem solving can take many forms and may involve the development of communication skills, assertiveness training, changing habits, or changing cognitions about stressful events in much the same way as cognitive strategies are used to change cognitions about symptoms. Again, data collection is important in establishing the relationship between events in a person's environment and the onset or exacerbation of abdominal pain.

Biofeedback and Relaxation Training

The onset of either stress or pain usually results in an increase in physiologic arousal and emotional lability which can serve to increase the perception of pain. Biofeedback and relaxation strategies are aimed at helping the individual with chronic pain learn to decrease physiologic arousal, and they provide an alternative (parasympathetic) response to both pain and the stressful events surrounding it. Biofeedback accomplishes this by providing information to the patient about the level of arousal in various biologic systems of the body. This information can then be used by the patient as a guide in learning to control physiologic activity. Relaxation techniques help the patient learn to voluntarily produce decreased levels of arousal through a set of systematic physical and cognitive exercises. These procedures often have the effect of decreasing pain perceptions, and many patients report being able to improve their symptoms by decreasing the physiologic and emotional arousal usually associated with their pain. Relaxation procedures also offer the patient a distracting activity which helps focus attention away from anxiety and pain. In addition, while biofeedback alone is often reported as being an effective form of pain management, its combination with relaxation training increases its usefulness and is a productive way of helping the patient maintain the gains associated with biofeedback once treatment is discontinued. It is also possible to get quite satisfactory results using relaxation strategies alone, and these techniques should not be overlooked because of the unavailability of biofeedback equipment.

While all of the cognitive and behavioral procedures mentioned above can be helpful for the patient, the most effective therapy is often obtained by combining many of these strategies in a fashion which meets the individual needs of the chronic pain patient. Unfortunately, it is not always readily apparent how one goes about implementing such a program. An example may help to illustrate a cognitive behavioral approach to the patient with chronic abdominal pain.

CASE REPORT

A 23-year-old obese woman was referred to the Gastrointestinal Pain Center of the Francis Scott Key Medical Center for chronic abdominal pain of 3 years duration. The onset of the patient's pain was sudden, but it was initially infrequent. At the time of her first experience of abdominal pain, the patient was working as a secretary and was enjoying a healthy and normally active life. Over the next several years, as episodes of abdominal pain became more frequent, she was evaluated by a number of gastroenterologists and given a variety of medications to try to reduce her pain. When this did not work a cholecystectomy was performed. When this also failed to provide relief, the patient began to become more and more anxious, quitting her job and restricting her activities. At the time of this patient's referral, she was taking Donnatal, Dilaudid, Tylenol 3, and Bentyl and had been to the emergency room ten times for her abdominal symptoms in the 8 weeks just prior to beginning treatment.

During the initial session, the patient stated that she felt she had been misdiagnosed by her doctors and that her symptoms were an indication that something was seriously wrong with her. She also indicated that her pain was constant throughout the day, but that at times it would become almost intolerable. When this occurred, the patient stated that she would begin to panic, and rush off to the hospital thinking she was about to die. This patient also revealed that her family was constantly asking her how she was feeling and her mother was telling her she should move home and not worry about going back to work.

Treatment was initiated based on the cognitive-behavioral model outlined above. Self-control strategies were employed to help the patient cope more effectively with her pain, and to reduce the panic she experienced at these times. In addition, the patient was asked to note her level of pain at hourly intervals throughout the day. Once these procedures had been initiated, the patient's symptoms were discussed with her in terms of a benign, chronic condition rather than an acute illness. Her symptoms were placed in the context of the irritable bowel syndrome and she was given an explanation of why her symptoms might occur and what they meant. The patient was then asked to think of her symptoms in this context whenever she began to panic and feel as if her life were threatened. In addition, the patient's family was instructed not to remind the patient she was in pain by inquiring or talking about her pain.

In this case data collection served two important functions. First, the patient began to realize that her pain was not constant all day long, but varied from periods of increased pain to times when she was almost pain free. Secondly, as therapy progressed, the patient was able to see that her symptoms were improving, even though she was not pain free. In reviewing her pain records, she began to realize that her episodes of pain always decreased in a short while, no matter how bad they seemed, and her panic about her symptoms began to disappear.

As the treatment program progressed, the patient's symptoms were reduced significantly to where she was entirely pain free an average of 2 days per week and rarely experienced pain on more than two occasions per day. Once her symptoms had begun to improve, the patient was encouraged to become more active, to go out with her family, become more involved with her 5-year-old son, and to move back into her apartment. Problem solving was also initiated at this time to help the patient find a job and become more self-sufficient. She was also weaned from her pain medications during this period and instructed to take only Tylenol is she felt she needed medicine for her symptoms.

This treatment program occurred over a 6-month period during which the patient was seen for 1-hour sessions on a weekly basis. She was then followed on a bimonthly and then a monthly basis for the next 5 months. During this period she obtained employment, moved out of her parents' house, and began to live a more normal life as she had before her symptoms began. In spite of the fact that her pain never entirely disappeared, the pain management program she participated in allowed this patient to reduce the amount of pain she experienced and to overcome the disability her symptoms had initially caused her.

REFERRAL

As can be seen from this example, working with the patient with chronic pain often requires a fair amount of patience and time. When frequent contact or increased time spent with a patient is not feasible, referral to a behavioral pain management program such as that described above may be the best course of action. However, even when it seems readily apparent that a patient might benefit from such a referral, the individual may resent or refuse such suggestions. This is especially true if the patient begins to feel that such a referral means that he is "crazy" or that the pain is imaginary. One way of avoiding this potential difficulty is to suggest to the patient that stress may be a factor in his symptoms and that the referral is for a pain managment program to help reduce the stress and anxiety associated with the patient's symptoms. This often allows the patient to feel more comfortable about participating in a behavioral pain management program and at the same time facilitates the maintenance of a good relationship with the patient.

CONCLUSIONS

Whenever chronic pain symptoms occur, whether they be of an abdominal nature or otherwise, the likelihood of psychological complications producing more pain and disability than may be necessary should be carefully examined. If illness behavior or disability out of proportion with physical findings is indicated, a cognitive behavioral pain management approach offers a good method of reducing pain as well as improving the ability to cope with a chronic medical condition. Components of such a program should include, but may not necessarily be limited to: (1) adequate medical diagnosis to rule out symptoms resulting from organic disorders; (2) behavioral assessment of the patient, including an evaluation of the individual's response to the pain as well as that of others; (3) systematic data collection to better identify the nature and frequency of the patient's symptoms and to help pinpoint stressors that may be contributing to or exacerbating the chronic pain condition; and (4) behavioral and cognitive psychotherapy to include individual and family therapy, as indicated.

A pain management program such as that described offers a good alternative for the patient who fails to respond to medical or surgical procedures. Clinical and research data suggest that one can expect from two-thirds to three-fourths of those participating in such programs to show improvement in their pain symptoms or the behavioral or emotional disability often associated with chronic pain.

CHRONIC INTRACTABLE ABDOMINAL PAIN

RICHARD G. BLACK, M.D.

The seriousness and frequency of the complaint of abdominal pain are recognized by every physician. It is when the patient's complaint becomes chronic in nature and the symptoms refractory to common treatment that this complaint becomes a diagnostic and therapeutic problem. Before the patient is labeled as a complainer, or with even more uncomplimentary terms, consideration must be given to the possible causes for such a complaint continuing beyond its expected time.

Possible causes of failure to respond to conventional therapy include wrong diagnosis, a long-term problem, incurable benign or malignant disease, or a presentation of the chronic pain syndrome. The patient with a continuing complaint of pain that is out of context with the physician's understanding of the presumed disease state is in danger of iatrogenic harm from well-intended but inappropriate therapy applied before the problem is thoroughly understood. This therapy is often derived from the specialty of the physician rather than the needs of the patient.

DEFINITIONS

Patients with chronic intractable pain problems require different management than patients with self-limiting health problems presenting with acute pain. Management as used herein implies a long-term process as contrasted with a procedure or cure. The first step in such managment is confirmation of the current diagnosis. Very often patients may carry the label of a disease for years without reevaluation, or a histologic diagnosis may be applied to explain the problem of pain. Most notorious is the diagnosis of cancer, which, although histologic in nature, may be used to explain the cause of pain related to myofascial problems, peptic ulcer disease, or constipation, resulting in inappropriate management, often with strong narcotics.

Another distinction must be made when discussing the complaint of "pain"; there is a significant difference between acute pain and chronic pain. These states represent two distinctly different diseases having in common only the complaint of pain. Unfortunately, the experiences of physicians and patients with acute pain are often carried over into areas of chronic pain with disastrous results. Hence the patient with a complaint of vague abdominal discomfort may be treated in the same manner as a patient with an acute pain problem. The usual drugs and operations known to be successful for the acute problem are applied and only briefly, perhaps for a few months, help the patient, who then becomes worse. With continuing complaints both the patient and the physician become desperate, seeking stronger medications and more mutilating surgery without success until each regards the other as being incompetent or psychologically disturbed. Referral is made to other specialists who have a try until the patient becomes firmly labeled with the regrettable terms of "crock" or 'crazy."

Many definitions of chronic pain have been attempted, some of which require that the pain be present for 6 months or longer. However, the duration of the pain complaint is not an important factor in defining the syndrome of chronic pain. The most significant factors differentiating chronic pain from acute pain are that the pain is no longer serving as a protective or warning signal but has become an end unto itself, and, most important, that the victim's life-style has been significantly altered, out of proportion to the disease state. Care must be taken, however, not to confuse chronic nonciception with chronic pain. Many sufferers of arthritis and other diseases have chronic nonciception but in no way can they be compared with the depressed, dependent victims of chronic pain with their high incidence of medication dependency and disturbed social function.

DE NOVO REASSESSMENT

A suggested approach to the patient identified as having either long-term or inappropriate complaints of abdominal pain is to reassess these patients de novo, as if they had just come under your care for the first time. The questions that must be addressed are the following:

1. Are the patient's pain complaints appropriate to a known disease state?
2. Are the patient's pain complaints in a location and of a quality that reasonably relate to abdominal body wall or intra-abdominal structures?
3. Do the patient's pain complaints suggest referral of pain from body structures outside the abdomen?
4. Is the patient's pain behavior in keeping with his physical activity and apparent state of health or does it appear to be exaggerated?
5. Does there appear to be excessive involvement of the patient's family and other support personnel?
6. Is there a long-term use of high levels of analgesic medications?

To help address these questions, the presentation of intra-, extra-, and referred abdominal nonciception will be briefly reviewed, together with the problem of medication abuse. It will be assumed that the reader is already very familiar with the presentation of the usual and unusual disease states of the abdomen. These are well reviewed in the other chapters in this book.

MECHANISMS OF ABDOMINAL PAIN

In most instances pain in the abdomen is due to disorders of the viscera contained within the abdominal cavity and pelvis. Pain referred into the abdominal region from disease of the chest or dorsal spine is the second most common type.

The somatic innervation of the lower thoracic cavity and the upper abdomen may be neurologically considered as one unit. The sensory and motor nerve supply of the lower half of the thoracic parietal pleura, the periphery of the diaphragm, and the upper four-fifths of the abdominal wall are supplied by the lower six or seven thoracic somatic spinal nerves. Moreover, the afferent nerves that mediate the sensory impulses from the upper abdominal viscera synapse in the same spinal cord segments as do the somatic nerves.

The abdominal viscera are innervated by sympathetic and parasympathetic nerves which supply viscerimotor fibers. The sympathetic fibers are usually derived from below the fifth thoracic ganglion bilaterally and reach the viscera via the greater, lesser, and least splanchnic nerves. Parasympathetic fibers are supplied by the vagus and the second through fourth sacral nerves. Sensation from the abdominal viscera reaches the central nervous system without interruption by conveniently accompanying the autonomic fibers in the above nerves. These visceral afferent fibers are not classified by some authors as autonomic fibers but as visceral afferents. They are cerebral spinal fibers having their roots in the posterior root ganglion and entering the central nervous system via the dorsal root, and they do ultimately reach consciousness. Afferent fibers accompanying the vagus, on the other hand, are concerned with subconscious reflex regulation of the viscera and therefore do not reach consciousness. The afferent fibers accompanying the splanchnic nerves and the sacral parasympathetics do, however, transmit painful sensation.

The phrenic and segmental spinal nerves mediate pain sensation from the diaphragm and parietal peritoneum. In addition, the phrenic nerve might be part of the nerve supply of the upper abdominal viscera in some individuals. This is often given as an explanation for sparing of upper abdominal pain sensation following total sympathetic ganglion destruction by surgery or lytic block. In addition, hiccups may accompany upper abdominal pathologic changes in the distribution of the phrenic nerves.

The number of pain fibers in visceral nerves is small in comparison with that in somatic nerves. The visceral endings also adapt more easily to stimulation than their somatic counterparts and are less specific in their ability to be stimulated. The visceral afferent fibers are larger, however, and more heavily myelinated than their motor fellow travelers, as evidenced by a higher concentration of blocking drug required to stop afferent conduction relative to efferent conduction. Adequate and necessary stimulation of the visceral afferent nerve endings may be sudden distention, contraction, or stretching and tearing of a hollow viscus or capsule of a solid viscus. Another potent stimulus is ischemia of the visceral musculature. This may be vividly seen in women undergoing sterilization by tubal banding in which a tight plastic band is used to occlude the fallopian tube and its blood supply. The relatively high threshold of irritability of the visceral afferent fibers can be reduced by inflammation, action of chemicals, toxins, and elevation of temperature, leading to nociceptive input out of proportion to local disease when these conditions are present.

Because of lack of experience of a clear body image of the viscera, the pain stimulation from this area is often diffuse and poorly localized. Therefore, afferent visceral input may produce somatic referred pain, cutaneous tenderness, hyperalgesia and hyperesthesia, muscular rigidity, and various autonomic manifestations—all without awareness of the primary visceral component.

Visceral Pain

In general, visceral pain is dull, poorly localized, and associated with excessive autonomic response, such as vomiting, nausea, and diarrhea. It is generally referred to the midline, reflecting the midline origin of the viscera in embryonic development.

Most diseases of specific abdominal visceral origin have relatively specific areas of reference. These are well documented in older diagnostic manuals written when modern technology was not available. In general, pain from the upper abdominal viscera may be felt in the midthoracic region; renal and pelvic nociception will be referred to the lumbosacral region. Caution must be exercised because of the phenomenon of "habit reference," in which pain from early visceral disease may be referred, not to it's predicted area of reference, but to some preexisting surgical scar or sensitized area.

Pain Localization

Abdominal pain with a general distribution may arise from acute and chronic peritonitis, acute intestinal obstruction, gastroenterocolitis, chronic ulcerative colitis, dysentery, early acute appendicitis or other focal disease, sickle cell crisis, lead poisoning, and other metabolic causes of ileus. Pain in the epigastrium can be related to lesions of stomach, duodenum, pancreas, lung, and heart. These may be accompanied, as noted, by hiccups. The most important causes are chronic or perforated ulcer, gastritis, biliary tract disease, cancer of the pancreas and chronic pancreatic disease, and congestive failure.

Abdominal pain referred to the right hypochondrium may arise from disease of the liver, gallbladder, or colon; from passive congestion, subphrenic abscess, or a kidney tumor. Pain in the left hypochondrium may indicate disease of the spleen, colon, left side of the chest, fecal impaction, splenic embolism, or thrombosis. *Umbilical* pain suggests a referral source in the midportion of the intestine, such as a hernia or diverticulitis. Superior mesenteric occlusion, rupture of graafian follicle, or salpingitis can produce a similar pain. Right iliac referral suggests the source may be the appendix, small intestine, cecum, ureter, ovary, a twisted ovarian cyst, or endometriosis. Left iliac pain referral signals disease of the sigmoid, female organs, hip, or sacroiliac joints, or iliac artery aneurism. If the pain is in the *hypogastrium* the bladder and internal genitals are implicated.

Somatic Pain

Pain referred to the abdominal area from outside sources is generally somatic in character. It is therefore described as superficial, bright, and well localized, as contrasted with deep, dull, and poorly localized. Reflex muscle spasm and sensory changes in dermatome patterns should be sought. The pain may be localized to a limited area. Some examples are postherpetic pain, generalized myositis, segmental neuralgia, thoracic spinal cord tumor, vertebral body compression, or an infected disk space. Often missed is the slipped costal cartilage and intercostal myositis.

Some visceral causes of referred pain are lobar pneumonia, diaphragmatic hernia, and cardiac disease. Less frequent causes of abdominal pain include postcordotomy syndrome, abdominal angina, abdominal epilepsy, porphyria, and generalized vascular disease, such as diabetes and polyarteritis nodosa.

INAPPROPRIATE DRUG USE

Abuse of short-acting analgesic medications is probably the primary factor responsible for sustaining a chronic pain state. It applies especially to chronic abdominal pain because of the gastrointestinal upset that often accompanies the heavy and chronic use of these medications. Patients and their families have been led to believe, through a constant bombardment of advertising by drug companies, that a simple taking of a pill will in some miraculous way solve all their problems. Many physicians who properly use analgesics for acute pain apply the same regimens to their patients with chronic abdominal pain and ultimately make the patient worse. Unfortunately, the long-term use of short-acting analgesics on a "PRN" or as-needed basis results in development of tolerance and escalation of their use. Depression from their effects on neurotransmitters and a resulting increase in reported intensity of pain occurs. Non-analgesic drugs, such as the tranquilizers, hypnotics, and muscle relaxants, also have cumulative toxic effects and play as important a role in this problem as do the analgesics. Confusion of the high thought processes, similar to an organic brain syndrome, which results from continued use of prescription and over the counter drugs is often missed by the examining physician even though it may contribute significantly to misdiagnosis and inappropriate therapy. Chronic users of analgesic medications report less pain after these medications are discontinued and the patients detoxified. So important, and sometimes subtle or even occult, is this problem that a basic principle in the managment of pain patients is that *whenever excessive or chronic use of medications is even suspected, all medications must be withdrawn before a meaningful diagnostic evaluation can be attempted.*

APPROACH TO THE PATIENT WITH CHRONIC ABDOMINAL PAIN

Detailed Pain History and Diary

Since these patients may be considered to have failed the conventional medical approach, some differences in the way they are reassessed may be helpful in solving their problem. Especially helpful is a detailed pain history starting with the onset of the pain and noting how each treatment applied in the past has altered the pain. A detailed questioning of the patient concerning all the factors affecting his pain and its daily, weekly, and monthly time course is more helpful if supplemented by a diary kept by the patient in which he notes pain severity, use of medications, and activity for each hour of the day. Examination of this diary can reveal excessive down time or show activities related to the pain. Interviewing the spouse can confirm activities and medication use. Occult alcoholism is always a consideration.

Evaluating Pain Site

The usual evaluation of the patient might be modified to allow examination when the patient is in pain and to permit more detailed examination of the area of the pain complaint. If the pain complaint is intermittent, the clues afforded by muscle spasm or sensory changes may not be present without the pain. This also applies to diagnostic procedures, such as roentgenographic contrast studies, urinalysis and thermography. A detailed sensory neurologic examination is helpful in isolating referred somatic pain, but unfortunately it is often passed over lightly unless some neurologic disease is present. The charts of patients with pain problems who are seen in consultation rarely have a detailed examination of the site of the pain documented, nor do they contain an adequate pain history. Correcting these deficiencies often leads to successful management of the patient.

ANALGESIC BLOCK IN MANAGEMENT OF ABDOMINAL VISCERAL PAIN

While pain due to visceral disorders of the abdomen can be treated by conservative medical measures or by surgical intervention, there are many disorders in which analgesic nerve block offers great diagnostic, prognostic, and possible therapeutic value. Nerve blockade can be used as a differential diagnostic tool with certainty only in those conditions in which the nerve supply carrying the pain is accessible in widely separated anatomic locations. Thus it can be helpful in determining whether epigastric pain is the result of disease of thoracic or abdominal viscera and may be of value in differentiating the pain of myocardial infarction from that of acute pancreatitis, pulmonary embolus from ruptured ulcer, and pneumonia from appendicitis.

More positive distinction can be made between visceral and somatic or abdominal wall pain. Relief of abdominal pain following intercostal or field block or local infiltration, neither of which interrupts visceral fibers, strongly suggests that the pain is not visceral. Caution must be exercised, since anesthetization of the site of referred pain sometimes relieves the symptoms of the visceral disease. Nerve blocks are an *aid* to diagnosis. It is necessary to correlate their results with the history and physical findings.

Prognostic Blocks

Nerve blocks can be used to prognosticate the effects of surgical or chemical interruption of nerve pathways. Since serious and irreversible surgical intervention may follow "prognostic" blocks, it is necessary that they be performed under optimal circumstances, i.e., after the patient is withdrawn from medications and, when indicated, with roentgenographic control. The results of the block should be interpreted by an expert. This may require prolonged observation of the patient during the time the block develops and wanes. At least two or three blocks should be done with consistent results. Very often, in the hands of a skilled physician, nerve blocks can reveal much about the psychological make-up of the patient and act as a measure of the severity of the pain being experienced.

Therapeutic Blocks

Therapeutic blocks fall into two categories. In the first category are nerve blocks performed with agents of relatively *short duration*. These often last much longer than the effect of the agent used, which is believed to be related to relief of sustained ischemia producing muscle spasm or else resetting of autonomic vascular tone. Often benign but troublesome abdominal pain will respond satisfactorily to three or four temporary celiac or lumbar sympathetic nerve blocks per year. It is characteristic that an emotional crisis may precipatate a recurrence of the pain, necessitating a repeat block.

In the second category are *long-term* nerve blocks performed with lytic agents, with the intention of interrupting nerve pathways by chemical destruction of the nerves or ganglia involved. These are appropriate only if the patient has a short life expectancy or in selected patients in whom a pure visceral block is done without any somatic involvement. The alcohol celiac plexus block, often performed on an outpatient basis, has a high success rate in completely relieving the pain of abdominal malignancies. It is a relatively benign procedure and should be done early in the course of the patient's disease before narcotic addiction, dehydration secondary to cachexia, and pain-related behavior develop. Unfortunately most patients are referred for this procedure late in the course of their disease and then only as a last resort, if at all. Percutaneous celiac or splanchnic blocks do not carry the high incidence of morbidity of surgical splanchnicectomy or ganglionectomy and have a high rate of success.

Analgesic block is useful in the management of pain referred to the abdomen from lesions of the dorsal spine ranging from collapsed vertebral bodies to, when not otherwise manageable, epidural spread of tumor. Site of block may be epidural, paravertebral, peripheral, or at the site of irritation. These procedures also are relatively benign but do require an individual skilled in their use.

TRANSCUTANEOUS ELECTRICAL NERVE STIMULATION

Transcutaneous electrical nerve stimulation (TENS), a technique that is likened to an electronic mustard plaster, has been in clinical use for more than a decade. It is effective for peripheral nerve-related pain and is particularly effective for visceral pain. Success in the long-term management of patients with porphyria has been demonstrated.

Contemporary TENS units are the size of a package of cigarettes and run many days on rechargeable batteries. They are relatively trouble-free and most insurance companies will pay for them on the basis of medical need. Rental units are generally available in larger cities and are suggested for a therapeutic trial. The stimulating electrodes must be placed on an innervated area of skin, preferably in the involved dermatome. For visceral pain, a paravertebral placement over the lower thoracic dermatomes is usually appropriate. Adequate instruction in their use is available and arrangements should be made to have the patient instructed in use of the unit if it is to be successful.

Complications of TENS are rare and generally limied to irritation of the skin by the electrodes or conductive jelly. Patients who complain that they are made worse by the stimulation should, in the absence of other findings, be suspected of having major psychosomatic problems.

CARBOHYDRATE MALABSORPTION

JAY A. PERMAN, M.D.

Malabsorption of carbohydrate results in a predictable set of symptoms, including diarrhea, gas, bloating, cramping, and borborygmi. These symptoms can be understood in light of the pathophysiology of sugar malabsorption. Passage of significant quantities of carbohydrate to the colon causes an osmotic diarrhea. In addition, fermentation of carbohydrate by colonic bacteria results in gas production and release of short-chain fatty acids, which contribute to the osmotic load and stimulate peristalsis.

Malabsorption of sugar may be secondary to a variety of conditions which have specific treatments. Therapy for the underlying condition is thus essential. For example, lactose malabsorption associated with gluten-sensitive enteropathy usually resolves within several months following institution of a gluten-free diet. Restriction of lactose alleviates symptoms during the recovery process, but is no longer necessary following regeneration of mucosa. In contrast, intolerance to lactose caused by primary or adult-onset lactase deficiency requires persistent restriction of lactose in the diet. Rapid alleviation of symptoms attributable to malabsorption of sugar depends on restriction of the offending sugar in both secondary and primary forms of carbohydrate malabsorption.

TABLE 1 Lactose-Free Diet

This diet is for the patient who must eliminate *all* sources of lactose from the diet. Lactose is the sugar found in milk, so all foods containing milk are to be excluded from the diet.

Read the label carefully. Avoid any food containing *milk, nonfat milk solids, skim milk, butter, cream,* and *lactose.*

FOODS ALLOWED		FOODS AVOIDED
MILK:	None	All milk, milk drinks—including whole, skim, low fat, dried, evaporated, and condensed milk—human breast milk Yogurt—any type Cream—sweet or sour Infant formulas other than those permitted Frappes, ice cream sodas
BEVERAGES:	Powdered, fruit-flavored drinks, ginger ale, carbonated beverages, cocoa without added milk solids, coffee, tea	Any made with milk, such as frappes, eggnog, hot chocolate
MEATS:	Any baked, broiled, roasted, and boiled, except those to be avoided	Creamed or breaded meat, fish, or poultry, and prepared meats that may contain dried milk solids, including bologna and cold cuts, frankfurters, salami, commercially prepared fish sticks, and some sausage
EGGS:	As desired	Any made with milk—use specific formula; do not prepare with butter
CHEESE:	None	
BREADS:	Breads made without milk only, such as French bread, Italian bread, water bagels, or "pareve" breads; saltines, graham, oyster, and soda crackers, Triscuits	Made with any form of milk Any baked product made with milk (muffins, biscuits, waffles, pancakes, donuts, sweet rolls) Commercial mixes
CEREAL:	Any made without milk, cooked or ready to eat (read labels). Macaroni, spaghetti, pasta, rice, all prepared without milk or cheese	Any prepared cereal that contains dry milk solids
VEGETABLES AND POTATOES:	All—cooked, canned, frozen, or fresh	Any vegetable prepared with milk, butter, milk solids, bread or bread crumbs; no cheese or cream sauces
FRUIT:	All	
DESSERTS:	Any made without milk or milk products, such as gelatin desserts, fruit crisp, snow puddings, fruit and water sherberts, pie with fruit filling, angel cookies, milk-free cookies (fig bars, ginger snaps, lemon snaps), tofu ice cream	All commercial cake and cookie mixes, ice cream, custard puddings, junket, ice milk, or sherberts that contain milk; frostings made with milk or butter, dessert sauces, cheese cakes
SOUP:	All prepared without milk or milk products; homemade or canned, e.g., chicken rice	All creamed soups, chowders; no cheese
FATS:	Milk-free margarine or "pareve" margarine; oils, nuts, peanut butter	Butter, margarine, some commercial salad dressings (check labels)
SUGAR AND SEASONINGS:	Sugar, honey, molasses, maple syrup, corn syrup, jelly and jam, hard candy, gum drops, marshmallows, hard peppermints, fondant Salt, pepper, spices, herbs, condiments, vinegar, catsup, relish, pickles, olives, tomato sauce, coconut, wheat germ Artificial flavoring and extracts	Any product made from milk, butter, cream, chocolate, toffee, cream mints, caramel candy, candy with cream centers, butterscotch
MISCELLANEOUS:	Coffee Rich, Coffee Mate	Medications that may contain lactose as filler or bulk agents; party dips; nonprescription vitamins, spice blends, Easter egg dyes; dietetic foods and foods advertised as "high protein" sometimes contain lactose or dry milk solids *Check all labels carefully*

LACTOSE INTOLERANCE

When lactose malabsorption is suspected as a basis for the patient's symptoms, I generally perform a lactose hydrogen breath test before instituting dietary therapy. In my experience, history sometimes, but not always, identifies the patient with lactose malabsorption. Confirmation of lactose malabsorption by breath hydrogen determination provides objective evidence to both the physician and the patient of inability to digest and absorb lactose, and allows both physician and patient to proceed confidently with dietary restriction.

The patient should understand that primary lactase deficiency is not a disease. I find it helpful to tell patients that this disorder occurs in the majority of the world's population, and those with normal lactase activity throughout life are in fact "abnormal." A distinction should be

TABLE 2 Lactose Content of Selected Milk, Milk Products, and Substitutes

Product	Unit	Lactose (Approx. g/unit)
Milk	1 cup–244 g	11
Low-fat milk, 2% fat	1 cup–244 g	9–13
Skim milk	1 cup–244 g	12–14
Chocolate milk	1 cup–244 g	10–12
Sweet Acidophilus	1 cup–244 g	9–10
Sweetened condensed whole milk	1 cup–244 g	35
Dried whole milk	1 cup–128 g	48
Nonfat dry milk, instant	1½ cup–91 g	46
Buttermilk fluid	1 cup–245 g	9–11
Whipped cream topping	1 tbs–3 g	0.4
Light cream	1 tbs–15 g	0.6
Low-fat yogurts	8 oz	8–15
Cheese		
Blue	1 oz–28 g	0.7
Camembert	1 oz–28 g	0.1
Cheddar	1 oz–28 g	0.4–0.6
Colby	1 oz–28 g	0.7
Cream	1 oz–28 g	0.8
Gouda	1 oz–28 g	0.6
Limberger	1 oz–28 g	0.1
Parmesan, grated	1 oz–28 g	0.8
Cheese, pasteurized, processed		
American	1 oz–28 g	0.5
Pimento	1 oz–28 g	0.5–1.7
Swiss	1 oz–28 g	0.4–0.6
Cottage cheese	1 cup–210 g	5–6
Cottage cheese, low-fat (2% fat)	1 cup–226 g	7–8
Butter	2 pats–10 g	0.1
Oleomargarine	2 pats–10 g	0
Ice cream		
Vanilla, regular	1 cup–133 g	9
French, soft	1 cup–173 g	9
Ice milk, vanilla	1 cup–131 g	10
Sherbert, orange	1 cup–193 g	4
Ice, orange	100 g	0

From Welsh JD. Carbohydrate Malabsorption. In: Bayless T, ed. Current therapy in gastroenterology and liver disease. Toronto: BC Decker, 1984, p 136.

made between lactose malabsorption and milk allergy. This distinction has therapeutic implications because the individual allergic to cow's milk protein will require strict elimination of dairy products from the diet. In contrast, the individual with lactose malabsorption need not strictly eliminate dairy products from the diet except for an initial diagnostic period.

Dietary modification should begin with strict avoidance of lactose for a short time. This interval is determined by the frequency with which the patient's symptoms occur. If the patient has symptoms daily, strict restriction of lactose for the purpose of determining whether lactose malabsorption is the basis for the symptoms can be limited to 1 or 2 weeks. On the other hand, strict elimination of lactose-containing products for a month's time is reasonable when symptoms attributable to lactose malabsorption occur only once or twice a week.

It is particularly important to reassure patients, especially children, that adherence to a strict diet will not be necessary once it is confirmed that elimination of all lactose from the diet ends the symptoms. The prospect of a life devoid of lactose-containing foods is dismal to most individuals, and it should be pointed out that the strict restriction is being undertaken for confirmation of diagnosis only. In my experience, most patients will accept a strict restriction on this basis.

I provide patients with a lactose-free diet including not only foods avoided but foods *allowed* (Table 1). This assists patients in accepting what might otherwise appear to be a very restrictive diet, and also helps to ensure that the resulting diet will be reasonably well balanced.

Upon confirmation of the symptomatic response to elimination of lactose from the diet, reintroduction of lactose-containing foods to the degree consistent with control of symptoms can be undertaken. The patient should be given information on the lactose content of various foods (Table 2).

A variety of strategies are available to the patient who is a lactose malabsorber, but who prefers dairy products in his diet. Microbial sources of lactase are available which may be added to milk or taken at the time that lactose-containing foods are ingested. LactAid (LactAid, Inc, Pleasantville, NJ) may be added to milk which is then refrigerated for 24 hours. This procedure results in hydrolysis of the bulk of lactose present, reducing the symptoms associated with lactose malabsorption. Some patients,

TABLE 3 Sucrose-Restricted Diet

FOODS ALLOWED	FOODS AVOIDED
Milk, unsweetened evaporated milk, and cream	Sweetened condensed milk and formulas containing sucrose
Asparagus, broccoli, Brussels sprouts, cabbage, cauliflower, celery, chard, chicory, cucumber, lettuce, mushrooms, spinach, tomatoes bamboo shoots, radishes, and potatoes (0.3 g/100 g)	Peas, dried beans, lentils, turnips, parsnips, and other vegetables not listed in foods allowed or those not tolerated
Grapes, fresh cherries, dried Kadota figs, blackberries, cranberries, currants (red and white), lemons, loganberries, and medium ripe strawberries (0.3 g/100 g)	Those not on the list of fruits allowed or those not tolerated
Fried, hard-cooked, soft-cooked, and poached eggs	
Fresh meat, fish, and ham	Check all commercially prepared meats and fish
All cheeses	
Bread (homemade), spaghetti, and macaroni (without sugar)	Breakfast cereals, wheat germ, rice, and bran
Butter, margarine, cooking oil, lard, and salad dressing (oil and vinegar)	Mayonnaise, salad dressing (French, Roquefort, Thousand Island, Russian)
Cocoa, coffee, tea (all unsweetened), and vegetable juice	Malted milk, milk shake, Kool-Aid, and pop
Salt, pepper, gravy, spices, herbs, and vinegar	Olives, pimento, and pickles (sweet and sour)
Chicken and beef broth, bouillon, and consommé	
Glucose (dextrose) and artificial sweeteners	Sugar (cane, beet, granulated, powdered, brown), jam, honey, jelly, candy, molasses, maple syrup, and frosting
Homemade cake, cookies, ice cream using glucose, gelatin, tapioca, and diabetic chocolate	Commercially prepared pies, cookies, cakes, diabetic products (unless mentioned elsewhere), ice cream, sherbert, and any food prepared with sugar
	Salad dressing, pickles, chutney, and medicines made up in syrup

From Perman JA, Watkins JB. Malabsorptive syndromes and intestinal disaccharidase deficiencies. In: Gellis SS, Kagan BM, eds. Current pediatric therapy 10. Philadelphia: WB Saunders, 1982, p 222.

however, will find the resulting milk too sweet for their taste. Capsules containing lactase (Lactrase, Kremers-Urban Co, Milwaukee, WI) or LactAid can be taken orally just before and during ingestion of dairy products or foods containing added milk solids. The dose is titrated upward until symptoms are controlled. Recent evidence indicates that yogurt containing active culture, i.e., not pasteurized, is an autodigesting source of lactose. Bacterial lactase present in the yogurt apparently survives passage through the stomach and is activated in the duodenum, thus substituting for the lack of endogenous lactase in individuals with low lactase activity.

Consideration should be given to supplementation of calcium and riboflavin in the diet of those patients who severely curtail their intake of dairy products. Calcium gluconate or other calcium-containing products can be used. For example, the individual can take calcium-containing antacids or wafers rich in calcium. Riboflavin can be economically given using a riboflavin-containing multivitamin.

SUCROSE MALABSORPTION

Isolated sucrase-alpha-dextrinase deficiency causes symptoms of carbohydrate malabsorption in early childhood. Occasionally, however, an adult previously thought to have an irritable bowel syndrome may be diagnosed as having the disorder. Despite the deficiency of alpha-dextrinase (isomaltase), starch is generally well tolerated by these individuals because of hydrolysis by other pathways. Restriction of sucrose is required to control symptoms. The patient is instructed on how to follow a sucrose-restricted diet which again emphasizes both foods allowed and foods avoided (Table 3). Some affected patients may demonstrate increasing tolerance to sucrose as they grow older.

Sucrose malabsorption may occur as a result of sucrase deficiency secondary to mucosal injury, short gut, or intestinal bypass. Since disaccharidase deficiency in these situations is not limited to sucrase activity alone, concomitant restriction of lactose-containing foods is also necessary.

MONOSACCHARIDE AND SORBITOL MALABSORPTION

Congenital glucose-galactose malabsorption is a well-established but fortunately rare inability to digest and ab-

TABLE 4 Fructose Content of Foods

Figs*	30.9 g†
Dates*	23.9 g†
Prunes*	15.0 g†
Grapes*	8.0 g†
Soft drinks containing high fructose-syrup	37.5 g‡

* Dried
† Per 100 g edible portion
‡ Per 18–19 oz of soda
From Ravich WJ, et al. Fructose: incomplete intestinal absorption in humans. Gastroenterology 1983; 84:26.

TABLE 5 Sorbitol Content of "Sugar-free" Products and Various Foods

"Sugar-free" gum	1.3–2.2 g/piece
"Sugar-free" mints	1.7–2.0 g/piece
Pears	4.6*
Prunes	2.4*
Peaches	1.0*
Apple juice	0.3–0.9 g*

* Expressed as grams of sorbitol per 100 g dry matter or per 100 g juice. Dry weight equals approximately 15% of fresh weight.
From Hyams JS. Sorbitol intolerance: an unappreciated cause of functional gastrointestinal complaints. Gastroenterology 1983; 84:30.

sorb all sugars other than fructose. This disorder presents in very early infancy. A mono- and disaccharide-free formula to which fructose can be added is utilized to manage these infants. In other infants, severe mucosal injury may result in transient inability to transport glucose. Continuous feedings of modular formulas permitting titration of the quantity of sugar, or parenteral alimentation is necessary for a variable period of time.

Recent evidence indicates that healthy adults may have symptoms associated with malabsorption of fructose. A dietary history indicating intake of large amounts of fructose-containing food or drink may suggest this diagnosis (Table 4). Since both the degree of malabsorption and associated symptoms are dose related, dietary counseling designed to decrease fructose intake will be useful to these individuals.

Similarly, healthy individuals malabsorb sorbitol. When diet history suggests considerable intake of sorbitol (Table 5) in individuals with symptoms suggesting carbohydrate malabsorption, a trial of a sorbitol-free diet is appropriate.

OTHER FORMS OF CARBOHYDRATE MALABSORPTION

Limited evidence indicates that some individuals with functional intestinal complaints will respond to a gluten-free diet despite the absence of gluten-sensitive enteropathy. Starch malabsorption may occur in healthy individuals ingesting foods containing both starch and gluten, e.g., breads made from wheat. Further study is required, but it appears that gluten restriction may reduce functional complaints attributable to sugar malabsorption in some otherwise normal individuals. Similarly, further study is required of carbohydrate malabsorption in the elderly. For the present, reduction of the total amount of carbohydrate ingested in a meal may be useful in some elderly individuals should the degree of symptomatology warrant intervention.

POSTPRANDIAL HYPOGLYCEMIA

ANGELIKI GEORGOPOULOS, M.D.
SIMEON MARGOLIS, M.D., Ph.D.

Postprandial hypoglycemia is a controversial disorder for several reasons. The adrenergic symptoms associated with it (palpitations, sweating, weakness, shakiness, and so on) are nonspecific and can be encountered in other situations; in addition, no specific level of plasma glucose universally produces these symptoms. Symptomatic postprandial hypoglycemia can follow sugar ingestion in some otherwise normal individuals in whom carbohydrate intake is very limited. Finally, many patients with postprandial hypoglycemia tend to be obsessive-compulsive persons who are tense and emotionally labile and can experience adrenergic symptoms during times of stress even with normal plasma glucose levels.

For all these reasons, when dealing with a patient whose history is suggestive of postprandial hypoglycemia, the physician must verify the diagnosis by establishing that adrenergic symptoms are present at the same time that the plasma glucose level is below 60 mg per deciliter. Moreover, he or she frequently has to assess the extent to which the patient's everyday symptoms can be attributed to hypoglycemia. This assessment is of particular relevance when dietary and drug regimens have failed to control the patient's symptoms.

DIAGNOSTIC APPROACH

As shown in Figure 1, a careful dietary history is necessary to confirm that symptoms are postprandial and to assess the carbohydrate content of the diet. The latter is important, since a low intake of complex carbohydrates, coupled with simple sugar ingestion, can provoke hypoglycemia in some otherwise normal individuals. Finding out if the patient's symptoms are associated with low blood sugar is also important. The patient is thus instructed in the use of a glucose oxidase strip reagent (Chemstrips BG) to measure blood glucose at the time of symptoms. The strips are brought to the office within a week and the reading verified by the physician or staff. Glucose levels greater than 80 mg per deciliter rule out the diagnosis. If the glucose level is below 80 mg per deciliter and the patient is on a low carbohydrate diet, the diet is modified to contain at least 50 percent of calories as complex carbohydrates, and simple sugars are severely restricted. If symptoms persist and are accom-

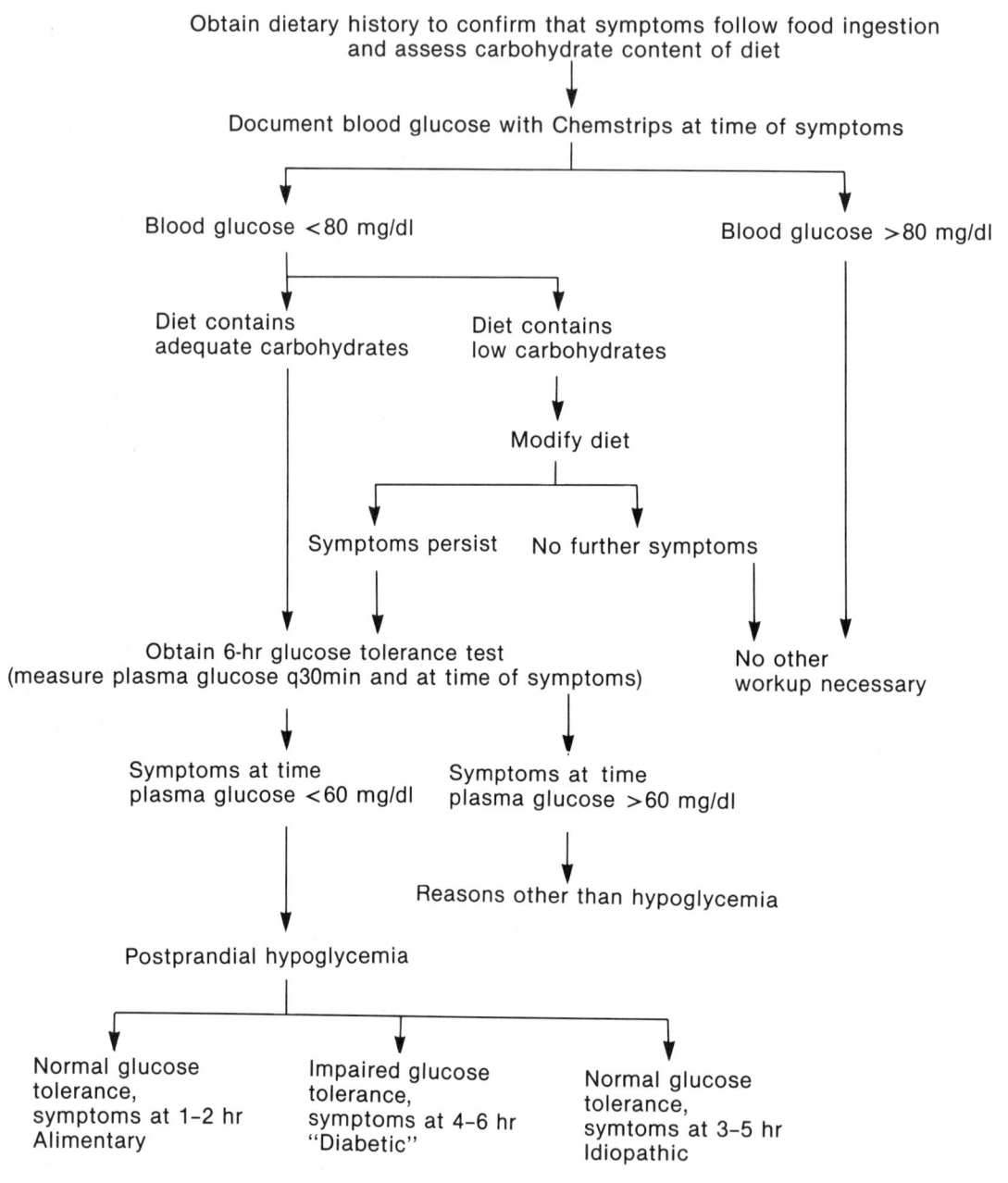

Figure 1 Diagnostic approach to postprandial hypoglycemia.

panied by Chemstrip glucose values less than 80 mg per deciliter, a 6-hour glucose tolerance test is performed following a 3-day preparation with 250 g carbohydrates daily.

The ideal method for diagnosis of hypoglycemia is continuous blood glucose monitoring. Since this is not readily available, plasma glucose should be measured every 30 minutes and at the time of any symptoms to avoid missing the often transient glucose nadir. The personnel drawing the blood should be trained to recognize adrenergic symptoms and signs and should instruct the patient to notify them when symptoms are experienced. The diagnosis is confirmed by the concurrence of appropriate symptoms with a plasma glucose level less than 60 mg per deciliter.

The results of the glucose tolerance test and the timing of symptomatic hypoglycemia will differentiate among the various forms of postprandial hypoglycemia, namely, alimentary, "diabetic," and idiopathic. The *alimentary* form, most commonly seen after gastric surgery, is characterized by rapid gastric emptying causing a precipitous rise in plasma glucose levels. The resultant dramatic insulin secretion causes symptomatic hypoglycemia 1 to 2 hours after glucose ingestion. (Note that dumping symptoms occur 15 to 20 minutes after food intake.)

"*Diabetic*" hypoglycemia is characterized by im-

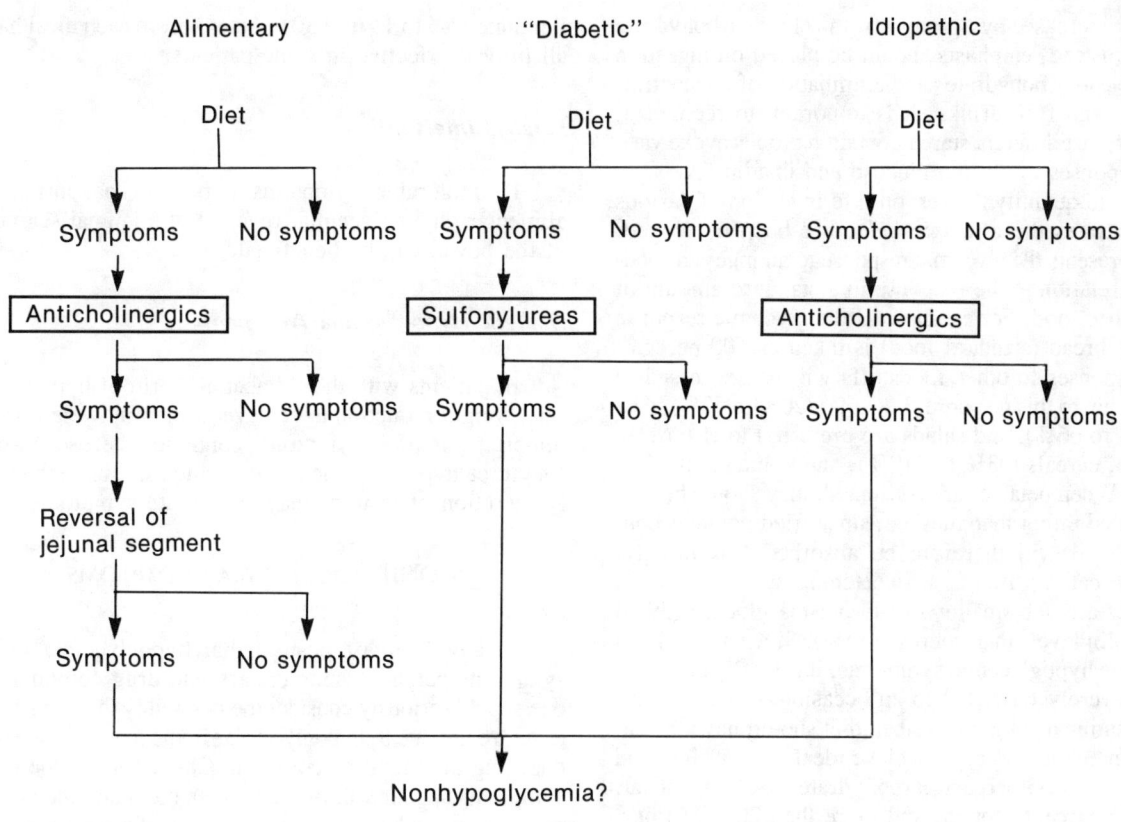

Figure 2 Treatment approach for postprandial hypoglycemia

paired glucose tolerance (normal fasting plasma glucose, but at least one plasma glucose level exceeding 200 mg per deciliter during the first 2 hours of the glucose tolerance test and a 2 hour value between 140 and 200 mg per deciliter) and symptomatic hypoglycemia 4 to 6 hours after glucose ingestion. The hypoglycemia is attributed to excessive and delayed insulin secretion.

The *idiopathic* form is characterized by normal glucose tolerance, heterogeneous and often delayed insulin secretion, and symptomatic hypoglycemia occurring 3 to 5 hours following glucose ingestion. Although elevated GIP levels have been reported in some of these subjects, the origin of the disorder remains unclear.

Other Forms of Postprandial Hypoglycemia

Two enzyme deficiency states may provoke postprandial hypoglycemia in children. These are deficiencies of galactose-1-phosphate uridyl transferase in galactosemia and fructose-1-phosphate aldolase in fructose intolerance. Elimination of galactose and fructose from the diet will alleviate postprandial hypoglycemia in these children.

Rarely, patients of any age with insulin-secreting tumors or deficiencies of counter-regulatory hormones (Addison's disease of panhypopituitarism) may experience symptoms of both postprandial and fasting hypoglycemia.

TREATMENT

Dietary Modification

Figure 2 summarizes the treatment approach for postprandial hypoglycemia. The first line of treatment of all adult forms of postprandial hypoglycemia is dietary modification. There have been no controlled clinical trials in the treatment of this disorder. Clinical experience shows, however, that in most cases dietary treatment alone is successful in relieving symptomatic hypoglycemia. The rationale of the proposed diet is based on the postulated underlying pathophysiology of the disorder. Generally recommended for all three forms of postprandial hypoglycemia are meals containing foodstuffs (such as fiber and fat) known to decrease gastric emptying, postprandial hyperglycemia, and insulin secretion. The prescribed diet should thus include fiber and some fat in every meal. Moreover, since overeating and undereating are frequently associated with abnormalities in glucose tolerance and insulin secretion, the diet should contain the appropriate amount of calories to achieve ideal body weight.

High protein, carbohydrate restricted diets were stressed in the past, but studies suggest little benefit, and possibly increased symptoms, from a low carbohydrate intake. Instead, emphasis should be placed on ingestion of complex carbohydrates and elimination of concentrated sugar and fruit drinks. It is important to recognize, however, that different starch-containing foods evoke variable responses in plasma glucose and insulin levels. In an effort to quantify the response to ingestion of various carbohydrates the *glycemic index* has been developed. This represents the glycemic response to an ingested foodstuff in relation to the response to a standard amount of a reference food. For example, if the glycemic response to white bread (standard food) is taken as 100 percent, then responses to other foodstuffs will be expressed in relationship to this response. Legumes (20% to 50%), pasta (61% to 66%), and salads are preferred to rice (83% to 96%), cereals (73% to 119%), and potatoes (81% to 135%). When potatoes are consumed, they should be prepared fried rather than mashed, since fried potatoes contain fat and will therefore be absorbed less rapidly. Fructose can be used as a sweetening agent because it produces a much smaller rise in plasma glucose (39%) and insulin levels than sucrose (86%). Since alcohol can aggravate hypoglycemic symptoms, it is totally eliminated or severely restricted to an occasional social drink.

In summary, the prescribed diet should have the caloric content necessary to achieve ideal body weight and contain 50 to 55 percent carbohydrates, 30 percent fat, 15 to 20 percent protein, and more than 20 g of fiber. The diet is divided into four to six meals, each containing some fiber and fat. The types of preferred complex carbohydrates are specified. Concentrated sugar, juice, and alcohol are severely restricted or eliminated.

Anticholinergic Drugs

If dietary treatment is not totally satisfactory, the addition of drugs can be tried. In alimentary and idiopathic hypoglycemia, anticholinergic drugs will further slow gastric emptying and intestinal motility and inhibit vagal stimulation of insulin release. Tincture of belladonna (10 to 15 drops), atropine sulfate (0.5 to 1 mg), or Pro-Banthine (7.5 to 15 mg) 30 minutes before each meal have all proved effective in some patients.

Surgical Intervention

If intolerable symptoms persist in patients with alimentary hypoglycemia, reversal of a jejunal segment of the bowel can be beneficial.

Diabetic Hypoglycemia Treatment

In patients with the "diabetic" form of hypoglycemia, weight reduction to achieve ideal body weight is an important goal. If symptoms continue, the use of sulfonylurea hypoglycemic agents, which stimulate the early secretion of insulin, may ameliorate symptoms.

"NONHYPOGLYCEMIA" SYMPTOMS

In any form of postprandial hypoglycemia when symptoms persist despite dietary and drug compliance, one should seriously consider the possibility that the symptoms are not due to hypoglycemia. In the majority of cases checking the blood glucose with Chemstrips at the time symptoms appear will prove to the patient and the physician that hypoglycemia is not the cause. Other causes for the symptoms can then be sought with greater confidence. In the absence of thyrotoxicosis, carcinoid, or pheochromocytoma, anxiety attacks are the most likely cause. Psychotherapy or the use of a mild tranquilizer could be very helpful.

In summary, we believe that postprandial hypoglycemia does exist, but it is far less common than the public has been led to believe by the lay press or "nutritional specialists" (physicians and others). In most referred patients, we cannot verify that hypoglycemia is responsible for their symptoms. Moreover, symptoms not related to hypoglycemia are frequently present even among the patients who have been correctly diagnosed as having postprandial hypoglycemia.

BACTERIAL OVERGROWTH SYNDROME

JOHN G. BANWELL, M.D., F.A.C.P.
PETER YANG, M.D.

The mucosal surface of the small intestine is the location for a limited growth of commensal microorganisms. In the proximal small bowel this consists of a predominantly gram-positive microflora (*streptococcus*, *staphylococcus*, diphtheroids, and fungi). Toward the distal small bowel, coliform organisms (*Escherichia coli*, *Klebsiella*) are found in increasing numbers near the ileocecal valve, and anaerobes increase prior to the development of their massive growth in the cecum and colon. A most important feature is that they are always in low concentration ($<10^5$ organisms per milliliter of intestinal fluid). *Bacterial overgrowth syndrome* is a clinical disorder directly attributable to an abnormal proliferation of the small intestinal microflora. *Tropical enteropathy, or tropical sprue* is a similar malabsorption disorder characterized by malaise, weight loss, and chronic diarrhea, which may be severe with acute fluid and electrolyte depletion or may be associated with abdominal distention, boborygmi, and voluminous pale, bulky stools. The number of small bowel bacteria is increased but the pathogenesis of its malabsorption is unclear. The abnormal bacterial flora is primarily aerobic, is not associated with overgrowth of anaerobic organisms or deconjugation of bile salts, and is less severe than in the bacterial overgrowth syndrome. Therapy for both disorders is nonspecific and includes treatment with broad-spectrum antibiotics.

BACTERIAL OVERGROWTH SYNDROME

Three major conditions may cause the bacterial overgrowth syndrome:

1. *Structural or anatomic abnormalities of the small intestine*, including strictures associated with Crohn's disease, radiation enteritis or associated with small bowel tumors such as carcinoids or lymphoma; enteric fistulas; duodenal or jejunal diverticula; surgical defects, such as afferent loops after gastrectomy, jejunoileal bypass operations for obesity, continent ileostomy, or enteroanastamoses
2. *Abnormalities of bowel motility*, such as systemic sclerosis, idiopathic pseudo-obstruction, diabetic enteropathy and old age
3. *Disorders of mucosal resistance*, such as acquired immunodeficiency syndrome (AIDS), congenital and acquired T and B cell deficiency, and IgA deficiency associated with abnormal bacterial colonization are also considered part of the syndrome.

The abnormal bacterial flora in persons with bacterial overgrowth syndrome is significantly different quantitatively and qualitatively, from normal bacterial flora. Concentrations of microorganisms are much higher (10^6 to 10^{11} organisms per milliliter), and the predominant flora is a mixture of coliforms and anaerobes (*Bacteroides, Clostridia*, and *Bifidobacterium*). Metabolic degradation and utilization of protein, cobalamin (vitamin B_{12}), and bile salts account for clinical features of hypoproteinemia, megaloblastic anemia, and steatorrhea. Mucosal injury and disaccharidase deficiency from damage by bacteria and their enzyme activity also occurs. Diagnosis is made by culture of intestinal secretions and breath analysis of $^{14}CO_2$ or H_2 following administration of ^{14}C-xylose, ^{14}C-glycocholate, or lactulose. The chapter *Carbohydrate Malabsorption* discusses breath hydrogen tests as a method for diagnosing bacterial overgrowth.

Therapeutic Approach

Therapy may require medical, nutritional, and/or surgical care. Their application will depend on a thorough appreciation of the clinical problem, the extent of underlying disease and its cause, and whether the lesion is amenable to surgical cure. Symptoms due to the abnormal bacterial overgrowth may be difficult to distinguish from those of the associated disease.

Antibiotic Management

Antimicrobial therapy is the most readily available option. Treatment with antibiotics should be instituted only where evidence of abnormal small bowel bacterial overgrowth has been detected. The choice of antibiotic to administer is frequently empiric because the flora is polymicrobial and sensitivity to any particular antibiotic is unknown. Nor is it known whether all, several, or only one resident bacteria require eradication, whether an anaerobicidal or aerobicidal antibiotic is best used, and what is the significance of resistant organisms which may develop. Despite such limited understanding, several antibiotics are effective in practice. *Tetracycline* is the antibiotic of choice. Striking clinical improvement is frequently noted within a few days. It is best used for a 10- to 14-day course at a dosage of 250 mg every 6 hours. Repeat courses of the same drug every 4 to 6 weeks may be instituted as symptoms recur. Chronic administration is less desirable, although some physicians prescribe courses of up to 6 weeks' duration.

Other effective alternatives are available. *Metronidazole*, because of its availability and low cost (as a generic drug), is useful. *Chloramphenicol*, although shown to be an effective treatment, should not be used unless other antibiotics fail because of its potential to cause aplastic anemia. *Combination therapy* with cephalosporins may be tried. Clindamycin, lincomycin, and erythromycin have been used less effectively. Ampicillin, neomycin, and penicillin are usually ineffective. Repeat courses of therapy consisting of 10- to 14-day courses of several different drugs in rotation is also a useful approach. Follow-up tests can include fecal fat, fasting breath hydrogen, or repeat $^{14}CO_2$ exhalation testing.

Nutritional Considerations

Improvement in nutritional status will often require early attention in patients with the bacterial overgrowth syndrome, and although severe diarrheal fluid loss is rare, it may occasionally require intravenous fluid and electrolyte treatment.

Minerals and Vitamins. Minerals and water- and fat-soluble vitamins should initially be replaced parenterally and later orally. There is no standard specific supplemental vitamin recommendation for persons with bacterial overgrowth. A suggested list (Table 1) provides reasonable dosages for mild nutritional deficiencies such as are encountered in the syndrome. A variety of proprietary multivitamin preparations usually provide 100 to 150 percent of the required dietary allowance for nutritional supplementation. Cobalamin deficiency should be treated by 50 μg daily for 2 weeks and continued malab-

TABLE 1 Bacterial Overgrowth Syndrome

Minerals (RDA)*	Available Preparations	Vitamins	Available Preparations
Calcium 800–1,200 mg	Calcium carbonate (40% calcium) Tablets: 500 mg (200 mg calcium); 625 or 1.25 mg calcium carbonate (250–500 mg calcium) with or without 125 U vitamin D available as Os-Cal (Marion Lab)	Vitamin B_1 25–50 mg	Thiamine hydrochloride Tablets: 5, 10, 25, 50 mg Elixir: 2.25 mg/5 ml
		Vitamin B_2	Riboflavin Tablets: 5, 10 mg
	Calcium lactate (13% calcium) Tablets: 325 mg (42.25 mg calcium), 650 mg (94.5 mg calcium)	Vitamin B_3 20–50 mg	Niacin Tablets: 25, 50 mg Elixir: 50 mg per 5 ml
	Calcium gluconate (6% calcium) Syrup: 1.8 g (115 mg calcium/5 ml)		Niacinamide (does not cause flushing) Tablets: 25, 50 mg
Phosphorus	Neutra-Phos-K Capsules: 250 mg phosphorus (7.125 mEq Na and K/capsule) Powder: reconstituted (same as capsule/75 ml)	Vitamin B_5 10–20 mg	Calcium pantothenate Tablets: 10 mg
		Vitamin B_6 10–25 mg	Pyridoxine hydrochloride Tablets: 5, 10, 25 mg
	Neutra-Phos-K Same preparations except potassium substituted for sodium	Vitamin C 50 mg	Ascorbic acid Tablets: 25, 50 mg Syrup: 20, 100 mg/ml
Magnesium 300–400 mg	Magnesium sulfate 50% solution: 202 mg magnesium/ml injectable. Magnesium chloride, 10% solution, 1 tbsp b.i.d.	Folic acid 1 mg	Folic acid Tablets: 0.1, 0.4, 1 mg
		Vitamin A 10,000–25,000 IU	Vitamin A (water miscible) Capsules: 25,000 and 50,000 IU Solution: 50,000 IU/ml
Zinc 50–150 mg	Zinc sulfate Capsules: 220 mg (50 mg zinc)		
Iron 10–18 mg	Ferrous sulfate (20% iron) Tablets: 300 mg (60 mg iron) Elixir: 200 mg (44 mg iron/5 ml)	Vitamin D 4,000–12,000 IU	Vitamin D Capsules: 25,000 and 50,000 IU Liquid: 8,000 IU/ml
	Ferrous gluconate (11.6% iron) Tablets: 325 mg (38 mg iron) Elixir: 325 mg (38 mg iron/5 ml)	Vitamin E 30–60 IU	Vitamin E (water miscible) Capsules: 30 IU Solution: 50 IU/ml
		Vitamin K 5 mg	Menadiol sodium diphosphate (K_4) Tablets: 5 mg Phytonadione (K_1) Tablets: 5 mg
		Vitamin B_{12} 200 µg IM monthly	Cyanocobalamin Injection: 30, 100, 1,000 µg/ml

* RDA = recommended dietary allowance

sorption of the vitamin by 100 µg intramuscularly each month. Vitamin K deficiency should be controlled with 5 to 10 mg intravenously or intramuscularly.

Nutrient Deficiency. With severe malnutrition, intravenous central hyperalimentation administered by Hickman or Broviac catheter may be life saving. Indeed, some patients with systemic sclerosis and intestinal pseudo-obstruction may require home intravenous alimentation. There is insufficient experience with enteral alimentation, however, dietary supplementation and adjustment are often sufficient to achieve an enhanced caloric intake and weight gain. Increased dietary calories (approximately 2,500 Kcal) can be provided as extra carbohydrate (>250 g) and protein (>80 g). Tolerance to fat may be limited, and diarrhea can be reduced by restricting long-chain triglycerides to 30 to 40 g per day. Medium-chain triglycerides (MCT) may be used as a dietary supplement at tolerated levels of 30 g 3 times daily as MCT oil or Portagen powder.

Specific Therapy for Individual Disorders

Infusion of plasma or constituent gammaglobulins on a regular basis (monthly) may be useful in treating diarrhea associated with *hypogammaglobulinemia*. Interferon and interleukin II therapy may be advantageous in treatment of *AIDS*. The most optimal timing and dosage for these agents have not been accurately defined. Motility agents—prostigmine, 25 mg 4 times daily, metoclopramide (Reglan), 10 mg 3 times daily, and indomethacin, 25 mg 3 times daily—may be useful in the management of *intestinal pseudo-obstruction*. Each of these disorders is discussed in separate chapters in this volume.

Symptomatic Therapy for Diarrhea

Loperamide (Imodium) is the drug of choice for treatment of chronic diarrhea in doses of 2 to 4 mg 3 times a day or as needed. Side effects of dependency have not been a problem with this antidiarrheal agent which does not cross the blood-brain barrier. Diphenoxylate plus atropine (Lomotil), 1 to 6 tablets a day, and codeine sulfate, 30 mg 3 times a day, are less desirable alternatives.

Surgical Management

Surgical cure may be possible for resection of intestinal strictures, localized areas of diverticula, fistulas, or tumors. Revision of jejunoileal bypass operation for obesity may ameliorate the arthropathy, bowel symptoms, and abnormal metabolic effects of D-lactic acidosis. Surgical cure of structural abnormalities associated with bacterial overgrowth have been described, however, the lesions amenable to surgical correction are but a few of all those causing bacterial overgrowth. Moreover, the general physical condition of the patient, often ill with chronic diseases such as Crohn's disease or recovering from prior abdominal surgery, may often preclude further surgical intervention. A useful additional surgical role is treatment of patients with postgastrectomy afferent loop syndrome. Such patients often have symptoms of bilious vomiting, weight loss, and chronic gastrointestinal bleeding which may also benefit from reconstructive surgery. The role of transplantation surgery in organ failure has expanded to include marrow transplant in a few patients with chronic immune deficiency states. In the future, intestinal transplantation may be available for repair of diffuse structural lesions of the small bowel, such as large resections and diverticula.

Usually, several of these medical or surgical measures may improve symptoms and well being in most patients with bacterial overgrowth even when the underlying intestinal disorder cannot be cured.

TROPICAL ENTEROPATHY

Definitive diagnosis of tropical enteropathy depends on documentation of malabsorption of fat, d-xylose, or cobalamin, and nonspecific morphologic abnormalities in biopsy specimens of the small intestine, and exclusion of other recognized causes of the malabsorption syndrome.

Therapeutic Management

Therapy is directed toward replacement of fluid and electrolyte loss, restoration of vitamin and mineral deficiency, and improvement in the underlying intestinal mucosal disorder.

Fluid and Electrolytes

Severe dehydration requires rapid rehydration. Several regimens provide effective fluid replacement of electrolyte loss in stool water. In some cases this can be achieved by *oral rehydration* utilizing a solution similar in composition to the World Health Organization rehydrated solution (sodium chloride, 3.5 g; sodium bicarbonate, 2.5 g; potassium chloride, 1.5 g; glucose, 20 g in 1 L of potable water). Assessment of the adequacy of rehydration is made by regular evaluation of clinical findings (skin tone, blood pressure and quality of pulse, and urine output). If severe carbohydrate malabsorption is present it may limit the initial usefulness of oral rehydration solutions. Intravenous fluid replacement, if necessary, can be achieved with Ringer's lactate solution or two parts isotonic saline to one part bicarbonate or lactate.

Response to Definitive Therapy

Tropical enteropathy patients improve dramatically with institution of therapy with folic acid, vitamin B_{12}, and antibiotics. Improved well-being of the patient is accompanied by a rapid reticulocyte response, and rise in hemoglobin and red cell count when megaloblastic anemia is present. The response of the malabsorption disorder is difficult to ascribe to a specific mode of therapy because it has been shown that intestinal function may improve spontaneously with hospitalization and change in diet alone, with folic acid therapy, with cobalamin therapy, and with use of antimicrobial agents. Since patients are often hospitalized when treatment is instituted or may have been moved out of an area endemic for tropical enteropathy, it is often difficult to define which factor(s) led to cure of the intestinal disorder.

Spontaneous improvement, when observed, usually occurs slowly over weeks or months with reduction in steatorrhea. It is less frequently encountered in patients from the West Indies and cannot be relied on to achieve rapid or complete remission of the disease.

Folate

Small doses (1 to 200 μg per day) may improve bowel function independent of the hematologic response. Usually, however, the hematologic response occurs without improvement in steatorrhea, even with a constant larger dose (5 mg per day). Approximately 50 percent of persons may be expected to lose their gastrointestinal symptoms on folate alone.

Cobalamin

Cobalamin therapy (100 μg per day IM) will improve bowel dysfunction in addition to curing cobalamin deficiency and instituting a hematologic response. Glossitis will usually improve greatly with vitamin B_{12} and/or folic acid therapy.

Antimicrobial Therapy

Tetracycline (250 mg every 6 hr), sulfamethazine (2 g per day), and chloramphenicol (500 mg every 6 hr) have each been shown to be effective in treatment. Intestinal absorptive function improves in 50 to 70 percent of all patients treated. As is the case for other bacterial overgrowth states, *tetracycline is the drug of choice*. The progression of healing of the intestinal lesion is very good in expatriates treated in the tropics or on return to temperate climates. Recurrence or relapses however, may require repeat therapy.

Optimal therapy should include use of *folate* (5 mg orally per day) and *tetracycline* (250 mg orally every 6 hr). A rapid response usually occurs, but it is empirically useful to continue therapy for 3 to 4 weeks or until absorptive parameters for d-xylose, the Schilling test, or morphologic findings in intestinal biopsy specimens are normal. In indigenous persons with tropical enteropathy, recurrence and relapse may occur even after migration to temperate climates. Moreover, continuous therapy may need to be maintained for much longer (approximately 6 months) in many instances to achieve maximum improvement in intestinal mucosal structure and function.

WHIPPLE'S DISEASE

RUSSELL D. KEINATH, M.D.
WILLIAM O. DOBBINS III, M.D.

CLINICAL AND DIAGNOSTIC FEATURES

Whipple's disease is an uncommon systemic bacterial illness that affects primarily middle-aged white males. The clinical hallmarks of the disease are abdominal pain, weight loss, diarrhea, and arthralgia.[1] Atypically, the patient may present with central nervous system (CNS) and/or ocular symptoms and signs. Rare, but clinically significant involvement of the endocardium, pericardium, pleura, and peritoneum has been observed. The disease is characterized pathologically by the presence of macrophages that are stained intensely by the periodic acid-Schiff (PAS) stain. These macrophages are found in virtually all organ systems. There is, however, a unique predilection for these macrophages to be found in the lamina propria of the small intestine, mesenteric lymph nodes, mitral and aortic values of the heart, and the CNS. Bacilli, appropriately called Whipple bacilli, with all the structural characteristics of bacteria, have been observed within the intestinal mucosa, Kupffer cells of the liver, mesenteric and peripheral lymph nodes, heart, central nervous system, eye, kidney, and lung. The uniform appearance of Whipple bacilli as determined by light and electron microscopy and the uniform antigenic structure of the bacilli as determined by immunofluorescence staining are imposing evidence that a single microorganism is the likely cause of the disease. This putative microorganism has not been cultured in vitro, however, and the disease has not been reproduced in animals. There may be an immune deficit that predisposes certain individuals to infection with the Whipple bacillus. The diagnosis of Whipple's disease is made by finding characteristic PAS-positive macrophages in the lamina propria in small bowel biopsy specimens, or by demonstrating the presence of characteristic bacilli on electron microscopy of other clinically involved tissues, or both.

The majority of patients with Whipple's disease respond, at least initially, to antibiotics. Whipple bacilli disappear from involved tissues following successful treatment with antibiotics. Prior to the antibiotic era, Whipple's disease was uniformly fatal. Treatment with adrenocorticotropic hormone, steroids, and radiation was not successful. In 1952 the first report of antibiotic usage in Whipple's disease was published. Since that time patients have been shown to respond to a number of antibiotics, including tetracycline (TCN), doxycycline, chloramphenicol, penicillin (PCN), ampicillin, streptomycin (STM), and trimethoprim-sulfamethoxazole (TMP/SMZ).[2] Although antibiotics are the treatment of choice for Whipple's disease, it has become increasingly evident that, in a certain number of cases, they are far from curative. This is evidenced by the alarmingly high number of patients who, following apparently successful treatment, have had a clinical relapse manifested by either a recurrence of their initial symptoms or the development of new symptoms in another organ system. Many of these relapses are neurologic, and the neurologic relapses are usually irreversible. The initial choice of antibiotic regimen may therefore be crucial to a successful long-term outcome.

PAST APPROACHES TO TREATMENT

Standard textbook recommendations for antibiotic treatment of Whipple's disease include three different regimens: oral tetracycline for 1 year, penicillin for 2 to 4 months, or parenteral penicillin and streptomycin for 10 days to 2 weeks followed by oral tetracycline for 1 year. Recently, we conducted a retrospective study of patients with treated Whipple's disease in an attempt to determine the optimal antibiotic regimen.[3] Long-term follow up was obtained in 88 treated patients. Thirty-one of these patients relapsed (Table 1). Eighteen of the 31 patients had non-CNS relapses, usually a recurrence of their original clinical, arthralgia, gastrointestinal, or cardiac symptomatology. Thirteen of the 31 patients had a CNS relapse, the clinical features of which are outlined in Table 2. Of the 49 patients who had been treated originally with tetracycline alone, 21 relapsed and nine of the relapses involved the CNS. The eight patients treated originally with penicillin alone had three relapses, two of which in-

TABLE 1 Initial Antibiotic Regimen and Relapse Data

Antibiotic(s)	No. of Patients	Total No. of Relapses	CNS Relapses
TCN* alone totals	49	21	9
All other regimens			
PCN + STM + TCN*	15	2	0
PCN/PCN*	8	3	2
PCN + STM	5	2	0
TMP/SMZ*	3	0	0
Other	8	3	2
Totals	39	10	4

* Oral therapy

CNS = central nervous system; TCN = tetracycline; PCN = penicillin; STM = streptomycin; TMP/SMZ = trimethoprim-sulfamethoxazole;

Modified from Keinath, et al: Antibiotic treatment and relapse in Whipple's disease. Gastroenterology 1985; 88:1867-1873.

volved the CNS. There were no CNS relapses following treatment with parenteral PCN and STM followed by oral TCN, PCN/STM alone, or with oral TMP/SMZ alone (see Table 1).

In view of these considerations, we believe that neither TCN given alone nor PCN given alone represents adequate treatment. Both TCN and PCN fail to cross the blood-brain barrier effectively in the absence of meningeal inflammation. Central nervous system Whipple's disease rarely results in evidence of meningeal inflammation. Therefore, the CNS may be a reservoir of Whipple bacilli that are not exposed to bactericidal concentrations of antibiotics in patients who are treated with TCN and PCN. We suspect that all patients with Whipple's disease have CNS involvement, even in the absence of evidence of meningeal inflammation and in the absence of clinically apparent neurologic symptoms.

RECOMMENDED TREATMENT

We recommend treatment with TMP/SMZ as the initial therapy for all patients with Whipple's disease. The agent penetrates the blood-brain barrier well. Indeed, two patients who presented with CNS Whipple's disease have responded to treatment with TMP/SMZ.[2] One double-strength tablet should be given twice daily for 1 year. If the patient is severely ill the double-strength tablet may be given 3 times per day for 2 weeks, and then given twice daily for 1 year. Folic acid deficiency is a potential complication of such therapy, especially in a malnourished individual. Folinic acid, 3 mg per day, should prevent this complication, and it should be administered routinely when patients are given 3 double-strength tablets on a daily basis.

Central nervous system relapses were not found in patients who had been treated with parenteral PCN and STM, with or without subsequent administration of oral TCN. Thus, one could argue that treatment with parenteral PCN and STM for 10 to 14 days, followed by oral TCN, is effective. However, patients so treated do not receive antibiotics that cross the blood-brain barrier. A reasonable alternative would be to treat with parenteral PCN (1.2 million units) plus streptomycin (1.0 g) daily for 10 to 14 days, followed by 1 year of TMP/SMZ (1 double-strength tablet twice a day). This regimen may be especially applicable to patients initially too ill to receive oral medications. In the patient allergic to sulfonamides, we recommend treatment with parenteral PCN and STM for 10 to 14 days, followed by oral PCN (penicillin VK, 250 mg 4 times per day) for 1 year.

TREATMENT OF RELAPSE

Once therapy is initiated and the patient improves clinically, there is no need for routine invasive diagnostic studies, such as an annual intestinal biopsy. The patient's progress may be monitored by routine clinical and laboratory procedures. If the patient clinically improves and his laboratory tests (hemoglobin, albumin, etc.) return to normal, a repeat small bowel biopsy is not necessary. It has been shown that PAS-positive macrophages in the lamina propria of the small bowel may persist for years in the clinically well patient, and we do not recommend monitoring their presence as a guide to therapy.

Relapses may be manifested by a recurrence of the patient's original symptoms or by the development of clinical symptoms in a previously uninvolved system. In our review of 88 patients we found that all cardiac and CNS relapses occurred at least 24 months after diagnosis. The clinical, arthralgia, and gastrointestinal relapses were more likely to occur less than 24 months after diagnosis. If relapse of any clinical type is suspected, a small bowel biopsy should be obtained and examined for presence of free bacilli using electron microscopy. Further, biopsy of other tissues should be seriously considered if clinical data indicate that they may be involved. This may include brain biopsy at sites in the brain indicated by the presence of computed tomography or magnetic resonance imaging scanning abnormalities. A lumbar puncture with examination of the cerebrospinal fluid for PAS-positive macrophages should be performed if CNS disease is sus-

TABLE 2 Neurologic Features of Central Nervous System Relapse

Feature	No. of Patients*
Dementia	11
Ataxia	8
Hypothalamic signs	5
Ophthalmoplegia	5
Seizures	3
Hemiparesis	2
Vertigo	1
Nystagmus	1
Psychosis	1

* Many patients had multiple neurologic features.

Modified from Keinath et al: Antibiotic treatment and relapse in Whipple's disease. Gastroenterology 1985; 88:1867-1873.

pected. Presence of free Whipple bacilli in any tissue clearly establishes relapse. If clinical evidence of relapse is strong, and especially if there is development of CNS symptoms and signs, treatment should be given in the absence of biopsy proof of relapse. The treatment of non-CNS relapse is usually effective regardless of the antibiotic chosen. In our review, we found that 19 of 20 patients with non-CNS relapse had an excellent response to a variety of antibiotics.[3] In contrast, the response of CNS relapse to antibiotic therapy was poor in ten of the 11 patients in whom data were available. One patient responded to oral TMP/SMZ after failing to respond to a variety of other antibiotics.

The treatment of relapse is the same as that outlined above for initial therapy. If the patient with CNS relapse fails to respond to TMP/SMZ, we recommend treatment with oral chloramphenicol, 1 g per day (250 mg 4 times a day) for 6 to 12 months. Chloramphenicol, like TMP/SMZ, results in relatively high CNS concentrations of the drug. Failure of the patient wtih non-CNS relapse to respond to TMP/SMZ may require trials of oral penicillin (PEN VK, 250 mg 4 times daily) or of oral tetracycline (250 mg 4 times daily).

Because patients with Whipple's disease may be severely malnourished, folate, vitamin B_{12}, vitamin K, iron, and other dietary supplements may be beneficial. Only time will tell whether initial treatment with TMP/SMZ will lower the incidence of late CNS complications in Whipple's disease. We believe that such treatment will decrease the rate of devastating CNS relapses.

This chapter was supported by funding from the Veterans Administration.

REFERENCES

1. Maizel H, Ruffin JM, Dobbins WO III. Whipple's disease. A review of 19 patients from one hospital and a review of the literature since 1950. Medicine 1970; 49:175–205.
2. Ryser RJ, Locksley RM, Eng SC, Dobbins WO III, Schoenknecht F, Rubin CE. Reversal of the dementia associated with Whipple's disease by antibiotics which penetrate the blood-brain barrier. Gastroenterology 1984; 86:745–752.
3. Keinath RD, Merrell DE, Vlietstra R, Dobbins WO III. Antibiotic treatment and relapse in Whipple's disease: long-term follow-up of 88 patients. Gastroenterology 1985; 88:1867–1873.

CELIAC SPRUE AND RELATED DISEASES

ADRIAN P. DOUGLAS, M.D., M.R.C.P.

The diseases covered in this chapter include gluten-sensitive enteropathy, so-called refractory or nonresponsive sprue syndromes, and lymphoma of the small intestine. These are characterized by abnormalities of small intestinal function, resulting in malabsorption, and by histologic abnormalities of the mucosa of the duodenum and jejunum. An additional feature may be partial or total improvement when gluten is excluded from the diet.

The definition of the role of dietary gluten exclusion in the management of children with celiac disease by Dicke in 1950 not only revolutionized treatment but also spawned intensive research into the etiopathogenesis of the disease. The exact chemical nature of the toxic fraction of gliadin remains undefined, as does the precise mechanism by which the intestinal mucosa is damaged. There are two major hypotheses for the latter. The first suggests that mucosal damage results from the direct toxic effect of a peptide which remains undigested by the celiac patient because of the inherent deficiency of a mucosal peptidase enzyme. The second hypothesis assumes that the damage is the result of immunologic reaction to the gliadin protein or a fraction thereof. Recently a third hypothesis has been advanced which postulates that the toxic moiety reacts with cell membrane glycoproteins as a lectin and thereby damages the function of the cells. It is now well recognized that the sensitivity to gluten varies among patients with the same characteristic mucosal abnormalities and may also differ in the same patient at different times of his life.

The essential diagnostic test is biopsy of the mucosa of the upper small intestine and demonstration of the characteristic lesion comprising loss of villi, flattening of the surface epithelial cells, crypt hyperplasia, and increased density of chronic inflammatory cells within the lamina propria.

GLUTEN-SENSITIVE ENTEROPATHY

Dietary Treatment

The gluten-free diet is the cornerstone of treatment and may be the only therapy necessary in upward of 70 percent of all patients with celiac disease. There is no way of predicting which patients are gluten-sensitive, but because of the serious and long-term commitment which may be necessary, I believe it is always essential to demonstrate histologic abnormality before embarking on this therapy. This is particularly important when one appreciates that many nonceliac causes of diarrhea and/or malabsorption may show an apparent initial clinical response to a gluten-free diet. The reason for this is uncertain but may represent a response to the elimination of a complex protein which is perhaps difficult to assimilate and digest. (Gluten is named for its glue-like and stickily tenacious nature which holds dough together when bread is being manufactured and which, when absent, results in the friable character of gluten-free breads.) A gluten-free diet represents a lifetime commitment for the patient. Because of the potential inconveniences to the other members of the family and those that may arise when the patient eats away from home, a precise pretreatment diagnosis is essential. Furthermore, not all malabsorption is due to celiac disease and other more precise therapeutic approaches may be necessary.

The patients who do respond to the introduction of a gluten-free diet improve rapidly. Such patients will feel better, lose their diarrhea, and begin to gain weight within 2 to 3 weeks. If they are anemic, a reticulocyte response to the dietary-induced improvement in absorptive function will occur by 4 weeks and steatorrhea will resolve within a couple of months. To confirm the diagnosis a repeat intestinal biopsy should be done after some 3 to 6 months of demonstrated clinical improvement. Some histologic improvement should be seen if there has been a true response to gluten withdrawal. At the very least the surface epithelial cells will be seen to have increased in height and to have assumed the normal columnar appearance. The reappearance of villi may take more than a year, and, in adults over the age of 45 to 50 years, true villi may never reappear.

In children there are many diseases which produce the same histologic lesion as seen in celiac disease and which result in transient gluten intolerance. Thus the resolution of clinical symptoms and histologic abnormality with a gluten-free diet is not sufficient to justify a lifelong interdiction of wheat products in children. For this reason it is recommended that gluten be reintroduced, preferably as a dose of gluten powder daily for a week, in an attempt to produce a relapse before confirming the diagnosis. Following this challenge, an additional intestinal biopsy should be done, since, just as the initial symptoms may be subtle, definition of a relapse requires demonstration of histologic abnormality which may precede clinical symptoms. In adults, by contrast, gluten challenge is rarely necessary and probably inadvisable. I have seen patients with a satisfactory clinical and histologic response to gluten withdrawal relapse after inadvertent reintroduction of gluten and then remain unresponsive to subsequent gluten withdrawal even to the point of death.

The essence of a gluten-free diet is very simple to describe. I point out to my patients and their relatives* that they can eat all the meat and potatoes and green vegetables and salads and rice and corn and (eventually) dairy products that they wish. They must eschew only foods containing flour made from wheat, barley, and rye. The jury is still out on the question of the toxicity of oat gluten. Certainly there are some celiacs who apparently relapse when exposed to oats, whereas others are able to tolerate that cereal with impunity. For this reason I generally recommend that oats also be avoided.

Milk and dairy products are permitted, but a word of caution must be provided for the newly diagnosed celiac. In these patients the severe mucosal damage often produces a degree of secondary lactase deficiency, so that diarrhea may be perpetuated or even exacerbated if too much milk is included in the diet initially.

TABLE 1 Gluten-containing and Gluten-free Items

Gluten-containing	Gluten-free
Wheat	Rice
Rye	Potato
Barley	Corn
Oat	Rice flour
Wheat flour	Rice polish
Enriched wheat flour	Corn flour
Wheat starch	Corn meal
Cake meal	Corn starch
Rye flour	Corn syrup
Oat flour	Potato flour
Rolled oats	Potato starch
Flour (unbleached)	Yeast
Graham	Hydrolyzed yeast protein
Malt	
Malted milk	Baking soda
Hydrolyzed vegetable protein*	Baking powder
	Tapioca
Hydrolyzed plant protein*	Arrowroot
	Agar-agar
Starch*	
Modified starch*	
Cereal*	
Millet*	

* Most likely contain gluten. Write to manufacturer for definite information.
Note: These are items likely to be mentioned in lists of ingredients. It is most important to read all labels.

Having written that the gluten-free diet is essentially simple, I must also acknowledge that there are major difficulties in applying the general principles to the standard Western diet. This diet contains a large proportion of processed foods, and wheat glutens are added to many canned, frozen, and convenience-type foods. Even dry cereals whose principal ingredient is rice or corn may contain wheat or barley, so adherence to the diet requires a major interest in the manufacturers' labeling of product ingredients. A listing of such potential "pitfall" foods is given in Table 1. It goes almost without saying that the diet is easiest in the home, where all-natural foods can be eaten and special flour used for baking bread and cooking. Difficulty arises most often in restaurants, as flour is so commonly used in many varied ways. Table 1 lists those food items that contain gluten and those that are gluten-free. Table 2 lists some foods that can be eaten and some that must be avoided. I have these lists available to give to my patients when they first begin the diet. I believe that the physician who treats celiac patients should have a good understanding of the dietary principles involved so as to be able to introduce the subject to the patient and help answer initial questions. A knowledgeable dietitian is a great help, and most hospital dietary depart-

---

* I mention relatives to make the point that it is often easiest for the newly diagnosed patient to adjust to a gluten-free diet when everyone in the home adheres to that same dietary restriction. This is true not only for the child with celiac disease but also for the adult, and it is probably no major hardship for the rest of the family to apply the same restrictions to themselves; it certainly will make food preparation easier when there is only one menu to be followed by the cook.

TABLE 2 Some Representative Allowed and Forbidden Foods

Allowed	Forbidden
Decaffeinated coffee, fruit juices, lemonade, coffee, tea, cocoa	Postum, Ovaltine, malted drinks, beer, ale
All meat, fish, and poultry that is not breaded, creamed, or served with thickened gravy	Bologna, canned meat and meat analogues, liverwurst, meat loaf made with bread crumbs

ments can advise on this subject. The close involvement of a relative in the early instruction sessions is extremely helpful. There are many useful and inexpensive books which contain instructions and gluten-free recipes, and there are a number of manufacturers who specialize in gluten-free products and who have helpful customer relation departments (Table 3).

The key to compliance with a gluten-free diet clearly is education about the underlying principles. In practice it is often extremely difficult to achieve complete elimination of gluten products even with the aid of a research dietitian doing home visits. A celiac patient must be both intelligent and obsessive to succeed in avoiding gluten completely. In teenagers the strong need for peer identification may often make total compliance difficult to achieve, and they are especially liable to stray from the pursuit of perfection. In these patients, particularly, the physician must often seek a reasonable balance between the requirements for dietary perfection and the needs of everyday living. Compromise, to maintain a good patient-physician relationship, is often necessary with adolescents. Communication and follow-up can thus be maintained and any complications that may develop in the future can be rapidly identified and treated with additional reinforcement of the need for strictness in the diet. It must be emphasized that the need for a gluten-free diet in the celiac is lifelong. Although the older pediatric literature is uniform in stating that a gluten-free diet, either by name or in essence, does not need to be maintained after puberty, this is no longer believed to be true. A celiac is always a celiac, and a gluten-free diet is the best permanent treatment for these patients. No vitamin supplements are necessary, and, as time passes, the occasional dietary relapse does not seem to be followed by clinical relapse or, as far as we know, by long-term mucosal damage.

Symptomatic Therapy

It is perhaps heretical to suggest that strict adherence to a gluten-free diet is not always necessary or practicable. In the elderly celiac the histologic response to complete interdiction of gluten may be minimal and clinically it may be unclear that any real improvement has occurred for a long time, if ever. For this reason I believe that a symptomatic approach to therapy is often most appropriate in the celiac patient first diagnosed after the age of 65 and in the patient who does not show a good clinical response to a gluten-free diet after about 6 months (after careful evaluation to confirm that a strict gluten-free diet has been followed).

One potential problem with the approach that I am suggesting is related to the propensity that patients with celiac disease have for developing lymphoma. Many gastroenterologists have a "gut feeling" that perhaps patients on a strict gluten-free diet may be less likely to develop lymphoma than those who are under no dietary restriction. There is no good evidence to support this view, and in its absence I believe that in some circumstances it is most appropriate to be somewhat lenient with regard to dietary restriction.

By symptomatic therapy I mean vitamin supplements with vitamins A and D and folic acid and the provision of appropriate iron- and calcium-containing compounds. I do not believe that these should be used in most patients at the onset of therapy with a gluten-free diet, since improvement in hematologic and biochemical parameters are common and are a useful yardstick for responsiveness. The severely ill patient, however, whose celiac disease is not recognized until there is diarrhea-induced dehydration and hypokalemia, abnormalities of coagulation due to vitamin K deficiency, or hypocalcemia or hypomagnesemia, will need appropriate correction. Rarely is anemia so profound that transfusion is necessary, but if this is so then it is essential to take appropriate samples for measurements of serum hematinic levels before transfusing blood. I do not give supplemental vitamin D and calcium to the patient who is on, and responding to, a gluten-free diet. In most parts of the United States, as distinct from overclouded Britain, sufficient sunlight is available to make vitamin D therapy unnecessary even in the nonresponsive patient. In addition to these measures, symptomatic therapy may also require use of low-fat diets and easily assimilable foods, such as medium chain triglycerides and predigested enteral nutrition products. For those patients in whom diarrhea remains a problem appropriate antidiarrheal agents may be necessary. Vitamin B-complex deficiency (with the exception of folic acid) is

TABLE 3 Suppliers of Gluten-free Products*

Anglo-Dietetics Ltd., 641 Lancaster Pike, Frazer, PA 19335
Chicago Dietetic Supply, Inc., 405 Shawmut Avenue, La Grange, IL 60525
El Molino Mills, 345 N. Baldwin Park Blvd., City of Industry, CA 91746
Ener-G Foods, Inc., P.O. Box 24723, Seattle, WA 98124
General Mills Chemicals, Inc., 4620 W. 77th Street, Minneapolis, MN 55435
Giusto's Specialty Foods, Inc., San Francisco, CA 94080
Shiloh Farms, P.O. Box 97, Sulphur Springs, AK 72768
Vita Wheat Baked Products, Inc., 1839 Hilton Road, Ferndale, MI 48220
Walnut Acres, Penns Creek, PA 17862
White Oaks Farm, 13 Lake Street, Sherborn, MA 01770

* Health food stores remain the best source of specialized gluten-free items.

very rare and the provision of these vitamins is unnecessary, since they are readily absorbed from the usual dietary sources.

UNRESPONSIVE MALABSORPTION SYNDROMES

Nonresponse is rare, if it in fact exists, in childhood celiac disease but is a well-recognized feature of some adult patients. Some workers have even suggested that the nonresponsive group consists of patients with a different disease or diseases such as collagenous sprue and unclassified or "refractory" sprue. While I do not deny this concept, there are well-documented examples of patients who have changed from responsiveness to nonresponsiveness during different periods of their lives. Furthermore, as mentioned earlier, it seems that the incidence of responsiveness among groups of celiac patients diminishes with increasing age at diagnosis (and presumably is related in some way to the duration of exposure to gluten).

By unresponsiveness I mean a continuation of malabsorption, either subclinical or overt, with failure of the intestinal mucosa to show histologic improvement. Diarrhea is not, of course, necessarily equated with malabsorption, and persistence of this symptom does not of itself imply unresponsiveness. When due to coexistent primary lactase deficiency it will often respond well to elimination of milk products from the diet, particularly in children. The most common cause of unresponsiveness is the continued ingestion, often inadvertent, of gluten. This possibility must be excluded by a careful dietary history which should include asking the patient to keep a diary of everything eaten over a 2-week period. If these measures do not reveal gluten ingestion it may be appropriate to admit the patient to hospital for careful dietary monitoring before concluding that the patient is truly unresponsive.

The incidence of unresponsiveness is about 20 percent of those initially diagnosed as having celiac disease. A very small proportion of these will have another cause of the mucosal lesion characteristic of celiac disease. Included among these are *tropical sprue*, which most often can be readily distinguished by the travel history and the clinical features in which distal small intestinal disease is more predominant than disease of the duodenum and proximal jejunum; and *lymphoma* whose clinical features are those of celiac disease only when the underlying cause of the lymphoma is celiac disease. Some patients become unresponsive as they develop singular or multiple small bowel ulcerations. Other causes of the mucosal lesion, such as intraluminal bacterial overgrowth in the *stagnant loop syndrome*, acid hypersecretion in the *Zollinger-Ellison* syndrome, and *eosinophilic enteritis*, may occasionally produce the clinical syndrome that characterizes celiac disease, but these are distinguished by diagnostic testing.

The simplest therapeutic approach to the unresponsive patient is by symptomatic therapy, as outlined above. In those who continue to lose weight, have a persistently low serum albumin, and perhaps severe steatorrhea and diarrhea, other approaches may be necessary. It has been known for many years that patients with adult celiac disease will respond clinically to oral corticosteroids and that a histologic response identical to that after gluten withdrawal can be produced by prednisolone. A gluten-free diet when the patient is receiving corticosteroids is not absolutely necessary but is probably desirable. (I have seen patients who were receiving 10 to 15 mg of prednisone daily for other reasons and who had a flat jejunal mucosa respond to a gluten-free diet.) The indication par excellence for steroid therapy is a low serum albumin level, which is usually due to protein loss from the intestine. A persistently low serum albumin level is a serious prognostic feature and in patients dying of unresponsive celiac disease appears to be the one common denominator. The usual practice is to commence therapy with 40 mg of prednisone (or equivalent) per day and reduce this gradually to the smallest dose compatible with a normal serum albumin. Usually the maintenance dose is between 10 and 15 mg of prednisone. A few patients may eventually be weaned off steroids. A small group of patients do not respond to a combination of a gluten-free diet and corticosteroids, and continue to lose weight and have a persistently low serum albumin level. Some will eventually die of inanition or superimposed infection. In these unresponsive patients a trial of other immunosuppressant drugs, such as cyclophosphamide or azathioprine, may be worthwhile, since there are isolated reports of their being beneficial: I have never had success with these agents, however. Total parenteral nutrition is a modality worth trying in this small group of patients using a central venous catheter and appropriate solutions of glucose, amino acids, and fat.

If there is an immune basis to the mucosal lesion, the unresponsiveness persisting after removal of gluten from the diet may be due to continued antigenic stimulation within the intestinal lumen. Bacterial flora are a possible source of such antigenic stimulation and it seems logical to treat these patients with broad-spectrum antibiotics. This approach has been successful in alpha-chain disease ("Mediterranean" lymphoma). Although I tried this in one patient with unresponsive celiac disease without success, there are some reports of improvement with antibiotic therapy. Pancreatic insufficiency also has been documented in a few unresponsive patients with celiac sprue.

LYMPHOMAS

Extranodal lymphoma arises in the small bowel in an estimated 10 percent of patients with celiac sprue. The majority of these are non-Hodgkin's lymphomas, most often a histiocytic lymphoma or reticulum cell sarcoma, and the usual symptoms are caused by bowel obstruction, although ulceration with bleeding and perforation may also occur. In such patients, with diffuse involvement of the small intestine, the mucosa adjacent to malignant tissue may be histologically indistinguishable from untreated celiac disease. As indicated earlier, however, the patient does not have symptoms of malabsorption or the other subtle features of celiac disease except when the lymphoma has arisen in the setting of preexisting celiac disease. There is clear evidence that the incidence of lymphoma (and also of malignancies involving embryologic foregut derived structures, particularly the esophagus) is increased in individuals with celiac disease. For this reason lymphomatous change has to be considered in the differential diagnosis of the unresponsive or relapsing celiac patient. Some patients with celiac sprue and apparently benign small bowel ulcerations are found at surgery to have lymphoma. Abdominal lymphadenopathy, as determined by CT scanning, may be difficult to evaluate in the celiac patient because this may, at times, occur in untreated actual celiac disease.

A particular variety of diffuse intestinal lymphoma has been described in patients from North and South Africa and Iran which is distinct from the "Western" variety described above. This "Mediterranean" lymphoma does not arise in the setting of celiac disease, primarily involves the upper small intestine, and is associated with the appearance of a plasma paraprotein which is the heavy-chain of immunoglobulin A. It may produce a celiac-like histologic lesion and often is associated with diarrhea, weight loss, steatorrhea, and abnormal xylose and Schilling tests, as well as with the more usual manifestations of diffuse lymphoma.

The treatment of small intestinal lymphoma requires surgical resection when the disease is confined to the bowel wall. When regional lymph nodes are involved, combination chemotherapy is required in addition to surgical resection. Unresectable and extensive disease is treated with both chemotherapy and radiation therapy. The combination of cyclophosphamide, Adriamycin, vincristine, and prednisone has been used for these diffuse intestinal lymphomas. Vincristine should be used with caution, since an acute paralytic ileus has been associated with its use. The prognosis in these instances is poor because the tumor is usually undifferentiated and the occult nature of the clinical presentation makes late diagnosis the rule rather than the exception.

PARASITES OF THE SMALL INTESTINE

THOMAS C. QUINN, M.D.

A wide variety of parasites are known to infect the small intestine of man. Over 2 billion people worldwide are estimated to be infected with small intestinal protozoans and helminths. In the United States increasing numbers of small intestinal parasitic infections are now being seen in specialized groups. These include inhabitants of major urban centers, rural areas in the Southeast and Southwest United States, homosexual men, travelers, and immigrant refugees from tropical countries. With this increasing incidence of parasitic infections, physicians must be aware of their associated clinical syndromes and specialized drug therapy. Many of these infections induce symptomatic disease and malabsorption syndromes, particularly if untreated. Several of these parasites, such as *Cryptosporidia* or *Isospora*, may result in a fatal diarrheal illness in immunocompromised individuals. Other small intestinal parasites cause few or no symptoms and are frequently diagnosed on routine stool examination. Treatment is now available for nearly all small intestinal parasitic infections except for several of the newly recognized organisms, such as *Cryptosporidia, Isospora*, and *Microsporidia*. The treatment of these infections requires careful follow-up examinations, since resistant infections, such as giardiasis, are increasing in frequency. This chapter will review the diagnosis and treatment of the protozoans, nematodes, and cestodes known to infect the small intestine of man (Table 1).

PROTOZOAN INFECTIONS

Giardiasis

Giardia lamblia is the leading protozoan cause of diarrhea in travelers and in water-borne outbreaks in the United States. Giardiasis is found throughout the world, with an average incidence of 7 percent worldwide and 4 to 7 percent in the United States. Giardiasis is frequently marked by persistent diarrhea and malabsorption, and is commonly found in areas with poor sanitation and among populations unable to maintain adequate personal hygiene. It has recently emerged as a major cause of diarrheal disease in homosexual men and patients with immunodeficiencies. Other outbreaks have occurred in nursery schools and in towns using contaminated water where water plant filtration systems have been defective. Individuals have also become infected by drinking water from contaminated streams and lakes where other mammals are known to be reservoirs for this infection.

Giardia lamblia is a multiflagellated protozoan with both a trophozoite and a cyst stage. Infection in man is initiated after ingestion of the cyst form. Excystation occurs within the stomach and upper gastrointestinal tract. The organism remains in the duodenum and upper jejunum where the alkaline pH is more favorable for survival. *Giardia* multiplies by longitudinal fission and the trophozoite firmly attaches to the intestinal epithelial surface by means of a powerful sucking disc. *Giardia* apparently incorporates the host's biliary lecithin into their membranes. As the trophozoites pass into the colon excystation occurs and the cysts are excreted from the body.

TABLE 1 Treatment of Small Intestinal Parasites

Parasite	Drug of Choice	Alternative Drugs
Protozoans		
Giardia lamblia	Metronidazole, 250 mg t.i.d. × 7 days	Quinacrine hydrochloride, 100 mg t.i.d. × 7 days
Cryptosporidia species	Immunocompetent: No drug treatment required	
	Immunosuppressed: No drug has been shown to be fully effective	Immunosuppressed: Spiromycin has been recommended, but no controlled trials
Isospora belli	As for *Cryptosporidia*	Immunosuppressed: Furazolidone has been recommended, but no controlled trials
Sarcocystis hominis	No treatment required	In severe cases, a trial of trimethoprim-sulfamethoxazole 160/800 mg q.i.d. × 10 days
Helminths		
Ascaris lumbricoides	Mebendazole, 100 mg b.i.d. × 3 days	Pyrantel pamoate, 11 mg/kg once (max 1 g) *or* Piperazine citrate, 75 mg/kg × 2 days
Hookworm (*Ancylostoma duodenale, Necator americanus*)	Mebendazole, 100 mg b.i.d. × 3 days	Pyrantel pamoate, 11 mg/kg once (max 1 g)
Strongyloides stercoralis	Thiabendazole, 25 mg/kg b.i.d. × 2 days	
Trichostrongylus species	Thiabendazole, 25 mg/kg b.i.d. × 2 days	Pyrantel pamoate, 11 mg/kg once (max 1 g)
Capillaria philippinensis	Mebendazole, 200 mg b.i.d. × 20 days	Thiabendazole, 25 mg/kg/d × 30 days
Anisakis species	Surgical removal	Thiabendazole, 25 mg/kg b.i.d. × 3 days
Cestodes		
Diphyllobothrium latum	Niclosamide, 4 tablets (2 g)	Praziquantel, 10–20 mg/kg once
Taenia species	Niclosamide, 4 tablets (2 g)	Praziquantel, 10–20 mg/kg once
Hymenolepis nana	Praziquantel, 15 mg/kg	Niclosamide, 4 tablets (2 g)

Cysts may remain viable and infectious in water for longer than 3 months.

Symptomatic disease varies widely in patients infected with *Giardia lamblia*. Symptomatic disease usually occurs 1 to 2 weeks after infection and is characterized by the sudden onset of watery, foul diarrhea, abdominal distention, flatulence, nausea, anorexia, and abdominal cramps. The stools are often malodorous, loose, and mixed with mucus. Blood and fecal leukocytes are rarely, if ever, present. This acute stage may last for 3 to 4 days and, if not treated, may progress to a chronic infection, which is associated with steatorrhea and malabsorption. For unknown reasons, many patients recover completely without treatment. Other persons who are infected fail to demonstrate any symptomatology. The parasite load detectable in these patients may be far less than that detected in symptomatic patients.

If the disease progresses to chronic infection, there may be periodic, brief episodes of loose bowels, stools may be yellowish and frothy, and are accompanied by increased abdominal distention and flatulence. Abdominal cramps are occasionally present, but anorexia, nausea, and midepigastric discomfort are more frequent complaints. Malabsorption studies are usually abnormal.

The diagnosis of giardiasis, which is based primarily on identification of the cyst or trophozoite on stool examination, is often difficult owing to variable cyst and trophozoite excretion. Some investigators claim that only 50 percent of cases can be confirmed by stool diagnosis, but others have shown that at least 90 percent of documented *Giardia* infections can be identified by two or three stool examinations on different days using a formalin-ether concentration. Duodenal intubation with aspiration of duodenal contents and duodenal biopsy may be useful in confirmation of the diagnosis. The Enterotest (Hedeco, Palo Alto, CA) is a gelatin capsule containing a string that can be used to sample the duodenal contents for *Giardia* trophozoites, thereby avoiding duodenal intubation and biopsy. Another diagnostic test is an enzyme linked immunoabsorbent assay for *Giardia* antigen in the stool. It is equally sensitive and specific for *Giardia* diagnosis as the above test and is far more applicable for larger epidemiologic studies.

All *Giardia* infections should be treated. Therapy for giardiasis consists of treatment with either metronidazole, 250 mg 3 times a day for 7 days, or quinacrine hydrochloride, 100 mg 3 times a day for 5 days. Either drug will result in elimination of the organism in 70 to 90 percent of cases. Other drugs effective against *Giardia* include furazolidone, tinadazole, and nimorazole, the latter two of which are not licensed in the United States. Furazolidone is recommended for children under the age of 5 and it is easy to give as a suspension. Pregnant women should receive therapy only if severely symptomatic, since the infection may be self-limited in many persons. For pregnant women paromomycin, 10 mg per kilogram of body weight 3 times a day for 1 week, is first recommended. If symptoms persist, metronidazole may be used in the second or third trimester. Metronidazole is not recommended for use during the first trimester because of teratogenicity.

As mentioned above, initial treatment may not succeed in 10 to 30 percent of cases. Hence, more than one course of treatment may occasionally be necessary, and close follow-up examination is required. Repeat treatment with metronidazole at a higher dosage, such as 500 or 750 mg 3 times a day, is recommended for more resistant cases. Examination of other family members and water supply should also be undertaken to rule out the possibility of reinfection rather than failure to respond to initial treatment. A post-*Giardia* lactose intolerance may also develop in patients from ethnic groups with a predisposition to lactose deficiency following apparent eradication of parasites with specific therapy.

Coccidian Parasites

The subclass of protozoal Sporozoa, Coccidia, contains a number of organisms that depend upon invasion of mucosal cells of the intestinal tract for completion of all or part of their life cycle. They are intracellular parasites with both sexual and asexual life cycles, and some require an intermediate host for a portion of the asexual cycle. The sexual cycle of all species usually occurs in the epithelial cells of the intestinal tract. *Toxoplasma gondii* has a nonobligatory two-host life cycle in which the organism undergoes sporogony in the intestinal mucosa of cats, and subsequently causes tissue infection within man. *Eimeria* infections of birds are of great economic importance because they induce inflammatory and destructive lesions in bird intestines, but infection of man has not been documented. *Cryptosporidia*, *Isospora*, and *Microsporidia* infect the small intestinal mucosa of man, leading to an illness characterized by diarrhea and malabsorption.

Cryptosporidia

Infection with *Cryptosporidia* has recently been recognized as a significant cause of morbidity and mortality, particularly in immunocompromised patients. *Cryptosporidia* have been known to cause diarrhea in a wide variety of animals, but human infection was not reported until 1976. Since then it has been described as causing a severe debilitating diarrheal disease frequently resulting in death, limited primarily to homosexual men with acquired immune deficiency syndrome (AIDS). Within the last 2 years, however, *Cryptosporidia* have also been shown to induce a self-limited intestinal infection in immunocompetent individuals who are exposed to infected animals or other persons known to be infected with *Cryptosporidia*.

The disease in normal, immunocompetent humans causes transient diarrhea with watery stools for a period of 2 weeks, associated with abdominal cramps, and occasionally fever and nausea. In the immunocompetent person, both the symptoms and shedding of oocysts stop spontaneously, but in the immunocompromised the infection becomes chronic and is associated with protracted watery diarrhea. Marked signs of malabsorption, fluid and electrolyte loss, and intermittent periods of severe diarrhea have characterized the infection in the immunocompromised.

Diagnosis is made by identifying the oocytes in the stool and by careful examination of small bowel biopsy specimens. The stool should be concentrated by sucrose flotation and the concentrate stained with a modified acid-fast stain for rapid identification of the oocytes. In diarrheal cases, the oocytes may be readily found in acid-fast stains of unconcentrated feces. Treatment of *cryptosporidia* in the immunocompetent requires only fluid replacement therapy, since this infection usually lasts only 2 weeks. In immunocompromised patients, such as those with AIDS, no specific effective therapy has been identified. In limited studies, spiromycin, an antiprotozoan drug, has been shown to ameliorate some of the symptoms in AIDS patients infected wtih *Cryptosporidia*, but further study on its effective eradication of the organism is required. Spiromycin is not available commerically and must be obtained by special permission from the Food and Drug Administration.

Isospora

Similar to *Cryptosporidia*, *Isospora* infect the intestinal mucosa of humans, leading to an illness characterized by diarrhea and malabsorption. One species, *I. belli*, has been reported as a cause of fatal diarrheal illness in immunocompromised patients. *I. hominis* infection has also been described in man, but this is probably identical to *Sarcocystis hominis*.

Isospora infection is acquired by contact with food or water contaminated by human feces, since it is apparently not a zoonosis. The major clinical signs and symptoms include watery diarrhea, abdominal cramps, nausea, vomiting, and signs of malabsorption, including weight loss and vitamin deficiencies. *I. belli* infection is usually self-limited in otherwise healthy individuals, resolving within 2 weeks. In the immunocompromised patient it follows course similar to that of *Cryptosporidia* infection, resulting in severe debilitation.

Diagnosis depends upon the identification of the oocytes on concentrated fecal material or on acid-fast stains of wet preps in severe diarrheal cases. No treatment is required for *Isospora* infections in the immunocompetent, but if symptoms are severe, treatment with antifolates, such as pyrimethamine, sulfadiazine, or furazolidone, has been recommended. Treatment of infections in immunocompromised patients is often unsatisfactory and the infection frequently results in death of the patient. As with *Cryptosporidia*, fluid and electrolyte replacement is the cornerstone of treatment of these infections in the immunocompromised patient.

Sarcocystis

Sarcocystis species are similar to *Toxoplasma* in that they have an asexual stage in the muscle of many mammals and a sexual stage in the mucosal epithelium of other mammals. The human intestinal infection is acquired by eating undercooked beef or pork that contains *Sarcocystis*. Identification of oocytes in the intestinal tract of patients with diarrhea and abdominal distress usually confirms the diagnosis. The infection is frequently confused with that caused by *Isospora* species and the illness is nearly identical to isosporiasis. Very little is known about the treatment of human infection with *Sarcocystis*, since the majority of these infections are considered accidental, zoonoic, and are usually asymptomatic. Treatment with antifolates has been recommended in symptomatic cases, but very little is known of their efficacy.

NEMATODES

Ascaris

Ascaris lumbricoides is known as the giant roundworm of man and it is indeed the largest of intestinal nematodes. *Ascaris* is the most common helminthic infection of man, with an estimated prevalence of 1 billion infections, 4 million in the United States. Adult worms are known to inhabit the lumen of the small intestine and to have a short life span of approximately 10 to 24 months. Eggs are excreted in the stool and gestate for 3 weeks or more in a moist environment. Following ingestion of eggs, the larvae hatch within the duodenum and pass into the venous circulation, where they migrate to the lungs and cross the pulmonary capillary beds. The larvae migrate up the respiratory bronchi and are swallowed to reach their final destination within the jejunum.

During the migratory phase of the larvae the nematodes may cause pneumonia characterized by marked eosinophilia, fever, cough, wheezing, and migratory pulmonary infiltrates (Löffler's syndrome). Intestinal symptoms may vary according to the quantity of worm burden. In heavy infections (between 500 and 2,000 worms), serious complications may occur including obstruction of pancreatic and bile ducts, appendicitis, intussusception, volvulus, intestinal perforation, and intestinal obstruction. *Ascaris* have also been shown to cause a modest degree of malabsorption of fat, protein, and carbohydrates. In rare cases, *Ascaris* may also migrate outside of the gastrointestinal tract when irritated by antibiotic therapy, fever, or other concurrent infections.

Diagnosis depends on the identification of the characteristic eggs present in the stool. Direct smear examination of the stool is sufficient for diagnosis because of the large quantity of eggs. Occasionally the worms can be seen as a filling defect on radiography of the small bowel. *Ascaris* infection should be treated with mebendazole, 100 mg orally twice a day for 3 days. In cases where intestinal or biliary obstruction is suspected secondary to *Ascaris*, piperazine citrate, 75 mg per kilogram daily for 2 days, is recommended. A third alternative drug is pyrantel pamoate, 11 mg per kilogram as a single dose. When mixed intestinal infections are present, *Ascaris* should be treated first, since noneffective drugs can sometimes induce migration of the worms within the intestine or extraintestinally.

Hookworm

Human infection with two species of hookworm, *Ancylostoma duodenale* and the *Necator americanus*, is estimated to affect one-quarter of the world's population. Hookworms reside predominantly in the upper small intestine attached to the mucosa by their strong buccal capsule. Human hookworms have a mean life span of approximately 5 years and the average daily blood loss secondary to hookworm ranges from 0.03 ml to 0.2 ml. Infection results from direct skin contact with the infectious filariform stage which may cause a pruritic cutaneous eruption. The larvae follow a migratory pattern similar to that of *Ascaris* and may cause an eosinophilic pneumonia.

Within the intestine, the clinical manifestations are directly proportional to the number of worms. The distinction between asymptomatic infection with relatively few worms and a disease produced by sizable worm burden is clinically important and can be roughly quantitated by fecal egg counts. Abdominal pain, diarrhea, and weight loss are noticed in heavy infections with hookworm. The chronic manifestations of hookworm disease include iron deficiency, anemia, and hypoalbuminemia. Direct fecal smear examination is adequate for diagnosis. Light hookworm infections require no treatment, whereas therapeutic intervention is required in moderate to heavy infection. Mebendazole is the drug of choice, administered as 100 mg orally twice a day for 3 days regardless of the patient's body weight. This regimen results in 95 percent cure rate and in 99.9 percent reduction of egg counts. The anemia secondary to hookworm infection should be corrected by iron administration. Alternatively, pyrantel pamoate, 11 mg per kilogram orally as a single dose, has also been shown to be adequate for treatment of hookworm.

Strongyloides

Strongyloides stercoralis is another common human intestinal nematode distributed widely in the tropics and subtropics. *Strongyloides* can survive and reproduce as parasitic forms in humans or as free living forms in the soil. Like hookworm, filariform larvae initially infect man via penetration of the skin that comes in contact with infected soil. The larvae are passed by the bloodstream to the lungs where they migrate through the alveolar space and are subsequently swallowed to their final habitat in the small intestine. Deposition of eggs begins approximately 28 days after initial infection. Larvae typically hatch within the mucosa and are passed in the feces. The larvae may molt and differentiate into free living adult males and females or metamorphose into filariform infectious forms. These filariform larvae may autoinfect man while they are passed in the feces, thus continuing the cycle.

Approximately one-third of the people with strongyloidiasis are asymptomatic. The skin and pulmonary symptoms resemble those encountered in hookworm disease described above. The more characteristic clinical features are those of the intestinal phase of strongyloidiasis. Burning or colicky abdominal pain, often epigastric, occurs and is associated with diarrhea and the passage of mucus. Some patients may complain of nausea, vomiting, and weight loss with evidence of malabsorption or a protein-losing enteropathy. Eosinophilia is a prominent feature of the infection. In debilitated immunosuppressed or steroid treated patients, massive autoinfection with widespread dissemination of larvae to extraintestinal organs, including the central nervous system, may occur. This hyperinfection is often associated with severe enterocolitis and gram-negative bacteremia which may occasionally lead to death.

Definitive diagnosis depends on the demonstration of *Strongyloides* larvae in feces or duodenal fluid or sputum. Frequently repeated examinations of purged stools may be necessary to exclude the diagnosis. Treatment consists of thiabendazole, 25 mg per kilogram twice a day orally for 2 days. Unfortunately, the drug is not always effective. Confirmation of effective therapy may be difficult, since worm burdens are often low before treatment and a partial reduction of worm numbers may make it almost impossible to detect any remaining parasites. One recent study suggests that up to one-third of patients may not be cured with a single course of thiabendazole and that patients should be reassessed 6 months after treatment. For disseminated strongyloidiasis, thiabendazole, 25 mg per kilogram twice daily for up to 1 week, should be given. Patients with intestinal obstruction may require intravenous fluids and suction plus intermittent administration of thiabendazole suspension via nasogastric tube. If possible, immunosuppressive agents should be eliminated or their dosage reduced at least temporarily.

Trichostrongylus

Trichostrongyloides are nematodes which are found to infect the mucosa of the duodenum and jejunum predominantly in inhabitants of Asia and Africa. Their life cycle is similar to that of *Ascaris*. Man is frequently infected because of ingestion of contaminated food or water. Most infections are asymptomatic, but heavy infections have been associated with ulceration and bleeding from the small intestine. Eosinophilia is frequently seen in heavy infections.

Diagnosis depends upon detection of the characteristic eggs, which are similar in appearance to hookworm eggs. Treatment consists of thiabendazole, 25 mg per kilogram twice a day for 2 days, or pyrantel pamoate, 11 mg per kilogram as a single dose.

Capillaria

Intestinal capillariasis is a chronic wasting disease of man caused by infection with the nematode *Capillaria philippinensis*. Infection is primarily limited to the inhabitants of the Philippines and Thailand, and may be seen in immigrants to the United States from these endemic areas. *Capillaria philippinensis* adults and larvae are found in the small intestine, especially the jejunum. The adults are partially embedded in the mucosa and small numbers are found free in the larynx, esophagus, stomach, colon, and rarely near the portal area of the liver. The initial symptom of borborygmus is followed by abdominal pain and diarrhea with numerous sprue-like stools daily. Infection is frequently associated with anorexia, malaise, nausea, and vomiting. In more advanced cases general muscle weakness, wasting, and hyporeflexia have been documented. A severe protein-losing enteropathy, malabsorption, hyperalbuminemia, hypocalcemia, and hypocholesteremia have also been documented. Death can occur after 2 to 4 months of illness without treatment.

Diagnosis is made by finding the adult worms or eggs in the feces. Treatment consists of replacement of fluid and electrolytes, a high-protein diet, and antihelminthic therapy. Mebendazole is the drug of choice at 200 mg daily for 20 days. Thiabendazole, 25 mg per kilogram daily for 1 month, continued on alternate days for up to 6 months, can also be used if mebendazole is not available.

Anisakis

Anisakiasis is an infection of the small intestine of man caused by ingestion of rare or poorly preserved marine fish, such as herring, cod, cuttlefish, mackerel, salmon, or whale. The larvae penetrate the mucosa of the stomach, small intestine, or colon, where they can induce an eosinophilic granulomatous tumor or sometimes cause perforation. Anisakiasis is seen frequently along the coasts of the Far East, Alaska, and the northern coastal areas of Europe. There are a few reports of inebriated fishermen eating their bait fish and getting acute anisakiasis. Signs and symptoms of anisakiasis vary depending on parasite location and the chronicity of infection. Most patients with anisakiasis develop gastric lesions, either acute or chronic. Acute lesions develop within 12 hours of eating infected fish or squid if the patient is complaining of nausea, vomiting, and epigastric pain. *Anisakis* larvae have also been identified in the stomach at gastroscopy; they cause a ring-like or serpiginous defect with a partially protruding larval worm which can be removed with biopsy forceps. An upper gastrointestinal series may show a characteristic 3-cm long serpiginous type of defect with a circular ring shape. Anisakiasis of the small bowel mimics appendicitis or regional enteritis, and the patient frequently undergoes laparotomy. Infection of the colon is rare.

Diagnosis is usually made by examining surgical specimens demonstrating a marked eosinophilic infiltrate. A leukocytosis with eosinophilia is often present. Serologic testing is not likely to be helpful, although IgG is elevated. Occasionally anisakiasis is diagnosed by identifying the larvae that are vomited or present in the biopsy specimens. Thiabendazole can be used for treatment in the rare patient in whom the diagnosis is suspected before surgery.

CESTODES (TAPEWORMS)

Tapeworms are highly prevalent in man and are cosmopolitan in distribution. These parasites also have complex life cycles in which they cause illness in man in either of two stages of their life cycle: the adult stage, which may cause signs and symptoms referable to the gastrointestinal tract where the adult tapeworms reside; or the larval stage, which may cause signs and symptoms secondary to enlarging larval cysts in various tissues of the mammalian host. Four tapeworms primarily cause gastrointestinal infections: *Taenia saginata*, *Taenia solium*, *Diphyllobothrium latum* and *Hymenolepis nana*. *T. solium* and *H. nana* may also infect man as an intermediate host, with survival of a larval form in tissue outside the gastrointestinal tract.

Diphyllobothrium

D. latum is referred to as the fish tapeworm. It has two intermediate hosts, a copepod crustacean and freshwater fish. The definitive hosts, which include man and fish-eating carnivores, become infected by ingesting the second stage larvae in undercooked fish. The adult tapeworm can measure 19 m and can have as many as 3,000 segments. It primarily inhabits the ileum and, less commonly, the jejunum. In North America, highly endemic foci have been found among Eskimos in Alaska and Canada. Endemic foci have also developed in the northern and central United States and in Canada, particularly in the small lakes of the Great Lakes region.

The adult tapeworms cause little damage of the mucosa and most carriers are asymptomatic. Often the infection is first recognized in asymptomatic patients as a result of stool examination carried out for other reasons. Occasionally patients report passing proglottids during defecation. Anemia is present in most infected people, since the tapeworm competes with the host for vitamin B_{12}. The anemia is thought to occur only if the tapeworm is located in the proximal part of the jejunum, but not if it is located more distally in the small bowel. Folate absorption by the host may also be diminished. Low levels of ascorbic acid, thiamine, and riboflavin have also been described. Approximately 40 percent of persons harboring the worm will have reduced serum vitamin B_{12} levels, but fewer than 2 percent will actually develop severe anemia. Neurologic findings, including weakness, numbness, parasthesias, and disturbances of motility and coordination, can also occur in the absence of hematologic abnormalities.

The diagnosis is made by finding the characteristic operculate eggs in the stool. Proglottids are occasionally passed in the feces, and their internal structure is diagnostic. Niclosamide is the treatment of choice, prepared as chewable tablets containing 0.5 g of the drug. The adult dosage is 4 tablets, 2 g; children weighing more than 34 kg are given 3 tablets; children weighing 11 to 34 kg receive 2 tablets. Niclosamide should be given in the morning on an empty stomach. The tablets must be chewed thoroughly and then swallowed with water. The patient may eat 2 hours later. The expected cure rate for *D. latum* infection with one course of treatment is 85 percent. Alternatively, praziquantel has also been shown to be effective. In three clinical trials, 96 percent of 246 patients infected with *D. latum* were cured after treatment with a single dose of 25 mg per kilogram of praziquantel. Antihelminthic therapy should be followed by administration of vitamin B_{12} and folic acid for anemia. Starting 3 weeks after treatment, stool should be examined for eggs three times at 3 week intervals.

Taeniasis

Taeniasis is an intestinal infection of humans caused by adult tapeworms of two species, *Taenia solium*, the pork tapeworm, and *Taenia saginata*, the beef tapeworm. Humans are the only definitive hosts of *T. saginata* and they acquire the infection by eating rare or poorly cooked infected beef. *Taenia solium* is very rare in the United States and is unique in that humans can be either the intermediate or the definitive host. When man ingests the eggs the cysticercal stage emerges, and the larvae penetrate the small bowel to disseminate in the bloodstream or lymphatics to various organs. When man ingests infected pork containing cysticerci, the larvae emerge and become adult tapeworms, which attach to the mucosa of the small intestine.

Symptoms due to *T. saginata* are minimal and consist of mild abdominal cramps and "hunger pains." Rarely, a large number of worms have caused intestinal or appendiceal obstruction. Intestinal symptoms with *T. solium* are similar to those of *T. saginata* or nonexistent. More prominent symptoms may occur, however, when man is infected with cysticercosis. Central nervous system involvement is commonly seen and manifested by headache, papilledema, hemiparesis, decreased vision, and seizures.

Diagnosis depends upon identification of the eggs or proglottids in stool. The treatment of *T. saginata* and *T. solium* infections is identical. The drug of choice is niclosamide, and praziquantel is the alternative choice, both at the recommended dosages given in the discussion on diphyllobothrium. Another drug is paromomycin, 1 g every 15 minutes for 4 doses for adults and 11 mg per kilogram every 15 minutes for 4 doses for children. This 1-day course of treatment commonly produces side effects of diarrhea, abdominal pain, nausea, and vomiting which can be reduced by giving the drug after meals.

In the treatment of *T. solium* infections precautions should be taken to prevent autoinfection or dissemination to others. In addition, treatment of *T. solium* has the potential for inducing cysticercosis. First, any drugs that induce vomiting should be avoided, since retrograde peristalsis may bring gravid proglottids into the gastroduodenal area, resulting in their subsequent digestion followed by egg hatching, penetration, and cysticercosis. Second, since niclosamide, praziquantel, and paromomycin kill the worm but do not kill the eggs released from disintegrating gravid segments, cysticercosis is theoretically possible following treatment. No cases of cysticercosis have been reported by this mechanism, however. As a precaution, many workers advise that in the treatment of *T. solium* an effective purge such as 15 to 30 g of magnesium or sodium sulfate should be given 2 hours after treatment to eliminate all mature segments before eggs can be released. The patient should be followed closely to ensure that prompt evacuation occurs. Follow-up examination of the stools for 3 to 4 months is recommended.

Hymenolepis

H. nana, the dwarf tapeworm, primarily infects humans, who are both the definitive and intermediate host for the parasite. *H. nana* is worldwide in distribution and children are more commonly affected than adults. Prevalence rates are highest under conditions of overcrowding and poor personal and environmental hygiene. Humans are the natural reservoir for the parasite, and transmission is generally directed from human to human by ingestion of eggs from feces of infected individuals.

The tapeworm resides in the small bowel of the intestine, and desquamation of epithelial cells and necrosis have been observed at the site of attachment. Small infections generally cause no significant mucosal damage and are either asymptomatic or cause vague abdominal complaints. Heavy infections are not uncommon, especially in children. These are associated with general symptoms of headache, dizziness, weakness and weight loss. Gastrointestinal symptoms of nausea, anorexia, epigastric pain, diarrhea, and vomiting may be present. Moderate eosinophilia in heavy infections has also been reported by several investigators.

Diagnosis is made by identifying the characteristic egg in the stool. The treatment of choice for *H. nana* is praziquantel, 15 mg per kilogram given once after a light breakfast. Of 286 persons, mainly children, treated with praziquantel, 88 percent were cured. Side effects, especially in children, are mild and transient. An alternative drug is niclosamide, given in the same doses as described in the section on *Diphylobothrium*. Paromomycin has also been used to eradicate *H. nana* infections but few studies have confirmed its effectiveness. It is given in a dosage of 45 mg per kilogram (maximum 4 g) once daily for 5 to 7 days and it has frequent but generally mild side effects. All patients should be reexamined several times over a 2- to 4-month period.

DETERMINATION OF CURE

Generally most intestinal parasitic infections are not 100 percent effectively treated with one course of treatment. Consequently, very careful follow-up with repeat stool examinations 1 or 2 months after treatment is required. Failure to respond to treatment may indicate drug resistance, poor compliance, reinfection, or infection with another parasite.

SHORT BOWEL SYNDROME

ELLIOT WESER, M.D., F.A.C.P.

The degree to which a patient has symptoms and disability after small bowel resection depends upon the site and extent of small intestine removed. Much can be done to improve the consequences of small bowel resection in the adult, particularly if more than 3 to 4 feet of residual small bowel remains and is in itself healthy tissue. Resection of mid small intestine or loss of jejunum is better tolerated than resection of either duodenum or ileum. Loss of the ileocecal valve adds to the detrimental effects of ileal resection. Most often, small bowel resection involves the terminal ileum, which is the specific site for active reabsorption of conjugated bile salts and active absorption of vitamin B_{12}. Thus, loss of this area results in malabsorption of these important compounds. Failure to reabsorb bile salts from the ileum results in increased amounts of bile salts entering the colon, where they are deconjugated and dehydroxylated by bacteria and partly reabsorbed by colonic mucosa. During this process they increase water and electrolyte secretion by activating the adenyl cyclase system and thus produce watery diarrhea, referred to as "choleretic diarrhea." More severe bile salt malabsorption results in a depletion of the circulating bile salt pool with a decrease in bile acid secretion in bile. This increases the lithogenicity of bile and the incidence of gallstone formation. In addition, small bowel luminal bile salt concentrations are decreased, resulting in reduced bile salt micelle formation and steatorrhea.

Bacterial action on unabsorbed fat in the colon will produce hydroxy fatty acids which also interfere with water and electrolyte absorption from the colon. Malabsorption of fat-soluble vitamins will increase with increasing steatorrhea. Also accompanying fat malabsorption are losses of calcium, magnesium, and zinc in the stool that may lead to deficiencies of these cations. The ileum and right colon are important sites for the conservation of electrolytes and water. Their removal tends to worsen diarrhea, dehydration, electrolyte losses, and hypovolemia; hence the importance of special attention to fluid and electrolyte balance in such patients. The large bowel is also a major site of absorption of soluble luminal oxalate usually derived from dietary sources. Normally, most of the oxalate eaten in food reacts with luminal calcium to form insoluble calcium oxalate which is not absorbed. Patients with steatorrhea bind luminal calcium with unabsorbed fatty acids and fats, allowing more oxalate to remain in soluble form and be absorbed from the colon. Increased absorption is followed by increased urinary excretion of oxalate, placing these patients at higher risk for developing calcium oxalate kidney stones. Severe malnutrition may also be accompanied by reduced pancreatic function, which can further contribute to malabsorption. Patients with short bowel may also not produce sufficient enteric hormones, such as secretin and cholecystokinin, which normally are synthesized in the small intestine and play an important role in pancreatic secretion. Finally, the residual small intestine has the capacity to undergo adaptive changes that may lead to improvement in function in many patients with varying lengths of small bowel resection. The management of patients with short bowel logically follows from an understanding of the pathophysiology.

GENERAL CONCEPTS

Treatment of short bowel syndrome involves both nutritional or dietary manipulation and the use of drugs or medications. Table 1 outlines those agents, which alone or in combination, may be necessary for successful management, depending on the extent of resection and severity of short bowel consequences. Most patients will require parenteral nutritional in the early postoperative period. Some may have been malnourished prior to surgery and should have parenteral nutrition started preoperatively.

Parenteral nutrition via a central line is accomplished by providing 2,000 to 3,000 Kcal per day using amino acids and glucose solutions. It is also necessary to provide Intralipid once or twice weekly. These calories are delivered in 2,000 to 3,000 ml of fluid daily with electrolytes adjusted to the patient's needs. There is a separate chapter on parenteral alimentation. In patients with less extensive resections, usually with much of the jejunum remaining, enteral feedings may be started (and tolerated) fairly rapidly, often in the first week following surgery. Parenteral nutrition should be continued, albeit reduced, until it is clear that the patient will tolerate enteral nutrients. Formula defined diets may be useful in implementing enteral feeding. They may be given orally, but because of their low fat content they are relatively unpalatable and may require administration via a small nasogastric feeding tube. In full strength these solutions are hyperosmolar and may cause diarrhea; therefore, they should be diluted to one-third strength and 600 to 700 ml given daily, if necessary by slow continuous 24-hour drip, with gradual increases in solution volume and strength over a 5- to 7-day period. Thereafter, a gradual increase in volume to 2,000 ml or more is usually well tolerated and provides 1 Kcal per milliliter. As it becomes clear that the patient can tolerate these enteral loads, parenter-

TABLE 1 Useful Agents in the Treatment of Short Bowel

Drugs

  Antidiarrheal drugs
    Codeine sulfate, 30–60 mg, up to 4 times daily
    Diphenoxylate hydrochloride and atropine, up to 20 mg daily in divided doses
    Loperamide hydrochloride, 4–16 mg daily in divided doses
    Deodorized tincture of opium, 10 drops 2–3 times daily
  Cholestyramine, 4–16 g daily (ileal resections less than 100 cm)
  Cimetidine, 300–600 mg 4 times daily
  Ranitidine, 150 mg twice daily
  Anticholinergic drugs (not usually used)
    Propantheline bromide, 15–30 mg intramuscularly
  Pancreatic enzyme supplements
    Pancrelipase (USP), 3–4 capsules with each meal (12–16 capsules daily)
    Pancrease (enteric coated microspheres of pancrelipase), 1–3 capsules with each meal
    Pancreatin, 3–4 tablets with each meal (12–16 tablets daily)
  Broad-spectrum antibiotics (in divided doses, 7–14 days)
    Tetracycline, 1 g daily
    Ampicillin, 2–4 g daily

Nutrients

  Fat-soluble vitamins
    Vitamin A, 25,000–50,000 IU daily. Larger doses may be necessary intermittently. If steatorrhea is present, may need water-miscible form, Aquasol A.
    Vitamin D, 30,000–50,000 USP daily—depends upon initial deficiency. Carefully determine maintenance dose—avoid hypercalcemia. If steatorrhea is present, may need water-miscible form, Drisdol in propylene glycol, 10 drops daily.
    Vitamin K (menadione, USP), 4–12 mg daily; vitamin K (Mephyton), 5–10 mg daily
  Water-soluble vitamins
    Vitamin B_{12}, 100–1,000 μg IM monthly (ileal resections)
    B-complex (containing daily requirements), 2–3 tablets daily or liquid equivalent
    Vitamin C, 500 mg daily
    Folic acid, 5–10 mg daily
  Mineral supplements
    Calcium gluconate, 3–15 g daily
    Magnesium sulfate, 1–6 g daily (may worsen diarrhea)
    Ferrous gluconate or sulfate, 1.8 g daily
    Zinc sulfate, 110–220 mg daily

al nutrition may be gradually decreased. The chapter on enteral feedings contains information on various commercial preparations.

All patients should be given a trial of solid foods with some degree of fat restriction. This certainly adds to the quality of life if solid foods are tolerated reasonably well.

RESECTION OF TERMINAL ILEUM

Vitamin B_{12}

All patients should be treated prophylactically with monthly intramuscular injections of vitamin B_{12} (100 μg). This is inexpensive and will prevent vitamin B_{12} deficiency over the ensuing years.

Bile Salt Malabsorption

The clinical difficulties with resection of the terminal ileum depend upon the extent of ileum removed. When less than 100 cm is removed and the remaining ileum is anastomosed to the colon, symptoms may be slight or transient, although some diarrhea is likely. These patients can still reabsorb some bile salts and increase hepatic bile acid synthesis, so there is only a minimal, if any, reduction in their circulating bile salt pool. However, enough bile salts can escape into the colon to cause choleretic diarrhea. Such patients have only minor degrees of steatorrhea and usually minimal problems with weight loss. Resins capable of binding bile salts have proved very helpful in managing these patients. Cholestyramine is usually given in a dose of 4 g with each meal and with a bedtime snack (16 g per day) and then titrated downward to the lowest effective dose. Some patients may do well on a single dose of cholestyramine taken with the morning meal, possibly because after an overnight fast, the gallbladder contains more bile acids with which the resin can bind. In patients with limited ileal resection and an ileostomy, choleretic diarrhea is obviously not a problem. Rarely, diarrhea worsens with cholestyramine. Under these circumstances aluminum hydroxide or bismuth-containing antacids may be tried as bile salt binding agents.

Patients with more extensive ileal resections (>100 cm) and ileocolic anastomoses lose a much greater quantity of bile salts, which results in a decrease in the bile salt pool, severe steatorrhea, weight loss, and loss of fat-soluble vitamins. The diarrhea is caused by reduced water and electrolyte absorption, as well as long chain unsaturated fatty acids which are hydroxylated by bowel bacteria and particularly irritate colonic mucosa. These patients generally do better on a limited fat diet below 40 g per day. It is usually impossible to reduce fat content below 20 g daily without using liquid formula diets. It may be helpful to give most of the fat with breakfast, since a full gallbladder may provide some bile salts necessary for the digestion of the fat. Since these patients generally have a reduced bile salt pool with lowered concentrations of bile salts in the intestinal lumen, treatment with cholestyramine does not help their diarrhea and may even make it worse. Spacing out meal ingestion to five or six feedings daily may also improve diarrheal losses. Sometimes a trial of either nonabsorbable or absorbable antibiotics is helpful in reducing diarrhea.

Depending upon the length of proximal ileum removed, digestion of fat may be aided by administering pancreatic extracts, 3 or 4 capsules with each meal. There also is some evidence that excessive gastric secretion may occur in patients with short bowel, particularly early in their course after starting oral feedings. The increase in volume and acid secretion may worsen diarrhea, and particularly steatorrhea, by lowering small bowel intraluminal pH, which results in reduced pancreatic enzyme function. Use of H_2 receptor blocking agents such as cimetidine or rantidine may be helpful and should be tried in doses adequate to reduce secretory volume or increase pH to permit improved pancreatic enzyme action (as judged by decreased steatorrhea).

Water and Electrolyte Balance

Water and electrolyte balance requires the utmost attention, particularly in the early adaptive phase following resection. Parenteral supplementation often is necessary until diarrhea is brought under better control. The use of potent antidiarrheal agents given in effective doses tailored for the individual patient can be most helpful. I have found that some patients do better on liquid codeine preparations; other preparations that can be used are loperamide (Imodium), diphenoxylate and atropine (Lomotil), or deodorized tincture of opium. The use of medium chain triglycerides as an oral supplement—in salads and cooking oil or spreads—provides additional calories and appears to improve fluid absorption, although the mechanism is unknown. Some patients have also successfully controlled their diarrhea by intramuscular injections of propantheline or other anticholinergics. Some patients with an ileostomy retain a portion of the colon. If necessary, this segment of retained colon can be used to help maintain fluid balance. Saline solutions with added potassium chloride have been used, either as a retention enema or as an infusion through a colonic mucous fistula.

Consequences of Steatorrhea

Along with steatorrhea, which may follow extensive ileal resections, malabsorption of fat-soluble vitamins and extensive losses of calcium, magnesium, and zinc may occur. Patients should have vitamin K status assessed by measuring the prothrombin time and should be treated appropriately with parenteral or enteral vitamin K preparations. To maintain or replace vitamin D losses, most patients are treated with oral doses. Water-soluble forms, such as Drisdol in prophylene glycol, 10 cc daily, may be preferable. Vitamin A can be measured in the blood and given when deemed appropriate. Aquasol A, 25,000 units per day is a water-miscible source of vitamin A. There are no good methods routinely available to measure vitamin E, although vitamin E deficiency rarely occurs and the early ocular neurologic defects are reversible.

Calcium Malabsorption

Unabsorbed fatty acids in the intestinal lumen will bind calcium and magnesium, resulting in excessive losses and depletion of these cations. The insolubility of these bound cations makes them unavailable to bind dietary oxalate, permitting increased absorption of soluble oxalate in the colon and subsequent hyperexcretion in the urine, with increased risk of renal stone formation. A low fat diet, avoidance of high oxalate foods (Table 2), and perhaps an increased calcium intake may help reduce the risk of hyperoxaluria. Occasionally, zinc and magnesium supplements may be required.

TABLE 2 High Oxalate Foods

Fruits
  Plums, strawberries, oranges, figs, Concord grapes, raspberries, gooseberries, cranberries, blackberries, red currants
Vegetables
  Spinach, beets, sweet and green peppers, carrots, celery, artichokes, green onions, parsley, okra, beet greens, endive, chards, sweet potatoes, yams, rhubarb, wax beans
Beverages and miscellaneous
  Tea, cocoa, Coca-Cola, chocolate

PROXIMAL SMALL BOWEL RESECTION

Patients with resection of proximal small bowel do fairly well over the long term, since the adaptive capacity of the ileum is remarkable and will eventually compensate for nutrient absorption. Immediately after surgery, patients will require careful parenteral support until enteral nutrition can be fully tolerated and adaptation occurs. Iron absorption may remain abnormal and require maintenance oral supplementation. Pancreatic function may also be decreased, since the major sites of cholecystokinin and secretin synthesis are lost with the removed intestine. Thus, long-term supplementation with pancreatic extracts may be required. Again, if gastric hypersecretion occurs, these patients may benefit from H_2 blockade.

MASSIVE BOWEL RESECTION

Although not commonly seen, massive bowel resection with only 50 to 80 cm of remaining proximal small bowel usually requires treatment with prolonged use of parenteral nutrition via a permanent central venous catheter under supervision of an experienced team. Rarely can such patients be managed by oral intake alone. With increasing technology, special vests containing infusion pump and solutions can be worn during the day, allowing the patient to carry out routine activities while the parenteral nutrient solution is infused. Over long periods of parenteral nutrient maintenance, care must be taken to avoid deficiencies of minerals (calcium, zinc, copper, cobalt) as well as vitamins and essential fatty acids. Some details are presented in the chapter on parenteral alimentation.

LACTOSE INTOLERANCE

With removal of substantial lengths of small bowel, the disaccharidases of the mucosa are also removed, and thus the ability to hydrolyze disaccharides, particularly lactose, may be impaired. This should be kept in mind in managing such patients, especially when diarrhea, excess gas, and cramping are troublesome. Trial of a lactose-free diet for several days will usually determine the degree to which lactose intolerance (lactase deficiency) contributes to the problem. Small amounts of milk may gradually be reintroduced into the patient's diet to see the extent of the intolerance or degree of recovery (as part of adaptive changes in remaining bowel). It has recently been shown that yogurt with active bacterial cultures contains lactase capable of autodigesting the yogurt lactose in a majority of subjects with lactose intolerance. This could be useful in patients with small bowel resection and might help provide needed calcium. In selected patients, the enzyme lactase (as LactAid) may be added to milk or taken with milk products (Lactrase) to help digest the lactose and ameliorate symptoms. Patients who remain on low-lactose or lactose-free diets also require calcium supplementation.

In summary, the management of patients with small bowel resection logically follows from an understanding of the pathophysiology of short bowel. Patient education is also important. Adherence to the treatment concepts outlined above will prove helpful to the patient and be gratifying to the physician.

HYPEROXALURIA AND NEPHROLITHIASIS

JOHN WHITBY DOBBINS, M.D.

Since the 1960s, patients with idiopathic inflammatory bowel disease have been noted to have an increased incidence of nephrolithiasis. The incidence of this condition has also increased since the advent of the jejuno-ileal bypass for obesity. The overall incidence of nephrolithiasis in inflammatory bowel disease is not great, probably only in the 2 to 3 percent range; however, prior surgical treatment increases the risk of nephrolithiasis. The incidence of nephrolithiasis in patients with Crohn's disease, who have undergone an ileal resection, is approximately 10 percent; the majority of stones, when analyzed, are composed of calcium oxalate. The incidence of nephrolithiasis in patients with ulcerative colitis who have undergone an ileostomy is also approximately 10 percent; however, in these patients uric-acid stones make up a significant proportion of the calculi. The incidence of nephrolithiasis in patients who have undergone jejuno-ileal bypass for obesity is the highest, the incidence being in the 20 percent or greater range.

URINARY CONSTITUENTS IN INTESTINAL DISEASE

Examination of the urine in patients with stone formation reveals a number of abnormalities (Table 1). The urine volume is low as is the sodium and chloride content. This indicates dehydration and extracellular volume deficit. The urine citrate, the pH, and the carbon dioxide content is low and the ammonia concentration is high. This is indicative of a metabolic acidosis, although, as will be discussed later, other factors control urinary citrate levels. Magnesium and pyrophosphate levels are also low. Magnesium, pyrophosphate, and citrate are considered inhibitors of calcium-oxalate stone formation because they either chelate the calcium or form stable complexes with the calcium or the oxalate. Urinary oxalate excretion is normal in patients who have undergone a total colectomy or who have had an ileostomy, whereas excretion is elevated in patients who have undergone an ileal resection, have either all or part of the colon in the alimentary stream, or have undergone a jejuno-ileal bypass for obesity. As a general rule, all of these urinary abnormalities, except for oxalate levels, are attributable to the malabsorption of water, electrolytes, and alkali thereby accounting for the acidosis and hypocitraturia. The increased absorption of oxalate is the sole exception and, as will be discussed, is primarily attributable to the increased absorption of dietary oxalate. In the following sections I will discuss how intestinal disease, resection, or bypass can result in the urinary abnormalities listed in Table 1.

ENTERIC HYPEROXALURIA

Oxalic acid is an organic acid composed of two molecules of carboxylic acid; it is a strong acid that is ionized at the physiologic pH. The calcium salt of oxalic acid is only slightly soluble in water. Oxalate is a metabolic end-product in man and serves no known purpose. Oxalate is excreted almost exclusively by the kidney.

In normal individuals, approximately one-half of urinary oxalate is derived from the endogenous catabolism and one-half from the absorption of oxalate in the diet. In a normal diet oxalate is present in many foods; however, less than 10 percent is absorbed. In hyperoxaluria resulting from intestinal disease, there is increased absorption of dietary oxalate; this is designated enteric hyperoxaluria. Hyperoxaluria can also result from increased endogenous production of oxalate (primary hyperoxaluria), or present as secondary to a number of conditions such as ethylene-glycol poisoning (where ethylene glycol is converted to oxalate), pyridoxine deficiency, or excessive intake of oxalate-containing foods (rhubarb "poisoning"). Primary hyperoxaluria and secondary or acquired hyperoxalurias, other than enteric hyperoxaluria, are rare.

The mechanism of enteric hyperoxaluria is twofold. First, when intestinal disease results in steatorrhea, there is an increased *solubility* of oxalate. Normally, dietary calcium binds to dietary oxalate, forming an insoluble precipitate which prevents oxalate from being absorbed—better to form the stone in the intestine than in the kidney. When intestinal disease, resection, or bypass surgery results in malabsorption of fat calcium will bind to fatty acids more avidly than to oxalate, thereby leaving oxalate in solution and allowing more to be absorbed. Second, when bile acids and fatty acids are not absorbed in the small intestine because of disease, resection, or bypass, and spill into the colon, the *permeability* of the colon to oxalate is increased. This increased permeability is probably the result of bile acids and fatty acids chelating calcium in the tight junctions, thus making them loose or more permeable to small molecules like oxalate.

Of interest is that patients who have had a total colectomy or an ileostomy do not exhibit increased absorption of dietary oxalate or hyperoxaluria (Table 1). This suggests that increased colonic permeability to oxalate is important in the genesis of enteric hyperoxaluria. Bile acids and fatty acids do *not* appear to increase the permeability of the small intestine to oxalate. Recent evidence suggests that oxalate can be actively transported by the colon. However, the clinical significance of these observations remains to be determined. It is known that dietary protein contributes to hyperoxaluria in patients who have had a jejuno-ileal bypass for obesity; however, this contribution is small at best. In these patients, dietary protein may be converted to oxalate by bacteria in the colon.

HYPOCITRATURIA

Profound hypocitraturia has been noted in patients who have had an intestinal resection and bypass. Hypocitraturia is multifactorial in origin. Acidosis is known to decrease urinary-citrate excretion, and patients with hypocitraturia develop a metabolic acidosis secon-

TABLE 1 Urinary Constituents Important in Stone Formation

Urinary Constituents	Small Bowel Resection or Bypass	Ileostomy
Volume	Normal or ↓	↓
pH	Normal or ↓	↓
NH_4	↑	↑
CO_2	↓	↓
Na,Cl	Normal or ↓	↓
K	↓	↓
Calcium	Normal or ↓	Normal
Mg	↓	↓
Pyrophosphate	↓	↓
Citrate	↓	↓
SO_4	↓	Normal
PO_4	↓	↓
Oxalate	↑	Normal
Urate	Normal	Normal

↓ value lower than normal
↑ value higher than normal

dary to bicarbonate loss in diarrheal stool. Urinary magnesium excretion has a profound effect on urinary-citrate excretion, and since hypomagnesuria is common in these patients, hypocitraturia is undoubtedly related to this problem. It was once thought that malabsorption of dietary citrate may play a role in hypocitraturia; however, removal of citrate from the diet has no effect on urinary citrate excretion in normal subjects; thus it appears that dietary citrate is unnecessary for the maintenance of a normal citrate excretion.

HYPOMAGNESURIA

The mechanism of normal magnesium absorption is not well understood; therefore, our understanding of the role of the intestine in hypomagnesuria associated with intestinal resection and bypass is limited. However, it is known that fatty acids and bile acids can precipitate magnesium and that some magnesium malabsorbtion probably occurs on this basis. It appears likely that when there is extensive resection or bypass that some magnesium is malabsorbed because of the loss of intestinal surface area. Some magnesium malabsorption may be obligatory simply because of the volume of diarrheal stool.

TREATMENT

Calcium Oxalate Nephrolithiasis

Increase Urine Volume. In general, the goal of

TABLE 2 Oxalate Content of Common Foods*

Oxalate Content	Foods	Serving Size	Serving Weight (g)	Oxalate Content	Foods	Serving Size	Serving Weight (g)
>100 mg/serving:	Beets	½ cup	83	10-20 mg/serving (continued):	Rutabagas	½ cup	100
	Chard	½ cup	90		Turnip greens	½ cup	90
	Rhubarb	½ cup	100		Blueberries	½ cup	120
	Spinach	½ cup	90		Blackberries	½ cup	70
	Cocoa	Tbsp.	7		Currants	½ cup	100
70-100 mg/serving:	Collard	½ cup	90		Strawberries	10 large	100
	Leeks	½ cup	90		Oranges	½ small	120
	Okra	8-9 pods	100		Fruit cake	1 slice	60
	Gooseberries, raw	⅔ cup	100		(WW) Allison's bread	1 slice	30
	Peanuts	½ cup	75	5-10 mg/serving:	Corn on the cob	1 small ear	100
40-70 mg/serving:	Raspberries	¾ cup	100		Mustard greens	½ cup	90
20-40 mg/serving:	Beans, green and wax	½ cup	62-100		Potato	1 small	100
					Parsnips	⅔ cup	100
	Carrots	⅔ cup	100		Parsley	1 Tbsp.	3.7
	Onion, fresh	½ cup	100		Tomato	½ cup	100
	Grapes	½ cup	100		Grapefruit	½ cup	100
	Squash, summer	½ cup	90		Prunes	5 large	50
	Chocolate	1 oz	28		Biscuits	1 small	30
10-20 mg/serving:	Beans, pinto	½ cup	100		Kidney	3 oz	90
	Eggplant	½ cup	100		Liver	3 oz	90
	Celery	½ cup	100		Sponge cake	1 slice	60
	Dandelion greens	½ cup	100		Orange peel	1 Tbsp.	4
	Fruit cocktail	½ cup	100		Lemon peel	1 Tbsp.	4
	Pepper, green	2 cups	100				

		Beverages					
Oxalate Content	Beverage		Serving Size (oz)	Oxalate Content	Beverage		Serving Size (oz)
10-20+ mg/serving:	Tea		8	0-5 mg/serving:	Apple juice		6
	Cola (Coke)		12		Grape juice		6
5-10+ mg/serving:	Coffee (ground)		8		Orange juice		6
	Coffee (instant)		8		Pineapple juice		6
	Ovaltine		8		Tomato juice		6
	Red Wine		6		White wine		6
					Milk		8

Foods With Little If Any Oxalate				
Apple	Cucumbers	Mango	Plums	Sugar, salt
Avocado	Grapefruit	Melons	Radishes	Turnip
Cauliflower	Grapes	Nectarines	Squash	Flavoring extracts
Cherries	Lime, lemon	Olives, pickles	Starches (except potato)	

* The following table presents dietary constituents according to oxalate content per average serving. Oxalate content was obtained from standard reference sources. Foods not listed have either less than 5 mg oxalate/serving *or* the oxalate content is uncertain. The standard serving is presented as both volume and weight. Foods containing more than 10 mg oxalate/serving should be avoided, and those containing 5 to 10 mg/serving used only sparingly. (From: Earnest DL. In: Bayless TM ed. Current therapy in gastroenterology and liver disease. Toronto: BC Decker 1984:176.)

therapy in nephrolithiasis should be to reverse all the urinary abnormalities that increase the likelihood of stone formation (Table 1). This can be difficult in a patient with an extensive ileal resection that results in the short bowel syndrome. Urine volume should be increased by increasing fluid intake and by decreasing diarrhea. Since most of the urinary abnormalities in Table 1 are attributable to diarrhea, considerable attention should be directed toward decreasing it. In general, diarrhea is treated by reducing the malabsorption of fat and carbohydrates as much as possible and by using antidiarrheal agents (codeine, loperamide, etc).

Low Oxalate Diet. If hyperoxaluria is present, a low oxalate diet should be instituted (Table 2). This will significantly reduce urinary oxalate excretion in most patients. Foods with a high oxalate (>40 mg per serving) should be avoided and even foods with a moderate oxalate content (>10 mg per serving) should be limited.

Decrease Steatorrhea. If there is significant steatorrhea (>20 g per day), then a low fat diet should be instituted. A low fat diet decreases fatty-acid concentration in the colon resulting in a decrease in fatty-acid-mediated alteration in colonic permeability. There is also less calcium-fatty-acid soap formation, and more calcium will be available to precipitate oxalate, thus preventing the absorption of oxalate. Unfortunately dietary fat cannot be decreased below approximately 50 g per day without making the diet unpalatable. This problem can be overcome somewhat by using medium-chain triglycerides. Medium-chain fatty acids neither increase the permeability of the colon to oxalate nor do they chelate calcium; thus, they do not affect the permeability or the solubility of oxalate.

Anion Binding Agents. "Anion binding agents" work by binding to bile acids and fatty acids, thereby decreasing bile acid and fatty-acid induced diarrhea. Thus they prevent the increase in colonic permeability induced by these acids, which bind to oxalate, and prevent its absorption. Anion-binding agents that can be used include cholestyramine, calcium, aluminum, magnesium, and bismuth. Cholestyramine however, can make the steatorrhea worse and should not be used if fecal-fat excretion is greater than 20 g per day. Also cholestyramine should be used with caution if the fecal fat excretion is greater than 10 g per day. The usual dose is 4 g (one packet) up to 4 times a day; however, this varies from patient to patient. Cholestyramine is also expensive. To avoid making the aluminum phosphate depletion significantly worse, aluminum hydroxide must be used with care (Table 1). Likewise, one must keep an eye on urinary-calcium excretion when administering this agent. Patients with significant small-bowel resection or bypass, however, usually have hypocalciuria. Of the alkali-metal preparations, I prefer Camalox, which is a combination of calcium carbonate, aluminum hydroxide, and magnesium hydroxide. The calcium, magnesium, and aluminum bind to oxalate, bile acids, and fatty acids. Magnesium is provided to help correct hypomagnesuria and alkali is provided to help increase urinary pH and to correct any hypocitraturia. Camalox usually does not worsen the diarrhea. I begin

TABLE 3 Treatment of Nephrolithiasis Associated with Intestinal Disease

Modality	Amount
Calcium Oxalate Nephrolithiasis	
Increase urine volume	
Increase fluid intake	
Decrease diarrhea	
Low oxalate diet	<75 mg/day
Low fat diet	50 g/day
Anion binding agents	
Cholestyramine	Up to 4 g q.i.d.
Calcium ⎫	Variable, must monitor urinary
Magnesium ⎬ Camalox	oxalate excretion
Aluminum ⎭	
Bismuth	
Pepto Bismol	
Magnesium	
Camalox	Enough to normalize urinary
Mg oxide	citrate excretion
Mg gluconate	
Citrate	
NaHCO$_3$	Enough to normalize urinary
Polycitra	citrate excretion
Urate Nephrolithiasis	
Increase urine volume	
Increase urine pH	
NaHCO$_3$	Increase until urine pH is in the
Polycitra	6.5 range

with 1 tablespoon (3 tablets) 3 times a day with meals, and I adjust the dose until urinary oxalate excretion is less than 50 mg per 24 hours.

Increase Urinary Magnesium Excretion. Urinary magnesium is important because it increases the solubility of oxalate and helps prevent hypocitraturia. Hypomagnesium can be difficult to correct because magnesium-salt ingestion can make the diarrhea worse. Diarrhea may be less of a problem when magnesium is administered along with calcium (i.e., Camalox). Some investigators have claimed success with magnesium oxide and magnesium gluconate. Various preparations can be tried. The amount of magnesium administered should be increased until urinary magnesium excretion is normal or a significant increase in diarrhea occurs. When using Camalox, administer it as already described. If using magnesium oxide, begin wtih 150 mg 4 times a day and increase until urinary magnesium excretion is normal or diarrhea is significantly worse.

Increase Urinary Citrate Excretion. To correct hypocitraturia it is necessary to restore urinary magnesium excretion to a level as close to normal as possible and to give alkali, such as calcium carbonate or sodium bicarbonate. Citrate can be given, but this is expensive. One advantage of citrate is that it comes in fairly concentrated forms. One ounce of Polycitra is equivalent to a 60 milliequivalent of bicarbonate, and it takes eight 650-mg sodium bicarbonate tablets to give the same amount of bicarbonate. I start with a half ounce of Polycitra twice a day or 2 tablets of sodium bicarbonate 4 times a day and increase the dose until urinary citrate levels are in the normal range. Alternatively, one can monitor serum bicarbonate and urinary pH. Keep in mind that dehydration can result in a contraction alkalosis, thereby making serum bicarbonate levels difficult to evaluate.

Urate Nephrolithiasis

Uric acid stones are seen primarily in patients with an ileostomy, and generally speaking, these patients do not have increased excretion of uric acid in the urine (Table 1). Uric acid stone formation in these patients is attributable to decreased urine volume and low-urine pH; low-urine pH is the most important factor. Urinary volume can be increased as described previously. Urinary pH should be increased by administration of bicarbonate or citrate in amounts sufficient to keep the urinary pH consistently in the 6.5 range; patients should be given nitrazine paper so they can monitor their own urinary pH. Allopurinol should be used only if urinary urate excretion increases or if the patient continues to form uric acid stones after correcting volume and pH changes as much as possible.

Approaches to the treatment of nephrolithiasis associated with intestinal disease are summarized in Table 3.

DIABETIC DIARRHEA

KONRAD H. SOERGEL, M.D.

Diarrhea associated with longstanding insulin-dependent diabetes mellitus usually appears when other complications of this metabolic disease already are manifest. The typical patient with diabetic diarrhea suffers from occlusive atherosclerosis, retinopathy, cataracts, glomerulosclerosis, and peripheral neuropathy. Signs of autonomic neuropathy are present in the vast majority and include orthostatic hypotension, neurogenic bladder, anhidrosis or dyshidrosis, erectile impotence, and a diagnostically useful sign, reduced cardiac beat-to-beat variations with respiration. Some patients exhibit other symptoms of gastrointestinal dysfunction, particularly fecal incontinence and vomiting. The diarrhea appears about 9 years after the onset of diabetes, and it occurs more frequently in males than in females. Many patients, depressed about their poor health, no longer follow medical advice. Thus, diabetic diarrhea occurs in the setting of a multisystem disease which significantly complicates the treatment of this disorder.

In one survey of consecutive diabetic outpatients, 22 percent reported diarrhea and 20 percent fecal incontinence with considerable overlap between these two groups. On the other hand, fewer than 1 percent of diabetics seek treatment for diarrhea and fewer still for fecal incontinence. This implies that the diarrhea usually is not perceived to be severe and that incontinence frequently goes unreported by the embarrassed patient unless a perceptive physician asks about it.

The cause of diabetic diarrhea remains unclear. There is no intestinal microangiopathy, mucosal morphology is normal, and there are no reproducible alterations in water, salt, and sugar absorption from the perfused jejunum; the ileum and colon have not yet been studied in this regard. Disordered intestinal motility has been demonstrated in both the fasted and the fed state. Bacterial overgrowth in the small intestine can rarely be documented, but excessive bacterial growth may occur in the stomach in the presence of gastric retention. Altered release of enteric hormones remains a possibility and increased plasma motilin levels have indeed been demonstrated. Histologic evidence of axonic and dendritic damage in the sympathetic trunks and paravertebral ganglia and of decreased numbers of adrenergic fibers and reduced catecholamine content in the wall of the ileum suggest a disorder of sympathetic innervation of the intestine involving mainly the ileum. These observations, coupled with the fact that stimulation of alpha$_2$-adrenergic receptors situated on the basolateral wall of the enterocyte increases sodium and chloride absorption, provide the rationale for recent attempts at treating diabetic diarrhea with alpha$_2$-agonists.

Clinically, diabetic diarrhea does not cause progressive weight loss. The course is intermittent with diarrheal episodes lasting from 2 weeks to 8 months. The daily stool weight rarely exceeds 800 g. Mild to moderate steatorrhea is found in one-fourth to one-third of patients without associated malabsorption of vitamins and minerals. Postulated causes of this steatorrhea include decreased enterohepatic circulation of bile acids due to "sluggish" gallbladder emptying, bacterial overgrowth, and pancreatic insufficiency. I favor the latter explanation because pancreatic exocrine function is impaired in most insulin-dependent diabetics and because we have demonstrated painless chronic pancreatitis in several patients with diabetic diarrhea and steatorrhea. There is no need to treat steatorrhea, however, unless sustained weight loss or vitamin and/or calcium deficiency appear.

DECISION TO TREAT

When may the diagnosis of diabetic diarrhea be considered established with sufficient certainty to begin treatment of this condition? Three points need to be kept in mind:

First, is diarrhea present? Whereas diarrhea is operationally defined as a stool weight of more than 250 g per day in the absence of excessive fiber intake, patients tend to report both increased stool frequency and fecal incontinence as diarrhea. Most patients are able to collect their stools for 48 hours at home, to be submitted for weighing and quantitative fat analysis. Only after measuring the severity of the diarrhea and inquiring about the existence and frequency of fecal incontinence should the physician decide which of these two disorders requires treatment. The therapeutic approach to fecal incontinence is described in a separate chapter.

Second, diabetic diarrhea is a diagnosis of exclusion. This implies that other causes of chronic intermittent diarrhea must be excluded. As a minimum I order two stools for ova and parasites, a small bowel series, prothrombin time and measurement of serum folate, vitamin B_{12}, calcium, and iron levels. If any of these are abnormal, another diagnosis should be suspected. Keep in mind that pernicious anemia is relatively common among diabetics and may present as isolated vitamin B_{12} deficiency. Further, diarrhea in a diabetic patient without peripheral and automonic neuropathy should raise serious doubts about the diagnosis of "diabetic diarrhea." Because diabetics frequently receive antibiotic therapy for urinary tract infection, their stools should be checked for *Clostridium difficile* and the cytotoxin elaborated by some strains of this anaerobe.

Third, the diabetic patient with diarrhea after renal transplantation presents special diagnostic problems. Here, a small bowel biopsy is indicated to rule out the presence of giardia, cryptosporidium, cytomegalovirus, and other opportunistic infectious organisms. Intubation of the upper small bowel for biopsy or aspiration of contents is often difficult, particularly in the presence of gastric hypomotility. Metoclopramide (Reglan), 10 mg IV administered over 10 minutes, or bethanechol chloride, (Urecholine), 5 to 10 mg subcutaneously may help the passage of an intestinal biopsy tube through the pylorus. Alternatively, adequate biopsy particles and fluid samples can be obtained from the distal duodenum more quickly through the endoscope equipped with a large biopsy channel.

ASSOCIATED CONDITIONS

Malabsorption

When blood tests suggest a malabsorptive disorder or when steatorrhea is present, three diseases need to be considered:

Celiac Sprue. There appears to be a greater than chance association between celiac sprue and type 1 diabetes mellitus; both diseases exhibit an increased prevalence of the HLA-B 8 histocompatibility antigen. The question is settled by obtaining several small bowel biopsy specimens and by observing the clinical response to a gluten-free diet if villi are absent from the mucosal biopsy. The D-xylose test is useless in this situation because abnormally low urinary excretion of this test sugar may be caused by gastric stasis, bacterial overgrowth, or renal insufficiency.

Pancreatic Exocrine Insufficiency. While pancreatic enzyme output is decreased in most type 1 diabetics, the problem is to identify those patients in whom lipase secretion is sufficiently reduced to account for steatorrhea. Indirect approaches have to be used because routine clinical methods are not available to quantify pancreatic enzyme secretion directly. Among these, a clearly abnormal pancreatogram obtained at endoscopic retrograde cholangiopancreatography, and/or marked decreases in pancreatic volume and bicarbonate output during a standard secretin test persuade me to initiate a trial with therapeutic doses of pancreatic extract (see chapter on *Chronic Pancreatitis: Exocrine and Endocrine Insufficiencies*.)

Bacterial Overgrowth. Bacterial contamination of the small bowel has been demonstrated in only a small number of diabetic patients with diarrhea. Hence, I view bacterial overgrowth as an alternative diagnosis to diabetic diarrhea rather than as a cause of this condition. The diagnosis continues to rest on direct demonstration of large numbers (more than 10^5 per milliliter) of viable bacteria in small intestinal aspirates by the laborious method of quantitative aerobic and anaerobic culture. Although increased excretion of $^{14}CO_2$ in the breath following an oral dose of 1 g of ^{14}C-D-xylose may be a more sensitive and certainly simpler indicator of bacterial overgrowth in the intestine, this test is not always available. In view of the cost and potential risks of broad-spectrum antibiotic therapy for the "blind loop syndrome" and of the intermittent natural course of diabetic diarrhea, such therapy should be reserved for patients in whom bacterial overgrowth has actually been documented.

THERAPY FOR DIABETIC DIARRHEA

Effective symptomatic management is challenging for patient and physician alike. Dietary restrictions have no place in the treatment of diabetic diarrhea. The patient should, however, avoid "diet" candy and soda and "sugarless" gum if these contain sorbitol as a sweetener. This polyalcohol is poorly absorbed and acts as a cathartic. Medications that patients may be receiving for other diabetic complications should be reviewed for their potential to contribute to or cause diarrhea: loop diuretics, some antihypertensives,—especially guanethidine—antacids, cimetidine, and bethanechol belong to this category. Patients treated with the dopamine antagonists metoclopramide (Reglan) or domperidone (not yet released in the United States) for gastric retention frequently develop increased diarrhea and abdominal cramping; in these patients, the decision has to be made which is worse, vomiting or diarrhea.

Opioids

Opioid antidiarrheal agents are the mainstay of therapy. While the dose schedule has to be individualized, these medications should be taken at regular times, rather than "prn" after each bowel movement. The aim is to prevent diarrhea, not to treat after it has occurred. In principle, these drugs are best taken one-half to 1 hour before diarrhea usually appears according to the patient's experience.

Three effective agents are available: *codeine phosphate or sulfate* available as 15-, 30-, and 60-mg tablets and as codeine sulfate solution, 30 mg per milliliter; *diphenoxylate hydrochloride with atropine* (Lomotil) as 2.5-mg tablets and solution, 2.5 mg per 5 ml; and *loperamide hydrochloride* (Imodium) as 2-mg capsules and solution, 1 mg per 5 ml. Dosage ranges from 15 to 60 mg 3 or 4 times daily for codeine, 5 to 7.5 mg 3 or 4 times daily for Lomotil and 2 to 8 mg twice a day for Imodium. The higher doses may result in abdominal cramping and constipation. All three retard transit through the intestinal tract and decrease stool volume. Loperamide may also stimulate water and electrolyte absorption directly and may aid continence by increasing anal sphincter pressure and by dampening the rectoanal inhibitory reflex. Codeine produces central opiate effects, Lomotil only when given in large doses, and Imodium essentially none. Although the known actions of these drugs on the intestine are similar, failure to respond to one does not necessarily predict failure of response to the others. I usually prescribe Imodium first because of its long duration of action (8 to 12 hours) and its lack of central nervous system effects. Codeine is my next choice despite its sedative action and addictive potential; Lomotil helps only rarely when the first two are ineffective.

Alpha$_2$-Agonists

Preliminary reports suggest that alpha$_2$-agonists are highly effective in diabetic diarrhea, probably by direct action on the enterocyte to stimulate sodium and chloride absorption. *Clonidine hydrochloride*, (Catapres), available as 0.1-, 0.2-, 0.3-mg tablets, as well as the experimental drug *lidamidine hydrochloride,* has been used in a few patients. Clonidine therapy is started at 0.1 mg every 12 hours and is advanced to 0.5 to 0.6 mg ever 12 hours over a few days. No hypotensive effects have been reported so far, presumably because the drug acts centrally to increase sympathetic outflow in the face of peripheral sympathetic arteriolar denervation in patients with autonomic neuropathy. Nonetheless, each patient should be checked for the appearance or worsening of orthostatic hypotension during initiation of this therapy. The major side effect is drowsiness. Withdrawal of the drug should be gradual over a period of 1 to 2 weeks to avoid rebound hypertension.

Other therapeutic agents have occasionally been recommended but have proved to be ineffective. These include bile acid binders (cholestyramine, aluminum hydroxide), bismuth subsalicylate (Pepto-Bismol), corticosteroids, psyllium mucilloid (Metamucil), wheat bran, and the indiscriminate use of broad-spectrum antibiotics and pancreatic extract therapy.

GASTROINTESTINAL DISORDERS IN THE IMMUNODEFICIENT STATE

MARVIN EARL AMENT, M.D.

The normal gastrointestinal tract contains numerous immunocompetent cells derived from the B and T cell lymphocyte series. These lymphocytes are involved in the defense of the gastrointestinal mucosa against antigens gaining entrance through the lumen. Any alteration in the barrier between the immune mechanisms of the gastrointestinal tract and the luminal environment of the intestine may lead to intestinal disease. IgA-, IgM-, IgG-, and IgE-producing plasma cells are found in the lamina propria along the entire gastrointestinal tract; however, the IgA plasma cells dominate and are found in a ratio of 20:3:1:0.5 (IgA, IgM, IgG, and IgE). The most important gammaglobulin found in the intestinal secretions is secretory IgA. This is an 11S gammaglobulin in which a secretory piece, which is produced in the mucosal epithelium, becomes attached to the IgA molecules as they diffuse from the lamina propria to the mucosal surfaces between and through the enterocytes. The "J" piece interconnects two IgA molecules; it is also produced in the mucosal cells. It is believed that the IgA-containing secretion of immunoglobulin is the one most responsible for the protection of the mucosal barrier from foreign antigens. It is only part of the protective mechanism, however. Cellular immunity in the gastrointestinal tract is very important to the maintenance of its integrity, but it is not understood how the cellular protective systems work within the digestive tract.

CLASSIFICATION OF PRIMARY IMMUNODEFICIENCY SYNDROMES AND EVIDENCE FOR GASTROINTESTINAL DISEASE IN THESE SYNDROMES

Primary immunodeficiency syndromes are a heterogeneous group of diseases characterized by impairment of the B cell system (humoral immunity), the T cell system (cell mediated), or both. Impairment of the normal development of functioning B cells will lead to deficiency in immunoglobulin synthesis. Failure to generate an effective T cell system results in defective cell mediated immunity. Repeated bacterial, severe viral, or fungal infection are the most common findings in immunodeficiency syndromes. Chronic gastrointestinal disease is characteristic of only certain immunodeficiency syndromes.

Antibody (B cell) Defects

X-linked Infantile Hypogammaglobulinemia

The main features of this immunological disorder are an IgG level of less than 0.3 g per deciliter and reduced or absent IgA, IgG, IgE, and IgM levels. Plasma cells are either absent or markedly decreased in number, and B lymphocytes are not found in the bone marrow and peripheral blood of these patients. Cellular immune function is intact in this defect. These patients usually develop recurrent pyogenic infections by 6 months of age, when maternally transferred IgG antibody disappears from the blood. This condition is believed to have developed because the mammalian equivalent of the avian bursa of Fabricius fails to develop, resulting in lack of the correct environment for the differentiation of primitive stem cells into B lymphocytes. These patients differ from those with transient physiologic hypogammaglobulinemia because they lack B lymphocytes and plasma cells throughout the gastrointestinal tract.

This group of patients demonstrates that the role of cellular immunity is quite important in the protection of the gastrointestinal tract. Individuals with X-linked agammaglobulinemia do not typically have chronic gastrointestinal disease as one of their major symptoms. Chronic diarrhea is not a typical feature of X-linked agammaglobulinemia. The causes of diarrhea, when it occurs, are no different than in the general population. Giardiasis has been reported to occur in individuals with X-linked agammaglobulinemia, but it is not common. The patients who get this infection, if untreated, have persistent diarrhea and malabsorption. They do respond to treatment and can have total reversal of any damage to the mucosa. Lactase deficiency can develop secondary to the injury caused by *Giardia* or viruses.

Although bacterial overgrowth can be found in the proximal small intestine in X-linked agammaglobulinemia, it cannot be correlated with morphologic damage to the small intestinal mucosa, nor with defects in absorptive function or symptoms.

Although overt clinical colitis is not typically seen, there may be microscopic evidence of colitis in biopsy specimens from these asymptomatic patients. They show early crypt abscesses with polymorphonuclear leukocytes scattered through the lamina propria. I have seen clinically apparent colitis secondary to antibiotic use with overgrowth of *Clostridium difficile*. These patients do respond to the use of vancomycin to eradicate the *C. difficile* and/or the use of cholestyramine to bind the toxin. When patients fail to respond to either mode of treatment, metronidazole may be used. Only if *C. difficile* and the other bacteria recognized to cause colitis have been excluded can ulcerative colitis be diagnosed. Crohn's disease has not been reported in any patient with X-linked agammaglobulinemia.

Recently, *maloplakia* of the colon with recurrent strictures has been reported in X-linked agammaglobulinemia. Its cause is unknown, but it is suspected of being infectious in origin.

Recurrent purulent *triaditis* should be considered in patients with agammaglobulinemia and fever of unknown origin. Biopsy and culture of the liver must be done to establish diagnosis and start appropriate antibiotic therapy. Primary sclerosing cholangitis has also been reported.

Selective IgA Deficiency

Selective IgA deficiency is characterized by serum IgA level of less than 0.05 g per deciliter and normal cell-mediated immunity. It is associated with recurrent sinopulmonary infections, autoimmune disease, and a variety of gastrointestinal and hepatic disorders. This is the most common primary immunodeficiency in man and occurs in between 1 in 500 and 1 in 700 individuals. The condition can occur sporadically but also as an autosomal dominant, and in other families as an autosomal recessive, condition.

An undetectable serum IgA level usually exists in conjunction with the absence of secretory IgA from body secretions such as saliva and jejunal fluid. Individuals with this condition have a reduction in IgA containing plasma cells in the gastrointestinal tract. A very few individuals, however, may have normal secretory IgA production with normal numbers of IgA fluorescing cells in their intestines but have deficient serum IgA. Alternatively, a selective deficiency of secretory IgA may be found in the presence of normal serum IgA concentration. This suggests that IgA deficiency may result from the failure of B lymphocytes to differentiate into IgA cells, from the IgG or IgM precursors, or from the arrested development of IgA cells due to metabolic abnormalities or disturbances in factors exrinsic to the B lumphocyte. These factors are essential in normal production of plasma cell maturation. In general, IgA deficiency appears to be found in association with, rather than as the cause of, gastrointestinal disease. It is becoming increasingly clear that IgA deficiency is linked, in a majority of patients, with deficiency of IgE. Recent studies have also shown that patients with IgA deficiency may also have defects in their synthesis of IgG subclasses II and IV. In addition, many patients with IgA deficiency will also have T cell defects.

Malabsorption syndromes typically occur in 10 percent of those with IgA deficiency. The etiologic agent of the malabsorption syndrome can be infectious, protozoan, or, in a rare case, gluten enteropathy. Celiac sprue, or gluten-induced enteropathy, is linked only to IgA deficiency. No other immune deficiency syndrome has the increased association between it and gluten.

Intestinal biopsy specimens of patients with selective IgA deficiency and celiac disease is similar to those seen in patients with celiac disease and normal IgA levels. Significant differences are found in the number of IgM-stained cells in the intestinal mucosa. In patients with selective IgA deficiency and celiac disease, almost all the plasma cells in the lamina propria stain for IgM. In patients who are not immunoglobulin deficient, there are increased numbers of plasma cells in the lamina propria that stain for IgA. Patients with IgA deficiency and celiac sprue have increased levels of IgM in their blood, whereas nonimmunoglobulin deficient individuals have increased IgA levels. Ulcerative colitis and regional enteritis, or Crohn's disease, have been reported in association with selective IgA deficiency. Their course and responsiveness to therapy have not been recognized to be different from those in patients who are not immune deficient. Pancreatitis, diabetes mellitus, and malabsorption secondary to exocrine pancreatic insufficiency have been described in a child with IgA deficiency.

X-linked Immunodeficiency with Hyper-IgM

This syndrome is characterized by X-linked recessive inheritance; recurrent bacterial infections; and decreased or absent serum levels of IgG, IgA, and IgE, but elevated IgM. Neutropenia, lymphadenopathy, hypertrophic tonsils, and splenomegaly are part of this syndrome. Although this condition occurs predominantly in males, it has been reported in a few girls and adult females. The syndrome has been recognized to develop following congenital rubella infection. It is said that individuals may have a defect in the switch mechanism, preventing the generation of IgG and IgA; a lack of "feedback inhibition" by serum IgG, further increasing the level of IgM; and in some, a lack of helper T lymphocytes. Neutropenia in this condition is believed to stem from a defect in the stem cell series.

The cause of neutropenia in this syndrome is unknown. These individuals are susceptible to developing idiopathic stomatitis and mouth ulcers. Esophageal ulcers with stricture formation, secondary to *Candida tropicalis,* have been reported in one patient who had neutropenia. This can be successfully treated with antifungal and antibiotic medications; however, healing may result in esophageal strictures. If this occurs, the esophagus may have to be dilated with mercury-filled bougies. *Cryptosporidium* have been described in patients with this syndrome who have chronic diarrhea and malabsorption. Treatment with sporocidin resulted in a reversal of the diarrhea, but the patient continued to malabsorb.

Immunodeficiency with Normal or Hyperimmunoglobulinemia

This syndrome is characterized by recurrent bacterial infections, onset during infancy, normal or elevated serum immunoglobulins, and defective antibody responses to certain antigens. This condition may actually represent a variety of immunodeficiency syndromes. In some of these patients the T cell defect may be responsible for the immune aberration. Chronic diarrhea and malabsorption have been described in this conditon, with severe injury to the intestinal mucosa. In the very few cases in which this has been recognized, no specific bacterial or viral agents have been successfully isolated from the intestinal tract.

Ataxia Telangiectasia with Immune Deficiency

This autosomal recessive disorder is typified by telangiectasia, progressive ataxia, sinopulmonary infections, immunodeficiency usually consisting of selective IgA and IgE deficiency, cutaneous allergy, and depressed but not absent in vitro lymphocyte responses. These patients have increased levels of autoantibodies against endocrine organs, liver, and parietal cells of the stomach and muscle. Patients with this condition have demyelinating and degenerative central nervous system lesions, which have been thought to be autoimmune in nature. Patients with ataxia telangiectasia also have elevated alpha-fetoprotein levels, which some say are evidence for basic defects in organ differentiation and maturation. Cells of patients with ataxia telangiectasia are said to be extremely sensitive to radiation. These patients undergo a progressive deterioration of the immune system.

Gastrointestinal symptoms in patients with ataxia telangiectasia are not common. The major problems these patients have are related to their sinopulmonary infections, which lead to bronchiectasis. Gastrointestinal disease, per se, is not a major factor in patients with ataxia telangiectasia, however, death of these patients can be attributed to carcinoma of the stomach and small intestine as well as to intestinal lymphoma in the stomach, small intestine, and colon. Virtually all of the malignancies described in this condition have developed by the third decade. Virtually all patients with ataxia telangiectasia have died by their third decade. Although studies have shown that patients with ataxia telangiectasia commonly have normal liver function tests, these patients have not been studied by serial biopsies. There is some evidence of injury to hepatocytes because of the elevation of their anti-smooth-muscle and anti-mitochondria antibodies. The titers of these antibodies, however, have never been correlated with histologic studies of the liver.

Death has come to patients with ataxia telangiectasia secondary to adenocarcinoma of the stomach and small intestine. Lymphomas of the small intestine and colon have also been reported as early as the second and third decade. Diagnostic studies should be done at the onset of any gastrointestinal symptoms.

Transient Hypogammaglobulinemia of Infancy

This is a self-limited syndrome which usually begins between 3 and 6 months of age and lasts from 6 to 18 months. It is usually associated with an increased susceptibility to infection resulting from an abnormal delay in the onset of immunoglobulin synthesis. Patients with transient hypogammaglobulinemia of infancy commonly present with a history of frequent bacterial infections of the skin, nose, meninges, and respiratory tract. Some patients have a decreased number of peripheral lymph nodes and a decreased volume of tonsillar tissue. Infants with this conditon may fail to gain weight and grow normally because of frequent infections. These individuals are not particularly susceptible to the development of thrush.

Placentally transferred immunoglobulins decline during the first months of life. These infants, however, fail to start synthesizing their own immunoglobulins until much later than normal. A spontaneous recovery usually starts between 9 and 15 months of age, and often the children reach 2 to 4 years of age before they are completely normal. There are normal or near normal numbers of circulating B cells in the intestine. A thymus can be seen on chest roentgenogram. The bone marrows of these children usually have a marked decrease in the number of plasma cells.

Patients with transient hypogammaglobulinemia of infancy have an increased incidence of chronic diarrhea. Ten to 15 percent of all infants with chronic diarrhea have transient hypogammaglobulinemia of infancy. Therefore, all infants with chronic diarrhea should have immunoglobulins measured. The causes of the diarrhea in these patients are not unique; they include giardiasis, *Campylobacter jejunii*, rotaviruses, and *C. difficile* and its toxin. Patients with transient hypogammaglobulinemia of infancy and chronic diarrhea have a far greater chance of having one of the infections listed above than individuals with normal immunoglobulins. Therapy includes gammaglobulin if the IgG level is less than 400 mg per deciliter. Protozoan and bacterial gastrointestinal infections should be treated as one would treat a patient who is not immune deficient.

There is no definite syndrome in which IgE deficiency alone has been linked to gastrointestinal disease.

IgG Subclass Deficiencies and Abnormalities

There are four types of IgG subclasses. In normal serum the percentages of subclasses are IgG_1, 66 percent; IgG_2, 23 percent; IgG_3, 7 percent; and IgG_4, 4 percent. Patients with common variable immune deficiency syndromes have a 20 to 25 percent chance of having imbalanced IgG subclasses. New studies have shown no correlation between IgG subclass concentration, a type of immune deficiency syndrome, and the presence or absence of gastrointestinal disease.

Common Variable Immunodeficiency Syndrome, or Acquired Agammaglobulinemia, Adult Agammaglobulinemia, Late-Onset Agammaglobulinemia

This is a heterogeneous group of patients who present some time after infancy, usually in the second or third decade. Patients are characterized by recurrent bacterial infections, decreased serum immunoglobulins, partial antibody responses to specific antigens, and either normal or partially defective cellular immunity. Most of these patients have a significant amount of gastrointestinal disease. The peripheral lymphocytes in this condition suggest a variety of immune defects. The B lymphocytes of some patients are markedly depressed or absent. The B lymphocytes of others are present in normal numbers but fail to divide and produce immunoglobulin when stimulated with a T cell mitogenic factor. In others, the B cells divide, transform, and produce immunoglobulin but fail to release de novo synthesized immunoglobulin. Other patients have serum factors that inhibit maturation of B lymphocytes, and still in others, the B lymphocytes are being suppressed by their own suppressor T lymphocytes.

Sinopulmonary infections are the most common presenting features in patients with common variable immunodeficiency syndrome. Ultimately these patients develop bronchiectasis. The three most common organisms implicated in respiratory tract infections are pneumococci, staphylococci, and *Hemophilus influenzae*. Tonsillar tissue and lymph nodes are present in most patients with this condition. Rarely, they will have hepatomegaly, splenomegaly, and adenopathy. Chest findings in those with chronic lung disease are not unusual and consist of rales, clubbing, and altered chest configuration.

Gastrointestinal abnormalities and disease are not unusual in common variable immunodeficiency syndrome. A generalized malabsorption syndrome characterized by steatorrhea, lactose intolerance, protein-losing enteropathy, generalized disaccharidase deficiency, and malabsorption of vitamin B_{12} and folic acid has been frequently described. It is typically associated with varying degrees of damage to the villous architecture. Such lesions have been described with giardiasis, cryptosporidiosis and strongyloidiasis. In most instances, treatment of *Giardia lamblia* with metronidazole or other antiprotozoan medications, and *Cryptosporidium* with sporicidin has resulted in eradication of the parasites and reversal of malabsorption and mucosal lesions toward normal. *Giardia lamblia* infections may be difficult to diagnose and require aspiration of duodenal contents or examination of multiple small bowel biopsies. *Crytosporidium* may be diagnosed most easily by multiple stool examinations and small intestinal biopsies. This is also true of strongyloidiasis.

Bacterial infections of the small intestine and colon appear more frequently and are prolonged in this group of patients. *Campylobacter jejunii* has been recognized to cause a chronic diarrhea syndrome, which may respond to treatment with erythromycin. Chronic enteroviral infections also occur in this group of patients.

Nodular lymphoid hyperplasia of the small intestine has been described in many patients with adult-onset immune deficiency syndrome. Microscopic examination shows large lymphoid follicles with germinal centers within the lamina propria. This causes protrusion of the overlying mucosa in a nodular, polypoid appearance. Plasma cells are either absent or diminished in the lamina propria.

Follicular lymphoid cells contain no detectable immunoglobulin on immunofluorescence. Patients with this condition are able to change from IgM to IgG antibody production. The nodules seen in nodular lymphoid hyperplasia are widespread in the large and small bowel but are predominantly in the distal small bowel. Nodular lymphoid hyperplasia is not typically seen in selective IgA deficiency but with common variable hypogammaglobulinemia. Colitis in patients with common variable hypogammaglobulinemia deficiency syndrome may be clinically similar to that in immune incompetent patients. The lesions may be typical of ulcerative colitis or Crohn's disease but not contain as many plasma cells. Recently, cases of colitis in which the rectosigmoid involvement was not typical for either ulcerative colitis or Crohn's disease have been described. Some have shown protein-losing confined to the rectosigmoid. Large, elongated masses of fibrous tissue have been seen on barium enema and during proctosigmoidoscopy. Biopsies show the lamina propria filled with macrophages which account for 80 to 90 percent of the cells in the lamina propria. Fortunately, these patients have responded to conventional management with 2 g of Azulfidine, 40 mg of prednisone, and hydrocortisone enemas.

Some patients with common variable immune deficiency syndrome and malabsorption have no recognizable cause of the malabsorption in small intestinal mucosal biopsy specimens. They do not respond to a gluten-free diet, and they fail to respond to antibiotic therapy for bacterial overgrowth.

Patients with common variable immune deficiency syndromes have an increased incidence of pernicious anemia characterized by its onset at young age and the presence of antiparietal cell antibodies. There is a link to gastrointestinal malignancy, since as many as one-third of adults with common variable immune deficiency syndrome and gastrointestinal disease ultimately develop adenocarcinoma or lymphoma of the stomach, small intestine, and/or colon.

Antibody Deficiency with Transcobalamin II Deficiency

This is an extremely rare syndrome, first described in an infant whose parents were first cousins. The infant had intractable diarrhea and megaloblastic anemia at 4 months of age. There was no antibody response to several antigens during the D_{12} deficient phase. T cell function was reportedly normal. The diarrhea was thought to be due to a malfunction or immaturity of the intestinal absorptive cells, which depend on a continuous supply of vitamin B_{12}. The problem seemed to resolve when the patient was given injections of vitamin B_{12}.

Immunodeficiency with Generalized Hematopoietic Hypoplasia

This exceedingly rare syndrome is seen only in infants and is characterized by a severe, congenital cellular antibody deficiency associated with agenesis of the granulocytic precursors of the bone marrow. Infants with this condition present with failure to thrive, vomiting, diarrhea, or localized infection. Most patients have died before 2 weeks of age. All have marked leukopenia. The gammaglobulin levels in the blood represent fully what has been transported transplacentally. At autopsy these patients appear very similar to those with combined immune deficiency disorders except that, in addition, they have absence or marked deficiency of the granulocytic precursors. The only treatment is a bone marrow transplantation. The etiologic agent of the diarrhea is unknown.

Thymic Hypoplasia

Thymic hypoplasia (DiGeorge's syndrome, or cellular immune deficiency with hypoparathyroidism) is a congenital immunodeficiency syndrome characterized by hypocalcemic tetany, congenital heart disease, unusual facies, and increased susceptibility to infection. These patients are typically recognized by their characteristic external facies, which include hypertelorism, antimongoloid slant of the eyes, low-set ears with notched pinnae, reduced helix formation, and micrognathia. The gastrointestinal symptoms that have nominally been associated with it are esophageal atresia and imperforate anus. If the infant survives the neonatal period, increased susceptibility to infection occurs, typically characterized by chronic rhinitis, recurrent pneumonia, oral candidiasis, and diarrhea. The diarrhea has never been well defined but could be linked to hypoparathyroidism. There is a known association between the two. Fetal thymus transplant is the recommended therapy, following correction of the hypoparathyroidism with calcium gluconate, low phosphorus diet, calcium supplements, and low doses of vitamin D. Heart disease in these patients may also be severe and can be fatal.

Combined Immunodeficiency Disease

Combined immunodeficiency disease is congenital and usually hereditary. It typically includes deficiencies of both the T and B cell systems and is associated with lymphoid aplasia and thymic dysplasia. The basic defect in this condition is, in most patients, secondary to a stem cell defect. In others there is a thymic helper defect or intrathymic defect. Recurrent septic episodes and severe bacterial pneumonia are the typical presenting symptoms, followed by chronic oral candidiasis which proves refractory to all forms of local therapy. The condition has also been reported to present as Letterer-Siwe disease. Some patients develop severe esophagitis. They typically develop overwhelming infections with *pneumocystis carinii*, cytomegalovirus, or rubeola.

Ninety percent of patients with combined immunodeficiency disease develop gastrointestinal disease. Typically, they first present with lactase deficiency and steatorrhea from mucosal injury. If no specific treatable cause is found, they progress to a generalized malabsorption syndrome with difficulty digesting and absorbing all nutrients, including monosaccharides and amino acids. Prolonged excretion of rotavirus is a recently described phenomenon that could account for the intractability of the diarrhea in these patients. Quite often, the damaging agent or agents cannot be isolated. Cryptosporidiosis has been described in patients with combined immune deficiency syndrome. Therapy with sporicidin should be tried to see if it eradicates this protozoan.

Fatal progressive adenovirus infection and hepatic necrosis have been described, as has diffuse cytomegalovirus involvement of the esophagus, stomach, and gastrointestinal tract. Experimental therapy with the drug DHPV is now being attempted. The effectiveness of such therapy in patients with cytomegalovirus is still unknown.

Survival in some of these patients may require total parenteral nutrition through a central venous catheter, until either a thymus or bone marrow transplantation can be performed. Patients who undergo successful transplants will experience reconstitution of their gastrointestinal tract, and reversal of their malabsorption.

Short-limbed Dwarfism with Immune Deficiency and Cartilage Hair Hypoplasia

This autosomal recessive, predominantly T cell immunodeficiency syndrome is associated with both metaphyseal and spondyloepiphyseal dysplasia. It is a variant of short-limbed dwarfism, in which fine, sparse hair is present. Short stature occurs as a result of disproportionate shortening of the extremities. Immunologically, these patients have either a T cell defect, a B cell defect, or a combined defect. Celiac sprue, malabsorption of unknown etiology, and Hirschsprung's disease have all been described in this condition. Celiac sprue is responsive to a gluten-free diet; Hirschsprung's disease must be managed surgically; and in cases of malabsorption of unknown etiology, the patients often have to be treated symptomatically.

Varicella has been the most common fatal infection. Rubeola and poliovirus vaccine are also potentially lethal to these patients. Bone marrow transplantation in one child reversed the malabsorption, chronic diarrhea, and regenerative anemia with growth failure.

Wiskott-Aldrich Syndrome

Wiskott-Aldrich syndrome is an X-linked recessive immunodeficiency syndrome characterized by thrombocytopenia, eczema, and recurrent infection. Its gastrointestinal manifestations include hematemesis, melena, and chronic diarrhea. These patients often have difficulty tolerating standard infant feedings with intact protein. They develop malabsorption syndromes but respond to elemental formulas such as Vivonex, Pregestimil, and Nutramigen. They often have difficulties throughout infancy and beyond in tolerating intact protein. They frequently have diets limited to fruits, vegetables, and a select group of proteins. Patients with Wiskott-Aldrich syndrome die from bleeding and malignancy unless they undergo bone marrow transplantation. Bone marrow transplantation to reconstitute these individuals has been successful. The malignancies seen in Wiskott-Aldrich syndrome are lymphomas.

Chronic Mucocutaneous Candidiasis

Chronic mucocutaneous candidiasis is a cellular immunodeficiency syndrome that may be associated at times with a B cell defect and is characterized by a persistent *Candida* infection of the mucous membranes, scalp, skin, and nails. It is typically associated with Addison's disease, hypoparathyroidism, thyroiditis, and diabetes mellitus. Acute and chronic hepatitis and cirrhosis have been reported. Some cases of mucocutaneous candidiasis may be associated with hepatitis B surface antigen. Chronic active hepatitis, at times progressive, has been described but can be arrested by the use of corticosteroids and 6-mercaptopurine. Candidiasis is typically present on the oral mucous membranes. Fingernails and toenails are frequently involved, as is the skin of the face, hands, and feet. These patients may have increased pigmentation secondary to Addison's disease, and they may have tetany and seizures secondary to hypocalcemia.

Hypoparathyroidism is present in 70 percent of such patients, Addison's disease in 37 percent. Hypothyroidism, diabetes mellitus, and pernicious anemia are less commonly found. The endocrine dysfunction in this condition may be treated by supplying the deficient hormone whenever possible. Some patients have dysphagia secondary to *Candida* infection of the mouth, pharynx, and esophagus. This can be successfully treated with ketoconazole and, in some instances when this fails, with intravenous amphotericin.

Acquired Immune Deficiency Syndrome

This unfortunate group of patients has a variety of gastrointestinal disorders, some or all of which may be present simultaneously. The recognized causes can be treated using therapy prescribed for those who do not have acquired immune deficiency syndrome (AIDS).

Mucositis secondary to candidiasis with or without esophageal involvement can lead to difficulty chewing and swallowing solid food. The buccal mucosa may be involved independent of esophageal involvement, and vice versa. Treatment of choice is mycostatin or ketoconazole, in that order.

Idiopathic aphthous ulcerations may also cause significant difficulty chewing and swallowing. Cytomegalovirus may at times be isolated from these lesions. They should always be cultured for viruses and examined for fungi. Patients with cytomegalovirus infections can be treated with new experimental but specific therapy.

Acid reflux can also occur in AIDS. I believe it occurs in a disproportionate number of these patients, and it can be quite severe, leading to large ulcerations of esophageal mucosa.

Diarrhea with or without malabsorption is a major problem. Many AIDS patients have significant nutritional wasting because of the severity of their problem. Malabsorption can be generalized and severe and involve all nutrients. Patients may require placement of central venous lines, if their malnutrition and malabsorption warrant it, to provide the necessary nutrients intravenously.

The origin of the diarrhea and malabsorption may involve the common organisms that affect immune competent patients, as well as ones typically seen in AIDS patients. Stools should be examined for *Giardia lamblia, Strongyloides, Cryptosporidium,* and *Isospora.* All of these may respond to appropriate antiparasite medications. Rotaviruses, adenoviruses, and cytomegaloviruses all may damage the small intestinal mucosa, with the latter affecting the colon as well. All should be tested for and cultured in instances in which this is the mode of diagnosis. There is currently no effective treatment for chronic rotavirus and adenovirus infection of the gastrointestinal tract.

Cytomegalovirus may be treatable with a new but still experimental antiviral agent, HHPV, but this would not offer a long-term cure unless the immune status could be improved. Although there are a few suggestions of overgrowth of bacteria in the proximal small intestine this is not a consistent finding. Unfortunately, there is not a good correlation between overgrowth and response to treatment with antibiotics. I would, however, recommend a trial of broad-spectrum antibiotics.

In some patients, the cause of the mucosal injury is never determined and never improves. Even in some patients treated appropriately, symptoms improve but bowel function does not return to normal.

Kaposi's sarcoma can involve the gastrointestinal tract from mouth to anus and can be a cause of gastrointestinal bleeding.

Colitis in these patients may be secondary to the usual pathogenic organisms in the colon. The difference in these organisms in the AIDS patient is their persistence and failure to clear spontaneously if not treated. *Clostridium difficile, Campylobacter, Shigella, Salmonella* and amebae should be considered as possible causes of colitis.

In addition, patients shoud be assessed for *Neisseria gonorrhoeae* in stool cultures. *Chlamydia* and cytomegalovirus may also be found in ulcerations in the colonic epithelium and be a cause for the destructive changes in the colon. The chapter *Sexually Transmitted Intestinal Disease* includes additional information on AIDS and AIDS-related conditions.

White Blood Cell Killing Defects

In addition to the immunodeficiency syndromes, there is a group of diseases which occur as a result of defects in the function of polymorphonuclear leukocytes and macrophages. The illnesses caused by the defects in these cells are of a different and distinguishable nature from those based on immune deficiency disorders.

In some instances, patients have been described who have both immunoglobulin deficiency and phagocytic cell disorders. The immunoglobulin deficiency syndromes, in which phagocytic cell dysfunction and gastrointestinal disease have been described, include hyper-IgE syndrome, X-linked agammaglobulinemia, nodular lymphoid hyperplasia, selective IgA deficiency, and combined immunodeficiency syndrome.

Disorders of Phagocyte Killing in which Gastrointestinal and Hepatic Disease Are Prominent

The most extensively studied disorder of intraleukocytic metabolism is chronic granulomatous disease of childhood. It is X-linked in inheritance in 85 percent of cases and autosomal recessive in the remainder. Patients are unable to produce hydrogen peroxide because of defective oxidative metabolism in their leukocytes. They are very susceptible to infections with *Staphylococcus aureus, E. coli, Serratia marcescens, Candida albicans, Nocardia,* and *Aspergillus.*

Such patients may develop an illness similar to Crohn's disease in its distribution and manifestations and they may present with draining perineal fistulas and perianal ulcers. Diarrhea, rectal bleeding, abdominal pain, and nonbilious vomiting may be among their gastrointestinal symptoms. A contracted edematous antral duodenal area with poor distensibility may be seen on upper gastrointestinal and small bowel series. The small bowel may show loss of normal distensibility, loss of mucosal pattern, fistula formation, and intra-abdominal abscesses. Similar changes, as well as microulcerations, may be identified in the colon by barium enema.

Patients should initially be treated with metronidazole, 1 to 1.5 g per day, if they are febrile. Corticosteroids could be used first if the patient's symptoms are primarily obstructive in nature, or if bleeding from the terminal ileum or colon is the major symptom.

Occasionally surgical resection must be done, especially if the patient has abdominal abscesses or enterofistulas. Liver abscesses may require both antibiotic treatment and subsequent drainage. Initially, aspiration to culture the responsible organisms aids antibiotic selection.

BONE MARROW TRANSPLANT: GASTROINTESTINAL CONSIDERATIONS

PAUL C. SCHROY III, M.D.
SIDNEY J. WINAWER, M.D.

Bone marrow transplantation has emerged as a tremendous advance in the treatment of a number of hematologic disorders, immunodeficiency syndromes, and malignancies. Despite the overall success of this approach, serious and potentially fatal complications are frequently encountered. This is particularly true of the gastrointestinal system, where toxicity due to intensive conditioning, graft-versus-host disease (GVHD), and infections account for considerable morbidity and mortality. The following discussion will outline a rational approach to the management of these problems. There is a separate chapter, *Liver Transplantation: Gastroenterologic Considerations*, which also contains useful general information regarding transplantation.

EFFECTS OF CONDITIONING

Successful bone marrow engraftment in a relatively immunocompetent host requires intensive pretransplant conditioning to prevent graft rejection. Since bone marrow toxicity is not a problem, near-lethal doses of cyclophosphamide are given to all patients prior to marrow infusion. In patients with malignancies, especially acute leukemia, total body irradiation is also given to ensure disease ablation. These regimens are extremely toxic to a number of organ systems, including the gastrointestinal tract and liver.

Gastrointestinal Toxicity

Small bowel and colonic mucosa are particularly vulnerable to the damaging effects of these regimens. Anorexia, nausea and vomiting, diarrhea, and crampy lower abdominal pain are extremely common and may persist for up to 2 weeks after conditioning. Standard antiemetic therapy with phenothiazines, cannabinoids, or metoclopramide is given but is usually only partially effective. Similarly, opiate-based antidiarrheal drugs, such as diphenoxylate with atropine (Lomotil), have limited efficacy but remain the only available treatment. Because of poor oral intake and painful mucositis, caloric support in the form of parenteral hyperalimentation is given to all patients. Intravenous administration of medications whenever possible is also advised because of erratic intestinal absorption. Rectal manipulation or manipulation of drugs should be avoided in patients with neutropenia or thrombecytopenia because of the risk of infection and bleeding.

Liver Toxicity

Veno-occlusive disease (VOD) of the liver occurs in approximately 5 percent of marrow transplant recipients. Obliteration of centrilobular and sublobular veins caused by the toxic effects of high-dose chemotherapy and irradiation during the conditioning stage is responsible for the rapid development of hepatomegaly, ascites, and marked hepatic dysfunction which characterize this disorder. Clinical manifestations typically occur within the first 4 weeks after transplantation but may occur later. Differential diagnoses include hepatic vein obstruction (Budd-Chiari syndrome), pericardial tamponade, GVHD, intra-abdominal sepsis, liver abscess, and pancreatic ascites. Diagnosis is generally made on clinical grounds, since coagulopathy usually precludes percutaneous liver biopsy. Prognosis is poor, with mortality in the range of 30 to 50 percent. Since there is no specific therapy for VOD, survival depends on vigorous supportive care and prompt recognition and treatment of complications. Management is the same as for other causes of hepatic failure, which is discussed in detail in the chapter *Fulminant Hepatic Failure*.

GRAFT-VERSUS-HOST DISEASE

Graft-versus-host disease is a major cause of morbidity and mortality in patients undergoing bone marrow transplantation. It results from reactivity of engrafted immunocompetent donor T lymphocytes against recipient (host) tissues. Acute and chronic forms exist which differ not only in their time of onset but also in their clinical features, pathophysiology, and treatment. Because of these differences, each warrants a separate discussion.

Acute Graft-Versus-Host Disease

Acute GVHD typically develops 20 to 100 days after transplantation. It occurs in 30 to 70 percent of patients receiving a human leukocyte antigen (HLA)-identical marrow graft and in nearly 100 percent of those receiving HLA-incompatible grafts. Factors associated with an increased risk include greater host age, marrow grafts from female donors, and the presence of normal to increased natural killer cell activity in the recipient prior to transplantation. Although the pathophysiology remains incompletely understood, engrafted alloreactive T lymphocytes appear to initiate an immunologically mediated process resulting in damage to certain target organs, primarily skin, liver, and gut. The relative roles of the conditioning regimen, infectious agents, and other immune effector systems are not well established.

The most common gastrointestinal manifestation of acute GVHD is watery diarrhea, which in severe cases may be bloody. Associated symptoms may include crampy abdominal pain aggravated by eating, nausea, anorexia, and/or a protein-losing enteropathy. In addition, several

TABLE 1 Clinical Stage of Acute Graft versus Host Disease

Stage	Skin	Liver (mg/dl)	Gut (ml/day)
+	Rash covering <25% of body	Bilirubin 2–3	Diarrhea 500–1,000
+ +	Rash covering 25–50% of body	Bilirubin 3–6	Diarrhea 1,000–1,500
+ + +	Generalized erythroderma	Bilirubin 6–15	Diarrhea > 1,500
+ + + +	Desquamation, bullae	Bilirubin > 15	Diarrhea with pain or ileus

cases of pneumatosis intestinalis have been reported. Since gastrointestinal damage secondary to irradiation, drugs and infection can produce a similar clinical picture, rectal biopsy has been advocated in questionable cases. Histologic features include crypt cell necrosis, crypt abscesses and drop-out, and mucosal denudation. Although similar changes may be induced by the conditioning regimen, resolution should be complete by the third week after transplantation unless acute GVHD is present. It should also be noted that a subacute syndrome characterized by anorexia, mouth ulcers, abdominal pain, and diarrhea has been described which appears to be distinct from the usual patterns of either acute or chronic GVHD.

Liver involvement is also common in acute GVHD. Its actual incidence, however, is unknown, since other factors such as infection, irradiation, drugs, and veno-occlusive disease (VOD) may contribute to the high frequency of abnormal liver function tests observed during the first several weeks after transplantation. Both hepatocellular and cholestatic enzyme elevations are common. Hepatocyte necrosis, bile duct atypia, and lymphoid infiltration of the portal tract are the usual histologic features. Although progressive liver dysfunction may be seen in severe cases of acute GVHD, fulminant hepatic failure is uncommon.

Prognosis is closely linked to disease severity. Since the clinical manifestations correlate with disease activity, clinical staging and grading systems have been established (Tables 1 and 2). Patients with advanced disease, i.e., grades II through IV, have a mortality in the range of 30 to 40 percent, which is two to four times greater than in patients with grade I disease. Because of the profound immunosuppression associated with GVHD and its treatment, however, sepsis rather than end-organ failure is the usual cause of death.

TABLE 2 Clinical Grade of Severity of Acute Graft versus Host Disease

Grade	Organ Involvement
I	+ to + + rash; no liver or gut involvement; normal clinical performance
II	+ to + + rash; liver and gut involvement (or both); mild decrease in clinical performance
III	+ + to + + + rash; + + to + + + liver or gut involvement (or both); marked decrease in clinical performance
IV	Similar to grade III but with + + to + + + + organ involvement and extreme decrease in clinical performance

Treatment

Immunosuppression and supportive care are the mainstays of current therapy for acute GVHD. Various agents have been used, including antithymocyte globulin (ATG), cyclosporin A, and corticosteroids. Of these, corticosteroids appear to be the most effective, but responses tend to be variable and only occasionally satisfactory. Each has been reported to decrease the clinical severity of the disease, especially the skin and gut manifestations, but afford little, if any, improvement in overall survival. High-dose methylprednisolone has been advocated in severe cases, but, as with all immunosuppressive therapy, potential benefits may be outweighed by the risk of fatal infection.

At our institution, systemic corticosteroids are the treatment of choice for grades II through IV acute GVHD. Generally, high-dose methylprednisolone (2 mg per kilogram per day) is given until an objective clinical response is seen, at which point the dosage is tapered and prednisone (1 mg per kilogram per day) is substituted. Therapy is continued with tapering doses until resolution is complete. In those in whom corticosteroids are ineffective, ATG is used, but the overall response has been poor. The major complications have been opportunistic infections and interstitial pneumonia, both of which are often fatal.

Prophylaxis

Because of the relative ineffectiveness of available therapeutic regimens, current interest is centered on prevention. Two major approaches have evolved. The first and most widely used has been post-transplant immunosuppression with methotrexate, ATG, cyclosporin A, and corticosteroids, either as single agents or in combination, for periods of 3 to 6 months. Despite the reported success in animal models, none has been successful in eliminating GVHD in humans. Cyclosporin A has attracted the greatest attention based on the results of early non-randomized trials in which both the incidence and severity of acute GVHD were significantly reduced when compared with historical controls. Recent randomized trials comparing cyclosporin A with methotrexate have shown some increased efficacy in decreasing the incidence and severity of acute GVHD in select patients but have failed to demonstrate significant improvement in long-term survival. Current studies are investigating the efficacy of cyclosporin A combined with prednisone or methotrexate.

The second and most promising approach involves the elimination of T lymphocytes from the donor marrow prior to transplantation. Several methods have been employed, including (1) physical separation on the basis of density or volume; (2) agglutination with soybean lectins followed by rosette formation with sheep erythrocytes; and (3) anti-T-cell monoclonal antibodies with or without other effector systems such as complement or toxins. Preliminary clinical studies have reported marked success in decreasing both the incidence and severity of acute GVHD, with several institutions reporting complete elimination. Unfortunately, some have also noted increased rates of graft rejection and early leukemic relapse. Thus, although the overall impact on survival is unclear, donor T cell depletion appears to show great promise as an effective means of preventing acute GVHD.

Both approaches are currently under investigation at our center. Preliminary work with lectin separation has shown a marked decrease in the incidence of acute GVHD in both HLA-identical and HLA-nonidentical transplants. There has been a small number of graft rejections, however, a problem infrequently encountered in the transplantation of HLA-identical unseparated marrow for patients with leukemia. Since rejections are known to occur in a significant percentage of unseparated marrow grafts in patients with aplastic anemia, these patients are not generally candidates for T cell elimination and instead receive prophylaxis with methotrexate.

Use of a protective environment (intestinal decontamination with oral, nonabsorbable antibiotics, laminar air flow, sterile food) has also been advocated based on favorable results from both animal and human studies. Unfortunately, total decontamination is difficult to achieve, expensive, and poorly tolerated by patients, and cannot be recommended in the routine management of bone marrow transplant recipients.

Management of Specific Problems Due to Acute Graft-versus-Host Disease

Bleeding

Bleeding is a frequent complication of severe gastrointestinal GVHD. The site of bleeding is often difficult to determine because of the diffuse nature of the underlying process. Management includes immunosuppressive therapy with high-dose corticosteroids, packed red cell transfusions, and correction of any superimposed coagulopathy with irradiated HLA-matched platelets and fresh plasma as indicated. Most patients also receive empiric antacids and antifungal therapy to treat other possible causes. Histamine$_2$ blockers are generally avoided because of their potential bone marrow suppressive effect.

In those who remain refractory to these measures or in whom there is strong suspicion of causes other than acute GVHD, endoscopy and/or localizing techniques such as tagged red-cell scans are performed. Unfortunately, the lesion is usually diffuse, thus precluding successful endoscopic or angiographic therapeutic interventions. Both vasopressin and prostaglandins have been tried in this situation but have been ineffective. Surgery has not been helpful in patients with localized bleeding refractory to maximum medical therapy.

Diarrhea

Although acute GVHD is the most common cause of diarrhea in the early post-transplant period, infectious causes must be ruled out. Once these are excluded, therapy is primarily supportive and includes bowel rest, intravenous fluid and salt replacement, and total parenteral nutrition. Anticholinergics and long-acting opiates should be avoided because of the risk of ileus. Oral feedings with lactose- and gluten-free, low-osmolality liquids are started once the diarrhea improves. Diet can later be advanced when tolerated by the patient. Agents possibly useful for secretory diarrhea are discussed in a separate chapter.

Nausea and Vomiting

Nausea and vomiting are extremely common problems in the early post-transplant period. Etiologic possibilities are numerous and may include acute GVHD, infection, liver disease, drugs, or cystic duct obstruction, to name only a few. If these symptoms are secondary to acute GVHD, standard antiemetic therapy is given in conjunction with systemic corticosteroids. Antiemetics possessing potent anticholinergic or potential cholestatic properties should be used with caution.

Ileus and Distention

Paralytic ileus can occur as a result of acute gastrointestinal GVHD. More often, however, it is precipitated by the use of opiates and anticholinergics in the treatment of diarrhea and cramps. Infectious enteritis, intraabdominal sepsis, and pancreatitis should also be considered in the differential diagnosis. Perforation is an uncommon complication but can occur and should be excluded in all cases of abdominal pain and ileus. Barium studies and laxatives should usually be avoided. Treatment is directed at the underlying disease. Nasogastric suction with a sump tube should also be used to decompress the bowel and relieve discomfort. If colonic distention is prominent, the long tube intubation and rotating patient position technique described in the chapters *Fulminant Colitis and Toxic Megacolon* may be useful.

Jaundice

Hepatic failure as manifested by ascites, encephalopathy, and prolongation of the prothrombin time is rarely caused by acute GVHD of the liver alone. Its presence should heighten suspicion of other possible problems discussed above. Treatment is directed at the underlying disease as well as the usual supportive measures employed in the management of hepatic failure secondary to other causes.

Chronic Graft-versus-Host Disease

Chronic GVHD is a heterogeneous, autoimmune-like process which generally develops 3 to 12 months after transplantation and affects approximately one-third of long-term survivors of allogeneic bone marrow transplantation. Increasing grade of prior acute GVHD, increased host age, and nonirradiated donor buffy-coat transfusions have been identified as risk factors. A number of immunologic abnormalities have been described, suggesting a complex immunopathogenesis involving both cellular and humoral immunity.

The clinicopathologic elements of chronic GVHD have select features of several different autoimmune disorders, such as scleroderma, systemic lupus erythematosus, Sjögren's syndrome, lichen planus, and primary biliary cirrhosis. Clinical manifestations vary depending on sites of organ involvement and may include localized or generalized skin disease, generalized sicca syndrome, severe oral and esophageal mucositis, malabsorption, chronic liver disease, pulmonary insufficiency, polymyositis, recurrent bacterial infections, and generalized wasting. Pathologic findings are similar to those seen in several of the collagen-vascular diseases mentioned above.

Prognosis primarily depends on the extent of organ involvement. Limited disease characterized by localized skin involvement and/or liver involvement carries a favorable prognosis, while extensive disease characterized by generalized skin and/or multiorgan involvement carries a much poorer prognosis. Mode of onset also appears to be of prognostic value; patients with prior acute GVHD, especially if "progressive" (i.e., direct continuation of acute GVHD), have an unfavorable prognosis compared to those with "de novo" onset. Persistent thrombocytopenia beyond post-transplant day 100 has also been identified as a poor prognostic sign. As in acute GVHD, infection rather than end-organ failure is the major cause of death.

Treatment

Treatment of chronic GVHD is usually more successful than that of acute GVHD, if initiated prior to the development of fibrosis. Currently, combination immunosuppressive therapy with prednisone (1.0 mg per kilogram per day on alternate days) and azathioprine (1.5 mg per kilogram per day) appears to be most beneficial. Prednisone in combination with cyclophosphamide was shown to be equally effective but associated with greater toxicity, particularly hemorrhagic cystitis. Whether prednisone alone is equally efficacious is currently being evaluated by the Fred Hutchinson Cancer Research Center in a double-blind trial of placebo and prednisone versus prednisone and azathioprine. Duration of treatment varies depending on response but is frequently long term, as in other autoimmune disorders. Supportive measures, including prophylactic trimethoprim-sulfamethoxazole, sun-blocking creams, vigorous oral hygiene, and artificial tears are also recommended.

Prophylaxis

The role of prophylaxis in chronic GVHD has been inadequately studied. To date, neither corticosteroids nor thymic tissue transplantation has demonstrated reproducible efficacy in its prevention.

Treatment of Gastrointestinal Involvement

Chronic liver disease is the most frequent gastrointestinal manifestation of chronic GVHD. Because of the absence of pathognomonic features, diagnosis rests on the presence of persistent elevations of alkaline phosphatase (5 to 10 times normal), characteristic histologic findings resembling those of primary biliary cirrhosis, and other clinical manifestations of chronic GVHD. In patients in whom chronic GVHD involves only the liver, the diagnosis becomes more ambiguous and other etiologic agents, such as viral and fungal infections, sepsis, drugs, and recurrence of the underlying disease, should be considered. Treatment strategies are based on the extent of the chronic GVHD. Those with extensive disease generally receive immunosuppressive therapy as outlined above, whereas those with disease confined to the liver receive only supportive care. Such measures may include nutritional supplementation, cholestyramine for pruritus, and vitamin K when indicated.

Esophageal involvement is characterized by a desquamative esophagitis which, if left untreated, can progress and result in stricture and web formation. Early aggressive therapy with azathioprine and prednisone is effective in treating the inflammatory component and in preventing the fibrotic complicatins. Additional measures, such as antacids, H_2 blockers, and head-of-bed elevation may afford more rapid symptomatic relief than immunosuppressive therapy alone. Patients remaining unresponsive to this approach should be evaluated for other possible causes, especially infection. Strictures and webs are managed in the usual manner with peroral dilation.

Malabsorption with steatorrhea is another problem occasionally encountered in these patients. Its pathogenesis, however, remains an enigma. In contradistinction to acute GVHD, mucosal damage is not a prominent feature of intestinal involvement in chronic GVHD, as demonstrated by normal histologic findings and tests of mucosal integrity, such as the D-xylose absorption assay. Infectious causes, including bacterial overgrowth, should be excluded in all cases. Management is primarily supportive unless a specific treatable etiologic agent is found.

GASTROINTESTINAL INFECTIONS FOLLOWING TRANSPLANTATION

Infectious complications are a formidable problem in the management of bone marrow transplant recipients. The gastrointestinal tract plays an integral role, since it is not only a common site of localized infections but also the source of many systemic infections. Decreased host resistance due to mucosal damage, neutropenia, and profound immunosuppression is responsible for this heightened susceptibility. This discussion will focus on the treatment of specific infections involving the gastrointestinal tract.

Bacterial Infections

Bacterial infections confined to the gastrointestinal tract are relatively uncommon, with the exception of *Clostridium difficile* enterocolitis. Esophageal infections caused by *Corynebacteria* species, which are gram-positive cocci, are occasionally encountered but usually in the setting of coincidental oropharyngeal corynebacterial infections or superinfection of viral ulcerations. Common enteric pathogens are not a problem because of isolation and decontamination measures, including sterilization of food.

C. difficile toxin enterocolitis is treated as in the immunocompetent host. Oral vancomycin (500 mg orally every 6 hours for 7 to 14 days) is the treatment of choice. Alternative therapies include bacitracin (25,000 units orally every 6 hours) and metronidazole (500 mg orally every 8 hours). Cholestyramine, a resin which binds the toxin, is occasionally used in mildly ill immunocompetent hosts but should be avoided in immunocompromised patients. In non-neutropenic patients with adynamic ileus, vancomycin can be given by enema (1 g in 1 L of saline every 6 hours) alone or in combination with systemic vancomycin, metronidazole, or both.

Other bacterial infections should be treated as indicated by culture sensitivity results.

Fungal Infections

Candidiasis is the most common fungal infection of the gastrointestinal system. These infections may be localized to the esophagus and/or stomach or involve the entire gastrointestinal tract. Endoscopic and radiographic findings are generally nonspecific, since viral infections can produce similar abnormalities. Accurate diagnosis generally requires histologic demonstration of invasive mycelia on biopsy specimens since the presence of yeast forms without mycelia, or positive oropharyngeal or stool cultures may represent colonization only. Regardless, aggressive therapy is warranted in all neutropenic patients with any of these findings, since there is good correlation between colonization and the subsequent development of invasive disease with dissemination. Systemic therapy with amphotericin B is indicated in all such patients. Although "low-dose" (0.3 mg per kilogram per day) therapy is advocated by some, we prefer full-dose (1.0 mg per kilogram per day) therapy, since disseminated disease is difficult to document. Combination therapy with Amphotericin B and 5-Fluorocytosine (50 mg per kilogram per day) may be indicated for infections caused by *Candida tropicalis*. In non-neutropenic patients, oral therapy with nystatin, ketoconazole, or miconazole may be adequate.

Viral Infections

Herpes viruses including cytomegalovirus (CMV), herpes simplex virus (HSV), and varicella zoster viruses (VZV) are responsible for the majority of gastrointestinal infections in transplant recipients. Acyclovir (250 mg per m^2 every 8 hours) has repeatedly demonstrated efficacy in the prevention and treatment of HSV and VZV infections but is ineffective in the management of CMV infections. To date, there is no effective prophylaxis or treatment for CMV infections. Prophylactic hyperimmune globulin has been touted as a potentially effective prophylactic measure but, at present, requires further investigation. Vaccination is another approach currently under investigation.

Viral gastroenteritis has also been a common problem following transplantation. Adenovirus and coxsackievirus are the usual causative organisms. Treatment is primarily supportive because no effective therapy exists. Antidiarrheal agents should be avoided in this setting. Persistant viral enteritis, as evidenced by stool ELISA assays, has been a poor prognostic sign in at least one center.

Parasitic Infections

Sporadic cases of cryptosporidiosis have recently been reported in bone marrow transplant recipients. The illness is characterized by severe, life-threatening watery diarrhea, malabsorption, and fever, similar to symptoms in patients with acquired immunodeficiency syndrome. Person-to-person transmission has been implicated. Spiramycin (3 g per day in divided doses), an experimental macrolide antibiotic, has had anecdotal success but has generally been ineffective. Supportive care remains the mainstay of treatment.

ALLERGIC GASTROENTEROPATHY

DANIEL G. MALONE, M.D.
DEAN D. METCALFE, M.D.

The term *allergic gastroenteropathy* in this chapter will be used to refer to those diseases of the gastrointestinal tract, exclusive of gluten-sensitive enteropathy, which appear due to abnormal responses to food substances. These include *food protein-induced gastrointestinal disease of newborns and infants, eosinophilic gastroenteritis*, and *transient IgE-mediated immediate hypersensitivity reactions* in which the initial target organ is the gastrointestinal tract. These disorders cause a wide spectrum of signs and symptoms, not necessarily limited to the gastrointestinal tract. Principles of diagnosis and therapy are generally similar in these disorders. Since the choice of therapy depends on the mechanisms underlying the symptoms, it is important to recognize the additional nonimmunologic types of adverse reactions due to food, and the terminology that has been formulated to classify them (Table 1). Immediate reactions to foods, and some forms of eosinophilic gastroenteritis and adverse reactions to foods in infants are due to type I, or anaphylactic, immune reactions. Such responses are mediated by chemicals released from blood-borne basophils or tissue mast cells after interactions on the cell surfaces between antigen-specific IgE (affixed to the mast cell/basophil by the Fc receptor) and the antigen against which the IgE is directed. The other types of immune reactions to food antigens are thought to result from mechanisms not primarily involving IgE, and may account for some of the manifestations of food protein-induced gastrointestinal diseases of newborns and infants. Non-IgE-mediated reactions cause a wider range of symptoms than the rather easily recognized type I reactions. For example, children sensitive to milk and/or soy proteins may present not only with signs and symptoms consistent with immediate hypersensitivity responses, but also with enterocolitis with severe diarrhea, dehydration with electrolyte imbalance, and even failure to thrive due to malnutrition. In the latter case, colonic mucosa may show ulceration, inflammation, and villous atrophy. Immune complex deposition and activation of the complement cascade are two non-IgE-mediated immune mechanisms proposed as culpable in this disorder.

TABLE 1 Definitions Relative to Adverse Reactions to Foods

Term	Definition
Adverse reaction to a food	Clinically abnormal response believed caused by an ingested food or food additive
Food hypersensitivity (allergy)	Immunologic reaction resulting from the ingestion of a food or food additive
Food anaphylaxis	Classic allergic hypersensitivity reaction to food or food additives involving IgE and release of chemical mediators
Food idiosyncrasy	Quantitatively abnormal response to a food or food additive; response differs from its physiologic or pharmacologic effect and resembles a hypersensitivity reaction but does not involve an immune mechanism; anaphylaxis-like reaction may be called "anaphylactoid"
Food intolerance	General term describing an abnormal physiologic response to an ingested food additive that is *not* proved to be immunologic in nature; category includes idiosyncratic, pharmacologic, metabolic, or toxic responses to food or food additives
Food toxicity (poisoning)	Term implying an adverse effect caused by direct action of a food or food additive on host recipient without the involvement of immune mechanisms; nonimmune release of chemical mediators may take place; toxins may be either from the food itself or from microorganisms; anaphylaxis-like reaction may be called "anaphylactoid"
Anaphylactoid reaction to a food	Anaphylaxis-like reaction to a food or food additive as a result of non-immune release of chemical mediators
Pharmacologic food reaction	Adverse reaction to a food or food additive as a result of a naturally derived or added chemical that produces a drug-like or pharmacologic effect in the host
Metabolic food reaction	Adverse reaction to a food or food additive as the result of the effect of the substance on the metabolism of the host recipient

DIAGNOSIS

Although the public generally perceives hypersensitivity reactions to foods as a major cause of morbidity, the scientific literature suggests that most disorders blamed on abnormal responses to foods are in fact due to other causes. Table 2 is a partial list of possibilities to be considered in the differential diagnosis of allergic gastroenteropathy. A careful history and a physical examination are essential to identify the cause of an often baffling array of symptoms. Careful scrutiny may reveal inciting substances such as gluten or sulfiting agents in processed foods, often to the surprise of both doctor and patient.

The initial diagnosis of any allergic gastroenteropathy may be supported by a variety of dietary manipulations and laboratory tests, the use of which must be tailored to each patient. Eliminating suspected foods from the diet is one method of identifying offending substances. When judged safe, a careful reintroduction of such foods resulting in a return of symptoms is reasonable confirmatory evidence.

If removal of one or several foods from the diet fails to eliminate symptoms, if multiple food sensitivities are

TABLE 2 Differential Diagnosis of Food Hypersensitivity*

I. Additives and contaminants
   A. Dyes
      1. Tartrazine
   B. Flavorings and preservatives
      1. Nitrites and nitrates
      2. Monosodium glutamate
      3. Sulfiting agents
      4. Sodium benzoate
   C. Toxins
      1. Bacterial
         a. Botulism
         b. Staphylococcal intoxication
      2. Mushroom toxins
      3. Mycotoxins (aflatoxins)
      4. Seafood-associated
         a. Saxitoxin (shellfish)
         b. Scombroid poisoning (histamine)
         c. Ciguatera poisoning (fresh reef fishes as grouper, snapper)
   D. Infectious organisms
      1. Bacteria
         a. Salmonellosis
      2. Parasites
         a. Giardiasis
         b. Trichinosis
         c. Diphyllobothriasis
      3. Viruses
         a. Hepatitis
   E. Insect parts
   F. Mold antigens
   G. Accidental contaminants
      1. Heavy metals
      2. Pesticides
      3. Antibiotics

II. Gastrointestinal diseases
   A. Structural abnormalities
      1. Hiatal hernia
      2. Internal obstruction
   B. Enzyme deficiencies
      1. Lactase deficiency
      2. Glucose-6-phosphate dehydrogenase deficiency
      3. Galactosemia
   C. Malignancy
   D. Other
      1. Peptic ulcer disease
      2. Gallbladder disease
      3. Cystic fibrosis
III. Endogenous pharmacologic agents
   A. Caffeine
   B. Theobromine
   C. Histamine
   D. Tyramine
   E. Tryptamine
   F. Dopamine
   G. Norepinephrine
   H. Serotonin
   I. Phenylethylamine
   J. Alcohol
   K. Hallucinogenic alkaloids
IV. Psychological reactions
V. Other
   A. Collagen-vascular diseases
   B. Endocrine disorders

* The list is not comprehensive. Examples only are given.

suspected, or if symptoms are thought not to be due to food sensitivities, initiation of a severely limited diet under a physician's supervision may be indicated. If symptoms persist while the patient is on the limited diet, the possibility that the disorder is related to an adverse reaction to food can be eliminated.

Severely limited diets, especially in children, are employed for only short periods of time (7 to 14 days). For infants under 3 months of age, these regimens may include breast milk or milk substitute (Table 3) alone; for infants 3 to 6 months of age breast milk or rice cereal plus milk substitute; for children 6 months to 2 years milk substitute with vitamin supplements, rice cereal, applesauce, pears, carrots, squash, and lamb; and for older children and adults lamb and rice (Table 4) or the use of an elemental diet (e.g., Vivonex). Care must be taken to ensure that the individual takes nothing by mouth except foods specified in the diet, and avoids oral and topical medications when possible.

Skin testing is also of value in diagnosis of IgE-mediated transient adverse reactions to foods, since persons with negative skin tests to a particular antigen are usually found not to be sensitive to that antigen (that is, false negative skin tests are uncommon). In patients with a history of anaphylactic reactions, for whom food challenge or skin testing is felt to be too risky, testing the serum for antigen-specific IgE by the enzyme-linked immunoabsorbent assay (ELISA) or radioallergosorbent test (RAST) may be helpful, although neither is as sensitive as skin testing. Challenge of the patient's peripheral blood basophils in vitro with the suspected allergen to determine the amount of histamine release is expensive, time-consuming, difficult to perform, and generally no more reliable than the other methods mentioned above. There are insufficient convincing data to support the use of in vitro cytotoxicity testing (in which the putative allergen induces death of the patient's white blood cells in vitro), or sublingual or subcutaneous challenges with suspected allergens, in the diagnostic work-up of allergic gastroenteritis.

TABLE 3 Substitute Formulas for Cow's Milk Allergy

Breast milk

Soy-based formulas, such as
Isomil, ProSobee, Neo-Mull-Soy

Elemental formulas, such as
Vivonex, Pregestimil

TABLE 4 Lamb and Rice Diet

Foods allowed

Brown rice—natural, long grain, short grain; par boiled
White rice—enriched, converted; cook without added fat
Brown or white rice flour
Brown rice cakes—containing *only* brown rice and salt (if desired)
Puffed Rice Cereal—containing only brown rice
Lamb
Water
Salt

All food must be prepared without added fat. Rice, lamb, salt, and water are the only allowable foods. No food containing any other ingredients is to be eaten. Check labels. Salt or baking soda should be used to brush the teeth.

Eliminate

All foods not listed above, especially coffee, tea, soft drinks, juices, chewing gum, toothpaste, vitamins, aspirin, and any medication not ordered by a doctor must be eliminated.

Possible Menu

Breakfast	*Lunch*	*Dinner*	*Snack*
Rice mush	Rice patties	Rice and lamb sauté	Rice cakes
		Pan-fried lamb chops	

Instructions

Stay on basic diet for ____ days.
Then, on ____ add ____ all by itself, first thing in A.M.
Then, on ____ add ____ all by itself, first thing in A.M.
Then, on ____ add ____ all by itself, first thing in A.M.
Next, on ____ add ____ all by itself, first thing in A.M.
Next, on ____ add ____ all by itself, first thing in A.M.

Continue food additions one at a time at ____ day intervals until most or all other foods in the diet have been tested. Keep a diet diary as indicated. Add foods in large amounts, and eat them several times a day during addition period.

TREATMENT

Young patients with mild, non-life-threatening symptoms from food sensitivity, such as those seen in food protein-induced gastrointestinal disease of infants and newborns or acute transient IgE-mediated reactions, are best treated by preventive measures and avoidance of the offending food. In infants this may require the use of one of the elemental formulas in Table 3. Since milk protein sensitivity appears to be more common in children from atopic families, mothers of newborn infants from such families should be advised to breast feed their infants when possible. Also, the mothers themselves should minimize ingestion of more highly allergenic foods, such as soybean products, codfish, peanuts, crustaceans, cow's and goat's milk, and egg proteins, as allergenic substances may be transferred in breast milk. If the disorder has resulted in severe malnutrition, total parenteral nutrition may be indicated. In milk-sensitive patients, goat's milk should be avoided, since children sensitive to cow's milk are often sensitive to similar antigens in goat's milk as well. In children who present with severe disease, a short course of oral corticosteroid therapy (e.g., prednisone, 1 mg per kilogram per day) is occasionally necessary, care being taken to minimize the dose and duration of steroid therapy. When the child's clinical status has improved, gradual restoration of foods to the diet while watching for the return of symptoms is a good way simultaneously to normalize the diet and identify further offending allergens. As the child grows older, the offending food itself may be carefully reintroduced, as some children who are sensitive to food allergens at early ages outgrow the condition and are able to tolerate the food without undue incident later in life.

In all age groups, generalized life-threatening IgE-mediated acute hypersensitivity (anaphylactic) reactions caused by ingestion of food allergens may occur in patients with allergic gastroenteritis. These are treated in the same way as other anaphylactic reactions. The identity of the causative allergen has little bearing on the management of the reaction. Epinephrine, intravenous fluids, pressor drugs, and H_1 histamine receptor antagonists such as diphenhydramine are the mainstays of treatment. Intravenous administration of H_2 histamine receptor antagonists, such as cimetidine and ranitidine, may be useful in combating hypotension resistant to fluid therapy and first line pressor agents in anaphylactic shock. Prevention should be stressed in patients who suffer these types of life-threatening reactions, and knowledge of what foods contain the offending allergen is essential. A dietician can be quite helpful in providing educational materials and instruction to these patients, and the importance of such instruction cannot be overemphasized. Since inadvertent ingestion of allergen is by no means uncommon, sensitive individuals should carry preloaded syringes of

TABLE 5 Common Food Groupings*

Animal

Crustacea	Pelecypoda	Cephalopoda	Osteichthyes
Shrimp	Oyster	Octopus	Sardine
Crab	Clam	Squid	Trout
Lobster	Scallop		Salmon
Crayfish	Abalone		Whitefish

Vegetable

Bromeliaceae	Gramineae	Leguminosae	Rutaceae
Pineapple	Barley	Kidney bean	Lemon
Chenopodiaceae	Corn	Lima bean	Grapefruit
Spinach	Oats	String bean	Orange
Compositae	Rye	Pea	Solanaceae
Lettuce	Wheat	Peanut	White potato
Cruciferae	Rice	Soybean	Chili pepper
Horseradish	Juglandaceae	Liliaceae	Tomato
Cabbage	English walnut	Garlic	Sterculiaceae
Mustard	Pecan	Onion	Chocolate
Cucurbitaceae	Lauraceae	Asparagus	Cola
Squash	Cinnamon	Palmaceae	Umbelliferae
Cantaloupe	Bay leaf	Coconut	Carrot
Watermelon		Polygonaceae	Caraway seed
Cucumber		Buckwheat	Dill
Drupaceae		Pomaceae	Celery
Almond		Apple	
Plum		Pear	
Peach		Rosaceae	
Apricot		Strawberry	
Cherry			

* Examples only

epinephrine on their persons at all times and be taught how to self-administer the drug. In addition, they should carry an identification bracelet or card clearly stating the particulars of their allergic condition.

In adults, as in children, the most important form of therapy for acute IgE-mediated reactions to foods is dietary avoidance. Care must be taken to ensure that the diet delivers palatable, optimal nutritional intake while completely eliminating the causative allergen. The patient should be given a working knowledge of botanic families as well as the classification of foods from animal sources, since cross-reacting antigens may be found among foods in the same group (Table 5). Learning to recognize foods that may contain allergen in a "hidden" form is also useful in minimizing symptoms. For example, a primary ingredient in mayonnaise is egg.

Gastrointestinal symptoms may improve with orally administered H_1 receptor antagonists, although some experts feel that symptoms in the lower gastrointestinal tract do not respond as well as do symptoms in the mouth and oropharynx. Short-term systemic corticosteroid therapy may be used to control severe gastrointestinal symptoms of food allergy (distinctly rare in adults). Such treatment is reserved for patients with *eosinophilic gastroenteritis*, a rare disorder in which oral corticosteroids are usually effective, or *protein-losing gastroenteropathy* (discussed in another chapter). In such instances, a short course of therapy is usually given, and the medication is discontinued after the dose has been carefully tapered from 60 mg per day as symptoms resolve. It is advisable to switch to an alternate-day dosage program as early in the course of treatment as possible.

Some patients with eosinophilic gastroenteritis have IgE-mediated hypersensitivity reactions to multiple (up to 15) foods. The use of elimination diets in these individuals is usually unsuccessful owing to the complexity of design and the difficulty of compliance with such intricate diets.

While there is some evidence suggesting that inhibitors of prostaglandin synthesis, such as indomethacin, ibuprofen, and so on, are useful in the treatment of gastrointestinal symptoms of food allergy, more definitive studies are needed before such agents can be recommended for routine use. Much the same can be said for the use of disodium cromoglycate, especially since no formulation of the drug for oral ingestion is available in the United States, and the Food and Drug Administration has not approved its use in allergic gastroenteropathy of any kind. In addition, the capsules dispensed for use in inhalers contain lactose, which could exacerbate gastrointestinal symptoms.

Drug therapy is also used to treat IgE-mediated systemic symptoms that may also accompany the inadvertent ingestion of the allergen, or as a prophylactic measure, although evidence in support of the latter is less clear cut. The choice of agents depends in large part on which organ system is affected. Urticaria, conjunctivitis, rhinitis, and angioedema caused by food allergens often respond to orally administered H_1 receptor antagonists such as chlorpheniramine (4 mg 3 to 4 times daily) and diphenhydramine hydrochloride (25 to 50 mg 3 to 4 times daily). Topical steroid preparations are useful in treating eczema which occasionally accompanies food allergy.

Treatment of food allergen-induced bronchospasm is identical to that of bronchospasm induced by any other allergen, whether inhaled, injected, ingested, or absorbed through the skin. Inhaled beta-adrenergic agents are an acceptable and effective therapy for this condition. One must be aware, however, that inhalant beta-agonists may contain sulfiting agents as preservatives, with obvious ramifications in sulfite-sensitive patients.

The use of immunotherapy in the treatment of any form of allergic gastroenteropathy cannot be recommended at present, since there is as yet no evidence that significant benefit is derived from oral desensitization or injection immunotherapy. More detailed studies using proper control groups and proven methods of evaluation are needed before the value of immunotherapy can be judged.

PROTEIN-LOSING ENTEROPATHY

DANIEL W. THOMAS, M.D.

The gastrointestinal tract plays an integral role in normal protein catabolism. There is a large endogenous pool of approximately 35 to 100 g of protein that is recycled through the gut each day. These endogenous proteins are derived primarily from sloughed cellular debris and intestinal secretions. Transmucosal leakage of serum proteins into the gut occurs normally and also contributes to protein turnover. It has been estimated by radiolabeled albumin studies that enteric loss of serum protein accounts for less than 10 percent of daily protein catabolism. Bacterial and intestinal proteases digest intraluminal proteins, regardless of their source, and the nitrogenous end products are then available for metabolic utilization after being absorbed from the gut. Intestinal absorption of the end products of dietary and endogenous protein degradation is usually very efficient, as less than 2 g of nitrogen per day is excreted in the stool of healthy individuals.

Protein-losing enteropathy (PLE), sometimes termed exudative enteropathy, refers to a condition in which there is excessive transmucosal leakage of serum protein into the gastrointestinal tract. Such exudative losses can eventually lead to hypoproteinemia if synthesis of new serum proteins does not compensate for these deficits. All classes of serum protein are lost in exudative enteropathies; however, the serum levels of the proteins with the longest half-lives, such as albumin, are the most profoundly reduced. Severe hypoproteinemia can occur if patients with PLE have a concomitant hypercatabolic state, inadequate nutritional intake, intestinal malabsorption of dietary and endogenous protein, or other sites of serum protein loss.

Protein-losing enteropathy is frequently associated with a wide variety of gastrointestinal disorders (Table 1). The mechanism of exudative loss is not known in every case, but it is generally thought that at least three different processes may be responsible. Abnormal transmucosal protein efflux is possible when there is mucosal erosion, epithelial cell alteration, or impairment of lymphatic flow. Hence, PLE is an important, albeit nonspecific, sign of gastrointestinal mucosal dysfunction.

RECOGNITION

Several techniques have been employed in an attempt to detect PLE. Assay of fecal nitrogen excretion is inadequate because azotorrhea as a consequence of dietary

TABLE 1 Established Causes and Mechanisms of Protein-Losing Enteropathy

Mucosal Erosion
   Crohn's disease
   Chronic ulcerative colitis
   Enterocolitis (radiation, milk allergy, infectious, parasitic, vasculitic)
   Carcinomas

Mucosal Alteration
   Gastrointestinal polyps
   Hypertrophic gastritis/enteritis
   Celiac disease
   Allergic gastroenteropathy
   Parasitic infestations
   Tropical sprue
   Whipple's disease
   Graft-versus-host disease
   Vasculitic disorders

Impaired Lymphatic Dynamics
   Primary lymphangiectasia
   Secondary lymphangiectasia:
     Lymphoma
     Abdominal tuberculosis
     Graft-versus-host disease
     Crohn's disease
     Radiation enteritis
     Congestive heart failure
     Superior vena cava/venous obstruction
     Constrictive pericarditis
     Lymphenteric fistula
     Scleroderma
     Retroperitoneal fibrosis/tumors
     Mesenteric tumors/inflammation
     Parasitic infestation

Note: Some disorders may result in protein-losing enteropathy by more than one mechanism.

protein malabsorption cannot be distinguished from exudative enteropathy. Also, fecal nitrogen excretion may remain in the normal range despite the presence of exudative protein loss. This occurs because of rapid intraluminal proteolysis of the exuded protein into the gut and subsequent reabsorption of constituent amino acids. For the same reason, direct quantitation of specific serum proteins in the intestinal secretions and feces of patients suspected of having PLE has not been successful until recently.

The diagnosis of PLE in the past was most often the result of esoteric curiosity in the evaluation of patients with "idiopathic hypoproteinemia." Cumbersome and impractical radiolabeled protein excretion studies actually restricted the number of patients in whom PLE could be used as a clinical tool in the recognition and management of gastrointestinal diseases. Intravenous administration of ^{51}Cr-albumin and scintillation assay of fecal excretion has been the method of choice for demonstrating exudative enteropathies for almost 20 years. This technique has numerous disadvantages which make it impractical for routine patient screening and serial clinical assessment, including high cost, required hospitalization, the use of radioactive materials, and tedious stool collections. Since the availability of ^{51}Cr-albumin currently is restricted, there is a need to develop other techniques to diagnose PLE.

Exudative enteropathies can now be reliably detected by measuring fecal alpha$_1$-antitrypsin (FA$_1$AT) excretion. Alpha$_1$-antitrypsin (A$_1$AT) is a serum protein that is an antiprotease. When it is leaked from the serum into the intestine, it is excreted into the stool undegraded. Approximately 4 percent of the total serum protein content is comprised of A$_1$AT under normal conditions. It has a molecular weight of about 50,000 daltons, which is similar to that of albumin. Thus, FA$_1$AT excretion should parallel enteric loss of albumin. This has been confirmed by performing concomitant FA$_1$AT and ^{51}Cr-albumin excretion assays in patients with PLE. Abnormal FA$_1$AT concentrations have been found in a wide range of gastrointestinal disorders previously known to cause exudative enteropathies.

Determination of FA$_1$AT excretion can be accomplished by measuring random stool concentrations or intestinal A$_1$AT clearance. The following formula is used to calculate intestinal A$_1$AT clearance:

$$\text{daily A}_1\text{AT clearance (ml serum/day)} = \frac{\text{FA}_1\text{AT (mg/g stool)} \times \text{stool wt/day (g stool/day)}}{\text{serum A}_1\text{AT concentration (mg/100 ml)}}$$

Only a small aliquot of stool (less than 5 g) is required to quantitate FA$_1$AT concentration. Our laboratory performs random FA$_1$AT determinations by first lyophilizing the stool to eliminate variation in water content. Lyophilized stool samples are extracted in saline (in a given volume to weight ratio) and then centrifuged. A small aliquot of the resultant supernatant is assayed for A$_1$AT content by radial immunodiffusion. Fecal A$_1$AT concentrations to be used for deriving daily clearance are assayed on aliquots taken from 24- to 72-hour stool collections.

Slight variation in the range of values for FA$_1$AT concentrations has occurred between different laboratories but there have been no major discrepancies. These differences most likely represent minor variations in technique. Some investigators determine FA$_1$AT content on unlyophilized stool samples and others have used different methods of quantification, such as rocket electrophoresis. One should first standardize the method to be used within one's own laboratory and then establish the range for normal FA$_1$AT excretion before applying the assay to routine clinical use.

In our laboratory, normal individuals excrete approximately 1 mg of A$_1$AT per gram dry weight of stool. This value holds true for all ages except for children under 1 year. Young breast-fed infants tend to have higher random FA$_1$AT concentrations, but this difference is probably not of biologic importance. Total daily FA$_1$AT excretion for infants receiving human milk is similar to that for infants receiving other types of milk feedings. The small amounts of FA$_1$AT normally excreted by healthy individuals is probably derived from bile and/or low levels of transmucosal protein efflux from the gut.

Fecal A$_1$AT assays are simple and inexpensive to perform, noninvasive, suitable for serial patient assessment, and do not require hospitalization. Additionally, A$_1$AT is stable in stool samples for long periods. Almost 92 percent of the A$_1$AT content is retained in stool incubated at 37 °C for three days. Specimens can be frozen and saved indefinitely for later analysis.

One might argue that FA$_1$AT determinations on random fecal specimens are suboptimal and subject to variability due to differing stool patterns. Utilizing our particular method of determination, however, random FA$_1$AT concentrations in healthy persons are surprisingly constant and reproducible from day to day. There is a high degree of direct correlation between random FA$_1$AT concentration and intestinal A$_1$AT clearance. This suggests that random determinations are adequate for detecting PLE.

Nevertheless, many investigators have preferred to express FA$_1$AT excretion as intestinal clearance. There are some theoretical flaws in utilizing clearance. Since A$_1$AT is an acute phase reactant for which deficiency states occur, serum concentrations could potentially be affected and result in falsely altered intestinal clearance values. It is implied that A$_1$AT clearance from the serum to the gut is a passive process, but this may not necessarily be the case. Patients with very high serum A$_1$AT concentrations due to systemic illnesses usually have normal random FA$_1$AT concentrations. As one might suspect, there is little correlation between serum and fecal A$_1$AT concentrations. Normal A$_1$AT clearance has been found to be less than or equal to 12 ml per day. This value is somewhat different than the calculated normal intestinal albumin clearance of less than or equal to 40 ml per day.

Abnormal FA_1AT excretion is indicative of intestinal mucosal dysfunction caused by one of the mechanisms already mentioned. Patients with intraluminal malabsorption have normal FA_1AT excretion. Thus, dietary sources do not contribute to FA_1AT excretion. This is attributable in part to inactivation of A_1AT in the acid environment of the stomach. Individuals with protein-losing gastropathies usually do not have abnormal FA_1AT excretion unless they also have achlorhydria.

MANAGEMENT

There is no uniform therapy for patients with exudative enteropathy, since it is a nonspecific indicator of intestinal mucosal dysfunction with numerous potential etiologies. The value of the diagnosis of PLE is in the recognition of the existence of a gastrointestinal disorder and its availability as a tool by which to follow the clinical course and response to therapy.

Patients with unexplained hypoproteinemia or who are suspected of having intestinal mucosal dysfunction, whether due to mucosal damage or impaired lymphatic flow, can easily undergo initial screening by measuring FA_1AT excretion. Some patients without hypoproteinemia have abnormal FA_1AT excretion. Hence, a normal serum albumin concentration does not rule out the existence of an exudative enteropathy. Mucosal versus intraluminal digestive defects can be first examined by obtaining both fecal fat and FA_1AT excretion tests. A normal FA_1AT assay in the presence of steatorrhea is suggestive of an intraluminal cause of malabsorption. This is an example of how recently developed noninvasive screening tests can aid in the detection of gastrointestinal disorders and provide an indication for performing more specifically directed diagnostic procedures.

The remainder of this chapter is devoted to the evaluation and management of two disorders which commonly result in exudative enteropathy: Crohn's disease and intestinal lymphangiectasia. Emphasis will be placed on diagnostic evaluation. A more detailed approach to therapy of Crohn's disease is presented in chapters: *Crohn's Disease of the Small Bowel, Growth Failure in Inflammatory Bowel Disease*, and *Crohn's Disease: Surgical Treatment*.

CROHN'S DISEASE

Despite its relatively common occurrence, the recognition of Crohn's disease is often delayed because of the variability and unpredictability of the clinical manifestations. This is especially true in children and adolescents, when this disease is often confused with other illnesses and functional bowel disorders. While invasive procedures and intestinal radiographs are usually necessary to confirm the diagnosis, a few simple noninvasive screening

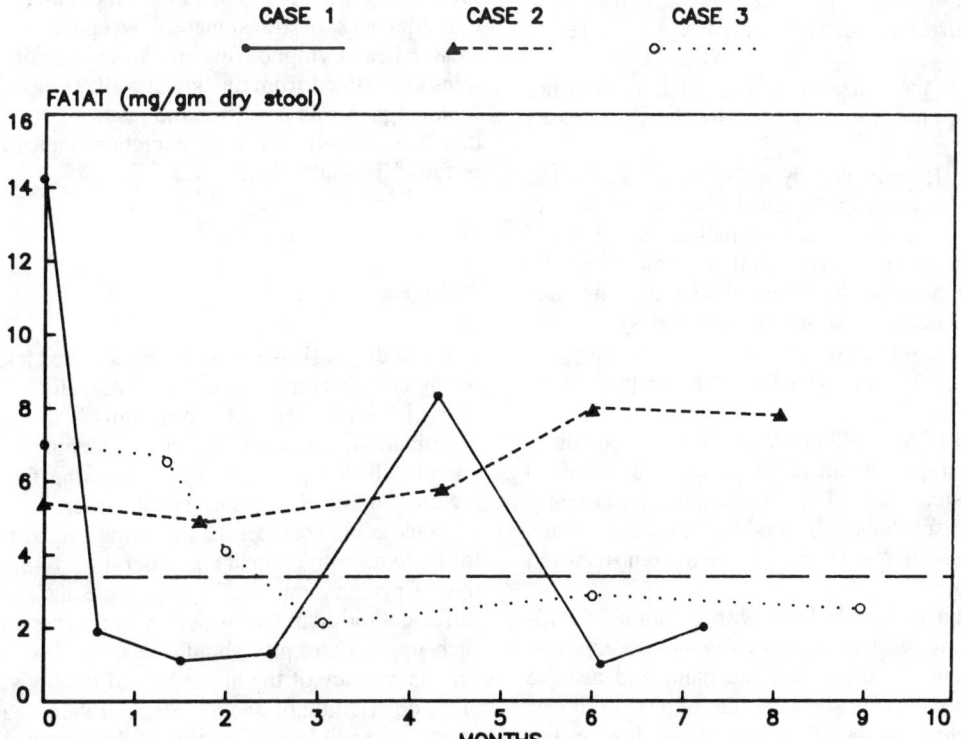

Figure 1 Serial fecal alpha$_1$-antitrypsin (FA_1AT) concentrations are shown for three adolescents with Crohn's disease. The dashed horizontal line at a FA_1AT of 3.4 mg per gram dry stool is representative of the mean value +3 SD for a group of normal subjects. See text for case descriptions.

tests are helpful in selecting patients who warrant further studies.

Exudative enteropathy is one of the most common functional abnormalities of the bowel in patients with Crohn's disease. We have found that measuring FA_1AT excretion is an invaluable diagnostic tool. Seventeen of the first 18 patients with Crohn's disease whom we tested had abnormal FA_1AT concentrations. In fact, Crohn's disease is unlikely in the absence of one of the following findings: anemia, hypoalbuminemia, an elevated erythrocyte sedimentation rate, occult fecal blood loss, stool leukocytes, change in growth velocity, or abnormal FA_1AT excretion. Colonoscopy and/or intestinal radiographs are appropriate if the clinical and laboratory findings are consistent with this diagnosis.

Monitoring Therapeutic Response

Measurement of FA_1AT is also useful in monitoring therapeutic response. Since FA_1AT excretion reflects active intestinal disease, it is also a useful guideline by which to rate disease activity. There is a high degree of correlation between the presence of clinically active disease and abnormal FA_1AT excretion. A direct linear correlation has not been evident, however. This may well be attributable to the frequent discordance of clinical disease activity and severity of intestinal inflammation. Disease activity scores are comprised of subjective criteria (abdominal pain and general well-being) and laboratory tests indirectly indicative of active intestinal inflammation (elevated erythrocyte sedimentation rate, leukocytosis, and anemia) which make direct correlation with FA_1AT excretion difficult.

Examples of the utilization of FA_1AT in monitoring therapeutic response are illustrated by the three cases shown in Figure 1.

Case 1 is a 15-year-old boy with Crohn's ileitis and short stature. He underwent surgical resection of the terminal ileum and had subsequent normalization of FA_1AT excretion in association with clinical remission. His FA_1AT excretion was again abnormal 4 months after surgery. This preceded the onset of intestinal symptoms. Recurrent disease was demonstrated in the remaining ileum and proximal colon. His flare was responsive to prednisone.

Case 2 is a 17-year-old boy with Crohn's ileocolitis. Rapid clinical improvement occurred after he began to receive prednisone but his FA_1AT remained persistently abnormal. He discontinued the prednisone after 6 months of therapy because he "felt well." His symptoms recurred a short time later.

Case 3 is an 11-year-old girl with Crohn's ileocolitis. Her symptoms resolved while on low-dose prednisone and sulfasalazine. Fever, abdominal pain, and malaise were noted 4 months after she went into remission. It was initially suspected that she had a flare of her disease, but her FA_1AT was normal. It was soon discovered that she had a urinary tract infection which was successfully treated. Her symptoms then resolved.

INTESTINAL LYMPHANGIECTASIA

Primary intestinal lymphangiectasia occurs infrequently and is thought to result from a generalized congenital disturbance of the lymphatic system. It is sometimes associated with other inherited disorders, such as Turner's and Noonan's syndromes. Varying degrees of both visceral and limb lymphatic abnormalities are apparent in affected individuals. Clinical manifestations usually are present before 10 years of age but may be delayed until early adulthood. Typical findings include growth failure, intermittent diarrhea, abdominal distention, hypocalcemic tetany, malabsorptive stools, and asymmetric, nonpitting edema of the extremities. Reversible blindness is present occasionally in individuals with associated macular edema. Chylous effusions are not uncommon in severely affected patients. The course is unpredictable, as spontaneous relapses and remissions are frequent.

The most common form of intestinal lymphangiectasia usually occurs later in life and is secondary to other diseases. Acquired intestinal lymphangiectasia can result from impediment of venous flow to the heart, localized intra-abdominal lesions, retroperitoneal lymphatic obstruction, or acquired diseases of the bowel itself. These disorders are listed in Table 1.

The pathogenesis of intestinal lymphangiectasia is due to obstruction of the lymphatics at any level of the bowel. Lymph is lost from dilated mucosal lacteals into the gut. Mucosal absorption of long-chain fatty acids and glycerides is also impaired. The laboratory findings reflect the consequences of transmucosal weeping of lymph and steatorrhea. Lymphocytes and all classes of serum proteins are exuded from the bowel wall. Hypocalcemia and hypomagnesemia are often the result of steatorrhea and diarrhea. Abnormal FA_1AT excretion, indicative of PLE, is found in most cases.

Diagnosis

The diagnosis of secondary or acquired intestinal lymphangiectasia is usually inferred after the causative disease is identified. A thorough history, physical examination, and a few selected screening tests are frequently all that is necessary in directing the evaluation toward finding the underlying disorder.

One could consider the following diagnostic approach for patients with clinical and laboratory findings suggestive of primary intestinal lymphangiectasia. A dynamic sulfur-colloid scan performed by intravenous injection of each upper extremity should be done first to establish venous patency of the upper half of the body. Unrecognized obstruction of one of the major veins leading to the heart can result in malfunction of the thoracic duct. If no venous obstruction is found, then a dynamic sulfur-colloid lymphatic scan should be done. The subcutaneous tissue of one of the interdigital spaces of the foot is injected for the scan. This procedure, unlike conventional lymphangiograms, is not uncomfortable and does not require specific localization of a lymphatic vessel for injection. The use of other radiolabeled macromolecules, such as dextran, may significantly shorten the time required for sequential imaging. Lymphatic scans are useful in recognizing aberrant or impaired flow. This technique is also capable of detecting lymphatic ectasia. The diagnosis of primary intestinal lymphangiectasia can then be confirmed by intestinal biopsy.

Other diagnostic procedures are useful in unusual cases. Computerized axial tomography is generally not helpful in examining the lymphatic system. Lymphatic cysts and other isolated lesions are rare but may be identified by this method. The use of intraoperative mesenteric lymphangiograms has been reported and could potentially be helpful in rare individuals with only a short segment of lymphangiectatic bowel.

Therapy

Therapy for intestinal lymphangiectasia depends on the cause. Management should be directed at the underlying disease in cases of secondary lymphangiectasia. Surgical correction is possible only in a few patients. Lesions amenable to surgery include rare cases of localized bowel involvement, isolated lymphatic cysts, neoplasms, and lymphenteric fistulas; surgery is also possible in patients with cardiovascular causes of impaired lymphatic flow. The successful creation of a lymph-venous fistula has been reported but is not yet a proven procedure. We have successfully inserted peritoneal-venous shunts in a small number of patients with refractory disease and complications due to chylous fluid collections, such as respiratory compromise. Peritoneal-venous shunts may be more widely utilized in the future.

Medical management includes dietary restriction of long-chain fats and sodium, supplemental fat-soluble vitamins if there is significant steatorrhea, and the occasional use of diuretics. Some patients with severe diarrhea require additional calcium and magnesium. Infants with intestinal lymphangiectasia can be fed Portagen, a 67 Kcal per deciliter formula in which the fat content is primarily medium-chain triglycerides (MCT). Intestinal absorption of MCT is via the portal system and is not dependent on normal lymphatic function. Adults can also be maintained on Portagen at a caloric density of up to 100 Kcal per deciliter. Many older children and adults do very well on a low-fat diet alone. It is inappropriate to repeatedly tap and discard chylous fluid collections. Repeated intravenous administration of colloids, especially plasma, is not recommended and is ineffective in managing this disorder.

A few patients who have severe intestinal lymphangiectasia with an inflammatory component are responsive to steroid therapy. Clinical improvement should occur soon after steroid therapy is initiated. Prolonged treatment with steroids is unwarranted if clinical improvement is not observed after a short period of time.

A fat-free diet is sometimes necessary in individuals with severe disease. Vivonex, an elemental formula which is almost fat-free, is well suited for use under these circumstances. Resolution of chylous fluid collections can be achieved and essential fatty acids may then gradually be added to the diet. Essential fatty acids can be given enterally in the form of safflower oil. It is necessary to provide about 3 percent of fat calories as essential fatty acids. A few patients require prolonged dietary restrictions or a period of total parenteral nutrition. Any form of enteral nutrition in these unfortunate individuals seems to result in the reaccumulation of chylous effusions.

Most patients respond to medical management and eventually tolerate a fairly liberal diet. It is common for affected children to undergo clinical remission as they become older. We have also seen transient relapses after several years of apparent well-being.

PARENTERAL NUTRITION

C. RICHARD FLEMING, M.D.

Parenteral and enteral nutrition are not mutually exclusive techniques with which to feed our patients. There are many patients with patent intestinal tracts who simply cannot or will not eat enough; therefore, parenteral nutrition as supplemental rather than the sole nutrition is appropriate.

The terminology available to describe various forms of parenteral nutrition is confusing, and there is no uniformly accepted nomenclature. Hyperalimentation, parenteral alimentation, total parenteral nutrition, central parenteral nutrition, peripheral hyperalimentation, and protein-sparing therapy are terms which do not convey the same meaning to all readers. We will use central parenteral nutrition (CPN) to mean the use of a large-diameter central vein through which to administer hypertonic formulas. Peripheral parenteral nutrition (PPN) will refer to the use of small-diameter peripheral veins to infuse isotonic or hypotonic solutions.

QUALITY CONTROL

The assignment of one person, rather than a committee, to oversee the day-to-day supervision of parenteral nutrition is ideal. That individual is usually a nurse, dietitian, or pharmacist who works very closely with physicians and other health care professionals who comprise a nutritional support group. Specifics that require close supervision include the following:

Flow monitors for all patients on CPN. The use of either a pump or drip regulator reduces metabolic complications and optimizes nutrient utilization.

Catheter care should be carefully controlled either by continuing education of floor nurses or, if the hospital size permits, one nurse managing all catheters placed in large-diameter central veins.

Flow sheets with which to record serial chemistries that allow early detection of nutrient excesses or deficiencies.

A *monograph* for hospital staff which details the basic information needed for day-to-day patient care.

Incompatibilities between specific nutrients or between drugs and nutrients.

A nutritional support team is active in most large medical centers. Most are run on a consultative basis, but a few hospitals make a consultation mandatory for any patient started on enteral or parenteral nutrition.

NUTRIENTS

The basic nutrients delivered in parenteral nutrition are fat, carbohydrates, amino acids, electrolytes, macroelements, trace elements, and vitamins. Table 1 lists the usual composition of 1 L of CPN.

Fat

Intravenous fat emulsions are available as emulsions of soybean or safflower oils, egg phospholipid, and glycerol. Ten and 20 percent concentrations of isotonic fat emulsions can be administered with PPN or CPN. All patients on parenteral nutrition more than a week should receive at least enough fat each week (e.g., 1 to 1.5 L of 10% fat emulsion for the average adult) to prevent biochemical evidence of essential fatty acid deficiency.

Carbohydrate

Dextrose is a safe and efficiently used caloric source. Solutions of alcohol, sorbitol, xylitol, and fructose have all been tested and proved to be less safe or more expensive (or both) than dextrose.

The use of dextrose as the only nonprotein energy source in CPN solutions is associated with several problems. Infusion of dextrose in excess of that which is readily oxidized results in net synthesis of body fat and water accumulation. Complications observed in patients receiving excess glucose are fatty liver and mild elevations in serum amino transferase and alkaline phosphatase values, and, in patients on respirators, an increase in carbon dioxide production with only minimal increase in oxygen consumption. The dual energy system (dextrose and fat) appears more efficient than glucose alone in replenishing protein and avoiding water retention. The apparent advantage of using the dual energy system in all patients must be weighed against the disadvantage of the added expense of the fat emulsions.

Protein

Synthetic crystalline amino acids are available in concentrations of 3 to 10 percent, with and without electrolytes. Most amino acid preparations consist of approximately two-thirds nonessential and one-third essential amino acids. These preparations are very efficiently used; the mean nitrogen retention when 1 g per kilogram of body weight per day of a 10 percent amino acid mixture was given was equivalent to high biologic value protein given orally to healthy adults.

Electrolytes

Single package electrolyte solutions added to parenteral nutrition will meet most patients' needs. There are exceptions when alterations are needed, such as in patients with cardiac, renal, or hepatic disease or when there are large gut losses of electrolytes as can occur in patients with short bowel syndrome or high output, proximal enterocutaneous fistulas.

Trace Elements

Commercial solutions with multiple trace elements (e.g., copper, zinc, chromium, and manganese) are available; however, some of these trace elements, such as chromium and manganese, are often not needed. Also, patients with large stool losses may lose zinc in excess of what the multitrace element formula will contain (4 mg zinc). Vials containing single trace elements allow for adequate

TABLE 1 Central Parenteral Nutrition with Standard Electrolytes*

	Final Concentration			
Dextrose	☐ 10%	☐ 15%	☐ 20%	☐ 25%
Amino acids		4.25%		
Sodium		36.5 mEq		
Potassium		30.0 mEq		
Calcium		4.8 mEq		
Magnesium		5.0 mEq		
Chloride		35.0 mEq		
Phosphorus		15.0 mmol		
Acetate		67.5 mEq		
Grams nitrogen		7.15 g/L		
Total kilocalories	510	680	850	1,020
Approx. osmolarity	1,090	1,340	1,595	1,845
Approx. volume		1,000 ml		

*One liter of standard central parenteral nutrition. The standard adult multivitamin injection is added to one bottle daily. Generally, a standard adult trace element injection is added to one bottle daily (4 mg of zinc, 1 mg of copper, 500 μg of manganese, and 10 μg of chromium/ml).

flexibility in nutrient mixing and for maintaining normal blood levels.

Iron is not routinely added to parenteral nutrition solutions. Iron dextran can be added in small amounts to daily CPN, or it can be given by a bolus infusion designed to replace body stores. Parenteral iron has been associated with anaphylaxis or a constellation of symptoms including myalgias, fever, and headache. A small test dose of parenteral iron should be given prior to initiating the replacement of larger amounts of iron. Preliminary reports that parenteral ferrous gluconate was safer than iron dextran have not yet been followed by its commercial availability.

Vitamins

There are vitamin preparations with both water-soluble and fat-soluble vitamins. Vitamin K is not routinely added, but it can be supplemented either orally or parenterally. The multivitamin preparation MVI-12 (Armour Pharmaceutical, Kankakee, IL) results in normal blood levels of almost all vitamins when added to 1 L of CPN each day.

Most hospital pharmacies provide dextrose, amino acids, vitamins, electrolytes, and macroelements (calcium, phosphorus, and magnesium) in a "standard" CPN formula. This formula is not "total" as implied in the label *total* parenteral nutrition because several nutrients are not routinely added, including vitamin K, essential fatty acids, iron, and trace elements. The likelihood of deficiencies of each of these nutrients increases with the duration of nutritional support.

TYPES OF PARENTERAL NUTRITION

Peripheral Vein Parenteral Nutrition

The advent of safe, isotonic fat emulsions in 10 and 20 percent concentrations created great hope that one could meet the needs of most patients requiring parenteral nutrition by PPN. These hopes, however, have been tarnished by frequent episodes of phlebitis and soft tissue infiltrations, with the end result being the inability to feed the patients adequately. The addition of small amounts of heparin and corticosteroids to PPN solutions decreases the incidence of phlebitis and thrombosis. A double-blind, prospective study showed that the use of a $0.22-\mu$ filter decreased the incidence of phlebitis by approximately two-thirds compared to that in patients receiving PPN without filters. This latter study suggested that the phlebitis is caused by microparticulate components present in the infusion fluids which are removed by in-line filtration.

Peripheral vein nutrition should be reserved for patients whose nutritional status is near normal and in whom the treatment goal is to maintain and not to replace lean body mass. Such patients may be undergoing elective surgery, in which case one can anticipate a 3- to 7-day period of nothing by mouth. Several alternatives exist:

First, dextrose-in-water, 100 to 150 g daily, with multivitamins and 20 to 30 mEq potassium chloride per liter. This is usually given as 2 or 3 L of 5 percent dextrose in water. The administration of dextrose and the stimulation of insulin, the premier anabolic hormone, will decrease urinary nitrogen losses by 50 percent compared with the administration of saline without calories. This mainstay has served patients well and remains the usual short-term postoperative nutrition for patients undergoing elective surgery.

Second, crystalline synthetic amino acids can be given as isocaloric replacements for dextrose. This "protein-sparing therapy" was initially promoted as a better alternative than dextrose-in-water because amino acids decrease urinary nitrogen losses by 50 percent when compared with isocaloric amounts of 5 percent dextrose. This response is independent of insulin and glucagon secretion, and the critical ingredient for "protein sparing" appears to be the administered protein itself—in this case, amino acids. The response is dose dependent—1 g per kilogram ideal body weight per day results in a cumulative nitrogen loss in patients undergoing elective surgery whereas 2 g per kilogram ideal body weight per day promotes a cumulative nitrogen retention. Although it provides a good lesson in nutritional metabolism, the use of intravenous amino acids alone has little clinical use. There are no data to show that there is clinical benefit (such as reductions in hospital stay, postoperative complications, and rehabilitation time) to justify the extra expense of amino acids instead of hypotonic dextrose for the uncomplicated patient undergoing elective surgery.

Third, combinations of hypotonic dextrose, amino acids, and fat emulsions plus vitamins, minerals, and trace elements can meet the average patient's basal energy and protein needs provided that 50 percent of the calories are given as fat calories. The dextrose and amino acids have traditionally been mixed together along with the micronutrients and given through the main line while the fat emulsions are given through a Y-connector placed downstream from the filter. Table 2 itemizes the usual components in 1 L of peripheral parenteral nutrition solution used in our hospitals. Most adult patients will receive 2 or 3 L of PPN and 500 ml of a 10 percent fat emulsion each day.

More recently, three-in-one mixtures have been marketed. These allow the mixture of dextrose, amino acids, and fat emulsions in the same bag. At least one control study has shown a significantly higher rate of catheter occlusion when the three-in-one system was used compared with the conventional system of dextrose and amino acids in one bottle and the fat emulsion in another.

Central Vein Parenteral Nutrition

Catheter Placement and Care

Generally, the infraclavicular approach to the right subclavian vein is used in adults. In small children, the jugular vein is often catheterized and the proximal end

TABLE 2 Peripheral Parenteral Nutrition with Standard Electrolytes*

	Final Concentration
Dextrose	5%
Amino acids	4.25%
Sodium	36.5 mEq/L
Potassium	30.0 mEq/L
Calcium	4.8 mEq/L
Magnesium	5.0 mEq/L
Chloride	35.0 mEq/L
Phosphorus	15.0 mEq/L
Acetate	67.5 mEq/L
Grams nitrogen	7.15 g/L
Total kilocalories	340 kcal/L
Approx. osmolarity	835 mOsm/L
Approx. volume	1,000 ml

* The standard adult multivitamin injection is added to one litre of standard peripheral parenteral nutrition daily. Generally, a standard adult trace element injection is added to one bottle daily (4 mg of zinc, 1 mg of copper, 500 μg of manganese, and 10 μg of chromium/ml).

of the catheter is tunneled subcutaneously to exit through an incision behind the ear. Dressings should be changed 3 times a week, using the same aseptic techniques that were followed when the catheter was inserted. A filter, either 0.22 or 0.45-μ pore size, is inserted between the intravenous tubing and catheter; the tubing and filter are changed daily. Careful taping at tubing connections and/or Luer locks are used to prevent accidental disconnections and the potential for air embolism. Intravenous drugs, colloid, and blood should not be given through the central line except under unusual circumstances when no other venous access is available.

Indications

Rigid guidelines as to when and in whom to use CPN often disintegrate on hospital wards, but most patients for whom enteral nutrition is impossible or inadequate for more than 10 days and who have lost 10 percent or more of their usual weight are candidates. Most such patients have gastrointestinal diseases or conditions (Table 3). Although the usual CPN formulas are applicable to most, specialized solutions have been marketed for patients with renal or hepatic failure and "stress formulas" for those experiencing marked catabolism. Of these special formulas, the high branched chain preparations for trauma patients appear to have the soundest and most reproducible results.

Fistulas. The combination of CPN and bowel rest for traumatic or surgically induced fistulas will result in nonoperative, permanent closure in 70 to 80 percent of cases. The same treatment for fistulas arising in cases of Crohn's disease, radiation enteritis, or malignancies may result in temporary closure, but the fistulas will usually reopen soon after resumption of oral food. Although CPN and bowel rest rarely result in a "cure" in the latter circumstances, they are important adjuncts to optimize nutrition prior to surgery.

Unresolving Pancreatitis. These patients should probably not be fed with tube enteral infusions placed downstream from the pancreas. Instead, CPN and bowel rest interrupt the predictable sequence of oral food → postprandial pain → ↓ oral intake → malnutrition. One must monitor plasma glucose levels at least once each day, because marked hyperglycemia may occur. If hypertriglyceridemia is present at presentation, I do not use intravenous fat emulsions. In the absence of elevated serum triglycerides, fat emulsions are used to give 20 to 30 percent of nonprotein calories and minimize the risk of severe hyperglycemia. Intravenous fat emulsions have not been shown to increase pancreatic enzyme outputs through pancreatocutaneous fistulas or alter the course of experimental pancreatitis in animals.

Diffuse Motility Disorders. Patients with pseudo-obstruction from scleroderma or amyloidosis are extremely difficult to manage over long periods with CPN because of their multisystem involvement. The chronic idiopathic intestinal pseudo-obstruction syndromes, however, are relatively easy to manage and patients usually fare well with normal body weights and periods of less severe symptoms when some enteral nutrition is possible.

Radiation Enteritis. Most patients who experience pain, diarrhea, and rectal bleeding following abdominal radiation have self-limiting symptoms and minimal long-term morbidity. Another group who undergo total abdominal radiation develop diffuse submucosal edema and subsequent fibrosis, which results in chronic small bowel obstruction at multiple sites, often requiring long-term home parenteral nutrition. Yet a third group are those who develop a picture of subacute intestinal pseudo-obstruction following total abdominal radiation for which CPN for several months is necessary.

Inflammatory Bowel Disease. Central parenteral nutrition with or without "bowel rest" is often used in patients with inflammatory bowel disease as an adjunct to conventional medical or surgical treatment, to prepare the debilitated patient for surgery, or as primary therapy for patients with extensive Crohn's disease and gut failure.

TABLE 3 Common Indications for Central Parenteral Nutrition

Gastrointestinal Diseases
  Fistulas
  Unresolving pancreatitis
  Intestinal pseudo-obstruction
  Radiation enteritis
  Inflammatory bowel disease
  Prolonged postoperative ileus
  Severe diarrhea in infants

Specially Designed Formulas
  Hepatic failure
  Renal failure
  "Stress" high branched chain amino acid
    formulas for catabolic patients

Dickinson and colleagues conducted the only randomized trial of CPN and bowel rest in patients with acute colitis, most of whom had chronic ulcerative colitis. Control patients were fed an ad lib oral diet and the treatment group received CPN and bowel rest. Controls and CPN treated patients were taking comparable amounts of prednisone. Half of each group required surgery during the same hospitalization. Among those not requiring surgery, the duration of medical treatment required to induce clinical remissions was comparable in the two groups. Thus, there was no difference in the outcome in the controlled and CPN groups with regard to frequency of surgery or duration of medical therapy. These data should not discourage the use of CPN in malnourished patients with chronic ulcerative colitis for whom enteral nutrition is inadequate.

Uncontrolled data suggest that 60 to 70 percent of patients with *Crohn's disease* who are refractory to medical treatment and are treated with CPN and bowel rest undergo an initial in-hospital remission, but only 50 percent of those followed for 3 months remain in clinical remission. These observations need to be tested in a randomized trial comparing CPN and bowel rest with other means of nutritional support, such as tube enteral and peripheral parenteral nutrition. Lochs and associates conducted a randomized trial comparing CPN with bowel rest to CPN without bowel rest in 20 patients with Crohn's disease. There was no apparent advantage by clinical scores or nutritional indices in the patients with complicated Crohn's disease with 12 weeks of CPN and bowel rest. No medications were given. Although surgery was initially avoided in 25 to 30 patients, the cumulative relapse rate was 60 percent after 2 years and 85 percent after 4 years. This was compared with the results of resection, obtained from a 10-year period before CPN was begun at the same hospital, showing the cumulative recurrence rates after CPN to be four times higher than after resection. The available data on CPN in adults with Crohn's disease punctuates its importance as an adjunctive tool to reverse the frequent protein-calorie malnutrition; however, it is not a substitute for corticosteroids and surgery, which are the mainstays of treatment.

Thirty percent of children or adolescents with Crohn's experience growth retardation. Adequate nutritional supplementation alone, regardless of the form, stimulates growth. The calorie and protein requirements revert to those of the newborn infant—75 to 100 Kcal per kilogram and 2 g of protein per kilogram per day. Although most of these patients can be managed with aggressive enteral nutrition, CPN is necessary in some of the most severe cases.

Complications

Discussion of the major metabolic complications in patients receiving TPN, shown in Table 4, is beyond the scope of this chapter. Sequential measurements of blood and/or urine concentrations of most of these nutrients will alert one to evolving deficiencies or excesses.

TABLE 4 Major Metabolic Complications in Patients Receiving Total Parenteral Nutrition

Nutrients	Presentations
Excess of:	
Glucose	Hyperglycemia, polyuria, polydipsia
Amino acids	Hyperammonemia in patients with liver disease Azotemia in renal failure
Calcium	Hypercalcemia, pancreatitis, renal stones
Vitamin D	Hypercalcemia, negative calcium balance, osteopenia, long bone pain (reported in long-term home parenteral nutrition patients)
Deficiency of:	
Copper	Neutropenia, anemia, scorbutic bone lesions, ↓ ceruloplasmin
Zinc	Nasolabial and perineal acrodermatitis, alopecia, ↓ T cell function, ↓ alkaline phosphatase
Chromium	Glucose intolerance
Selenium	Myalgias, cardiomyopathy, ↓ glutathione peroxidase
Molybdenum	Amino acid intolerance, tachycardia, tachypnea, central scotomas, irritability, ↓ uric acid
Essential fatty acids	Eczymoid dermatitis, ↑ 20:3/20:4
Vitamin A	Night blindness, ↓ dark field adaptation
Vitamin K	Easy bruising, hypoprothrombinemia
Vitamin E	In vitro platelet hyperaggregation and H_2O_2-induced red blood cell hemolysis
Vitamin D	Osteomalacia, long-bone pain, low serum 25-OH vitamin D
Biotin	Dermatitis, alopecia, hypotonia
Thiamine	Wernicke's encephalopathy
Taurine	Impaired vision, abnormal retinogram
L-carnitine	Inadequate data

One of the most common mistakes made is *overfeeding* the cachectic patient—too much nutrition in too short a period of time. Sudden deaths have been reported in this setting. Although the exact cause of such deaths is unknown, the most likely possibilities include cardiac arrhythmias and/or severe hypophosphatemia. When refeeding the severely protein-calorie malnourished patient, one should start at approximately one-third the estimated maintenance calories and slowly (every third day) increase the caloric load to the maintenance level.

Patients with hypoalbuminemia who are started on parenteral nutrition will frequently reduce their serum albumin levels even lower during the first 1 to 2 weeks. This reduction usually reflects only rehydration and should not be managed by increasing the amino acids infused. The half-life of albumin is approximately 19 days; therefore, serum albumin levels are not good indicators of protein synthesis over a shorter period of time.

The malnourished patient who is hypoproteinemic and edematous will frequently lose weight shortly after starting CPN. This initial weight loss is accompanied by a diuresis and mobilization of edema fluid. This may be interpreted as inadequate parenteral nutrition and the volume or concentration of CPN (or both) will inappropriately be increased. Weight gain in hospitalized paients on TPN is often erratic. For instance, patients who are adequately fed may not gain for several days and then the weight may suddenly increase by 1 pound per day. Only after a stable course of 2 weeks do we see a desirable, steady weight gain of ¼ to ½ pound per day.

HOME PARENTERAL NUTRITION

Patients with gut failure from any cause are candidates for home parenteral nutrition (HPN). Most such patients suffer from severe short bowel syndrome, extensive Crohn's disease of the small bowel, extensive radiation enteritis, chronic adhesive small bowel obstruction, or intestinal pseudo-obstruction. Because of the complexity of our HPN cases, we organize our efforts by means of a multispecialty team consisting of physicians, nurses, a pharmacist, dietitians, and a social worker. Venous access is achieved with a subcutaneously tunneled catheter that is inserted in the operating room. The training of patients in the hospital takes approximately 2 weeks and is done by HPN nurses and a pharmacist who rely heavily on our HPN training manual. A home health care company delivers supplies to patients' homes at monthly intervals according to our prescription. After discharge, patients return to see us at 3-month intervals initially; the frequency of visits lessens as stabilization occurs. Almost all of our HPN patients eat, but their intakes are often limited by fear of diarrhea or increased abdominal pain.

HPN has significantly improved the quality of life for gut failure patients. Nutritional repletion is dramatic and approximately 70 percent return to active routines as students or homemakers, or to gainful employment. Only 4 percent of the total HPN days (656/15,035) of our 41 active patients in 1983 were spent in the hospital.

One-third of patients will experience a catheter-related septicemia at some time during their course of HPN. Considering that our patients have been on HPN for an average of 30 months, the frequency of these infections is one for every 3.5 patient years of HPN. A small cluster of patients have repeated infections, perhaps due to faulty aseptic technique. The most common problem is damage to the external segment of the catheter, which is easily repaired with a repair kit. Catheter occlusions are surprisingly rare and can usually be managed by instillation of streptokinase into the catheter.

The estimated average daily price for HPN in 1984 was $200 (or $73,000 per year for a patient who infuses nightly), compared with $25 per day ($9,125 per year) 10 years ago. Our patients' HPN bills range from $35,000 to $70,000 per year and depend on the number of nights they infuse, their formulas, and the vendor. Most third-party carriers will pay 80 percent of the HPN expenses, but most patients cannot realistically pay the remaining 20 percent.

ENTERAL FEEDING: LIQUID FORMULA DIETS

ROLANDO H. ROLANDELLI, M.D.
JOHN L. ROMBEAU, M.D., F.A.C.S

Enteral feedings by tube have been used for many centuries. Until the advent of safe techniques for parenteral nutrition in the late 1960s, enteral feeding was the only means to nourish patients who were unable to eat. As parenteral nutrition became popular, the use of enteral nutrition declined. A major factor in this decline was that enteral feeding was commonly associated with complications and was poorly tolerated by the patient.

Parenteral nutrition was advocated as a better method of alimentation for the critically ill because it eliminated the "lag time" produced by intestinal and hepatic processing of nutrients. Furthermore, because of the theoretical advantage of bowel rest, parenteral feeding was recommended as the primary treatment for some gastrointestinal diseases. Recent reports, however, have shown that bypassing the digestive system via parenteral nutrition is not entirely innocuous. Complications, such as fatty liver, occur frequently in parenterally fed patients. Moreover, several controlled clinical studies have failed to show an improvement in clinical outcome with the use of parenteral nutrition for patients in need of bowel rest for inflammatory bowel disease.

While the hypothesis of parenteral feeding was being clinically tested, remarkable advances were made in the development of feeding techniques and dietary formulas for enteral nutrition. Thin, soft, radiopaque feeding tubes were developed that allowed longer periods of isoenteric intubations with less discomfort. New enteral diets were formulated for specific nutrient needs, and they were delivered efficiently via the soft tubes. New feeding methods, such as continuous, pump-assisted feeding into the jejunum, were developed for the patient at high risk of aspiration. Finally, and perhaps most importantly, a significant reduction in dietary costs due to the use of enteral feeding was documented. Although the costs of parenteral nutrition have undergone a marked reduction in the last few years, they are still significantly greater than those for enteral feedings.

These new enteral feeding techniques are currently available in almost every hospital, and they are being used more frequently as better life-sustaining methods and treatment become available. The availability of these improved techniques makes the use of the gastrointestinal tract more efficient and less risky. "Starving" the hospitalized patient is considered today to be malpractice. For all of the aforementioned reasons a new trend in clinical nutrition has evolved which reemphasizes an old concept: "If the gut works, and can be used safely, use it." This chapter will discuss the rationale, indications, routes of access, formula composition, delivery methods, monitoring techniques, and complications of the delivery of liquid formula diets by tube.

RATIONALE

A major rationale for the use of enteral feeding is the physiologic benefit that accrues from the influence of food on the gastrointestinal tract. This benefit results from increased hormonal secretions and direct trophic effects on the intestinal mucosa. Enteral diets stimulate the secretion of diverse enterohormones, such as gastrin, gastric inhibitory polypeptide (GIP), and enteroglucagon. Some of these enterohormones, e.g., gastrin, are essential to maintain the structure and function of the intestinal epithelium. Other enterohormones, e.g., GIP, participate in the metabolism of absorbed nutrients. GIP, also called "glucose insulinotropic polypeptide," because of its effect on insulin secretion, may mediate the greater insulin response when carbohydrates are delivered enterally as compared to parenterally.

The intestinal mucosa itself is an active cellular mass that requires continuous nutrition. Mucosal cells have selective needs for fuels, such as glutamine for the small bowel and short-chain fatty acids for the colon. These fuels are utilized preferentially when present in the lumen of the gut rather than in the bloodstream. When the intestine lacks enterohormonal stimuli and luminal nutrients, villous atrophy occurs; digestive enzyme secretion is reduced and absorption is impaired.

As noted previously, the role of the gastrointestinal tract in nutrition is more than a mode of passive transference of metabolic substrates to the bloodstream. Nutrients delivered enterally are processed in the intestinal wall and the liver before reaching the systemic circulation. The induced hormonal secretion that results from enteral feeding provides a more efficient utilization of metabolic substrates.

INDICATIONS

Our selection of enteral feeding methods is based on an algorithm, as shown in Figure 1. Before initiating nutritional therapy, one must first obtain baseline nutritional data via a thorough medical history, dietary review, complete physical examination, and laboratory evaluation. To establish the need for enteral feeding, it must be demonstrated that the patient's volitional intake is insufficient to meet his nutrient needs.

The objectives of enteral feeding must be clearly identified. Enteral feedings by tube can be used as primary treatment for various gastrointestinal disorders, or secondarily for conditions causing impaired oral intake, surgery, chemotherapy, and radiotherapy (Table 1).

ROUTES OF ACCESS

Enteral feedings are delivered through nasoenteric tubes or tube enterostomies. For one to decide on the appropriate route, the duration of feeding and the risk of aspiration need to be considered. If enteral feedings are to be given for less than 6 weeks, a nasoenteric tube should be used. If the patient is at potential risk of aspiration, a nasojejunal tube should be placed.

Several small-bore tubes are available for transnasal passage into the stomach, duodenum, or jejunum. These tubes are placed in the stomach with the aid of a stylet. Passage into the duodenum and jejunum is accomplished by gastrointestinal propulsion of the weighted tip. Positioning of the patient in the right lateral decubitus position and the intravenous administration of metoclopamide help promote passage across the pylorus. The tube can be manipulated into the duodenum with the aid of fluoroscopy or endoscopy if the weighted tip does not advance in 48 hours. If gastric contents cannot be aspirated with a syringe after initial placement of the tube, radiographic confirmation of the position of the tube in the stomach is mandatory before infusion of the diet. This will identify inadvertent intubation of the tracheobronchial tree. Once the correct position is confirmed, the tube is secured to the malar skin. In instances of repeated accidental removal of the feeding tube, a special bridle can be constructed to secure the tube to the nasal pharynx.

Feeding tube enterostomies can be placed by surgical procedures in several locations in the gastrointestinal tract. The most common types are pharyngostomies, gas-

TABLE 1 Indications for Enteral Feedings

Primary Treatment[*]
  Malabsorption syndromes
  Inflammatory bowel disease
  Short bowel syndrome
  Fistulas
  Oropharyngeal disorders
  Esophagogastric obstructions

Secondary Treatment
  Anorexia nervosa
  Neurologic disorders
  Burns
  Renal failure
  Hepatic failure
  Cardiac disease
  Respiratory insufficiency
  Perioperative
  Cancer

[*] It is acknowledged that enteral feeding may also be used as a secondary modality for some of these indications.

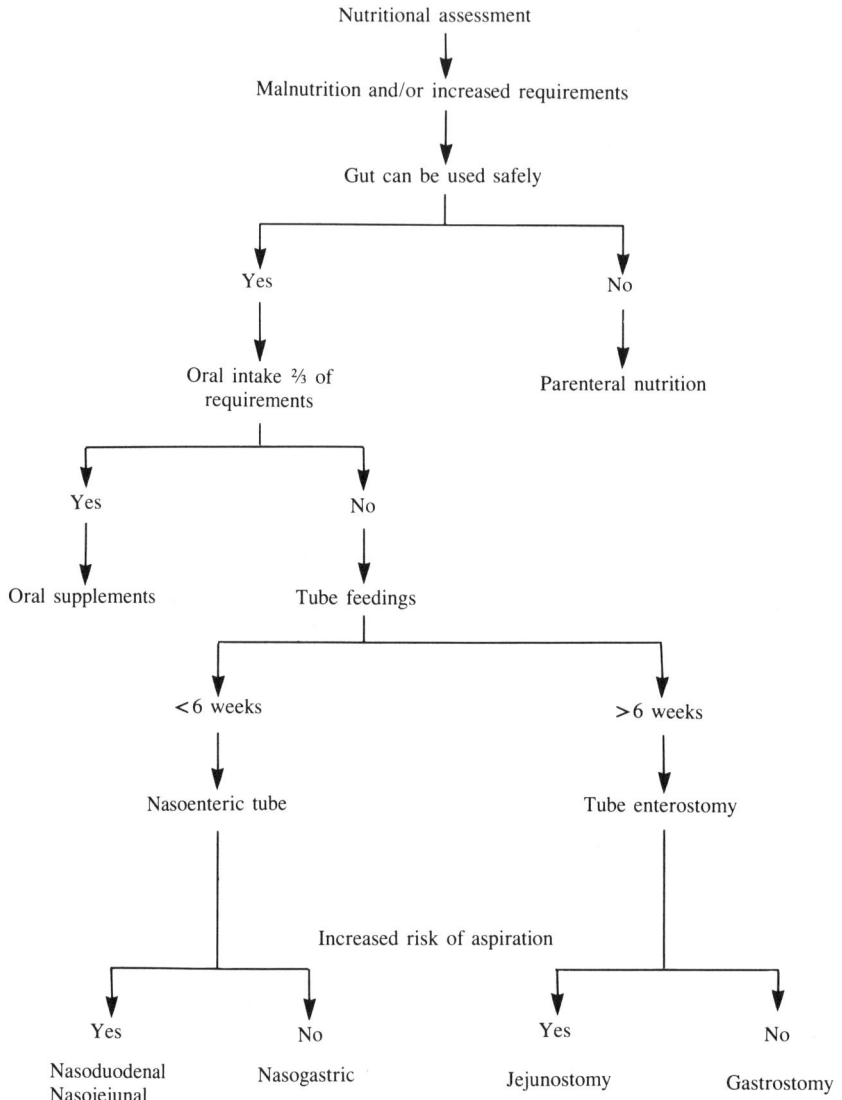

Figure 1 Decisions for enteral feeding route access.

trostomies, and jejunostomies. Pharyngostomy is a useful adjunct to head and neck surgery and has also been recommended as an easy technique for any patient requiring long-term tube feedings.

Gastrostomies are the most common type of tube enterostomies. They are performed via different surgical techniques, such as those described by Stamm and Janeway. The Stamm technique is used for temporary needs and the Janeway is a permanent gastrostomy. Recently the *percutaneous placement of a feeding gastrostomy* by endoscopic technique has gained in popularity.

Pulmonary aspiration of gastrostomy feedings is a potential complication in high-risk patients. For these patients a new tube has been devised which combines a decompression gastrostomy with a feeding jejunostomy (Fig. 2). When the risk of aspiration is overcome, the gastric port of the tube can be used for feedings or medications. As with the other temporary gastrostomies, the tube is easily replaceable.

There are two basic types of feeding jejunostomies: the Witzel and the Delany techniques. A sutured tunnel is created in the Witzel technique, and a 14-gauge needle of the type used for subclavian vein catheterization is used in the Delany method. The Delany method is an easier technique with fewer surgical complications, but its limitation is that a No. 15 French catheter is used, while a No. 16 French tube is used for the Witzel jejunostomy. The resultant diameter, 1.5 mm versus 5 mm, mandates the use of low-viscosity (expensive) elemental diets for needle catheter jejunostomy feedings.

FORMULAS

Many liquid diets for enteral feeding are currently available in the United States. Several classifications of these diets have been proposed, but unfortunately, none is completely satisfactory. The problem with existing clas-

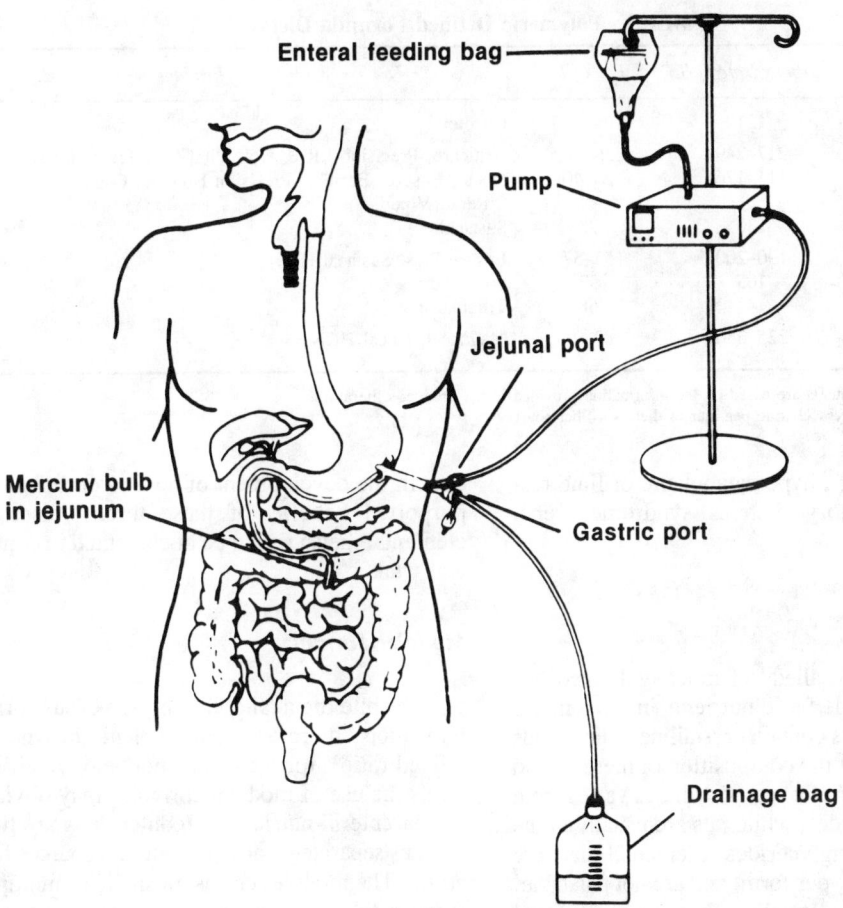

Figure 2 Enteral feeding with combined decompression gastrostomy and feeding jejunostomy. With permission from Delrio et al. Enteral Nutrition. California: Medical Specifics Publishing; p. 133.

sifications is that the dietary categories are often intermingled as to both composition and clinical use. We have chosen the following classification which is based on nutrient composition: (1) polymeric, (2) elemental, and (3) modular.

Polymeric Diets

In polymeric diets the three basic nutrients—proteins, carbohydrates, and fats—are in complex forms, i.e., polymers. Carbohydrates are present in the form of oligosaccharides, maltodextrins, or polysaccharides; fats consist of medium- or long-chain triglycerides. The protein source is a natural protein which may be intact or partially hydrolyzed. In general, these diets are isotonic, lactose-free, "ready to use," and available in liquid form. Many polymeric diets can be used either for tube feedings or for oral supplementation. Selection of these diets is made on the basis of calorie, protein, and fluid requirements. Polymeric diets can be further divided according to their caloric density (Table 2). The caloric density of polymeric formulas is 0.6, 1.0, 1.5, or 2.0 Kcal per milliliter. The group with 1 Kcal per milliliter includes the largest number of commercially available diets. The nonprotein caloric content in these diets is derived from either carbohydrates or lipids. Polymeric diets formulated with carbohydrates as the main caloric source have higher osmolality than isocaloric diets containing lipids. Hypertonic diets, which are carbohydrate based, are well tolerated when infused intragastrically and reasonably well tolerated when administered directly into the small bowel. Carbohydrate based diets are advantageous for patients with steatorrhea and hyperlipidemias. Polymeric diets, which are fat based, may be more appropriate for patients who have diarrhea associated with tube feedings, especially when the feedings are infused directly into the small bowel. High-fat diets are useful for patients on mechanical ventilatory assistance, since they reduce the carbon dioxide production and thereby facilitate ventilator weaning. Most polymeric diets are formulated to provide approximately 6.25 g of protein (1 g of nitrogen) for every 150 Kcal. The concomitant provision of sufficient calories at this ratio promotes the utilization of nitrogen for synthesis of structural compounds, i.e., visceral and muscle protein. If the caloric content of the diet does not meet the patient's requirements, the protein content is utilized as an energy source and the nitrogen intake results in increased ureagenesis. Diets with high calorie:nitrogen ratios are recommended for patients with renal and hepatic insufficiency. Diets with higher caloric density, 1.5 and 2.0 Kcal per milliliter, are used for patients with increased

TABLE 2 Polymeric Defined Formula Diets*

Kcal/ml	Protein (g/L)	Carbohydrate (g/L)	Fat (g/L)	Product
0.66	40	121	1.7	Citrotein
	26–45	217–249	1.3–13.5	Criticare, Precision LR & HN, Vital HN, Travasorb HN & STD
1	25–49	115–176	25–40	Isocal, Ensure, Enrich,† Precision Isotonic, Osmolite, Travasorb MCT, Renu, Vipep
	60	130	23	Sustacal
1.5	55–61	190–200	53–57	Ensure Plus, Sustacal HC
	62	105	92	Pulmocare
	83	143	68	Traumacal
2.0	70–75	225–250	80–91	Magnacal, Isocal HCN

* Caloric density and nutrient contents are based on the information provided in the product's literature.
† Enrich includes 21 g of soy polysaccharide per liter of diet as a fiber source.

energy requirements, e.g., hypercatabolism, or fluid restrictions, e.g., respiratory distress syndrome, renal failure, and so on.

Elemental Diets

Elemental diets, also called "chemically defined" or "synthetic" diets, include basic nutrients in monomeric forms. All elemental diets contain crystalline amino acids as the protein source, but the composition of these amino acids is variable. The source of carbohydrates varies from dextrose to oligosaccharides, while fats are usually in the form of medium-chain triglycerides. Elemental diets are hypertonic, usually in powder form, and are not palatable. Because of this lack of palatability, they are rarely used for oral supplements. Elemental diets were initially formulated with a ratio of essential:nonessential amino acids of 35 percent:65 percent, as recommended by Rose. These ratios were chosen because they resembled the high biologic value of proteins such as egg albumin and human milk.

In addition to this standard formulation of amino acids, new elemental diets have been developed with different compositions of amino acids (Table 3): (1) *stress* formulas enriched in the branched-chain amino acids (leucine, isoleucine, and valine); (2) *hepatic* formulas containing increased branched-chain amino acids and decreased aromatic amino acids (phenylalanine, tryptophan, and tyrosine) and the sulfur amino acid methionine, and (3) *renal* formulas containing all essential amino acids and histidine and lacking the other nonessential amino acids. These three types of elemental diets consist of crystalline amino acids, monosaccharides, and low amounts of fats in the form of medium-chain triglycerides. "Stress" formulas have been developed from metabolic studies on hypercatabolism which demonstrate that branched chain amino acids may improve nitrogen balance by serving as the precursors of muscle protein. Renal formulas have been used to nourish non-dialysis patients with renal failure to promote the re-utilization of urea nitrogen for synthesis of nonessential amino acids by transamination in the liver. The hepatic formulas were initially formulated to reduce the availability of precursors of neurotransmitters (aromatic amino acids) synthesized in excess in the development of hepatic encephalopathy. The purported benefits of these three "disease-specific" elemental diets need to be documented in controlled clinical trials.

Modular Formulas

Despite the availability of numerous formulated enteral diets, there are some patients in whom standard, "fixed ratio" formulas may not be optimal. In these patients the use of modular formulas may obviate the need for parenteral nutrition. Modular diets are those formulated as separately packaged nutrient sources for each substrate. The modules consist of single or multiple nutrients that can either be combined to produce a nutritionally complete feeding or used individually to enhance an existing "fixed ratio" formula, i.e., polymeric or elemental diets. The modular system allows the physician to alter the ratio of a constituent nutrient without affecting the concentration of other constituents. One can select not only the amount of each nutrient, substrate, mineral, vitamin, etc, but also the type of nutrients most appropriate for the patient, e.g., whole protein versus partially hydrolyzed versus crystalline amino acids.

It is often difficult to select the appropriate enteral formula, although choices may be limited because of an incomplete selection at any one institution. Our decision process is summarized in Figure 3. Polymeric diets are the first choice for patients with normal intestinal function and without dietary restrictions and in whom standard-sized feeding tubes have been placed. Elemental diets usually have specific disease-related indications, such as impaired enzymatic digestion, reduced absorptive surface, renal or hepatic failure, and hypercatabolic states. Modular diets are reserved for the rare patient who cannot be fed with the two previously mentioned formulas.

DELIVERY METHODS

Once the optimal diet and access site are selected, it must be decided whether to infuse the diet intermittently or continuously. Advantages of *intermittent feedings*

TABLE 3 Elemental Diets*

Formula	Total	Essential Total	B–C	A	Nonessential	CHO (g/L)	Fat (g/L)	Kcal/g N	Kcal/ml	Product Name
Standard (stress)	38	20.1	12.6 (33%)	3.8	18.2	206	3	164	1.0	Vivonex T.E.N.
Stress	37	23.2	16.4 (44%)	3.4	14.0	140	23	90	1.2	Stresstein
	28	18.4	13.9 (50%)	2.7	9.6	166	12	87	1.0	Traum-Aid HBC
Renal	19	18.3	6.4 (33%)	6.0	0.6	366	19	380	1.9	Amin-Aid
	23	14.5	5.9 (25%)	3.9	8.4	274	18	362	1.3	Travasorb Renal
Hepatic	43	24.4	13.8 (32%)	1.3	18.5	289	36	215	1.7	Hepatic-Aid
	29	20.7	12.5 (43%)	0.8	7.8	210	15	218	1.1	Travasorb Hepatic

Amino Acids (g/package)

* Nutrient contents and caloric density are based on the information provided by the product's literature.
B–C = branched amino acids. The numbers in parentheses refer to the percentage of essential amino acids provided as B–C. The amount given for nonessential amino acids includes histidine, which may be regarded as essential amino acid for renal patients.
A = aromatic amino acids and includes methionine.

are that a pump is not required for their administration and they may be more physiologic, since they resemble the periodicity of normal alimentation. Experimental evidence suggests that nutrients delivered intermittently are more efficiently converted into storage forms of energy than when delivered continuously. This improved utilization of nutrients appears to be mediated by the increased activity of hepatic enzymes that are involved in the conversion of carbohydrates into lipids. Intermittent feeding is also associated with improved nitrogen balance and protein synthesis. In patients with normal gastric emptying and intestinal transit, we prefer to feed intermittently into the stomach. This is particularly advantageous if the patient has a large-bore feeding tube and needs to continue enteral feedings at home. In these patients, viscous formulas or blenderized foods can be infused intermittently. Disadvantages of intermittent feeding include an increased risk of gastroesophageal reflux and aspiration. Furthermore, it is difficult to feed intermittently via a jejunostomy, especially when using hyperosmolar diets.

Advantages of *continuous feedings* include a reduction in side effects such as diarrhea and abdominal cramps. Continuous feedings are preferable for patients with delayed gastric emptying, accelerated intestinal transit, or need for hyperosmolar diets. The disadvantages of continuous feedings include the physical and psychological "attachment" of the patient to the pump and the expenses involved with the use of the pump.

MONITORING TECHNIQUES

Patients who receive enteral feedings require the same careful monitoring as those who receive parenteral nutrition. A protocol should be established and followed to ensure that the specified nutritional goals are met. This is especially relevant in institutions where individuals with varying experience are responsible for writing orders.

Most patients who require enteral feedings are malnourished. Malnutrition per se or other underlying conditions may be the cause of gastrointestinal intolerance to enteral diets. Therefore, it is essential to start infusing small volumes of the diet with a gradual increase in the rate of delivery according to the tolerance of the patient. When increasing the rate of continuous feedings into the jejunum, we prefer to increase the volume prior to increasing the concentration of the diet. Continuous feedings can be started at a rate of 50 ml per hour and increased by 25 ml per hour daily in the absence of gastrointestinal side effects. When feeding intermittently into the stomach, volumes of 200 ml can be administered every 4 hours over a period of 15 minutes and increased by 50 ml per feeding. If the caliber of the feeding tube is sufficient, gastric residuals are checked before each feeding or every 6 to 8 hours with continuous feedings. If the residual is greater than 150 ml the patient must be evaluated for delayed gastric emptying and the feeding withheld temporarily.

COMPLICATIONS

There are two major types of complications of enteral feeding: tube-related—improper placement, dislodgment, or occlusion of the feeding tube—and gastrointestinal—delayed gastric emptying, diarrhea, and constipation. The improper placement or dislodgment of the feeding tube may lead to aspiration. The gastrointestinal complications are important. Diarrhea is the most common gastrointestinal complication and its cause is often multifactorial. Hypertonic liquid diets may cause diarrhea by an osmotic mechanism that is aggravated if

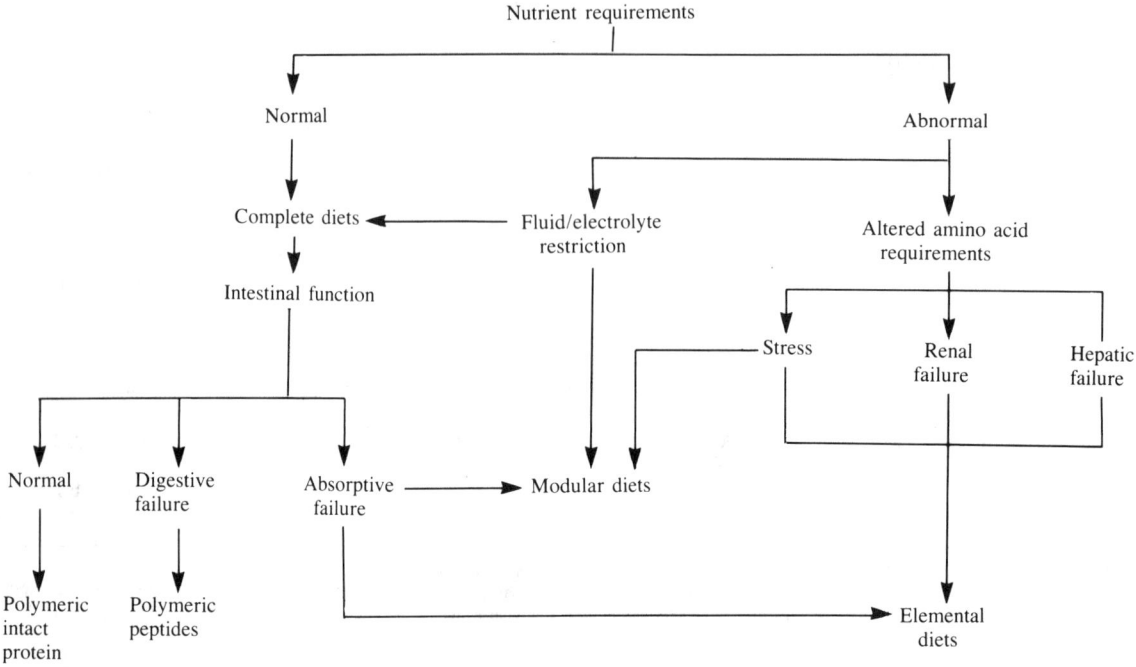

Figure 3 Selection of enteral feeding formula.

the patient is hypoalbuminemic. After long periods of malnutrition and/or diminished oral intake the activity of digestive enzymes may decline. Acquired disaccharidase deficiencies may cause malabsorptive diarrhea. Perhaps the most important cause of diarrhea is the administration of antibiotics concomitantly with enteral feedings. Broad-spectrum antibiotics cause perturbation of the colonic flora, which in turn reduces the production of short-chain fatty acids. Bacterially produced short-chain fatty acids are required for sodium absorption, and when the colon is deprived of them the luminal concentration of sodium increases, thereby leading to watery diarrhea. Contamination of enteral diets has also been implicated as a cause of the diarrhea in tube feedings.

Several measures may help in the treatment of diarrhea. If the patient is receiving hyperosmolar diets the concentration should be reduced. If diarrhea is reduced the solute deficit may be compensated for by increasing the volume of the diluted diet or by switching to an iso-osmolar diet. If malabsorption is suspected in a patient receiving a diet containing polymeric nutrients, the formula should be changed to an elemental diet. The deleterious effect of antibiotics on the colonic flora may be partially overcome by adding a noncellulosic fiber such as pectin to the enteral diet. Maintenance of the colonic flora depends on the availability of energy substrates in the form of fiber polysaccharides. One percent pectin can be added to enteral diets without impairment of formula delivery. Antidiarrheal agents such as paregoric (1 ml per 100 ml formula) can be used if diarrhea becomes severe. Enteral feedings should be discontinued in patients with diarrhea who are resistant to all of these therapeutic measures.

Constipation may be a serious problem in patients receiving elemental diets. The addition of bulk agents such as soy polysaccharide or mucilage (Metamucil) may improve colonic emptying.

SUGGESTED READING

Greene HL (ed). Enteral nutrition. Mead Johnson Symposium Series No. 2. Princeton NJ, Excerpta Medica, 1984.

Heimburger DC, Weinsier RL. Guidelines for evaluating and categorizing enteral feeding formulas according to therapeutic equivalence. JPEN 1985; 9:61.

Rombeau JL, Barot LR. Enteral nutritional therapy. Surg Clin North Am 1981, 61:605.

Rombeau JL, Caldwell MD (eds). Clinical nutrition, vol I. Enteral and tube feeding. Philadelphia: WB Saunders Co, 1984.

Torosian MH, Rombeau JL. Feeding by tube enterostomy. Surg Gynecol Obstet 1980; 150:918.

FOOD FADS AND ALTERNATIVES

SIMEON MARGOLIS, M.D., Ph.D.

One dictionary defines a fad as "a practice or interest followed for a time with exaggerated zeal." Food fads are also characterized by their divergence from the dietary practices of the general population, and often, by the belief of the faddist that the diet provides health benefits despite the lack of scientific evidence to support this viewpoint. Among the more common fad diets are vegetarian and macrobiotic diets and those employed for weight reduction. Alternative dietary practices include an emphasis on the use of organic or natural foods, as well as supplementation of the diet with specific nutrients, such as vitamins, minerals, protein, lecithin, or fiber.

Many factors contribute to the popularity of food fads and alternative dietary patterns. Some individuals follow vegetarian diets because of philosophical or religious convictions opposing the ingestion of animal foods. Others have adopted fad diets in an attempt to control problems, such as obesity, which have not been successfully managed by more conventional dietary or medical approaches. Common motivations for the use of alternative dietary practices are the widespread beliefs that the usual American diet is nutritionally inadequate and that the American public is slowly being poisoned by food additives and by the agricultural use of fertilizers and pesticides. These misconceptions foster the intake of nutritional supplements and the purchase of organic or natural foods.

Abetting these factors is the enormous proliferation of books, newspaper and magazine articles, radio and television shows, and advertisements concerning nutritional issues. Although some of this outpouring disseminates worthwhile nutritional information, the majority contains misinformation, at times because the author is well meaning but poorly informed. All too often, however, the promotion of nutritional fallacies is motivated by the profit from sales of books or nutritional products.

I am convinced that the usual American diet is nutritionally adequate and that organic or natural foods add no health benefits. In fact, a healthy adult in the United States who can afford to buy enough food and is not an alcoholic would have to follow a most unusual diet to become significantly deficient in any nutritional requirement, with just a few exceptions in women. Nutritional needs are increased during pregnancy and lactation; moreover, many women need iron supplementation prior to menopause and additional calcium intake following, and for at least a decade before, menopause. Although the contamination of our food with pesticides and other environmental pollutants is deplorable, organic foods do not contain smaller amounts of these undesirable substances. Food additives have been carefully tested for safety and most are essential to prevent food spoilage.

Some disadvantages and health risks are associated with fad diets and alternative food habits. Nutritional supplementation and the purchase of specially grown or prepared products add unnecessary expense to the food budget. Some patients may rely upon ineffective nutritional measures rather than seek or follow medical advice for treatable illnesses. Finally, toxic side effects may result from excessive amounts of some nutritional supplements and from the use of some exotic foods. The dangers of a fad diet depend upon the magnitude of its nutritional imbalance and how long the diet is followed. Fortunately, most fad diets are monotonous or unpalatable enough to limit their use to a relatively short time.

FAD DIETS

Vegetarian Diets

The health risks of vegetarian diets vary with the degree of avoidance of animal foods. Partial vegetarian diets, which eliminate only specific animal foods such as red meats, pose no risks and may indeed provide some health benefits. The most common vegetarian diets limit the intake of animal foods to dairy products (*lactovegetarian*) or dairy products and eggs (*lacto-ovo-vegetarian*). Such diets are usually adequate in nutrients other than iron. Bioavailability is greater for heme iron, which is present only in animal foods, than for the nonheme sources of iron found in other foods. Strict vegetarians, or *vegans*, consume no foods of animal origin. Vegan diets require careful planning to avoid nutritional deficiencies of calories, protein, minerals and vitamins.

Caloric needs may not be met, particularly in children, because vegan diets are high in bulk. Although vegans can easily ingest enough protein to meet the recommended daily allowance (RDA), many plant proteins are deficient in one or more of the essential amino acids. Therefore, meals must include an appropriate combination of foods that contain proteins which together provide all of the essential amino acids. For example, an adequate intake of essential amino acids can be achieved by the combination of cereal proteins, which are high in methionine and relatively deficient in lysine, with legumes, which contain ample lysine but are low in methionine. It is possible to avoid shortfalls in calcium and iron by careful selection of foods, but the inclusion of fortified soybean milk or an iron supplement may be necessary to ensure adequate intakes. Most vegan diets contain enough vitamins except for vitamin B_{12}. Fortified meat substitutes or a vitamin supplement should be used.

The potential risks of vegan diets are considerably increased in infancy, pregnancy, lactation, and when individuals are ill. It is also important to recognize that some vegetarians ingest large amounts of unconventional nutrient supplements and employ unorthodox sources of health care and advice. Vegans who also have the irritable bowel syndrome may be quite uncomfortable with the gas-producing legumes that are a major part of that diet.

Macrobiotic Diets

Adherents of macrobiotic diets move through a series of rice-rich diets that are progressively more limiting in nutritional content. The ultimate macrobiotic diet consists almost exclusively of unpolished rice. The obvious nutritional dangers of such diets are compounded by their being advocated to treat diseases in lieu of standard medical care. Complications of strict macrobiotic diets include scurvy, anemia, hypoproteinemia, renal dysfunction, severe emaciation, and death.

Reducing Diets

Nutritionists recommend low-calorie diets that are well balanced with respect to their content of carbohydrate, fat, and protein. The effectiveness of such diets depends upon controlling the quantity of food intake rather than restricting its variety. The popularity and frequent short-term success of fad diets for weight reduction are due to the common inability of obese individuals to limit food quantity without a concomitant restriction in food variety.

A bewildering array of fad diets has been tried for weight loss, and new formulas for weight reduction grace the best-seller lists almost every year. The central features of these fad diets involve a wide assortment of ways to limit food variety. Most are low in carbohydrate, but some high carbohydrate diets have been recommended. Some low carbohydrate diets emphasize the use of certain foods, such as grapefruit and even wine; others are high in fat or protein content. Although the risks and benefits of these diets have not been studied carefully, it is *not* evident that they have caused serious ill effects, because most are only moderately unbalanced and the "single food" diets are followed for a short time. Of greater concern are a widely used group of diets that employ a form of protein-sparing modified fasting. Such diets, limited to 200 to 800 calories daily, can be dangerous because of their severely restricted nutrient intake. The underlying principle of these diets is to avoid the protein breakdown and negative nitrogen balance that accompany total starvation by using hydrolyzed protein as the exclusive source of calories. In addition to moderate complications of orthostatic hypotension and attacks of gout, more than 50 deaths, due to myocardial degeneration and arrhythmias, have been reported in patients utilizing protein-sparing modified starvation. These deaths were generally attributed to the use of protein hydrolysates deficient in essential amino acids. Even with a nutritionally adequate source of protein, however, such diets should be undertaken only with close medical supervision and for periods no longer than 2 months. The diet must provide supplemental vitamins, minerals, and fluid.

ALTERNATIVE DIETARY PATTERNS

Organic and Natural Foods

Although neither term is formally defined, organic foods are those grown without the use of chemical fertilizers, herbicides, or pesticides, while natural foods undergo no processing and contain no synthetic ingredients or additives. The purveyors and users of these special foods claim that they are more nutritious, better tasting, and safer than regular foods. Food analyses and blind taste tests have shown no differences from regular foods in either the composition or the taste qualities of organic and natural foods. Two studies in New York, a decade apart, demonstrated that organic and regular foods had similar contents of pesticides. This finding, attributed to the widespread contamination of American soil with environmental pollutants, suggests that it is now difficult to avoid their presence in food products by organic farming. The use of organic or natural foods poses no health hazard, but these products are significantly more expensive than ordinary foods.

Most food additives are used to prevent spoilage from the growth of bacteria or molds and to slow the development of rancidity due to the oxidation of unsaturated fats. The geographic separation between the producers and consumers of food products in this country fully justifies the employment of preservative substances. Some additives, such as artificial sweeteners and synthetic dyes used as food colorings, are not essential to protect the food supply. The safety of such additives has been thoroughly tested, however, and the Food and Drug Administration has banned cyclamates and food dyes when animal studies suggested health risks for humans.

The ultimate example of the avoidance of food additives is the diet recommended initially by Feingold for the management of children with the hyperactivity syndrome. This diet restricts not only all foods with artificial coloring or flavoring but also a number of fruits and vegetables that contain natural salicylates. The severe limitations of the diet have created difficult problems for parents trying to follow this recommendation, and there is no valid evidence for the effectiveness of the diet.

Nutritional Supplementation

Supplementation of the diet with vitamins and other nutrients is widespread in this country. Some estimates indicate that almost half the elderly population regularly uses some form of nutritional supplement. With the exception of calcium and iron in women, healthy individuals do not need such supplements. At best, such practices are an added expense, but not harmful. The costs of vitamin supplements are compounded by claims that "natural," more costly forms are more effective than synthetic vitamins. Dangers arise when the diet is supplemented with megadoses (10 to 100 times the required daily allowances) of certain vitamins. Excessive intake of the fat-soluble vitamins, *A* and *D*, has long been recognized as a cause of toxic manifestations that may persist for many months because of the tissue storage of these vitamins. More recently, toxic manifestations have been identified from the consumption of more than a gram daily of *pyridoxine* (RDA = 2 mg per day) for a period exceeding 2 months. Side effects of megadoses of *niacin* were

TABLE 1 Side Effects of Megavitamin Use

Vitamin	Side Effects
A	Headaches due to increased intracranial pressure; nausea, vomiting and anorexia; fatigue and somnolence; petechiae and epistaxis; skin desquamation and hair loss; hypercalcemia; bony tenderness. Chronic toxicity may also cause papilledema and fibrotic changes in the liver.
C	Hemolysis in individuals with glucose-6-phosphate dehydrogenase deficiency; diarrhea; possibly kidney stones.
D	Hypercalcemia; polyuria and polydipsia; anorexia, nausea, vomiting, constipation; headaches, fatigue, weakness, confusion; nephrocalcinosis and renal failure.
Niacin	Cutaneous flushing, pruritus, urticaria; peptic ulcer; impaired glucose tolerance; hyperuricemia and gouty arthritis.
Pyridoxine	Progressive sensory ataxia; impaired position and vibratory sensation.

recognized from its use in the treatment of patients with hyperlipidemia. The untoward effects of each of these vitamins, as well as *vitamin C*, are listed in Table 1. Physicians must be aware of the toxic manifestations of these vitamins and routinely determine the vitamin intake of their patients. It is ironic that individuals risk the side effects of these vitamins either unwittingly, because of the high content of vitamin A in some multivitamin preparations, or in the unproven expectation that large doses of vitamin C prevent colds and cancer or that megadoses of pyridoxine ameliorate the premenstrual syndrome or hyperactivity or are useful in body-building regimens.

Other nutritional supplements are equally ineffective but relatively harmless. For example, lecithin and vitamin E have no proven efficacy in preventing the complications of atherosclerosis even though the former is widely used for that goal and the latter is probably the most common nutritional supplement. Many *fiber-containing* pills and other products are available, but any benefits of a high fiber diet should be obtained through the appropriate selection of food products rather than by adding supplements to the diet.

RECOGNITION, ASSESSMENT, AND THERAPEUTIC INTERVENTION

Physicians frequently obtain inadequate nutritional data from the history and physical examination. The usual questions about dietary practices are perfunctory and superficial. Instead, physicians should always obtain certain salient information about a patient's nutritional status, including weight changes, appetite, alcohol history, and problems that may interfere with the ingestion or absorption of food, such as difficulty in chewing, loss of taste, dysphagia, vomiting, diarrhea, or prior abdominal surgery. Anthropometric measurements and detection of specific signs of malnutrition are important parts of the physical examination. Physicians should also take the time to discover whether the patient follows a fad diet or alternative dietary habits. In many instances patients are reticent about mentioning unusual dietary habits and do not recognize the relevance of their diet unless the physician asks about it directly. The presence of most unusual dietary practices will be uncovered by asking the questions presented in Table 2. Identification of unusual dietary habits is worthwhile because they may have significant diagnostic and therapeutic implications. Moreover, most patients on fad diets have an intense interest in nutrition and great faith in the health benefits of their particular diet, and therefore they may doubt the interest and skills of a physician who does not even ask about their diet.

Once unusual dietary habits are discovered, the physician must decide what to do about them. This decision depends on the extent of variance of the diet from sound nutritional practices and the likelihood that the patient's diet has, or will have, serious adverse health effects. It is especially important to consider the health consequences

TABLE 2 Questions to Ask Patients to Determine Whether They Are At Risk from Unusual Diets

Question	Rationale
Has your doctor prescribed any special diet?	The special diet may need modification or more detailed explanation by a nutritionist.
Are you on any other special diet, such as a vegetarian or weight loss diet?	Such diets are apt to be nutritionally inadequate unless well planned.
Do you take any vitamins, minerals, or other supplements such as fiber?	Very large doses of vitamins may be toxic.
Do you exclude any types of foods (animal foods, processed foods, convenience foods) or food groups from your diet?	Restrictions on types of foods, especially entire food groups, raise the possibility of nutritional shortfalls and imbalances.
How long have you adhered to this diet?	In general, the longer the patient has been on the regimen, the greater are the health risks.
Do you indulge in fasting, self-induced vomiting, or extreme use of enemas?	These practices suggest anorexia nervosa or bulimia.
Why have you adopted special dietary practices?	Exploring the rationale for the use of the diet often permits insight into other health beliefs and provides clues to acceptable dietary advice.

of unusual diets during adolescence, pregnancy or lactation, and when the presence of disease, such as diabetes, dictates specific dietary measures.

In many instances the physician can easily assess the nature and extent of the unusual practices by asking a few more questions about the diet. Time spent in discussion may help to establish patient rapport and later compliance with nutritional and other therapeutic measures. A more detailed dietary history, with the assistance of a trained nutritionist, is recommended to ensure the adequacy of the diet when patients have followed, or plan to follow, a fad diet for a considerable period. Depending on the type and duration of the diet, the physician may choose to perform laboratory tests to assess current nutritional status. Thus, measurements of serum albumin or transferrin levels may be indicated to determine adequacy of protein intake in patients on a strict vegetarian diet.

Physician intervention to alter unusual dietary habits may be difficult. Patients are quite confident of the health benefits of their diets and of their own knowledge of nutrition, though much of it may be faulty. Even physicians well versed in nutrition may be unable to convince patients that their dietary practices are not beneficial and may be harmful. When the dietary habits are unnecessary, but safe, such as modest supplements with vitamins, minerals, lecithin or fiber, I point out the economic disadvantages and make no serious effort to alter the diet. I do not intervene when patients are on most fad diets for weight reduction, but rather insist on close follow-up with the anticipation that the diet will be discontinued before the occurrence of serious consequences. Although I may not agree with these dietary choices, prolonged battles with the patient are not worth the risk that he will abandon medical follow-up.

In contrast, more firm measures must be taken to interrupt or control dietary practices with serious health implications. Patients taking megadoses of vitamins or minerals are informed of the toxic effects of vitamins A and D and pyridoxine and are strongly urged to discontinue their use. Those on reducing diets containing fewer than 800 calories per day are warned of their nutritional inadequacies and told to stop the diet. If they refuse, this group of patients, along with those committed to strict vegetarian diets, are referred to a nutritionist for more complete evaluation of the diet and for detailed advice on measures to minimize the dangers of their diet.

CROHN'S DISEASE OF THE SMALL BOWEL

STEPHEN B. HANAUER, M.D.

Crohn's disease is a chronic variant of inflammatory bowel disease for which neither the cause nor the cure has been identified. Hence, when making therapeutic decisions, the physician must consider the short- and long-term consequences of the actual illness as well as the potential benefit and "cost" of medical therapy. Furthermore, since surgery is almost never curative for Crohn's disease, one must constantly balance the less immediate rewards of continuing medical therapy against the short-term benefits of surgery followed by almost certain recurrence.

In initially managing the patient with Crohn's disease, it is important to confirm the diagnosis and to exclude complications such as intercurrent enteric infections, lactose intolerance, or bile-acid-induced diarrhea. A review of the original diagnosis and, if necessary, an update of studies to assess the current location and extent of the inflammatory process are essential.

The diagnosis of active Crohn's disease can be confirmed by the presence of inflammatory symptoms and signs (fever, night sweats, abdominal tenderness and so on) supported by laboratory findings of an increased white blood cell count, elevated sedimentation rate, fecal leukocytes, an increase in fecal alpha$_1$-antitrypsin and radiographic or endoscopic evidence of mucosal edema or ulceration. Any patient presenting with a sudden exacerbation of symptoms should have stool cultures for enteric pathogens, a fecal smear for ova and parasites, and an assay for *Clostridium difficile* toxin. More chronic or progressive symptoms require a review of the current therapy for possible adverse consequences, or postsurgical or noninflammatory complications. The latter may range from partial obstruction in areas of scarred bowel with poor motility and bacterial overgrowth to the short bowel syndrome with profuse diarrhea and malnutrition.

A thorough evaluation (or reevaluation) of each patient is essential to determine the site of activity of the Crohn's inflammation, and to exclude superinfection or additional complications. A review of the dietary history and an updated nutritional profile are important whenever new or changing symptoms arise. The extent of the evaluation will depend upon the complaints and the previous history of the individual patient.

MEDICAL APPROACH TO TREATMENT

The potential medical therapy for small intestinal Crohn's disease ranges from changes in diet to immunosuppressant medication. Many of the therapeutic alternatives, including steroids, are nonspecific and are directed at symptoms rather than the actual disease process. The ultimate goal of treatment often is supportive, aiming to control symptoms and to maintain an active lifestyle until the disease activity is brought under control.

Each patient will require an individualized program of therapy incorporating dietary modifications, medications, and recommendations regarding necessary changes in lifestyle. A complete nutritional assessment and dietary plan must ensure replacement and/or maintenance of essential nutrients which are administered in a manner to minimize adverse symptoms. Antidiarrheal agents and additional adjunctive medications should be prescribed to reduce symptoms. Antibacterial agents are indicated for such complications as bacterial overgrowth or abscess or, in a more general role, to supplement or spare steroid therapy. Sulfasalazine presumably has specific gut-related anti-inflammatory activity and is often used as a first-line therapy or combined with steroids to treat mild to moderate intestinal Crohn's disease. Steroids remain the mainstay of medical therapy for more moderate to severe small bowel Crohn's disease, but they require judicious monitoring of the cost-benefit ratio. *Specific objectives of therapy* should be identified prior to administering steroids, immunosuppressant agents or hyperalimentation.

Nutritional Therapy

Diet and nutritional factors are of the utmost importance in the management of patients with intestinal ailments. In small intestinal Crohn's disease in which the normal absorptive mechanisms have been disrupted, nutritional evaluation and planning are indispensable. Whether the patient complains of weight loss, abdominal pain, diarrhea, or nonintestinal symptoms, a review of the dietary history is an important first step. Lactose intolerance should be ruled out by breath hydrogen or blood sampling. A nutritional profile including the assessment of iron stores, folate, vitamin B_{12}, and fat-soluble vitamins is important, as are the more routine measurements of electrolytes, calcium, magnesium, phosphate, and serum albumin. Trace mineral deficiencies should be considered in patients with protracted, severe diarrhea or malnutrition.

While no dietary factors are known to cause or activate intestinal inflammation, modifications in the diet can provide relief from a variety of symptoms, and a dietary plan for the individual patient is an important practical measure.

Most patients can be managed with an oral dietary program. Sufficient calories and protein to maintain body weight and replenish intestinal losses are essential. Milk products should be withheld or modified by one of the available lactase products (e.g., LactAid or Lactrase) for patients with lactose intolerance. In either case, sufficient calcium (1 g daily) should be provided. Replacement of diminished vitamin stores by either the enteral or parenteral route will depend on the deficient factors and the patient's tolerance of these compounds. The amount of fat allowed in the diet will depend on the individual's tendency to develop steatorrhea.

In most patients with small bowel Crohn's disease I institute a modified low-residue diet that avoids large amounts of "hard roughage" such as raw fruits and vegetables, nuts, and seeds in favor of cooked, canned, or peeled fruits and vegetables. Highly seasoned foods also are proscribed in patients prone to diarrhea.

More refined or elemental diets have been useful as an adjunct in patients with more severe disease. While controversy still exists regarding the ultimate role of highly modified diets, there is no question that a change to elemental feedings can markedly reduce the symptoms of patients with active disease or luminal narrowing. Unfortunately, the lack of palatability of the available preparations over prolonged periods limits the length of time that most patients will tolerate this modification. In some situations, such as children with growth retardation, nocturnal enteral elemental feedings via a nasoenteric feeding tube may be a useful supplement to the daily oral intake.

Parenteral nutritional support may be useful to (1) provide supplemental feedings in patients unable to tolerate sufficient oral calories, (2) improve the nutritional status in malnourished patients scheduled for elective surgery, (3) reduce symptoms in patients with active disease, (4) reverse growth retardation in children, and (5) provide maintenance therapy for the short bowel. The role of total parenteral nutrition and bowel rest is the subject of continued controversy. A regimen of complete bowel rest often is of symptomatic benefit in situations in which the added caloric intake cannot be tolerated without aggravating symptoms. Fistulas and perianal suppuration often improve with the reduction in intestinal output, although permanent closure of fistula tracts unfortunately is rare. It also has been speculated that the reduction in orally derived antigens may beneficially alter the local gut immune response and allow healing. I have observed marked reductions in inflammatory masses and have avoided surgery in patients with complicated courses by the prolonged (3 to 6 months) use of hyperalimentation. tation.

Adjunctive Medications

Medications often are administered to reduce symptoms. Antispasmodics may be effective in alleviating abdominal cramps and pain. Anticholinergic agents can be administered safely in patients with luminal narrowing, although they should be closely monitored and warned to discontinue antimotility agents in the presence of progressive or severe pain or abdominal distention. I tend to prescribe such drugs on a continual rather than "as needed" basis to maintain control of the symptoms. Antidiarrheal drugs also are of benefit in patients with small (and large) bowel Crohn's disease. Again, these agents should be discontinued in the presence of toxic symptoms, severe abdominal pain, or suspicion of obstruction.

$Histamine_2$ receptor antagonists may help relieve symptoms in patients with Crohn's disease of the upper gastrointestinal tract. Sucralfate may be similarly helpful, although neither has been studied in a controlled clinical trial.

Cholestyramine is useful in patients who have undergone surgery with bile-salt-induced diarrhea. In this setting, the dose is titrated to the point of maximal symptomatic benefit. One may begin with one-half packet or one-half scoopful (2 g of resin) administered twice daily and adjusted upward to three to four packets daily.

I often note benefit at lower doses, and higher doses may actually worsen symptoms if the bile salt pool becomes depleted. Care should be taken to avoid administering this resin with other medications, levels of fat-soluble vitamins need to be monitored, and the drug should be discontinued in the presence of partial obstruction, as formed contents may worsen or complete the blockage.

Sedatives or anxiolytics have a role in individual patients but should be carefully regulated because of the hazard of possible drug dependency. Accordingly, I *almost never* prescribe narcotic analgesics. Pain severe enough to require narcotics should be evaluated for more sharply focused therapy. Cramps may be treated with antispasmodics, partial obstruction with a more refined diet, abscess by drainage, and so on. Partial obstruction may be aggravated by narcotics (increased intraluminal pressure) and, conversely, can be eased by dietary adjustments and antispasmodics. Other causes of chronic pain are never resolved by narcotics. Many patients are referred who are already addicted to narcotics and thus require inpatient admissions for detoxification. In these situations, I emphasize the alternative approaches to the treatment of pain (biofeedback, transcutaneous electrical nerve stimulation, physiotherapy, and so on) and withhold potent analgesia for the perioperative setting. There are two separate chapters on *Chronic Abdominal Pain: A Cognitive Behavioral Treatment Approach* as well as a chapter on *Hypochondriasis, Hysteria, and Depression* and on *Functional Illness*.

Patient support measures include literature from the National Foundation for Ileitis and Colitis (NFIC), 444 Park Ave. South, New York, 10016 as well as local NFIC chapter support groups.

"Specific" Medications

Sulfasalazine. Many experienced clinicians have found sulfasalazine therapy useful to reduce enteric inflammation and to maintain patients once the active phase has subsided. Although sulfasalazine had only limited but significant benefit in small intestinal Crohn's disease in the National Cooperative Crohn's Disease Study (NCCDS), I have found the drug helpful in some patients with mild to moderate small bowel disease even in the absence of active colonic inflammation. For mild symptoms, the drug may be administered as the solitary "specific" medication in quantities of 2 to 4 g daily in divided doses. If symptoms improve, a maintenance dose of 2 g daily may be continued almost indefinitely. Here again, little benefit in preventing relapses was observed in the NCCDS; however, I frequently observe flare-ups in patients when sulfasalazine therapy is suddenly withdrawn. In the presence of more severe inflammatory symptoms, sulfasalazine may be administered in conjunction with corticosteroids and maintained as the steroids are gradually withdrawn. Sulfasalazine (or other antibiotics, see below) may behave as a "steroid-sparing" agent, and can maintain quiescent symptoms as the steroids are tapered.

The mode of action of sulfasalazine in inflammatory bowel disease has not been elucidated (see the chapters *Ulcerative Colitis and Proctitis* and *Crohn's Disease of the Colon*). Although once regarded mainly as an antibacterial drug, the 5-aminosalicylic acid moiety is the more active component, at least for colonic disease. Both the parent compound and 5-aminosalicylic acid interact at various levels within the arachidonic cascade of inflammatory mediators.

Sulfasalazine is best tolerated when taken with meals to avoid the side effects of headache and nausea. A gradual dose increment is useful to initiate therapy, at which time patients can be observed for intolerance. Allergic side effects, such as skin rashes or drug fever, are not uncommon and can be overcome by a desensitization program beginning with very low doses of sulfasalazine suspension (1 to 50 mg initially), with doubling of the dose every 3 days. More severe allergic reactions, such as hepatitis, agranulocytosis, or hemolytic anemias, are less common and require discontinuation of the drug. Sulfasalazine is known to inhibit the absorption of folic acid from the diet; hence, 1 mg daily of folic acid is added to the regimen of patients receiving chronic therapy.

Antibacterial Agents. Antibiotics also have been found to be useful either alone or in conjunction with steroids. *Metronidazole* has been used extensively lately, following reports of its value in the treatment of perianal Crohn's Disease. Subsequently, the European Cooperative Crohn's Disease Study found metronidazole to be as effective as sulfasalazine for colonic Crohn's disease and somewhat better than sulfasalazine for the treatment of ileal Crohn's disease. The optimal dose of metronidazole has not been determined, although a cooperative study of metronidazole as the sole treatment of Crohn's disease in the United States in evaluating both 10 and 20 mg per kilogram per day, while 20 mg per kilogram per day has been recommended for perianal disease.

Most patients will tolerate between 500 and 1,500 mg daily. The common side effects include a metallic taste in the mouth, a coated tongue, and occasional nausea. Peripheral neuropathy has been the most troublesome complication of metronidazole. In my experience this occurs more commonly in malnourished patients. Therefore, I prescribe supplemental vitamins for all patients taking metronidazole with a warning to discontinue the drug should they develop any signs of tingling or numbness in the extremities. The neuropathy seems reversible in most instances, although there have been a few reports of persistent changes. Patients also should be warned of the interaction between metronidazole and ethanol producing an Antabuse-like effect. Potential tumorigenicity and mutagenicity in laboratory animals have been observed, causing concern over the long-term use of this drug in humans. The potential benefit (response) in this chronic illness needs to be weighed against reports of animal toxicity, although no such effects have been described in humans. I maintain patients on the lowest possible dose of metronidazole (assuming an initial response) and warn women against becoming pregnant while on the drug.

Alternative antibiotics have not been extensively studied in clinical trials, although most gastroenterologists who treat Crohn's disease utilize antibacterials in a nonspecific manner. Individual practitioners have favored regimens which employ either a single drug or alternating antibiotics in a serial fashion (as one might treat bacterial overgrowth). The *tetracyclines, sulfonamides, ampicillin, erythromycin,* and *sulfamethoxazole-trimethoprim* each have proponents. Again, I tend to prescribe a single antibiotic as primary therapy either alone or in combination with steroids for patients who have failed to improve with or are tolerant of sulfasalazine. These drugs also are indicted for treatment of suspected bacterial overgrowth or evidence of an abscess or septic focus and may be of benefit for patients with enteric arthropathies or cutaneous manifestations of Crohn's disease.

Corticosteroids. Steroids have been the most consistently effective agents for the treatment of active small bowel Crohn's disease in all clinical trials. Unfortunately, the efficacy has been at the expense of a wide spectrum of adverse consequences. Furthermore, as with all drugs studied to date in Crohn's disease, corticosteroids have a palliative rather than curative action. Steroids appear to be of no benefit in maintaining remissions of quiescent disease or in preventing recurrences after surgical resection.

Nevertheless, steroids are the most commonly used (and often abused) medications for small bowel Crohn's disease. Steroids are indicated if sulfasalazine or antibiotic therapy has not been adequate to control symptoms of mild ileitis or ileocolitis and should be prescribed alone, or in combination with sulfasalazine or an antibiotic, as initial treatment for moderate or severe disease. One can expect a prompt reduction of symptoms and a return to a feeling of well-being with an improved appetite and associated weight gain. Corticosteroids are potent antidiarrheal agents in small intestinal Crohn's disease, can reduce inflammatory masses, will reduce luminal narrowings due to active disease (in the presence of mucosal edema and ulceration, but not fibrotic strictures, manifest by pseudo-diverticula and the absence of inflammation), may improve perianal disease (partially by decreasing diarrhea), but have not been effective in closing enteric fistula. These drugs may be hazardous in the presence of sepsis (abscess or peritonitis) unless they are administered in "stress doses" to patients with adrenal suppression from prior steroid therapy.

Adrenocorticotropic hormone injections or intravenous drip infusions may be of similar benefit for patients with flare-ups of Crohn's disease, and appear to be best suited for patients who have not been receiving other forms of steroids.

A variety of preparations are available for oral or parenteral use, and change from one form to another may be associated with clinical improvement in patients who seem to be no longer responsive to steroid therapy. The most widely used preparation is *prednisone,* usually prescribed as 40 to 60 mg daily in a single morning dose. The once a day schedule mimics the diurnal variation of endogenous cortisone, allows convenient tapering, and appears appropriate for alternate day dosing and an eventual return of adrenal function with gradual weaning. Alternatively, split doses may be necessary for patients with persistent nocturnal symptoms. *Prednisolone* and *methylprednisolone* are alternatives which can be used in a similar manner. *Hydrocortisone* may also be prescribed in divided doses (initially 50 mg 4 times daily) and may be of use in patients who fail to improve with prednisone, although at the expense of enhanced salt retention (as may be seen also with *triamcinolone*).

Once a clinical remission has been achieved, tapering should begin, but the exact schedule will depend upon the individual patient's response to the initial decrease in dosage. I find that the most frequent cause of referrals for active disease is an exacerbation of the disease due to too rapid tapering of steroids. In general, the weaning process correlates with the length and severity of symptoms and prior therapy. Patients with the acute onset of ileitis may have their dose decreased from 40 mg by 5 mg per week, whereas patients who have been under therapy for many months or years require a more gradual approach. In these patients a reduction by 5 mg per month down to a 20-mg dose and a 2.5 mg per month reduction thereafter, may be necessary to wean a chronically ill patient from steroids. Some patients may remain at a dose of 20 mg daily and have trouble with further tapering. In this situation, the addition or change to a different antibiotic and/or steroid preparation can be useful in renewing the tapering process.

Alternate day therapy may be useful in selected patients and has the benefit of lessened adrenal suppression. In children with small bowel Crohn's disease, alternate-day therapy can be effective in avoiding the problem of growth retardation. In adults it is presumed, though not tested in clinical trials, that alternate day therapy will reduce the adverse consequences of long-term steroid therapy. Unfortunately, this worthy goal is difficult to achieve in most adults, although some patients with chronic, low-grade symptoms can be maintained on alternate-day prednisone.

The adverse effects of steroid therapy are well known and need not be detailed in this review. There are, however, a few complications more characteristic of small intestinal Crohn's disease which should be emphasized. First, the physician should be cautious about initiating steroid therapy in a patient with a potential suppurative complication for which antibiotics and/or surgical drainage are likely to be more helpful. In children steroids can aggravate growth retardation, and we have found that in both children and adults steroid therapy is most beneficial in terms of a more rapid response if the nutritional status has been restored toward normal. Metabolic bone disease is seen without steroids in Crohn's disease, and the addition of steroids to regimens for patients with insufficient calcium, magnesium, and vitamin D intake may accelerate bone demineralization and osteoporosis. It is essential that vitamin D stores be maintained and adequate calcium supplemented as part of the nutritional program.

Immunosuppressant Agents. Immunosuppressive agents have been used sporadically for 20 years despite a number of clinical trials that have not as yet provided clear evidence of their efficacy in Crohn's disease of the small bowel. The acute and chronic course of Crohn's disease, the wide spectrum of clinical situations, and the length of time necessary to evaluate objectively a response to these drugs probably have made it difficult to document proof of benefit in randomized controlled trials. Hence, it is not surprising that the NCCDS was unable to identify improvement in the patients treated with azathioprine (2.5 mg per kilogram) as a single therapeutic modality over 17 weeks when steroid withdrawal was mandatory. Other investigators have recognized that azathioprine may have a role as an adjunct to steroid therapy or in the prevention of relapse of medically or surgically treated patients. Most recently, Present and Korelitz have utilized 6-mercaptopurine in a 2-year placebo-controlled, crossover protocol.[1] These two investigators were able to identify a favorable response in two-thirds of their patients manifested as significant improvements in symptoms, improvement in fistulas, and a reduction in the steroid dose. In this study and in subsequent reports, many patients required up to 6 months to respond, so that the short-term efficacy probably cannot be evaluated. Furthermore, many patients were receiving concurrent steroid treatment which was gradually tapered, compared with the NCCDS which demanded regular reduction of steroids and termination of azathioprine at 17 weeks.

The immunosuppressive drugs probably are effective in a subgroup of patients with Crohn's disease. The fears of long-term consequences, most notably susceptibility to malignancy, as yet have not been borne out in the large series of patients from New York. Nevertheless, patients must be followed closely for the development of neutropenia. Pancreatitis was observed in 5 percent of patients receiving azathioprine in the NCCDS and probably occurs with a similar frequency with 6-mercaptopurine. Possible hepatotoxicity and malignancy have yet to be confirmed in patients with Crohn's disease.

I reserve the use of immunosuppressants in small bowel Crohn's disease (1) for patients with refractory disease activity which persists despite steroids or recurs with tapering; (2) as adjunctive therapy for patients with postoperative recurrences in an attempt to avoid additional surgery; (3) in patients with diffuse small bowel Crohn's disease (jejunoileitis) in whom surgery would be impractical; (4) in patients with intractable perianal disease; (5) in patients with fistulas for whom surgery is not desirable; and (6) in patients with extra-intestinal manifestations of inflammatory bowel disease (arthritis, erythema nodosum, iritis and so on) out of proportion to the bowel disease. I begin with 50 mg daily of either azathioprine or 6-mercaptopurine and follow the complete blood count weekly for the first month. After 2 weeks the dose is increased to 100 mg daily and eventually to a total dose of 2 to 2.5 mg per kilogram per day. Blood counts are followed monthly after a stable dose has been achieved. Many patients respond to lower doses (e.g, 50 to 100 mg per day), which diminish the risk of neutropenia. Abdominal pain or nausea should be evaluated by measuring serum amylase or lipase, and liver function tests should be followed every 3 to 4 months. I generally begin to taper steroids after a stable clinical course has been achieved. Although up to 6 months may be required to determine efficacy, most patients tolerate these drugs well. Unfortunately, experience indicates that disease activity typically recurs after withdrawal of these medications, so that long-term therapy, albeit at reduced dosages, may be necessary.

ACUTE DISEASE

Patients presenting with new or recurrent disease should be assessed as described above for the location and activity of the Crohn's disease as well as for possible complications. Those with milder symptoms of diarrhea, abdominal cramping, limited weight loss and no abdominal mass or fistula may begin to receive sulfasalazine (2 to 4 g per day) alone or an alternate antibiotic and instructed as to a diet (usually low-residue with or without milk products according to their lactase status). Adequate protein, calcium, and vitamin supplements should be provided. If symptoms persist, a trial of mild antispasmodics, antidiarrheal agents, or both should be instituted prior to advancing to steroid therapy. Therapy is then continued until a complete response is achieved. Even though symptoms remit, I will maintain the initial dose of sulfasalazine for up to 5 to 6 months before beginning to taper down to a maintenance dose of 2 g per day.

Patients with moderate disease manifested by fever, significant weight loss, more severe diarrhea and abdominal pain and tenderness usually will require steroids. While the benefit of combination therapy remains controversial, I commonly prescribe both prednisone and an antibiotic (or sulfasalazine) beginning with 40 mg of prednisone until a complete response is achieved. At that point, the prednisone can be decreased rapidly by 5 mg every week or 2 (as tolerated) down to 20 mg, and by about 5 mg per month thereafter. While this schedule probably is slower than many physicians prescribe, I have been impressed by the frequency of incomplete responses or exacerbations with the rapid tapering schedules frequently employed. I maintain the antibiotic therapy while the steroids are tapered and often will change drugs if there is a worsening of symptoms prior to complete withdrawal. Dietary and nonspecific, symptomatic therapy are, of course, continued.

Patients with more severe disease manifested by malnutrition or a tender inflammatory mass or abscess, or those appearing septic require hospitalization. They should be stabilized with intravenous hydration and broad-spectrum antibiotics (after appropriate cultures of blood, urine, and so on), such as metronidazole and an aminoglycoside; clindamycin and an aminoglycoside; or cefoxitin. Steroids should be withheld (unless the patient has been taking adrenal suppressive doses) until a suppurative process has been excluded. Once an abscess or perforation has been ruled out, parenteral steroids should be administered in divided doses equal to 40 to 60 mg per day of prednisone. This can be changed to an oral regimen as the patient improves.

The decision whether or not medical therapy should be continued in acute disease will depend upon associated complications. Indications for an operation, in general, are the subject of another chapter (see *Crohn's Disease: Surgical Treatment*), but I consider evidence of an abscess, persistent obstruction, continuing hemorrhage, or complicated fistula (enterosigmoid, enterovesical, and so on) as indications for surgical intervention. Surgery usually is recommended as soon as the patient has been stabilized, rehydrated, and prepared with preoperative antibiotics.

Patients who respond to initial medical intervention may be considered for further medical and nutritional therapy. For severely malnourished individuals with significant abdominal pain, an inflammatory mass, or partial obstruction, a period of hyperalimentation and bowel rest will allow the steroids (and time) to determine whether surgery will be necessary. For those who respond the diet can be gradually advanced. Less ill patients who can tolerate oral feedings may be placed on elemental feedings or a low-residue diet as discussed previously. With clinical improvement, the diet then may be advanced as tolerated, with constant monitoring of weight, nutritional stores, and calorie counts. The patients then are gradually weaned off steroids as described for less severely ill individuals.

CHRONIC DISEASE

Chronically ill patients require a separate decision analysis because of their failure to respond completely to medical therapy, inability to eliminate steroids, a persistent mass, or recurrent obstruction. These patients are caught in a dilemma because medical treatment has been less than optimal, prior surgery has provided only temporary improvement, or the patient is a poor surgical candidate owing to diffuse or multifocal disease. The objectives of medical therapy in this setting are to create a less toxic, but effective long-term treatment regimen or to modify the intestinal inflammation to the point that a well-planned, elective operation will successfully eliminate a specific problematic segment of bowel.

Depending upon the individual situation, a modification of medical therapy will often shift the course in a more favorable direction. Often, a change in steroids (e.g., prednisone to methylprednisolone or hydrocortisone) as well as the use of an alternate antibiotic may be beneficial. Some small bowel symptoms may be related to bacterial overgrowth or malabsorption, which justifies the change in antibiotic and allows further dietary modifications. Elemental feedings or a period of total parenteral nutrition may provide a respite from symptoms, induce a more prolonged symptomatic remission, reduce the size of an inflammatory mass, or resolve the bowel narrowing resulting from active inflammation. This approach may require up to 3 to 6 months to produce a lengthy clinical response. Total parenteral nutrition is of little benefit (aside from nutritional repletion prior to elective surgery) in permanently closing enteric fistulas or in opening tight fibrotic strictures. While I have found TPN to be most useful in patients with chronic or unrelenting Crohn's disease, some patients will not improve sufficiently to resume total enteral diets. In many of these individuals the course of TPN will have further confined and delineated the small bowel inflammation sufficiently to limit the extent of a necessary surgical resection, or, rarely, patients may require long-term home TPN.

Another option for these patients is the introduction of an immunosuppressant drug to assist in steriod tapering or possibly to be used in conjunction with dietary modifications (elemental feedings or TPN). A few patients will be unable to eliminate steroids and they then should be transferred to an alternate day schedule to reduce the potential for long-term steroid toxicity.

The decision to recommend surgery in chronic Crohn's disease needs to be weighed against the likelihood of recurrence. Chronicity itself is a favorable feature, as extended intervals between operations appears to be a good prognostic indicator for prolonged remissions. By this time, the active disease has "burned out" and physicians and surgeons are dealing with problems related to scarring and fibrosis. Indications for surgery include stricture formation, suspicion of malignancy in a newly narrowed segment or excluded loop of bowel, and failure to wean patients of TPN or down to acceptable levels of steroids or immunosuppressants or both. The latter indication is, of course, the most subjective and often creates one of the most difficult decisions for experienced clinicians and their well-informed patients.

RECURRENT DISEASE

When patients present with symptoms after a surgical resection in Crohn's disease, it is necessary to determine whether the symptoms are related to active Crohn's disease or represent a complication of the surgery. Inflammatory symptoms, fever, extraintestinal symptoms, and an abdominal mass or new fistula indicate disease activity. Diarrhea, abdominal pain, and weight loss are less specific and warrant a reevaluation because of the possibility that the new symptoms are related to intercurrent infection of *Clostridium difficile,* malabsorption (lactose, and so on), a short-bowel syndrome, bacterial overgrowth, or bile salt induced enteropathy.

An examination of the stool for fecal leukocytes is a simple initial test that should be followed by a 72-hour collection for stool volume and fecal fat. Steatorrhea, with the daily excretion of more than 10 to 20 g of fat, usually responds to a low-fat diet (which can be supplemented with medium-chain triglycerides if necessary). Patients excreting less than 10 g of fecal fat often will respond to the introduction of cholestyramine to reduce the conversion of colonic bile salts to bile acids.

Loss of the ileocecal valve alone can lead to more frequent bowel movements. Additionally, many patients without inflammatory symptoms or signs will have symptoms of an irritable bowel which can be treated with dietary modifications, antispasmodics, and antidiarrheals.

The chapter on small bowel resection provides additional details of management.

Patients who present with recurrent Crohn's disease require a great deal of patience, understanding, and supportive therapy to deal with their disappointment over the need for reinstitution of medical therapy. Once again, all of the nonspecific supportive measures, including dietary adjustments and symptomatic medications, sulfasalazine or antibiotics, should be used prior to reinstituting steroids. If immunosuppressants have not previously been employed, then these agents may be useful to control extending or refractory inflammatory disease.

COMPLICATIONS

Many of the local complications of small bowel Crohn's disease have been discussed previously (inflammatory mass, fistula, strictures) or are the topics of other chapters (*Crohn's Disease of the Colon, Crohn's Disease: Surgical Treatment,* and *Idiopathic Inflammatory Bowel Disease and Neoplasia*). Crohn's disease of the upper digestive tract rarely occurs independently of intestinal Crohn's disease, but aphthous ulcerations in the mouth, esophagitis, and Crohn's ulcerations of the stomach and duodenum will occasionally produce symptoms requiring therapy in addition to that for small bowel disease. Usually, these manifestations improve as the intestinal disease is treated, especially with systemic steroids. *Oral ulcerations* can be treated topically with Kenalog in Orabase. *Esophageal involvement* tends to mimic peptic disease of the distal esophagus and may symptomatically respond to acid reduction therapy. Theoretically, liquid sulfasalzine therapy might be helpful because of the antiinflammatory action of the parent compound. *Gastroduodenal* Crohn's disease also is difficult to separate from peptic ulcer disease except for the increased tendency toward gastric outlet obstruction from either impaired motility and pyloric or duodenal narrowing. A low-residue or liquid diet may be beneficial and many patients will respond to H_2 receptor antagonists. Steroids are occasionally effective in improving the obstruction, which may require palliative (bypass) surgery. Crohn's disease *fistulas* involving the duodenum present some of the most complicated problems because of their intractabiltiy and the potentially serious surgical complications.

Exraintestinal Complications

Growth retardation and *hyperoxaluria* are topics of other chapters. *Ocular manifestations,* including iritis, iridocyclitis, and uveitis rarely occur with small bowel involvement and usually improve with topical steroids or with systemic steroids administered for the intestinal inflammation. Peripheral *arthritis* is more common with colonic disease and also responds to treatment of the bowel disease. In a few patients the arthropathy is more severe and troublesome than the intestinal inflammation but may improve with the *cautious* use of nonsteroidal antiinflammatory agents. Intra-articular injections of steroids or a brief course of systemic steroid therapy may improve the arthropathy. I have found immunosuppressives useful in a group of patients who would otherwise require maintenance steroids to control the joint manifestations. While symptoms of peripheral joint involvement frequently improve coincident with improving bowel disease, the HLA B27-related arthropathies of ankylosing spondylitis and sacroiliitis tend to run a course independent of the bowel disease. Occasionally, a course of antibiotics will improve these "enteric arthropathies."

The cutaneous manifestations of Crohn's disease, *erythema nodosum* and *pyoderma gangrenosum,* occur more often with colonic than small bowel Crohn's disease and usually improve with treatment of the intestinal disease, although pyoderma gangrenosum may require intensive local therapy with a combination of topical steroids and antibiotics and may occasionally benefit from oral high-dose antibiotics (tetracycline, erythromycin, or dapsone).

Pericholangitis requires no specific treatment. *Sclerosing cholangitis* has a rather unpredictable course which typically is unassociated with the intestinal manifestations. *Cholelithiasis* most often is related to bile salt malabsorption associated with ileal disease or resection. A number of patients have developed acute *cholecystitis* after a course of TPN and subsequent refeeding due to the formation of sludge in an atonic, unstimulated gallbladder. Protocols under investigation to avoid this complication include small, intermittent feedings interspersed with TPN, or daily injections of cholecystokinin.

Pregnancy and inflammatory bowel disease has been the topic of several recent reviews.[2,3] Despite the expected influence of a chronic illness and potent medications upon the menstrual cycle, it appears that women with Crohn's disease are as fertile as the general population, although in the presence of active disease there is an increased risk of a spontaneous abortion. Pregnancy does not seem to activate quiescent Crohn's disease and has little impact upon the overall course of Crohn's disease, although a number of women may have flare-ups subsequent to delivery. There is no increased risk to the fetus as a result of the inflammatory bowel disease, and most obstetricians are more concerned that the expectant mother be maintained under good control. Despite the theoretical effects of steroids and sulfasalazine upon the fetus, there have not been reports of significant effect upon the fetal outcome or significant birth defects. Because of the mutagenic and teratogenic potentials of metronidazole and the immunosuppressants, I continue to warn women taking these drugs against becoming pregnant and will attempt to taper off or change the medical regimen prior to conception. Some women may require TPN for nutritional support, which has been used successfully during pregnancy.[4] Sulfasalazine can affect sperm count and motility and can be a factor in male infertility.

Crohn's disease of the small bowel is a most challenging clinical problem for the physician, who must contend with a chronic, remitting, and as yet, incurable illness. Potent and effective, but potentially toxic medications can be used or, alternatively, surgery, but this can never be considered curative and has potential adverse consequences. The physician must approach each patient and consider the underlying pathophysiologic processes, in order to define an optimal diet, to prescribe supportive and specific medications, and to control problems unique to each individual. Throughout the course of treatment, the physician must maintain an optimistic attitude with the patient and his family; this will help preserve a positive outlook. For certainly, the underlying cause and the eventual cure of Crohn's disease will be discovered.

REFERENCES

1. Present, Korelitz. Treatment of Crohn's disease with 6-mercaptopurine. N Engl J Med 1980; 302:981–987.
2. Management of medicine problems in pregnancy—inflammatory bowel disease. N Engl J Med 1985; 312:1616–1619.
3. Crohn's disease in pregnancy. Gut 1984; 25:52–56.
4. Successfully completed pregnancy in patient maintained on home parenteral nutrition. Br Med J 1983; 286:602–603.

GROWTH FAILURE IN INFLAMMATORY BOWEL DISEASE

RICHARD J. GRAND, M.D.
KATHLEEN J. MOTIL, M.D., Ph.D.

Growth failure in children with inflammatory bowel disease is a common and ominous complication that is frequently overlooked in the course of medical management. Impairment of linear growth, lack of weight gain, retarded bone development, and delayed onset of sexual maturation are seen in 10 to 40 percent of patients under 21 years of age with inflammatory bowel disease. In our own population of recently studied patients, linear growth delay was present in approximately 40 percent and occurred in those individuals whose heights deviated below the third percentile. Only one-fourth of the children and adolescents with growth failure were prepubertal. Weight for age deficits were also apparent in 49 percent of the patients; however, weight for height deficits were seen in only 19 percent, which suggested that this group fit the criteria for nutritional dwarfism. Growth failure was much more common in children with Crohn's disease (40%) than in those with ulcerative colitis (20%).

For clinical purposes, growth failure is defined as cessation of linear growth for more than 6 months, a decrease of one standard deviation in height percentiles, or bone age delay of greater than 2 years or both. Growth data may be obtained from the clinical history and from assessment of growth and development milestones, as well as family history, particularly the patient's height in relation to parents' height. The pediatricians's records or school data may be an important source of growth information, and yearly height and weight should be plotted on an appropriate growth chart to assess the characteristics of growth prior to onset of inflammatory bowel disease.

Abnormalities in body composition in our patients were demonstrated by combined height and weight deficits in almost half of the children and adolescents. Midarm circumference and arm muscle area measurements were less than the fifth percentile in 10 percent of the group, and the triceps skin fold thickness was reduced in 5 percent of the patients. Serum total proteins and albumin levels were depressed in nearly 20 percent of these individuals.

These observations suggest that alterations in body composition are a prominent feature of chronic inflammatory bowel disease in children and adolescents, and represent the consequences of long-term nutritional deficiencies.

Additional clinical correlation may be made in children with inflammatory bowel disease and growth failure (Table 1). As shown in Figure 1, growth failure may precede clinical illness, often by years. Furthermore, growth failure may occur when clinical disease is quiescent. Under these circumstances, it must be assumed that the chronic demands placed on the body by the presence of undiagnosed inflammatory disease account for chronic nutritional debility. Growth failure is rarely, if ever, associated with endocrine abnormalities. Tests of hormonal function have generally been normal. Recent reports have demonstrated that some children with growth failure have low serum somatomedin-C levels. Somatomedins are dependent on protein intake, however, and serum levels rise quickly after repletion of protein nutriture. Furthermore, some children with growth failure and inflammatory bowel disease have normal somatomedin levels. Thus, this potential mediator requires further study before it is identified as the final common pathway for growth failure in inflammatory bowel disease.

TABLE 1 Correlations of Growth Failure with Inflammatory Bowel Disease

Growth failure a common complication of inflammatory bowel disease

May precede clinical illness by months or years

May occur when clinical disease is quiescent

Associated with malabsorption or nutritional deficiencies in some patients

Rarely, if ever, associated with endocrine abnormalities

May occur in the presence or absence of steroid therapy

Reduced energy intake a major factor in poor growth

Cost of catch-up growth greater than normal

Adequate nutritional repletion can reverse malnutrition and stimulate growth

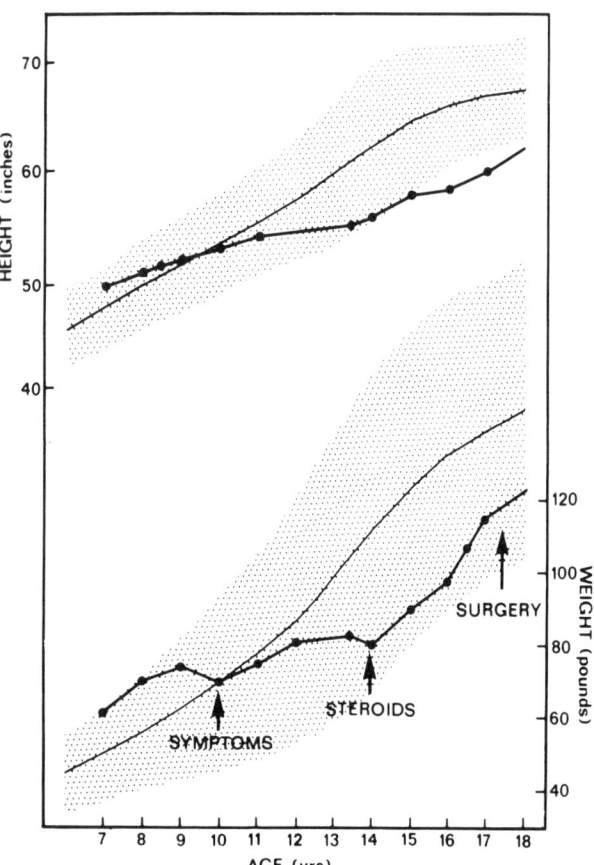

Figure 1 Example of extreme growth failure in a patient with Crohn's disease. Note onset of poor weight gain and linear growth occurring prior to the onset of symptoms. The solid line represents the fiftieth percentile pattern for a normal individual.

ETIOLOGY OF MALNUTRITION AND GROWTH FAILURE

The cause of malnutrition in patients with inflammatory bowel disease is multifactorial and generally cannot be ascribed to a single agent. The major factors include inadequate dietary intake, excessive gastrointestinal losses, malabsorption, and increased nutritional requirements (Table 2).

Inadequate dietary intake in patients with inflammatory bowel disease may occur as a result of the anorexia associated with chronic illness or recurrent bouts of inflammatory activity. Often children refuse to eat because of increased diarrhea or abdominal pain associated with the ingestion of food. Excessive losses of nutrients may originate from the gastrointestinal tract or through the kidneys. Hematochezia, protein-losing enteropathy, and increased fecal losses of cellular constituents are associated with chronic inflammation and damage to the intestinal mucosa. Bile salt losing enteropathy and subsequent fat malabsorption result from ileal disease, resection, or fistulas. Large doses of corticosteroids or the stress-induced response to acute inflammation may lead to increased urinary nutrient losses.

TABLE 2 Etiology of Malnutrition in Inflammatory Bowel Disease

Inadequate dietary intake
    Anorexia
    Altered taste
    Abdominal pain
    Diarrhea
Excessive intestinal losses
    Protein-losing enteropathy
    Hematochezia
    Bile-salt-losing enteropathy
Malabsorption
    Protein
    Carbohydrate (xylose, lactose)
    Fat
    Minerals (Ca, Mg, Fe, Zn)
    Vitamins (folate, B_{12}, D, K)
    Bacterial overgrowth
    Drug inhibition (folate)
Increased requirements
    Fever
    Fistulas
    Repletion of body stores
    Growth

Malabsorption is more common in patients with Crohn's disease, particularly in individuals with small bowel involvement, and less common in patients with ulcerative colitis. These abnormalities are summarized in Table 3.

It is apparent that the potential for nutritional deficiencies on the basis of nutritional malabsorption and enteric losses is present in patients with inflammatory bowel disease and warrants frequent evaluation.

Increased nutritional requirements may occur in response to increased inflammatory activity, fever, intes-

TABLE 3 Prevalence of Malabsorption in Crohn's Disease

	Prevalence (%)	
Nutrient	Adults	Children
Protein		
Protein loss (^{51}Cr)	70	70
Serum albumin (< 3.3%)	52	52
Carbohydrate		
Xylose	40	16
Lactose	10	17
Bacterial overgrowth	30	——
Fat		
Serum carotene ↓	94	——
Fecal fat ↑	43	29
Vitamins and minerals		
Serum folic acid ↓	77	60
Vitamin B_{12} (abnormal Schilling)	58	55
Vitamin K (abnormal prothrombin time)	30	——
Serum iron ↓	58	70
Serum calcium ↓	17	18
Negative calcium balance	13	18

tinal fistulas, or periods of rapid growth, particularly during adolescence. Inflammation leads to negative energy and nitrogen balances as a result of decreased dietary intake and increased metabolic activity. Additional nutrient requirements also occur as a consequence of the demands of growth in children. With a peak weight gain of 7 kg per 6-month interval during puberty and at an energy cost of up to 4.4 calories per gram of tissue gained, an additional energy intake of 170 kilocalories per day may be needed during the adolescent growth spurt. Therefore, the stress imposed by inflammation and growth is an important factor in the development of chronic malnutrition in children with inflammatory bowel disease.

NUTRITIONAL ASSESSMENT

It is obvious that regular evaluations are necessary to assess the initial impact of nutritional failure on the child with inflammatory bowel disease and growth failure, and also to measure the success of therapy over time. Recommendations for nutritional assessment are shown in Table 4. The use of this sequential assessment allows the clinician to maintain close surveillance not only over nutritional status but also over measurements of linear and ponderal growth. Alterations in therapy must be made to

TABLE 4 Evaluation of the Nutritional Status of Children with Inflammatory Bowel Disease

History
  Appetite, extracurricular activity
  Type and duration of inflammatory bowel disease, frequency of relapse
  Severity and extent of current symptoms*
  Medications
Three-day diet record
Physical examination
  Height, weight, arm circumference, triceps skinfold measurements
  Loss of subcutaneous fat, muscle wasting, edema, pallor, skin rash, hepatomegaly
Laboratory tests
  Complete blood count and differential, reticulocyte and platelet count, sedimentation rate, urinalysis
  Stool guaiac, cultures for bacteria, smears for ova, parasites, and fat
  Serum total proteins, albumin, transferrin, retinol binding protein, orosomucoid, immunoglobulins
  Serum electrolytes, calcium, magnesium, phosphate, iron, zinc
  Serum folate, vitamins A, E, D, B_{12}
Special tests
  Xylose absorption, 72-hour fecal fat, fecal alpha$_1$-antitrypsin, lactose breath test, Schilling's test
Radiology
  Upper gastrointestinal series with small bowel follow-through
  Air-contrast barium enema
Colonoscopy with biopsies

* Crohn's Disease Activity Index (Gastroenterology 1976; 70:439) or Lloyd-Still Clinical Scoring System (Dig Dis Sci 1979; 24:620) may be useful in the assessment.

TABLE 5 Commonly Used Drugs in Treatment of Inflammatory Bowel Disease

Drug	Daily Dose	Comment
Sulfasalazine	50 mg/kg	May increase to 75 mg/kg or standard adult dose
Steroids		
Prednisone Prednisolone	1–2 mg/kg	Single AM dose when possible Dose depends upon severity Not to exceed standard adult dose
Adrenocorticotropic hormone	1.6–2.0 U/kg	Administer as a continuous infusion
Azathioprine	2 mg/kg	Not to exceed standard adult dose
Metronidazole	20 mg/kg	Not to exceed 1 g

achieve and maintain normal expected growth rates. Carefully maintained growth and nutritional data are mainstays of treatment of children with growth failure and inflammatory bowel disease.

TREATMENT OF GROWTH FAILURE

Medical Treatment

In the routine management of inflammatory bowel disease with or without growth failure, *control of inflammatory activity is the first goal of medical treatment*. Medications currently used in children with inflammatory bowel disease are listed in Table 5. Sulfasalazine (50 to 75 mg per kilogram per day, maximum of 3 to 4 g per day) is recommended for the treatment of mild acute attacks and maintenance of remission when the colon is involved. Some patients with small bowel Crohn's disease will also respond to sulfasalazine therapy, but less predictably so. In contrast, prednisone (1 to 2 mg per kilogram per day, maximum 60 to 80 mg per day) is more effective in treating moderate to severe disease activity.

Corticosteroids are effective in inducing remissions but do not prevent relapses and may increase overall morbidity when used in a maintenance fashion. Therefore, corticosteroids are generally recommended in courses. A single morning dose is recommended when the severity of the disease permits this form of therapy. Twice daily oral doses are sometimes necessary.

When intravenous therapy is required, methylprednisolone should be used (1 to 2 mg per kilogram per day) in 2 or 3 divided doses. Adrenocorticotropic hormone (ACTH) (1.6 to 2.0 units per kilogram per day) is recommended for treatment of newly diagnosed active disease or recurrent disease when oral steroids are not being used. If therapy has been initiated with intravenous steroids or ACTH, oral prednisone may be given when symptoms abate, first using the twice daily schedule and then switching to a daily morning dose. Therapy is main-

TABLE 6 Surgical Treatment of Growth Failure in Crohn's Disease

Author	Year	Journal	Number of Patients Growing 2–5 Years After Surgery		Pubertal Status
McCaffery	1970	Pediatrics	3/11	(27%)	?
Homer	1977	Pediatrics	2/15	(14%)	Prepubertal
			0/23		Pubertal
Gryboski	1978	Gastroenterology	8/45	(18%)	Prepubertal
			0/12		Pubertal

tained for 4 to 6 weeks with tapering to an alternate-day regimen by decreasing the dosage 5 mg every other day at 5- to 7-day intervals. If necessary, prolonged alternate-day therapy may be maintained. In most patients, this regimen allows for gradual decrease of medication without flare-up of disease. Low-dose, alternate-day steroid therapy is an acceptable alternative form of long-term treatment.

Pharmacologic doses of corticosteroids have been associated with urinary excretion of nitrogen and have been implicated in linear growth delay in chronic disease. Nevertheless, some patients with inflammatory bowel disease demonstrate accelerated linear growth despite high-dose steroid therapy, presumably because of suppression of inflammatory activity. An improvement in appetite however, may account in part for the growth response owing to increased dietary protein and energy intakes associated with corticosteroid use. This may be particularly true when alternate-day steroid therapy is used for a prolonged period.

Other medications may be valuable in bringing disease activity under control. Azathioprine and 6-mercaptopurine may allow reduction in the dosage of steroids required, prolong remission, obviate the need for surgery, and allow prolonged maintenance in patients who would not be candidates for other forms of therapy. Metronidazole is valuable for perianal disease, and vancomycin may be helpful in those patients whose disease flare-ups are associated with *Clostridium difficile* overgrowth. (See the chapters on Crohn's Disease and *Ulcerative Colitis and Proctitis*.)

Surgical Treatment

Surgical resection of disease has been considered as an alternative in the management of growth failure in patients with inflammatory bowel disease, but the results of this approach have not supported its routine use for this purpose (Table 6). In most studies, children with Crohn's ileocolitis have only limited response to removal of active disease, with only 14 to 28 percent of patients showing postoperative catch-up growth. Virtually *all* children who have had *catch-up growth after surgery were prepubertal at the time of operation*. In general, pubertal patients have shown no catch-up growth after surgery. These patients have either ceased to grow or have grown at the same rate as they did prior to surgery.

At the present time surgical intervention should be reserved for those patients in whom there is a clear indication other than growth failure. In selected *prepubertal* children in whom medical and nutritional therapy have failed to alter growth arrest, surgical treatment may be beneficial.

Nutritional Treatment

Even in the absence of nutrition failure or growth retardation, the indications and benefits of nutritional therapy in inflammatory bowel disease have become apparent. The indications for nutritional therapy are listed in Table 7. With respect to disease activity, nutritional regimens have been advocated as primary modes of therapy in newly diagnosed cases of Crohn's disease, and there is adequate documentation that clinical, biochemical, and nutritional abnormalities are reversed by nutritional therapy alone. Even in patients who have been maintained on corticosteroid treatment, with adequate nutritional support, it is often possible to reduce or discontinue entirely

TABLE 7 Indications for Nutritional Therapy in Patients with Inflammatory Bowel Disease

Primary therapy for disease activity
    Newly diagnosed inflammatory bowel disease
    Chronic disease unresponsive to medical management
    Short bowel syndrome
    Closure of fistulas
    Small bowel obstruction
    Ostomy care

Supportive therapy for disease activity
    Inoperable diffuse disease
    Preoperative nutritional rehabilitation

Drug-nutrient interactions
    Sulfasalazine/folic acid

Abnormalities of specific laboratory test
    Anemia (microcytic, macrocytic)
    Hypoproteinemia
    Fat malabsorption
    Lactose intolerance
    Serum mineral deficiencies (Fe, Ca, Mg, K^+)
    Serum vitamin deficiencies (folate, B_{12}, A, D)
    Prolonged prothrombin time (vitamin K)
    Depressed alkaline phosphatase (Zn)

Complications of inflammatory bowel disease
    Malnutrition
    Growth failure

the dosage of steroids administered. In terms of growth failure, both chronic enteral and parenteral nutritional regimens have produced nutrition repletion in children and adolescents with this complication of inflammatory bowel disease. Improved linear and ponderal growth rates have been observed in adolescents with Crohn's disease who received continuous enteral feedings by the nasogastric route for 6 weeks, and a dramatic rehabilitation of nutritional status and stimulation of growth have been achieved using total parenteral nutrition with or without enteral feedings as well.

In our own clinics, programs of long-term nutritional supplementation have been initiated for severely growth retarded adolescents with Crohn's disease. These patients received a daily protein and energy intake of 3.2 g per kilogram and 95 Kcal per kilogram per day, respectively. Results of supplementation in these patients are shown in Table 8. After 3 weeks of nutritional supplementation, a weight gain of 4 kg occurred, nitrogen balance improved fourfold, and total body potassium increased significantly. After 7 months of nutritional supplementation, average height and weight velocities were at least five times greater than those observed during the 10 months prior to supplementation, and equaled or exceeded velocities of normal adolescents. These observations demonstrate that the abnormalities in the nutritional status of adolescents with Crohn's disease, malnutrition, and growth failure were not related to intrinsic defects in the metabolic pathways, and that with appropriate supplementation, nutritional rehabilitation and stimulation of growth occurred. Moreover, neither the presence of chronic inflammation nor the use of corticosteroids interfered with the ability to rehabilitate these patients nutritionally.

In clinical situations in which abdominal symptoms, such as severe diarrhea, abscesses, or fistulas, prevent enteral rehabilitation, parenteral nutritional therapy can reverse nutritional failure and stimulate growth.

Goals of Nutritional Therapy

In the nutritional management of children with growth failure and inflammatory bowel disease the major aim is to replace the nutrient losses associated with the inflammatory process, to correct body deficits, and to provide sufficient nutrients to promote energy and nitrogen balance for normal metabolic function. In children, additional nutrients must be provided to restore normal growth and to produce catch-up growth. To accomplish these aims, appropriate assessment of nutritional status should be performed routinely as described above. The frequency and extent of nutritional assessment will vary for each individual and should be reviewed frequently.

The methods available for treatment of nutritional disorders in inflammatory bowel disease include the enteral and parenteral routes (Table 9). The easiest way to provide nutritional supplementation is to increase dietary intakes by the enteral route using standard table foods. No specific diet has been shown to alter the course of ulcerative colitis or Crohn's disease in patients who are in remission. There is also no clear evidence that the consumption or avoidance of specific foods influences the severity of disease or the frequency of relapse, or induces remission. Accordingly, patients are encouraged to eat a well-balanced adequate diet and to avoid food fads. In children and adolescents, it is preferable to allow the intake of favorite foods and beverages rather than force a limited energy intake. When disease is active, when specific foods exacerbate symptoms, or when laboratory tests suggest specific abnormalities, such as lactose intolerance, the diet should be modified accordingly. In the presence of severe postprandial pain, a low-residue diet administered as frequent small meals is often recommended. In children with watery diarrhea due to hydroxy-fatty acid or bile acid excretion, a low-fat diet supplemented with medium-chain triglycerides or the use of cholestyra-

TABLE 8 Effect of Nutritional Supplementation on Body Composition, Protein and Energy Metabolism, and Growth in Adolescents with Inflammatory Bowel Disease

Measurement	Dietary Interval (Data)	
	Presupplementation	Postsupplementation
Body composition		
Weight (kg)	37	41
Nitrogen retention (mg/kg/day)	36	137
Total body potassium (g)	80	87
Whole body protein and energy metabolism		
Amino acid incorporation (mg/kg/day)	269	447
Amino acid oxidation (mg/kg/day)	262	154
"Basal" oxygen consumption (ml/min/m^2)	156	206
Growth velocity		
Height (cm/6 mo)	0.6	3.0
Weight (kg/6 mo)	1.3	7.3

TABLE 9 Nutritional Therapy for Inflammatory Bowel Disease

Well-balanced, high protein and energy diet
  ± Low residue
  ± Lactose-free
  ± Low fat, medium chain triglyceride (MCT), and cholestyramine supplemented

Enteral supplementation (140% to 150% of Recommended Daily Allowances for height age)
  Continuous or intermittent nasogastric tube feeding
  Feeding gastrostomy, continuous, or intermittent

Total parenteral nutrition (140% to 150% of Recommended Daily Allowances for height age)
  Peripheral
  Central

Vitamins and Minerals
  Supplemental
    Multivitamins with minerals (daily)
  Therapeutic
    Folate — 1 mg daily
    Iron
      Ferrous sulfate (20% Fe) — 6 mg elemental Fe/kg/day, divided in 3 oral doses
      Ferrous gluconate (11.5% Fe)
    Iron dextran (IM) (Imferon) — Follow directions on package insert
    Magnesium — 200–400 mg elemental mg/day IV
    Vitamin B_{12} — 1,000 g at 3-month intervals, (SC or IM)
    Zinc sulfate (22% Zn) — 50–100 mg elemental Zn/day divided into 3 oral doses

---

mine may be helpful in controlling symptoms. Care must be taken however to ensure adequate energy intakes when patients are provided with instructions for a low-fat diet.

Multivitamins with minerals should be administered routinely to replace deficits in the diet. Oral iron and folic acid therapy should be provided when laboratory findings are consistent with a deficiency state. Parenteral administration of vitamin B_{12} may be necessary in patients with extensive small bowel disease or ileal resection. Despite an association between serum zinc levels and linear growth delay, very few patients with growth failure have low serum zinc levels. Those who have this abnormality are generally treated with oral zinc supplments.

When the patient is unable to increase dietary protein and energy intakes with larger meals or palatable snacks, oral supplementation with a commercially available liquid formula should be attempted. Successful supplementation of dietary intake may be achieved with such formulas; however, many patients will experience early satiety when taking these formulas and will not increase their total nutrient intake significantly. Under these circumstances, nutritional supplementation can be accomplished by intragastric feedings or parenteral alimentation.

Nasogastric infusions used either continuously or intermittently have been effective in reversing metabolic imbalances and improving nutritional status, linear and ponderal growth rates, and the clinical well-being of patients with inflammatory bowel disease. With this method, a silicone rubber nasogastric tube of small diameter may be passed through the nose into the stomach and left in place for continuous slow drip or pump feedings. Alternatively, the nasogastric tube may be passed in the evening for an overnight liquid infusion and removed when the patient awakens. We prefer the latter method because it does not interefere with school attendance or the social development of the adolescent. If the patient does not tolerate this form of therapy, a gastrostomy may be performed for either continuous or intermittent tube feedings in the same manner as the nasogastric regimen. The gastrostomy tube is advantageous in that it is cosmetically acceptable, and it is easily cared for. In our experience, the only complication associated with intragastric tube feedings has been reversible diarrhea secondary to too rapid administration of the nutritional supplement.

The amount of nutritional supplementation administered via the nasogastric or gastrostomy tube will vary, depending upon the nutritional requirements and tolerance level of the individual. In our adolescent patients, 1,500 ml of a commercial formula, administered nightly for 8 to 10 hours, was well tolerated. This volume of supplemental formula, in addition to usual meals and snacks, provided protein and energy intakes of 3 g per kilogram per day and 95 kcal per kilogram per day, respectively. We also recommend that commercially prepared formulas be used as adjuncts rather than as the sole source of long-term nutritional intake to avoid potential nutrient imbalances. The chapter *Parenteral Nutrition* contains additional useful information.

When patients with inflammatory bowel disease are unable to tolerate adequate amounts of enteral alimentation because of disease activity or diarrhea, parenteral alimentation may provide substantial benefits. Peripheral nutrition with standard solutions providing 10 percent glucose, 2.5 percent amino acids, vitamins and minerals may be an acceptable primary or supplemental form of therapy for short periods. Under these circumstances, peripheral alimentation must be accompanied by an intravenous lipid preparation to provide adequate energy and essential fatty acid intakes. Alternatively, central venous parenteral nutrition may provide long-term support. It appropriately improves nutritional status as demonstrated by linear and ponderal growth rates, lean body mass deposition, and postoperative recovery. Parenteral alimentation may also induce a clinical remission. Home parenteral alimentation is available for those patients who require long-term nutritional support for active disease, short bowel syndrome, or growth failure.

In general, the nutritional recommendations have been similar to those used for enteral nutrition support. Patients may be monitored by their own hospital programs or by a commercial nutritional maintenance company. (See the chapter *Parenteral Nutrition*.)

Portions of this chapter are reproduced with permission of WB Saunders from Pediatr Clin North Am 1985; 32:447–469.

CROHN'S DISEASE: SURGICAL TREATMENT

ARTHUR H. AUFSES, Jr., M.D.

Granulomatous inflammatory bowel disease, now known worldwide as Crohn's disease, was originally described by Crohn, Ginsburg, and Oppenheimer as involving only the terminal ileum. Descriptions of involvement of other segments of the gastrointestinal tract followed rapidly, and it is now accepted that Crohn's disease can involve the entire gastrointestinal tract from mouth to anus, including the esophagus. Involvement of extraintestinal sites such as ovary, skin, and respiratory tract by granulomatous inflammatory lesions suggests that the disease may actually be systemic and not limited to the intestinal tract. Although true surgical rates are difficult to obtain except in those countries where all patients are registered, it appears that the majority of patients with Crohn's disease will eventually require a surgical procedure.

Because we do not know the etiology, because of the ubiquitous nature of the disease, and because of its almost inexorable tendency to recur, the surgeon can never speak of cure in managing Crohn's disease. We may eradicate infections, palliate symptoms, restore good health, and improve the quality of life, but we do not cure.

WHEN TO OPERATE

With the exception of the rare patient whose first manifestation of Crohn's disease is a catastrophic complication, all patients being seen by a surgeon for consideration of operation will have had some form of therapy for a varying period of time.

Although difficult to prove, it appears that the longer a patient has had Crohn's disease prior to operation, the more favorable will be the postoperative prognosis. As a result of longstanding disease, however, with elements of intestinal obstruction and/or diarrhea, infection, and the influence of steroids or immunosuppressive therapy, patients may require surgery at a time when they are malnourished, debilitated, and immunologically compromised. In recent years, though, patients for the most part are being referred for surgery before severe debility ensues, a most commendable trend from the surgeon's viewpoint.

The factors involved in surgical decision-making include the length of time the patient has had the disease, the extent of disease as identified radiographically and/or endoscopically, the current symptomatology and complications leading to the consultation, and a detailed knowledge of any prior operative procedures. I always involve the patient and his family in the decision-making process and invariably ask the patient, "Have you had enough?" It will usually be very evident when the answer is going to be yes, and patients should never be pushed into accepting surgery. Once the decision has been made to operate, a frank discussion must be held which should include the options open to the surgeon at the operating table, the problems likely to be encountered postoperatively, and the likelihood of recurrence. Unfortunately, the patient with Crohn's disease is a patient for life, and the time to establish an appropriate relationship is at the first visit.

The indications for surgery tend to follow the "patterns of disease" outlined at the Cleveland Clinic. Patients with gastroduodenal Crohn's disease usually require surgery because of obstruction or hemorrhage. Seventy-five to 80 percent of patients with primarily small bowel involvement will be operated upon because of the complications of either obstruction, fistula, or abscess, while a significant number of patients with predominantly colonic disease will require operation because of chronic debility and inadequate response to nonoperative therapy.

Patients with diffuse ileocolitis or diffuse ileojejunitis are usually not considered candidates for surgical therapy. This also holds true for the patient who has had multiple prior operations and is now considered to have a "short bowel" syndrome. Nevertheless, should these patients have a localized stricture with obstruction, or abscess with infection, they too can be helped by appropriate surgical management. The management of perianal disease is discussed elsewhere in this volume but this too can require abdominal surgery to divert the fecal stream to give relief. Unfortunately, the patient with severe perianal disease will usually end up with a permanent ileostomy, especially if the rectum is involved.

PREOPERATIVE PREPARATION

Patients entering the hospital for elective surgery can usually be operated upon within 36 hours of admission.

Needed investigations can be carried out before admission. If there is a lower abdominal mass, I believe that the patient should have an intravenous pyelogram, since the incidence of hydronephrosis or hydroureter is significant in these patients. Computed tomographic scans may also help define tender abdominal masses in the febrile patient. Because of the high incidence of cholelithiasis in patients with longstanding inflammatory bowel disease, it has been suggested that these patients have gallbladder sonography preoperatively. If cholelithiasis is present, cholecystectomy is indicated at the time of laparotomy, but only if the procedure has gone well to that point.

Since most patients have an element of obstruction, I place them on clear fluids for 48 hours prior to hospitalization. In patients with inflammatory bowel disease I depend upon dietary restriction as a major element in bowel preparation. Cathartics should not be given and enemas should only be given in the hospital to cleanse the colon before operation. Patients receiving steroid therapy must be maintained before, during, and after surgery. My regimen is 100 mg of hydrocortisone intravenously before surgery, 100 mg during operation, and then this dose is continued every 8 hours through the first postoperative day. At this point the intravenous dose is tapered and maintained until the patient is on oral intake, at which time the preoperative oral dose is reinstituted. This is then tapered so that the patient leaves the hospital taking 15 mg or less of prednisone per day. If the patient is on long-term steroid therapy, it may be several months before steroids can be withdrawn.

There is no question but that *preoperative oral antibiotics* are of value in the prevention of wound infection following intestinal surgery. My own preference is to use *neomycin* and *erythromycin base*, giving three doses of 1 g each on the day before operation. I also give 1 g of an intravenous *cephalosporin* 1 hour before surgery, 1 g intraoperatively, and continue it for 24 hours postoperatively.

The patient who is already hospitalized and then requires surgery for continuing or progressive symptoms may present a different problem. This individual may be severely debilitated, anemic, dehydrated, and suffering from acute and chronic infection. Every attempt should be made to stabilize the patient and try to bring him to the operating room in optimal condition. This may require a series of transfusions, and it is in this type of situation that total parenteral nutrition may be of great value. Utilizing total parenteral nutrition, a severe catabolic state can be reversed in as short a time as 5 or 6 days. This may make the difference between the surgeon being able to perform only a diverting procedure or being able to proceed with a complete and definitive operation.

INTRAOPERATIVE MANAGEMENT

A thorough exploration of the entire abdomen should be carried out in all patients. The length of the small bowel should be measured as accurately as possible and note should be made of all areas suspected of harboring inflammatory bowel disease. I do not hesitate to leave areas of Crohn's disease in situ if they do not appear to be causing symptoms, but their location should be noted for future reference.

Resection is the procedure of choice whenever feasible, but in all instances the amount of bowel resected should be kept to a minimum. The most accurate guide to the extent of gross bowel disease is the extent of "creeping fat." This is the term given to the pathologic finding of abnormal fat accumulation on the bowel wall extending from the mesenteric fat toward the antimesenteric border of the bowel. One need only resect 4 to 5 cm proximal and distal to this area. Several studies have shown that, provided the bowel at the line of resection is pliable and will hold sutures, the presence or absence of nonspecific inflammatory changes or actual Crohn's disease will have no bearing on immediate postoperative morbidity or long-term recurrence. A major problem in resecting a segment of bowel containing Crohn's disease may be the markedly thickened, indurated, and infected mesentery which must be divided. The blood supply must be carefully controlled. In resecting the terminal ileum, the ascending colon should be divided just above the ileocecal valve to preserve as much of the right colon as possible.

The management of the patient with colonic disease represents a greater intraoperative therapeutic dilemma. Preoperative colonoscopy can be of great help in this regard by providing accurate information as to the location of areas of colonic involvement. If the patient has ileocolitis with involvement of the terminal ileum and right colon only, then ileocolic resection is indicated with ileotransverse colon anastomosis. Many patients with ileocolitis, however, will have "skip areas" of disease in the region of the splenic flexure, descending colon, or sigmoid. While multiple segmental resections are technically possible, I believe that this situation is best handled by a subtotal colectomy with resection of the involved terminal ileum and an anastomosis of the new terminal ileum to the mid- or distal sigmoid. When the entire colon is involved but the rectum has been spared (as occurs in about 20% of the cases of colonic involvement) ileorectal anastomosis is the procedure of choice. One must recognize, however, that these patients do have a high incidence of recurrence and that some recurrences will happen promptly after the operation.

The patient who has total colonic involvement with rectal disease will require total proctocolectomy. I feel that patients with Crohn's disease should not undergo ileoanal pull-through because of the dangers of recurrence in the ileum and the difficulty in performing a mucosal stripping in the presence of transmural disease of the rectum. These patients appear to do best with a standard Brooke ileostomy. If there is severe perianal disease with sepsis the surgeon may wish to stop short of proctocolectomy. Following subtotal colectomy and ileostomy, the perianal disease will improve significantly so that at a subsequent time abdominoperineal resection can be performed with much less risk of postoperative perineal sepsis and failure of healing of the perineal wound.

Although largely superseded by resection, bypass still

has a role in the surgical management of Crohn's disease. Numerous studies have shown that diversion of the fecal stream will lead to subsidence of the inflammatory process and allow restoration of health. Whether performed "internally" by the usual technique of ileotransverse colostomy with exclusion of the bowel, or "externally" by the formation of an ileostomy, the major indication for the procedure is in the severely ill patient with either widespread retroperitoneal infection, multiorgan involvement, multiple fistulas, or, as mentioned earlier, severe perianal disease. It must be remembered that the bypassed loop may be at increased risk for the development of *malignant disease* if left in situ indefinitely. As a consequence, thought may have to be given to eventual excision of the bypassed loop.

Strictureplasty

In recent years "strictureplasty" has become part of the surgeon's armamentarium. This procedure is accomplished by incising the bowel longitudinally in a narrowed area and then closing it transversely to widen the lumen. Strictureplasty is best utilized in a short segment of involved bowel where the disease would appear to be of relatively short duration, when inflammation, spasm, and edema play a major role in the narrowing as opposed to dense fibrosis. In the latter situation, when the bowel is markedly thickened and the lumen is pencil-thin, resection is the favored technique in my opinion.

GASTRODUODENAL DISEASE

Approximately 20 percent of all patients with Crohn's disease will have some radiologic abnormality in the antrum or duodenum. Endoscopy is indicated to try to distinguish Crohn's disease from peptic ulcer disease. Slightly less than 10 percent of all patients will have significant abnormalities, but only a few of these patients will require surgery. The indications for operation in this group are usually duodenal or gastric outlet obstruction and occasionally massive hemorrhage. The preferred operation is a *gastroenterostomy*, and *vagotomy* should be included to prevent marginal ulceration. Selective vagotomy has been suggested to preserve the celiac and hepatic branches of the vagus nerves in an attempt to reduce the incidence of diarrhea and cholelithiasis. By and large the results of bypass are good, but a recent report suggests that involvement of the gastroenteric stoma or jejunum by Crohn's disease may lead to further difficulty. Almost all of these patients will have disease distally in the intestinal tract and this too may require surgery at a later date.

I have recently seen a patient with duodenal Crohn's disease and pancreatitis, the latter thought to be due to involvement of the ampulla of Vater by the inflammatory reaction in the duodenum. This patient, who also had severe duodenal obstruction, has remained well after gastroenterostomy and vagotomy, but the follow-up is only of a few months duration.

MANAGEMENT OF FISTULA

The presence of an enteroenteral or other fistula is *not* in and of itself an indication for operative intervention. It is, however, an indication that disease has perforated from one loop of bowel into another loop or into an adjacent viscus. It has been suggested that, since most fistulas occur immediately proximal to a stenotic segment, this is "nature's way" of bypassing an obstructed segment. The most common fistulas are from ileum to cecum or ascending colon, ileum to ileum, or ileum to sigmoid. When surgery is necessary and the fistula is either ileoileal or ileocecal, it is usually resected en bloc with the specimen. When the fistula is ileum to sigmoid it becomes imperative to know whether the sigmoid is intrinsically normal or whether it is also involved with Crohn's disease. If the colon is intrinsically normal, it is almost always possible to separate the ileum from the sigmoid, close the sigmoid, and proceed with the resection of the diseased ileum. On the other hand, if the sigmoid is also involved, a double resection may be necessary. *Ileovesical fistula* is treated by separating the ileum from the bladder and closing the latter. An indwelling catheter must be left in the bladder for 7 to 10 days following surgery to ensure healing of the bladder wall.

MANAGEMENT OF EMERGENCY SITUATIONS

During exploration for suspected acute appendicitis, an inflamed, thickened, edematous ileum will be found on rare occasions. The lesion may be Crohn's disease with acute inflammation, but in children an almost identical picture can be caused by *Yersinia*, and in adults the disorder can be produced by *Campylobacter, Shigella,* or *Salmonella* infection. In my view the management is the same. If the *base* of the cecum appears normal, appendectomy is indicated. If the cecum is involved in the inflammatory process, appendectomy should not be performed. Of the patients who have Crohn's disease, about one-fifth will develop an *enterocutaneous fistula* following appendectomy. At reoperation, these fistulas almost never come from the site of the appendix stump, but arise from the mesentery of the diseased ileum. If appendectomy is not performed, a similar number of patients will also develop an enterocutaneous fistula. Appendectomy therefore removes a potential source of confusion in differential diagnosis should right lower quadrant pain recur at a later date. Following operation, stool cultures should be obtained immediately to look for specific bacterial infection.

Acute appendicitis very rarely develops in a patient with known Crohn's disease. Crohn's disease of the appendix, however, does occur. It is usually associated with ileal or colonic Crohn's disease but may appear as an isolated entity. When it does occur without other intestinal involvement, preoperative diagnosis is nearly impossible and will only be made by pathologic examination of the appendix.

Toxic Megacolon

Toxic megacolon occurs in Crohn's disease but is less common than in ulcerative colitis. For the most part the treatment is *nonoperative*. Almost all patients with toxic megacolon due to Crohn's disease will respond to a combination of intravenous alimentation, antibiotics, intravenous steroids, intestinal decompression, and frequent change of position to redistribute the colonic gas. These patients must be watched jointly by a gastroenterologist and a surgeon, and with any deterioration of general status, operation should be performed. My preferred procedure is an ileostomy and subtotal colectomy.

Perforation

Free perforation occurs rarely but is a catastrophic complication. If the perforation is through the bowel wall, resection is mandatory. If the lesion is in the distal small bowel, anastomosis should not be attempted, and after resection a double-barreled ileostomy is created. If the lesion is in the proximal jejunum, then anastomosis must be performed despite the presence of peritonitis. Most perforations, however, represent the *rupture of a mesenteric abscess* into the peritoneal cavity. This is best managed by drainage of the abscess cavity and the creation of a ileostomy proximal to the abscess to divert the fecal stream. These patients are usually desperately ill and resection is a hazardous undertaking.

Abscess

From time to time simple drainage of an abscess will be necessary, and this is usually followed by an enterocutaneous fistula. Although the fecal drainage may be copious at first it usually decreases rapidly. These fistulas rarely close and subsequent resectional surgery will usually be necessary.

POSTOPERATIVE MANAGEMENT

The postoperative care of the patient following surgery for Crohn's disease is similar to that after any intestinal surgery. Oral intake is withheld until gastrointestinal function has been restored. Antibiotics are used if the patient has sepsis at the time of surgery. Because of the inflammatory and infectious nature of the disorder, the vast majority of complications are related to sepsis and wound infection. If pus was encountered at surgery I prefer to leave the skin and subcutaneous tissue of the wound open and perform a delayed primary closure if the wound remains clean. As most of the patients are in the younger age group, cardiovascular or pulmonary complications are unusual. Patients frequently have moderate diarrhea when gastrointestinal function returns but it usually slows down after solid intake is provided. I make no attempt to control the diarrhea until after the patient is well on his way to recovery and eating a normal diet.

Recurrent Disease

Unfortunately, at least 50 percent of patients operated on for Crohn's disease will develop a recurrence within 15 years. This recurrence may be either radiographic, symptomatic, or proven pathologically because of a need for a second operation. The management and indications for surgery in recurrent disease are the same as in the primary case.

For the most part patients undergoing surgery for Crohn's disease are extremely grateful in the postoperative period. Following a prolonged period of disability, they have been restored to symptomatic good health, and although they are aware that further troubles may be in the offing, they are overwhelmingly pleased with the restoration of satisfactory quality of life.

INTESTINAL OBSTRUCTION

GREGORY B. BULKLEY, M.D., F.A.C.S.

Acute obstruction of the small or large intestine is a common problem. It may be defined as a partial or complete anatomic blockade of the intestinal lumen by an intrinsic or extrinsic lesion. This discussion will therefore exclude paralytic ileus, primary mesenteric ischemia, and similar conditions from which mechanical obstruction must often be distinguished in a clinical setting. The predominant cause of small bowel obstruction is adhesions from a previous laparotomy, but it can also be caused by a number of other lesions, benign and malignant (Table 1). Colonic obstruction may be due to cancer, diverticulitis, Crohn's disease, or volvulus. Although the particular underlying lesion is often suspected, and should always be kept in mind, the initial approach to bowel obstruction should be a more generic one, based more upon the degree and site of the obstruction than upon the primary cause.

DIAGNOSIS

The approach to diagnosis should be systematic, and may be divided into four steps, each of which will be addressed sequentially (Fig. 1).

Recognition of Mechanical Obstruction

The initial problem is to recognize bowel obstruction in the first place. In most cases recognition is based upon

TABLE 1 Causes of Intestinal Obstruction

Cause	Approximate Incidence (%)
Small Intestine	
Adhesions	60
Malignancy	20
(⅓ primary; ⅔ metastatic)	
Hernia	10
(⅘ abdominal wall; ⅕ internal)	
Inflammatory bowel disease	5
Volvulus	3
Miscellaneous	2
Large Intestine	
Cancer	30
Diverticulitis	50
Crohn's Disease	5
Volvulus	5
Other	10

the characteristic symptoms, physical signs, and the flat and upright plain abdominal x-ray films. Indeed, this aspect of the diagnostic problem is usually straightforward, and the assessment completed within a few mintues. It should not require waiting for the results of laboratory tests or the scheduling of special diagnostic studies. Two types of patients may present a problem, however. The first is the occasional patient who presents with a complete mechanical small bowel obstruction, but with minimal gas on the abdominal x-ray film. This condition may be indicative of a closed loop obstruction but cannot be considered as an invariable sign of this condition. In these patients the characteristic dilated small bowel loops will not be visible and there may be no air fluid levels. A casual viewing of these films can result in missing the diagnosis altogether. A careful study, however, usually reveals a "ground glass" haze in the midabdomen, and the effect of a central mass on the adjacent, air-outlined stomach, colon, and/or proximal small intestine. If serious doubt persists, a contrast study should be performed, as discussed below, except in those patients in whom there is a serious suspicion of primary mesenteric ischemia. In these patients, angiography should be performed prior to the use of barium. Patients who develop acute small bowel obstruction in the postoperative period may also present a real problem with respect to recognition (see below).

Distinguishing Partial from Complete Obstruction

Because I believe that management of complete mechanical bowel obstruction is primarily operative, while that of a partial obstruction is, at least initially, nonoperative, this distinction is critical, and represents the next logical step in management. It is therefore important to determine the completeness of obstruction as definitively and as quickly as possible. A number of clues from the history and physical examination may be helpful, and the gas pattern on the plain films is often useful. The correlation of the duration of symptoms with the quantity of distal gas on the x-ray film is often the most revealing.

(Although colonic gas may be introduced by sigmoidoscopy, the introduction of air by a digital rectal examination, except with the patient in the knee-chest position, is an unlikely proposition.) Serial abdominal radiographs can be helpful as well. This emphasizes the importance of obtaining the initial radiographs as soon as possible after the patient is first seen. As in the management of all patients with an acute abdominal problem, repeat examinations by the same physician over time remains the most reliable means of clinical diagnosis. In some patients it will still be difficult to distinguish partial from complete obstruction. For example, abdominal x-ray films from patients with partial small bowel obstruction are virtually indistinguishable from those of patients with early complete small bowel obstruction. In these cases, it is best to proceed to the use of a contrast x-ray examination as soon as possible after the initial presentation. This approach is rapid, cheap, readily available, safe when applied appropriately, and is therefore quite efficient. It is first important to distinguish colonic from small bowel obstruction. In cases where the level of obstruction is thought or even suspected to be in the colon, a barium or gastrografin enema should be performed beforehand to answer this question definitely. In cases of near total colonic obstruction, barium is best avoided to preclude the production of complete obstruction from proximal barium impaction.

Once colonic obstruction has been ruled out, 50 to 100 ml of dilute barium should be introduced from above, usually via a nasogastric or intestinal tube in these nauseated patients. The tube is then clamped for an hour, or for a shorter period if the patient begins vomiting. Abdominal x-ray films are then retaken and suction resumed. Even if most of the contrast material has been aspirated by the tube, enough will remain to pass distally to reveal the degree and level of small bowel obstruction. This should be followed by sequential films, often in conjunction with the positioning of an intestinal tube. With the exception of those patients with a severe ileus, the answer is usually obtained within 24 hours. Complete small bowel obstruction can be recognized or ruled out with a fair level of confidence. In patients with partial small bowel obstruction, the degree and level of obstruction is usually demonstrated. It is not necessary to fluoroscope the patient for this particular form of upper gastrointestinal examination, nor is it necessary to obtain perfect cleansing of the gastrointestinal tract. The recognition of these facts by both the physician and the radiology department will help avoid delays in the examination, which does not necessarily require the presence of a radiologist.

Despite a great deal of published experience with the use of barium in small bowel obstruction, this issue is controversial in some circles. The safety of barium is undisputed, however, in cases of *small* bowel obstruction. Unlike the colon, the small bowel does not absorb enough water to create proximal impaction. Moreover, it is unwise to use large volumes of contrast material, as this will only tend to obscure the image. If large volumes are avoided, the risk of significant barium contamination of the peritoneum at the time of surgery is minimal. I do not

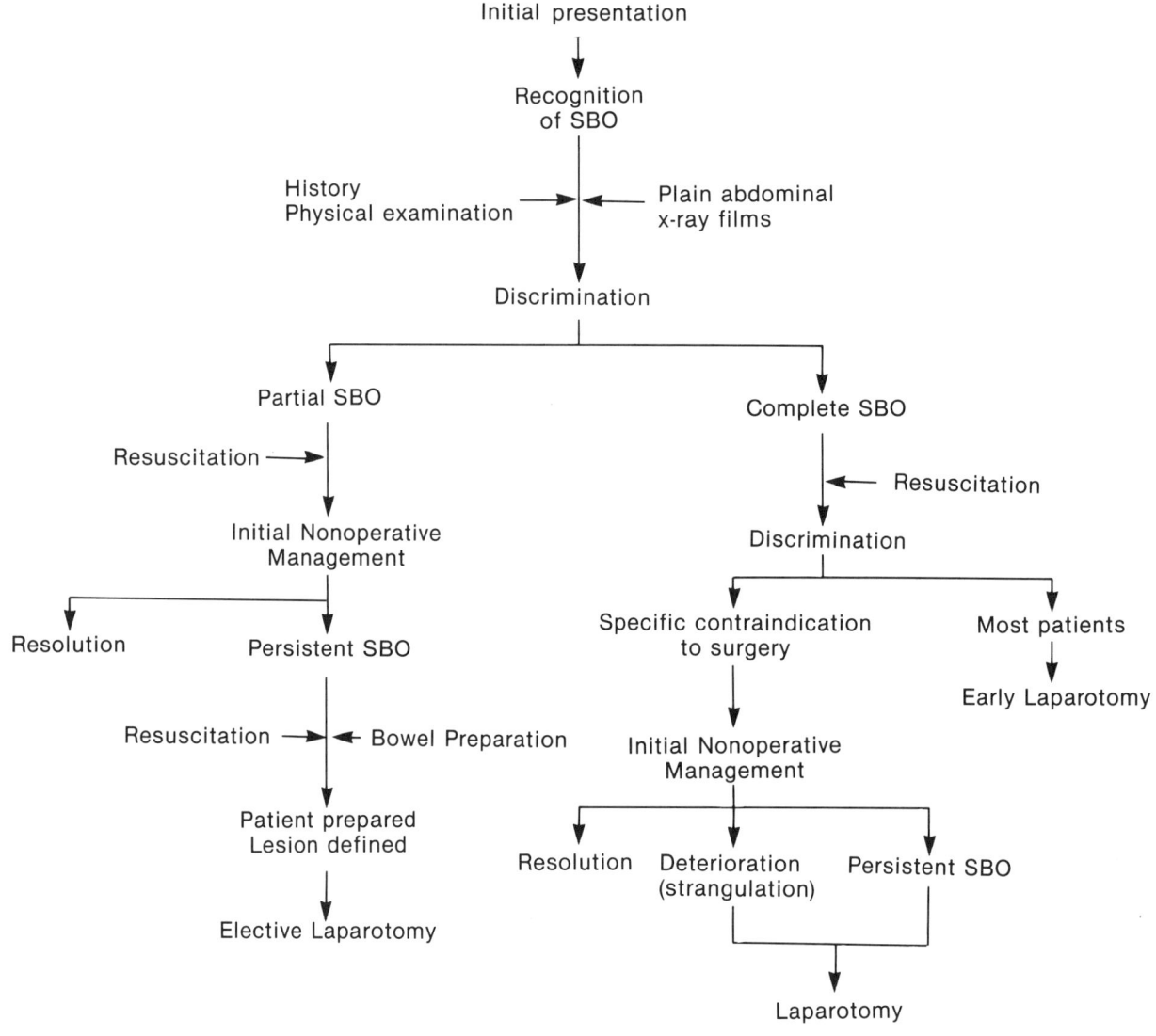

Figure 1 Management of small bowel obstruction (SBO).

like to use water-soluble contrast media in this situation. It provides significantly poorer images, especially after the contrast has passed more distally and becomes diluted with secretions. Furthermore, it presents a substantially increased risk for pulmonary injury in the event of aspiration from vomiting or when anesthesia is induced. Finally, its osmotic properties tend to increase the sequestration of "third space" fluid within the intestinal lumen, and to stimulate peristalsis. This may increase the risk of perforation and certainly increases the level of the patient's distress.

Recognition of Vascular Compromise (Strangulation)

The early recognition of strangulation in patients with mechanical small bowel obstruction has been a great source of controversy over the years. Perhaps because every physician has been indoctrinated as to the "classic signs of strangulation" at some time during training, the myth persists that such a distinction is possible, despite overwhelming evidence to the contrary. The issue has been greatly confused by published series which have mixed patients who have partial obstruction with patients who have complete obstruction. It is therefore essential to determine the degree of the obstruction first, as outlined above. Except for the rare patient with a strangulated Richter's hernia that has not been detected on physical examination, any patient with partial obstruction can be considered to have a negligible risk for strangulation and be managed accordingly (see the following).

Any patient with *complete obstruction*, however, is at substantial risk for strangulation. In operative series this risk has been consistently reported at 30 percent, but it is probably lower in series that include patients managed nonoperatively. In patients with complete small bowel obstruction, several retrospective studies and our own prospective study have demonstrated unequivocally that the accurate recognition of early vascular compromise is simply *not* possible on clinical grounds. Traditional criteria, such as continuous (as opposed to colicky) pain, fever, tachycardia, signs of peritonitis, leukocytosis, or the elevation of any of a number of serum electrolytes (potassium, phosphate) or enzymes (alkaline phosphatase, serum aminotransferase, alanine aminotransferase, lactic dehydrogenase, creatine phosphokinase), are simply not sensitive, specific, nor predictive of strangulation. Furthermore, no combination of these factors can accurately predict vascular compromise. Of primary importance, we found that the physician's clinical impression of the presence or absence of strangulation was equally unreliable: The diagnosis of simple obstruction (no strangulation) was correct only 70 percent of the time. When the overall incidence of strangulation (30%) was taken into account, the clinical diagnosis proved to be no better than would have been achieved by chance alone. Moreover, only one of the six patients in this series with early, *reversible* ischemia (viable intestine) was identified preoperatively. Retrospective series have reported a similar experience. This is because the signs that have been used to identify strangulation are a reflection of the body's response to de facto tissue necrosis. Therefore, to wait for signs of strangulation is to wait for the presence of irreversible damage and attendant ongoing sepsis. This factor probably contributes substantially to the fact that the mortality for patients with strangulation is more than double that of simple obstruction in most reported series. Therapeutic decisions (see below) in patients with *complete* small bowel obstruction must be based upon the 30 percent chance of the presence of strangulation, despite there being no indication of it whatsoever.

Identification of the Primary Lesion

In most patients with small bowel obstruction, initial management and the decision for or against surgery is made on the basis of the factors discussed above, without regard to the underlying cause of obstruction. In other cases, however, important clues from the history and physical examination will suggest an underlying lesion that may modify the therapeutic approach from the outset. Radiation enteritis, peritoneal carcinomatosis, incarcerated hernia that has been reduced, intra-abdominal abscess, and multiply recurrent adhesive obstruction often argue for initial nonoperative management. These conditions are discussed individually further on. In most cases, however, the obstructive process is initially dealt with on its own terms, while underlying lesions are managed secondarily, on an individualized basis.

Likewise, most patients with colonic obstruction require early relief of the obstruction, regardless of the primary lesion, although some with partial obstruction may be amenable to the pursuit of a definitive primary diagnosis, by endoscopy, for example. In either case, the approach to the primary lesion is secondary to ensuring early relief of the obstruction.

GENERAL TREATMENT MEASURES

Systemic Factors

Patients with small bowel obstruction are invariably dehydrated owing to lack of oral intake, vomiting, and the sequestration of fluid in the bowel lumen. Fluid should be replaced aggressively with an isotonic saline solution such as Ringer's lactate, following standard guidelines for the replacement of deficits. Many patients will require additional monitoring of intravascular volume with a Foley and a central venous or even a Swan-Ganz catheter. Because the fluid losses are often substantial, it is important not to underestimate the needs of these patients, particularly just prior to the induction of general anesthesia.

All patients with mechanical bowel obstruction are at risk for portal and systemic bacteremia due to the lost intestinal barrier to bacteria. This is true for patients with simple as well as strangulation obstruction. For this reason, and because of the significant risk of the occult presence of ischemia (strangulation), I prefer to treat all patients with acute bowel obstruction with *broad spectrum antibiotics* (penicillin, gentamycin, and clindamycin) until the condition has been resolved. This is true whether or not the patient requires surgery.

Tube Decompression

Virtually all patients with bowel obstruction require a nasoenteric tube to allow decompression of the gastrointestinal tract proximal to the obstruction. This provides symptomatic relief from the nausea and vomiting and, to some degree, the abdominal pain. It allows the proximal administration of contrast material when appropriate, as discussed above. A nasoenteric tube helps prevent aspiration at the induction of anesthesia in the event the patient requires surgery and also greatly facilitates the surgical exploration and the subsequent abdominal closure. Sometimes it may provide a splint at the time of operation in the hope of preventing recurrent obstruction. In some situations, it will provide definitive treatment in lieu of surgery, particularly in cases of partial small bowel obstruction. The decision for or against surgery, however, must be made on its own merits.

I much prefer the use of a *Cantor tube* with the apical bag filled with about 7 ml of mercury. I ignore the instructions on the package and pass the tube nasogastrically with the patient sitting upright. I then place the patient in the right lateral decubitus position and send him to have a plain x-ray film taken. (Often this film will coincide with the 1-hour postbarium film discussed above.) I do this immediately to ensure placement of the tube tip in the distal antrum, before waiting for it to pass through the pylorus. I continue to have x-ray films taken and aggressively reposition the tube and/or patient until the mercury bag has passed the ligament of Treitz. (During this period, I leave the other end of the tube untethered and connected to straight drainage.) This aggressive approach will almost always result in the tube reaching the jejunum within an 8- to 12-hour period. Up to this point, decisions about the patient's position based upon assumptions of tube position related to elapsed time are invariably wrong unless the patient is monitored radiographically. Thereafter, I attach the tube to low, intermittent suction and allow it to pass distally at its own rate, with films initially at 12- then at 24-hour intervals.

Although well-documented clinical experiences at some institutions have demonstrated equivalent decompression with a nasogastric tube, a long intestinal tube greatly facilitates decompression at the operating table. When using such a tube, it is important to remember to evacuate the stomach separately with a nasogastric tube prior to the induction of anesthesia to avoid the danger of aspiration.

Operative Versus Nonoperative Management of Small Intestinal Obstruction

The most controversial aspect of the management of small bowel obstruction is the role of surgery. On one hand, there is the substantial risk, discussed above, of delaying treatment of unrecognized, indeed *unrecognizable*, intestinal ischemia. On the other hand, there are numerous large series, albeit retrospective and poorly controlled, that report success with initial nonoperative management, with surgery being reserved for selected patients who deteriorate or fail to improve.

This issue has been greatly confused by failing to distinguish partial from complete obstruction. Many of the aforementioned series mix these two groups of patients, and the interpretation of their results is thereby obscured. Clearly, patients with *partial* obstruction should be managed initially without surgery, as discussed below, and there seems to be little disagreement on this point. Patients with *complete* small bowel obstruction can then be considered separately, in light of the substantial risk of occult strangulation. Because of this risk, my usual approach to these patients is to proceed to laparotomy within 12 to 24 hours, after the patient has been rehydrated, has achieved therapeutic tissue levels of antibiotics, and after decompression is well under way. I do not believe that an initial therapeutic trial of nonoperative management is justified or advantageous on a routine basis. Nevertheless, there is frequently justification for a 12- to 24-hour delay while an unstable patient is resuscitated. Moreover, a number of special clinical circumstances justify serious consideration of a trial of primary nonoperative treatment. These include documented carcinomatosis, multiply recurrent adhesive obstruction, radiation enteritis, and a number of other conditions. Whether early use of computed tomography scans with oral contrast material will help resolve some of these questions has not yet been determined. This decision, therefore, not unlike any other difficult decision in clinical medicine, should be made after weighing the risks and benefits of the nonoperative approach with those of the operative. One of the major risks (30%) of nonoperative management is that one is delaying the treatment of occult intestinal ischemia. When the benefits of nonoperative management are great enough to justify this risk, this choice is a reasonable one. Under most circumstances, however, and particularly in patients with a routine presentation of complete small bowel obstruction, this risk is simply not justified. On this basis, my own choice for the routine management of *complete* small bowel obstruction is early laparotomy.

MANAGEMENT OF SPECIFIC SMALL BOWEL LESIONS

Strangulation Obstruction

The preoperative diagnosis of strangulation has been addressed above. When strangulated bowel is encountered at operation, the underlying cause is removed simply and easily by reduction, combined with lysis of the adhesion or repair of the hernia. A determination must then be made as to intestinal viability. Nonviable bowel is resected, while viable intestine can be left in situ with no adverse effects. There is a discussion of bowel viability in the chapter on *Intestinal Ischemia*.

Adhesions

Patients with an initial presentation of acute small bowel obstruction due to adhesions will usually benefit from early operative lysis. Even patients with partial obstruction from this cause will often require surgery (see below), although the procedure is facilitated by an initial trial of tube decompression.

Patients with multiply recurrent adhesive obstruction present an exceedingly difficult, but fortunately uncommon, problem in management. I usually try to treat such patients nonoperatively whenever possible, for it is unusual for these patients to have the residual intestinal mobility to allow the formation of a strangulated loop. Moreover, there is less likelihood that a definitive cure will be effected surgically, although many patients will require surgery to relieve the current bout of obstruction.

The prevention of recurrence is a more difficult proposition. Aside from the normal measures of good surgical technique, there is no specific treatment to prevent adhesions. Agents such as steroids which inhibit adhesion formation also inhibit healing, and there is at present no practical way to approach this aspect of the problem. The surgeon must therefore focus on minimizing the operative trauma to the serosa and on trying to position the bowel to avoid its kinking when adhesions do form, as they inevitably will. Plication procedures have not been demonstrated to be beneficial. It is important to remember, however, that the majority of patients who undergo laparotomy for adhesive small bowel obstruction will not suffer recurrence.

Incarcerated Hernia

When an incarcerated abdominal wall hernia is the cause of obstruction, the obstruction itself can often be managed by simple manual reduction. After reduction of the hernia, these patients should always be admitted for observation to avoid sending a patient home with occult dead bowel. They should be observed in the hospital for at least 24 to 48 hours to preclude this possibility. This opportunity can be employed to effect elective hernia repair if no signs of intestinal ischemia appear.

Malignancy

Small intestinal obstruction due to a primary malignancy is usually caused by a lesion of another abdominal organ, often the colon. These patients are managed no differently than other patients with simple small bowel obstruction, combined with resection of the primary lesion whenever feasible.

Patients with documented carcinomatosis present a more difficult problem, however, and can sometimes be managed successfully over the short term with tube decompression. When this is unsuccessful, I do not hesitate to offer lapraotomy to all but the most terminal of patients. The benefits of local control of intestinal obstruction to avoid pain and an indwelling intestinal tube usually more than justify the discomfort of surgery, although the management of these patients should be individualized. At the operation, a bypass of the obstructed area is often preferable to a primary resection that would necessitate an extensive dissection.

Patients with a history of treatment of a prior malignancy, often of the breast or within the abdominal cavity, are sometimes assumed to have carcinomatosis as the basis for obstruction. This is an error, less common today that it was a decade ago, for about a third of these patients will have obstruction due to an unrelated lesion, and about two-thirds will have a resectable or bypassable lesion. Overall, fewer than a third will have unresectable, disseminated carcinoma. To write off a patient with a history of prior malignancy based upon an unconfirmed suspicion of peritoneal carcinomatosis is inexcusable.

Crohn's Disease

Patients with primary inflammatory disease of the small intestine can present with partial or complete small intestinal obstruction. These patients can often be managed successfully by tube decompression, combined with a pharmacologic assault on the primary inflammatory process. This is particularly true when the obstruction is due to acute inflammation early in the course of the illness, and an initial trial of nonoperative management here is usually justified. On the other hand, when the obstruction is due to scarring as the result of the body's attempt to heal a longstanding inflammatory process, the patient will usually require surgical resection or bypass. This fact does not preclude initial nonoperative management to effect decompression and perhaps reduce inflammation. In many cases, the obstructive component due to irreversible scarring proves to be only partial as the phlegmon resolves. In most of these situations, the patient can then undergo elective resection or bypass, often after parenteral treatment of concurrent nutritional depletion. During the period of nonoperative management, radiographic, computed tomographic and endoscopic measures are used to obtain as complete a picture as possible of the bowel anatomy, including fistulas and possible abscesses.

Abdominal Abscess

Regardless of its cause, an acute abdominal abscess can produce a clinical picture indistinguishable from complete, mechanical bowel obstruction, although at operation it is often found that the lumen is anatomically patent adjacent to the abscess. The mechanism is probably an intense local ileus, exacerbated somewhat by external compression. In any case, drainage of the abscess itself is usually sufficient to relieve the obstruction, and the patient will often not require a full-scale laparotomy to effect this. If the obstruction persists, laparotomy can be performed later when the patient is no longer septic.

Radiation Enteritis

Radiation enteritis is best managed by avoidance, by working with well-trained radiotherapists who carefully design their ports and who do not treat those abdominal malignancies in which there is little potential for benefit. Careful patient positioning and the assurance of small intestinal mobility prior to pelvic radiation are particularly important. In these situations, it is helpful if the surgeon has carefully closed the pelvic floor after the resection of a pelvic malignancy. When enteritis is encountered acutely, within a few weeks of radiation therapy, it is usually not obstructive and will often respond to local or systemic steroids. In these situations surgery can usually be avoided. More often, however, intestinal obstruction due to radiation enteritis presents years after the completion of therapy, and at this point there is no effective treatment for the primary disease process. Moreover, the condition will almost certainly progress. Patients with partial obstruction can sometimes avoid surgery for a time, but most of them will require laparotomy. The surgeon then has the choice of resection or bypass of the affected bowel. Contrary to the conventional approach, I prefer to resect when possible, particularly when a relatively short intestinal segment is involved. The dissection is sometimes not as difficult as anticipated, particularly when one realizes that there is no harm in injuring the intestine to be excised. Whether one resects or bypasses the involved area, it is essential to avoid the anastomosis of radiated intestinal tissue. When the involved bowel cannot be resected, it is sometimes necessary to bring out ends of irridiated loops as defunctionalized stomata. If continuity can be restored for a sufficient length of unradiated intestine, these patients can do well, whether or not the affected loops can be resected.

Partial Obstruction

When the barium study confirms the diagnosis of *partial* small bowel obstruction, the patient should be managed initially with a trial of tube decompression. Most of these patients will open up, and many will not suffer a recurrence, particularly if the underlying lesion is an adhesion. Surgery is reserved for those patients who fail to open up sufficiently to allow normal oral alimentation, and for those suffering from recurrent bouts of partial obstruction.

Enteroclysis Study. In either group of patients, the location, degree, and anatomy of the lesion can often be defined preoperatively by an enteroclysis study. A Cantor tube is passed down to a point just proximal to the obstruction, if possible. Residual barium from previous studies should be evacuated as efficiently as possible, by suction from above and by enemas from below. (Cathartics are inhumane in patients with any degree of bowel obstruction.) A small volume of dilute barium is then introduced under fluoroscopic control by a radiologist experienced in this technique. The quality of the imaging obtained in the specific area of interest is often superb, greatly facilitating the decision for or against surgery, and often providing useful clues as to etiology. Once the decision has been made to proceed with surgical resection, the operative approach is no different than that for complete obstruction and will be influenced primarily by the nature of the underlying lesion.

Acute Postoperative Obstruction

Small bowel obstruction appearing in the immediate postoperative period presents a challenging and often mismanaged problem. In the first place, it is difficult to recognize, since its primary symptoms, pain and vomiting, can often be attributed to the incision and to postoperative ileus, respectively. A careful history that reveals increasing colicky, as opposed to constant aching, pain and which pays particular attention to the time course of symptoms, signs, and the abdominal x-ray films is often revealing. Here again, repeated evaluation by the same observer over a period of time is invaluable. When the diagnosis is suspected, it can be confirmed by *barium contrast* given through a nasoenteric tube as discussed above, as long as there is no danger of proximal perforation or suture line leakage. Indeed, this is the best means of distinguishing mechanical obstruction from postoperative ileus.

Once small bowel obstruction has been recognized, its management is controversial. When partial obstruction is confirmed or strongly suspected, a trial of nonoperative management is clearly preferable. Even when the condition fails to resolve, the opportunity to stabilize the acute situation temporarily and to delay surgery a short while further into the postoperative period is usually worthwhile.

Complete obstruction presents a more serious problem, however. Many cite this situation as one in which they would prefer an initial trial of primary nonoperative management. This position, while understandable in light of the clinical situation, is more emotionally than scientifically based. Several series have reported a higher incidence of missed strangulation in acute postoperative patients than was found in the studied population as a whole. Consequently, I believe that *complete* mechanical small bowel obstruction in the acute postoperative period, when confirmed as described, is a relatively clear indication for *early reexploration*. As in other clinical situations, the concurrent presence of substantial risk factors is not necessarily a contraindication to surgery. It is instead a compelling obligation that the physician make the correct therapeutic decision, the one that maximizes benefit and minimizes what might be substantial risks. In many of these situations, the choice that optimizes this cost/benefit ratio is early surgery.

MANAGEMENT OF LARGE BOWEL LESIONS

Complete Obstruction

Patients with *complete* obstruction of the large intestine represent an urgent situation, and the physician should strive to complete diagnostic studies and provide *decompression* within the first 24 hours. The diagnosis is usually obvious on the plain films but can easily be confirmed by a contrast enema. Sigmoidoscopy or colonoscopy will often be helpful in obtaining a tissue diagnosis and ruling out concurrent distal lesions, but this is not essential. Particularly if the patient has a competent ileocecal valve, suggested by a dilated cecum without dilated small bowel loops, there is real danger of perforation if decompression is not provided quickly. This is a difficult distinction to make on clinical grounds, however, and a delay of treatment based upon an incorrect assumption of ileocecal valve incompetence is a serious error.

For the most part, surgery will be required to provide adequate decompression. Often this can be combined with definitive management of the underlying lesion by primary resection. Even patients with acute diverticulitis as the cause of obstruction can often undergo primary resection. In all cases, however, it is too dangerous to attempt a primary anastomosis of obstructed colon, and a proximal colostomy should be fashioned, with the end of distal colon brought out as a mucous fistula, if there is sufficient length, or closed over to form a defunctionalized Hartmann's pouch. In some patients, owing either to sytemic instability or extensive local disease at the sight of obstruction, a primary resection at the time of initial operation is not safe. In these patients, a proximal loop colostomy will provide adequate decompression and allow preparation for a subsequent definitive procedure. In severly ill patients, this can even be performed under local anesthesia, if necessary. Primary cecostomy for decompression is an uncommon procedure today but may be appropriate in a rare patient who is too ill to undergo even a formal colostomy. Once diversion has been achieved, the patient may resume normal feeding and can even return home to recover before undergoing definitive resection. During this period, sepsis can be controlled, nutrition supplemented, and the bowel then prepared to allow the elective resection to take place under optimal circumstances.

Partial Obstruction

Unlike the patient with total colonic obstruction, the patient with a *partial* obstruction can usually be managed in such a way that the initial operative procedure, if needed, can take place under optimal conditions. These patients should immediately cease oral intake, and they will often require a nasogastric tube to reduce the volume of swallowed air that is passed downward from above. Although cathartics should usually be avoided, the colon can often be cleansed with enemas, relieving the acute obstructive component and facilitating diagnosis. Endoscopy should be employed early to attempt to define the nature of the lesion, the status and length of distal colon, and the presence or absence of more proximal lesions when it is possible to pass the colonoscope beyond the point of partial obstruction. A diagnostic enema with a water-soluble contrast material can also be helpful, especially in cases of suspected diverticulitis. Computed tomographic scans have been quite helpful in defining the problem in patients with diverticulitis and painful obstruction. Barium should usually be avoided in cases of partial colonic obstruction to preclude formation of a proximal impaction. For this reason, endoscopy is usually more revealing. Following diagnostic studies and bowel preparation, the patient can undergo elective surgery.

Patients with primary carcinoma, as well as those with completely obstructing inflammatory lesions, clearly require resection. In some cases of Crohn's disease and diverticulitis, however, a vigorous medical regimen, combined with cessation of oral intake, can result in substantial relief of the obstruction. It is sometimes possible to avoid surgery altogether. The difficulty with this approach is the possibility of missing a carcinoma masquerading as an inflammatory lesion. This is unusual in cases of Crohn's disease, but not at all unlikely in patients diagnosed as having diverticulitis. The well-known radiologic guidelines to distinguish obstructing diverticulitis from cancer are helpful but not reliable. If a flexible endoscope can be passed the entire length of the lesion to the proximal, unobstructed bowel, it will afford a high level of diagnostic accuracy to an experienced endoscopist, aided by biopsy. If any doubt remains after colonoscopy, however, the patient should be presumed to have cancer unless proven otherwise, and a resection planned.

INTESTINAL ISCHEMIA

MARC COOPERMAN, M.D.

Despite significant advances in the care of the critically ill patient, intestinal ischemia continues to be associated with distressingly high morbidity and mortality. Recent reports have noted the mortality of mesenteric embolism and thrombosis to be as high as 75 to 100 percent and the mortality of strangulated intestinal obstruction as high as 70 percent. The most important single factor responsible for this mortality rate is a delay in diagnosis. Often the diagnosis is not made until peritonitis develops due to either migration of bacteria across the wall of the injured bowel or perforation and fecal soilage of the peritoneal cavity.

To improve patient survival every effort must be made to make the diagnosis and intervene therapeutically before the ischemic damage becomes irreversible and infarction of the involved bowel occurs. Otherwise, as is too often the case, the surgeon is faced with the need to perform a massive intestinal resection in a severely septic patient. Even if the length of infarcted bowel is relatively limited, as in strangulated obstruction secondary to adhesions and strangulated hernias, septic complications due to peritoneal contamination by intestinal organisms may preclude a successful outcome.

Early diagnosis will be achieved only if there is a high index of suspicion on the part of the clinician. He or she must be aware that the clinical picture is often unclear until infarction has taken place and the resultant peritonitis and sepsis leads to a belated diagnosis. The reason for this confusion is the frequent absence of physical findings early in the course of intestinal ischemia. The physician is typically confronted with a patient with complaints of severe abdominal pain and diarrhea, which may contain blood, in whom the examination of the abdomen is either normal or demonstrates mild nonspecific findings. The discrepancy between the severity of the symptoms and the absence of physical findings often serves to reassure the physician falsely. In fact, the findings of marked abdominal tenderness, guarding, rebound, and absent bowel sounds indicating the presence of peritonitis are often late in developing and are present only after intestinal ischemia has progressed to a point where the bowel is usually no longer salvageable. The difficulty in diagnosis is often compounded by nonspecific laboratory and radiologic findings that contribute to a delay in instituting effective treatment.

Intestinal ischemia and infarction are the final common pathway from a variety of diverse pathologic processes interrupting the normal intestinal blood supply. These include arterial embolism and thrombosis, venous thrombosis, strangulating obstructions and hernias, low cardiac output, neoplasms, and trauma. Common to all of these entities is the difficulty of recognizing intestinal ischemia while the process is still reversible and the intestine viable. Only a high index of suspicion and an aggressive diagnostic and therapeutic approach will avoid intestinal infarction and reduce mortality; mortality has been shown to double if surgery is delayed beyond 36 hours after the onset of the symptoms.

Laboratory Diagnosis

There currently is no specific accurate laboratory test available for the early diagnosis of intestinal ischemia. Although experimental studies have suggested that certain enzyme determinations may have clinical applicability, none has yet found widespead use.

The white blood and hemoglobin counts are usually abnormal in patients with ischemic intestine. Although the white blood count is elevated in 75 percent of cases, it is of little specific diagnostic use, since a wide variety of intra-abdominal pathologic processes also cause a leukocytosis. Similarly, an elevated hemoglobin count due to third space fluid losses occurs in such a wide variety of conditions as to be of limited value.

Acidosis in a patient with abdominal pain should suggest the diagnosis of ischemic bowel. Acidosis is not uniformly present, however, and often is a late occurrence when the ischemic process is far advanced.

Hyperphosphatemia and elevation of peritoneal fluid phosphate levels in association with ischemic intestine have been demonstrated both in the experimental laboratory and the clinical setting. Elevations of serum phosphate have been reported in up to 70 percent of patients with long segments of ischemic intestine. The test, however, is difficult to interpret in the presence of renal disease or lactic acidosis.

A large number of enzymes, including amylase, lactic dehydrogenase, transaminases, alkaline phosphatase, creatine kinase, and diamine oxidase, have been studied as possible markers for intestinal ischemia.

Clinical experience has proved that while amylase, lactic dehydrogenase, and the transaminases are occasionally elevated, they are far too nonspecific to be diagnostically useful. For example, elevations of serum amylase, which occur in approximately 20 percent of patients with intestinal ischemia, are usually due to either pancreatitis or biliary tract disease. More exciting is the possibility that intestinal alkaline phosphatase, creatine phosphokinase BB, diamine oxidase, or one of the intestinal dissacharidases may be more specific for ischemic intestinal injury. Although experimental studies have been encouraging, as have isolated clinical reports, further clinical studies need to be done to evaluate the diagnostic accuracy and specificity of these tests.

Radiologic Evaluation

Plain abdominal films should be taken in any patient suspected of having intestinal ischemia but will be helpful in making the diagnosis in only about 50 percent. In the other half, findings will either be absent or nonspecific. The classic finding of ischemic bowel is "thumbprinting." This is a scalloped appearance of the lumen secondary to submucosal hemorrhage. As the ischemic process progresses, further changes include separation of bowel loops with dilation and loss of peristalsis. The presence of gas in the wall of the bowel or the portal vein indicates advanced ischemia and carries a poor prognosis.

Whether or not plain films are positive, angiography should be done immediately if ischemia in the distribution of the superior mesenteric artery is suspected. Angiography will identify superior mesenteric arterial occlusion if embolus or thrombosis has occurred and also allows for treatment of nonocclusive disease by intra-arterial infusion of papaverine. It is thought that vasospasm plays an important role in occlusive disease as well, and there have been reports of improved survival if an intra-arterial infusion of vasodilator is continued after the occlusion has been corrected surgically.

General Preparation of the Patient

Aggressive resuscitation of these patients with the view toward preparing them for surgery should be carried out while diagnostic studies are under way. The two major problems which must be addressed are hypovolemia and sepsis, which may be present even in the absence of transmural infarction.

Hypovolemia occurs secondary to massive third space fluid losses and should be corrected prior to induction of anesthesia. The amount of fluid replacement required is often surprisingly high, and in the presence of significant cardiovascular disease or renal impairment, a Swan-Ganz catheter is often extremely helpful. In the absence of renal failure, restoration of adequate urine output is the best indicator that hypovolemia has been corrected. Prior to surgery, the patient's electrolyte status should also be determined and normalized to the extent possible. It is important to be aware that patients with intestinal ischemia may manifest a marked metabolic acidosis. Blood gas determinations should be performed in all patients suspected of having intestinal ischemia, and acidosis should be corrected to the extent possible by administration of sodium bicarbonate. Correction of hypovolemia with improvement in cardiac output and tissue perfusion will also help to correct the acidosis.

A nasogastric tube should be inserted to decompress the bowel. Studies have clearly shown that intestinal distention will significantly reduce blood flow within the bowel, adding to the ischemia.

Sepsis is an invariable accompaniment of transmural infarction and often precedes it as the ischemic, but still viable, intestine loses its mucosal integrity with bacterial contamination of the peritoneal cavity. As a result, the clinical picture may be complicated by multisystem failure. All patients should receive broad-spectrum antibiotics, including anaerobic coverage. The cardiovascular, respiratory, and renal manifestations of multisystem failure should be treated vigorously, but should not excessively delay surgery, as the single most important factor in treating the multisystem failure is correction of the underlying intestinal ischemia or resection of nonviable bowel.

INTESTINAL OBSTRUCTION

When strangulation complicates a simple intestinal obstruction mortality is dramatically increased. Whereas the mortality rate of uncomplicated intestinal obstruction is well below 10 percent, mortality rates exceeding 50 percent have been reported with strangulation. Therefore, the goal of surgical therapy is to intervene before strangulation occurs. Unfortunately, the classic findings of strangulation, which include fever, leukocytosis, guarding, rebound, severe constant pain, palpable mass, and bloody diarrhea, are not invariably present and frequently do not develop until the bowel becomes gangrenous. Numerous studies have shown that attempts by experienced surgeons to differentiate between uncomplicated and strangulated obstructions preoperatively are incorrect in a significant percentage of cases. For this reason most surgeons advocate an aggressive approach to all such patients with prompt fluid resuscitation, administration of antibiotics, nasogastric decompression, and laparotomy. Delaying laparotomy beyond the time required to resuscitate the patient adequately will only increase the incidence of irreversibly ischemic bowel.

Decompression of the distended bowel is an important part of the management of patients with intestinal obstruction. Nasogastric intubation should be performed in all patients. By decompressing the intestinal tract, the risk of aspiration with the induction of anesthesia is reduced and the component of ischemia secondary to distention of the bowel is decreased. Studies have shown that simple distention of the intestine can reduce intestinal blood flow by as much as 75 percent. As a result of marked distention, ischemia and necrosis may develop in the distended bowel at a point remote from the point of obstruction. For this reason the surgeon must be careful to inspect the entire bowel at the time of operation to avoid overlooking an area of significant ischemia.

At operation the surgeon must first relieve the cause of obstruction. The remainder of the operation is predicted on whether the intestine is viable. As discussed below, the clinical indicators of viability are often misleading, and objective methods of determining viability are available. A period of 10 minutes should be allowed to elapse before the bowel's viability is assessed; placing warm, moist packs over the bowel and injecting lidocaine into the root of the mesentery may serve to augment blood flow. All nonviable intestine must be resected. A primary anastomosis is almost always preferable in cases involving the small bowel. Proximal enterostomies are difficult to manage in terms of fluid losses and pose major problems in nutritional management. If an accurate determination of viability is made, the complication rate for performing an anastomosis should be low. On the other hand, when necrotic obstructed colon must be resected, as in the case of sigmoid volvulus, then a primary anastomosis should be avoided and a colostomy performed.

Two causes of intestinal obstruction require separate discussion. These are *incarcerated inguinal hernias* and *volvulus*. As with other causes of intestinal obstruction, both can result in intestinal ischemia and infarction. As with other causes of obstruction, early recognition and management are essential to preserve intestinal viability.

Incarcerated Inguinal Hernia

The nonoperative reduction of incarcerated inguinal hernias is controversial because of the possibility of reducing gangrenous bowel back into the peritoneal cavity. Studies have shown, however, that strangulated hernias can usually be recognized clinically and that, surprisingly, the reduction of nonviable bowel does not increase mortality. Conversely, mortality is increased when no attempt at nonoperative reduction is made and patients with nonstrangulated hernias and other significant medical illnesses undergo unnecessary emergency operation. For this reason, an attempt at nonoperative reduction should be made in the absence of strangulation. Approximately 50 percent of incarcerated hernias can be reduced nonoperatively with the use of narcotics or muscle relaxants. If reduction is successful, the patient should be observed closely for signs of peritonitis indicating that nonviable bowel was reduced. In the absence of this complication, associated medical problems can be corrected and the patient can undergo elective operation with markedly improved safety.

In contrast, the patient with a strangulated hernia should be operated on as soon as adequate intravenous fluids and broad-spectrum antibiotics have been given. Complications will be reduced if contamination of the peritoneal cavity is avoided. Therefore the abdomen is not opened unless contents of the hernia sac are unintentionally lost into the peritoneal cavity. Once the hernia sac has been opened and the constricting band at the neck divided, a determination of the viability of the involved bowel is made. Nonviable bowel is resected and an anastomosis performed. The bowel is then returned to the peritoneal cavity and the hernia repaired.

Volvulus

Volvulus accounts for slightly less than 5 percent of cases of intestinal obstruction. A volvulus occurs when the bowel twists around a fixed point. The sigmoid colon, followed by the cecum, are most commonly involved. Volvulus of the transverse colon or small intestine is quite rare. The diagnosis is usually suggested by typical findings on plain films of the abdomen and can be confirmed with barium enema.

As with other causes of intestinal ischemia, early therapeutic intervention is essential to avoid intestinal gangrene with the resultant increase in morbidity and mortality. Studies have shown that the mortality of sigmoid or cecal volvulus increases to approximately 40 to 50 percent in the presence of gangrenous colon, compared with mortality figures of 10 percent or less when the colon is still viable.

In the absence of peritoneal signs indicating intestinal infarction, the initial management of sigmoid volvulus is nonoperative. Sigmoidoscopic decompression will be successful in almost 80 percent of patients. If sigmoidoscopy is unsuccessful, then immediate laparotomy is indicated. Simple detorsion of the volvulus is followed by a high recurrence rate, and most surgeons favor resection of the involved segment with creation of a colostomy and mucous fistula. Intestinal continuity is restored in a second operation. If sigmoidoscopy is successful, and there is no strong medical contraindication, the patient should undergo elective resection of the redundant sigmoid, as the likelihood of recurrent volvulus is high.

Cecal volvulus, which presents as a distal mechanical small bowel obstruction, is not amenable to nonoperative decompression. These patients should undergo immediate laparotomy. Once the bowel has been untwisted, its viability is determined. If infarction has occurred, the involved segment is resected and a primary anastomosis may be performed. If the bowel is viable, cecopexy is the procedure of choice. Cecostomy, which is advocated by some authors, is unnecessary and, by opening the bowel, increases the risk of septic complications.

MESENTERIC ARTERIAL THROMBOSIS AND EMBOLUS

A successful outcome in the patient with acute mesenteric arterial occlusion is critically dependent on prompt diagnosis and treatment to avoid infarction of the majority of the small intestine and proximal colon. Once infarction occurs, even if the patient is salvaged by resection of the gangrenous bowel, there is rarely sufficient viable bowel remaining to avoid the need for permanent parenteral nutrition.

The diagnosis of acute mesenteric arterial occlusion should be suspected in the patient with the onset of severe steady periumbilical pain in whom physical findings are conspicuously absent. Vomiting may occur and there may be bloody diarrhea. The onset of symptoms is more sudden in patients with embolus than in those with thrombosis. In the latter group there is frequently a history of intestinal angina preceding the thrombosis.

If the diagnosis is suspected, the patient should undergo emergency angiography. After a flush aortogram is performed, a selective superior mesenteric arteriogram is obtained. Usually embolus can be differentiated from thrombosis. The occlusion produced by emboli is typically distal to the origin of the middle colic artery and a meniscus suggesting an embolus may be seen. In contrast, thrombosis usually occurs within 2 cm of the origin of the vessel and prominent collaterals may be present.

Once the diagnosis is established, it may be helpful to begin an infusion of papaverine, as studies have shown that vasoconstriction is an important contributor to the ischemic process and may persist for several hours after surgical relief of the arterial occlusion. Laparotomy should be performed as soon as possible. In the case of mesenteric embolus, embolectomy can be performed through a longitudinal arteriotomy using a standard Fogarty embolectomy catheter. The arteriotomy is then closed with fine vascular suture; a patch angioplasty is rarely necessary. The treatment of mesenteric thrombosis consists of an aortomesenteric bypass graft using a segment of saphenous vein. Thromboendarterectomy has been largely abandoned because of the high failure rate.

Once blood flow to the bowel has been restored, the viability of the affected segment of intestine is determined and any nonviable bowel is resected. Even with aggressive surgical management, however, the mortality of acute mesenteric arterial occlusion approaches 50 percent.

NONOCCLUSIVE MESENTERIC ISCHEMIA

Nonocclusive mesenteric vascular insufficiency, once thought to be quite rare, is now being recognized with increasing frequency and may account for 50 percent of cases of mesenteric ischemia. The underlying vasospasm is almost always associated with states of low cardiac output. Digitalis has also been implicated as a causative agent.

Nonocclusive mesenteric vascular insufficiency should be suspected in a patient who develops the clinical picture of intestinal ischemia in the setting of low cardiac output. The best results have been obtained in centers where an aggressive approach utilizing selective mesenteric angiography is employed early in the course of the disease. Once the diagnosis is established, a direct infusion of papaverine into the superior mesenteric artery is begun at a dose of 30 to 60 mg per hour. The infusion is continued for up to 5 days, depending on the clinical response of the patient and the results of angiograms repeated at 24-hour intervals. The development of signs of peritonitis are an indication for immediate surgical exploration.

Even with this aggressive approach mortality rates approximate 40 percent. This is probably a reflection of the severity of the underlying condition producing the low cardiac output as well as the intestinal ischemia itself.

MESENTERIC VENOUS THROMBOSIS

Mesenteric venous occlusion is a relatively uncommon cause of intestinal ischemia. In more than 50 percent of cases, an underlying cause for the thrombosis can be determined. These include *intra-abdominal sepsis, neoplasms, trauma, portal hypertension,* and *hypercoagulable states,* such as the thrombocytosis which may follow splenectomy.

In contrast to the sudden onset of severe abdominal pain which characterizes mesenteric arterial occlusion, the development of symptoms is often gradual, complicating the diagnosis. Pain tends to be vague, and physical examination often shows only mild abdominal tenderness. Often the diagnosis is not made until infarction with peritonitis develops. Barium studies of the intestinal tract may be very helpful, demonstrating severe edema of the involved segment of bowel.

The surgical treatment of this disorder depends on the length and viability of involved bowel. If only a short segment of intestine is involved or if the bowel is gangrenous, then surgical resection is the treatment of choice.

Venous thrombectomy, if performed early enough, may be successful in preventing intestinal infarction or may limit the extent of resection necessary. Recurrent thrombosis occurs in approximately 30 percent of patients, however, leading some to advocate routine second look laparotomies 24 hours later.

Anticoagulation has been shown to be important in reducing mortality and preventing recurrent thrombosis. Heparin should be started in the early postoperative period. Patients should be discharged on Coumadin, which is continued for 3 to 6 months.

ISCHEMIC COLITIS

Ischemic colitis may occur as a spontaneous event or as a complication of aortic surgery. In either case transmural infarction is associated with mortality rates in excess of 70 percent. The most common sites of involvement are the splenic flexure and the sigmoid colon, areas where important vascular anastomoses may be inadequate or absent.

The best form of treatment for ischemic colitis encountered following aortic surgery is prevention. The preoperative angiogram often gives important information about the intestinal blood supply. The presence of an enlarged meandering artery of Drummond, filling from the inferior mesenteric artery, should alert the surgeon to significant stenosis or occlusion of the superior mesenteric artery. Ligation of the inferior mesenteric artery in such patients during the course of surgery for aortic aneurysm or aortic occlusive disease may be expected to produce intestinal ischemia.

Even in the absence of angiographic abnormalities, the surgeon must be certain that the viability of the left colon is not compromised if sacrifice of the inferior mesenteric artery is necessary. The artery should be ligated as close to the origin from the aorta as possible to avoid interruption of collateral flow to the vessel. Simple inspection of the colon may be misleading following inferior mesenteric artery ligation, because changes in the appearance of the bowel may not develop with sufficient rapidity. Some authors have advocated inspection of the divided inferior mesenteric vessel to assess back bleeding. If pulsatile back bleeding is present, it is presumed that sufficient collateral flow to the colon is present to maintain viability. Objective indicators of viability, including Doppler ultrasound, fluorescence, and measurement of inferior mesenteric artery stump pressures, are available, however, and one of these should be used routinely to ascertain that colonic viability has not been compromised. If the bowel is not clearly viable, then the inferior mesenteric artery should be implanted into the prosthesis or an aortomesenteric graft performed and the viability then retested. If the ischemia cannot be corrected, the segment of bowel must be resected once all graft materials have been reperitonealized.

If ischemic colitis does develop, either following aortic surgery or as a spontaneous event complicating atherosclerosis, the hallmarks are lower abdominal pain, tenderness, and diarrhea, which may become bloody. If the diagnosis is suspected, colonoscopy should be performed to establish it and assess the severity of the ischemic damage.

Unless the bowel appears gangrenous, initial management of ischemic colitis consists of nasogastric suction, intravenous fluids, and broad-spectrum antibiotics. The patient must be followed closely for signs of sepsis with frequent vital signs and physical examinations of the abdomen. If evidence of peritonitis develops, the patient should undergo immediate laparotomy and resection of all nonviable intestine. Serial colonoscopies provide an excellent means of following the disease process. It is important, however, in these patients to avoid over-inflating the colon with air and to limit the extent of colonoscopy to minimize the risk of perforation. If serial examination demonstrates disease progression, then surgical resection is indicated before perforation occurs.

In the majority of patients with ischemic colitis, resolution occurs. Follow-up barium examination of the colon is important in these patients, as a high percentage will develop strictures. Elective one-stage resection is the treatment of choice if this late complication develops.

DETERMINATION OF VIABILITY

Regardless of the origin of intestinal ischemia, successful surgical treatment is predicated on the ability to assess accurately the viability of the involved intestine at the time of surgery. The clinical indicators of intestinal viability, i.e., the appearance of the bowel, presence of pulsations and peristalsis, and the amount of bleeding from the cut edge of the bowel, are not always dependable. They are subjective by nature and changes may be late enough in developing as to not be helpful at surgery. Clinical experience, as well as experimental studies, has shown the unreliability of subjective assessment of intestinal viability.

As a result, numerous techniques have been developed in an attempt to provide an objective means of determining intestinal viability. Currently, two have gained widespread clinical use and have established their reliability: Doppler ultrasound and fluorescein dye injection. The two techniques should be viewed as complementary since each has advantages and disadvantages.

Doppler ultrasound will detect arterial and venous flow within the small vessels of the intestinal wall. The audible signals produced by arterial and venous flow are easily differentiated, and only the arterial signals are important in measuring viability. The gas-sterilized Doppler probe is lightly applied to the surface of the intestine; acoustic contact is enhanced by coating the probe tip with a sterile water-soluble gel. If arterial flow signals are detected, the bowel is judged viable. One of the advantages of the technique is that it is an all or none phenomenon; subjective interpretation of the quality of the signals is unnecessary. Experimental studies and extensive clinical use have shown it to be an extremely reliable method of determining intestinal viability. It has the advantages of being technically simple to perform, easy to interpret, and does not require expensive equipment. Its major drawback is that it is cumbersome when long segments of bowel are ischemic. It is important to be certain that arterial flow signals are present at 2-cm intervals, a process that can be time-consuming if the viability of the entire small bowel is in question, as in acute mesenteric arterial thrombosis. In cases such as this, fluorescein dye, as described below, should be used initially, and any questionable areas identified checked with the Doppler probe.

Fluorescein dye injection has also been shown to be a reliable means of assessing intestinal viability. The technique is also simple to use and the required equipment is inexpensive. Fluorescein dye, 1,000 mg, is injected intravenously. A 3600 A Woods lamp is then used to illuminate the bowel. The presence of fluorescence indicates viability. Failure to stain with the dye indicates that irreversible ischemia is present. This technique is particularly well suited to study long segments of intestine, where use of the Doppler would be excessively time-consuming. Occasionally, however, the fluorescence pattern seen is not clear and requires subjective interpretation. Patchy staining of the bowel or speckling may be inconclusive. If this occurs, the Doppler should be used. The other major disadvantage is that fluorescein can be used only once in a patient, since a second injection is uninterpretable due to prior staining of tissues.

Surgeons operating on patients with ischemic intestine should be familiar with both techniques and should employ one or both whenever bowel viability is in question.

SECOND-LOOK LAPAROTOMY

The practice of routinely reexploring patients operated on for mesenteric arterial occlusive disease 24 hours after the initial operation was based on problems in accurately predicting intestinal viability. Frequently these procedures were helpful, with a high incidence of positive findings. The practice of routine second-look procedures, however, also exposes seriously ill patients to what may be an unnecessary major surgical procedure.

The development of accurate objective methods of predicting the viability of ischemic intestine, Doppler ultrasound and fluorescein, has reduced the need to routinely reexplore these patients. If Doppler ultrasound or fluorescein indicates that segments of intestine are nonviable, there is no justification for not resecting them at the initial operation.

Conversely, if the intestine is clearly shown to be viable, then the decision to reexplore a patient should be based on his clinical course. A second-look laparotomy should be performed only in those patients suspected on clinical grounds of having developed recurrent ischemia.

CONCLUSION

In summary, intestinal ischemia may be the end result of a diverse group of pathologic processes resulting in diminished blood flow to the bowel. Regardless of the cause, all have in common the problem of making an early diagnosis when therapeutic intervention can prevent intestinal infarction. Morbidity and mortality will be reduced only when there is a high index of suspicion on the part of the clinician, who must take an aggressive diagnostic approach to these often confusing patients.

SECRETORY DIARRHEA

KIERTISIN DHARMSATHAPHORN, M.D.

Secretory diarrhea results from the stimulation of water and electrolyte secretion in the intestine. In most cases, secretion of chloride ions is the primary driving force for water secretion by the epithelial cells. Inhibition of electrolyte absorption may also cause secretory diarrhea, but it is probably a less frequent cause. The clinical features of secretory diarrhea include excessive watery stool, more than 225 g per day (most patients with severe secretory diarrhea have stool volume greater than 1,000 g per day); and a stool osmolarity essentially equal to the concentration of its ions, i.e., stool $(Na^+ + K^+) \times 2$ approximately equals stool osmolarity. This chapter omits the discussion of acute secretory diarrhea and the two major types of chronic secretory diarrhea, those induced by bile salts or fatty acids, which are discussed in other chapters in this volume. Diarrhea associated with inflammatory bowel disease is also discussed in other chapters. This leaves us with chronic secretory diarrhea due to endocrine tumors, laxative abuse, and secretory diarrhea of unknown cause. Recently the profile of chronic secretory diarrhea has changed with the increased prevalence of patients with acquired immune deficiency syndrome (AIDS). Until now, it was the general rule that infections did not lead to chronic secretory diarrhea, but the unusual infections associated with AIDS have changed this rule.

Therapy for secretory diarrhea focuses on fluid and electrolyte replacement, along with treatment of the specific cause, should the latter be feasible. For example, exclusion of fat in the diet is essential for treatment of diarrhea associated with fat malabsorption, and cholestyramine is useful for diarrhea induced by bile salts, as are gluten-free diets for celiac sprue, and proper antimicrobial agents for infectious diarrhea. In many cases of chronic secretory diarrhea, however, specific treatment may not be available or possible. Such patients may benefit from antidiarrheal drug therapy in addition to fluid and electrolyte replacement.

FLUID AND ELECTROLYTE REPLACEMENT

Fluid and electrolyte management is most critical when stool volume exceeds 1 to 2 L a day. Dehydration and sodium, chloride, and potassium depletion in these patients usually requires immediate attention. First, it must be emphasized that the absorptive and secretory mechanisms of the intestine are two separate and unrelated processes. When the secretory process is stimulated by exogenous toxin or endogenous secretagogues, the intestinal cells can still absorb glucose, sodium, and water normally. Second, glucose, together with sodium, is avidly and actively absorbed by the intestinal epithelial cells via the sodium glucose cotransport mechanism. Therefore, in the presence of glucose (sugar or starch), electrolytes and water are absorbed at an accelerated rate. Sustaining the absorptive mechanism for water and electrolytes should improve the water-electrolyte balance and prevent dehydration, despite the ongoing secretion. Despite the ability to restore fluid and electrolyte balance, carbohydrate/electrolytic solutions usually do not decrease the stool output, and may even make the symptoms worse.

The composition of oral replacement solutions varies from one institution to another. Balanced salt/carbohydrate solutions containing potassium are generally used. The World Health Organization recommends a replacement solution containing the following (in grams per liter): glucose, 20; sodium chloride, 4; potassium chloride, 2; sodium bicarbonate, 2. This results in a solution containing (in millimoles per liter): glucose, 111; sodium chloride, 60; potassium chloride, 20; sodium bicarbonate, 30; with an osmolarity of about 331. The electrolyte content of the different replacement solutions varies mainly in the sodium concentration, which does not appear to be critical in patients with normal kidney function. In patients with impaired kidney function, however, the composition of electrolytes should be modified accordingly, depending on the fluid and electrolyte status of the patient. For these patients, a lower sodium concentration in the replacement fluid may be needed. On the other hand, patients with short bowel syndrome may need a replacement solution with a higher sodium content. When a higher sodium content is necessary, glucose is best given as glucose polymer to prevent hypertonicity of the solution. Glucose polymers are available commercially as Polycose (Ross Laboratories, Columbus, OH), Moducal, (Mead Johnson, Evansville, IN), or Caloreen, (Roussel Limited, Wembrey Park, England). A solution containing (in grams per liter) glucose polymer, 20; sodium chloride, 7; and potassium chloride, 1, is recommended.

Some patients may not be able to tolerate the excessive amount of oral intake necessary to keep up with the diarrhea. It may be necessary to use a feeding jejunostomy tube or total parenteral nutrition in these patients. At our institution, total parenteral nutrition has proved to be a very useful method to compensate for severe loss in diarrheal fluid. This technique should be considered early in patients with AIDS whose diarrhea does not respond to conventional management.

PHARMACOLOGIC INTERVENTION IN SECRETORY DIARRHEA

Reversal of the electrolyte secretion, either by limiting the receptor-mediated process or by interrupting the intracellular events (secondary messengers) leading to secretion, is the key to pharmacologic intervention. Knowledge regarding the regulation of water and electrolyte transport by peptides and neurotransmitters can be applied to the treatment of diarrhea: opiates, alpha-adrenergic agents, and somatostatin interfere effectively at the receptor sites; chlorpromazine and its derivative, trifluoperazine, interfere with the intracellular events. Alternate approaches that may be possible in the future include prevention of the binding of toxin to the receptor, and blockage of the chloride exit pathway on the luminal membrane of the intestinal epithelial cells. Table 1 is a summary of pharmacologic options.

Opiate Agents

Since ancient times, opiates have been the mainstay in the treatment of diarrhea. Endogenous opiates both inhibit water and electrolyte secretion and stimulate water and electrolyte absorption by epithelial cells. These compounds also stimulate contraction of the circular smooth muscle to delay gastrointestinal transit. Although the high doses of synthetic opiates normally used in clinical practice can stimulate water and electrolyte absorption, the efficiency of synthetic opiates is mainly due to their antimotility action. Currently, the commercially available opiates include *diphenoxylate with atropine* (Lomotil), *loperamide* (Imodium), and *codeine*. These compounds are quite effective; however, their clinical utility is limited by the possible side effects at high doses, specifically the central nervous system side effects. Most notable among these is a depressed mental status; other central nervous system side effects include nausea, vomiting, respiratory depression, and the possibility of developing physical dependence with prolonged use. The toxicity of atropine is a limiting factor when a high dose of Lomotil is needed. Imodium is more expensive than codeine or Lomotil. Because Imodium does not cross the blood-brain barrier well, it produces fewer central nervous system side effects than the other opiates and can be administered in high doses; Imodium may also have less tendency to cause physical dependence. There are few, if any, data, however, suggesting that codeine or Lomotil causes physical dependence. The usual dosage of Lomotil is 1 to 2 tablets (each contains 2.5 mg diphenoxylate) four times a day; that of Imodium, 1 to 2 capsules (each contains 2 mg) twice a day; and that of codeine, 30 to 60 mg four times a day.

It is worthwhile to try Imodium at a very high dose in patients who fail to improve after treatment with the

TABLE 1 Summary of Pharmacologic Options

Drug	Effectiveness	High Doses Tolerated?	Side Effects	Comments
Opiates	Quite effective	Usually	Drowsiness, nausea	First choice drug
Alpha-adrenergic agonists	Good	Usually not	Postural hypotension, drowsiness	Combined with an opiate and/or verapamil
Prostaglandin synthetase inhibitors	Good in selected patients	Follow manufacturer's recommended dose	Vary with drug	Need testing, still not widely used
Chlorpromazine and trifluoperazine	Good	Yes but not commonly used	Retinopathy, movement disorders, blood dyscrasias, abnormal liver function tests	Monitor all patients closely
Verapamil	Not good as a single drug	Follow manufacturer's recommended dose	Cardiovascular	Combine with an opiate and/or an alpha-adrenergic agonist (use only if no heart disease)
Lithium	Good	Yes	Cardiovascular, neuromuscular, CNS	Relatively safe
Glucocorticoids	Good in selected patients with VIPoma	Not well	Many side effects of steroid, particularly at high dosage	Decrease dose to smallest effective dose
Somatostatin	Good	Unknown	Steatorrhea, abnormal glucose tolerance	Must be given subcutaneously

usual doses of synthetic opiates. In our clinic these patients are started on 16 capsules (32 mg) of loperamide per day. Doses up to 64 mg per day have been used without significant side effects, however, the patients who do not respond to 32 mg of loperamide per day, in general, do not respond to a higher dose.

Alpha-Adrenergic Agents

Alpha-adrenergic agonists represent a new class of antidiarrheal agents. They inhibit water and electrolyte secretion as well as slow the gastrointestinal transit. *Clonidine* is an alpha-adrenergic agent which is readily available, but it crosses the blood-brain barrier readily and has many side effects. The cardiovascular side effects, in particular, limit its clinical application to relatively mild disorders such as diarrhea. Newer alpha-adrenergic agonists developed for their intestinal action may have less severe side effects. One of these, *lidamidine* (William H. Rorer, Inc., Fort Washington, PA), may become available in the near future. At the present time, alpha-adrenergic agents should be used to control diarrhea only in patients who are either unresponsive to synthetic opiates or are unable to use the opiate compounds because of the side effects. I recommend that an ECG be done, and I usually exclude patients who have significant cardiac disease.

Clonidine should be given in combination with loperamide, starting with 0.1 mg per day and slowly increasing the dose every 4 to 5 days. When clonidine is used alone it is usually effective at a dose of 0.3 to 0.4 mg or higher per day. Postural hypotension is invariably detected at these effective doses and may be very troublesome, though it usually becomes more tolerable as time passes. About half of all patients are able to tolerate the drug after being on it for approximately 1 week; the other half unfortunately do not experience a significant decrease in this side effect. Some patients with diabetic diarrhea tolerate the medication well, and doses up to 1.2 mg per day have been used without significant side effects. Their diabetic neuropathy may cause them to have less or no postural hypotension. Some patients with diabetic diarrhea are paradoxically sensitive to the medication, however, and may not be able to tolerate a dose of clonidine as small as 0.1 mg per day. Therefore, I always start the patient on 0.1 mg per day for at least a couple of days and then gradually increase the dose. To avoid troublesome withdrawal symptoms, the medication should not be discontinued abruptly. A gradual tapering off over 4 to 5 days is recommended, even when the side effect is the reason for discontinuing the medication. Lidamidine is effective at 8 to 16 mg per day given in divided doses four times daily. The side effects of lidamidine are similar to those of clonidine; however, the medication appears to have a wider therapeutic window.

Prostaglandin Synthetase Inhibitors

Interest in these agents stems from the fact that prostaglandins stimulate water and electrolyte secretion. Therefore, inhibition of prostaglandin synthesis may result in less water and electrolyte secretion. Indomethacin has proved useful in some selected patients with secretory diarrhea who have an increased prostaglandin production. Salicylates may also be effective as judged by the fact that bismuth subsalicylate (Pepto Bismol) can prevent traveler's diarrhea, and 5-aminosalicylic acid is effective in inflammatory bowel disease. The effectiveness of indomethacin and salicylates in differential diarrheal diseases remains to be tested. If these medications are to be employed, the manufacturer's recommended dose should be used.

Chlorpromazine Derivatives and Verapamil

Altering the intracellular events that lead to intestinal secretion is another approach to the effective treatment of diarrhea. After binding of the hormone or toxin to the receptor, the critical intracellular events involve either an increase in cellular cyclic adenosine monophosphate, cyclic quanosine monophosphate, or calcium. Chlorpromazine derivatives inhibit water secretion and lessens diarrhea possibly by binding to and inactivating the calcium-calmodulin complex, a probable mediator in intestinal secretion. Clinically, *trifluoperazine* has been used successfully in patients with watery diarrhea due to VIPoma. Adverse effects are relatively common, however. Therefore, trifluoperazine should be started at a small dose, 2 or 4 mg per day, and increased to 30 mg per day over a period of about 1 week while the patient is monitored closely. I recommend an eye examination because retinopathy has been reported with phenothiazines. The medication should be discontinued if the patient develops any movement disorder (e.g., parkinsonism, tardive dyskinesia), abnormal blood count, or an abnormal liver function test. The effectiveness of *chlorpromazine* has been observed at 1 to 4 mg per kilogram of body weight in patients with cholera. Similar precautions outlined for trifluoperazine also apply to chlorpromazine.

Verapamil, a calcium channel blocker, inhibits calcium entry into the cells, inhibits water secretion, and decreases diarrhea. I usually combine verapamil, 80 mg three times a day, with Imodium and clonidine in patients with severe secretory diarrhea who do not have a cardiac disease.

Other Medications

Lithium carbonate, glucocorticoids, and somatostatin are effective in patients with VIPoma and chronic idiopathic secretory diarrhea. The mechanism of action of *lithium* is not well understood. At the usual dose, 300 mg twice a day, the medication appears to be relatively safe. Troublesome side effects may involve the cardiovascular, neuromuscular and central nervous system.

Glucocorticoids stimulate the absorption of water and electrolytes, and may improve diarrhea in some patients with pancreatic cholera. Prednisone should be started at 60 mg per day. If it is effective one can gradually decrease the dosage and keep the patient on the smallest dose possible to maintain effectiveness.

Somatostatin is a peptide hormone that inhibits water and electrolyte secretion in the intestine. It has been used successfully to inhibit diarrhea in patients with carcinoid tumors, VIPoma, and short bowel syndrome. The side effects are relatively few, despite the concern that somatostatin affects many organ systems. Abnormal glucose tolerance and steatorrhea are the major side effects, and theoretically gallstones may develop with prolonged usage. A number of somatostatin analogues have been developed for clinical use, including some long-acting analogues. However, at the present time, the medications are available only in the injectable form. The lack of oral drugs makes somatostatin an impractical medication for diarrheal diseases, except in the most severely affected patients who are unresponsive to other medications. The dosage of the long-acting analogue, SMS 201–995 (Sandoz Laboratory, East Hanover, NJ) is 100 µg subcutaneously twice a day.

SPECIAL CONSIDERATIONS

Pancreatic Cholera Syndrome

Pancreatic cholera syndrome is also known as watery diarrhea, hypokalemia, achlorhydria syndrome (WDHA), VIPoma, or Verner Morrison syndrome. The large volume of watery diarrhea results from intestinal secretion secondary to the high circulating levels of vasoactive intestinal polypeptide (VIP) or other endogenous secretagogues which may be secreted along with the VIP. The tumor usually originates in the pancreas, but it can also arise from the stomach or upper duodenum. Bronchogenic carcinoma, ganglioneuroma, or ganglioneuroblastoma can also secrete VIP and cause this syndrome.

Despite the fact that about one-third of these patients have metastases at the time of diagnosis, total excision of the tumor should be the objective if it proves feasible. When complete resection is not possible, the surgeon may decide to excise some tumor mass to reduce the source of endogenous secretagogues. Hepatic artery embolization has also been attempted. Chemotherapy with streptozocin or 5-fluorouracil is effective in some patients. When resection is not possible, a therapeutic trial of antidiarrheal agents should be carried out. Normally, patients with advanced disease will not respond adequately to a single drug. When Imodium at a high dose (16 mg twice a day) is not effective, I recommend the addition of clonidine and verapamil. Verapamil is given in a dosage of 80 mg three times a day, while clonidine is gradually titrated upward as tolerated, starting with 0.1 mg per day. If these drugs in combination do not control diarrhea, or the patient is unable to tolerate the side effects of the medication, a trial of other drugs—such as lithium carbonate (300 mg twice a day) or trifluoperazine (gradually increasing dose to 30 mg per day) or indomethacin (25 to 50 mg three times a day)—is indicated. Finally, if all the oral medications fail, one may try the long-acting somatostatin analogue, which has to be administered as subcutaneous injections. Combination of two partially effective medications may result in better control than the use of either drug alone. It has been suggested that overhydrating such patients can lead to increased diarrhea and thus cause a vicious circle of increased replacement and increased diarrhea.

Malignant Carcinoid Syndrome

Diarrhea in this syndrome results from excessive

secretion of serotonin and other peptides or neurotransmitters which are secreted along with it. Surgery should be considered, but in most patients this is not feasible because of the advanced, although slow growing, metastases. For medical therapy, the same guidelines as those outlined for pancreatic cholera syndrome apply to carcinoid syndrome. Most patients show some response to opiates or other medications. In addition, serotonin antagonists, such as methylsergide, cyproheptadine, or ketanserin, a selective $5HT_2$-antagonist (Janssen Pharmaceuticals, New Brunswick, NJ), are useful. Chemotherapy with 5-fluorouracil, streptozocin, and adriamycin may result in some objective responses, but in general, the side effects make me hesitate to recommend them. I am all the more hesitant because the symptoms of most patients can be well controlled with an opiate or with other antidiarrheal drugs and a serotonin antagonist.

Zollinger-Ellison Syndrome and Medullary Carcinoma of the Thyroid

Diarrhea in Zollinger-Ellison syndrome results from the excessive delivery of acidic gastric fluid to the small bowel as a result of a gastrin-secreting tumor. Should resection of the tumor not be feasible, an H_2 blocker, such as cimetidine or ranitidine, usually is quite effective in controlling the diarrhea. Should the H_2 blocker prove inadequate, other medications can be added as outlined for pancreatic cholera syndrome. Medullary carcinoma of the thyroid leads to excessive release of calcitonin, a hormone that causes intestinal secretion. Again, resection of the tumor is the primary treatment; should this be inadequate or unfeasible, the treatment is that outlined for pancreatic cholera syndrome. Debulking the tumor theoretically should lessen the amount of circulating secretagogue.

Other Chronic Secretory Diarrhea

Chronic idiopathic secretory diarrhea may be diagnosed in patients with chronic secretory diarrhea in whom a tumor cannot be found and laxative abuse is not suspected. The treatment follows the same guidelines as for pancreatic cholera syndrome, except that surgery is discouraged. Many patients in this group already have undergone a laparotomy. Repeat investigations generally are not very productive and probably should be delayed for 6 months to 1 year. Under these circumstances, it is more appropriate to treat the patient symptomatically. In a number of these patients, persistent diarrhea may improve several months or years later; alternatively, a malignant tumor may be found.

Surreptitious laxative ingestion is the most common cause of chronic diarrhea, according to the experience of some major medical centers. It occurs almost exclusively in females. The diagnosis of laxative abuse can be established either by the detection of laxative contents in the stool, or by the discovery of laxatives in a room search. Once the diagnosis is made, an honest discussion with the patient is in order. Every effort should be made to be considerate and gentle with the patient, as well as with the family, and to obtain psychiatric help for the patient. Unfortunately, one can expect a number of patients to deny their laxative abuse persistently and to discharge themselves from the hospital.

Finally, tumors of the distal colon may cause secretory diarrhea. This is especially true for secreting villous adenoma, but carcinoma may also give the same clinical picture. The therapy of choice is, of course, surgical resection.

CONSTIPATION

ALASTAIR M. CONNELL, M.D.
ALVIN M. ZFASS, M.D.

To be normal is to be "regular." While gastroenterologists have traditionally minimized the need for "a stool a day," epidemologic studies have suggested reasonably convincing benefit associated with a large daily stool! But what is a "normal" stool, and precisely what is the definition of "normal bowel habits?" What is meant by constipation?

Constipation can be defined according to frequency of the stool and/or consistency of the stool. Most surveys show that "a stool a day" is most commonly experienced in healthy populations, but the frequency varies. For example, in the United States, approximately 5 percent of healthy subjects report two or fewer stools per week; others consider three stools per day as "regular" or healthy.[1]

As noted, constipation is also a term used to describe the consistency of stool. A hard or desiccated stool contains little water, usually 50 percent. Normal stools contain 70 percent water, and "liquid" stools contain more than 95 percent water.

In summary, terminology is confusing. Hard, infrequent stools that are associated with straining represent a consensus example of constipation. However, there are unusual examples where definitions fail. Consider the soft effortless stool that happens every 4 days or the pellet-like stool that is passed only with considerable straining! A working definition of constipation is often best provided by the patient: any change in defecation, due to a decrease in frequency and/or an increase in the consistency, may be considered "constipation."

PHYSIOLOGY

Constipation usually represents a disordered function of the colon or of the anorectal region. For example, transit through the upper gut in patients with constipation has been shown to be only slightly prolonged, and this is of no clinical significance.[2]

The precise abnormalities in colonic function that result in constipation have not been satisfactorily identified. Three major normal functions of the colon have been identified: (1) the extraction (conservation) of water, which is a function of the colonic epithelial cell, (2) the maintenance of an abundant intraluminal bacterial population, and (3) the capacity to control the delivery of feces (colonic motility and the act of defecation). The constipated patient has been poorly studied, and it is not possible in any given case to assess which of the aforementioned functions is abnormal.

Careful observation of colonic contraction and flow of intraluminal colonic contents suggests that the colon is broken into three distinct functional segments. In the proximal part of the colon, there is little regular propulsive movement, and the colonic content tends to remain in the cecum for long periods. This type of motility results in a longer contact time of intraluminal contents and increased water absorption.

In the transverse and descending colon, the major muscular activity is segmenting contracting caused by contraction of the circular muscle. This results in a to-and-fro movement of the content with a gradual forward progression toward the sigmoid and rectum.

Occasional strong contractions occurring in the colon move the fecal mass caudad. These movements occur infrequently, but the fecal mass, when moved, is transported over long segments. One such contraction occurring approximately once daily results in defecation.[3]

Although the process of defecation is incompletely understood, it is generally accepted that distention of the sigmoid or rectum by stool entering it stimulates pressure receptors. This stimulus causes forward movement of a bolus of stool and a reflex relaxation of the internal anal sphincter accompanied by the "urge" to defecate. Continence is ensured by a variety of mechanisms, including a reverse gradient of contraction in the sigmoid and the existence of the internal anal sphincter. The external anal sphincter also maintains continence. This striated muscle sphincter is under voluntary control and provides the appropriate "emergency" squeeze when necessary. When the rectum is suddenly distended, the internal anal sphincter relaxes involuntarily and defecation is imminent. The area of mucosa proximal to the anal margin acts on a sensory zone and can discriminate between water or solid. It is response to the sensory discrimination that provides input for voluntary consent to defecation.

The rectal vault is also important in maintaining continence since it may act as a reservoir. Its ability to do so is related to rectal compliance and the ability of the rectum to allow an increase in volume without a concomitant increase in pressure. Although not adequately studied, this "receptive relaxation" may be similar to that observed in the gastric fundus.

CONTROL MECHANISMS

Control of the movement of colonic contents is poorly understood. A brief overview of the important factors follows.

Myogenic Factors

Myogenic factors include electrical activity of smooth muscle cells (periodic depolarization and repolarization) of the colon. This activity is irregular, but conforms to the basic "slow waves" and "spike bursts" described in the stomach and small intestine. A relationship between slow waves, contractions, and movement of intraluminal contents has been suggested in man. Slow wave frequencies occur over a range of 2 to 12 cycles per minute and frequently occur irregularly. Slower frequencies have been described in constipation, but the data are not convincing. It is probable that myogenic control mechanisms play a more important role in the proximal colon than in the distal colon. Exercise has an important role in preventing constipation and has an effect on colon motility, but the exact mechanism is not clear.

Neuro-endocrine Factors

The motor nerves to colonic muscle can be broadly classifed as (1) excitatory nerves, which are both cholinergic and noncholinergic, and (2) inhibitory nerves, which are adrenergic and nonadrenergic. Lesions of the spinal cord, especially destruction of the lumbosacral cord, cause severe and sometimes intractable constipation. Recently, the classic model of the autonomic nervous system with only cholinergic or adrenergic neurotransmitters has been greatly expanded, and noncholinergic and nonadrenergic regulatory peptides have been identified not only in the gut, but in the brain and other tissues. These peptides are released from specialized endocrine cells in the gut or from autonomic nerves. In the human colon, enteroglucagon, gastric inhibitory polypeptide, and neurotensin are confined to the specialized endocrine epithelial cells. Vasoactive intestinal polypeptide (VIP), substance-P, and bombesin-like peptides have been demonstrated exclusively in nerves. VIP is likely to be the most important "relaxant" or inhibiting neurotransmitter in the gut.

The gastrocolic responses, which result in increased motor activity during or following eating certain foods and may contribute toward bowel regularity, are mediated in part by gastrointestinal hormones. It is important, but may prove difficult, to identify the specific roles of these peptides in constipation. In Hirschprung's disease (aganglionosis), however, there is a depletion of VIP- and substance-P-containing nerves in the myenteric plexus. The absence of the inhibitory neurotransmitters is related to the segment of contracted bowel, and this area of contraction, which does not relax, leads to the development of megacolon.[4] Recent studies have demonstrated abnormalities in the myenteric plexus in idiopathic pseudo-obstruction.[5] In another study, women with severe intractable constipation were also found to have abnormalities of the myenteric plexus.[6]

Water Absorption

Mucosal absorption of water by the colon determines the consistency of stool at the time of defecation. Mucosal surface area, mixing, contact time, and intraluminal pressure are important factors. An increased "avidity" for water absorption has not been demonstrated in constipation, although carefully designed studies have not been reported.

Transit-Pressure Alterations

In constipated subjects, transit (radiopaque markers, barium, telemetering devices) through the colon is delayed. The usual pattern of prolonged transit is a uniform delay in passage throughout the entire colon so that intraluminal contents remain in each segment of the colon for longer than normal periods of time. In some patients, especially the young and elderly, delay occurs in the rectal segment. Persistent fullness of the rectum is abnormal and used to be known as dyschezia. Addition of fiber to the diet decreases transit time by as much as 50 percent, but the precise factors that promote this acceleration have not been elucidated. Gastrointestinal hormones may be implicated.

Pressure studies using small balloons as sensors or open-tipped catheters have demonstrated higher than normal resting pressure in the left colon (10 to 30 cm from the anal verge) in some constipated patients. Although exaggerated colonic response (increased pressure) after food or other stimuli has been reported, it has not been noted consistently. In general, the overall motility responses of groups of constipated subjects are not significantly different from those of subjects with normal elimination.

CLINICAL CONSIDERATIONS

Constipation with No Structural Abnormalities Identifed

Deficient bulk. This deficiency is probably the most common cause of constipation in western countries. Dietary changes designed to increase fecal bulk and fecal water are helpful. Wheat bran, oatmeal, certain fruits, and root vegetables such as carrots are beneficial.

Poor Defecation Habits. During the rush of daily life, the suppressed urge to defecate or disagreeable toilet facilities result in continued filling of the rectal ampulla or vault. The need to defecate is suppressed and normal anorectal sensation diminishes. The stool becomes desiccated while remaining in the rectum. This hardened stool makes subsequent defecation difficult and uncomfortable. Management consists of behavioral modification by the patient. Use of simple glycerin suppositories help to restore rectal sensation, lubricate the stool, and facilitate emptying of the rectum. Rarely, operant conditioning (biofeedback) with rectal training programs are needed to restore normal rectal reflexes.

Irritable Colon Syndrome with Constipation. Treatment in this disorder is for the underlying irritable bowel syndrome. An adequate explanation of the pathophysiology of constipation in conjunction with a high fiber diet is usually effective. Stool bulking agents such as psyllium seed can help. Occasionally, antispasmodics such as mebeverine or dicyclomine are useful.

Idiopathic (Slow Transit) Constipation of Women. In this interesting group of patients, transit time is strikingly prolonged, and as noted, the constipation is most common in women. Abdominal distention, pain, and laxative abuse are also commonly noted. Treatment is unsatisfactory and, specifically, dietary fiber supplementation may increase or aggravate the symptoms. Frustration with all forms of medical management may lead to consideration of colonic resection.

Constipation with Structural Disease of the Colon

Laxatives are rarely necessary for treatment of constipation and should always be used under supervision. Laxative abuse, especially with phenolphthalein, has become a major problem, particularly with elderly persons or young females.

Anal Pain. Any disease of the anus associated with pain may interfere with defecation. Common disorders include anal fissures or hemorrhoids. Medical management is effective and includes stool softeners, sitz baths, and application of local anesthetic ointments or suppositories. Anal dilation under general anesthesia may be required in some cases.

Aganglionosis. This disease is usually diagnosed in childhood, but may be recognized for the first time in adult life. Anal manometry and rectal biopsy establish the diagnosis with certainty. Surgery is indicated.

REFERENCES

1. Connell AM, Hilton C, Irvine G, Lennard-Jones JE, Misiewicz JJ. Variation of bowel habit in two population samples. Brit Med J 1965; 2:1095–1099.
2. Eastwood HDH. Bowel transit studies in the elderly:radio-opaque markers in the investigation of constipation. Gerontol Clin 1972; 14:154–159.
3. Christensen J. Motility of the colon. In: Johnson LR, ed. Physiology of the gastrointestinal tract. New York: Raven Press, 1981, Chapter 14, pp 445–471.
4. Tsuto T, Okamura H, Fukui K, Obata HL, Terubayashi H, Iwai N, Majima F, Yanaihara N, Ibata Y. Immunohistochemical investigation of vaso active intestinal polypeptide in the colon of patients with Hirschsprung's disease. Neurosc Letter 1982; 34:57–62.
5. Schuffler MD, Jonak Z. Chronic idiopathic pseudo-obstruction caused

by a degenerative disorder of the myenteric plexus: the use of Smith's method to define the neuropathology. Gastroenterology, 1982; 82:476–486.

6. Krishnamurthy S, Schuffler MD. Severe idiopathic constipation is caused by a distinctive abnormality of the colonic myenteric plexus. Gastroenterology 1983; 84:1218.

CHRONIC INTESTINAL PSEUDO-OBSTRUCTION

SINN ANURAS, M.D., F.A.C.P.

Chronic intestinal pseudo-obstruction is a syndrome in which the patients have recurrent symptoms and signs of intestinal obstruction without actual mechanical obstruction. It is caused by ineffective propulsion of intestinal contents because of disease of the smooth muscle or myenteric plexus. Table 1 lists the diseases that can cause chronic intestinal pseudo-obstruction. Although chronic intestinal pseudo-obstruction implies difficulty only in the small intestine, patients usually have difficulty in other parts of the digestive tract as well. Atonic dilated esophagus, gastroparesis, and/or megacolon may be seen in these patients, depending on the underlying disease. It is interesting that lesions caused by a given disease are usually similar and tend to differ from those of other diseases. It is beyond the scope of this chapter to discuss the typical lesions seen in the various diseases listed in Table 1, and readers are referred to several recent reviews on this topic. In practice, I first determine the extent of small bowel involvement, then identify the abnormalities of other parts of the digestive tract. Diseases that can cause intestinal pseudo-obstruction are then sought with such tests as antinuclear antibody, fasting blood sugar, creatine phosphokinase and isoenzymes, triiodothyronine and thyroxine and so on. The treatment plans are based on these findings.

SHORT SEGMENTAL SMALL BOWEL DYSFUNCTION

The patients who have short segmental involvement of the small bowel have a better prognosis, because the dysfunctional segment can be resected or bypassed.

In the most common type of familial visceral myopathy, the patients have megaduodenum that causes intestinal obstructive symptoms. Side-to-side duodenojejunostomy with resection of the anterior wall of the duodenum usually gives symptomatic relief. Patients must take a clear liquid diet and antibiotics, such as tetracycline or neomycin, for a few days before the operation to sterilize the megaduodenum because there are large amounts of retained food and bacteria in the dilated duodenum. Subtotal colectomy and ileoproctostomy have also been performed with good result in patients with this type of familial visceral myopathy who have severe obstipation from a redundant colon. Colectomy must not be performed in patients who have dysfunction of the entire small bowel, because excessive ileal output of up to 8 L per day has been observed.

If the dysfunctional segment is distal to the ligament of Treitz, a resection can be performed. A patient who had multiple diverticula of the first 18 inches of the jejunum has been asymptomatic for over 4 years since the resection of the first 2 feet of the jejunum.

TABLE 1   Causes of Chronic Intestinal Pseudo-obstruction

Primary Chronic Intestinal Pseudo-obstruction
   Familial types
      Familial visceral myopathies
      Familial visceral neuropathies

   Nonfamilial types
      Visceral myopathies
      Visceral neuropathies
      Undetermined causes (normal pathologic examination)

Secondary Chronic Intestinal Pseudo-obstruction
   Diseases involving the intestinal smooth muscle
      Collagen vascular disease: scleroderma, dermatomyositis, systemic lupus erythematosus
      Muscular dystrophies: myotonic dystrophy, Duchenne's muscular dystrophy
      Amyloidosis

   Neurologic diseases
      Parkinson's disease
      Hirschsprung's disease
      Chagas' disease
      Ganglioneuroma of intestine

   Endocrine disorders
      Myxedema
      Diabetes mellitus
      Hypoparathyroidism
      Pheochromocytoma

   Pharmacologic causes
      Phenothiazines
      Tricyclic antidepressants
      Antiparkinsonian medications
      Ganglionic blockers
      Clonidine
      Narcotic analgesics
      Amanita (mushroom) poisoning

   Miscellaneous
      Nontropical sprue
      Jejunoileal bypass
      Jejunal diverticulosis
      Porphyria
      Eosinophilic gastroenteritis
      Radiation enteritis
      Paraneoplastic syndrome

LONG SEGMENTAL SMALL BOWEL DYSFUNCTION

This group of patients has a poor prognosis, because palliative surgery cannot be performed. In addition to long segmental small bowel involvement (usually the entire small bowel), the patients frequently have an atonic dilated esophagus, gastroparesis, and megacolon. In this group of patients resection of any part of the bowel is contraindicated, because the patients may have more difficulty from adhesions or other complications. I have seen two patients on referral who had dysfunction of the entire digestive tract and who had undergone colectomy and ileostomy for severe constipation. Postoperatively, both had ileal output of 3 to 8 L per 24 hours and it was difficult to keep up with fluid loss because they could not take large amounts of fluid by mouth. Therefore, the colon must not be removed if the small bowel function is not known. Two studies, small bowel x-ray films and small intestinal manometry, can be used to detect severe small bowel motility disturbances. The small bowel x-ray films will show marked dilatation of the entire small bowel and markedly delayed transit of the barium. It may take more than 24 hours for the barium to reach the cecum. Small intestinal manometry is the most sensitive method to detect abnormal small bowel motility, and it should be performed in assessing the small bowel function if available.

Only nonsurgical treatment can be used in this group of patients. We will divide the discussion of the treatment into two parts: symptomatic and supportive treatments, and specific treatments.

Symptomatic and Supportive Treatments

I will discuss the treatment of intestinal obstructive symptoms (abdominal pain, abdominal distention, nausea and vomiting) together. Obstructive symptoms in most patients occur intermittently; however, in a few patients (approximately 10%), these problems may be persistent. The obstructive symptoms are directly related to eating. Therefore, by manipulating the amount, the nature, and the frequency of meals, patients with intermittent symptoms can reduce their symptoms. The important point is to give the patients enough calories without overloading the inefficient bowel. A rule of thumb is to give approximately 25 calories per kilogram of ideal body weight per day. Adults should consume 1,500 to 1,800 calories per day divided into three or four equal feedings. At least half of the calories should come from total feeding formulas such as Ensure, Isocal, Vivonex, and so on, because liquid empties faster from the stomach than a solid meal and probably progresses more easily through the small bowel. These formulas are lactose free and contain enough daily requirements of vitamins and minerals. I prefer Vivonex because it is very low in fat content and does not require any digestion. Therefore, it is readily absorbable in the small bowel and it may be more suitable for patients who also have gastroparesis. Milk should not be used because it contains lactose and it forms a tough curd in the stomach. A dietitian should educate the patients about the caloric content in each type of food. The patients should try various types of the feeding formulas to find a few that are palatable to them. They must avoid carbonated beverages to prevent adding excessive gas to the digestive tract, and they should be encouraged to drink fruit juice instead. When patients still feel full several hours after the first meal and have no appetite, it is important that they not force themselves to eat subsequent meals, because symptoms will increase if they do. Some fluid may suffice for that day. Occasionally, nasogastric suction and intravenous fluids are needed when the patients have severe obstructive symptoms. When the obstructive symptoms and pain persist or occur several times a week despite dietary manipulation, long-term parenteral hyperalimentation is the only treatment that will improve the patients' symptoms and nutrition.

Abdominal pain unrelated to an obstructive episode is uncommon in patients with chronic intestinal pseudo-obstruction. During episodes of obstruction, patients may require parenteral injection of narcotics such as morphine or meperidine. Long-term narcotic use must be discouraged because the patients will become addicted to them and narcotics may further disturb gastrointestinal motility.

Constipation is common in patients who also have colon involvement. It is important to make certain that the patients have a good bowel movement at least once every few days, because constipation tends to increase symptoms of intestinal obstruction. I use 1 to 2 oz of milk of magnesia a day, and tap water enemas if the patients have no bowel movement for 3 days. Bulk forming laxatives should be avoided because they just add more load to an inefficient organ.

Diarrhea is usually due to bacterial overgrowth and malabsorption. I try several kinds of antibiotics, such as tetracycline, ampicillin, Bactrim, and Metronidazole, until I find the one that works best, and I treat patients on a long-term basis in cycles of 1 week on and 1 week off.

Specific Treatment

A few types of secondary chronic intestinal pseudo-obstruction, such as myxedema and drug-induced ileus can be treated with thyroid replacement and discontinuation of the offending drugs, respectively. These situations are uncommon. In most cases there is no specific treatment.

Several gastrointestinal motility stimulants, e.g., bethanechol and neostigmine, have been tried, and the results are disappointing. Metoclopramide does not help in most cases. I have, however, observed a dramatic symptomatic improvement in one patient who had active small intestinal motility demonstrated by intestinal manometry for the past 4 years. It is encouraging that a small subset of patients with chronic intestinal pseudo-obstruction may respond to this drug. A serious side effect of metoclopramide, in my experience, is severe depression. I observed severe depression in three patients who took

30 mg of metoclopramide per day for over a month for abdominal bloating. Two patients committed suicide. Metoclopramide must be discontinued immediately when the patient complains of depression.

URINARY PROBLEMS

Megacystis may occur in patients with chronic intestinal pseudo-obstruction. The majority of patients with megacystis have no symptoms, while dysuria may be the complaint in some male patients. Asymptomatic microscopic hematuria is commonly seen, but cystitis is uncommon. Urine culture should be obtained in patients with cystitis, and then the appropriate antibiotic(s) is given.

Dysuria improves in some patients with bethanechol, 10 mg three times a day. In other patients, subtotal cystectomy (80%) and Y-V plasty of the bladder neck may improve symptoms.

ACUTE INFECTIOUS DIARRHEA

GAIL L. BONGIOVANNI, M.D.
RALPH A. GIANNELLA, M.D.

Acute infectious diarrhea is an extremely common clinical problem throughout the world. In the developing world, acute infectious diarrhea is a major cause of mortality, particularly in children; in fact, it is the leading cause of death in children under the age of 5. Although it is an unusual cause of mortality in the United States, acute infectious diarrhea is a major cause of morbidity, being second only to the common cold.

The causes of acute infectious diarrhea are varied and include bacterial, viral, and parasitic organisms. Evaluation and treatment should be directed toward identifying the specific causative agent and providing supportive care as well as toward providing specific treatment when warranted.

DIAGNOSTIC GUIDELINES

Infectious diarrhea is usually abrupt in onset and may be associated with systemic signs and symptoms. Invasive microorganisms injure the intestinal mucosa, are associated with an inflammatory process (fecal leukocytes), and may produce bloody diarrhea or dysentry. Invasive enteropathogens include *Shigella, Salmonella, Campylobacter jejuni,* and *Yersinia enterocolitica.* Other bacteria elaborate tissue-destroying cytotoxins, which can result in an inflammatory process, fecal leukocytes, and bloody diarrhea. These include *Clostridium difficile,* and enteropathogenic *Escherichia coli.* Bacteria that cause diarrhea by production of an enterotoxin, on the other hand, generally result in a watery, nonbloody diarrhea unassociated with intestinal inflammation (no fecal leukocytes). Enterotoxin-producing bacteria include *Vibrio cholerae, V. parahemolyticus,* and other *Vibrio, E. coli* and other coliforms, *Staphylococcus aureus, C. perfringens,* and *Bacillus cereus.* Thus, fever and copious fecal leukocytes associated with diarrheal symptoms usually suggest an invasive or cytotoxin-producing organism.

Viral agents, Norwalk-like viruses in adults and rotaviruses in children, generally cause a watery diarrhea associated with fever but without fecal leukocytes. The illness generally is mild and self-limited, requiring only supportive therapy.

Acute diarrhea may result from the ingestion of contaminated food or water and give rise to a "food-poisoning" syndrome. Table 1 reviews the relevant features of acute bacterial food posioning.

A specific evaluation of the patient presenting with acute diarrhea is best made based on the individual clinical setting. Certain general recommendations, however, can be made. First, if diarrhea is massive or prolonged, patients should be evaluated for dehydration and electrolyte and acid-base alterations. Second, patients should submit stool samples for examination and culture. The finding of fecal leukocytes on Wright's stain suggests an invasive or cytotoxin-producing pathogen. Stools should be cultured for *Shigella, Salmonella, C. jejuni,* and *Y. enterocolitica.* In patients who have recently taken antibiotics, stools should also be cultured for *C. difficile* and the stool sent for detection of *C. difficile* toxin. Examination for parasites should especially be done in patients with recent travel history or homosexual practices. Third, except in cases of acute bloody diarrhea, proctosigmoidoscopy is unnecessary if symptoms subside within a week. Sigmoidoscopy should not be done if there is colonic dilatation on plain abdominal roentgenogram. Toxic megacolon may be precipitated. Finally, radiologic studies are not required in most cases of acute infectious diarrhea. They should not be performed during the acute phase of the illness. All stool samples for culture and examination should be obtained prior to radiologic investigation.

THERAPY

The goals of therapy include (1) prevention of dehydration, (2) rehydration if necessary, (3) relief of symptoms, and (4) shortening the course of the illness if possible, i.e., with antimicrobial agents.

Most cases of acute infectious diarrheal disorders are brief, self-limited, and spontaneously resolve in a few days. Thus, most episodes are improving by the time a

TABLE 1 Acute Bacterial Food Poisoning

Organism	Contaminated Sources	Incubation Period (hr)	Features	Duration	Treatment
Staphylococcus aureus	Mayonnaise, milk, and milk products	1-6	Preformed enterotoxin Prominent vomiting	10 hr	Fluids, no antibiotics
Clostridium perfringens	Meats, poultry and poultry products, legumes	6-12	Enterotoxin made by proliferating C. perfringens in intestine Small, cluster outbreaks Crampy abdominal pain common	24 hr	Fluids, no antibiotics
Bacillus cereus (Type I)	Improperly cooked rice	2	(Like S. aureus) Preformed enterotoxin Prominent vomiting	9 hr	Fluids, no antibiotics
Bacillus cereus (Type II)	Improperly cooked rice	6-14	Toxin produced in host Prominent abdominal cramps	20 hr	Fluids, no antibiotics
Vibrio parahemolyticus	Improperly prepared fish Utensils used with contaminated food source	6-48	Enterotoxin is produced (relationship to symptoms unclear)	24-48 hr	Fluids, no antibiotics
Salmonella species	Virtually all foods, dairy products, small animals, especially chickens	8-48	Headache, fever Occasional chills Sudden onset watery diarrhea Abdominal cramps	2-5 days	Fluids, no antibiotics

Modified from: Bacterial infections of the gastrointestinal tract. In: Bongiovanni GL (ed). Manual of clinical gastroenterology. New York: McGraw Hill, 1983: p 364.

physician is consulted or by the time a specific diagnosis is made. As a consequence, in most patients specific therapy, i.e., antimicrobial agents, is neither possible nor necessary. The indiscriminate use of antibiotics in treatment of acute infectious diarrheal disorders is not warranted and is to be condemned.

Dietary Modification

Since most episodes of acute infectious diarrhea are brief, major modifications of diet are seldom necessary. Formerly it was customary to stop all dietary intake during acute diarrheal disease. This practice is no longer physiologically tenable and should not be recommended. Avoidance of all oral intake is especially detrimental in infants, and even a few days of avoidance of nutrition can result in long-lasting intestinal malfunction and resumption of diarrhea on refeeding. With severe vomiting, however, all oral intake may have to be briefly curtailed.

If diarrhea is severe or persists beyond 24 hours, fat and lactose-containing products should be avoided. This recommendation is made because lactase deficiency and lactose intolerance may be unmasked or induced anew by the infection. This is especially true in infants and children. Continued ingestion of lactose-containing food can thus worsen the symptoms and prolong the illness. If such dietary curtailment is necessary, adequate oral hydration and nutrition should be maintained. In some patients, especially infants and children, prolonged lactose intolerance can result from acute infectious diarrhea and persist for many weeks. In this circumstance, ingestion of lactose-containing foods may provoke abdominal cramps and diarrhea.

Fluid Therapy

Avoidance of dehydration and maintenance of hydration should be the major goals of treatment of patients with acute infectious diarrheal disorders. Only in the face of severe vomiting should the patient be advised to take nothing by mouth. Continuation of oral fluid and electrolyte intake should be encouraged and emphasized, and patients should be specifically instructed in the details of maintenance of hydration and replacement of fluid and electrolytes lost in diarrhea and vomitus.

Avoidance of dehydration and rehydration in most instances can be done orally by the ingestion of a variety of liquids. The ideal diarrheal replacement fluid for the adult is the World Health Organization Oral Rehydration Solution (WHO-ORS). This solution is ideally formulated to replace electrolytes lost in diarrheal fluid and to maximize the intestinal absorption of salt and water by the inclusion of sodium, bicarbonate, and glucose in appropriate proportions. Solutions containing an appropriate concentration of glucose markedly enhance the absorption of sodium and thus water. The WHO-ORS is not readily available in prepackaged form in the United States but can be easily made by most pharmacists. Two very similar formulations are available in prepackaged form and are available in most parts of the United States. These are Pedialyte-RS (Ross Laboratories, Columbus, OH) and Infalyte (Pennwalt Pharmaceutical, Rochester, NY). The composition of these three solutions is shown in Table 2.

Patients with mild dehydration may be rehydrated by oral ingestion of one of these solutions. The solutions are well tolerated and can, if necessary, be easily ingested by most adults at the rate of as much as 8 oz per hour.

TABLE 2 Composition of Oral Rehydration Solutions

	Infalyte	Pedialyte-RS	WHO-ORS
Na$^+$ (mEq/L)	50	75	90
K$^+$ (mEq/L)	20	20	20
Cl$^-$ (mEq/L)	40	65	80
HCO$_3^-$ (mEq/L)	30	·/·/·	30
Citrate (mEq/L)	·/·/·	30	·/·/·
Glucose (mmol/L)	111	139	111

These solutions are also surprisingly well tolerated in patients who have nausea and occasional vomiting. Patients with severe dehydration are best hospitalized and rehydrated with intravenous fluids. The absolute rate of fluid administration is best monitored by the degree of dehydration and by an estimate of the continuing losses in diarrheal fluid and in vomitus. The adequacy of rehydration can usually be easily monitored by clinical signs such as skin turgor, axillary sweat, and urine output.

Should these ideal oral treatment solutions not be available, a variety of home beverages and other solutions are superior to tap water. These include carbonated beverages, apple juice, clear soups, Karo Syrup with water, or Gatorade. These solutions, however, are markedly hypotonic, poor in electrolytes, and do not replace ongoing stool losses. Although Gatorade is ideal for replacing water and electrolytes lost in sweat, it is not formulated as a replacement for water and electrolytes lost in the proportions seen in diarrheal fluid.

Should intravenous fluid therapy be required, the composition of such fluids should approximate the composition of diarrheal fluid. Isotonic saline alone is inadequate, since it replaces neither potassium nor base (bicarbonate) lost in fecal output. Solutions of the following composition are recommended: sodium, 120 to 130 mEq per liter; potassium, 20 to 40 mEq per liter; chloride, 80 to 95 mEq per liter; and bicarbonate, 40 to 50 mEq per liter. This composition can be achieved by using half normal saline to which 30 to 40 mEq of potassium and a 50-ml ampule of 7.5 percent sodium bicarbonate (45 mEq Na$^+$ and 45 mEq HCO$_3$) have been added.

Symptomatic Therapy (Antidiarrheal Agents)

In general, most cases of acute infectious diarrhea do not *require* symptomatic therapy, which is designed to lessen the frequency of or change the character of the bowel movements. However, such therapy is *appropriate* depending upon the duration and severity of the diarrhea and the presence of associated symptoms. In general, we agree with the recommendations of DuPont and associates that symptomatic therapy should be given depending upon the severity of the process. For example, if there are merely one to three loose bowel movements per day without other associated symptoms, either no antidiarrheal therapy need be given or the adsorbent, bulk-forming agents may be used. If the patient is experiencing three to five bowel movements per day with some associated symptoms, the antimotility synthetic opiate alkaloid, loperamide (Imodium) can be given. If the diarrhea is severe, prolonged, or frankly bloody, symptomatic therapy should be given while a specific etiologic agent is sought so that specific antimicrobial therapy can be instituted.

In the usual case of only mild diarrhea, bulk-forming agents such as Kaolin-Pectin mixture generally suffice. Kapoectate can be administered in a dosage of 2 to 4 tablespoons every 4 hours or, if Kaopectate concentrate is used, 1 or 2 tablespoons every 4 hours. An alternative bulk-forming agent is calcium polycarbophil (Mitrolan), which can be administered as 2 tablets four times a day up to a maximum of 12 per day. These tablets should be thoroughly chewed before being swallowed. Bismuth subsalicylate (Pepto-Bismol) is also suitable. The adult dosage for the liquid is 2 to 4 tablespoons every 4 hours, or if the tablets are used 2 tablets every 4 hours. Since the salicylate in these formulations is absorbable, they should be administered with caution in patients already on salicylate therapy.

In the more severe cases of diarrhea, especially when associated with abdominal cramps, more potent antidiarrheal agents can be used. These include Lomotil, Imodium, paregoric, and tincture of opium. For most cases either Imodium or Lomotil is preferable. Lomotil should be administered in a dosage of up to 2 tablets every 4 hours and Imodium as 2 capsules initially and then 1 capsule every 4 hours until the diarrhea subsides.

It has been stated that use of agents that alter intestinal motility may be harmful in "invasive" bacterial diarrheal disorders and actually prolong and intensify the illness. Although this might occur, it is rare and should not prevent the use of such agents when the diarrhea is severe, prolonged, or associated with severe abdominal cramps.

Specific Antimicrobial Therapy

In general, antibiotics are not to be used in a routine case of acute diarrheal disease. This recommendation is made because in most cases the illness will be of short duration and will spontaneously abate. In this circumstance, antibiotics will not significantly abbreviate the duration of the illness or make the patient feel better sooner. In addition, inappropriate use of antibiotics may prolong the fecal excretion of the organisms and render such organisms antibiotic-resistant. Furthermore, many of the most common causes of acute diarrheal illness are not amenable to antibiotic therapy. These include food poisoning syndromes (*C. perfringens, S. aureus, B. cereus,* or *V. parahemolyticus*) and viral diarrheal disorders.

Antimicrobial therapy is indicated for certain acute diarrheal disorders of specific bacterial etiology or in certain circumstances in which the diarrhea is severe or prolonged, or the physician is concerned with the possibility of superimposed complications. These will be specifically enumerated below. In general, our specific recommendations are listed in Table 3 in which the various causes of acute infectious diarrhea are listed alpha-

TABLE 3 Specific Treatment of Acute Infectious Diarrheas

Pathogen	Primary Treatment	Alternative Treatment
Amebiasis	Metronidazole (Flagyl), 750 mg PO t.i.d. × 10 days *or* Diiodohydroxyquin (Yodoxin), 650 mg PO t.i.d. × 21 days	./././.
Campylobacter species	Erythromycin, 250 mg PO q.i.d. × 5 days	Tetracycline, 500 mg PO q.i.d. × 5 days *or* Clindamycin, 300 mg PO q.i.d. × 5 days
Clostridium difficile (antibiotic-associated colitis)		
Mild	Discontinue antibiotic if possible Cholestyramine (Questran), 1 packet (4 g) PO t.i.d. × 7 days	./././. ./././.
Severe or persistent	Vancomycin, 500 mg PO q.i.d. × 10 days *or* Metronidazole (Flagyl), 500 mg PO t.i.d. × 10 days	Bacitracin, 25,000 U PO q.i.d. × 10 days
Cryptosporidiosis	None available	
Food Poisoning *Staphylococcus* *Clostridia* *Bacillus cereus*	No antibiotics	Oral fluids and antidiarrheal drugs
Giardia	Metronidazole (Flagyl), 250 mg PO t.i.d. × 7 days *or* Quinacrine (Atabrine), 100 mg PO t.i.d. × 7 days	Furazolidone, 100 mg PO q.i.d. × 7 days
Salmonella*		
Acute gastroenteritis	Usually none	./././.
Bactermia/enteric fever	Chloramphenicol, 500 mg q6h IV × 10 days *or* Ampicillin, 1 g q4h IV × 10 days *or* Trimethoprim-sulfamethoxazole (Septra or Bactrim), 2 DS tablets q12h × 10 days	./././.
Shigella	Trimethoprim-sulfamethoxazole (Septra or Bactrim), 2 DS tablets q12h × 5 days	Ampicillin, 500 mg PO q.i.d. × 5 days *or* Tetracycline, 500 mg PO q.i.d. × 5 days
Unknown	No antibiotics	Oral fluids and antidiarrheal agents
Vibrio cholerae	Tetracycline, 500 mg PO q.i.d. × 2 days	Chloramphenicol, 500 mg PO q.i.d. × 2 days
Viral	No antibiotics	Oral fluids and antidiarrheal agents
Yersinia enterocolitica	Tetracycline, 250 mg PO q.i.d. × 7 days	Trimethoprim-sulfamethoxazole (Septra or Bactrim), 2 DS tablets q.i.d. × 7 days

* Does not include *S. typhi*.

betically, followed by both a primary treatment recommendation and an alternative treatment recommendation.

Campylobacter diarrhea is an extremely common disorder and is frequently associated with severe abdominal cramps and dysentery (bloody mucoid stools). As stated above, however, in most cases the diarrhea and other symptoms are already improving at the time of bacteriologic diagnosis. Should this not be the case, antibiotic therapy is recommended. In this case the agent of choice is erythromycin administered at a dosage of 250 mg orally four times a day for 5 days.

Most cases of *C. difficile* or antibiotic-associated colitis do not require specific antimicrobial therapy. If antibiotics can be discontinued this is frequently all that is required, especially if antibiotics are discontinued early in the course of the illness. Should this not be possible and the diarrhea is mild, therapy with cholestyramine (Questran) in the dosage given in Table 3 is recommended as initial therapy. If diarrhea is severe or persistent, then therapy with either vancomycin or metronidazole (Flagyl) should be instituted.

Nontyphoidal salmonellosis generally does not require antibiotic therapy. Fortunately, most cases of salmonellosis present as uncomplicated, self-limited gastroenteritis. In such cases, antibiotic therapy does not shorten the duration of the illness, but unfortunately does prolong the fecal excretion of the organisms and enhances the appearance of antibiotic resistant strains. Under certain circumstances, however, antibiotic therapy should be given. If diarrhea is severe or prolonged, if the patient is immunocompromised, if there is any suspicion of either bacteremia or enteric fever, or if the patient appears "toxic" with high fever, leukopenia, or striking leukocytosis, antibiotic therapy should be instituted promptly after fecal and blood cultures are taken.

In shigellosis, antibiotic therapy has been shown to diminish the length of the illness. Accordingly, antibiotic therapy should be administered. Trimethoprim-sulfamethoxazole is the treatment of choice.

Other illnesses that benefit from antibiotic therapy include diarrhea due to *V. cholerae* fortunately rarely seen in the United States, and disease due to *Y. enterocolitica*.

Several additional comments should be made. Since metronidazole is recommended for a variety of bacterial and nonbacterial causes of acute infectious diarrheal disease, its potential for causing an antibuse reaction should be appreciated. Patients treated with metrondiazole should therefore be advised not to consume alcohol.

Hospitalization

In general, most patients with acute infectious diarrhea can be treated at home and as outpatients. In certain circumstances, however, it is wise to hospitalize such patients initially or after 24 hours if the illness is not improving. Such patients include the immunocompromised host, those with intestinal disorders (short bowel syndrome, ileostomy, ulcerative colitis, or Crohn's disease), or elderly and debilitated patients. Should any of these patients appear to be dehydrated on initial presentation to the physician, they should be immediately hospitalized and procedures to rehydrate promptly instituted.

TRAVELER'S DIARRHEA

CHARLES E. McQUEEN, M.D.
EDGAR C. BOEDEKER, M.D.

Next year 16 million people will travel to developing countries, and the most common illness they will experience is traveler's diarrhea (TD). This is a syndrome caused by ingestion of defined bacterial pathogens, the majority of which can be identified in prospective studies, although such identification is not usually achieved or required to treat individual travelers safely and effectively. Inadequate waste disposal together with breaks in sanitation in the chain of food preparation are thought to be the major contributors to the incidence of TD. The illness occurs primarily in individuals traveling from areas where sanitation is good to developing countries where sanitation is poor, so the occurrence of TD is highly dependent on the destination of travel. High-risk areas in which attack rates approach 50 percent include the developing countries in Latin America, Africa, the Middle East, and Asia. In contrast, among travelers to Northern Europe, Canada, New Zealand, the United States (as well as Puerto Rico, Bahamas, and Virgin Islands), the incidence is 5 percent or less. This chapter discusses prevention and treatment of TD.

TD is a syndrome characterized by the abrupt onset of loose or watery bowel movements occurring at a frequency greater than twice normal. Most cases are mild to moderate (typically four to five bowel movements per 24 hours) and without high fever or frankly bloody stools, although associated symptoms include mild fever, abdominal cramps, nausea, bloating, rectal urgency, and malaise. Onset is usually 3 to 7 days after the traveler arrives in a developing country, and more than one episode may occur per trip, since different enteric pathogens may produce similar symptom complexes. Duration is less than 7 days (median, 3 to 4) in 90 percent of cases, and fewer than 2 percent of cases persist longer than 30 days. A retrospective study based on insurance claims of several hundred thousand Swiss travelers failed to implicate TD as either a primary cause of or contributing factor to death. Although not life-threatening, TD may cause significant disruption of schedules, decreased productivity, and general unpleasantness, particularly if toilet facilities are unavailable or not up to usual Western standards.

Although many questions remain to be answered, the usual causes of traveler's diarrhea are no longer a mystery. TD is caused by pathogenic microorganisms, usually bacteria, which are transmitted through fecal contamination of food or beverages. When the best available laboratory techniques are used, a pathogen can be identified in up to 80 percent of cases. Even in the remaining 20 percent of cases, the favorable response to antibiotics indicates that most of these undiagnosed cases are also caused by bacteria. Noninfectious factors such as fatigue, anxiety, drugs, and special foods are not well supported as causes of TD.

Enterotoxigenic *Escherichia coli* (ETEC) are the most frequent organisms causing TD in all countries surveyed. Despite the insensitive and technically difficult laboratory methods that are currently required for their identification, ETEC can be identified as the etiologic agent in at least 40 percent of cases of TD. Other bacteria that are consistently but less frequently isolated include *Salmonella, Shigella, Campylobacter, Vibrio parahemolyticus* and *Yersinia enterocolitica*. Potential pathogens that are sometimes isolated in populations with TD include *Aeromonas hydrophila* and *Plesiomonas shigelloides*. Although rotavirus can be found in stools of travelers, and serologic conversion to the Norwalk agent can occur during travel, viral agents do not appear to be frequent causes of the TD syndrome in adults. Parasites are infrequent causes of the syndrome of TD, but *Giardia lamblia* and *Entamoeba histolytica* are occasionally found. These agents should be considered primarily in the returning tourist with persistent diarrhea. Giardiasis may not become symptomatic until after the traveler returns home. Multiple pathogens can be identified in a significant percentage of travelers with diarrhea. This probably indicates the high degree of fecal contamination in the traveler's environment, rather than actual microbial synergy.

PREVENTION

Preventive measures fall into four major categories: (1) dietary discretion, (2) nonantimicrobial drugs, (3) prophylactic antimicrobials, and (4) vaccines (Table 1). Of these, the first is most highly recommended. Prophylaxis with available drugs, although of demonstrated efficacy, cannot be recommended with enthusiasm. Effective vaccines are not currently available.

Dietary Discretion

Avoidance of contaminated foods and beverages is prudent, inexpensive, and has the added advantage of preventing other food-borne illnesses. To practice dietary avoidance, travelers must know which foods and beverages are likely to be contaminated. The adage "If you cannot boil it, cook it, or peel it, forget it," provides generally sound advice. Untreated tap water, ice, improperly cooked or inadequately preserved foods, fresh vegetables, and salads should be considered unsafe. Foods that have been cooked, allowed to stand, and then have been partially reheated pose a special hazard which may be difficult for the traveler to recognize. Perhaps for this reason, people are more likely to get TD from food served by street vendors than in private homes.

Practicing dietary discretion is possible but difficult. Few studies have shown clear benefit from attempts at dietary avoidance, and perhaps this is because "mistakes" are often made by knowledgeable people who have limited choices, are hurried, or whose purpose for travel is to experience different cultures. One study revealed that 98 percent of informed travelers made at least one dietary "mistake" while vacationing.

Carbonated beverages, bottled beer and wine, and well-cooked foods served hot are usually safe. Noncarbonated bottled water cannot always be relied upon. If tap water must be used, it should first be disinfected. Methods for disinfecting water include boiling or treating with iodine or chlorine. These methods may be as important for the elimination of enteric viruses, including those such as hepatitis A which do not usually cause diarrhea, as for bacterial pathogens commonly associated with TD. The method involves adding 1 tablet of iodine (tetraglycine hydroperiodide) to 1 quart of clear water (7 ppm) or 2 tablets per quart if the water is cold or cloudy, indicating the presence of particulate matter. Similarly, chlorine tablets (calcium hypochlorite) can be added so that a level between 5 and 10 ppm is reached (as determined by a portable colorimetric test kit). Both iodine and chlorine are effective in killing most bacteria or viruses, but iodine appears to be more effective against *Giardia* or *Amoeba*. Recently, a water purification kit that permits a glassful of water at a time to seep through an iodine resin has become available in many sporting goods stores. Toxicity appears to be rare with these methods, but the chemicals do affect the taste of the water and they may be inconvenient. Water boiled 15 minutes is safe. If it is necessary to drink where the water may be unsafe and water purification systems are unavailable, drinking water obtained from the "hot" tap may provide a degree of protection if temperatures of 140° to 160° F are maintained, but this is clearly a less than optimal approach.

Nonantimicrobial Drugs

Bismuth subsalicylate (BSS) (as Pepto-Bismol liquid, 60 ml four times daily, or 2 300-mg tablets four times

TABLE 1 Prevention of Traveler's Diarrhea

Category	Agent	Recommendation		Comment
		NIH 85 Consensus	Ours	
Diet	Ice, tap water	Avoid	Avoid	"Boil it, cook it, peel it, or forget it"
	Vegetables, salads	Avoid	Avoid	
	Street vendor food	Avoid	Avoid	
	Carbonated beverages	Safe	Safe	Noncarbonated bottled water may not be safe
	Bottled beer and wine	Safe	Safe	
	Hot, well-cooked food	Safe	Safe	
	Iodine and chlorine water	·/·/·	Useful	
Nonantimicrobials	Bismuth subsalicylate, 60 ml liquid *or* 2-300 mg tablets q.i.d.	Not recommended	Qualified recommendation	Avoid in patients on aspirin, with renal failure, or if elderly
Antimicrobials	Trimethoprim, 200 mg daily	Not recommended	Not recommended	Prophylactic antibiotics *not recommended* because of possible extreme risk
	Trimethoprim, 160 mg/sulfamethoxazole, 800 mg daily	Not recommended	Not recommended	
	Doxycycline, 100 mg b.i.d. on day 1, then daily	Not recommended	Not recommended	If elected: duration not to exceed 2 weeks to begin on day of travel and continue 2 days after return
Vaccines	Not available for usual causative organisms	·/·/·	·/·/·	See text for recommendations re: hepatitis, cholera, and typhoid

daily) taken throughout the period of travel reduces the incidence of TD by 40 to 60 percent. Although we do not unqualifiedly recommend BSS for prophylaxis, it is probably the safest, most effective nonantimicrobial drug for prophylaxis and is available without prescription in liquid or tablet form. There are several potential drawbacks to BSS. It turns stools black, the liquid form is bulky for the traveler, and unfortunately, the minimal effective amount for prophylaxis is not known. Of more serious concern is potential salicylate intoxication, particularly in patients who are elderly, have renal failure, or are on other medications containing salicylates. Neurologic side effects from bismuth intoxication are a theoretical problem, but it seems unlikely that sufficient amounts of bismuth could be absorbed to reach neurotoxic levels. Because of these uncertain risks, and because effective treatment for TD (including BSS) can be made available, BSS was not recommended for prophylaxis at the 1985 National Institutes of Health (NIH) Consensus Development Conference on TD. We feel, however, that use of BSS, particularly in tablet form, can be an acceptable prophylactic measure to limit TD and that adverse reactions are unlikely to occur if care is taken not to administer this medicine concomitantly with other salicylates.

Antimotility agents, such as loperamide or diphenoxylate, should definitely not be given prophylactically, as these agents have been shown to increase the incidence of TD and may predispose to development of serious illness by inhibiting the normal protective action of peristalsis.

Other agents that should not be recommended because they are of unproven or minimal benefit include activated charcoal, kaolin, pectin, and lactobacillus preparations.

Antimicrobial Drugs

Several antimicrobial drugs have been shown to be effective in decreasing the incidence of TD, specifically the combination of trimethoprim-sulfamethoxazole (TMP/SMZ), trimethoprim (TMP) alone, or doxycycline. Despite the efficacy of these drugs, we *cannot* recommend them for prophylaxis, and in this we agree with the statement from the recent NIH Consensus Development Conference. The reasons for not recommending prophylactic antibiotics are as follows. On one hand, TD is usually a mild to moderate illness for which rapid, effective treatment can be made available in advance of travel. On the other hand, serious side effects from antibiotic therapy do occur (e.g., Stevens-Johnson syndrome, aplastic anemia, other idiosyncratic reactions, or antibiotic-induced colitis) and, however rare, reach a statistical likelihood when one considers the number of travelers that would be at risk if antibiotics were given routinely. It is difficult to justify the risk of a potentially fatal illness for prophylaxis of an illness that is seldom, if ever, fatal.

Some researchers have maintained that special classes of travelers could be identified for whom the risks of prophylaxis would be justified by the importance of their travel or by the possibility of occurrence of medical illnesses that would be worsened by dehydration. In general, however, we believe it is difficult to define categories of travelers for whom antibiotic prophylaxis is justified. The argument that special groups, such as businessmen on important trips, are more deserving of prophylaxis than the vacationer spending his own hard-earned money is hard to support. Similarly, the wisdom of prescribing prophylactic antibiotics to those with preexisting illness must be judged on a case by case basis. Nevertheless, since many travelers know of studies showing prophylactic efficacy of antibiotics, and may define themselves as deserving prophylaxis, they may demand such protection from their physicians or else plan to obtain antibiotics in the countries to which they travel. In these situations, it is important for the physician to discourage prophylactic antibiotic use by carefully informing the patient of the extreme, if uncommon, risks of antibiotic therapy. Other less severe side effects, such as tetracycline-associated photosensitivity in the case of doxycycline, which occur with more predictable frequency, should also be mentioned. We would also emphasize to the patient that in the event of illness, rapidly effective therapy is available and will be provided. If the patient elects prophylactic antibiotics, he should be advised that such use should not be continued for more than 2 weeks.

Our major concern with regard to use of prophylactic antibiotics is increased risk to the individual patient. The possibility that prophylactic antibiotics taken by travelers could significantly contribute to an increase in resistant organisms in the environment should also be considered, but may not be a major concern. This is not to deny that antibiotic resistance is definitely increasing among enteropathogens isolated in developing counries where the use of antibiotics is widespread and often unrestricted. Nevertheless, antibiotic use by travelers has probably not been a major selective pressure in this developing resistance, since it represents only a small proportion of antibiotic use in these countries. Moreover, it has been shown that the fecal flora of travelers quickly acquires the resistance pattern of the indigenous population of the developing countries, even though the travelers do not ingest antibiotics. Such emerging resistance is definitely a cause for concern, and may be expected to influence the effectiveness of antibiotics currently recommended for treatment.

Vaccines

Two vaccines against enteric pathogens are currently available, but neither is directed against organisms responsible for usual cases of TD.

The present *cholera* vaccine, a killed preparation, gives short-lived (less than 6 months) protection, and this protection may be less for travelers from nonendemic areas than for residents of endemic areas. Unless the traveler is going to a cholera-infected area, however, and will be subsequently entering a country where a certificate of cholera vaccination is required, he is unlikely to need this vaccine. A listing of cholera-infected areas as identified by the World Health Organization can be found in the biweekly "Summary of Health Information for International Travel" published by the Division of Quarantine, CDC, Atlanta, GA 30333 and available from the Superintendent of Documents #017-023-001736, United States Government Printing Office, Washington, DC 20402.

The current *typhoid* vaccine is a killed bacterial preparation administered intramuscularly which gives significant protection against *Salmonella typhosa*, but it is frequently associated with systemic and local side effects such as nausea, vomiting, and muscle soreness. An oral attenuated typhoid vaccine (strain Ty21a) has been tested with success in Egypt and Chile and may soon be available.

Prophylaxis against *hepatitis A* in the form of immune serum globulin is recommended for travelers outside the usual tourist routes in areas where sanitation is poor. Two ml IM is recommended for stays less than 3 months or 5 ml for longer visits. Vaccination against hepatitis B is not generally recommended for travelers except to protect against transmission by sexual contact in endemic areas of Africa and southeast Asia.

There is an intense effort to develop effective vaccines against other enteric infections. One promising approach involves use of the oral attenuated *Salmonella* strain Ty21a, which lacks the enzyme galactose-epimerase and has limited survival in the host intestine, as a carrier for antigens of other enteropathogens. Genetic material encoding for attachment factors or other immunogens present on the surface of pathogenic bacteria (such as *Shigella* or ETEC) can be inserted into this short-lived, self-destructive strain which can then express these antigens. While preliminary data on immunogenicity and protection look hopeful in the case of a Ty21a/*Shigella* vaccine candidate, it is unlikely that this or similar vaccines will be available for protection of travelers in the next 2 or 3 years.

A discussion of all currently available immunizations for travelers (including measles, meningitis, plague, polio, rabies, tetanus and diphtheria, and yellow fever) is beyond the scope of this chapter, but updated information can be found at intervals in publications such as the Medical Letter.

TREATMENT

Treatment of TD (Table 2) falls into three major categories: (1) maintaining adequate hydration and replacement of electrolytes, (2) symptomatic treatment, and (3) specific antimicrobial therapy.

Maintenance of Hydration

The only essential treatment of any diarrheal illness, including TD, is maintenance of adequate hydration. The tendency to stop oral fluids when diarrhea occurs is still distressingly common. Travelers should be advised that fluid replacement should be initiated at the onset of diarrhea and that it should at least exceed stool losses and be sufficient to ensure the usual flow of urine. Fortunately, severe dehydration does not usually occur in the course of TD in adults. Therefore, in this setting, any acceptable source of fluids with some readily available, palatable source of salt (such as saltine crackers) will suffice. Commercial products such as Gatorade, although hypotonic, are usually adequate for adults. Equally useful solutions can be formulated by adding a pinch of salt, a pinch of bicarbonate, and a tablespoon of sugar to each liter of water. The World Health Organization and several com-

TABLE 2 Treatment of Traveler's Diarrhea

Category	Agent	Recommendation		Comment
		NIH 85 Consensus	*Ours*	
Fluid and electrolyte replacement	Gatorade	Usually adequate	Usually adequate	Increase to maintain urine output
	Seven-up, Coca-Cola, etc.	Usually adequate	Usually adequate	
	Homemade solutions: Pinch of salt, pinch of bicarbonate, 1 tbsp sugar per liter water	Usually adequate	Usually adequate	Avoid caffeinated beverages and alcohol
	Oral rehydration solution	Best	Best	
Symptom relief	Diphenoxylate, 2 tablets q.i.d. then taper	Useful	Useful	Both agents are rapidly effective at relieving cramps and decreasing stools, but: Do not use more than 36 hrs; avoid with temperature over 101 °F or frankly bloody stools
	Loperamide, 2 tablets at onset, 1 after each stool (no more than 8 per 24 hr)	Useful	Useful	
	Bismuth subsalicylate, 30 cc every 30 min for 8 doses	Recommended	Recommended	Slower onset of action; turns stools black; watch for ASA toxicity
Antimicrobials	Trimethoprim, 200 mg b.i.d.	Recommended	Recommended	Provide travelers with a 3-day supply to begin after 2 to 3 loose stools
	Trimethoprim, 160 mg/sulfamethoxazole, 800 mg b.i.d.	Recommended	Recommended	
	Doxycycline, 100 mg b.i.d.	Alternative	Alternative	

ASA = acetylsalicylic acid

mercial companies produce packets of an oral rehydration salts (ORS) powder that can be easily mixed with water and used in cases with more severe purging. These packets can be purchased in the United States, but they are also widely available in developing countries. Initially, ORS solution should be given to replace cumulative estimated diarrheal losses volume for volume; later, during the maintenance phase of diarrheal illness, ORS intake should be alternated with equal volumes of water to replace continued losses in the stool. It is rare that the oral route does not provide adequate rehydration in cases of TD. Because they may aggravate dehydration, alcoholic beverages as well as coffee and other caffeinated beverages are best proscribed if other acceptable fluids are available.

Symptomatic Treatment

In mild to moderate cases of TD, treatment with synthetic opiates or BSS should provide adequate control of diarrhea and relief of symptoms.

The synthetic opiates, diphenoxylate plus atropine (Lomotil), initially 2 tablets four times a day, then tapered to a minimal maintenance dose; and loperamide (Imodium), 2 capsules followed by 1 capsule after each unformed stool, not to exceed 8 capsules in 24 hours, are rapidly effective at relieving cramps and decreasing frequency of stools. There has been considerable debate concerning the advisability of using these preparations for treatment of TD, since they may hinder the clearance of invasive pathogens. As stated in the preceding section, these agents should not be used for prophylaxis, and in the presence of fever (greater than 101 °F) or frankly bloody diarrhea indicating invasive pathogens, the antimotility agents should not be used for treatment. There is no evidence, however, that in the usual case of TD caused by ETEC or other noninvasive pathogens these agents worsen or prolong disease. Therefore, they can be recommended as reasonably safe and effective symptomatic therapy for uncomplicated TD, provided that their use is not continued beyond 36 hours. In choosing between the synthetic opiates, loperamide has the theoretical advantage of not crossing the blood-brain barrier and should therefore cause fewer central nervous system side effects. Neither loperamide nor diphenoxylate should be used in children under 2 years old.

As an alternative, for symptomatic relief in mild to moderate cases, BSS in liquid form (30 ml every 30 minutes for eight doses in adults) has also been shown to be effective (decreasing stools by 43% of nontreated levels). This is safe therapy but takes somewhat longer than the synthetic opiates (more than 4 hours, or not until the complete therapeutic dosage has been administered) to demonstrate its effect.

Antibiotic Therapy

For more severe cases, prompt antibiotic therapy is recommended. Although extensive laboratory studies have defined the causative agents of TD, it is impractical in the clinical setting to attempt to identify the causative organisms in uncomplicated cases of TD. Antimicrobial therapy should be given empirically, based on our current knowledge of antibiotic sensitivity of the responsible pathogens and on empirical field trials. Such antimicrobial therapy appears to be safe and effective.

Several studies have shown that TMP/SMZ or TMP alone decreases the duration of illness from 3 to 5 days to 1½ days. We recommend (as did the panel at the NIH Consensus Conference) that travelers at risk (without known contraindications) be provided with a supply of TMP (200 mg twice daily) or TMP/SMZ (160 mg/800 mg twice a day) sufficient to continue for a 3-day period. This treatment should be started after the third loose stool occurring in an 8-hour period. Nausea and vomiting without diarrhea are not indications for these drugs. Travelers should be cautioned to seek medical attention for severe or persistent illness, which could indicate resistant organisms. Unused drugs should be disposed of at the end of the trip.

Doxycycline (100 mg twice a day) also appears to be effective treatment for TD and would be a good choice for patients with known reactions to sulfonamides or TMP. Special cautions with regard to doxycycline include the likelihood of permanent staining of teeth, contraindicating its use in children; drug photosensitivity; fungal or bacterial overgrowth (e.g., *Candida vaginitis, Candida esophagitis,* pseudomembranous colitis); and idiosyncratic reactions.

Furazolidine has been suggested as an alternative treatment in areas of epidemic giardiasis, since it will cover most bacterial pathogens as well as the *Giardia* parasite, but it is not yet approved for use in the United States. We do not recommend furazolidone because of the unacceptable number of adverse reactions, such as an Antabuse effect, monoamine oxidase inhibitor effect, and G-6-PD unmasking. In one study involving 80 children this drug was stopped in 23 percent because of side effects.

CONCLUSION

Traveler's diarrhea is usually a mild to moderately severe illness for which rapidly effective therapy can be made available. Other than prudent dietary discretion, and possibly BSS, no other specific prophylactic measures should be routinely recommended. The patient should understand that there is almost always complete recovery even in the absence of therapy and that all prophylactic and therapeutic measures carry some risk.

For relief of symptoms in mild cases, diphenoxylate or loperamide has demonstrated efficacy in decreasing stools and relieving cramps. Bismuth subsalicylate (30 ml every 30 minutes for eight doses) also decreases stools but is less effective in that it is slower in onset.

For more severe illness, or if it is important to shorten the course of diarrhea, antimicrobials may be taken. After three loose stools in 8 hours with associated symptoms, a 3-day course of TMP/SMZ or TMP alone should be prescribed. Doxycycline may be used in those who cannot take TMP or SMZ. The risks of antibiotic or other therapy must be considered by the patient when instituting treatment for what almost always is a mild, self-limited disease.

If diarrhea is associated with fever greater than 101 °F or frankly bloody stools, or if it persists despite recommended antibiotic treatment, the traveler should seek medical attention. In all cases, strict attention should be given to maintaining adequate hydration.

The views expressed herein are those of the authors and not necessarily those of the United States Army or the Department of Defense.

PARASITIC DISEASES OF THE COLON

FRANCIS JOSEPH TEDESCO, M.D.

Intestinal parasitic infections in man are important worldwide health problems. With the expansion of international travel and changes in lifestyle, including sexual activities and the overcrowding in institutions, an increased recognition of parasites in the United States has occurred. This chapter deals with several important parasitic infections of the colon (Table 1), but recognizes the overlap between large bowel and small bowel parasites.

ENTAMOEBA HISTOLYTICA

Amebiasis is an acute and chronic disease caused by *Entamoeba histolytica*. Although multiple organs may be involved, the colon is the usual site of initial disease. Approximately 5 percent of the untraveled population of the United States is infected with *E. histolytica*. The increased occurrence of amebiasis associated with the homosexual population has recently become a major clinical dilemma.

In discussing the treatment of amebiasis, it is probably most reasonable to classify patients as asymptomatic cyst passers, those with mild to moderate intestinal disease, and those with severe intestinal disease. The treatment of amebic liver abscesses also will be described in this section.

Asymptomatic Entamoeba Histolytica Passers

This probably constitutes the largest group of individuals with amebiasis. The usual clinical setting varies from completely asymptomatic to a picture consistent with the irritable bowel syndrome, with intermittent diarrhea, constipation, and anorexia. Ameba cysts are discovered on stool examination for ova and parasites in these patients. In this clinical setting many clinicians would not treat at all. If treatment is to be undertaken, diiodohydroxyquin (iodoquinol), 650 mg three times a day for 20 days, is recommended in adults and 30 to 40 mg/kilogram of body weight per day in three doses for 20 days is recommended in children. Although side effects are not common, iodine reactions and occasionally optic atrophy and peripheral neuropathy have been reported after prolonged use. An alternative treatment could be diloxanide furoate (Furamide), 500 mg three times a day for 10 days in adults, and 20 mg per kilogram per day in three divided doses for 10 days in children. This is a highly effective treatment in more than 90 percent of intestinal cyst carriers. Its major side effects include nausea, anorexia, flatulence, and diarrhea. Metronidazole (Flagyl) had initially been disappointing as an effective treatment in asymptomatic cyst passers; however, recent work has demonstrated that metronidazole, given in a single 2-g dose for 2 days, has a cure rate of approximately 90 percent. In my experience patients are reluctant to take such a large dose because of the unpleasant metallic taste, headache, anorexia, and epigastric distress. Patients should also be warned to avoid alcohol because the combination of metronidazole and alcohol leads to the same effects as alcohol and disulfiram (Antabuse). Paromomycin (Humatin) can be used in a dosage of 25 to 30 mg per kilogram per day in three doses for 7 days in both children and adults.

Mild to Moderate Intestinal Amebiasis

Metronidazole, 750 mg three times a day for 5 to 10 days in adults, and 35 to 50 mg per kilogram per day in three doses for 10 days in children, followed by diiodohydroxyquin, 650 mg three times per day for 20 days in adults and 30 to 40 mg per kilogram per day in three doses for 20 days in children, is effective treatment for mild to moderate intestinal amebiasis. Less effective therapy which is still used in adults is tetracycline, 250 mg four times daily for 10 days, followed by a course of diiodohydroxyquin as above; or diloxanide furoate, 500 mg three

TABLE 1 Parasites Involving the Colon

Entamoeba histolytica
Dientamoeba fragilis
Trichuris trichiura
Enterobius vermicularis
Strongyloides stercoralis
Balantidium coli
Cryptosporidium species
Schistosoma species

times daily for 10 days in adults or 20 mg per kilogram daily in three doses for 10 days in children; or paromomycin, 25 to 30 mg per kilogram daily in three doses for 7 days for adults and children.

Severe Intestinal Amebiasis

In severe intestinal amebiasis for which a well-absorbed, tissue-active drug is needed, the drug of choice is metronidazole, 750 mg three times daily for 5 to 10 days for adults, and 35 to 50 mg per kilogram per day in three doses for 10 days in children, followed by diiodohydroxyquin, 650 mg three times a day for 20 days in adults, and 30 to 40 mg per kilogram daily in three doses for 20 days for children. If severe vomiting and/or ileus is present, metronidazole can be given intravenously as a loading dose of 15 mg per kilogram infused over 1 hour followed by 7.5 mg per kilogram every 6 hours. Alternatively, emetine, 1 mg per kilogram per day, or dehydroemetine, 1 to 1.5 mg per kilogram per day intramuscularly for 5 days, can be used. This is followed by diiodohydroxyquin as above. The usual maximum daily dose of dehydroemetine is 90 mg, and for emetine the maximum dose is 60 mg per day.

Hepatic Amebiasis

The liver is the most commonly involved extraintestinal organ. Amebic abscesses, if untreated, often are fatal. In patients with an amebic liver abscess the treatment is metronidazole, 750 mg three times daily for 10 days, followed by diiodohydroxyquin, 650 mg three times daily for 20 days. An alternative treatment would be the use of dehydroemetine or emetine as above, followed by chloroquine phosphate, 1 g daily for 2 days, then 500 mg daily for 2 to 3 weeks, plus diiodohydroxyquin as described above.

DIENTAMOEBA FRAGILIS

Dientamoeba fragilis is a protozoan parasite that is frequently unappreciated and unrecognized as a cause of intestinal disease. The usual clinical features are abdominal pain, nausea, vomiting, and diarrhea. Eosinophilia is found in more than half the patients with this parasite. Treatment is diiodohydroxyquin, 650 mg three times daily for 20 days in adults, and 40 mg per kilogram daily in three doses for 20 days in children. Tetracycline can be used as an alternative therapy in adults, 500 mg four times daily for 10 days. In children, tetracycline in a dose of 10 mg per kilogram four times a day with a maximum dose of 2 g per day for 10 days has been used, but I prefer to avoid using tetracycline in children less than 10 years old because of dental staining.

TRICHURIS TRICHIURA

Trichuris trichiura is a roundworm and is commonly found in the tropics and in areas of poor sanitation. This parasite is frequently unappreciated, since many of the infections are asymptomatic; however, in children it may cause severe and persistent diarrhea. The treatment is mebendazole (Vermox), 100 mg twice daily for 3 days. The dose for children over 2 years old is the same as the adult dose. Alternative treatments, such as flubendazole, 100 mg twice daily for 3 days, or albendazole, 400 mg as a single dose, have been used for light to moderate infections. At times, pretreatment with an antidiarrheal agent such as loperamide, 2 mg three times daily for 3 days, followed by mebendazole has increased the cure rate in patients with severe infections.

ENTEROBIUS VERMICULARIS

Infections with *Enterobius vermicularis* are extremely common in the United States, with an estimated 42 million cases occurring yearly. The treatment of choice is mebendazole as a single 100-mg dose, repeated in two weeks for adults and children older than 2 years. This retreatment is to eliminate reinfection acquired from eggs that have remained in the environment. Pyrantel pamoate (Antiminth) has also been used in an 11 mg per kilogram single dose regimen with a maximum dose of 1 g, repeated in 2 weeks.

Alternative treatments include piperazine citrate (Antepar) in a 65 mg per kilogram single dose to a maximum of 2.5 g daily for 7 days, with a repeat course in 2 weeks for pyrvinium pamoate in a 5 mg per kilogram single dose to a 350-mg maximum single dose repeated in 2 weeks.

STRONGYLOIDES STERCORALIS

This nematode usually involves the small intestine, although colonic involvement may occur. Symptoms include intermittent diarrhea and flatulence. With distal colon involvement, tenesmus and rectal pain are noted. Thiabendazole (Mintezol), 25 mg per kilogram twice daily for 2 days with a maximum of 3 g per day, is utilized. This medication should be given with meals to minimize nausea, vomiting, and anorexia. Patients should likewise be advised that their urine will develop an asparagus-like odor. Reexamination of the stool is recommended 2 weeks after treatment, and retreatment is recommended if larvae are found. With disseminated infections longer treatment periods may be required. An alternative treatment is cambendazole, 5 mg per kilogram single dose for adults.

Balantidium Coli

Balantidium coli infections, although frequently asymptomatic, may cause mild diarrhea or acute dysentery symptoms. Institutional living and/or swine contact have been associated with this infection. Tetracycline, 500 mg four times daily for 10 days in adults, and 10 mg per kilogram four times daily with a maximum of 2 g daily for 10 days in children, is considered the treatment of choice. Diiodohydroxyquin, 650 mg three times daily for 20 days in adults, and 40 mg per kilogram in three daily doses for 20 days in children, has likewise been effective. Metronidazole, 750 mg three times daily for 5 to 10 days, also has been effective.

CRYPTOSPORIDIUM SPECIES

Cryptosporidium infection has been recognized as a cause of diarrheal disease in man only in the past 10 years. *Cryptosporidium* species have recently been recognized as a cause of both small and large intestine disease in immunodeficient patients as well as in the homosexual population. The usual clinical presentation is profuse watery diarrhea and the diagnosis is made on intestinal biopsy with the recognition of the small parasites on the outer border of the intestinal crypts. The diagnosis has been enhanced by the use of a modified Kinyoun acid-fast stain and Sheather's sugar flotation method on stool examinations. Although there is no uniformly successful drug regimen, spiramycin, 1 g three times daily for 21 days in adults, and 1 g daily for 21 days in children, has been used with some success. At present there are no alternative choices.

SCHISTOSOMA SPECIES

The three principal species of *Schistosoma* affecting man are *S. mansoni*, *S. japonicum*, and *S. haematobium*. Schistosomiasis, although a world health problem, is not commonly encountered in the United States. With worldwide travel so commonplace, an awareness of this disease is important.

For *S. mansoni* infection, oxamniquine (Vansil), a single 15 mg per kilogram dose after the evening meal, has been used.

Niridazole (Ambilhar), 25 mg per kilogram per day in two divided doses for 5 to 7 days, has been effective. This drug is recommended for *S. japonicum* but is an effective alternative drug for *S. mansoni* and *S. haematobium*. It is available from the Centers for Disease Control for hospitalized patients. Other alternatives include praziquantel, 40 mg per kilogram in a single dose, for *S. mansoni*, *S. haematobium*, and *S. japonicum*.

For treatment of *S. haematobium* the preferred drug is metrifonate (Bilarcil), 10 mg per kilogram in three doses every other week. This drug, however, is available only from the Centers for Disease Control, Atlanta, Georgia (404) 329-3670.

SEXUALLY TRANSMITTED INTESTINAL DISEASE

PETER SPEELMAN, M.D.
WALTER E. STAMM, M.D.

The gastroenterologist may be confronted with sexually transmitted intestinal diseases (STIDs) either when patients present with symptoms and clinical manifestations of these infections or when signs of STID are evident on routine examination of the patient for an unrelated disease. Anorectal infections and several enteric infections have a high incidence in homosexual men and are less often seen in women who engage in receptive anal intercourse. The physician must therefore be aware of the patient's sexual practices and must be familiar with the causes and manifestations of anorectal and intestinal infections in homosexual men. The high risk of acquiring STID in homosexual men arises from several factors, including multiple sexual partners, anonymous partners, frequent asymptomatic infections, and specific sexual practices, particularly those involving direct or indirect oral-anal contact and rectal intercourse. Anorectal infections are usually acquired by direct inoculation of pathogens during rectal intercourse, while enteric infections are generally acquired via the fecal-oral route. The gastroenterologist must also be aware of the frequent enteric manifestations of the acquired immune deficiency syndrome (AIDS), which may be associated with either opportunistic infections, Kaposi's sarcoma, or AIDS itself. In this chapter we will review the diagnosis and treatment of common sexually transmitted intestinal infections, including those associated with AIDS (Fig. 1).

CLINICAL APPROACH

Assessment of the patient's sexual preference and practices is an essential part of the history. The number of recent sexual partners, illness in sexual partners, and a past history of sexually transmitted diseases are important data in evaluating the present risk of STID. The patient's presenting complaints should be classified into one of three syndromes: proctitis, proctocolitis, or enteritis

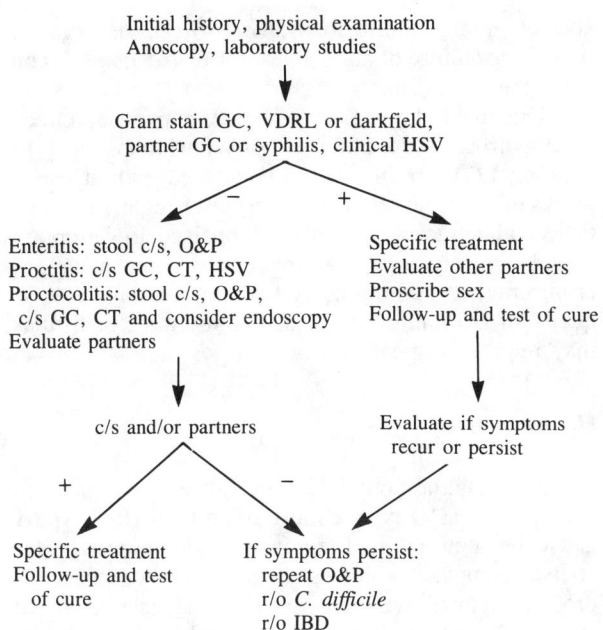

Figure 1 Management of sexually transmitted intestinal diseases.

(Table 1). Anorectal pain, mucopurulent or bloody rectal discharge, tenesmus, and constipation are symptoms associated with proctitis. Symptoms of enteritis include diarrhea, abdominal pain, bloating, and cramping; anorectal symptoms are absent in these patients. Proctocolitis produces overlapping symptoms of both proctitis and enteritis.

Physical examination should include the abdomen, the genitalia, the perianal area, the anal canal, and the rectum. A digital rectal examination and anoscopy or sigmoidoscopy are essential to classify patients into the three diagnostic categories. Patients with proctitis and proctocolitis usually have rectal exudates or rectal bleeding on anoscopy. Sigmoidoscopy may help to differentiate patients with proctitis from those with proctocolitis (see Table 1). In patients with proctitis, the disease is limited to the rectum, whereas in patients with proctocolitis the disease extends into the sigmoid colon. Anoscopy and sigmoidoscopy in patients with enteritis is normal.

When evaluating patients with possible STID, selected rapid diagnostic tests should routinely be performed during the initial examination, including a rectal gram stain for the evaluation of numbers of polymorphonuclear leukocytes and intracellular gram-negative diplococci, a darkfield examination of suspicious lesions, and an RPR test in patients with possible syphilis. Other routine tests should include urethral, rectal, and pharyngeal cultures for *Neisseria gonorrhoeae* and rectal cultures for *Chlamydia trachomatis*. Further diagnostic tests, such as stool tests for ova and parasites or bacterial cultures for enteric pathogens, should be selected based upon the suspected clinical syndrome. *N. gonorrhoeae*, herpes simplex virus, non-lymphogranuloma venereum (non-LGV) strains of *C. trachomatis*, and *Treponema pallidum* are associated with signs and symptoms of proctitis (see Table 1). Infections with *Campylobacter jejuni*, *Shigella* species, LGV strains of *C. trachomatis*, *Entamoeba histolytica*, and *Clostridium difficile* usually produce symptoms and signs of proctocolitis, while *Giardia lamblia* is usually associated with enteritis. Symptomatic patients frequently have two or more pathogens detected. Other, noninfectious causes of intestinal symptoms in homosexual men should also be considered.

Given the diversity of possible infecting agents, we prefer to withhold treatment in patients with mild symptoms until microbiologic results are available. In patients with severe symptoms and a great likelihood of an infectious cause, empiric treatment should be considered. We prefer a single dose of ceftriaxone 250 mg IM or a single dose of aqueous procaine penicillin G, 4.8 million U IM, plus probenecid, 1.0 g orally, followed by tetracycline, 500 mg orally four times a day, or doxycycline, 100 mg orally twice a day for 1 week, for patients with proctitis or proctocolitis. For patients with enteritis, metronidazole, 250 mg orally three times daily for 1 week, may be considered. All patients should have a test of cure. If symptoms persist after appropriate treatment, other pathogens should be sought. If no other pathogens can be found, inflammatory bowel diseases and other noninfectious processes should be considered. The sexual partners of patients with gonorrhea or syphilis should be examined and treated empirically. With other infections, partners should be treated only for specific identified infections.

TABLE 1 Syndromes of Sexually Transmitted Intestinal Diseases

	Proctitis	Proctocolitis	Enteritis
Pathogen	N. gonorrhoeae C. trachomatis T. pallidum HSV	C. jejuni Shigella species C. trachomatis LGV E. histolytica	G. lamblia
Symptoms	Anorectal pain, discharge, tenesmus	Symptoms of proctitis plus enteritis	Diarrhea, abdominal pain, nausea, bloating, cramps
Anoscopy	Abnormal	Abnormal	Normal
Sigmoidoscopy	Normal above 15 cm	Abnormal above 15 cm	Normal

Neisseria Gonorrhoeae

Rectal *N. gonorrhoeae* infection is the most common cause of proctitis in homosexual men; it is usually acquired by anal intercourse with an infected partner. The infection may produce either symptomatic or asymptomatic disease. Symptoms include mild anorectal pain, itching, mucopurulent discharge, and in some cases tenesmus and constipation. Anoscopy usually shows mucopus in the anal canal and sometimes mucosal friability. A rectal gram stain, showing polymorphonuclear leukocytes with intracellular gram-negative diplococci, may be helpful if positive but is only 20 to 40 percent sensitive compared with culture. Culture confirms the diagnosis. Preferred treatment of anorectal gonococcal infection in homosexual men is a single dose of ceftriaxone 250 mg IM or aqueous procaine penicillin G, 4.8 million U, plus probenecid, 1.0 g orally.

Penicillin-allergic patients can be treated with a single dose of spectinomycin, 2.0 g IM. Tetracycline should be avoided in the treatment of rectal infection with *N. gonorrhoeae* because of increasing resistance in rectal isolates from homosexual men. Penicillinase-producing strains of *N. gonorrhoeae* (PPNG), isolated in the United States since 1976, have been cultured infrequently from homosexual men. The recommended treatment of anorectal PPNG infection is spectinomycin 2.0 g IM once or a single dose of ceftriaxone 250 mg IM. Infection of the pharynx with *N. gonorrhoeae* can be treated with ceftriaxone 250 mg IM once or with a single daily dose of 9 tablets of trimethoprim-sulfamethoxazole 80/400 mg for 5 days. Test of cure cultures, contact tracing, and treatment of partners should be performed for either rectal or pharyngeal infection.

Chlamydia Trachomatis

The spectrum of disease resulting from *C. trachomatis* rectal infection ranges from absence of symptoms to severe granulomatous proctitis. *C. trachomatis* can be divided into two major serogroups, LGV and non-LGV. LGV serotypes cause more severe disease, usually an acute proctocolitis with severe tenesmus, bloody diarrhea, fever, malaise, and weight loss. Inguinal adenopathy, often not as prominent as with genital infections, may be present. Anoscopic findings often include edema, erythema, friability, and erosions or ulcers. Rectal biopsy specimens from patients with LGV infection can histologically mimic those seen with Crohn's disease. In LGV strain infection, antichlamydial antibody titers, as determined by the complement fixation test available in most state laboratories, are typically greater than or equal to 1:64.

Non-LGV strains are usually associated with a mild proctitis much like rectal gonorrhea or with asymptomatic infection. Non-LGV infections, which are acquired by direct inoculation via anal intercourse, usually involve the distal rectal mucosa and anal crypts as do *N. gonorrhoeae* infections. A diagnosis of *C. trachomatis* rectal infection should be suspected when symptoms of mild proctitis are present, a rectal gram stain shows polymorphonuclear leukocytes, and a culture for *N. gonorrhoeae* is negative. A positive culture or antigen test for *C. trachomatis* confirms the diagnosis.

Treatment of non-LGV infections consists of tetracycline hydrochloride, 500 mg orally four times a day for 1 week; LGV strains should be treated with at least 2 weeks of the same regimen. Alternative regimens for patients with tetracycline intolerance or fixed drug eruptions include doxycycline, 100 mg orally twice a day, or erythromycin, 500 mg oraly four times a day. Late sequelae of LGV infections, such as strictures or fistulas, may require surgical intervention.

Herpes Simplex Virus

Anorectal herpetic infection, caused by herpes simplex virus (HSV) type 2 more often than HSV type 1, is usually acquired by direct inoculation via rectal intercourse. Compared with those of gonococcal or chlamydial proctitis, symptoms are severe and include intense anorectal pain, tenesmus, hematochezia, and rectal discharge. Systemic symptoms such as fever, chills, malaise, and headache may be present. Rarely, patients complain of a stiff neck or photophobia. Neurologic symptoms, specifically urinary retention, S4-S5 dysesthesias, and impotence, occur in up to 50 percent of primary rectal HSV infections, distinguishing HSV from other forms of proctitis. In some cases clusters of perianal vesicles and/or shallow painful ulcers can be found. Since the patient may have severe pain, anoscopy or sigmoidoscopy may be difficult to perform. The rectum may appear edematous with discrete focal vesicular or ulcerative lesions occasionally present. Histologic examination shows microulcerations, intranuclear inclusions, or perivascular lymphocyte cuffing. The diagnosis can often be made based on the clinical picture alone. A culture, preferably taken from the base of one or more freshly opened vesicular lesions, confirms the diagnosis. Rectal herpes infection is usually a self-limited disease with manifestations which in most cases resolve in 2 to 3 weeks. The frequency of recurrences is unpredictable, but recurrent attacks are milder and resolve more quickly. Treatment of most recurrent attacks and milder primary infections is supportive, consisting of analgesics, sitz baths, stool softeners, and catheterization in the case of urinary retention. Preliminary data suggest that treatment with acyclovir, 400 mg orally five times a day for 10 days, decreases viral shedding significantly and may shorten the duration of symptoms. Acyclovir should be used in immunocompromised patients with rectal HSV or in immunocompetent patients with severe disease. Patients should be advised not to have intercourse when sores are present.

Anorectal Syphilis

An increasing proportion of men with early syphilis acknowledge homosexual or bisexual contacts. Currently, nearly half of the reported cases in the United States occur in homosexual men. Anorectal chancres usually appear two to six weeks after exposure by rectal intercourse. Symptoms are frequently absent but may include mild pain, constipation, rectal bleeding, and occasionally rectal discharge. The primary lesion is frequently overlooked in homosexual men if a careful rectal and anoscopic examination is not done, or if recognized, is misdiagnosed as a traumatic lesion, fissures, or hemorrhoids.

Primary anorectal syphilis may present as single or multiple perianal ulcers or ulceration within the anal canal or rectum. In secondary syphilis discrete polyps, smooth lobulated masses, mucosal ulcerations, and erythema and friability may be found in the rectum.

Condylomata lata, lesions of secondary syphilis, may be found near or within the anal canal and can be easily confused with anal warts. If in doubt, wart-like lesions should be examined by darkfield microscopy, since condyloma lata lesions are teeming with spirochetes. Late syphilis may involve any area of the gastrointestinal tract. The involvement varies from infiltrative constrictive polypoid masses in the stomach mimicking linitis plastica to lesions of the colon.

The diagnosis of anorectal syphilis is based on anorectal and perianal examination, anoscopy, darkfield examination, and serology. Anorectal and perianal lesions should be examined by darkfield examination for the presence of motile treponemes. Nonpathogenic treponemes may be present in the rectum, however, making the darkfield examination less specific for rectal lesions than for genital lesions. Biopsy specimens of rectal lesions should be examined by silver staining or by specific immunofluorescence. Histopathologic examination typically shows an infiltrate of predominantly plasma cells, lymphocytes, and histiocytes. Plasma cell infiltration is characteristic of syphilitic lesions.

Early syphilis, which includes primary, secondary, and early latent syphilis of less than one year's duration, should be treated with benzathine penicillin G, 2.4 million U IM at a single session. Patients allergic to penicillin may be treated with tetracycline hydrochloride, 500 mg orally four times a day for 15 days. Because of the superiority of the penicillin treatment regimen, persons with a questionable allergy to penicillin should be skin tested to ascertain their allergy status. All contacts should be examined, screened, and treated.

Condylomata Acuminata

Rectal warts or condylomata acuminata are caused by human papillomaviruses and are commonly found in patients practicing receptive anal intercourse. Anal warts may present as clusters of raised pink-to-brown papules and are commonly discovered on anoscopy for unrelated conditions. Patients with anal warts may be asymptomatic or may complain of anorectal pain and pruritus ani. More frequently, however, warts are psychologically disturbing to the patient. Condylomata lata, the moist, flat papules of secondary syphilis, should be differentiated from condylomata acuminata as outlined above.

The behavior of warts is unpredictable and they may regress spontaneously. The most commonly prescribed initial therapy is topical podophyllin (20% to 25% concentration in tincture of benzoin). Podophyllin has to be applied at least once weekly until the warts disappear. The treated area should be carefully washed by the patient 4 to 6 hours after the application to avoid chemical dermatitis. Podophyllin is contraindicated in pregnant women and is potentially oncogenic. It is not always effective, and the best alternative regimen for external anal warts is cryotherapy, i.e., freezing with liquid nitrogen, for a period of 10 to 30 seconds, to be repeated weekly for 3 weeks. Large warts should be treated surgically.

Treatment with antimetabolites, 5-fluorouracil, and laser therapy has yielded encouraging results in the treatment of genital warts. Immunotherapy is now being assessed. Patients should abstain from rectal sex during the treatment period.

ENTERIC PATHOGENS

Bacterial infections with *Shigella* and *Campylobacter* and parasitic infections with *G. lamblia* and *E. histolytica* can be sexually transmitted through fecal-oral contact. Most of these pathogens are transmitted by an inoculum as small as 10 to 100 organisms. In several cities in the United States 30 to 50 percent of the reported infections with these pathogens have been acquired through sexual contact. Bacterial diarrhea is also discussed in a separate chapter.

Shigella

Classically, shigellosis produces a clinical syndrome characterized by frequent passage of small volumes of bloody, mucoid stools with fever, abdominal cramps, and tenesmus. Usually fever occurs earliest, followed by watery diarrhea and sometimes by dysentery. In its milder form shigellosis may present as a nonspecific, afebrile diarrheal illness or may be entirely asymptomatic. Sigmoidoscopic examination shows erythema, edema, loss of vascular pattern, focal hemorrhages, mild friability, and adherent grayish-white mucopurulent layers. A wet preparation of the stool usually shows many white and also some red blood cells. Cultures of stool (preferably) or of rectal swabs confirm the diagnosis. Untreated, shigellosis in otherwise healthy men is usually a self-limited infection with symptoms resolving in seven to ten days. Since an infected person may excrete shigellae for weeks and may therefore infect sexual partners, antibiotic treatment of shigellosis in homosexual men is recommended. Treatment includes hydration and antibiotics. Trimethoprim-sulfamethoxazole 160/800 mg (double strength) orally twice a day for 5 days is the treatment of choice. Ampicillin can also be used, but many strains exhibit in vitro resistance in some parts of the country. The dosage of ampicillin is 500 mg orally four times a day for 5 days. The value of treating sexual contacts of infected homosexual men is not known, but it seems reasonable to screen and treat infected sexual partners.

Salmonella

Presumably because a larger inoculum is required to establish the infection, Salmonella is not sexually transmitted as often as Shigella. Clinical manifestations of Salmonella gastroenteritis include fever, headache, vomiting, abdominal pain, and diarrhea, following an incubation period of 24 to 36 hours. The diagnosis is confirmed by stool cultures. In most circumstances Salmonella gastroenteritis should not be treated, since antibiotics may prolong the carrier state. In cases of bacteremia or sepsis secondary to intestinal infection, antibiotic therapy with trimethoprim-sulfamethoxazole, 160/800 mg orally twice a day for 10 days, or ampicillin, initially 1.0 g IV every 4 hours followed by oral therapy up to 10 days, should be given.

Campylobacter

Campylobacter jejuni, C. coli, and closely related organisms are the leading bacterial causes of acute diarrhea in many communities. Campylobacter infection is generally acquired by ingesting contaminated food or water but may also be sexually transmitted among homosexuals by fecal-oral contact. Campylobacter jejuni has been isolated from symptomatic and asymptomatic homosexuals more often than from matched groups of heterosexuals. A group of newly described Campylobacter-like organisms may also produce diarrhea in homosexual men. Symptoms and signs of C. jejuni infection in homosexual men include diarrhea, abdominal cramps, bloating, and blood-tinged mucoid rectal discharge. The anoscopic and sigmoidoscopic appearance may be indistinguishable from shigellosis. The infection is confirmed by culture, using selective culture media to prevent overgrowth of other fecal flora and to provide the necessary microaerophilic environment at 42 °C optimal for C. jejuni. Campylobacter infections are usually self-limited. Infections in homosexual men should be treated with erythromycin, 500 mg orally four times a day for 5 days. Early treatment may shorten the duration of symptoms and decrease the period of excretion of C. jejuni in the stool. Sexual partners should be screened and treated if infected.

Giardia Lamblia

Infections with G. lamblia are highly prevalent among homosexual men in the United States. The high rate of asymptomatic infections and sexual practices involving direct or indirect fecal-oral contact contribute to the hyperendemicity of the infection. The spectrum of Giardia disease ranges from asymptomatic infection and mild diarrhea to severe disease with abdominal cramps and chronic diarrhea with malabsorption. G. lamblia affects the duodenum and upper jejunum. Anoscopy and sigmoidoscopy are therefore normal unless concomitant infection with other agents is present. Diagnosis requires identification of cysts and/or trophozoites by microscopic examination of stool specimens, but because Giardia are not shed continuously, multiple stool examinations may be required. Concentration techniques should be used to increase sensitivity. Duodenal or jejunal mucus obtained by a string test may also be helpful. Treatment regimens include quinacrine hydrochloride, 100 mg three times a day for 7 days, or metronidazole, 250 mg orally three times a day for 1 week. A course of metronidazole, 2 g orally per day in one dose for 3 consecutive days, is also highly effective. Another nitroimidazole derivative, tinidazole, 2 g orally as a single dose is very effective and has fewer side effects but is not approved in the United States. There is additional information in the chapter *Parasites of the Small Intestine*.

Entamoeba Histolytica

Most individuals infected with E. histolytica are asymptomatic, while others develop a mild gastrointestinal illness with loose stools, cramps, flatulence, and malaise which may continue for weeks or months. If bowel wall invasion occurs, symptoms of colicky pain, diarrhea with or without blood and mucus, and tenesmus may develop. Findings on sigmoidoscopy may be normal or include diffuse inflammation; classically, shallow ulcers covered with yellowish exudate surrounded by a rim of erythema may be present with a normal mucosal appearance between the ulcers.

The diagnosis of amebiasis requires identification of cysts and/or trophozoites in a direct fresh smear of rectal mucus or stool. Stool examination should also include flotation and staining methods. The findings of motile trophozoites with ingested red blood cells is indicative of invasive amebiasis. Symptomatic patients should be treated with metronidazole, 750 mg orally three times a day for 5 days, followed by diloxanide furoate, 500 mg orally three times a day for 10 days. Alternative treatment regimens include paromomycin, 25 mg per kilogram of body weight per day in three divided doses for 7 days. Asymptomatic cyst passers and sexual partners of proven cases should be treated with a 10-day course of diloxanide furoate. The importance of treating cyst passers is still unclear, since E. histolytica strains isolated from homosexual men were largely nonpathogenic by zymodeme typing. Treatment seems reasonable, however, from a public health point of view. The chapter *Parasitic Diseases of the Colon* also discusses amebiasis.

ACQUIRED IMMUNE DEFICIENCY SYNDROME

The acquired immune deficiency syndrome is an epidemic immunosuppressive disease that predisposes to life-threatening infections with opportunistic organisms such as *Pneumocystis carinii* or to tumors such as Kaposi's sarcoma. The majority of cases (73%) have occurred among homosexually or bisexually active men. Intravenous drug users (17%), hemophiliacs (0.7%), other recipients of blood transfusions (1.4%), heterosexual contacts of AIDS patients (0.8%), and children born to mothers with AIDS are also at risk. Recent studies have indicated a close association between newly discovered human retroviruses (LAV and HTLV-III) and AIDS. LAV has been found to be identical to HTLV-III. The virus can be recovered from more than 90 percent of patients with early stage AIDS but not always from patients with late-stage fulminant AIDS. The virus has also been recovered from seminal fluid and saliva of AIDS patients. Most patients with AIDS have antibodies to HTLV-III, whereas the frequency of antibodies to the virus among heterosexual controls is less than 1 percent. The virus infects T-cells with the OKT4 (helper/inducer) phenotype, resulting in absolute lymphopenia with a depletion of T helper cells and a reversal of the normal ratio of T helper/T suppressor lymphocytes (normal >1.2; AIDS <1). Other immunologic abnormalities include cutaneous anergy, an abnormal lymphocyte blastogenesis response to nonspecific mitogens and specific antigens, abnormalities of immunoregulation, hyperglobulinemia, and circulating immune complexes.

Patients may present with overt AIDS or with the so-called AIDS-related complex (ARC). Overt AIDS may manifest as *Pneumocystis* pneumonia (50%), Kaposi's sarcoma (30%), both (7%), or as other opportunistic infections (13%), including systemic infections with *Mycobacterium avium-intracellulare, M. tuberculosis, Cryptosporidium* species, *Candida* species, and many other viral, fungal, and parasitic organisms. The ARC includes persistent generalized lymphadenopathy (PGL), non-Hodgkin's lymphoma, other hematologic disorders, signs of cellular immunodeficiency, and a "wasting syndrome" with or without PGL.

Gastrointestinal symptoms, especially diarrhea and weight loss, are frequently present in patients with AIDS or ARC. In a minority of AIDS patients with diarrhea a specific agent may be found. Bacterial infections with *Shigella, Salmonella,* and *Campylobacter*, protozoan infections with *G. lamblia* and *E. histolytica*, and infections

TABLE 2 Treatment Regimens for Sexually Transmitted Intestinal Infections

Pathogen	Treatment Regimen	Alternative
N. gonorrhoeae	Procaine penicillin G 4.8 million U IM + 1.0 g probenecid PO or Ceftriazone 250 mg IM	Spectinomycin HCl, 2.0 g IM
C. trachomatis	Tetracycline, 500 mg PO q.i.d. × 7 days (14 days for LGV strains)	Erythromycin, 500 mg PO q.i.d. × 7 days (14 days for LGV strains)
HSV	Primary infection: Acyclovir, 400 mg PO 5 times daily × 10 days; nonprimary infection: supportive	
Early syphilis	Benzathine penicillin G, 2.4 million U IM	Tetracycline, 500 mg PO q.i.d. × 15 days or erythromycin, 500 mg PO q.i.d. × 15 days
Shigella species	Trimethoprim-sulfamethoxazole, (160/800 mg) 1 tablet PO b.i.d. × 5 days	Ampicillin, 500 mg PO q.i.d. × 5 days
Campylobacter species	Erythromycin, 500 mg PO q.i.d. × 5 days	Tetracycline, 500 mg PO q.i.d. × 5 days
Salmonella species (non-typhi)	None; in case of bacteremia or sepsis: trimethoprim-sulfamethoxazole, (160/800 mg) 1 tablet PO b.i.d. × 10 days	Ampicillin, 1 g IV q4h × 10 days
G. lamblia	Metronidazole, 2.0 g PO as single dose on 3 successive days or 250 mg PO t.i.d. × 7 days	Quinacrine, 100 mg PO t.i.d. × 7 days
E. histolytica (symptomatic)	Metronidazole, 750 mg PO t.i.d. × 5 days followed by diloxanide furoate, 500 mg PO t.i.d. × 10 days	Paromomycin, 25 mg/kg/day PO in 3 divided doses × 7 days
E. histolytica (asymptomatic)	Diloxanide furoate, 500 mg PO t.i.d. × 10 days	Diiodohydroxyquin (embequin), 650 mg PO t.i.d. × 10 days

with intestinal coccidia (*Isospora* and *Cryptosporidium,*) may lead to severe enteritis or enterocolitis.

Frequently, however, no organism can be identified despite thorough evaluation. Recent studies have shown that patients with AIDS or ARC who have diarrhea may have distinct histologic abnormalities seen in jejunal and rectal biopsy specimens. Abnormalities in the jejunum included partial villous atrophy with crypt hyperplasia and high intraepithelial lymphocyte counts. The most distinctive findings in the rectum were focal epithelial cell degeneration, mast cell infiltrates in the lamina propria, and viral inclusions near the base of the rectal crypts suggestive of infections with DNA-viruses such as CMV and HSV. Steatorrhea and d-xylose malabsorption were present in most patients with diarrhea. It seems likely that a specific but unknown process occurs in the small intestine and colon of these patients, leading to a wasting syndrome with malaise, weight loss, and chronic diarrhea.

Other gastrointestinal involvement in patients with AIDS includes infections with *Candida* species. Manifestations may include oropharyngeal infection (thrush) and severe esophagitis. *Candida* esophagitis may occur simultaneously with herpes in immunocompromised patients. HSV infection in AIDS patients may also cause perianal ulcers, colitis, and pneumonia.

Kaposi's sarcoma may affect the digestive tract and may disseminate throughout the intestines. Infections with tuberculosis and nontuberculous mycobacteria may infiltrate the lamina propria. The histologic picture of these lesions can mimic Whipple's disease. Suspicion of AIDS or ARC should prompt a clinician to assess the patient's immunocompetence and to check a serum sample for the presence of HTLV-III antibodies.

At present, no specific treatment is available for AIDS. Opportunistic infections should be aggressively evaluated and treated with specific therapy, even though they may prove to be relatively resistant to therapy or relapse. The treatment of infections with *Salmonella, Shigella, Campylobacter, E. histolytica,* and *G. lamblia* has been discussed earlier and is summarized in Table 2. In patients with AIDS, however, these infections may be unusually severe and may be complicated by bacteremia and relapses. Parenteral therapy may thus be necessary. *Salmonella typhimurium* has recently been recognized as an important opportunistic pathogen in this patient group. Usually the maximum dose of the antibiotic has to be given, duration of therapy has to be prolonged, and in cases of *Salmonella* infections even long-term suppressive therapy should be considered. Trimethoprim-sulfamethoxazole should not be the first choice of treatment for these infections in AIDS victims, considering the high frequency of side effects in these patients. Treatment of infections with *M. avium-intracellulare* is complicated by the fact that many strains are resistant to most antituberculous drugs. Treatment with four to six oral drugs plus one parenteral agent probably offers the best chance for success. The antileprosy agent clofazimine and a rifampin-like compound, ansamycin, may be helpful in these patients. In vitro susceptibility tests should be performed. No specific treatment is available for patients infected with *Cryptosporidium* species. Some patients have been cured with spiramycin, 3 g per day for a period of 3 days to 3 weeks. Infection with *Isospora,* has been treated with pyrimethamine plus sulfadiazine (7-week course); with trimethoprim-sulfamethoxazole (80/400 mg), 2 tablets four times a day for 10 days, followed by 2 tablets twice a day for 3 weeks; and with metronidazole. Herpetic esophagitis, colitis, and perianal ulcers may be treated with acyclovir, 250 mg/m² IV over 1 hour three times daily for 7 days. Oral thrush may be treated with nystatin, 100,000 U/ml 4 to 6 ml four times a day, or clotrimazole troches, 10 mg orally three times daily. Alternatively, ketoconazole may be used. *Candida* esophagitis should be treated with amphotericin B, 10 to 20 mg per day IV until improvement is seen.

Supported in part by grant A1-17805 from the National Institutes of Health.

INTRA-ABDOMINAL SEPSIS

JOHN GILL BARTLETT, M.D.

GENERAL PRINCIPLES

Microbiology

Infections of the abdominal cavity may be classified as monomicrobial or polymicrobial based on the number of bacterial species recovered from the infected site. Examples of monomicrobial infections are biliary tract infections and spontaneous or primary peritonitis. Most cases of intra-abdominal sepsis are polymicrobial, and involve both aerobic and anaerobic bacteria derived from the normal intestinal flora. Difficulties in treating these infections are that complete bacteriological data is not available at the time therapeutic decisions are required, valid specimens other than blood cultures are often difficult to obtain, cultures of exudate are arduous to perform, extended periods are often required to separate and identify individual isolates, and the organisms recovered may simply reflect the technical expertise and resources devoted to the exercise. Nevertheless, repeated studies have shown that predominant isolates in these cases are rather predictable: coliforms, especially *E. coli*, are the dominant aerobes while Bacteroidaceae, especially *B. fragilis*, are the dominant anaerobes.

Antibiotic Selection

The presence of multiple bacteria at the infected sites poses problems regarding antibiotic selection since it is uncertain which organisms represent true pathogens and require treatment. Most authorities consider both coliforms and anaerobes to be important in the pathogenesis of these infections and select antibiotic agents accordingly. Commonly advocated regimens which are considered equally meritorious are the following:

1. *An aminoglycoside directed against coliforms*
   a. Gentamicin, 2.0 mg per kilogram, then 1.7 mg per kilogram IV every 8 hours
   b. Tobramycin, 2.0 mg per kilogram, then 1.7 mg per kilogram IV every 8 hours
   or
   c. Amikacin 7.5 mg per kilogram, then 5.0 mg per kilogram IV every 8 hours

2. *Plus a second agent directed against anaerobes*
   a. Clindamycin, 600 mg IV every 8 hours
   b. Cefoxitin, 2 g IV every 6 hours
   c. Metronidazole 1 g IV, then 500 mg IV every 6 hours
   or
   d. Ticarcillin, mezlocillin or pipericillin, 3 to 5 g every 4 to 6 hours (usually 18 g per day)

The following factors may influence the regimen selected:

1. The aminoglycosides are considered equally effective against susceptible coliforms although sensitivity profiles within the institution may influence the choice within the group. Serum creatinine levels should be monitored regularly during treatment and dose adjustments should be made accordingly. Peak serum levels obtained at 30 to 45 minutes after intravenous infusion should show concentrations of 4 to 8 μg per milliliter for tobramycin and gentamicin, or 20 to 40 μg per milliliter for amikacin.

2. Cefoxitin may often be used as a single agent owing to its activity versus both coliforms and anaerobes. However, this approach is advised only for patients who acquired their infection prior to hospitalization and who have not received other forms of antibiotic treatment during the preceding 2 weeks. Other drugs potentially useful as monotherapy are moxalactam, timentin, and imipenem. These will be discussed later.

3. The only regimens just advocated that have activity against enterococci are those with an antipseudomonas penicillin and imipenem. Many consider enterococci to be relatively hapless in these mixed infections, although there are exceptions and some authorities recommend the routine addition of ampicillin to other regimens, e.g., "triple therapy." Treatment directed against enterococci is best justified when it is recovered in blood cultures, when it is recovered from exudate in pure culture, and when the patient fails to respond with no likely alternative explanation.

4. The national hospital study of in vitro sensitivity tests of 1,800 strains of *B. fragilis* from eight U.S. hospitals showed that all were sensitive to metronidazole and chloramphenicol; resistance rates to clindamycin, cefoxitin, pipericillin and moxalactam were 5 percent, 9 percent, 9 percent, and 13 percent, respectively. Pipericillin may be considered as prototypic for other antipseudomonad penicillins that are similar in activity versus anaerobes; these include carbenicillin, ticarcillin and mezlocillin.

5. Of the new antibiotics, the "third generation" cephalosporins have extraordinary activity versus aerobic gram-negative bacilli, but they are not as active as cefoxitin or many other alternative agents versus anaerobes. A possible exception is moxalactam, but this drug suffers the disadvantage of a potential bleeding diathesis that has disuaded usage. Imipenem also appears to be an exception and although clinical experience is limited, this drug is highly active against anaerobes including *B. fragilis*, aerobic gram negative bacilli, and enterococci as well. The combination of ticarcillin and clavulanic acid ("Timentin") has improved activity versus betalactamase producing strains of *B. fragilis* and also versus some aerobic gram negative bacilli when compared to ticarcillin alone. This may be used as a single agent in a dosage of 3 g of ticarcillin every 4 to 6 hours although again, experience is limited.

Timing of Antibiotics

Therapeutic guidelines and expectations are largely governed by the time during the evolution of the infection in which antimicrobial agents are initiated. Three phases of drug treatment are:

Prior to Infection. Recommendations for prophylaxis may be unique, as exemplified by the oral regimen of erythromycin and neomycin used for elective colon surgery. This combination has documented efficacy for preventing postoperative septic complications in patients undergoing elective colon surgery, but it certainly cannot be advocated for patients with established intra-abdominal sepsis.

Inflammatory Phase. This stage is characterized by an inflammatory response which, in the peritoneal cavity, may be diffuse with "generalized peritonitis," or localized as a "phlegmon." In each instance, there is no collagen wall of encapsulation with abscess formation. It is during this phase of an established infection that antibiotics have their maximum potential utility, and the earlier appropriate agents are given the better the therapeutic response.

Abscess Phase. This is the late sequelae of generalized or localized peritonitis in which there is a purulent collection entrapped by a collagen wall. Most intra-abdominal abscesses require drainage. The role of antibiotics during this phase is less clearly defined, although most advocate these agents to prevent bacteremia and local extension.

Failure to Respond

Patients with intra-abdominal sepsis who fail to respond to antibiotics should be evaluated for the following:

Inadequate Drainage or Debridement. Some patients will have persistent fever and leukocytosis or even positive blood cultures despite appropriate antibiotics, e.g., "breakthrough bacteremia."

Adverse Drug Reaction Such as Drug Fever or Antibiotic-Associated Colitis. Patients with drug fever often appear well despite elevated temperatures. Additional signs of an adverse drug reaction such as rash or eosinophilia are usually absent. Proper therapy is to withdraw the agent that is responsible; this should be accompanied by defervescence within 48 to 72 hours. Beta-lactam agents are most common and should be discontinued first. Patients with antibiotic-associated colitis almost invariably complain of diarrhea. These individuals should have a *C. difficile* toxin assay with or without endoscopy.

Inadequate Dose of Antibiotics. This is most likely with aminoglycoside administration in young patients when using the usual recommended doses, or when the unfortunately common practice of giving these agents in 80 mg doses is used as a routine. The adequacy of the dose selected can be readily verified by measuring the peak serum levels.

Superinfection. These are most likely to involve microorganisms that are resistant to the agents given, and in these situations a change in the antibiotic regimen is required. With the regimens advocated, the most likely are aminoglycoside-resistant gram-negative bacilli, methicillin-resistant *S. aureus, C. albicans,* and enterococci.

Untreated Pathogen. This is a surprisingly infrequent explanation when using the regimens advocated although substitution regimens are often tried. Bacteriology studies (especially blood cultures) with in vitro sensitivity tests provide guidelines if this information is available. Ampicillin or pipericillin may be added to treat the enterococcus if this was not included in the original regimen. Other considerations are amikacin in place of tobramycin or gentamicin, or metronidazole in place of clindamycin or cefoxitin.

Infection at Another Anatomical Site. Examples of these sites include the intravenous infusion lines, lungs (pneumonia), or the urinary tract.

Inability to Respond. Some patients are simply inadequate hosts and cannot mount a satisfactory response despite the use of appropriate medical and surgical modalities.

PERITONITIS

Secondary Bacterial Peritonitis

The implication of the appellation is that peritonitis is caused by perforation of a hollow viscus within the abdomen. The pathophysiology of ensuing complications depends on the nature of the insult, which can be chemical (gastric acid or bile) or bacterial. Secondary bacterial peritonitis usually involves the fecal flora which includes an imposing array of bacteria. Fecal spillage with free perforation of the colon causes generalized peritonitis with large collections of fluid in the abdomen, hypotension (hypovolemia and/or endotoxemia), shock, and rapid death. Therapy is directed at stabilizing the hemodynamic status, appropriate antibiotics, and early surgical intervention. Localized peritonitis is far more subtle, but may involve the same bacteria and is treated with the same antibiotics.

Immediate supportive measures in generalized peritonitis include aggressive volume replacement to prevent stagnant anoxia and lactic acidosis. Fluids should be given as colloid (plasma, albumin or blood) or crystalloid (electrolyte solutions such as saline). There are some controversial issues in the management of septic shock and these are outlined here. *Corticosteroids* are advocated by some authorities, but controlled clinical trials show disparate results. If given, the usual regimen for corticosteroids is a high dose, such as methylprednisone 30 mg per kilogram given once or in 2 doses separated by 4 to 6 hours. *Naloxone,* an opiate receptor antagonist, reverses septic shock in animals, although the initial clinical trials have been disappointing. If used, the dose is 0.4 to 1.2 mg, usually 1.2 mg, as an intravenous bolus. *Human antiserum to endotoxin* is obtained by immunizing healthy donors with heat-killed *E. coli* J5 or using plasma that is preselected on the basis of high titers of antibody to endotoxin-core glycolipid. The problem with this is that efficacy is best documented with antiserum to *E. coli* J5 and this material is not commercially available. It should be noted that corticosteroids may cause leukocytosis, decreased fever, and an altered mental status, thus distorting some of the parameters used to monitor response. The most important parameters to guide fluid administration are vital signs, urinary output, and central venous pressure or preferably, pulmonary wedge pressure using a Swan-Ganz line. The most useful tests for evaluating hematologic changes with disseminated intravascular coagulation (DIC) are platelet count, total hemolytic complement, fibrin split products, and prothrombin time. Patients with generalized peritonitis often have an ileus requiring a nasogastric tube or a long intestinal tube to decompress the bowel. Sedatives and analgesics are avoided or used sparingly until the diagnosis is established.

Antibiotics should be instituted following the collection of two blood cultures and instituting intravenous fluid support. Recommended agents are the dual drug regimens noted above. The usual loading dose is used for all agents regardless of the renal function; reduced total daily doses are appropriate in patients with compromised renal function primarily for aminoglycosides and to a lesser extent, for ampicillin and cefoxitin. No dose adjustment is necessary for clindamycin or metronidazole in patients with renal failure.

Surgery is conducted as soon as the diagnosis is established and the patient is sufficiently stabilized. The major goal is to control the source of contamination.

Spontaneous or Primary Peritonitis

This is a relatively common complication of ascites found primarily in children with nephrosis and adults with cirrhosis. The presumed mechanism is seeding of a susceptible nidus (ascites fluid) from a hematogenous source (portal bacteremia, remote infection, or transient bacteremia). Most cases in adults involve a single microbe, usually coliforms, followed by a variety of streptococci; *S. pneumoniae* is most common in children. Anaerobic bacteria are distinctly unusual. Antibiotic selection is best guided by culture results. Suggested regimens for empiric use while cultures are either pending or negative are use of an aminoglycoside such as gentamicin, 2 mg per kilogram, then 1.7 mg per kilogram every 8 hours plus either pipericillin, 4 to 5 g every 6 hours, or a cephalosporin, such as cefazolin, 2 g IV every 8 hours. Another option is to give a second- or third-generation cephalosporin as a single agent, such as cefamandole, 2 mg every 6 hours or cefotaxime, 1.5 to 2 g every 6 hours. Essentially all antibiotics diffuse well into the peritoneum so that direct inoculation into the abdominal cavity is unnecessary. There is an anticipated problem with aminoglycosides since these agents are distributed in the free-body water which may be increased by several liters in patients with ascites. Thus, therapeutic levels may be particularly difficult to achieve, serum levels must be followed, and alternative agents should be used when feasible.

Peritonitis Associated With Shunts or Peritoneal Dialysis

These infections represent medical complications of medical progress in which the key therapeutic decisions are these: (1) the decision to treat, (2) the propriety of local versus systemically administered antibiotics, and (3) the necessity to remove the foreign body. Treatment is advocated on the basis of clinical and laboratory findings. Most patients have abdominal pain or tenderness; cloudy ascitic or dialysate fluid with over 250 cells per milliliter and a predominance of polymorphonuclear cells; and positive cultures on primary isolation plates. As a general rule, all antibiotics penetrate into peritoneal fluid, and so there is no compelling need to deliver antibiotics locally. However, this approach is often advocated with aminoglycosides in patients receiving peritoneal dialysis since the desired serum levels are more easily attained by using dialysates containing the drug. The decision to remove the foreign body is always influenced by the necessity of the device and the response to treatment.

Peritonitis complicating peritoneal dialysis usually involves *S. aureus* or *S. epidermidis*. Less common isolates are streptococci, diphtheroids, coliforms, and Candida. Antibiotics are selected on the basis of in vitro sensitivity tests. A commonly used drug for infections involving gram-positive bacteria (staphylococci, streptococci, diphtheroids) is vancomycin since virtually all gram-positive bacteria are sensitive and a single intravenous dose of 1 g provides a complete 7 to 14 day course in the absence of renal function. When antibiotics are added to the dialysate the appropriate concentrations are nafcillin, 10 mg per liter; ampicillin, 20 mg per liter; ticarcillin, 100 mg per liter; penicillin G, 1,000 to 2,000 units; cephalothin, 20 mg per liter; gentamicin or tobramycin, 5 mg per liter; amikacin, 25 mg per liter; and clindamycin, 10 mg per liter. About 10 to 20 percent of patients require removal of the dialysis catheter due to catheter malfunction with poor flow or refractory infection with persistently positive cultures after 5 to 7 days or relapse when treatment is discontinued.

Peritoneovenous shunts which become infected require antibiotics directed against the isolated organisms. Most shunts that become infected require antibiotics directed against the isolated organisms. Most patients have a suboptimal response to therapy or relapse when antibiotics are discontinued. Definitive cure usually requires removal of the shunt, although a trial of systemic antibiotics followed by a prolonged course of oral agents may be attempted. An example is a 2 week course of intravenous cephalothin for a sensitive coliform followed by cephalexin for several months on an outpatient basis.

The treatment of peritonitis associated with ventriculoperitoneal shunts follows similar guidelines in that cure is difficult to achieve as long as the shunt is in place. The most common pathogen is *S. epidermidis* which must be treated according to sensitivity profiles, usually using nafcillin, cephalothin, or vancomycin. Initially, the antibiotics may be instilled into the shunt and given systemically as well. Local instillations are made into the reservoir daily using a 25-gauge needle after aspiration of 2 ml for cell count, chemistries and cultures, and an additional 2 ml for measurement of antibiotic levels. Representative doses advocated are gentamicin 1 to 8 mg, cephalothin 25 to 100 mg, nafcillin 50 to 100 mg, and ampicillin 50 to 100 mg. Meticulous sterile technique is required in preparing the injection site. Local instillations are continued until 2 to 3 consecutive cultures are sterile. Delayed response with persistently positive cultures or relapse after therapy is discontinued indicates the necessity for shunt removal. In some instances the antibiotics are administered intraventricularly and intravenously for 2 weeks; the shunt is then replaced regardless of the response, and then 2 additional weeks of antibiotics are given. The decision regarding the routine removal of the shunt versus a therapeutic antimicrobial trial is influenced by the necessity for the shunt and the technical difficulties with replacement counterbalanced by the clinical experience showing that medical treatment alone is often unsuccessful.

Candida Peritonitis

This is an increasingly recognized complication of peritoneal dialysis or intestinal surgery. Therapy with corticosteroids and antibacterial agents are contributing factors. In most cases, there is no evidence of disseminated candidiasis but the prognosis with this localized form is poor. *Candida* species are common isolates from a variety of specimen sources and usually represent contaminants making the diagnosis elusive to establish. Factors which influence the decision to treat *Candida* species recovered from peritoneal fluid are the reproducibility of culture results, semiquantitative assessment, cell count, and response to antibiotics. Preferred criteria are repeatedly positive cultures, recovery on primary isolation plates to the exclusion of other organisms, and a cell count exceeding 250 per ml. Most patients are febrile and have failed to respond to the traditional antibacterial agents. The preferred treatment is Amphotericin B, 200 to 1,000 mg IV. A test dose of 1 mg is given intravenously over 6 hours, and subsequent doses are increased in increments of 5 mg daily until a maintenance dose of 20 to 30 mg per day (0.3 to 0.5 mg per kilogram) is attained. Response is monitored by clinical signs (fever, leukocytosis, abdominal tenderness), peritoneal fluid cell counts, and follow-up cultures. For patients who fail to respond with repeatedly positive cultures the therapeutic possibilities include increasing the daily dose of amphotericin B to 1 mg per kilogram per day, or the addition of flucytosine to the regimen. An alternative approach to treatment of those receiving peritoneal dialysis is systemic amphotericin B combined with the addition of amphotericin B to the dialysate fluid in the concentrations of 2 to 5 μg per milliliter. The problem with this approach is the local pain which often precludes continued treatment by local administration. Many dialysis patients fail to respond and require removal of the dialysis catheter.

Tuberculous Peritonitis

The diagnosis is based on the detection of mycobacteria in peritoneal fluid, or peritoneal biopsy, or from any distant site in association with clinical evidence of chronic peritonitis, i.e., otherwise unexplained fever and peritoneal leukocytosis with a predominance of mononuclear cells. A presumptive diagnosis is made on the basis of the findings of mononuclear peritonitis or preferably, this is coupled with a peritoneal biopsy or pleural biopsy that shows granulomatous changes. These findings are sufficient to initiate antituberculous treatment pending mycobacterial cultures assuming there is no other readily apparent diagnosis. The purified protein derivative (PPD) skin-test is of little value. The preferred agents are isoniazid (INH), 300 mg per day combined with rifampin, 600 mg per day. These drugs are continued for 9 to 24 months depending on response. This regimen is usually supplemented in the initial 2 to 8 weeks with streptomycin, ethambutol, or pyrazinamide. Several factors may modify this approach:

1. Some authorities feel corticosteroids are beneficial in tuberculous peritonitis to reduce adhesions.
2. Patients who are unable to receive oral drugs should be treated with parenteral INH and streptomycin.
3. Patients who have been previously treated for tuberculosis should receive two drugs, which have not been previously given.
4. Suspected or established primary drug resistance is the major justification for using more than two first-line agents.
5. Patients with hepatic failure with encephalopathy or persistent elevations of SGOT or SGPT up to 6 to 8 × normal should be treated initially with streptomycin and ethambutol; a third drug will eventually be required. An alternative is cautious use of INH and rifampin in lower doses with frequent monitoring of liver function tests.

INTRA-ABDOMINAL ABSCESS

Virtually all intra-abdominal abscesses require drainage. The only exceptions are amoebic liver abscesses, some hepatic abscesses, and about 70 percent of tuboovarian abscesses.

The usual method for drainage is surgery, but an alternative possibility is percutaneous drainage using ultrasound or computed tomography (CT) scan guidance. This has the advantage of avoiding general anesthesia and postoperative complications. In experienced hands, percutaneous drainage has been accomplished with reduced mortality, reduced recurrence rates, reduced hospital stays, and reduced costs when compared to the reported experience with surgery. Despite justified enthusiasm, this is a relatively new procedure that challenges traditional therapeutic modalities. Thus it requires particular caution and the application of stringent criteria. Factors influencing the decision for percutaneous drainage are as follows:

1. Technical expertise is required.
2. Drainage is generally restricted to single, unilocular abscesses with a well-defined outer wall. CT scanning is the preferred method for anatomical definition. The demonstration of multiple abscesses, walled off loculations within an abscess, or poorly defined boundaries represent contraindications.
3. There must be a safe percutaneous drainage route as indicated by needle placement under CT, ultrasonic, or fluoroscopic guidance. These procedures should also confirm the diagnosis by the aspiration of purulent drainage.
4. There must be immediate operative capability in the event of failure or a complication.
5. Percutaneous drainage is especially favored in patients with intra-abdominal abscesses who have contraindications to surgery; in abscesses following recent abdominal surgery; and in abscesses which are easily approached due to large size and superficial location. Failures and complications are most common with pancreatic abscesses, abscesses within bowel loops, subphrenic abscesses and abscesses associated with intestinal fistula. Echinococcus cysts and multiple small abscesses are absolute contraindications.

Technical aspects of the aspiration and drainage procedure are used at the discretion of the person performing it. General principles are as follows:

1. The catheter may be inserted over a guide wire (Sel-

dinger technique) using a 8 to 14 F catheter; alternatively a 12- or 16-gauge Argyle catheter may be inserted into a trochar. The latter is preferred for large and superficial abscesses.
2. Extraperitoneal drainage and dependent drainage are desired, but neither is essential.
3. Irrigation of abscesses is usually not required.
4. Response is usually followed by the clinical parameters, amount of drainage and abscess size as determined by CT scan or ultrasound. Sinograms are generally unnecessary except with suspected enteric fistula. Hemorrhage from pancreatic vessels has occurred after sinograms into inflammatory pancreatic cavities.
5. Defervescence is anticipated in 2 to 4 days, drainage usually subsides in 7 to 14 days and follow-up scans usually show resolution of the abscess within 3 weeks. Surgery may be performed at any time that drainage appears to be inadequate.

INTRA-ABDOMINAL SEPSIS ASSOCIATED WITH SPECIFIC SITES

Appendicitis

Proximal obstruction of the appendix is the usual cause of appendicitis and prompt surgery is the mainstay of treatment. Antibiotics have no clearly established benefit in uncomplicated cases, but are uniformly endorsed for gangrenous or perforated appendicitis. Three options are usually advocated:

1. Antibiotics are initiated preoperatively in all cases and routinely continued for 3 to 5 days.
2. Antibiotics are initiated preoperatively and continued 3 to 5 days postoperatively, only if a gangrenous appendicitis or perforation is found.
3. Antibiotics are initiated preoperatively, only if perforation is specifically suspected.

The preferred antibiotic regimens are gentamicin or tobramycin, 1.7 mg per kilogram IV every 8 hours, combined with one of the following—clindamycin 600 mg IV every 8 hours, cefoxitin 2 g intravenously every 6 hours, or metronidazole 500 mg IV every 6 hours.

Pancreatic Infections

Cultures of the pancreatic secretions in patients with pancreatitis often yield coliform bacteria. Nevertheless, antibiotics have no demonstrable benefit for acute edematous, acute hemorrhagic, or chronic pancreatitis. These agents are not advocated for the usual nonsuppurative forms of pancreatitis, although they are frequently given with acute hemorrhagic pancreatitis simply because the patients are so ill.

Pancreatic abscesses are almost invariably fatal if drainage is not performed. The usual procedure is surgical debridement with external drainage using soft-sump or closed-suction drains. The most common pathogens recovered are coliforms such as *E. coli* and *Klebsiella*; anaerobic bacteria are uncommon. Antibiotics suggested for empiric treatment pending bacteriologic studies from operative specimens are an aminoglycoside, i.e., gentamicin or tobramycin 1.7 mg per kilogram IV every 8 hours, combined with ampicillin 2 g IV every 6 hours, a cephalosporin, such as cefamandole or cefoxitin, 2 g IV every 6 hours, or clindamycin 600 mg IV every 8 hours.

Liver Abscess

Liver abscesses are classified by etiologic agent as pyogenic or amebic, although the physician is often confronted with the situation in which therapy is required before results of diagnostic studies are available. Most liver abscesses are either pyogenic or amebic, although about 4 percent of amebic abscesses also harbor bacteria. Preferred studies to distinguish these possibilities are *E. histolytica* serology (complement fixation, indirect hemagglutination, and gel-diffusion-precipitin tests), blood cultures (pyogenic), and liver aspiration for microscopic examination and culture.

Amebic abscesses are treated medically using metronidazole given orally 750 mg three times a day, or intravenously 500 mg IV every 6 hours for 5 to 10 days. The drug is almost completely absorbed in the gastrointestinal tract so that the oral route is considered adequate. Follow-up liver scans should show complete resolution in 30 days after initial treatment, but this exam is unnecessary in patients who are doing well clinically. Alternatives to metronidazole include emetine given intramuscularly in a dose of 1 mg per kilogram per day to maximum of 65 mg for 10 days or chloroquine 250 mg four times a day for 7 days followed by 250 mg twice a day for 3 to 4 weeks. Use of emetine must be accompanied by cardiac monitoring with daily electrocardiograms (ECGs). A luminal amebicide such as diiodohydroxyquin should be given concurrently to eliminate cysts. Emetine is often combined with metronidazole for the first 2 to 3 days in patients who are seriously ill or have complications such as peritonitis secondary to abscess rupture. Needle aspiration is not indicated except to facilitate establishing the diagnosis, for very large abscesses (>10 cm in diameter), for imminent rupture, and for failure to respond after 5 days. Open drainage is reserved for patients who have failed to respond after 4 to 5 days of medical therapy, primarily in patients with abscesses which are inaccessible to needle drainage.

The management of pyogenic liver abscesses includes three fundamentally different approaches. These are:

1. The use of antibiotics alone. This approach is advocated by some for all pyogenic liver abscesses, but I use it only for patients who have multiple, widely-distributed liver abscesses or a solitary abscess in

which there is an impressive response to antibiotic treatment during diagnostic evaluation.
2. The use of antibiotics combined with needle aspirations that are performed at laparotomy, or percutaneously with CT, ultrasound, or fluoroscopic guidance. The aspiration provides a useful specimen source for microbiological studies, but this is not considered an important factor in treatment except for the aspiration of large volumes in patients with large solitary abscesses. Hence, this approach is endorsed for the indications noted earlier and is used with enthusiasm, primarily, for the opportunity to identify pathogens and/or decompress very large abscesses. Some authorities advocate repeated aspirations.
3. The use of antibiotics combined with surgical drainage is the time-honored approach advocated for solitary, pyogenic liver abscesses. This is still favored for most patients, the only recent change being that the method for placing drains may be either by operative approach (either transperitoneal or extraserosal), or by percutaneous insertion using CT or ultrasound guidance.

The dominant bacterial isolates are *E. coli, Klebsiella*, other coliforms, streptococci, anaerobic, microaerophilic, *S. milleri*, enterococci, *B. fragilis*, Fusobacteria and *S. aureus*; approximately half involve anaerobic bacteria. Appropriate antibiotic regimens for empiric use are an aminoglycoside, tobramycin or gentamicin 1.7 mg per kilogram IV every 8 hours, combined with a cephalosporin, such as cefoxitin 2 g IV every 6 hours, or clindamycin, 600 mg IV every 8 hours. Penicillin, 2 million units every 6 hours, or ampicillin, 2 g IV every 6 hours may be added to provide activity versus enterocci. Metronidazole, 500 mg IV every 6 hours may be desired for inclusion in cases where *E. histolytica* is a diagnostic consideration. The drug would also be appropriate for anaerobic bacteria, but it should be combined with an aminoglycoside and a penicillin to provide activity against coliforms and aerotolerant streptococci (enterococci, *S. milleri* and microaerophilic streptococci).

Hydatid Cyst

Echinococcal cysts of the liver should be surgically excised. Great care should be exercised to remove the entire cyst since any spillage may cause infection in the entire peritoneal cavity. This is accomplished by walling off the operative field, aspirating the cyst fluid, and then injecting a solution to kill the parasites using 2 percent formalin, 30 percent saline, povidone-iodine or absolute alcohol. If there is accidental spillage, the peritoneum should be irrigated extensively and the patient should be treated with mebendazole 400 to 600 mg orally three times a day for 3 to 4 weeks.

Splenic Abscess

The most prevalent bacteria are *S. aureus*, streptococci, coliforms, and anaerobes. Antibiotic recommendations for empiric use are an aminoglycoside combined with a cephalosporin or clindamycin. The usual definitive treatment is splenectomy, although occasional cases are managed by percutaneous needle aspiration under ultrasonic guidance. Patients who undergo splenectomy should receive pneumococcal vaccine preferably given at least 3 weeks prior to surgery.

Tubo-Ovarian Complex

This term refers to acute salpingitis and tubo-ovarian abscesses which appear to represent a continuum in cases of pelvic inflammatory disease. The three recognized agents of acute salpingitis are *N. gonorrhoeae*, anaerobic bacteria from the normal genital flora and *Chlamydia trachomatis*. Recommended treatment is that according to the most recent Centers for Disease Control (CDC) guidelines for patients who are hospitalized with this diagnosis and have no identified pathogen is as follows:

1. Cefoxitin, 2 g IV every 6 hours and doxycycline, 100 mg IV every 12 hours followed by oral doxycycline, 100 mg orally twice a day.
2. Clindamycin, 600 mg IV every 8 hours, and tobramycin or gentamicin, 1.7 mg per kilogram every 8 hours, followed by oral clindamycin, 450 mg orally every 6 hours.

Both recommendations include an initial regimen to be given parenterally for at least 4 days and until the patient is afebrile for at least 48 hours. This is followed by an oral regimen for outpatient treatment given to complete a total 10 to 14 day course of antibiotics. All patients with gonococcal infections should have test-of-cure cervical cultures at 4 to 7 days after treatment. Any sexual contacts of women with gonococcal infections should be treated with a penicillin. Sexual contacts of women with nongonococcal pelvic inflammatory disease (PID) should receive tetracycline, 500 mg orally four times a day or erythromycin, 500 mg orally four times a day for 7 days. Failure to respond to the suggested regimens usually indicates either the wrong diagnosis (acute appendicitis, ectopic pregnancy, ovarian cyst, ovarian tumor, mesenteric adenitis, diverticulitis, or corpus luteum hematoma) or a tubo-ovarian abscess which requires drainage. Drainage may be done percutaneously with ultrasound or CT guidance but surgery is preferred unless there is a medical contraindication. In the past, Crohn's disease was, at times, misdiagnosed as PID.

ENDOCARDITIS PROPHYLAXIS

FRANCOIS AUCLAIR, M.D.
GERALD T. KEUSCH, M.D.

The rationale for prophylaxis of infective endocarditis (IE) is based on definition of certain groups of patients at higher risk of acquiring the disease (Table 1) and on the demonstration that antibiotics can prevent endocarditis in experimental animal models. The uncertainties regarding prophylaxis include the relative risk of acquiring the disease after bacteremia and the validity of extrapolating data from animal models to humans.

RISK OF ENDOCARDITIS

Bacteremia is an essential prerequisite in the pathogenesis of IE. The presence of underlying cardiac lesions increases the risk of endocarditis. The incidence of IE in patients with rheumatic heart disease or prosthetic heart valves is approximately 0.4 to 1 percent per year, respectively. In patients with mitral valve prolapse (MVP), the relative risk of IE is increased at least threefold compared with that in subjects without MVP. It is much more difficult to estimate the risk of IE following procedures known to cause bacteremia. The risk is certainly quite low, since procedures like dental extractions cause transient bacteremia in up to 88 percent of subjects but rarely result in IE. The risk following gastrointestinal (GI) procedures is probably even lower because the incidence of transient bacteremia is lower. Indeed, we found only a few, isolated, well-documented cases of endocarditis in which a GI procedure was the likely portal of entry of the microorganism, in spite of the prevalence of cardiac lesions in the general population (e.g., up to 8% with MVP) and the frequency with which GI procedures are done. The principal organisms causing IE in these patients are streptococci, including Viridans streptococci in upper GI procedures and enterococci in lower GI procedures.

TABLE 1 Conditions Associated with Increased Risk of Endocarditis

High Risk
    Prosthetic valve
    Arteriovenous fistulas
    Patent ductus arteriosus
    Tetralogy of Fallot
    Ventricular septal defect
    Coarctation of aorta
    Mitral stenosis and/or insufficiency
    Marfan's syndrome
    Intra-atrial alimentation catheter
    Previous infective endocarditis

Intermediate Risk
    Mitral valve prolapse
    Tricuspid or pulmonic valve disease
    Asymmetric septal hypertrophy

Low Risk
    Arteriosclerotic plaques
    Coronary heart disease
    Atrial septal defect
    Cardiac pacemakers
    Surgically corrected lesions without prosthesis

PREVENTION OF INFECTIVE ENDOCARDITIS

The efficacy of antibiotic prophylaxis for IE has been demonstrated in animal models. These models require a high bacterial inoculum to induce endocarditis following direct trauma to the valve with a foreign body. The conditions and the timing of infection and antibiotic administration are strictly controlled. None of these factors pertains to the human disease.

Even with "adequate" prophylactic regimens, failures have been reported in humans. Moreover, since the introduction of antibiotic prophylaxis, there has been no dramatic decline in the incidence of IE attributable to this intervention. This may be because only a small

TABLE 2 Transient Bacteremia Associated with Gastrointestinal Procedures

Procedure	No. of Patients	Range (%)	Mean (%)
Upper GI endoscopy	742	0–8	4
Esophageal sclerotherapy	87	5–50	23
Esophageal dilatation	52	5–100	50
Rigid sigmoidoscopy	409	0–9.5	7
Flexible sigmoidoscopy	100	1	1
Colonoscopy	317	0–27	4
Barium enema	251	0–23	10
Liver biopsy	158	3–13.5	9
ERCP	534	0–14	3
Hemorrhoidectomy or sclerotherapy	97	8–9	8.5
Rectal examination	124	0–4	2.4

proportion of patients with endocarditis had previously recognized cardiac abnormalities and an antecedent manipulation known to cause bacteremia as a reason for administering antibiotics. In these circumstances, only a minority of cases of endocarditis could be prevented, even with perfect prophylactic therapy.

Despite these uncertainties, prophylaxis is recommended before certain procedures in susceptible patients, because such manipulations have been reported as the probable source of bacteremia in at least 15 percent of patients presenting with IE, and because the risk of antibiotic toxicity for an individual patient is considered to be significantly lower than the risk of morbidity and mortality associated with the disease.

TRANSIENT BACTEREMIA ASSOCIATED WITH GASTROINTESTINAL PROCEDURES

Virtually all GI procedures are associated with transient bacteremia (Table 2). Direct comparisons between studies is difficult because of different protocols for blood sampling, culture, and patient selection. In general, however, we can conclude that the risk of bacteremia is relatively low, that when bacteremia occurs it is during or shortly after the procedure (within 30 minutes), and that the density of bacteremia is low (usually less than 50 CFU per milliliter of blood). There is no documented correlation between biopsy and bacteremia in upper GI endoscopy, sigmoidoscopy, or colonoscopy.

The risk of bacteremia during upper GI endoscopy is approximately 4 percent. Streptococci, especially Viridans streptococci, are the single most frequent type of organisms isolated. Other isolates are predominantly upper respiratory tract commensals, although aerobic gram-negative rods and *Staphylococcus aureus* may occasionally be recovered. In many instances, the interpretation of positive blood cultures may be difficult because of possible contaminants from the skin, such as *S. epidermidis*, which are isolated in up to 17 percent of the cases (Table 3). Sclerotherapy for esophageal varices carries

TABLE 3 Organisms Causing Transient Bacteremia in Gastrointestinal Procedures

Organism	Incidence (%)
Upper GI Procedures (Endoscopy, Esophageal Sclerotherapy, or Dilatation)	
Streptococci and penicillin-sensitive oral flora	63
Staphylococcus epidermidis	17
Staphylococcus aureus	10
Gram-negative rods	7
Enterococci	3
Lower GI Procedures (Sigmoidoscopy, Colonoscopy, Barium Enema)	
Gram-negative rods	29
Enterococci	28
Bacteroides species and other anaerobes	27
Other streptococci	7
Miscellaneous	9

TABLE 4 Recommended Regimens for Endocarditis Prophylaxis in Gastrointestinal Procedures*

Regimen	Drugs and Adult Dosage
Standard	
Patients with prosthetic heart valves undergoing any GI procedure and other high-risk patients undergoing GI surgery, esophageal dilation, or sclerotherapy	Ampicillin, 2 g IM or IV, plus gentamicin, 1.5 mg/kg IM or IV, ½–1 hr before and 8 hr after
Special	
Oral regimen for minor or repetitive procedures in high-risk patients (see text)	Amoxicillin, 3 g PO 1 hr before and 1.5 g PO 6 hr after
Patients allergic to penicillin	Vancomycin, 1 g IV over 1 hr plus gentamicin, 1.5 mg/kg IM or IV 1 hr before (this may be repeated once, 8–12 hr later)

* Adapted from American Heart Association Recommendations
Note: Pediatric doses: Ampicillin, 50 mg/kg; gentamicin, 2.0 mg/kg; amoxicillin, 50 mg/kg; vancomycin, 20 mg/kg.

a similar risk, although the incidence may be higher when the procedure is performed on an emergency basis. Esophageal dilation appears to cause bacteremia more frequently than simple endoscopy, even when well-disinfected bougies are used. This may be secondary to the more severe trauma associated with the procedure.

The risk of bacteremia following sigmoidoscopy varies between 0 and 9.5 percent in different studies and appears to be significantly lower with flexible sigmoidoscopy. The risk following colonoscopy is intermediate between rigid and flexible sigmoidoscopy. In contrast, the incidence of bacteremia following barium enema has been reported to be as high as 23 percent and does not appear to be related to the nature of the underlying disease. Introduction of bacteria during barium studies may be secondary to abrasion of the rectal mucosa and/or increased intraluminal pressure in the colon. The organisms cultured from blood during these procedures are predominantly enterococci and aerobic gram-negative rods, which together comprise more than 50 percent of isolates. *Bacteroides* species and other anaerobes have been recovered in approximately 25 percent of cultures.

Liver biopsy is followed by transient bacteremia in approximately 9 percent of cases. The risk is increased in the presence of cholangitis. Gram-negative rods predominate, particularly *Escherichia coli*, and enterococci and anaerobes have been infrequently recovered, even though such organisms are often present in infected bile. The overall risk of bacteremia during endoscopic retrograde cholangiopancreatography (ERCP) is around 3 percent, but most positive cultures occur in patients with obstructive disease. Although bacteremia usually occurs early during ERCP, in some cases a positive blood culture is not detected for 1 to 3 days and thus may be unrelated to the procedure. Again, gram-negative rods and especially *E. coli* predominate. There are only isolated reports of bacteremia following peroral jejunal biopsy, rectal biopsy, or transhepatic cholangiography.

RECOMMENDATIONS FOR PROPHYLAXIS IN GASTROINTESTINAL PROCEDURES

Prophylactic regimens following GI procedures should be designed to be effective against the most commonly isolated bacterial causes of IE, namely Viridans streptococci and enterococci. Patients with prosthetic heart valves should also be protected against aerobic gram-negative rods. The protocol should consist of no more than one dose approximately 1 hour before and one dose several hours after the procedure; extending the regimen beyond this has not been shown to be more effective and could select resistant organisms as well as subject the patient to an increased risk of toxicity.

Recommendations for prophylaxis, recently revised by the American Heart Association[1] can serve as the basis for treatment guidelines (Table 4). We recommend that patients at high risk of IE because of prosthetic valves or previous endocarditis receive intravenous prophylaxis during any GI procedure likely to cause bacteremia, whether therapeutic or diagnostic. The risk of developing IE may not be higher than in other "high-risk" patients; however, the mortality and morbidity associated with prosthetic valve endocarditis justify the administration of parenteral antibiotics. Other high-risk patients should receive intravenous prophylaxis for GI surgical procedures such as gallbladder surgery, colon surgery, or hemorrhoidectomy. Although the clinical significance of the bacteremia associated with esophageal dilation and sclerotherapy is unknown, we feel it is reasonable to treat these patients before such procedures as well.

The American Heart Association recommends intravenous prophylaxis before colonoscopy and upper GI endoscopy and sigmoidoscopy with biopsy in high-risk patients, but accepts oral prophylaxis or none at all when biopsy is not done. The available data, however, do not support an increased risk of bacteremia during procedures with biopsy. Moreover, colonoscopy is not associated with a higher rate of bacteremia than sigmoidoscopy or even barium enema. For these reasons we cannot distinguish regimens based on whether or not biopsy is performed. We believe that prophylaxis is warranted during these procedures, although an oral regimen (amoxicillin) is probably both sufficient and more cost effective.

There is insufficient evidence to conclude that prophylaxis is mandatory in liver biopsy, ERCP, or barium enema, even in patients with mitral valve prolapse. At most, an oral regimen with amoxicillin could be implemented, especially if the procedure will have to be repeated.

REFERENCE

1. American Heart Association. Circulation 1984; 70:1123A–1127A.

ULCERATIVE COLITIS AND PROCTITIS

MARK A. PEPPERCORN, M.D.

Ulcerative colitis is a recurrent inflammatory process of unknown etiology involving predominantly the mucosa and submucosa of the colon. The disease may be limited to the rectum or rectosigmoid, involve the left colon to the splenic flexure, or in a continuous fashion extend to the cecum with associated mild superficial changes in the terminal ileum (backwash ileitis). Although worldwide in distribution, ulcerative colitis tends to be a disorder of developed countries, with about 10,000 new cases diagnosed yearly in the United States. Its peak incidence is between ages 20 and 40 years, although it can occur at any age. Approximately 20 percent of patients afflicted have a close relative with either ulcerative colitis or Crohn's disease. More common in whites than nonwhites, it also has a greater incidence in Jewish than in non-Jewish populations. The disease is characterized by its chronicity, with repeated attacks of bloody diarrhea, tenesmus, and abdominal pain with a potential for complications (perforation, massive bleeding, intractability) leading to colectomy. Patients with extensive longstanding colon involvement are at increased risk for the development of carcinoma of the colon. Ulcerative colitis can usually be distinguished from acute forms of colitis (bacterial, amebic, ischemic) by appropriate investigations, and from the other major cause of chronic colitis—Crohn's disease—which often spares the rectum, is predominantly right-sided, involves the colon transmurally, and may show granulomas microscopically on colonic biopsy.

THERAPEUTIC ALTERNATIVES

Drugs form the mainstay of any therapeutic program for patients with ulcerative colitis and proctitis. Topical therapy with corticosteroids and systemic therapy with oral sulfasalazine, prednisone, or parenteral corticosteroids are the major alternatives. Immunosuppressive agents, metronidazole, antibiotics, and nonspecific antidiarrheal drugs also may be part of the therapeutic program at a given time for such patients. New studies based on sulfasalazine's metabolism suggest that we are on the threshold of discovering new topical and systemic agents containing 5-aminosalicylate. In addition, new, rapidly metabolized forms of topical steroid therapy should soon be available. Other aspects of medical therapy may include dietary manipulations, psychiatric intervention, and behavior modification. When medical therapy fails to provide a satisfactory result or when the disease becomes rampant, surgery can be life-saving and curative. Before any therapeutic program can be satisfactorily devised, however, a number of factors must be assessed, including extent of disease, severity of symptoms, nutritional status, and the emotional make-up of the patient.

Extent of Disease

Ulcerative colitis always involves the rectum, although on occasion the severity of the rectal disease may be less prominent than that of more proximal areas. Ulcerative proctitis refers to disease limited to the distal 12 cm of colon, while distal colitis or proctosigmoiditis does not extend more proximally than the sigmoid colon. A high percentage of patients whose initial presentation is proctitis or proctosigmoiditis will progress with subsequent flares to more extensive disease. Most patients whose disease involves only the rectum or rectosigmoid have limited symptoms, are not at increased risk for carcinoma, and are candidates for topical forms of therapy.

Although many patients eventually have evidence of disease beyond the sigmoid, it is not unusual for the disease process to stop at the splenic flexure (left-sided colitis). These patients can have a range of symptoms from mild to severe, are at some increased risk for colon cancer, and usually require some form of systemic drug, although they may also be helped by topical agents.

The remainder of patients with ulcerative colitis have disease involving the transverse colon often extending to the cecum (universal colitis). Such patients tend to have more severe symptoms, are at a high risk for colon cancer when the disease is present for more than 8 years, and almost always will require one of the systemic treatment alternatives.

Since the most important initial determination with regard to extent of disease is whether the process is limited to distal involvement or extends proximal to the sigmoid colon, flexible sigmoidoscopy should be considered as part of the early evaluation of all patients with ulcerative colitis. Total colonoscopy, on the other hand, need not be done initially, since information gathered from the procedure rarely contributes to the initial therapeutic approach, and in the setting of active disease may increase the risk of megacolon or perforation. Once the disease quiets down, colonoscopy should be considered, since documentation of universal colitis will likely influence subsequent cancer surveillance. The barium enema can also contribute to morbidity in the acutely ill patient and often does not provide as much information as a flexible sigmoidoscopy.

Severity of Smyptoms.

In choosing from a variety of therapeutic alternatives, it is convenient to classify patients' symptoms as mild, moderate, or severe. Patients with mild symptoms may have only occasional rectal bleeding and/or mild diarrhea with fewer than four bowel movements per day. Tenesmus and mild cramping are common in such patients but severe pain, fever, and poor nutrition are not part of the spectrum of mild disease. These patients usually have more limited disease, although on some occasions active universal colitis can be associated with minimal symptomatology. When the symptoms are mild and the disease limited in extent, topical forms of therapy are usually desirable as an initial approach. If the disease is more extensive systemic therapy may be necessary, but the risks of side effects of the available systemic agents have to be weighted against the degree of morbidity from the mild symptoms.

Patients with moderate symptoms may have up to ten loose stools a day with frequent bleeding and mild anemia, but they usually do not need transfusion. Abdominal pain though often present, is not severe. Fever, if any, is low grade (less than 100°F), and although weight loss is common, the overall nutritional status is adequate. Most such patients will require some form of systemic drug therapy, although on occasion patients with distal colitis may present with moderate symptoms and a trial of topical therapy can be initiated. Moreover, topical therapy may be added to the regimen of systemic drugs for such patients. Although patients with moderate symptoms can usually be managed as outpatients the symptoms are such that some form of treatment is usually indicated, and when the disease is refractory hospitalization has to be considered.

Patients with severe symptoms who have more than ten bowel movements per day, bleeding often requiring transfusion, severe pain, fever at times as high as 103°F, and poor nutritional status almost always require hospitalization and therapy with parenteral agents. Patients who are toxic with or without magacolon will require early surgery if they fail to improve on medical therapy.

Nutrition

Perhaps in recognition of its being one aspect of their disease that they themselves might control, patients usually want dietary instructions. It is often discouraging for them to be told that there is no evidence that specific diets (e.g, low roughage, bland) are of significant help in ulcerative colitis. Although I usually suggest eliminating products that might contribute to diarrhea, gas, and cramps when symptoms are active (e.g. fresh fruits and vegetables, nuts, seeds, caffeine, monosodium glutamate, diet gum). I try to emphasise normalization of diet and adequate caloric intake to guard against excessive weight loss and nutritional depletion. Lactose intolerance, on the other hand, is worth considering in such patients, and it should be documented or excluded if there is any question. In lactose-intolerant patients supplemental calcium should be prescribed. Multivitamins are often part of a general therapeutic program, although their efficacy is dubious except in specifically documented deficiencies. Since chronic blood loss is a feature in many patients with ulcerative colitis and proctitis, iron replacement is often indicated.

Patients with unrelenting chronic disease activity may gradually become seriously nutritionally depleted (20 percent below optimal body weight). Such malnutrition alters the immune system and puts the patients at greater risk should surgery be needed. Although the nutrition of most such patients cannot be significantly improved until their disease is controlled, on occasion they will benefit from dietary supplements with an elemental diet.

For severely ill patients who require hospitalization, appropriate replacement of fluid and electrolytes is essential. If I suspect the hospitalization may be short I will try to temporize by placing such patients on peripheral hyperalimentation, usually with total bowel rest or clear liquids. This form of therapy does not provide adequate caloric repletion and is not tolerated for long periods because of discomfort due to phlebitis. For most seriously ill patients total parenteral nutrition (TPN) is indicated. In all such patients TPN will maintain and improve the nutritional status. The benefits of such therapy are reflected in reduced postopertive morbidity and mortality. This form of therapy, however, has no role as a primary treatment modality in ulcerative colitis and does not seem to influence the course of active disease.

Emotional Make-up

There is little evidence to support the concept that psychic disorders are etiologic factors in ulcerative colitis or that intervention with psychotherapy benefits the patient's course. On the other hand, some patients will manifest overt evidence of severe psychoneurosis, depression, or even psychosis and will require psychiatric consultation and psychotropic drug therapy. I have recently found behavior modification, usually with relaxation techniques, helpful for certain patients who themselves feel that stress and tension exacerbate disease activity. Some patients have a coexistent irritable bowel syndrome that had developed previously. All patients with ulcerative colitis seem to need, and benefit from, a caring physician who is willing to answer questions, be available at all times, and show a sincere interest in all aspects of their care.

PREFERRED APPROACH TO THE USE OF SPECIFIC DRUGS

Sulfasalazine

Sulfasalazine, which consists of sulfapyridine linked to 5-aminosalicylate via an azo bond, was first used for patients with ulcerative colitis in the late 1930s. Subsequent studies have shown that it will benefit 80 percent of patients with active mild or moderate disease whether the disease is limited to the rectum or rectosigmoid or involves the entire colon. It is not known whether the drug is of any benefit in severe colitis, but it is almost never used alone in such situations. Patients should begin therapy with 500 mg twice a day with gradual advancement of the dose to 3 or 4 g per day over a 1-week period. Most patients will respond within 2 to 3 weeks. Some will show a striking early response while others may take up to 2 to 3 months to show the full benefit of the drug. On occasion patients not responding to 4 g per day will respond to 5 or 6 g per day; such high doses, however, are not well tolerated by most patients.

Although sulfasalazine is often used adjunctively with both topical and oral steroid preparations, there are no data to support or refute such a role in ulcertive colitis and proctitis. In my own practice, although I often use sulfasalazine in combination with other agents, I try to stop the drug if it seems clear that it is having no therapeutic benefit on the course of the patient's illness.

A major role for sulfasalazine is in preventing relapses of ulcerative proctitis and colitis in patients who have gone into remission on some form of medical therapy. About 75 percent of patients maintained on 2 g of sulfasalazine per day will stay in remission for an idefinite period, compared with 35 percent of patients treated with placebo therapy. Four grams per day is actually a more effective prophylactic dose than 2 g per day but less well tolerated and therefore not usually used as a maintenance level.

Once patients have a clinical and sigmoidoscopic remission on standard therapeutic doses of sulfasalazine the drug can be tapered and maintained at the 2 g per day maintenance level. In those instances when the remission has been induced by corticosteroids, sulfasalazine is usually introduced at a maintenance level once the prednisone has been tapered to a range of 20 to 30 mg per day.

Does every patient in remission after an initial episode of ulcerative proctitis or colitis need to receive prophylactic sulfasalazine? If the episode has been moderate or severe with an extent of disease beyond the rectosigmoid, my own answer is yes. For such patients I tend to continue the drug at maintenance levels indefinitely, although there are no available data showing prophylactic benefit beyond 3 years. For patients with mild distal disease it is often worth a period of observation, and for those with early or frequent recurrences institution of prophylactic sulfasalazine once remission again is achieved may be helpful.

Because sulfasalazine and its metabolites cross the placenta and are secreted into breast milk, there has been valid concern over the use of the drug during pregnancy and nursing. Several large clinical studies suggest that the drug has no adverse effects on the fetus or on the pregnancy. Moreover, since its sulfa metabolite is a weak competitor for biliribin binding to albumin, jaundice does not seem to be a problem. Sulfasalazine, therefore, can be initiated and/or maintained in pregnancy as in the nonpregnant patient with ulcerative colitis, and can be continued during the nursing period.

One of the drawbacks of sulfasalazine is a high rate of intolerance and untoward reactions. Almost 20 percent of patients will experience nausea, headache, anorexia, or dyspepsia. A smaller percentage will have evidence of hemolysis and neutropenia. Mild allergic reactions characterized by fever and rash are seen as with other sulfa-containing drugs, but serious idiosyncratic reactions such as hepatitis, pancreatitis, alveolitis, and a serum-sickness-like illness are fortunately very uncommon. Two recently recognized adverse effects include an *exacerbation of the underlying ulcerative colitis* and reversible *infertility* in males. Although sulfasalazine may interfere with dietary folate absorption, routine folate replacement usually is not necessary.

The common untoward effects as well as hemolysis correlate with serum levels of the sulfapyridine moiety. These effects, as well as mild degrees of neutropenia, can be reversed simply by lowering the dose of the drug. Dyspepsia can be averted at times by the use of an enteric-coated prepartion. In patients with infertility, exacerbation of colitis, or the more serious systemic reactions the drug shoud be discontinued. It has been shown, however, that many patients who experience mild allergic reactions, such as fever and rash, can be desensitized to the drug. Although several desensitization schema have been proposed, two are particularly convenient for patients. One involves stopping the drug for a period of 1 to 2 weeks with reinstitution at a dose of 250 mg to 500 mg per day for 7 to 10 days and a gradual increase by 250 mg a week until maintenance or therapeutic levels of the drug are reached. However, the use of a new liquid oral suspension of sulfasalazine should make desensitization even easier than it has been. Another regimen begins with one-eighth of a 500-mg tablet daily with doubling of the dose every 3 to 7 days until therapeutic levels are reached. Clearly patients have to be monitored closely during this period for recurrence of their prior symptoms and laboratory abnormalities.

Despite its clinical availability for more than 45 years little was known about sulfasalazine's pharmacology until the past decade. Now studies of the drug's metabolism and distribution along with information about its toxicity have led to the development of a new generation of related drugs. The parent drug is partially absorbed from the proximal small intestine and then partly excreted unchanged in the urine, importing to the urine a strong yellow or light orange color. The remaining absorbed portion is excreted unchanged in the bile, and together with the unabsorbed drug reaches the distal ileum and colon where intestinal bacteria split sulfasalazine into its two components, sulfapyridine and 5-aminosalicylate. The sulfapyridine moiety is absorbed, metabolized by the liver, and excreted in the urine. The 5-aminosalicylate portion is largely unabsorbed and excreted in the stool.

The observation that 5-aminosalicylate is largely unabsorbed after sulfasalazine degradation and stays in contact with distal colonic mucosa led to the suggestion that it might actually be the active moiety of the parent drug, with sulfasalazine serving merely as the vehicle for delivery of the 5-aminosalicylate to distal disease sites. This speculation, coupled with the known findings about sulfapyridine's role in the drug's toxicity, led to the development of agents that deliver 5-aminosalicylate by itself to diseased areas of bowel. There are now several controlled trials which show convincingly that 5-aminosalicylate enemas and suppositories are efficacious in the treatment of mild and moderate distal ulcerative colitis and proctitis. Moreover, many such patients whose disease is refractory to conventional therapy with both sulfasalazine and topicl corticosteroids will respond to 5-aminosalicylate. An analogue of 5-aminosalicylate, 4-aminosalicylate, appears to be equally effective in these clinical settings. The hoped for safety of these agents has been realized, since patients previously allergic or intolerant to sulfasalazine can usually take topical aminosalicylate preparations without adverse effect.

In addition, there are currently four oral forms of 5-aminosalicylate under study in patients with inflammatory bowel disease. Disodium azo-disalicylate links two 5-aminosalicylate molecules via an azo bond. Balsalazide, on the other hand, links 5-aminosalicylate to an inert carrier molecule, aminobenzoylalanine, again via an azo bond. Asacol is a delayed release preparation wich coats 5-aminosalicylate with an acrylic-based resin which breaks down at pH 7. Finally, Pentasa is another slow-release preparation in which 5-aminosalicylate in microgranules is coated with a semipermeable membrane of ethylcellulose. Bioavailability, toxicity, and early efficacy studies suggests that one or more of these agents will be clinically effective and useful in patients with more proximal ulcerative colitis in whom topical agents are less likely to be effective. They may also be useful in patients with Crohn's disease of the ileum. Although there are no currently available commercial preparations of 5-aminosalicylate or 4-aminosalicylate in the United States, it seems clear that in the near future enema and oral forms of the drug will become available and emerge as front-line therapy for patients with inflammatory bowel disease.

It is hoped that an understanding of sulfasalazines and 5-aminosalicylate's modes of action might shed light on the pathogenesis of ulcerative colitis itself. Both sulfasalazine and 5-aminosalicylate are weak inhibitors of the cyclo-oxygenase pathway of arachidonic acid metabolism leading to prostaglandin synthesis inhibition. Although levels of prostaglandins are increased in active ulcerative colitis and diminished after successful therapy with sulfasalazine, other more potent inhibitors of prostaglandin synthesis are not efficacious in treating the disorder. In fact, indomethacin therapy actually may be associated with worsening of active colitis. An alternative explanation for sulfasalazine action suggests that sulfasalazine and 5-aminosalicylate, by inhibiting the lipoxygenase pathway of arachidonic acid metabolism, decrease the formation of leukotrienes and certain fatty acids which are potent chemotactic agents in recruiting polymorphonuclear leukocytes to sites of inflammation. At present, however, the actual mechanism of action of these agents remains unclear.

Corticosteroids

Topical Agents For patients with ulcerative proctitis and proctosigmoiditis the therapeutic choice is usually between sulfasalazine and a topical steroid enema preparation. The latter becomes a clear choice if the patient has a known sulfa or salicylate allergy, wants to avoid the potential adverse effects of sulfasalazine, and can't tolerate pills. Steroid enemas in the form of hydrocortisone or methylprednisolone in 60 ml of water are efficacious in such patients; more than 80 percent achieve a remission or significant improvement with the use of one enema nightly over a 2- or 3-week period. Systemic steroid side effects are usually not seen over such short periods of therapy. Occasionally a partial response will be obtained and the enema may be continued for a longer period on a nightly or every-other-night basis. Some positive response is usually noted within the first 2 weeks of treatment. If not, a twice daily steroid enema regimen is worth trying, but therapy for longer than 1 month with no clear improvement is not warranted. Occasionally, in the most limited forms of proctitis, steroid foams or even suppositories may be helpful in the same manner as the enema preparations.

The issue of whether steroid enemas work locally or through limited systemic absorption has been subjected to some study over the years. It is clear that the absorbed portion of an administered dose can lead, in some patients, to the usual adverse effect associated with chronic steroid administration. There are two new forms of topical steroid, however, which do appear to act locally with avoidance of chronic adverse reactions. One agent, *beclomethasone dipropionate*, is as clinically effective as hydrocortisone in enema form, but because of gut wall and first pass liver metabolism avoids suppression of the pituitary-adrenal axis. Similarly, a non-glucocorticoid, nonmineralocorticoid steriod, *Tixocortal pivolate*, also has rapid first pass metabolism, avoids suppression of the adrenal glands, is not salt retaining, and appears to be as effective in ulcerative proctitis and proctosigmoiditis as standard steroid enema preparations. Although neither of these preparations is currently available commercially in the United States each should emerge as an important form of therapy for distal ulcerative colitis and proctitis.

Systemic Agents. Oral corticosteroids were introduced into clinical medicine in the mid 1940s and quickly established themselves as useful in the therapy of ulcerative colitis. Prednisone, the oral agent most often used, is most helpful clinically in patients with moderate symptoms and disease proximal to the rectosigmoid who either cannot take or do not improve with sulfasalazine. More than 75 percent of such patients will achieve a remission or significant improvement. The drug is started at 30 to 60 mg per day, depending on the level of symptoms, and continued at the initial dose for about 2 weeks. Should the hoped for response be noted as assessed by disappearance of diarrhea and bleeding and improvement in the sigmoidoscopic appearance then a progressive reduction in dosage can be attempted at a rate of 5 mg per week. Somewhat paradoxically, patients with more limited distal colitis and proctitis not responding to topical steroids or sulfasalazine usually do not respond to prednisone, and its use in such patients should be discouraged or minimized.

A small proportion of patients with ulcerative colitis will present with severe or even fulminant symptoms and require hospitalization. The major therapy for such patients is some form of parenteral corticosteroid. For patients already receiving oral steroids the treatment of choice is either hydrocortisone, given as a continuous infusion at a dose of 300 mg per day, prednisolone, 60 to 80 mg per day, or methylprednisolone, 48 to 60 mg per day. I favor the latter drugs because salt retention is less of a problem. On occasion a refractory patient seems to respond to a brief trial of extremely high doses of these agents (e.g., 200 mg per day of prednisolone). Although most investigators have found corticotropin (ACTH) to be similar in efficacy to corticosteroids, recent experience suggests that ACTH may be more effective for patients with severe colitis who have not recently received oral steroid therapy. Corticotropin can be given as a continuous infusion at a dosage of 120 units per day.

Most patients with moderate symptoms and many with severe disease will obtain remission with systemic corticosteroid therapy. Such patients should be gradually weaned off steroids while continuing to receive sulfasalazine when possible. Unfortunately, low daily doses of corticosteroid (e.g., 7.5 to 10.0 mg of prednisone) do not appear to be effective in maintaining a remission in patients with ulcerative colitis. A recent trial, however, found that prednisolone, 40 mg every other day, was more effective than placebo in preventing relapses. Although chronic adverse effects may still occur on an alternate-day regimen, this type of therapy may be effective for patients with frequent flares of disease who are either unable to tolerate sulfasalazine as a maintenance drug or who have flare-ups despite its use.

Immunosuppressive Agents

Although increasingly used in Crohn's disease, azathioprine and 6-mercaptopurine thus far have played a more limited role in ulcerative colitis. Indeed, it has been difficult to show that these agents are of any benefit when used as single drugs in patients with ulcerative colitis and proctitis. In my own experience their major use is in the patient who is only partially responsive to prednisone and repeatedly flares when the dose is tapered below 20 to 40 mg per day. For many such patients the addition of azathioprine or 6-mercaptopurine at a dose of 1.5 mg per kilogram per day will permit a lowering of the steroid dose or withdrawal of the drug while the patient's disease continues at a quiescent level. Some preliminary information suggests that, as in Crohn's disease, these agents may be helpful in maintaining a remission in ulcerative colitis. Because of concern over the potential for neutropenia and infection and the unknown long-term risk of malignancy, I tend not to use these agents in patients with ulcerative colitis beyond 1 year.

Antibiotics

Broad-spectrum parenteral antibiotics such as ampicillin and an aminoglycoside have to be considered in toxic patients with ulcerative colitis with and without magacolon. In the face of impending perforation an agent active against the anaerobic colonic flora is usually added. Standard oral agents (e.g., ampicillin, tetracycline, cephalexin) are not helpful in less severe forms of ulcerative colitis and at times seem to trigger flares of the disease even in the absence of positive *Clostridia difficile* toxin titers. Metronidazole, however, may be one such agent that will find a role in the outpatient management of ulcerative colitis as it has in treatment of Crohn's disease involving the colon and perineum. There are as yet no available controlled studies of metronidazole in ulcerative colitis, but I have used the drug with apparent success in a small number of patients who are not responding to other measures. Its routine use in ulcerative colitis cannot at this point, however, be recommended.

Nonspecific Antidiarrheal Agents

Drugs such as loperamide, diphenoxylate with atropine, codeine, deodorized tincture of opium, and belladonna are useful in the treatment of diarrhea in patients with ulcerative colitis with mild, well-established chronic symptoms. Although the addictive potential of such drugs is a concern, their limited judicious use can make the difference between multiple trips to the bathroom at night and a good night's rest. These agents should be avoided, however, in patients with acute symptoms and more severe forms of the disease because of the risk of precipitating ileus and even megacolon.

SURGICAL CONSIDERATIONS

Surgery can be life-saving for patients with unresponsive fulminant colitis, some of whom may have already suffered a perforation or be having an exsanguinating bleed. A subtotal colectomy in such instances may be preferable to a total colectomy, since it is a lesser procedure in the severely ill patient and preserves the options for an alternative to a permanent ileostomy. With severe bleeding or fulminant disease clearly involving the rectum, a total colectomy may be necessary. The chapter *Fulminant Colitis and Toxic Megacolon* includes a discussion of timing of colectomy in such patients.

Another group of patients in whom colectomy has to be considered includes those with severe dysplasia on mucosal biopsy. It is hoped that the regular use of surveillance colonoscopy in patients at high risk (extensive disease for more than 8 years) will have an impact on the cancer problem in ulcerative colitis. This is also the topic of a separate chapter.

The majority of patients requiring an operation are not those with fulminant disease or in whom cancer is an immediate threat, but rather those with chronic symptoms who are often steroid-dependent and have suffered the physical and emotional ravages of the disorder over a number of years. Although once in place the standard permanent ileostomy is well tolerated by most patients, the specter of an ileostomy bag keeps many patients from surgery long after it may have been medically advisable. Now the surgical alterntives to a permanent conventional ileostomy (see the chapter *Ileostomy Alternatives*), may make decision-making easier for such patients.

FULMINANT COLITIS AND TOXIC MEGACOLON

DANIEL H. PRESENT, M.D.

When faced with fulminant colitis the managing physician must be well versed in treatment so as to be able to "anticipate" problems. If surgery is to be avoided, it is incumbent upon him or her to understand the appropriate "timing" of the various therapeutic modalities. Treatment should be instituted quickly in an attempt to avoid the development of toxic megacolon and if megacolon occurs, one must act appropriately and decisively to decompress the bowel.

In this chapter, I will outline, in sequence, what a physician faces when presented with a patient with either fulminant colitis or toxic megacolon as well as the questions that should be asked and the answers that must be obtained from the beginning of management through either improvement with medical therapy or surgery.

It is important to know whether the patient has Crohn's disease or ulcerative colitis, in terms of manage-ment techniques and decisions of therapy, especially those relating to hyperalimentation and the timing and type of surgery. It often is not possible in this acute phase to distinguish between the two entities, and the physician must try to obtain all prior data that will help in the differential diagnosis.

PRESENTATION AND DIFFERENTIAL DIAGNOSIS

It is almost trite to point out that a thorough history is the first crucial information that must be obtained when managing a patient with fulminant colitis. If the patient has a recent onset of symptoms with no prior history of bowel problems, it is important that the physician exclude other causes of colitis. I have seen patients present in a fulminant fashion with either *Campylobacter, Salmonella, Shigella*, or amoebic colitis. All these have also been described as causing toxic megacolon and perforation. Adequate stool cultures and stool examination for ova and parasites must be performed quickly by a competent laboratory. Once cultures are obtained a clinical decision must be made as to whether to start antibiotics before the results are available. If *Campylobacter* is suspected, a course of erythromycin, 500 mg four times daily, can be initiated. Both *Salmonella* and *Shigella* will respond to ampicillin, 500 mg four times daily. Although all of these diseases are self-limited and may not require antibiotics, if the patient looks severely ill little is lost by instituting antibiotics.

I have seen other causes of fulminant colitis, such as ischemic colitis and colitis secondary to gold therapy, but fortunately they are rare. Another type of colitis, which may ultimately become fulminant, is *Clostridium difficile* colitis secondary to antibiotic administration. If this specific history is obtained, studies for the toxin should be performed. If the patient's colitis is severe, he can be empirically treated with metronidazole, 500 mg three times daily, while awaiting the results. It is also important to remember that patients who have had prior inflammatory bowel disease may also develop superimposed infections. If the patient has been in remission for a long period of time and now presents with an exacerbation, the physician would do well to have stools tested for ova and parasites in addition to cultures. I have personally managed a half dozen patients who have had *Salmonella, Shigella, Campylobacter*, and *C. difficile* colitis superimposed on preexisting inflammatory bowel disease. If the patient has well-documented inflammatory bowel disease prior to presenting with a fulminant process, the physician is faced with the important question of whether this is ulcerative colitis or Crohn's colitis. Reports of prior sigmoidoscopies and barium enemas, history of bleeding, or presence of fistulas can all help in this differential diagnosis. If a patient is unaware of the results of the prior tests, the physician who saw the patient last should be contacted immediately. If the patient has had a prior history of colitis, the physician should be alerted to look for possible triggering factors, such as antidiarrheal or anticholinergic medications, recent barium enema and/or colonoscopy, and electrolyte deficiencies.

After this complete history is obtained, a standard physical examination is indicated and should especially include documentation of signs of toxicity, including fever, tachycardia, hypotension, as well as abdominal distention and tenderness along the areas of the colon. There is no harm in performing a limited sigmoidoscopy (rigid or flexible). I do not believe the scope should be advanced farther than 5 to 6 inches, because the essential information to be obtained is whether or not the rectum is normal, which would indicate Crohn's disease, or involved in a classic symmetric inflammatory pattern, indicating ulcerative colitis. The severity of involvement must also be noted. Attempts to pass a scope higher might serve to worsen the process and/or trigger a megacolon, or, rarely, perforate an actively inflamed bowel. A flat plate and upright film of the abdomen to include the diaphragms should be done quickly in the patient who presents with a fulminant picture. This flat plate may serve to exclude free air under the diaphragms and impending or existing toxic megacolon and at least may help to clarify the extent of the colitis, especially in new patients. It has been a clinical trick of mine to have the flat plate performed within a few minutes of having passed the sigmoidoscope for 5 to 6 inches. During the procedure air should not be forcibly placed in the bowel, but it is inevitable that a small amount of room air may enter the bowel. In the performance of an obstructive series, this little bit of air will often outline the extent of the inflammatory process (i.e., left-sided or universal).

Blood studies should include complete blood count, erythrocyte sedimentation rate, electrolytes, and SMA 12. In fulminant colitis, the most important studies to be monitored would be the blood count, looking for a severe leukocytosis, severe anemia, and for a shift to the left which perhaps indicates a secondary infectious process. It would be unusual to have a sedimentation rate below 40 mm per hour in a fulminant condition. It has been my practice to monitor sedimentation rates throughout the entire course of therapy, as this is easily done and is very helpful in charting the progression or improvement of the process. A low serum albumin level would tend to indicate a severe or chronic process, and electrolytes may need correction (e.g., hypokalemia). In ongoing processes, serum magnesium and calcium measurements might also prove to be helpful, and if they are low, replacement should be instituted.

The next major question is whether or not to hospitalize the patient. This is a clinical judgment and I am inclined to hospitalize if the patient has been febrile for 3 days or more, has evidence of moderate anemia (hemoglobin less than 10 g per deciliter), is hypoalbuminemic, or has severe generalized weakness with inability to function at work. Other criteria include a sedimentation rate over 50 mm per hour in this clinical setting or evidence of air starting to accumulate in the colon as an air column in the transverse and/or descending colon area. Discretion is the better part of valor when dealing with potential fulminant colitis, and the physician should always err on the side of hospitalization if there is some doubt. If the physician feels that the clinical status is not that severe and the patient is sent home, then no anticholinergic or antidiarrheal agents should be given until the situation is clarified. The patient should return to the office at least every other day until there is clinical improvement.

EARLY HOSPITAL MANAGEMENT

It is obvious, but important, to point out that the management of the patient admitted to the hospital with fulminant colitis or toxic megacolon involves frequent and careful observation. The patient should be seen at least *three times daily* by either attending or house staff, and management plans should be updated as often as required on a 6- to 12-hour basis depending on the clinical condition of the patient. Vital signs should be monitored for evidence of worsening. Deterioration would be indicated by hypotension, persistent fever, persistent tachycardia, and/or severe localized pain in the abdomen. The nursing staff should be alerted to the potential for disaster and should play an active management role.

If not already performed in the office, baseline blood studies on admission to the hospital should include complete blood count, erythrocyte sedimentation rate, electrolytes, and SMA 12. Blood cultures, stool cultures (for *Salmonella, Shigella*, and *Campylobacter*, and for *C. difficile* if the patient has received antibiotics) should be obtained before antibiotic therapy is instituted. Intake and output should be carefully monitored and either the nurse or patient should fill out a stool chart documenting the number of stools, time of day, consistency, and presence or absence and amount of blood seen. In my experience, this chart is very helpful in monitoring the progress of the patients. An obstructive series, including chest roentgenogram, should be performed on admission to rule out either an impending or a frank toxic megacolon. The radiologist should be alerted to the condition of the patient and these films should be carefully scrutinized to look for free air or air in the wall of the bowel, both of which would indicate surgical intervention.

It is crucial that a surgical consultation be obtained on admission to the hospital. Although it is always the gastroenterologist's hope that the surgeon will not be needed, it is unfair to ask the surgeon to make a difficult decision, such as the timing of surgical intervention, if he or she has not been following the patient on a regular basis. I therefore always have the surgeon follow the patient with me until I am positive that he will be able to leave the hospital without colectomy. One should, if possible, choose a surgeon who is familiar with inflammatory bowel disease and has had experience with the types of surgical procedure that might need to be performed depending on the clinical situation.

SPECIFIC MEDICAL MANAGEMENT

If the patient is ill enough to be admitted to the hospital with fulminant colitis and/or megacolon, he should cease to receive oral feedings as well as oral medications. The duration without oral feeding will depend upon the patient's progress and will be discussed later in the chapter. If the flat plates of the abdomen demonstrate full-blown toxic megacolon or moderate retention of air in the colon, as represented by a column of air outlining and spanning the transverse and/or descending colon, or by significant air in the small intestine, a long tube should be passed. I feel that there are strong advantages over use of a nasogastric tube, although this is not well documented in the literature. I have experience with a large consecutive series of patients which seems to suggest that a long tube is effective in decompressing toxic megacolon. In a situation in which fulminant colitis may become megacolon at any point, with subsequent accumulation of air in the small bowel, it is advantageous to pass this type of tube (which does not irritate the nasal passages). Surgeons often have more experience than internists in passing long tubes. Once the tube is in place the patient should be immediately taken down to the x-ray department and the tube positioned in the distal antrum or duodenum by either the radiologist or gastroenterologist. Patients should be instructed to lie on the right side for approximately 2 to 3 hours and then another film should be taken to see if the tube is in the correct position to pass into the small bowel. It is not appropriate to pass a long tube and wait a long time before determining if the tube has reached the correct position in the stomach. Time is of the essence in decompressing megacolon, and it is important that the physician send the patient for placement immediately after passage of the tube.

Intravenous fluids should be started to correct any dehydration as well as to maintain adequate hydration. Intravenous fluid must be administered to replace that removed from either a long or nasogastric tube. Close attention should be paid to the monitoring of electrolytes, including potassium, calcium, and magnesium. There is some evidence that deficiencies of electrolytes may tend to maintain the megacolon or the ileus pattern. If the patient is anemic blood should be replaced, with the hematocrit maintained above 30 percent, since there is always risk of sudden and acute hemorrhage.

Symptomatic medications, including antidiarrheals (such as diphenoxylate and loperamide), anticholinergics, and analgesics (such as demerol, morphine, and codeine) should not be given during the first acute phase of hospitalization. These agents tend to promote hypomotility and abdominal distention and can worsen the process. If the patient's pain pattern is such that he requires frequent analgesic injections, the physician must strongly suspect a walled-off perforation, abscess, or even free perforation. It is my experience that severe pain does not persist in patients with fulminant colitis once they have stopped eating and had a tube placed in the intestine; if severe pain persists, the aforementioned complications must be strongly suspected. The use of antidiarrheal agents will become important later in the course if the patient improves.

It is now customary for most physicians to start parenteral alimentation when a patient with fulminant colitis is admitted to the hospital. This can be done through a peripheral line if the patient's veins are in good condition, but in most situations it is given through a central line. The rationale is that this will help nutrition during the course of management and will help the patient heal the fulminant colitis. In my experience, and thus far in the literature, in the few controlled and uncontrolled trials that have been reported, there is no evidence that parenteral alimentation will in any way help to heal fulminant *ulcerative colitis* with or without megacolon. In those few reported studies the duration of hospital time needed to promote healing is not shortened, nor is there any evidence of a greater percentage of patients avoiding surgery after having been treated with parenteral hyperalimentation. In patients with ulcerative colitis, parenteral nutrition is a short-term modality to help maintain nutrition, especially when the past and present clinical course tend to indicate that the patient will have to undergo surgery in the near future. It is a common error for physicians to wait too long in deciding upon surgical intervention with the undocumented hope that parenteral alimentation will heal the bowel of a patient with active ulcerative colitis. Therefore, if it looks as if the patient is improving quickly and surgery will not be required, I would tend to forgo this extra procedure with its small but definite risk. If it looks as though there will be a protracted hospital course, however, or if the patient is markedly depleted from a nutritional point of view and surgery will have to be performed, I would then start parenteral alimentation through a central line.

One of the reasons physicians start a central line is the tendency to mistakenly focus on the results of hyperalimentation in Crohn's disease, in which both hyperalimentation and oral alimentation have been shown to be effective therapeutic modalities. Fistulas, both intraabdominal and external (enteric fistula to the abdominal wall and perianal fistula), have been temporarily closed with the cessation of feeding and total alimentation by central line. Therefore, in acute fulminant Crohn's colitis, hyperalimentation will not only help to maintain nutrition but may also prove to be valuable in the long term by helping to heal the inflammatory process. If it is anticipated that long and intensive therapy will be required, the physician should not only place a central line, but it should be a Broviac catheter, so that alimentation may be continued at home. I have had very satisfying experience in the use of home alimentation following hospitalization in patients with Crohn's disease. This is an attempt to maintain clinical improvement while waiting for other medications to become effective (such as 6-mercaptopurine and metronidazole).

I institute antibiotics, in patients with fulminant colitis and toxic megacolon, with both ulcerative colitis and Crohn's disease. In many of the patients there may be a microperforation and/or secondary infection extending deep into the bowel wall. Many have leukocytosis and marked tenderness of the abdomen along the contour of the colon, and it is often difficult to determine if there is secondary infection. This is especially so when steroids are instituted and clinical signs are masked (as well as when the leukocytosis is associated with steroid administration). I feel that there is much to be gained and little to be lost by the institution of antibiotics. I prefer to give a combination of agents directed against anaerobic as well as aerobic bacteria, and I prefer either gentamicin or tobramycin combined with either clindamycin or metronidazole to cover anaerobes. Metronidazole, in addition to its anaerobic coverage, may be helpful in that it would also be treating possible concurrent amebiasis while the physician awaits the results of stool tests for ova and parasites. My colleagues, who specialize in infectious disease, often suggest the addition of ampicillin to the combination of the aminoglycoside and metronidazole in order to cover enterococci. Before this great variety of antibiotics was available I found the use of chloramphenicol effective; however, many physicians are cautious in view of bone marrow toxicity, despite the fact that this rarely occurs. I tend to maintain antibiotics for a full 7 to 10 days through the acute course of the illness.

As regards the use of corticosteroids, there is no question in my mind that they are essential to the management of fulminant colitis and toxic megacolon. Physicians are concerned that the steroids will mask the signs of perforation, peritonitis, or abscess, but these fears must be abandoned because steroids are the prime medication for healing the inflammatory process in the colon. If the patient has been ill enough to be admitted to the hospital then oral steroids should not be used. Patients will be receiving nothing by mouth and oral steroids are reserved for the time when the patient is to be taken off intravenous therapy. In ulcerative colitis, when the patient has previously been receiving steroids, intravenous hydrocortisone in the form of Solu-Cortef is given in doses of 100 mg every 8 hours. It has been my experience, although not documented in the literature, that a continuous drip of steroids is more effective than steroids given by pulse technique. In those patients with ulcerative colitis who have not previously received steroids, it has been our experience at Mt. Sinai Hospital in New York, and recently has been reported in the literature, that adrenocorticotropic hormone (ACTH) is more effective. ACTH is given in doses of 40 units every 8 hours, also in a continuous manner. In the patient who is acutely ill with colitis, rectal steroids are usually not administered; however, if the patient does show rapid improvement, then rectal steroids in the form of 100 mg of Solu-Cortef (such as that in Cortenema) should be administered nightly. This will help alleviate inflammation in the rectum and thereby improve tenesmus. The combination of ACTH and rectal enemas has been shown to be effective in early British studies.

There is little role for sulfasalazine in acute fulminant colitis. When the patient improves, however, and is taking food by mouth, this can be reinstituted if he has been taking the medication in the past. Dosages range from 2 to 3 g daily. If the patient has not been on sulfasalazine in the past, I do not institute this medication until the patient has clinically improved and left the hospital on a regimen of oral steroids. I wait until this time because I do not want to complicate the picture with a possible reaction to sulfasalazine, when steroids are the most important therapeutic modality at the time of severe illness. There is no role for immunosuppressives in the acute management of fulminant colitis and toxic megacolon. The earliest response to immunosuppressive therapy is 3 to 4 weeks, with the mean time to respond of slightly more than 3 months. Therefore, these drugs are reserved for chronic patients in whom there is time to obtain the therapeutic effect. Immunosuppressives should not be introduced in any patient who may have to undergo imminent surgery.

MONITORING THE HOSPITAL COURSE

The first 2 to 3 days will often predict the final outcome of fulminant colitis and/or megacolon. It is the preference of many gastroenterologists, especially Sidney Truelove in England, to send the patient to a surgeon if he has not improved within 5 days. This would certainly include patients with toxic megacolon and very often patients with fulminant colitis. I do not believe that decisions such as these can be made on a broad basis; each patient's case must be individualized. If this is the patient's first episode of colitis I find it very difficult to bring a patient to surgery unless I am sure all medical therapeutic options have been exhausted. In patients who develop these complications and have been feeling well and are not depleted nutritionally, I am inclined to take a longer time before I send the patient to a surgeon. In Crohn's colitis, where there is less fear of free perforation and where hyperalimentation and immunosuppressives are of great value in long-term management, I am particularly loath to recommend surgical intervention. I believe most, if not all, of these patients can improve significantly if therapy is intensive and persistent. The physician must also understand that a total colectomy in a patient with Crohn's disease in no way ensures the maintenance of health in the future. The percentage of recurrent ileitis, after an ileostomy, increases with the passage of time.

On the other hand if a patient has had the ulcerative colitis for many years, has been requiring frequent or chronic steroid therapy, has been nutritionallly and emotionally depleted, it would appear prudent to try to improve the fulminant colitis and then send the patient to surgery on an elective basis. If this type of patient does not improve rapidly it is probably wiser to perform surgery soon after admission. I must repeat that all patients who develop fulminant disease must be treated on a case-by-case basis and that it is improper to suggest a simplistic surgical solution in a very circumscribed amount of time.

As previously noted, many variables must be monitored, including vital signs (blood pressure, pulse, temperature), intake and output and the number and character of bowel movements. Roentgenograms, including a flat plate and upright of the abdomen (to visualize the diaphragms), are to be performed daily or every other day with immediate review of the films. A bad prognosis would be indicated by persistent tachycardia, hypotension, or both. When a patient is receiving high doses of steroids as recommended, even a small temperature jump up to 100.5 °F (rectally) often tends to indicate a localized or free perforation. In these cases hepatic dullness must be percussed at least 3 to 4 times daily and obstructive films must be reviewed carefully. I have seen two patients who developed seizures during fulminant colitis as the first manifestation of sepsis, which was masked by high doses of steroids.

When in the hospital the physician is often intensely involved in the specifics of these potentially dangerous complications; however, it is also important to pay attention to the social and personal aspects of the illness and to be in close contact with the patient and family. The anxiety produced by this intensive observation, the passage of a long tube, and daily blood studies and roentgenograms often creates great tension in all. Patients and family should have concisely and clearly explained to them what the physician is attempting to do and how the patient can be of help (such as monitoring his bowel movements and being alert to any clinical changes).

The patient is almost always fearful of surgery, especially if the disease is of recent onset and the patient does not understand what is entailed in colectomy. The middle course must be taken, in that the patient cannot be told that the knife is hanging closely over his head (or in this case, the abdomen), but the mention of surgery should not be put off until the very last minute. If the patient has had the disease for a long time, then both the gastroenterologist and surgeon must explain what types of surgery may be necessary if the patient does not improve. If surgery appears to be unavoidable and time permits, it is helpful to have other patients who have had ileostomies, or who have been this severely ill and subsequently recovered, visit the patient. I have found that just seeing a patient who has had an ostomy, who is in good health and has been through what the patient has been through, provides more relief of anxiety than repeated explanations and reassurances by the physician or nurse. Although we do not consider the more advanced surgical procedures, such as continent ileostomies and ileoanal anastomosis with proximal pouches, in acutely ill patients, it also can be helpful for the patient to meet another patient who has undergone these procedures, knowing that in the future they will also be available to him. Low doses of minor tranquilizers such as diazepam or meprobamate are useful in this situation, and more potent tranquilizers are usually not required. The latter are reserved for the infrequent psychoses induced by steroids. The National Foundation for Ileitis and Colitis (444 Park Avenue South, New York, NY, 10016, telephone 212-685-3440) is quite helpful to both patient and family in these situations. Literature, in the form of brochures, books oriented toward patients (*The Crohn's Disease and Ulcerative Colitis Fact Book* and *People Not Patients*), as well as educational films are available. The Foundation has also organized support and mutual help groups as well as hospital visiting groups. Literature can also be obtained from local and national ostomy associations. In this mechanized age we must continue to remember that the emotional needs of the patient are as important as the combinations of medications.

TOXIC MEGACOLON

Although the preceding information applies to either fulminant colitis or toxic megacolon, I believe a short section of this chapter should be specifically oriented toward megacolon. It is the teaching in the literature that toxic megacolon per se is an indication for surgery. It is stated that any delay in medical therapy beyond 48 hours will markedly increase the risk of perforation and subsequent mortality. If one carefully reads the literature, however, it is evident that the same facts are open to different interpretations. The mortality in both medical and surgical studies is quite similar, although the surgeons point out that mortality is due to delay because of prolonged medical management. Other studies in which all patients are operated on within 48 hours on an emergency basis do not show a much improved rate in terms of mortality. My experience, which is similar to that of a few other gastroenterologists, is that toxic megacolon can be managed medically and that ultimate surgical intervention is required in less than half the cases. My long-term data also indicate that patients with Crohn's colitis who develop megacolon rarely, if ever, need surgery, and that slightly less than 50 percent of patients with ulcerative colitis require surgery for further complications or activity. I treat all patients with megacolon as outlined above—with a few additions. The crucial points in management, as previously noted, are that a long tube is essential and should be passed early, with radiologic placement of the mercury-weighted tip. Parenteral antibiotics are used to cover aerobic and anaerobic bacteria. Parenteral steroids in continuous drip are started immediately. Daily obstructive series, as well as daily evaluation by the surgeon (who is called in immediately in consultation), are undertaken.

In addition, it has become evident to me that air accumulates in the transverse colon preferentially because the patient lies in bed with his head elevated, and air tends to accumulate in the most anterior position of the bowel, the transverse colon. We have demonstrated that if the patient rolls on his abdomen for 10 to 15 minutes every 2 to 3 hours the air redistributes through the colon. The patient is then encouraged to evacuate the air immediately following the rolling process. If the patient cannot evacuate the air, a soft, small-caliber rubber catheter is passed into the rectum while the patient is lying on his abdomen. We have demonstrated a marked decrease, both clinically and radiographically, in the diameter of the transverse colon with decreased retention of air soon after the rolling and evacuation procedure. While this procedure does not in itself improve the patient's colitis, it allows the gastroenterologist more time in which to treat the patient with steroids and antibiotics.

In a personal consecutive series of 19 patients, I have decompressed all of the megacolons and 13 of the 19 are doing well on a long-term basis without surgical intervention. On the other hand, it is not unique for us to be able to decompress the megacolon and yet have the patient ultimately require surgery because of persistently active colitis. Once again, the clinical gastroenterologist must individualize each case, and there is no universal panacea. For example, it is my experience, and is borne out in the literature, that one-third of all megacolons occur in patients during their first attack. It is psychologically difficult for a new colitis patient to accept surgery, and by our aggressive medical management we have saved the colon in three-quarters of patients who presented with megacolon as their initial episode of colitis.

I have been fortunate in being able to conduct these clinical trials demonstrating significant improvement in megacolon because I have excellent surgical colleagues who have a great deal of experience with colectomies in acute situations. We work closely as a team, with the surgeons not being overanxious to operate immediately and with the knowledge that we will not prolong medical management if there are clear-cut signs of deterioration. We have together managed megacolon patients for over a week with good long-term results.

SURGERY

The timing of surgery must also be determined on a case-by-case basis. Free air under the diaphragms or dissection of air into the wall of the colon are definite indications for emergency surgery. Exsanguination, although rare, is also a clear-cut indication. Signs of sepsis or abscess, as evidenced by persistent tachycardia, hypotension, and spiking fevers (often accompanied by peritonitis), are positive and definite signs. Decisions become more difficult when one is dealing with such subtle findings as recurrence of low-grade temperatures (up to 100.5 or 101 °F) after the patient has been receiving steroids and antibiotics for more than 4 or 5 days. There is no question in my experience that the patient who has been receiving continuous intravenous steroids and antibiotics for more than 10 to 14 days and has not markedly improved is headed for surgery. It is rare for the patient to show major improvement after that time if therapy has been ideal.

I recently saw a number of patients who were transferred to me after having had an episode of fulminant colitis. They were treated adequately with steroids and antibiotics but still had persistent severe diarrhea. These were all patients with ulcerative colitis who had been treated with hyperalimentation, and because the diarrhea was persistent, the physician allowed the patient no oral intake and continued the alimentation. In this situation, after noting that the sedimentation rate was not significantly elevated and there were no systemic signs, I started the patients on oral feedings and added low doses of antidiarrheals (codeine, 15 mg ½ hour before meals and sleep). Most patients improved with the resumption of feeding of solids. It appears that the bowel affected by ulcerative colitis, when kept empty for protracted periods, will continue to produce diarrhea, even if the inflammation is under control. If the patient is fed and given small doses of antidiarrheals, he will then become much less symptomatic. Again, before this is tried, it must be well documented that the patient's systemic symptoms are under control. This again points up the failure of parenteral nutrition to heal ulcerative colitis, and in truth, the managing physician often maintains this modality for too long without a trial of food. As noted before, if the patient has a long history of ulcerative colitis and has been undergoing long-term steroid treatment with chronic activity or infrequent remission, it is important to perform a colectomy when the fulminant colitis is under control.

The type of surgery performed for ulcerative colitis appears straightforward. A subtotal colectomy is usually performed if there are thoughts of a future ileoanal anastomosis. This is why it is important to individualize cases and have meaningful discussions with the patients and the family as to the types of surgery. I usually reserve the ileoanal anastomosis with a proximal pouch for those patients who are young (under 25) and who have the time to devote to this two-stage operation with its numerous complications and temporary diarrhea after hook-up. If it is decided in advance that this patient is not going to be a candidate for ileoanal anastomosis then a total colectomy is preferred. The total colectomy would prevent those occasional cases of postoperative bleeding from the rectum stump which can require an immediate second operation. It also still leaves the option of conversion to a continent ileostomy at a later date. If the patient is severely ill, markedly hypoalbuminemic, or there has been evidence of perforation or abscess, the surgeon may also elect to perform a subtotal colectomy and leave a small Hartmann pouch for removal at a later date (with potential ileoanal anastomosis). I believe that this is a decision to be made by the experienced colorectal surgeon. It is rare for the surgeon to perform an ileoanal anastomosis or continent ileostomy in the acutely ill patient; these procedures are reserved for those chronically ill patients who undergo surgery electively.

The rectum is normal in most patients with Crohn's colitis, and there are therefore numerous choices. These include subtotal colectomy and ileosigmoidostomy or ileoproctostomy which can be performed if the patient is not acutely ill. If the patient is a poor risk, the surgeon may elect to perform the anastomosis and do a temporary loop ileostomy above his suture line. When the patient improves, this temporary ileostomy is closed (usually 6 weeks or longer after the operation). In many patients who are severely ill, a subtotal colectomy and ileostomy is performed with the thought of going back and anastomosing at a later date. This is usually feasible, but the anastomosis should be performed soon after the first procedure (approximately 2 to 3 months). Early reattachment is done, because in my experience the rectum worsens when bypassed (so-called bypass colitis). I therefore feel little is to be gained from waiting, provided the patient has recovered nutritionally and psychologically from the first procedure. It is rarely necessary to perform a total colectomy in patients with Crohn's colitis unless the rectum is severely involved. In my experience, if the rectum is either not diseased or only mildly involved, a hook-up with a temporary ostomy can be performed and the patient can then be treated medically. Initial treatment is hyperalimentation, and, for the long term, I use immunosuppressives and most patients ultimately gain good functional control of their bowel symptoms.

In new patients who have had to undergo a subtotal colectomy in the hopes of ultimately re-establishing bowel continuity, it is often very difficult to distinguish ulcerative colitis and Crohn's disease despite having the colon pathologic findings to review. The acute fulminant picture tends to make both processes look the same in the surgical specimen. In these cases we must therefore rely on the prior clinical story as well as on careful evaluation of the rectum by gross examination and biopsy early in the postoperative period.

MANAGEMENT OF PATIENTS WHO HAVE RESPONDED TO MEDICAL MANAGEMENT

If we have been successful in improving either the fulminant colitis or toxic megacolon we still face numerous decisions as to medical management. After the patient has been improved for about 48 hours, I start liquids by mouth and progress on a daily basis from clear fluids to full fluids to soft diet. If the patient has had a long tube in place and there are no signs of dilation when symptoms are clinically quiescent, I usually clamp the tube and start clear liquids, with full fluids the next day. If there is no further distention with the tube clamped for 48 hours, it is removed. If dilation recurs or starts to recur, I leave the tube open to drainage for another 48 hours and then repeat the process. Occasionally patients with megacolon may have mild persistent dilation but are not systemically ill, and in those patients I will maintain the tube for about 5 to 6 days on a clamped basis while feeding the patient and observing for any worsening of the colitis.

Intravenous steroids should be used for approximately 7 to 10 days. I might be tempted to transfer to oral medication earlier, but only if the patient is doing well and there are no problems with fluid retention or severe hypokalemia. There is often some exacerbation of symptoms when the patient is transferred from intravenous steroids to oral steroids. When starting oral steroids, I usually prescribe 60 mg of prednisone (20 mg three times daily) and give supplemental Solu-Cortef, 50 mg IM twice daily for 48 hours. I then give 50 mg IM daily for another 24 hours. Although this transition technique has not been documented by controlled trials to be more effective, there is, in my clinical experience, a decreased frequency of exacerbation when coming off intravenous steroids.

If the patient has ulcerative colitis I usually discontinue the antibiotics in 7 to 10 days. If the patient has Crohn's colitis, however, and especially in the face of known fistulas, I tend to maintain the patient on either ampicillin, Keflex, or metronidazole by mouth for another 2 to 3 weeks. Metronidazole often may inhibit the appetite and produce nausea, and in those situations I use ampicillin or a cephalosporin. As noted above, in those patients with Crohn's disease who will require further long-term therapy, a Broviac catheter is placed during the acute phase with continued hyperalimentation at home. In those patients with dramatic improvement in whom hyperalimentation does not appear to be required, I will still discharge them with the line in place, knowing that if there is an exacerbation in the succeeding weeks parenteral feeding can always be restarted. Once the patient has improved, symptomatic medications such as antidiarrheals can be reinstituted (although this must still be done cautiously). It is not unusual to see a patient on referral who has been well treated during an acute episode with persistent diarrhea at home because the physician is leery of inducing another megacolon. If there are not systemic symptoms and the sedimentation rate has returned toward normal, careful clinical judgment will indicate that antidiarrheals can be used once again.

In this chapter, I have tried to point out that each patient with fulminant colitis and/or toxic megacolon must be treated aggressively with a variety of therapeutic modalities and in an individualized manner. In following the patient from the beginning of an episode to the end, I have tried not to create a cookbook technique of treatment but have rather provided only the essentials, with the hope that experience and clinical judgment will result in bringing the patient back to health. Surgical intervention is neither to be ignored nor is it to be considered inevitable. In the practice of gastroenterology, there are few cases more rewarding than those which allow the experience of taking care of an acutely ill patient (and his family) and of following the case through to improvement. If the patient goes into remission and subsequently leads a normal life, I believe the physician will feel that the rewards more than compensate for the intensity and time spend during the acute treatment period.

CROHN'S DISEASE OF THE COLON

BURTON I. KORELITZ, M.D.

The classic description of ileitis reported in 1932 concerned 14 patients with a granulomatous inflammatory process involving the terminal segment of the small intestine. It was established soon after, however, that this entity could cross the ileocecal valve, involve the colon in conjunction with the ileum—subsequently referred to as ileocolits—or involve the colon without associated ileitis—now called Crohn's disease of the colon.

DEFINITION

The diagnosis of Crohn's disease of the colon implies an inflammatory process with gross and histologic features characteristic of Crohn's disease, involving any amount of the colon from a short segment to the entire organ. The process may be continuous or characterized by skip areas of involvement. Since Crohn's disease is characteristically an asymmetric process, one wall of the colon may be clearly involved while the opposite wall appears normal. Involved areas may be the sites of transverse fissures, fistulas, and pseudodiverticula, while grossly uninvolved areas may be the site of microscopic inflammation. Most commonly, the rectal segment appears normal or at least relatively uninvolved when compared with the more proximal colon. Crohn's disease of the colon most often affects some combination of areas including the right colon. This may be cecum to ascending, transverse, descending, or sigmoid colon. It may be transverse alone or extending to some point more distal. It may involve the left colon alone, with or without extension to the rectum. When the cecum is involved there is usually at least microscopic involvement of the terminal ileum as well; despite this, lack of gross involvement of the terminal ileum serves to retain colonic involvement under the classification of Crohn's colitis. There are cases of Crohn's disease limited to the rectal segment. Technically these must be considered cases of Crohn's disease of the colon even though they are exceptional and should probably maintain their own identity.

Crohn's disease of the colon is the third most common form of Crohn's disease accounting for approximately 25 percent of cases, following ileocolitis (40%), and ileitis (30%). Cases of Crohn's disease manifested by perirectal abscesses and fistulas which remain unassociated with bowel involvement, and cases of Crohn's diseases of the stomach, duodenum, or more proximal tissues, unassociated with more distal bowel disease, must be extremely rare. Though Crohn's disease limited to the colon has the same peak age of onset, in the latter half of the second decade, as other distributions of the disease, in patients with onset after the age of 50 Crohn's colitis is more common than ileocolitis. This is accounted for mostly by cases of Crohn's disease of the left colon and the occasional cases of Crohn's proctitis previously mentioned. Crohn's disease is slightly more common in females than in males, and this is true of Crohn's disease of the colon as well as other distributions.

DIFFERENTIAL DIAGNOSIS

The differential diagnosis of Crohn's disease from ulcerative and other kinds of colitis is particularly difficult when the inflammatory process is limited to the left colon. An acute infectious colitis can usually be identified by history, culture, and the self-limited course. A postantibiotic or pseudomembranous colitis can be recognized by historical and endoscopic features aided by a positive *Clostridium difficile* titer. A parasitic colitis can be determined by historical features and stool examinations. Ulcerative colitis can easily be ruled out if the rectal segment is spared and the mucosa appears normal at sigmoidoscopy. If the rectal segment is involved, however, differential gross and microscopic features are helpful but not always absolute. The most difficult problems in differential diagnosis occur in older patients with inflammatory processes involving the left colon. One is diverticular disease, which commonly involves the left colon and is often blamed for the passage of blood rectally even though it might not be the cause. The occasional appearance of longitudinal fistulas from diverticulum to diverticulum in the presence of other features of a colitis will help to clarify the diagnosis of Crohn's disease of the left colon. The other process is ischemic colitis, in which the diagnosis is supported by a sudden onset, associated degenerative diseases, and progressive deterioration or a self-limited course.

HISTOLOGIC FEATURES

Biopsies of rectal and colonic mucosa are important in the diagnosis of Crohn's disease. Even in those cases of Crohn's disease of the colon in which the rectal mucosa appears normal, rectal biopsies show nonspecific acute and chronic inflammation in about 60 percent. They also reveal, however, indicators of inflammation more specific for Crohn's disease in about 40 percent. These include crypt abscesses, some with eosinophils or macrophages, preservation of the mucosal goblet cells; disproportionate inflammation in the submucosa; lymphoid nodules; and lymphangiectasia. In 20 to 35 percent of patients characteristic granulomas and less well developed microgranulomas are found. When multiple biopsy specimens are taken and serial sections are studied, the yield of these diagnostic lesions increases. They are more likely to be found when the mucosa appears grossly normal than when the biopsy specimen is taken from a site of obvious inflammation. On colonoscopy biopsy specimens have also shown inflammation in areas more proximal where the mucosa appears normal, increasing the extent of involvement beyond that seen on x-ray films. Since there is evidence that Crohn's disease involves the entire gastrointestinal tract, definition of extent should include the diagnostic modality used to determine it (roentgenography versus endoscopy). Granulomas and microgranulomas are found much less frequently in colonoscopic biopsies than rectal biopsies, whether the mucosa appears normal or inflamed.

CARCINOMA OF THE COLON

Carcinoma of the intestine occurs less commonly in bowel involved with Crohn's disease than with ulcerative colitis, but its incidence is statistically significant. The incidence of carcinoma of the colon complicating Crohn's disease is approximately six times as great as in the average population, and the risk increases with duration of disease and extent of involvement just as it does in ulcerative colitis. Crohn's disease of the colon does not lend itself to a surveillance program as readily as ulcerative colitis because of stricturing, shortening, and extensive deformity. Nevertheless, dysplasia is prevalent and signifies a premalignant state. Therefore, if the colonoscope can be passed through the colon it should be done on a regular surveillance basis after 10 years of disease with biopsies performed throughout. Multiple synchronous neoplasms have been disclosed in resected specimens of Crohn's disease of the colon.

PREGNANCY AND FERTILITY

The fertility rate for women with Crohn's disease is not statistically different from that of the general population. In women with active Crohn's disease, however, the ability to conceive is reduced. One report concluded that fertility was even more compromised in patients with Crohn's disease of the colon than with other distributions of the disease. Current evidence supports a program of drug therapy in anticipation of pregnancy to improve the likelihood of conception.

Once pregnancy occurs there is an increased rate of premature delivery and spontaneous abortion attributable to active Crohn's disease. Again, disease activity should be suppressed with drug therapy throughout pregnancy to reduce this risk. Treatment with corticosteroids and sulfasalazine has been shown to be safe in regard to fetal outcome and nursing. The most favorable outlook for pregnancy depends on keeping Crohn's disease activity suppressed.

Pregnancy does not serve to worsen the course of the Crohn's disease in the female patient. Should the need for surgical intervention arise, however, survival of the fetus is severely threatened and the risk to the mother increased. Vigorous drug therapy is warranted for control of the disease for the sake of both the mother and the child.

MEDICAL MANAGEMENT

No one drug has been shown to be indefinitely effective in controlling Crohn's disease. Many drugs, however, have demonstrated their effectiveness in some distribution or some phase of activity. These include corticosteroids and adrenocorticotropic hormone (ACTH), sulfasalazine, (6-mercaptopurine and azathioprine), metronidazole, and broad-spectrum antibiotics. In general, all of these drugs have been more effective in Crohn's disease of the colon than in other distributions of Crohn's disease.

Adrenal Corticosteroids

Corticosteroids or ACTH almost always work well in Crohn's disease of the colon. When the patient is overtly or acutely ill, these drugs are almost always required to effect a remission, which then creates a role for the chronic phase drugs which earlier had less opportunity to be effective. Steroids serve to reduce inflammation rapidly; eliminate fever, diarrhea, and pain; and increase appetite and well-being. In some instances the remission that follows will be long, but eventually there will be a recurrence if a chronic phase drug is not added to the program. In still more cases, the symptoms of Crohn's disease of the colon will recur soon after stopping the steroids or even while the dosage is being reduced. When steroids are used on an ambulatory basis, the initial dose should be higher than that calculated to be effective. If prednisone is chosen, at least 60 mg daily should be prescribed, preferably in four divided doses. Once the favorable response is evident, which occurs within 2 to 10 days, a formula is established for the rate of reduction as guided by the original severity of symptoms or physical findings and the rate of response. On the average, it should take about a month to eliminate the prednisone. This time should be utilized to plan chronic phase therapy and introduce the new drug or method of administration. Often it is necessary to reintroduce or raise the dose of steroids soon after their initial elimination or before the reduction schedule can be completed. Under these circumstances the dose should once more be brought to a level calculated to suppress the disease. Raising the dose by small increments involves the risk of not effecting a remission and permitting the disease to become more entrenched and more difficult to eliminate. The inflammation should be suppressed as early as possible to reduce the risk of chronicity and the temptation to administer steroids at some dosage level indefinitely. Steroids should not be considered maintenance drugs. When used for prolonged periods these drugs cause many complications of their own which then substitute for or add to the manifestations and infirmities of the primary bowel disease.

When Crohn's disease is severe enough to warrant hospitalization, intravenous ACTH should be favored over oral steroids. Crystalline ACTH may be administered continuously at a rate of 120 U given over 24 hours or as a bolus of 40 U given every 8 hours. Both forms seem to be equally effective. The volume of intravenous fluids in which the ACTH is given may vary with the degree of dehydration. If hydration is not clinically necessary, the ACTH may be given in 500 ml of fluid, preferably water rather than saline to minimize salt retention. Otherwise a volume of 1,000 to 3,000 ml may be used. Once a remission is secured, the dose of intravenous ACTH can be reduced and intramuscular ACTH or oral steroids or both can be substituted. Oral steroids can then be reduced according to the formula previously mentioned, and eventually eliminated. Meanwhile, time is available for the introduction of chronic phase therapy. The specific goals of ACTH or steroid therapy should be determined for each case.

Sulfasalazine

Sulfasalazine has been the chronic phase drug with the longest use history in the treatment of Crohn's disease. Although its effectiveness against active Crohn's disease in general has been questioned, its favorable role in treating Crohn's disease of the colon has been confirmed. This may best be explained by the need for colonic bacteria to split the diazo bond releasing the effective moiety, 5-aminosalicylic acid. Its effectiveness as a prophylactic agent in maintaining remissions of Crohn's disease of the colon, similar to its major role in ulcerative colitis, has not been clearly demonstrated but is most likely valid. Once remission is accomplished, whether attributable to sulfasalazine or not, this drug, again similar to the situation in ulcerative colitis, should be continued indefinitely unless it has been demonstrated in the individual case to be of no value. The maintenance dose of sulfasalazine is 4 g per day to be administered in divided doses with meals and at bedtime. The full dose should be achieved slowly, however, to avoid nausea, headaches, and less common side actions. Starting with 1 tablet (0.5 g) daily and adding 1 daily until the full dose is reached or a side effect occurs, has proved to be an effective method. Clinical experience must be drawn on to achieve patient tolerance for this drug and to provide every opportunity for it to work. Even allergic skin eruptions caused by sulfasalazine should not serve to eliminate this drug. Desensitization by starting with tiny doses ($1/8$ to $1/4$ tablet daily) and slowly increasing (every 3 to 7 days) has been successful in 80 percent of cases, and the drug can be effective therapeutically for extended periods thereafter.

Immunosuppressives

It has been proven that 6-mercaptopurine effects remission in 65 to 70 percent of patients with active Crohn's disease and should be used in selected patients as a chronic phase drug. This drug has been most effective in Crohn's disease of the colon. The mean time after its introduction until it takes effect is 3.1 months. Therefore, it is often necessary to use ACTH or corticosteroids to effect a remission and allow time for the 6-mercaptopurine to take effect. The drug has served to permit elimination or at least reduction of the steroid dose, to close or improve all varieties of fistula, and to eliminate or reduce the primary bowel manifestations of the disease. Its favorable effect occurs independent of steroid therapy. Although 6-mercaptopurine is considered an immunosuppressive drug, the manner in which it achieves its success is not yet known. Leukopenia is a known side effect of the drug and should be expected at some time in each case. The initial dose is 50 mg daily, and complete blood count and platelets are monitored once weekly for the first 3 weeks. When it is shown that the patient tolerates the drug well, the frequency of monitoring can be reduced. If the blood count permits, the dose can then be increased to 50 mg on one day alternating with 50 mg twice daily, or to 50 mg twice a day.

Many patients and managing physicians fear the use of 6-mercaptopurine, mostly because of the high incidence of lymphomas and other malignancies when other immunosuppressive drugs have been used as part of a program for renal transplantations or chemotherapy. In those instances, however, multiple immunosuppressive agents have been used simultaneously and doses have been larger than ever used in the treatment of Crohn's disease. Serious complications have been demonstrated infrequently coincident with the small doses of 6-mercaptopurine used in treating Crohn's disease. Pancreatitis has occurred in about 5 percent of patients but in all instances was reversible. Bone marrow depression has not occurred since experience has been acquired in management. The rate of important complications of all drugs used in the treatment of Crohn's disease, especially corticosteroids, has been higher. When 6-mercaptopurine has been used in intelligent patients, when compliance has been complete, when all information known and unknown about the drug has been shared, and when the course of uncontrolled Crohn's disease of the colon has been described, most patients want an opportunity to try 6-mercaptopurine and do so without mishap. The drug is continued for an arbitrary period of

2 years once its effectiveness and its ease of management are demonstrated. Thereafter, some patients prefer to continue and others to stop. Relapse is anticipated, the mean period being 6 months after stopping the 6-mercaptopurine, but the recurrence can be mild and amenable to other drugs, or it may not take place at all until much later. Normal childbirth has been experienced by women who become pregnant while taking 6-mercaptopurine. Nevertheless, women have been advised to avoid pregnancy and men have been advised not to impregnate their wives until 3 months after the drug has been stopped.

Metronidazole

Metronidazole has been demonstrated to be effective in reducing perirectal and perineal abscesses and fistulas. Unfortunately, a dose range of 1.5 to 2.0 g daily is required to accomplish this, a level at which drug toxicity in the form of peripheral neuropathy often occurs. Even after the drug is stopped the neuritis may persist for many months. Coincidentally, recurrence of the abscesses and fistulas occurs as the drug is stopped or reduced. Metronidazole has also been shown to have an effect approximately equivalent to sulfasalazine against the primary bowel symptoms at the lesser dosage of 250 mg 3 times a day.

Broad-Spectrum Antibiotics

In addition to their supplemental role in treating the secondary infection accompanying perirectal and intra-abdominal abscesses, broad-spectrum antibiotics occasionally will be effective in the treatment of Crohn's disease of the colon when all other drugs have failed. In my experience the one most responsible for long remission is ampicillin, which I have continued to administer for more than a year in some patients. I have also witnessed remissions attributable to its use. I have used cephalexin (Keflex) and tetracyclne also, initially as supplemental drugs followed by their achieving a primary role. Chronic antibiotic therapy is specifically warranted for ileovesical fistulas when the only clinical manifestation is pyuria.

OTHER CONSIDERATIONS IN MEDICAL MANAGEMENT

Drugs given for pain should be used reluctantly and sparingly. Drug abuse and addiction are common in young people with Crohn's disease and the situation is compounded during postoperative periods.

Nonspecific antidiarrheal agents may be used to supplement a treatment program, but care should be taken to minimize the risk of dependence, addiction, and contribution to the development of colonic dilation and megacolon.

A small bowel tube is often used to treat colonic obstruction contributed to by a stricture, an abscess, or a mass.

Parenteral nutrition may accelerate the healing of the primary bowel inflammation, obstruction due more to inflammation than fibrosis and even fistulas. If ACTH or a steroid is used at the same time, the value of stopping oral feedings is questionable. Parenteral nutrition does not lead to permanent reversal of the inflammatory process, and therefore the temporary period of improvement should be used to initiate a new mode of drug therapy.

Emotional factors do not seem to be causative in Crohn's disease but clearly serve to aggravate its course. Although no generalization should be made, many patients will profit by consultation with a therapist, whether a psychiatrist or psychologist, a family therapist, or a psychiatric social worker. In this regard the self-help groups offered by Chapters of the National Foundation for Ileitis and Colitis have been extremely helpful.

CONSIDERATIONS REGARDING SURGERY

In the natural course of Crohn's disease the extent of involvement originally demonstrated by roentgenography remains more or less stable independent of the severity of the local involvement. With clinical worsening the disease might extend distally but not proximally. Once the bowel is transected for purposes of resection or diversion, however, the Crohn's disease spreads proximally. The extension occurs earlier when the operation is performed for ileitis or ielocolitis, later for colitis involving the right colon, and still later for colitis grossly limited to the left colon. Regardless of the original extent, given enough time the proximal spread can be anticipated in all cases. By the time clinical symptoms of recurrent Crohn's disease occur, characteristic features are already present on x-ray films and have probably been visible there for varying periods of time. Should colonoscopy or ileoscopy be performed prior to recurrent symptoms, evidence of inflammation is frequently encountered in the new terminal ileum. If gross inflammation has not yet appeared, biopsy specimens are likely to show histological features of inflammation, sometimes including granulomas.

Despite the provocation by resection or transection, surgical intervention has been indicated in approximately 70 percent of patients with Crohn's disease during their lifetimes. When Crohn's disease is grossly confined to the colon, many surgeons have managed the disease like ulcerative colitis with ileostomy and total proctocolectomy. Studies by two groups showed that the rate of recurrent ileitis in the patients with ileostomy was no greater than in the patients with ulcerative colitis, even though ileostomy revisions might be required more often. Other investigations, including my own, have demonstrated that the ileostomy is no barrier to extension of the Crohn's disease proximally after transection. The issue is academic to the extent that if surgery, which includes ileostomy, must be done, then it must be done, but it should not be performed with the expectation that Crohn's disease of the colon can be cured in this manner.

The Kock, or continent, ileostomy is contraindicated for Crohn's disease because of the likelihood of recurrence in the pouch. Only with due regard for this high risk might this procedure be considered and then only in very special circumstances.

There are two alternatives to total proctocolectomy. When the rectal segment is grossly spared, resection with ileorectal anastomosis might be feasible. In some instances in which the distal extent of Crohn's disease of the colon is more proximal, an ileotransverse, or ileodescending colostomy, or an ileosigmoidoscopy might be considered. Surgeons are unwilling to perform an ileorectal anastomosis in the presence of grossly active disease in the rectal segment. Microscopic inflammation need not necessarily contraindicate an ileorectal anastomosis. Retention of the anal sphincter contributes to quality of life, even if the average number of stools per day increases with an anastomosis. Even if the Crohn's disease eventually extends to the previously normal or almost normal appearing rectal segment, the few additional years gained without need for an ileostomy warrant considering this option. Sometimes the clinical situation necessitating the colectomy is such that performing an anastomosis is contraindicated. The rectum under these circumstances is left in situ and an ileostomy is performed with the intention of either leaving the rectum as is or doing the reanastomosis at a later date. The rectum, however, is subject to the same diversion proctitis that occurs when a temporary colostomy is performed for obstructing cancer of the colon or diverticular disease. It has been shown that inflammatory changes that develop in the rectum can be reversed with reanastomosis. Whether the proctitis which occurs in the rectal segment is purely diversion or Crohn's disease accentuated by the diversion, a primary reanastomosis should be favored. If this is not feasible, then the reanastomosis should be performed as early as possible.

PROGNOSIS AND INDICATIONS FOR SURGERY

Crohn's disease of the colon will most often require total proctocolectomy with ileostomy if surgical resection is warranted. This situation contrasts with a limited ileitis, for which minimal resection can be performed with reanastomosis and preservation of bowel continuity and sphincter control. In addition to having to cope with an ileostomy, the patient cannot be given the satisfaction of cure of the disease, as would be the case with ulcerative colitis. Therefore, every effort should be made to bring the disease into remission once again with nonoperative methods and to maintain that remission.

Fortunately, almost all current programs of drug therapy have been more effective for Crohn's disease of the colon than for any other type of Crohn's disease. Once ACTH or corticosteroids has reduced or eliminated the inflammatory process, sulfasalazine has been effective in completing and/or maintaining the remission for long periods in many cases. Once it is clear that sulfasalazine has failed, mercaptopurine also has been more effective in Crohn's disease involving the colon than in ileal disease. Patients should be made aware of the opportunity to be treated with mercaptopurine for Crohn's disease of the colon, particularly as an alternative to a surgical resection that would include an ileostomy as well as the risk of recurrent ileitis in the stoma.

There are few remaining absolute indications for surgical intervention in Crohn's disease. These include:

1. Massive hemorrhage that cannot be reversed by large doses of intravenous ACTH or corticosteroids.
2. Perforation of the colon.
3. Toxic megacolon that cannot be reversed. In my experience and that of Dr. Daniel Present, dilatation of the colon in Crohn's disease responds even better than the same complication of ulcerative colitis to a nonoperative program of intravenous ACTH, broad-spectrum antibiotic coverage, small bowel tube and rectal tube decompression, and rolling the patient to both sides and into the prone position. (See chapter *Fulminant Colitis and Toxic Megacolon*.)
4. Carcinoma of the rectum or colon. This diagnosis is made preoperatively but it has been done by both sigmoidoscopic and colonoscopic examinations and by biopsies.

Other indications for surgery in the course of Crohn's disease of the colon are relative:

1. The primary bowel symptoms usually respond to drug therapy, particularly when all drugs of proven value are utilized alone or in combination.
2. Colonic-vesical fistulas respond to 6-mercaptopurine in most instances.
3. Colonic-gastric, duodenal, jejunal, and ileal fistulas respond to 6-mercaptopurine in most instances.
4. Colonic and rectovaginal fistulas respond to mercaptopurine in most instances. Surgical repair of a rectovaginal fistula without colectomy can be considered only in special cases, and even then it should be accomplished by a diverting ileostomy.
5. Colonic-abdominal wall abscess-fistula that does not respond to drainage, antibiotics, and a new program of drug therapy might require colonic resection.
6. Perirectal, perineal, vulval, and scrotal fistulas often improve with simple drainage, usually in conjunction with a drug program that emphasizes 6-mercaptopurine or metronidazole. When this approach is not satisfactory, a modified Park's procedure, with dissection of fistulas to their common source and eradication of the underlying intersphincteric abscess, has been effective in preventing recurrences in 75 percent of patients without the need to resort to bowel resection. Extensive and destructive abscesses and fistulas eroding the perineum and buttocks have been successfully handled in this way, even as a primary procedure, thereby giving a new program of drug therapy the opportunity to concentrate on the primary bowel disease. Diversion of the

fecal stream by either colostomy or ileostomy is not effective therapy for this problem and causes the additional risk of recurrent Crohn's disease proximal to the transection.

7. Rectal strictures, unless markedly advanced, can be dilated with the 11-mm rigid scope, the finger, or both. With an improved drug program and frequent dilations, colectomy can be avoided. Suppository preparations of corticosteroids often aid this process.
8. Colonic strictures can sometimes be dilated via the colonoscope but infrequently cause obstruction. Only when there is a strong suspicion that the colonic stricture masks a carcinoma and the region cannot be satisfactorily biopsied should colectomy be considered.
9. Pyoderma gangrenosum not responding to steroids or mercaptopurine might require colectomy.
10. Poor quality of life sometimes warrants no further pursuit of an effective drug program and mandates surgical resection despite the risk of extension of disease.

In the past 5 years, I can recall only four patients with Crohn's disease of the colon who required surgical resection. One had a carcinoma of the rectum disclosed by rectal biopsy, and colectomy revealed multiple neoplasms. The second had a segmental resection of the descending colon for a long stricture associated with a mass causing pain, weight loss, and poor quality of life; a diverting ileostomy was performed and then closed three months later. The third had a fistula from the splenic flexure to the abdominal wall which was eliminated by a successful segmental resection. The fourth had total proctocolectomy performed for ulcerative colitis, and pathologic examination of the resected specimen revealed histologic evidence favoring Crohn's disease of the colon.

IDIOPATHIC INFLAMMATORY BOWEL DISEASE AND NEOPLASIA

THEODORE M. BAYLESS, M.D.

Patients with ulcerative colitis involving the entire colon are, after 20 years, at a 20-fold increased risk of developing colon cancer as compared with age-matched control populations. The average age at cancer discovery is 46, compared with an average age of 62 for non-colitis-related colon cancer. Those with macroscopic left-sided colitis have a delayed onset of increased cancer risk, while patients with self-limited, albeit recurrent, proctitis are not more susceptible to colorectal malignancy. Crohn's disease in the colon and in areas of longstanding ileitis, especially if bypassed, predisposes some patients to adenocarcinoma.

The physician providing care for an individual with idiopathic inflammatory bowel disease (ulcerative colitis, Crohn's disease, or indeterminant colitis) must be aware of these increased risks and must plot a strategy for preventing malignant degeneration of the bowel in each such patient.

ULCERATIVE COLITIS

Risk Factors

Duration

Duration of colitis is the best recognized risk factor. After 8 years of pancolitis, one begins to encounter unexpected "premature" colon cancers. Butt et al calculated from three series of 2,258 patients that there was a cancer risk of one patient per 564 patient years during the first decade of "extensive" colitis[1]. Thus a doctor caring for 56 such patients would find one cancer. In the second decade after the onset of symptoms, 13 cancers were found in 922 patients, so that one in seven patients with extensive colitis would develop colon cancer. In the third decade, only 323 patients were observed and in nine a carcinoma was discovered. In this small sample, one in four patients had adenocarcinoma of the colon. This was more than a 30-fold increased risk over that in the general population. Removal of most of the colon via a subtotal colectomy does not eliminate the cancer risk in the retained rectum. Baker et al[2] cite a risk of one cancer per 117 patient years after 20 years of colitis.

Age of Onset of Colitis

The age at the onset of pancolitis seems to affect the colorectal cancer risk. Patients whose ulcerative colitis began before age 20 have, as shown in several series, a shorter lag time before cancer develops than those whose bowel inflammation starts after age 20. Since more patients with youthful onset have extensive colitis as opposed to proctitis, extent of disease may be a factor in this seemingly age-related risk factor.

Extent of Colitis

The extent of macroscopic bowel inflammation correlates directly with cancer development. As cited, patients with pancolitis or "extensive" colitis, at least retrograde up to the hepatic flexure are at greatest risk, perhaps 25 percent by 20 years. At the other extreme, patients with disease restricted to the rectum or sigmoid colon are reportedly at no increased risk. When cancers are found in patients with proctitis, they have usually already reached the age of noncolitis-related colorectal cancer, i.e., the seventh and eighth decade.

Left-sided colitis, as defined by macroscopic disease identifiable by single contrast barium enema, produces an increased risk of carcinoma, but this risk doesn't seem to rise until after 12 to 16 years or longer. It is not yet known if histologic evidence of extensive colitis, as determined by colonoscopic biopsies or as inferred by double contrast barium enemas, will move a patient from the seemingly delayed risk inferred by the left-sided colitis label into the same risk situation as patients with macroscopic evidence of pancolitis.

Colitis Activity

Colitis activity is not related to cancer risk. Although patients with continuously active forms of colitis garner much of our attention, it is those with long periods of quiescent disease who make up most of today's colitis–cancer population. This lack of symptoms, either spontaneously achieved or aided by long-term sulfasalazine administration, tends to give both the patient and physician a false sense of security. Diagnostic studies are not performed, and often patient-physician contacts diminish in frequency, regularity, and thoroughness. Patients with severe or chronic unremitting ulcerative colitis are often removed from the at-risk pool by early colectomy. Another factor leading to late cancer recognition is the similarity between the symptoms of colon cancer and those of the underlying colitis.

Mucosal Dysplasia

High-grade dysplasia consists primarily of dysplastic cytologic changes in the epithelium comparable to those found in preinvasive neoplastic transformation in the epithelium of other organs, such as the cervix or bronchus. Dysplasia is usually, but not always, seen in the context of a glandular or villiform growth pattern like that of noncolitis adenomas. This neoplastic transformation can be found in the colon of almost all patients with ulcerative colitis who have already developed colon cancer. The concept of dysplasia being premalignant or "precancer" is strengthened by its being found in at least 20 percent of colectomy specimens from patients with ulcerative colitis of more than 10 years duration who had no evidence of invasive cancer. After 25 years of extensive colitis, the cumulative frequency of dysplasia without cancer in patients who underwent colectomy had increased linearly up to 74 percent in one Scandinavian series[3].

It would be wrong to infer that dysplasia always culminates in cancer, since ulcerative colitis itself does not, to my knowledge, lead inevitably to colonic cancer. In most newly instituted "surveillance" colonoscopy programs, however, at least half of the patients undergoing colectomy because of biopsy-diagnosed "precancer" had one or more foci of invasive cancer somewhere in their colons. The cancers were of more advanced Dukes grades (B2 and C) if the dysplasia was associated with an endoscopically or radiographically demonstrable mass.

The question of how long it takes for an area of severe dysplasia to become invasive is difficult to answer because of the varying degrees of dysplasia found in ulcerative colitis, as well as the lack of evidence of an inevitable progression from low-grade to high-grade dysplasia to cancer. Also, the dysplastic areas are often distributed in a patchy fashion and may remain undetected even after very careful colonoscopic examination and randomly collected biopsies. In addition, the natural history of the process is now often interrupted by colectomy. There are some clues to the "lag time" between dysplasia development and the progression to invasive carcinoma. Patients with ulcerative colitis who have had a colectomy which shows only "precancer" have, on the average, had colitis for 7 or 8 years less than those with colonic cancer. For example, in the Scandinavian series cited the mean duration in 41 patients with "precancer" was 8 years, while in ten who had developed colonic cancer it was 16 years. One of our patients had unrecognized "precancer" in a random rectal biopsy 9 years before Dukes C colon cancer was detected in the left colon.

Based on our current knowledge, the patient with inflammatory bowel disease whose colon contains confirmed histologic evidence of dysplasia must be considered at higher risk of cancer already being present elsewhere in the colon or of developing in the next 5 to 10 years than the patient whose colon is repeatedly free of dysplasia after careful and complete colonoscopies with multiple biopsy specimens taken from six to eight separated areas of the colon.

Strategies for Managing Colon Cancer Risk

Prophylactic Colectomy

Since a total colectomy will not only cure ulcerative colitis but will also prevent colonic cancer, physicians caring for patients with severe, extensive, unresponsive, and longstanding ulcerative colitis should have a low threshold for recommending a colectomy. The availability of ileostomy alternatives, such as the Kock pouch or ileoanal pouch anastomoses, have made it easier to convince patients to have a total colectomy. The presence of confirmed high-grade dysplasia is now a well-accepted indicator for colectomy, as will be detailed in the section on colonoscopy surveillance in this chapter.

Prior to development and validation of surveillance methods, some writers were recommending prophylactic colectomy for cancer prevention in all patients with pancolitis, regardless of activity status, at some point before 10 years had elapsed. Others made this recommendation mainly for those patients with a childhood onset of ulcerative colitis. With the alternative of surveillance for dysplasia, the risk of cancer, perhaps 5 percent in the total colitis population after 20 years, does not seem high enough to justify routine proctocolectomy and ileostomy, with its associated morbidity, mortality, and inconvenience. Even for the high-risk population with panco-

TABLE 1 Suggested Patient Management Related to Classification of Dysplasia

Biopsy Classification	Management
Negative	Continued surveillance
Indefinite	
Probably negative	
Unknown	Short-interval follow-up
Probably positive	(3–6 months)
Positive	
Low-grade dysplasia	Short-interval follow-up (3 months); or colectomy if macroscopic lesion
High-grade dysplasia	Colectomy (after confirmation of dysplasia)

(Modified from Riddell et al. 1983.)

litis of more than 8 years duration, it seems to be reasonable and safe to rely on regular colonoscopy and biopsy surveillance for dysplasia. In some individuals, however, such as a person in his twenties who has already had pancolitis for 8 or 10 years and perhaps also has a family history of colon cancer, one could argue that a total colectomy is preferable to a lifetime of colonoscopies with their accompanying morbidity, cost, and regularly recurrent anxiety. Prophylactic colectomy may also be recommended for a patient with pancolitis who has developed an irreversible stricture or who cannot or will not be a candidate for a regular surveillance program.

Early Cancer Diagnosis

The diagnosis of colorectal cancer in a patient with ulcerative colitis is usually quite difficult, especially at an early stage when tumors are small or flat. Even a polypoid cancer can be mistaken for an inflammatory pseudopolyp. In my experience, most patients with colon cancer and ulcerative colitis who underwent colectomy only after the cancer became symptomatic have died because of metastatic malignancy. Barium enemas, even with double contrast techniques, may miss well-developed carcinomas or dysplasia in the setting of chronic inflammatory bowel disease. The risk of radiation exposure would be another point against the regular and repeated use of barium contrast studies to seek early neoplasms or dysplastic masses.

Proctosigmoidoscopy is of limited use because only about one-third of the cancers in patients with ulcerative colitis occur in the rectum. The use of a 60-cm flexible sigmoidoscope will probably prove to be a helpful adjunct to colonoscopy.

Biopsies through the proctosigmoidoscope, flexible sigmoidoscope, or colonoscope are the most useful methods of diagnosing dysplasia and adenocarcinoma. Nevertheless, there are sampling problems. Negative biopsy specimens of a mass or stricture do not rule out carcinoma or dysplasia. Also, invasive cancer may arise below the surface and not be reached by the usual superficial colonoscopic biopsies.

Serum colonic embryonic antigen (CEA) determinations are not useful as an early detection method because the CEA levels may not be increased in early localized (Dukes A) adenocarcinoma, and CEA levels can be elevated with active ulcerative colitis. Tests for occult blood are useful only if they become positive after a long period of disease inactivity.

Surveillance for Dysplasia

Patients who fall into a high-risk group should be entered into a surveillance program for dysplasia and early carcinoma. Such programs are based primarily on colonoscopic examinations and biopsies of multiple areas. An air contrast barium enema can be used at the outset of the program to draw attention to areas of thickened mucosa, subtle plaque-like areas of dysplasia, or strictures. I also use a double contrast barium enema if there is an unresolved question of a macroscopic lesion on colonoscopy, or occasionally as a mid-surveillance procedure in someone whose precolonoscopy preparations have been inadequate to examine the colon thoroughly.

Surveillance should be considered for all patients with ulcerative colitis or indeterminant colitis except those with proctitis or proctosigmoiditis. Since the latter patients do not seem to be at increased risk of cancer development, flexible sigmoidoscopy with biopsies for dysplasia every 3 to 5 years seems reasonable. Patients with extensive colitis who have had a partial colectomy sparing the rectum are definitely at the same risk as if their colon were intact, and they require regular surveillance.

Colonoscopic examinations should be started after seven years of extensive colitis. There is some evidence to suggest that the patient who has left-sided colitis may not be at increased risk until 12 or 15 years. I usually perform colonoscopy and multiple biopsies after eight or ten years to determine the histologic extent of colitis. If the biopsies are negative for dysplasia, one can perhaps study such patients at 2- or 3-year intervals and use flexible sigmoidoscopy for some examinations.

Rectal and sigmoid biopsies can be done in the intervals between colonoscopies, since dysplasia can occur in the rectum. However, there are enough patients who have had dysplasia and carcinoma in the colon with negative rectal biopsies to make this unreliable as the only surveillance procedure.

At colonoscopy or flexible sigmoidoscopy, biopsies should be taken from thickened plaque-like areas, nodular areas of mucosa, polypoid lesions including the sides and base of any polyps, and any strictured areas. Cytology brushing is added for strictures. Multiple random biopsy specimens (usually 2 or 3) are obtained from flat areas of mucosa every 10 to 15 cm from the rectum to the cecum. Areas of obviously active colitis may contain histologic evidence of regeneration and atypia that may be difficult to distinguish from neoplastic dysplasia. Extensive areas of inflammatory polyps may be a problem for the endoscopist in terms of where and how closely to sample. Large polypoid areas, and polyps with marked variation in coloration and size and in areas with no obvious active inflammation nearby should be biopsied. If large areas of presumed inflammatory polyps are not biopsied, one should make an effort to sample them at the next study, if they are still present. I believe it is sometimes quite difficult for the endoscopist to feel comfortable about some areas of presumed inflammatory polyps in a patient who hasn't had an obvious clinical relapse for many months or years. I have recommended colectomy in a few such patients whom I felt uncomfortable following in terms of being able to recognize dysplasia or cancer.

Biopsy specimens from different areas should be put in separate carefully labeled containers. A very detailed diagram and report of the gross findings is essential so that the pathologist can appreciate the macroscopic setting from which a particular specimen was taken. About half of the dysplasia-containing biopsy specimens taken from a mass have been associated with an underlying invasive carcinoma. Knowing that a specimen came from an obviously active area of colitis also helps the pathologist's interpretation. Close collaboration among the gastroenterologist, the pathologist, and the patient is essential if a surveillance program is to accomplish its goal of detecting dysplasia before carcinoma has become surgically incurable.

Interpretation of Dysplasia and Recommendations

A new classification system based on the extensive deliberations of an international panel of expert pathologists is helping to reduce the confusion as to terminology and interpretation which has plagued both clinicians and pathologists. A detailed atlas of this classification system is published in Human Pathology[4]. Reprints are available from the NFIC, 444 Park Avenue South, New York, NY 10016, Tel; (212-685-3440).

Negative for Dysplasia. When all biopsy specimens of six to eight areas are normal or show features of quiescent or active colitis, regular yearly surveillance should be continued. This assumes that the colonoscopic examination was complete and that the patient has no symptoms or roentgenographic changes that would raise the suspicion of carcinoma. Studies are still in progress to try to determine a safe interval before the next study if all biopsies are negative. Some physicians are discussing two- or 3-year lags with flexible sigmoidoscopy and biopsies interspersed. This could probably be considered in patients with purely left-sided colitis.

Indefinitive for Dysplasia. If the changes are "indefinite for dysplasia, probably negative," periodic surveillance is probably safe. If the interpretation is "indefinite for dysplasia" and/or either "unknown" or "probably positive," a repeat colonoscopy within 3 to 6 months is requested. If active inflammation caused the indecision, then repeat biopsy after several months of clinically effective therapy is appropriate.

Positive for Dysplasia. If a pathologist who is familiar with this classification system feels that low-grade dysplasia is present in a biopsy specimen from a mass or stricture, the slides are shown to another pathologist for confirmation and then colectomy is recommended. If the tissue containing low-grade dysplasia is definitely known to have come from a random specimen of a flat area of mucosa, repeat biopsy specimens from the same area and from the entire colon are obtained within 3 months. If dysplasia is found repeatedly in the same area or in other areas of the colon, then colectomy is recommended. Some authors recommend colectomy for any degree of dysplasia on one biopsy.

Some patients with a single focus of low-grade dysplasia in a flat mucosa have either been followed or have refused or delayed surgery. In a very small number no dysplasia was found at colectomy, while in some carcinoma was present in the flat area of dysplasia. In still others the dysplasia has persisted and they have refused surgery.

If the pathologist feels that high-grade dysplasia is present, I usually ask another pathologist to review the slides and then recommend colectomy. If there is any doubt, especially in a flat area, repeat biopsies can be done; however, colectomy should be given very serious consideration.

Adenomatous Polyp. Since adenomatous poyps of the colon are common in people over 45 years of age, it is to be expected that an occasional patient with ulcerative colitis will develop an adenomatous polyp. If the patient is under 45, this is usually considered evidence of dysplasia, especially if dysplasia occurs elsewhere in the colon or on the stalk of the polyp, and colectomy is recommended. In the older patient, a single adenomatous polyp without dysplasia on the stalk and without carcinoma in the polyp has not been considered an indication, in itself, for colectomy. I have not encountered this problem often but other groups are following such patients in their regular surveillance program.

Yield From a Surveillance Program

The cumulative prevalence of dysplasia increased linearly after 4 or 5 years of colitis in a study of a series of colectomy specimens cited earlier. After 25 years of colitis, dysplasia was found in three-fourths of the colectomy specimens. Certainly this is a selected series. It is not yet clear how frequently dysplasia will be found by rectal and colonoscopic biopsy in asymptomatic patients with extensive colitis or with left-sided colitis. Lennard-Jones and his colleagues at St. Mark's Hospital in London found dysplasia in the rectal biopsy specimens of 53 of 937 patients with ulcerative colitis (5.7%). The duration and extent of colitis were not well defined. Forty-two percent of the patients with dysplasia in the rectum or colon already had developed carcinoma.

The yield of dysplasia will be higher if one is performing colonoscopy for the first time in a series of patients with chronic ulcerative colitis. Some may be symptomatic, perhaps because of carcinoma. At the Lahey Clinic, 21 percent of the first 86 patients in their series had evidence of dysplasia on rectal and colonoscopic biopsy. Ten underwent colectomy because of the dysplasia, and four had unsuspected carcinoma which was already metastatic in two patients. At the University of Chicago, 7 percent of the first 91 patients had dysplasia.

A true surveillance program would include *follow-up* colonoscopies in patients who were asymptomatic with no indication of cancer development and no obvious masses on barium enema. In such a follow-up series, Nugent and Haggitt from the Lahey Clinic found a yield of about 1 percent per year in terms of additional dysplasia in more than 100 patients in such a surveillance program. It is probably fair to estimate that in a series of patients with pancolitis lasting more than 8 years, there will be a yield of 1- to 3-percent dysplasia per year. With patients whose disease is of longer duration, the yield will be higher.

There are no comparable data on patients with left-sided colitis but the yield would presumably be the same or less.

Sensitivity of Colonoscopic Biopsies for Dysplasia

It should be stressed that this type of surveillance program may not be infallible. Dysplasia may be patchy and may not always be obvious to the endoscopist. Since the random biopsies sample only a fraction of the mucosal lining, it may not always be easily found even when cancer is present in the colon. Although this is probably a rare problem, there have been a few reports of colon cancer with no dysplasia elsewhere in the colectomy specimen. The adequacy of bowel preparation, the completeness of the colonoscopic biopsy examination, the recognition of subtle gross changes by the endoscopist, and the interpretive ability of the pathologist are all factors that influence the sensitivity of this procedure. Sending the biopsy slides to a pathologist familiar with the dysplasia classification schema for another opinion is often quite helpful.

In a setting where attention is paid to all these details, it seems reasonable to assume that a patient with ulcerative colitis who has had two completely negative studies at yearly intervals can be safely followed for at least one additional year without undue concern of colon cancer developing.

CROHN'S DISEASE

With Crohn's colitis there is at least a sixfold increased risk of colon cancer development. As with ulcerative colitis, the cancers occur at a younger than expected age; however, the risk factors in terms of duration of disease and extent of involvement are not as clear-cut. In a recent review of ten patients with colon cancer and Crohn's disease at The Johns Hopkins Hospital, Hamilton found that in two patients the inflammatory bowel disease was not diagnosed prior to cancer discovery. Crohn's disease had been recognized only 4 years before the cancer was discovered in one patient. One had carcinoma in a chronic pericolic fistula and two others had cancer in bypassed rectal pouches. Interestingly, high-grade dysplasia was found in the cancer-containing colon resection specimen of all ten of these patients.

In terms of surveillance for dysplasia, the issue is not as clear as in ulcerative colitis. As stated, the onset of Crohn's disease may be more subtle and difficult to date. Also, patients with Crohn's disease may have colonic strictures which could prevent examination of much of the colon. Others have retained rectal stumps which have become strictured at the rectum, thus preventing adequate examination. A few patients with Crohn's disease who have had their colons bypassed experienced a bowel perforation at the time of colonoscopic evaluation of the bypassed defunctionalized colon.

There is almost no data on which to base strong recommendations for surveillance in Crohn's colitis. It seems reasonable to take multiple random biopsies and to biopsy some of the nodular and polypoid areas whenever colonoscopy is done, especially if the disease is chronic and relatively quiescent. This should become more important after ten years of known disease. As a generalization, patients with Crohn's colitis and colon cancer have had inflammatory bowel disease known for an average of 20 years. Since bypassed segments of bowel may harbor malignancies, one should try to avoid creating rectal pouches or bypassed loops of bowel and to consider having these bypassed areas resected if one cannot perform representative biopsies for dyplasia on a regular basis.

Since carcinoma of the small bowel has been found in bypassed segments of ileum, this type of operation is probably best avoided. Also, one should look for an opportunity to resect bypassed defunctionalized loops. It is impossible to predict the unexpected carcinoma found occasionally in a chronically narrowed segment of small bowel at the time of resection for obstruction.

ETIOLOGIC CONSIDERATIONS

In terms of the origin of bowel cancer and the occasional lymphoma or leukemia in inflammatory bowel disease, one wonders if the repeated radiologic examinations during the long course of inflammatory bowel disease could be a contributing factor. In an effort to lessen this radiation exposure, known to some as "silent violence," one should restrict the use of repeat x-ray studies to instances in which a therapeutic decision will be made based on the result. Also in the unknown category is the possible role that immunosuppressives and metronidazole may play in future malignancies in inflammatory bowel disease. One also wonders about the chronic stasis created in Kock pouches and ileal pouch-anal anastomoses. Since there are a few reports of carcinoma in an ileostomy occurring after colectomy for ulcerative colitis and colon cancer, I have urged against these stasis-producing operations in patients with ulcerative colitis who have colon cancer.

COLLAGENOUS COLITIS

Collagenous colitis is a seemingly new syndrome that has been described in the past decade. It is unrelated to ulcerative colitis or Crohn's disease and is characterized by watery diarrhea. The syndrome usually occurs in elderly white women who have diffuse microscopic colitis with a layer of collagen deposited under the surface epithelium, but not around the colonic crypts. The collagen layer is most obvious in the sigmoid colon. The watery diarrhea is caused by decreased colonic absorptive flux in the face of the usual secretory flux; this is usually reversible with sulfasalazine or adrenocortical steroid therapy. With therapy, the collagen layer decreases, but the chronic inflammatory infiltrate usually persists.

There is no evidence that collagenous colitis is premalignant, although one elderly patient had a coexistent cancer of the colon. A number of the approximately 40 patients known to us (via the literature and as patients) had preceeding adenomatous polyps; this, interestingly, did not contain excess collagen. Dysplasia has not been reported in collagenous colitis.

REFERENCES

1. Butt JH, Lennard-Jones JE, Ritchie JK. A practical approach to the risk of cancer in inflammatory bowel disease—reassure, watch or act? Med Clin North Am 1980; 64:1203-1220.
2. Baker et al. Brit J Surg 1978; 65:865-868.
3. Kewenter J, Allman H, Hultèr L. Cancer risk in extensive ulcerative colitis. Ann Surg 1978; 188:824-828.
4. Riddel RH, et al. Dysplasia in inflammatory bowel disease: standardized classification with provisional clinical applications. Human Pathology 1983; 14:931-968.

ANORECTAL DISORDERS

SANTHAT NIVATVONGS, M.D., F.A.C.S.,
STANLEY M. GOLDBERG, M.D., F.A.C.S.

HEMORRHOID

In the upper anal canal there are cushions of submucosal tissues which are composed of connective tissues containing venules and smooth muscle fibers. Usually there are three cushions: left lateral, right anterior, and right posterior. This anatomic arrangement is remarkably constant and bears no relationship, as previously thought, to the terminal branches of the superior rectal vessels which are quite inconstant. The function of these cushions is speculative. By their bulk, they aid in anal continence, and during the act of defecation when they become engorged with blood, they cushion the anal canal and support the lining. Hemorrhoid is the pathologic term for a downward displacement of the anal cushions causing dilation of the venules.

External skin tag is a redundant fibrotic skin at the anal verge. It is usually the result of a previous thrombosed external hemorrhoid or previous anal surgery. Excision is indicated only if it causes pain, irritation, or interferes with anal hygiene.

External hemorrhoids are dilated venules of the inferior hemorrhoidal plexus located below the pectinate or dentate line. Thrombosed external hemorrhoids are intravascular clots of these vessels. They cause extreme pain during the first 48 hours. Excision is the treatment of choice and usually is done under local anesthesia as an office or outpatient procedure (Fig. 1). Incision should be discouraged because the clots are multiloculated. If the pain starts to subside, excision is unnecessary and warm sitz baths will speed up resolution.

Internal hemorrhoids most commonly are manifested by painless, bright-red rectal bleeding associated with bowel movement. The patient commonly describes the bleeding episodes as "blood drips into the toilet bowl." In chronic prolapse, mucus frequently causes perianal irritation. A feeling of incomplete evacuation is also common with severe hemorrhoids. Pain is not a common symptom of internal hemorrhoids unless they are complicated by an anal fissure, stenosis, or thrombosis.

The severity of internal hemorrhoids is graded according to the degree of prolapse. In first degree hemorrhoids, the anal cushions slide down beyond the dentate line on straining. The most common symptom is painless rectal bleeding. Treatment consists of bulk-forming agents such as bran or psyllium seed. If bleeding persists, rubber band ligation should be done (Fig. 2). In second degree hemorrhoids, the anal cushions prolapse through the anus on straining but can be spontaneously reduced. Rubber band ligation is the treatment of choice, along with bran or psyllium seed. In third degree hemorrhoids, the anal cushions prolapse through the anus on straining or walking and require manual replacement into the anal canal. Hemorrhoidectomy gives the best results. In fourth degree hemorrhoids, the prolapse stays out all the time. Hemorrhoidectomy is indicated. The prolapse may become strangulated, which requires urgent or emergent hemorrhoidectomy.

Usually patients with *post-partum hemorrhoids* have had some problems with hemorrhoids before or during pregnancy. Prolonged straining during labor causes

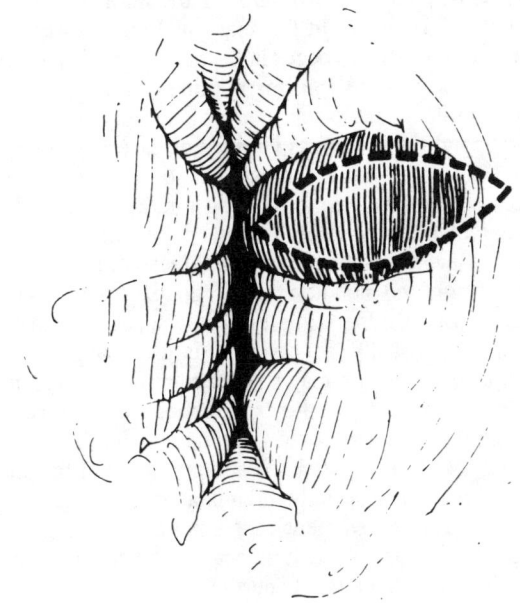

Figure 1 Excision of thrombosed external hemorrhoid.

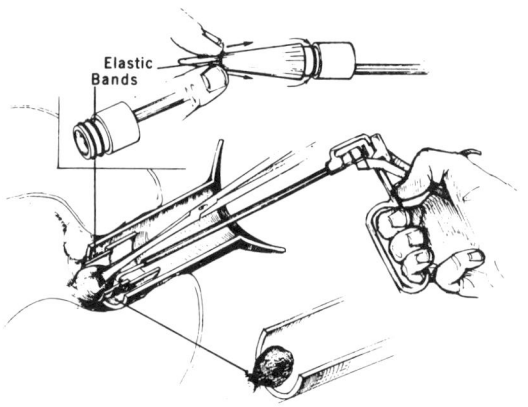

Figure 2 Rubber band ligation of an internal hemorrhoid.

thrombosis and/or strangulation to develop. Hemorrhoidectomy is the treatment of choice for most cases. If only a thrombosed external hemorrhoid occurs, excision is all that is necessary.

Although the portal system communicates with the systemic system via the superior rectal, middle rectal, and inferior rectal veins, the incidence of *hemorrhoids* in patients with *portal hypertension* is not higher than in the normal population. Active bleeding usually occurs from ulceration at the external or internal hemorrhoid. A "sticktie" at the bleeding site will solve the problem. In some cases a hemorrhoidectomy at the site of bleeding is necessary. Any bleeding diathesis must be corrected.

ANAL FISSURE

An anal fissure is a tear of the skin-lined part of the anal canal, i.e., the area from the pectinate or dentate line to the anal verge. It is usually a few millimeters in size and rarely larger than a centimeter. Most anal fissures are caused by passage of a large, hard stool. Owing to poor muscular support of the anal canal posteriorly, the majority of the fissures occur in the posterior midline and less frequently in the anterior midline. An anal fissure off the midline posterior or anterior is usually secondary to other conditions, such as Crohn's disease, chronic ulcerative colitis, syphilis, tuberculosis, or leukemia. Anal fissures occur mostly in young and middle-aged adults. The characteristic symptom is a sharp, burning pain during and after bowel movement. Another common complaint is bright red blood on the toilet paper upon wiping. The diagnosis is rather simple. Gentle separation of the buttock will usually reveal the fissure. Digital and anoscopic examination may be necessary to establish the diagnosis, provided that the examination does not cause too much pain. Proctoscopic examination should also be done to exclude any associated abnormalities of the anal canal and rectum, especially inflammatory bowel disease.

Conservative treatment consisting of anal hygiene, bulk-producing agents such as bran and psyllium seed, warm sitz bath, and a local anesthetic jelly will improve or heal many acute fissures. Once the fissure progresses to a chronic stage, surgical treatment is usually required. The treatment of choice is usually a lateral internal sphincterotomy. A fissurectomy may occasionally be indicated.

ANORECTAL ABSCESS

Anorectal abscesses are infections of the potential spaces around the anorectum. The primary source of the infection starts in the anal glands which lie between the internal and external sphincter muscles to form an *intersphincteric abscess*. The abscess may rupture into the anal lumen and the infection subsides. It may, however, extend into the perianal space to form a *perianal abscess*; extend through the external sphincter to form an *ischioanal* or *ischiorectal abscess*; or extend above the levator ani muscle to form a *pelvirectal* or *supralevator abscess* (Fig. 3).

Diagnosis

Patients with anorectal abscesses characteristically present with severe anal pain and tenderness, often accompanied by high fever. The diagnosis of the more common perianal and ischioanal abscesses is apparent by the tender swelling in the perianal area. The throbbing anal pain is acute and is aggravated by sitting, coughing, sneezing, and straining. The less common intersphincteric abscess causes dull aching or throbbing pain in the anorectum rather than the perianal area. The extreme tenderness usually precludes an adequate examination without anesthesia. Rectal examination reveals a soft or indurated mass in the wall of the upper anal canal, usually in the posterior quadrant. The rare supralevator abscess is difficult to diagnose. The patient may present with fever of unknown origin or signs of peritonitis mimicking an intra-abdominal process. Induration of the supralevator spaces suggests the diagnosis. Computed tomography scans are also helpful in localizing supralevator abscesses.

Treatment

The standard treatment of anorectal abscesses is incision and drainage even in the absence of fluctuation.

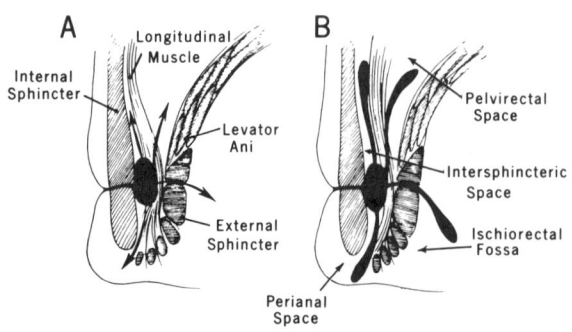

Figure 3 Avenues of extension in perianal abscess.

Antibiotics should never be the principal therapy but they may be used adjunctively. Most perianal abscesses can be drained under local anesthesia as an outpatient procedure (Fig. 4). Intersphincteric, ischioanal, and supralevator abscesses should be drained in the operating room under adequate anesthesia.

FISTULA-IN-ANO

Fistula-in-ano is a track lined by granulation tissue resulting from an incomplete healing of the drained anorectal abscess. The primary opening is in the cryptoglandular area of the anal canal at the dentate line, and the secondary opening is in the perianal skin where the abscess ruptured or drained.

Diagnosis

Most but not all patients with fistula-in-ano have a history of previous anorectal abscesses. Intermittent purulent or serosanguineous discharge is the main complaint. Pain is unusual but itching and irritation of the perianal area from the discharge are common. The external opening is usually apparent in the perianal area as a red elevation of granulation tissue with discharge on compression. The internal opening can be identified in the anal canal in most cases when examined in the operating room. In the simple fistula, the track can be palpated as an indurated cord.

Several disorders must be considered in the differential diagnosis of fistula-in-ano. It is important to rule out fistulas associated with Crohn's disease, in which case one would refrain from extensive operative procedures on the fistulas because of poor wound healing. The differential diagnosis may necessitate a complete gastrointestinal work-up. Sigmoid diverticulitis with perforation and fistulization to the perineum occurs rarely. Hidradenitis suppurativa (infection of sweat glands) is apparent by the presence of multiple openings in the perianal skin. Pilonidal sinus with perianal extension and infected perianal sebaceous cysts must be considered. Rarely, a carcinoma may develop in long-standing fistulas as occurs with Crohn's disease. Rectal and anal carcinomas rarely present as a fistula in the perineum.

Treatment

Once established, fistula-in-ano rarely heals spontaneously. The basic principle of treatment is to lay the fistulous track open. Deep or high fistulas may require a two-stage operation. To prevent anal incontinence a seton or a silk suture is placed around the sphincter muscle overlying the fistula to create fibrosis and fixation. The muscle is then cut 6 to 8 weeks later to lay open the fistulous track.

PROLAPSE OF THE RECTUM

Prolapse of the rectum (procidentia) is an uncommon condition in which full thickness of the rectal wall turns inside out, into, or through the anal canal. Typically, the extruded rectum is seen as concentric rings of mucosa (Fig. 5). This should not be confused with rectal mucosal prolapse or prolapsed hemorrhoids in which the radial folds of mucosa extrude through the anus. Although prolapse of the rectum can occur at any age, the peak incidence is between 60 and 70 years in women, but in men the age distribution is constant. Female to male ratio is 5:1. For years the theory of sliding hernia had been put forth, but more recently, with the use of cineradiography, intussusception has been demonstrated. The intussusception begins circumferentially 6 to 7 cm from the anal verge.

The early symptoms are minor, including anorectal pain or discomfort during defecation. Difficulty initiating bowel movements and the feeling of incomplete evacuation are also common. The diagnosis is easy if the prolapse comes through the anus. When the prolapse remains in the upper anal canal ("hidden prolapse"), the diagnosis can be difficult. Redness of the rectal mucosa, especially anteriorly at the 6 to 7 cm level, gives a clue. Straining of the anorectum with an anoscope in place is also helpful. In the advanced stage, fecal and urinary incontinence is common. Incontinence in long standing rectal prolapse is the consequence of entrapment or stretching of the pudendal or perineal nerve resulting in neuromuscular dysfunction. Therefore, it is essential to repair the prolapse before this mishap occurs.

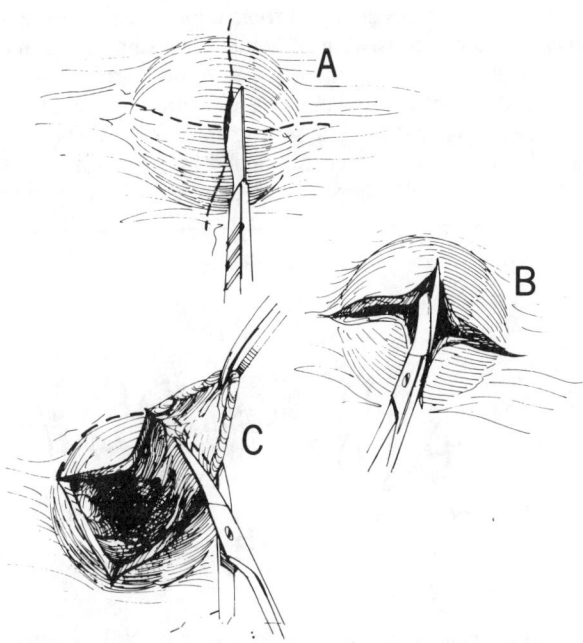

Figure 4 Drainage of perianal abscess with cruciate incision.

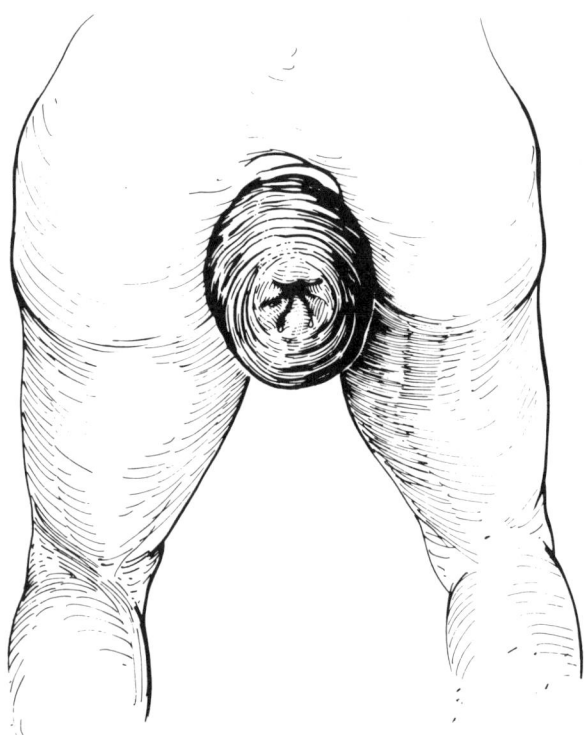

Figure 5 Concentric circular rings of mucosa in prolapse of rectum.

Treatment

There have been more than 100 methods for repair of rectal prolapse with variable success rates. The modern concept of the repair is to remove the intussusceptum or to prevent the occurrence of intussusception. Most methods of repair are by the transabdominal or transperineal approach.

The *rectal sling operation* was introduced by Ripstein and consists of a sling of Teflon or Marlex which fixes the fully mobilized rectum to the sacrum. The *Ivalon sponge wrap operation* was introduced by Wells and has been popular in the United Kingdom. The fully mobilized rectum is fixed to the sacrum with a rectangular sheet of Ivalon sponge (polyvinyl alcohol). *Anterior resection of the rectum* was first introduced by Muir in 1955 for the treatment of rectal prolapse. The technique consists of a full mobilization of the rectum as for abdominoperineal resection or low anterior resection for carcinoma of the rectum. The mid-rectum, along with the redundant sigmoid colon, is resected and an anastomosis made. *Transabdominal proctopexy* with or without sigmoid colon resection is another method of fixing the mobilized rectum to the sacrum but without the necessity of using a foreign material (Fig. 6). *Perineal rectosigmoidectomy* is a perineal approach in which the rectum and rectosigmoid colon are resected through the prolapse itself. It is very well tolerated by the patients, and general or regional anesthesia can be used (Fig. 7).

Our choice of procedure for good risk patients is the *transabdominal proctopexy*. For patients for whom an intra-abdominal procedure is not suitable but who can withstand general or regional anesthesia, perineal rectosigmoidectomy is the method of choice. In the elderly and those whose conditions preclude definitive repair, the Thiersch wire procedure may be used, i.e., the anus is encircled with wire or other suture materials under local anesthesia. The procedure is simple and is well tolerated but the success rate is poor, with a high incidence of recurrence, fecal impaction, and suture breakage. A modification of the technique using Marlex or a Silastic strip has been found to be superior.

PRURITUS ANI

Pruritus ani is a common problem but difficult to treat. The perianal skin is sensitive and any condition causing soiling or moisture in the area can produce itching. Pruritus ani may be a manifestation of local or systemic diseases. The surgically correctable conditions contributing to this condition are prolapsing hemorrhoids, ectropion, anal fissure, fistula-in-ano, condyloma acuminatum, and neoplasm of the anal canal and perineum. Other conditions include diarrhea, dermatitis, severe diabetes mellitus, severe jaundice, lymphomas, and leukemia. In children, *Enterobius vermicularis* (pinworm) is a common cause. In most cases no specific causes are found and the pruritus is called "idiopathic."

The diagnosis of pruritus ani is simple. In the acute and subacute stages, the anal and perianal skin is red, excoriated, and moist, frequently secondary to fungus infection, especially with *Monilia* and *Epidermophyton*. Clotrimazole (Lotrimin) 1 percent cream will rapidly improve the condition. When the condition has become chronic, the skin and the anoderm are thick, whitish in appearance, with multiple radial and irregular folds. There is no specific treatment for chronic idiopathic pruritus ani. Anal hygiene, consisting of gentle cleansing of the anal area with water-moistened tissue, is the cornerstone of successful control. Bowel habit regulation to prevent incomplete evacuation and soiling must be emphasized. Stool acidification is recommended by some clinicians. All other possible causes, such as sensitivity to certain

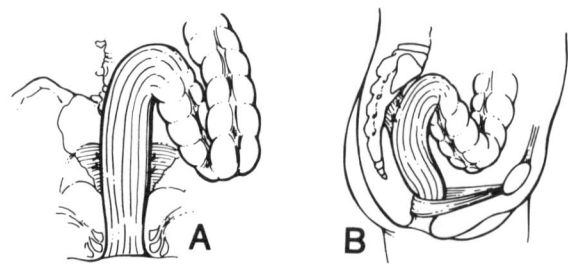

Figure 6 Transabdominal proctopexy. (A) The fully mobilized rectum is sutured to presacral fascia using 2-0 silk. Sigmoid colon is resected if it is redundant. (B) Lateral view.

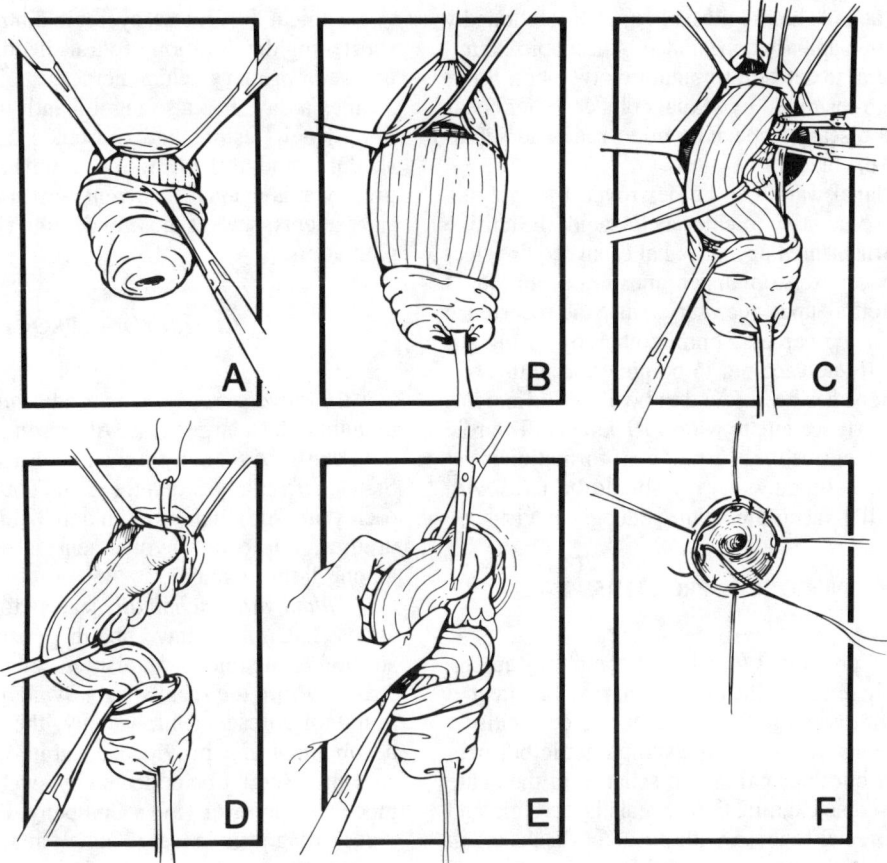

Figure 7 Perineal rectosigmoidectomy. (A) A circular incison is made 2 cm from the dentate line. (B) The anterior peritoneal reflection is opened. (C) The mesentery is divided. (D) The previously opened peritoneum is resutured to the anterior wall of the bowel. (E) The prolapse, along with the redundant bowel, is transected 2 cm distal to the anus. (F) Anastomosis is done using one layer of 4–0 polyglycolic acid (Dexon) or polyglactin (Vicryl) sutures.

kinds of toilet paper, various dyes in underclothing, and allergy to soap, cream, and ointment, should be excluded. Certain kinds of foods and beverages, such as coffee, tea, cola, beer, chocolate, and tomatoes, have been implicated as causing pruritus ani, although this is unproven.

Hydrocortisone, 0.5 percent preparation applied locally, gives temporary symptomatic relief. The undercutting operation, subcutaneous injection of alcohol, tattooing with mercury sulfate, and topical irradiation for chronic idiopathic pruritus ani have been abandoned. They are ineffective and achieve only transient relief.

PROCTALGIA FUGAX AND LEVATOR SYNDROME

Proctalgia fugax is a severe, spasmodic rectal pain lasting a few minutes or longer. The exact cause is unknown, but the condition may be due to levator ani muscle spasm. The characteristic history is that of severe pain awakening the patient. The pain usually is located in the mid-rectum and disappears spontaneously without residual symptoms. Proctoscopic examination is indicated to rule out anorectal diseases. Treatment to relieve the pain during an acute attack consists of firm pressure on the anus, warm sitz bath, or heating pad applied to the perineum. Since many of these patients are anxious and have cancer phobia, reassurance is an important aspect of therapy.

Another group of patients has chronic vague pain in the anorectum. Examination reveals tenderness of the levator ani muscle, more often on the left side. This is termed "levator syndrome." Digital massage of the tender muscle at weekly intervals may provide effective relief. Recently, electrogalvanic stimulation of the levator ani muscle by means of an intra-anal probe has been found to be effective.

CONDYLOMA ACUMINATUM

Anal condyloma acuminatum or wart, is caused by a papilloma virus. The condition is most commonly found in male homosexuals. In the majority of patients, the warts involve the perianal skin, anal verge, and anoderm. Occasionally, the lesions also involve the mucosa of the upper anal canal and the lower rectum. The extent of the disease varies from a few small warts to an extensive mass occluding the anus. The diagnosis is usually obvious by the characteristic papillary appearance. Anoscopic examination is essential to detect intra-anal involvement. Since most cases are transmitted by sexual contact, other coexisting venereal disease, especially gonorrhea and syphilis, should be excluded.

Small perianal warts can be destroyed by applying podophyllum solution or bichloracetic acid. Extensive warts in the perianal area or in the anal canal require electrocoagulation or excision under anesthesia. Frequent postoperative follow-up is necessary, since the recurrence rate is as high as 65 percent. Immunotherapy, using autogenous wart tissue vaccine, in conjunction with excision of the lesions has been found to be effective and has reduced the recurrence rate to within 10 percent. The role of immune mechanisms in recurrent wart formation is yet to be determined. Immunotherapy should be used with caution, since the vaccine contains oncogenic virus.

GONOCOCCAL PROCTITIS

Gonococcal proctitis is found most commonly among homosexuals. In females, the anorectum may be infected by the spread of discharge from gonococcal cervicitis or urethritis. Patients are generally asymptomatic but may have mild anal burning, pain, or discharge in the acute phase. Proctoscopic examination reveals hyperemic and edematous anorectal mucosa with purulent discharge in the anal crypts. In the chronic phase, the anorectum may appear normal. Diagnosis is confirmed by gram smears of the discharge and plating the cotton swabs of the discharge immediately onto Thayer-Martin media for cultures.

Penicillin remains the antibiotic of choice. When penicillin is contraindicated, oral tetracycline or intramuscular injection of spectinomycin hydrochloride may be used. In patients who fail to respond to penicillin, spectinomycin should be given. Repeat smears and cultures from the anorectum should be taken 1 week after the treatment to confirm the remission.

HERPES SIMPLEX

Anorectal herpes is caused by Herpes virus hominis type II, the same organism implicated in genital herpes. It is less common than gonorrhea but more common than syphilis. The clinical presentations usually begin with itching and soreness in or around the anus followed by severe anorectal pain. The pain may be so intense that the patient is reluctant to have a bowel movement, leading to constipation and impaction.

Examination reveals erythematous, red areas with small groups of vesicles which rupture and become ulcerated. The diagnosis is confirmed by viral culture of the vesicular fluid. There is no effective cure for herpes. The lesions should be kept clean by frequent sitz baths. Symptomatic relief is obtained with the use of analgesic drugs and the local application of soothing agents.

Topical 5 percent acyclovir ointment is effective in shortening the duration of viral shedding and the clinical course of primary genital herpes. Oral acyclovir, 200 mg 5 times a day, has also significantly reduced the formation of new lesions and shortened the duration of viral shedding and of the lesion. Systemic acyclovir is used as prophylaxis against recurrent activation in certain high-risk patients, such as those undergoing bone marrow transplantation.

CHLAMYDIAL PROCTITIS

Chlamydia trachomatis is a bacterium that was once thought to be a large virus. At present, it is the most common cause of sexually transmitted disease in the United States, striking between three and ten million Americans each year. Although most chlamydial infections affect the urethra, anorectal involvement is starting to emerge among homosexuals.

Chlamydia trachomatis is easy to treat once it is diagnosed. Until recently, the diagnosis required demonstration of the microorganism in cell culture, which took 2 days before the results were available. With the use of immunofluorescent microscopy, the diagnosis can now be obtained and provided accurately and rapidly. The specimen should be collected by swabbing the anorectal mucosa. Microtrak (Syva Company, Palo Alto, CA) provides a diagnosis in less than half an hour. The treatment is tetracycline, 500 mg 4 times a day for 7 days. The alternative regimen is erythromycin, 500 mg 4 times a day for 7 days. Because of the many patients with gonorrhea who also have chlamydial infection, at the present time it is recommended that anyone with a confirmed case of gonorrhea be treated for chlamydial disease as well.

ANAL AND PERIANAL CROHN'S DISEASE

Anal and perianal manifestations of Crohn's disease are very common—up to 90 percent if looked for carefully—but they usually cause only mild symptoms. Crohn's disease with the primary site being the anus and perianus occurs in about 5 percent of patients. It may precede the more proximal involvement by many years. When anal Crohn's disease is suspected, a complete gastrointestinal work-up is indicated.

Manifestations of Anal and Perianal Crohn's Disease

The most common anal finding is the edematous *skin tags*, which usually cause few problems or symptoms. *Fissures* are common. They are usually deep and indolent looking, but as a rule are not as painful as they appear. Severe pain in anal fissures of Crohn's disease may be a sign of an abscess formation and an abscess should be carefully sought. *Hemorrhoids* are not a common feature of anal Crohn's disease. What are usually regarded by patients or inexperienced physicians as hemorrhoids are actually skin irritations or anal fissures or ulcerations. *Stricture* or *stenosis* is a common complication of longstanding anal fissures or ulcers, or occurs as a result of anorectal surgery. *Perianal abscesses* in patients with Crohn's disease are more common than in the general population and tend to recur if not adequately drained. *Anal fistulas* in Crohn's disease can be single, multiple, simple, or complicated. Fistulas may come from the underlying active disease in the anal canal, rectum, or even colon or small bowel. *Anal incontinence* usually occurs because of diarrhea rather than from an involvement of the anal sphincter muscle with Crohn's disease. Destruction of the anal sphincter muscle is usually the result of aggressive surgery and contributes to the incontinence.

Treatment

The basic principles in the management of anal and perianal Crohn's disease are symptomatic and conservative. In many cases, anal hygiene and control of diarrhea are all that is required. Medical therapy includes the basic modalities of steroids, Azulfidine, and bowel rest with hyperalimentation or elemental diet. Some investigators have obtained good results using 6-mercaptopurine. Metronidazole has been used for anal and perianal Crohn's disease with variable success.

Skin tags may be excised if they become painful or interfere with anal hygiene. Anal fissures are best left alone unless there is an underlying abscess. Abscesses must be adequately drained. Simple fistulas can be left alone, or if necessary can be laid open like ordinary fistulas. Deep fistulas should never be divided. Instead, a seton suture should be placed. A No. 0 silk is loosely tied around the involved sphincter muscle overlying the fistula. In many cases, the seton suture can be removed a few weeks later without necessarily dividing the muscle. Anal stricture or stenosis is best treated by repeated dilation to one finger. In carefully selected cases, a rectovaginal fistula can be repaired if there is no active disease. The same principle is applied to anal incontinence.

In severe anal and perianal disease, particularly when there is active anorectal disease, proctectomy may be necessary. Most of the time this is done because of intolerable anal incontinence or pain. There is no evidence that resection of the proximal bowel with active Crohn's disease will cure or improve anal or perianal Crohn's disease.

INCONTINENCE

ARNOLD WALD, M.D.

Although not a life-threatening disorder, fecal incontinence can be devastating in terms of social disruption and damage to self-esteem. Because of their embarrassment, patients often do not volunteer their distress unless directly questioned by their physician. In addition, many physicians are unaware that effective treatment is now available for many patients.

A number of abnormalities of anorectal function may contribute to fecal incontinence. The rectum is richly innervated with sensory nerves, and rectal fullness or an urge to defecate occurs whenever the rectum is distended. In addition, rectal distention (i.e., with stool) results in reflex inhibition of the internal anal sphincter and temporary relaxation of the anal canal. Rectal contents then come into contact with sensitive nerve endings in the anal canal, which normally can differentiate gas, liquid, and solid. The continent person can voluntarily contract the puborectalis muscle and external anal sphincter, thus narrowing the anorectal angle and increasing resistance of the anal canal. Bowel control is thus dependent on at least four critical factors: (1) rectal sensation (the ability to perceive rectal distention); (2) the ability to contract the external anal sphincter, puborectalis, and/or gluteal muscles; (3) motivation to make the appropriate response; and (4) the ability of the rectum to serve as a reservoir for feces through adaptive compliance and accommodation. Most patients with fecal incontinence have abnormalities of one or more of these factors (Table 1).

Evaluation includes consideration of possible contributing factors, careful examination of the anorectum, and focused neurologic testing. The finding of a fecal impaction, rectal prolapse, or evidence of anorectal disease may be important. Anal "gaping" on posterior traction of the puborectalis suggests sphincter denervation, but, in general, digital estimation of rectal tone and strength correlates poorly with objective tests. Psychosocial assessment is particularly important at both ends of the age spectrum. Proctoscopy, barium-contrast roentgenography, and work-up for chronic diarrhea, if present, may be appropriate prior to referral. These studies can be supplemented by anorectal manometry, studies of rectal compliance, and by other measurements of anal sphincter integrity when indicated.

TREATMENT OF ADULTS WITH FECAL INCONTINENCE

Fecal Incontinence Associated with Rectosphincteric Abnormalities

Patients with rectosphincteric abnormalities include those with sphincter surgery, disease, or trauma and most patients with idiopathic fecal incontinence. Such patients may present with or without diarrhea.

TABLE 1 Rectosphincteric Abnormalities Associated with Fecal Incontinence

Groups	Motivation	Reservoir	Sensory	Sphincter
Adult				
Ileoanal anastomosis	N	A	N/A	N
Inflammatory bowel disease	N	A	N	N
Neurogenic	N	N	N/A	A
Diabetes mellitus	N	N	N/A	A
Sphincter surgery	N	N	N	A
Idiopathic	N	N	N	A
Pediatric				
Encopresis	N/A	N	N/A	N
Spina bifida	N/A	N	N/A	A
Imperforate anus	N/A	N/A	N	N/A

N = Normal most or all of the time; A = abnormal most or all of the time; N/A = may be normal or abnormal or findings are controversial.

Incontinence Without Diarrhea

Biofeedback based upon the techniques of Engel and associates is a simple and effective treatment for patients in this category. The method utilizes the manometer that is used for diagnostic studies; the recording apparatus provides information (feedback) about anorectal responses so that the patient can tell whether anal sphincter responses are being performed appropriately. thus, biofeedback is a trial-and-error learning process using a visual display to monitor anal sphincter responses.

After evaluation and acceptance into the program, an explanation of the importance of the external sphincter to fecal continence is provided and patients are shown how their response differs from normal ones. Biofeedback conditioning is then carried out in three phases.

Phase 1. Patients watch the recording of the sphincteric responses and are asked to contract the external anal sphincter. A normal response is illustrated and patients are praised if they can produce an appropriate contraction. The ability to make an appropriate contraction is achieved through trial and error; the first phase ends when the subject produces that response repeatedly.

Phase 2. The appropriate contraction response is then synchronized with rectal distention (and, therefore, internal sphincter relaxation). Responses are monitored by having patients watch the recording to ensure appropriate synchronization with internal sphincter relaxation.

Phase 3. Patients are weaned from the instrument by blocking their view of the recording. During this phase, patients are informed by the instructor when sphincteric responses are appropriate. When this occurs repeatedly, the training session is completed; sessions last from 45 to 60 minutes.

Subsequently, patients are instructed to practice contraction exercises three to four times daily and to contract the sphincter whenever they sense rectal distention or urgency. Routine reinforcement sessions are generally not needed for adults and are reserved for patients whose initial response is suboptimal or in whom relapses occur.

Prerequisites for successful biofeedback include appropriate motivation and the ability to comprehend and follow directions, to sense rectal distention in the normal range, and to contract the external anal sphincter or gluteal muscles. Success has been achieved in more than 70 percent of patients meeting these requirements.

Incontinence With Diarrhea

In many patients, fecal incontinence develops only after the occurrence of diarrhea. Liquid stool may be more difficult to perceive and, particularly when associated with urgency, more difficult to retain. Thus, diarrhea may uncover underlying abnormalities of anorectal continence mechanisms which result in fecal soiling. Rarely, massive diarrhea may overwhelm normal continence mechanisms.

The sphincter biofeedback program is often effective in controlling incontinence when there are demonstrable rectosphincteric abnormalities. In colonic motor disorders such as irritable bowel syndrome, which are associated with low volume diarrhea, fiber supplementation may regulate bowel habits and improve continence. If biofeedback fails or is only partially successful, antidiarrheal agents are often effective. Based upon recent trials, I employ loperamide in dosages up to 4 mg 4 times a day, adjusted according to clinical response, rather than administered after each episode of diarrhea. I prefer diphenoxylate as a second line agent and avoid codeine for long-term control because of its potentially addictive properties.

Diabetes-Associated Fecal Incontinence

Fecal incontinence occurs in up to 20 percent of diabetic patients, most of whom have diarrhea as well as peripheral and autonomic neuropathy. Many of these patients have rectosphincteric abnormalities and impaired continence mechanisms similar to nondiabetics with idiopathic incontinence. In addition, more than 50 percent have impairment of conscious rectal sensation.

We have modified the biofeedback process in diabetic patients by including rectal sensory conditioning in those patients with abnormal conscious rectal sensation. We attempt to decrease the threshold of conscious rectal sensation in the following manner: Once the smallest volume of rectal distention sensed by the patient is determined, progressively smaller distention volumes are administered in decrements of 1 to 5 cc of air. When a given distention volume is sensed repeatedly, the volume is decreased and the process is repeated until no further improvement can be achieved.

Following sensory discrimination training, the biofeedback program proceeds in an identical manner to that for patients with normal rectal sensation. Loperamide may be helpful in some of those who fail to respond to biofeedback. Good to excellent results have been obtained in more than 70 percent of a relatively small number of diabetic patients[1].

Fecal Incontinence Associated with Impaired Reservoir Capacity

Patients with impaired reservoir capacity include those with idiopathic inflammatory bowel diseases involving the rectum, radiation proctitis, chronic rectal ischemia, subtotal colectomy with ileoanal anastomosis, and sphincter-saving procedures for rectal lesions. Therapeutic approaches depend upon underlying disease processes. Rectal urgency and incontinence due to proctitis often respond to steroid retention enemas. These may be supplemented with loperamide or diphenoxylate to control diarrhea and cramping. Patients with soiling associated with subtotal colectomy and ileoanal anastomosis often lack localizing rectal sensation in addition to having reduced capacity. Therapeutic approaches include reducing fecal volume through carbohydrate and fiber restriction, use of loperamide or diphenoxylate to prolong transit and promote fluid and electrolyte intestinal absorption, and planned defecation after known stimulants such as meals. With time, rectal or ileal capacity may improve and restore continence in some patients.

Neurogenic Incontinence

Neurologic incontinence can occur with damage to the sacral cord or plexus, with injury to the spinal cord above the sacrum, or with disease of the frontal cortex or subcortical pathways. Rectal sensation is frequently lost and sphincter denervation is common, particularly with involvement of sacral cord or nerves.

Treatment consists of combining planned regular defecation with constipating agents. Patients should be seated on a commode during and after breakfast and encouraged to defecate, taking advantage of the "gastrocolic reflex." In addition, I recommend loperamide or diphenoxylate two to four times per day to decrease stool frequency. A weekly enema followed by a bisacodyl suppository (Dulcolax 10 mg) to promote colonic evacuation should be administered to prevent fecal impaction.

Fecal Incontinence Associated With Constipation

Incontinence associated with constipation is not infrequent in elderly patients, especially those who are physically immobilized. Soft, poorly formed stools seep around the obstructing fecal bolus which may be misdiagnosed as diarrhea. The correct diagnosis is made on rectal examination. The importance of a rectal examination to rule out impaction before treating diarrhea or incontinence in an elderly or debilitated patient is worthy of reemphasis.

Treatment begins with a series of phosphate enemas (Fleet). This should be done once or twice daily until there is no fecal return. The failure to evacuate the colon completely with repeated enemas is the most frequent reason for treatment failure. If the impaction is hard and cannot be evacuated with simple enemas, a mineral oil enema (Fleet) to soften the stool should be administered. Digital removal, an unpleasant task, is rarely necessary.

Once evacuation is complete, preventive measures should be taken, especially if the patient remains relatively immobile. Once a week, a phosphate enema followed by bisacodyl suppositories will ensure periodic colonic evacuation and prevent recurrence of the problem.

TREATMENT OF CHILDREN WITH FECAL INCONTINENCE

Encopresis

The vast majority of children with encopresis have constipation and overflow soiling, often associated with megarectum or megacolon. The correct diagnosis is made by rectal examination or abdominal x-ray films. As with adults, the key to initial management is colonic evacuation with enemas. I administer twice daily enemas (4½ oz disposable phosphate or 1 quart of warm tap water administered by bag drip) for at least 3 days; occasionally, children must be hospitalized to accomplish this critical task.

Following colonic evacuation, 1 or 2 tablespoons of lactulose (Chronulac) are given twice daily to produce one or two soft, formed stools per day. This is combined with a bowel training program in which the child is instructed to sit on the toilet 20 minutes after a selected meal (preferably breakfast) to take advantage of the "gastrocolic reflex." A footstool should be used so that the child's legs are firmly supported. A calendar is kept to record the patterns of defecation and soiling. Punishment is forbidden at any time. The lactulose can be tapered 6 to 12 months after continence is established and eventually discontinued.

Office counseling is generally sufficient if individual or family problems are uncovered, but more formal psychotherapy may be necessary in some cases. Fecal incontinence in children without constipation or fecal impaction responds poorly to treatment and suggests severe underlying psychopathologic factors.

Spina Bifida

Fecal incontinence is often associated with constipation in children with spina bifida. Sphincter denervation and decreased anal tone occur in most children and rectal sensation is often impaired. With good bowel programs, megarectum, megacolon, and fecal impactions can be avoided and satisfactory continence can often be achieved.

Toilet training should be started at age 2 or 3 years by placing the child on a commode 20 to 30 minutes after a meal. Rectal evacuation can be aided by manually increasing abdominal pressure or by the Valsalva maneuver. Insertion of a glycerin suppository shortly after the child eats may promote defecation. If such measures are unsatisfactory, a 2¼ oz disposable phosphate enema can be administered 30 minutes after meals to evacuate the distal colon.

In some patients, successful toilet training cannot be accomplished or diarrhea is a problem. A constipating diet low in fiber and lactose (in lactose-intolerant children), supplemented by loperamide or diphenoxylate to reduce stool frequency, may be helpful. Phosphate or warm tap water enemas once or twice a week will prevent fecal impaction. Laxatives and cathartics should be avoided and Colace is not helpful.

Some children with spina bifida have been successfully treated with biofeedback techniques in which gluteal muscle contraction substitutes for the external sphincter. Although only a few children are eligible, a successful outcome can be gratifying in terms of independence and control over a bodily function. Potential candidates should be strongly motivated and able to learn, capable of standing or ambulating without full leg braces, and have normal rectal sensation by objective testing. An average of four to six reinforcement sessions at 2-week intervals is required, unlike biofeedback training in adult patients.

Imperforate Anus

Fecal incontinence may be variously associated with a decrease in rectal compliance, anal sphincter weakness or dysfunction due to poor surgical placement, and occasional stricture with fecal impaction and overflow incontinence. A full diagnostic evaluation is necessary, since treatment approaches will differ according to the specific abnormalities present. Biofeedback may be effective for external sphincter dysfunction alone; anal dilation, bowel cleansing, and bowel training as previously detailed are effective if constipation and impaction are present. Decreased rectal compliance or capacity is difficult to correct surgically. Measures to reduce stool volume combined with constipating drugs and weekly or twice weekly enemas may be employed in such patients.

REFERENCE

1. Wald A, Tunuguntla AK. Anorectal sensorimotor dysfunction in fecal incontinence and diabetes mellitus. N Engl J Med 1984; 310:1282–1287.

OSTOMY CARE

VICTOR W. FAZIO, M.B., B.S., F.R.A.C.S., F.A.C.S.
IAN T. JONES, M.B., B.S., F.R.A.C.S., F.R.C.S.

Over the past few years, major innovations in colorectal surgery have been directed at sphincter preservation and the avoidance of a permanent stoma. Nevertheless, the conventional intestinal stoma retains a crucial role in the management of intestinal disease.

Successful stoma care depends on a sound knowledge of surgical technique, the management of complications, patient education, and routine daily care supervised by a trained enterostomal therapist.

ILEOSTOMY

Indications

An ileostomy may be constructed as an end, a loop, or a loop-end stoma. A permanent end ileostomy is made following proctocolectomy for inflammatory bowel disease or familial polyposis coli. If primary anastomosis is contraindicated after resection, e.g., a perforated ileal segment in Crohn's disease, a temporary end ileostomy can be constructed.

A loop ileostomy is most frequently used to protect a distal anastomosis or pelvic ileal reservoir, to provide fecal diversion above an enterocutaneous fistula, or combined with a transverse colon decompression stoma for toxic megacolon. Occasionally it is useful as the first stage of management of acute colitis in a debilitated patient. In the obese patient, an end stoma may become ischemic and a loop end ileostomy is a useful alternative, since this complication is less likely if no mesenteric vessels to the stoma are divided. If a definitive stoma becomes necessary where a loop ileostomy already exists, it is a simple matter to resect the efferent limb and create a loop end ileostomy.

Surgical Techniques

Preoperative Considerations

Preoperative stoma marking is essential. With the patient in the sitting position, an indelible mark is made on the summit of the infraumbilical fat mound away from the umbilicus, bony prominences, and existing or planned incision sites. A standard faceplate acts as a guide to ensure that there is no encroachment on these areas and that the selected site is easily visible to the patient. Occasionally an obese patient requires a supraumbilical site to fulfill this last requirement. The stoma must be constructed within the boundaries of the rectus abdominis muscle to prevent parastomal herniation.

Surgery

At the operation a circular incision 3.5 cm in diameter is made around the selected site and the disk of skin is excised, carefully preserving subcutaneous fat to prevent dead space formation. The fat and anterior rectus sheath are incised vertically by cautery and the fibers of the rectus abdominis are separated by a hemostat and held apart with short retractors. With the posterior rectus sheath exposed, an incision is made with cautery onto a small sponge held up against the peritoneum. the aperture should accommodate two fingers appearing at skin level at the distal interphalangeal joints; a larger aperture predisposes to prolapse. The site is checked for bleeding, especially from the inferior epigastric vessels. The terminal ileum, previously transected and closed with a linear stapler, is brought through the stoma site so that the mesentery lies in a cephalad direction and can be sutured to the anterior abdominal wall and falciform ligament to prevent internal hernia formation or volvulus. Sutures of 4–0 catgut are placed between the ileum (seromuscular bites) and the cut edge of peritoneum at the inner aspect of the aperture, and the abdominal incision is then closed. A curvature of the exteriorized ileum at the mesenteric edge is eliminated by ligating and partially dividing the mesentery at skin level. Sutures placed between subcutaneous fat and the ileum about 1 cm above skin level eliminate a tendency toward formation of a mucocutaneous depression or "moat," and excess ileum is then trimmed away, leaving sufficient bowel to create a stoma protruding 2 to 3 cm from the abdominal wall. Pulsatile arterial bleeding from the cut edge indicates an adequate blood supply and requires hemostasis. Radial sutures of 4–0 catgut are placed through the full thickness of the cut ileal end and the dermal layer of skin. Avoiding full-thickness bites of the skin with this stitch prevents mucosal island implantation in the skin which causes mucus discharge and leakage under the faceplate. All sutures are first placed and then tied to produce an everted stoma.

In making a loop ileostomy, any tension on the loop of bowel must be avoided, which requires careful selection of the loop to prevent the stoma from being flush with the skin. A tape is passed through a window in the mesentery, avoiding the bowel edge and marginal vessels, and each side of the loop is tagged with a suture of a different color to facilitate subsequent identification of afferent and efferent limbs. this ensures that any rotation will be prevented. The loop is brought out through the aperture using the tape for gentle retraction. A straight forceps is applied to one end of the tape and twisted several times so that it can "unwind" through the mesenteric window without tissue injury and to enable a stoma rod to be brought through the window. After the abdominal wound is closed, an incision is made along four-fifths of the circumference of the efferent limb (lying cephalad) about a centimeter above skin level, stopping 5 mm short of the mesentery. Catgut sutures are placed through the full thickness of the bowel edge and the dermis, creating an everted, caudad limb and a recessive, cephalad limb.

Postoperative Period

In the postopertive period, a transparent pouch is placed over a karaya disk to allow easy inspection of the stoma and patient education begins. The contribution of modern enterostomal therapy to the education and supervision of stomal management cannot be overstated and is supported by self-help community groups.

Patients are instructed in the use of fat solvents, deodorants, skin barriers such as karaya washers and Stomahesive wafers, and application of the pouch. Where possible, patients are encouraged to use cost-effective, reusable systems.

Complications

Early Postoperative Period

Several problems may be encountered early in the postoperative period. *Ileostomy dysfunction*, a functional bowel obstruction due to serositis of exposed ileum, has been largely eliminated by immediate mucocutaneous maturation of the stoma. *Ischemia* ranges from relatively harmless mucosal sloughing to frank gangrene that requires urgent laparotomy and refashioning of the stoma using viable bowel. When there is some doubt about adequacy of the stomal blood supply, the pinprick test is helpful in determining viability as evidenced by bright bleeding from the stoma after pricking.

Mucocutaneous separation is rarely a major problem, but gross separation may lead to serositis and stricture. *Parastomal abscesses* may be drained through the mucocutaneous junction, but when large, a separate radial incision and tube drainage is required. If a suture is placed through the entire thickness of the ileum, or tears out because of attachment to the rigid rectus sheath rather than the flexible subcutaneous fat, a *fistula* may appear. Beyond the immediate postoperative period, this may be a sign of recurrent Crohn's disease, best demonstrated by stomal injection studies. When this state of affairs exists, segmental resection and stomal reconstruction are required.

High Output

A high ileostomy output may have many causes, including the simple resolution of postoperative ileus, which is characterized by a thin, watery, greenish effluent with flecks of mucus. However, raised output may also be seen with intra-abdominal sepsis, gastroenteritis, recurrent Crohn's disease, and the short bowel syndrome. All patients with an ileostomy suffer from mild and subclinical water and sodium depletion, which can rapidly become symptomatic and even lead to serious dehydration and electrolyte disturbance when one of the above conditions is present.

Bowel Obstruction

Unfortunately, bowel obstruction is common after colectomy and ileostomy and is usually due to adhesions of loops of small bowel that fill the pelvis. Internal herniation or volvulus may also cause bowel obstruction but can be prevented by careful obliteration of the mesenteric defect. In the first 6 months or so after surgery, the ingestion of high-residue foods such as peanuts or popcorn may precipitate bolus obstruction, and this requires repeated stomal irrigation to clear the intestinal lumen.

Ileostomy Recession

Because of the liquid nature of its effluent, an ileostomy needs to protrude from the abdominal wall to prevent leakage under the faceplate and the inevitable skin damage that follows. Ideally, an appliance can be used for 5 to 7 days before changing is needed. Therefore, if recession occurs with leakage and premature pouch separation, correction is necessary and is usually possible by local revision and mobilization of an adequate length of terminal ileum. A bidirectional myotomy (Fig. 1) disrupts peristalsis and overcomes further tendencies toward recession. Excessive weight gain or poor stoma siting may also predispose to recession. Intra-abdominald tethering of the stoma may mandate a formal laparotomy to permit ileal exteriorization.

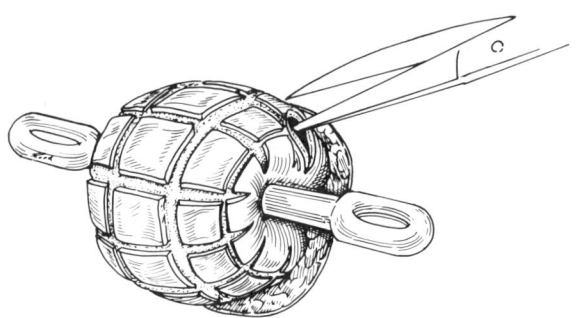

Figure 1 Bidirectional myotomy (in a loop ileostomy in this case) eliminates peristalsis and prevents stoma recession.

Parastomal Hernia or Prolapse

If the stomal aperture is too large or placed outside the rectus sheath, a parastomal hernia or prolapse may occur. This is always more likely in the presence of obesity or multiple abdominal incisions. Minor cases may be managed conservatively, but for more serious cases, laparotomy, stomal relocation, and repair of the old stoma site, often with a mesh implant, is the treatment of choice. Occasionally a local resection of redundant ileum is successful in treating prolapse.

Parastomal Ulcer

Local sepsis, trauma, or recurrent prestomal Crohn's disease accounts for most parastomal ulcers. Typically, these ulcers are undermined and the unhealthy skin edge covers a larger ulcer than is thought to be present on immediate inspection. Debridement and curettage under local anesthesia reveals the full extent of the lesion; if it is less than 2 cm in diameter, a patch of Telfa over the ulcer allows the placement of a Stomahesive wafer. If the ulcer is larger, this system will not prevent leakage and secondary skin damage will occur. The Perry Model 51 system overcomes the problem and consists of an absorbent paper pad, with a central aperture, which is soaked in Domeboro's solution (aluminum acetate) and placed directly on the skin. A snug latex sleeve fitted over the stoma, a plastic flange, pouch, and double belt complete the system, which can be changed as often as every few hours if necessary. Although it may take some weeks, most ulcers, except those due to recurrent Crohn's disease, will heal and surgery will be avoided. A linear ulcer on the inferior aspect of the stoma is caused by a faceplate aperture that is made too small and cuts into the stoma, and it can be easily corrected. Aphthous ulcers on the stoma are typical of Crohn's disease and need to be distinguished from surface irritation or hypertrophied polyps which can be dealt with by silver nitrate sticks. Surface contact bleeding from any of the above conditions needs to be carefully differentiated from intraluminal bleeding, which demands the usual investigation for any major upper gastrointestinal hemorrhage.

Parastomal Skin Damage

As already mentioned, parastomal skin damage and excoriation due to leakage of ileal content are seen with a recessed stoma, mucosal island implants, prolapse, hernia, or simply poor siting of the stoma. There are many minor problems that may contribute, however, including tape or skin barrier allergy, melting of the skin barrier when body temperature rises, psoriasis, or candidiasis. These and similar problems are particularly well managed by the experienced enterostomal therapist.

COLOSTOMY

Indications

As with an ileostomy, a colostomy may take the form of an end or loop stoma. An end iliac colostomy is made after proctectomy or in the management of diverticulitis, radiation proctitis, rectal trauma, or incontinence. When there is distal obstruction or inflammation in a retained rectum, a loop colostomy is preferable. A loop transverse colostomy is usually a temporary stoma and the first stage in the management of an obstructing left-sided lesion.

Surgical Techniques

The principles of ileostomy construction are applicable to colostomies but there are some points of difference. Unless the stomal output is expected to be watery, e.g., in radiation enteritis, a 1-cm everted stoma is adequate. In the obese patient, the internal aperture can be enlarged to facilitate stoma construction, and heavy nonabsorbable sutures are placed in the extended incision and tied after the colon has been brought through at skin level. Ensuring an adequate blood supply and obliteration of the lateral space defect remain important considerations. We do not use an extraperitoneal tunnel for our colostomy construction. A recent innovation that we are currently assessing is the continent colostomy device designed by Prager. This consists of an intra-abdominal silicone ring sutured to the inner aspect of the abdominal wall around the aperture and an inflatable slicone plug that occludes the colonic lumen proximal to the implanted ring. This may prove to be an improvement over the regular incontinent end colostomy. Early results are promising.

Since the transverse loop colostomy is temporary, placing it in the upper end of the abdominal incision is acceptable and avoids a separate incision. In this situation, all fascial sutures of the main wound are placed before tying, allowing accurate assessment of the number of sutures required to leave a snug closure around the stoma. A rod is placed through a mesenteric window beneath the loop and the colon is opened longitudinally over haustral sacculations parallel to the taenia coli. After maturation, a karaya washer is placed around the stoma and over the rod and a transparent pouch applied.

Although placement of a stoma in an abdominal incision has been criticized in some centers, it is clearly advantageous for a temporary stoma and we have not observed any increase in wound sepsis or incisional hernias.

Early in the postoperative period the patient may be instructed in the technique of colostomy irrigation, which frees him of unpredictable bowel activity and often obviates the need for an appliance. A 2-pint washout held in an enema reservoir is delivered into the lumen of the stoma through a blunt cone tip. The returned lavage fluid drains down an attached irrigation sleeve into the toilet bowl. Most patients (90%) are very pleased with irrigation and only require placement of a square piece of gauze over their stoma, although many wear an appliance or safety pouch for security, particularly at night. Some patients are unlikely to achieve satisfactory results with this method including those with irritable bowel syndrome or watery stools after prior irradiation. For these patients irrigation should be avoided.

For those who do not irrigate, many excellent types of manufactured appliances are available. The Squibb Sur-Fit consists of an adhesive faceplate incorporating a Stomahesive wafer to which a pouch can be snapped at the plastic connecting piece; the pouch can be replaced several times before the faceplate needs changing. Other systems incorporate one-piece disposable appliances consisting of faceplate and pouch in one unit and open and closed pouches, with or without belts.

Complications

Immediate Postoperative Period

Most of the complications described for ileostomy can be seen with a colostomy, but as the effluent is solid stool, leakage and skin excoriation are much less of a problem. Mobilization of the colon and careful preservation of marginal vessels should prevent ischemia, but if gangrene of the stoma does occur, urgent laparotomy and revision are necessary. Lesser degrees of ischemia may manifest themselves later as a stomal stricture; unfortunately, dilation is usually ineffective and revision is required.

Parastomal Hernia

Parastomal hernia may require surgery in as many as 15 percent of patients, especially the obese and when the stoma has been placed in the less well supported tissues outside the rectus sheath. As with paraileostomy hernias, troublesome or symptomatic hernias require stomal relocation and repair of the abdominal defect.

Prolapse

Prolapse is much more common with a colostomy and usually occurs in the distal limb of a loop stoma. In a temporary stoma, this state of affairs may be acceptable until the scheduled time for closure, but a large prolapse or hernia in a permanent loop stoma demands correction. After stomal mobilization, the prolapsed distal limb can be stapled closed after the loop is divided. The remnant is returned to the abdominal cavity. The proximal end is then sewn to the skin after narrowing the stomal aperture in the fascia. For an end colostomy prolapse, reduction of redundant bowel accompanie by tightening the aperture with sutures may suffice, although in some cases relocation will be necessary.

Parastomal Sepsis

Parastomal sepsis is uncommon but may occur because of imperfect hemostasis or obesity. Usually a pocket of pus will drain through the mucocutaneous junction and the condition is self-limiting. Minor trauma is common with poor stoma care, but serious injuries can occur with any type of instrumentation, e.g., ill-advised use of a rigid catheter rather than a cone tip for irrigation. For perforations, urgent laparotomy and resection are mandatory to prevent serious sequelae.

Patient Support Systems

The prospect of a permanent stoma will dismay most patients. However, meticulous attention to the principles of sound stoma construction, frank discussion with the patient and family, and the services of a trained enterostomal therapist will allow the patient to achieve a near normal life in most cases. In many communities ostomy societies can be a useful support system.

ILEOSTOMY ALTERNATIVES

KEITH A. KELLY, M.D.

A Brooke ileostomy, while simple and safe to construct, is completely incontinent of both gas and stool. An appliance must be worn day and night to collect the output from the stoma. The appliances are unsightly, uncomfortable, and odoriferous. Embarrassing noises may issue from the stoma during times of fecal discharge. There is also the ever-present danger of leakage at the site of attachment of the appliance to the skin. In addition, the appliances are expensive. Some patients estimate the cost of maintaining the appliance and servicing the ileostomy to be in the neighborhood of $400 to $500 per year. Thus, an alternative to the incontinent Brooke ileostomy would be well received.

Until recently, few alternatives were available. Today, however, a number of continence-preserving operations are available, the most attractive of which are the ileal pouch-anal anastomosis, the continent ileostomy (Kock pouch), and the continent ostomy device.

These newer operations are performed mainly for patients with ulcerative colitis and polyposis coli. The operations are not advised for patients with Crohn's disease, because of the risk of recurrence of Crohn's disease in the small bowel remaining after operation. They are done for the intestinal or extraintestinal complications of the colitis and polyposis coli, and to treat or prevent the development of cancer of the large intestine.

ILEAL POUCH-ANAL ANASTOMOSIS

My current preferred operative approach to ulcerative colitis and polyposis coli is colectomy, mucosal rectectomy, and ileal pouch-anal anastomosis.

Rationale

The rationale behind the operation is that it removes the disease via the colectomy and mucosal rectectomy, yet preserves anal sphincter function, voluntary transanal defecation, and anal continence. No permanent ileostomy is required. The ileal pouch provides a reservoir adequate enough to prevent excessive stool production. Moreover, because the mucosal rectectomy is done from the luminal side of the rectum, operative injury of the perirectal nerves to the bladder and genitalia is minimized. There is thus little likelihood of postoperative urinary or sexual dysfunction. In addition, because the anus and rectum are not excised, no perineal wound is present after the procedure, a wound which is sometimes difficult to heal.

Type of Patient

This operation can be done in children, young adults, or middle-aged adults. Patients older than 55 years are less likely to be candidates, because their anal sphincters may be less competent than those of younger patients. Patients should have good anal sphincteric function and good continence prior to operation and should not be obese. Also, the operation is more likely to be successful if there is no perianal disease, such as an abscess or an anal fistula, and if there has been no previous anal surgery. Severe illness, inanition, and the taking of corticosteroids do not, however, prevent use of the procedure.

Preoperative Preparation

The patients are placed on a clear liquid diet the day before operation and given an oral antibiotic preparation of neomycin sulfate, 250 mg 4 times a day, and tetracycline hydrochloride, 250 mg four times a day. Cephalothin sodium, 0.5 g, is administered intravenously just before the operation, during the operation, and in the immediate postoperative period.

Operative Technique

The patient is anesthetized and placed in a modified lithotomy position to provide access to both the abdomen and the perineum. A vertical, midline abdominal incision is made, the abdominal contents inspected, and the presence of ulcerative colitis or polyposis coli verified. The large intestine is mobilized from the cecum to the levator ani and its blood supply divided. The mid-rectum is stapled closed and transected at a point about 7-cm proximal to the levator ani. The cecum, colon, and proximal rectum are removed.

The surgeon then positions him- or herself at the perineum, everts the distal rectum onto the perineum, and strips the diseased distal rectal mucosa from the underlying tunica muscularis using the cautery. The dissection begins at the dentate line and extends to a point 5-cm orad to the line. At this point, the rectal wall is transected, and the rectum proximal to the transection is removed. The everted distal 5 cm of rectal tunica muscularis is then repositioned in its usual anatomic location.

The surgeon returns to the abdominal side where an ileal pouch is constructed from the terminal 30 cm of ileum. The 30 cm are fashioned into the shape of a J, and the anterior and posterior layers of the J are anastomosed using two layers of continuous 2-0 chromic catgut or stainless steel staples. The bottom of the J is then brought down endorectally and anastomosed to the dentate line with continuous 2-0 chromic catgut suture. A suction drain is placed through a left flank incision and positioned in the perirectal space to drain it during the postoperative period. A proximal diverting loop ileostomy in the right lower quadrant completes the initial operation.

The patient is allowed 2 months to recover from the initial procedure, at which time proctoscopy, roentgenographic studies of the ileal pouch and the anastomosis, and sometimes anorectal manometry are performed to ascertain the degree of healing and anorectal function. With a well-healed anastomosis, no sign of intrapelvic sepsis or fistulas, and a good anal sphincter, the diverting ileostomy is ready for closure at a second operation.

Postoperative Care

After closure of the ileostomy, the patients are placed on loperamide hydrochloride and a psyllium preparation until thickening of the enteric content is obtained and stool frequency is satisfactory. These medications can usually be gradually decreased over a 3-month to 4-month period.

Side Effects

The patients are completely continent during the day, but they do pass larger quantities of stool after operation than do normal individuals. The fecal output of the patients averages about 650 ml per day, a quantity passed as four to six bowel movements during the day and perhaps one at night. The discrimination of gas from feces is generally satisfactory but not quite as good as in health. In addition, during sleep there may be some minor fecal leakage because of the decrease in the reservoir function of the distal bowel after the colectomy, the more fluid nature of the enteric content, and the propulsive force of the distal ileal contractions.

Complications

The main complications of the operation are perianastomotic sepsis and intestinal obstruction. Perianastomotic sepsis can be minimized by using the preoperative preparation outlined above and by constructing the diverting loop ileostomy. Obtaining excellent hemostasis prior to closure and the use of the pelvic drain to remove serum and blood in the area of operation minimizes abscess formation. The drain should be placed well away from the ileal-anal anastomosis so as not to hinder healing of the anastomosis.

Intestinal obstruction is combated by careful hemostasis prior to closure; intra-abdominal irrigation to remove necrotic material, debris, and blood; and construction of the ileostomy in the right lower quadrant using the loop method. The proximal ileum is positioned intra-abdominally to the left of the stoma, and the distal ileum is placed to the right of the stoma and laterally. This positioning of the bowel helps to prevent herniation of the proximal bowel into the space lateral to the ileostomy. An intestinal tube is also placed into the proximal bowel via the stoma at the operation. The tube prevents kinking and volvulus of the proximal bowel in the early postoperative period, after which the tube is removed.

Outcome

The procedure does achieve its objective of maintaining fecal control without the need for permanent ileostomy and with voluntary transanal passage of fecal content. The main disadvantages of the procedures are frequent bowel movements, occasional leakage of stool at night, and an associated perineal or perianal irritation when leakage does occur. A few patients also develop a bacterial overgrowth in the ileal pouch, sometimes with unusual organisms such as *Clostridium difficile* or *Campylobacter*. The overgrowth of bacteria may result in diarrhea, fever, weakness, and malaise. It can usually be treated satisfactorily with an antibacterial agent, such as metronidazole, 250 mg 4 times a day.

THE CONTINENT ILEOSTOMY (KOCK POUCH)

The continent ileostomy, or Kock pouch, consists of three parts: a pouch made of distal ileum, a valve made of terminal ileum interposed between the pouch and the exterior, and an efferent ileal limb leading from the valve to the stoma. For patients who require an ileostomy, the Kock pouch provides fecal continence and eliminates the need for an ileostomy appliance.

Rationale

The rationale behind the procedure is that the pouch collects and holds fecal content until it is emptied by passing a catheter through the stoma and valve into the pouch. The content then drains through the catheter directly into the toilet bowl, after which the catheter is removed. The catheter is rinsed after its use and placed in a purse to be carried with the patient during the day. A small dressing is placed over the stoma to prevent mucus secreted by the surface epithelium of the ileum from soiling the clothes. In between intubations, no gas or stool leaks, and so no ileal appliance need be worn. The patient has complete control over the fecal discharge.

Type of Patient

This operation is suitable for young or middle-aged adults who already have an incontinent Brooke ileostomy after proctocolectomy for colitis or polyposis coli or who require proctocolectomy and do not wish to have the increased number of stools associated with the ileal pouch-anal anastomosis. Patients must have sufficient understanding, intelligence, and physical capabilities to deal with catheterization and care of the pouch. Thus, children or patients over 70 years of age are often not candidates. Also, construction of a Kock pouch is difficult in obese patients.

Operative Technique

The operation is done in one stage and is performed with the patient in the modified lithotomy position. The proctocolectomy is accomplished, after which the pouch is fashioned from the terminal 45 cm of ileum. The anterior and posterior walls of the pouch are constructed with two layers of continuous 2–0 chromic catgut. The terminal ileum is intussuscepted into the newly formed pouch for a distance of 5 cm to form the valve. The intussuscepted ileum is anchored in place with four cartridges of stainless steel staples, while additional sutures of 4–0 Dacron are taken at the exit of the efferent limb from the pouch to further anchor the valve in place. The efferent ileal limb leading to the stoma is made as short as possible, and the stoma is placed just above the hairline in the right lower quadrant. The pouch is sewn to the anterior abdominal wall just beneath the stoma, again with interrupted 4–0 Dacron sutures. The ileostomy is made flush with the skin. The space lateral to the pouch is closed by approximating the ileal mesentery to the parietal peritoneum of the right lower quadrant of the abdomen. This obviates volvulus of the pouch and peripouch herniation of the more proximal small intestine.

Postoperative Care

The pouch is intubated for a period of one month postoperatively to ensure that the pouch and valve remain in the appropriate position while the fibrous tissue of healing fixes the structures in place. The tube is then removed and the patient begins intermittent intubation of the pouch. At first, the intubations are done every 2 hours during the day, while the catheter is left in place continuously overnight. The interval between intubations is increased gradually, until after a second month the patient is intubating the pouch four times a day but not at night. The patients require no medication and can eat a general diet, provided that they masticate thoroughly. Poorly masticated, indigestible materials, such as mushrooms, kernels of corn, string beans, and cabbage plug the catheter during intubations and delay emptying.

Outcome

The procedure does achieve its objective of providing complete control over fecal discharge. The patients, however, do have an ileostomy, and they must intubate the ileal pouch to empty it. In addition, two complications of the Kock pouch have appeared: malfunction of the valve and diarrhea.

Malfunction of the valve occurs because the intussusceptum of terminal ileum which forms the valve sometimes reduces partially, resulting in a tortuous tract leading from the pouch to the exterior. The patient then has two problems: difficulty intubating the pouch and leakage of content from the pouch. Reoperation is usually required, at which time the valve must be replaced within the pouch and reanchored with stainless steel staples and sutures. Reoperation is necessary today in about 15 to 20 percent of patients and is usually successful. Reoperation does not guarantee, however, that the valve will function perfectly henceforth. A second reoperation may be required in an additional 15 to 20 percent of patients.

Diarrhea, which occurs in about 5 percent of patients, likely results from bacterial overgrowth in the pouch. The diarrhea, when symptomatic, can usually be managed satisfactorily with antibiotics.

ILEOSTOMY OCCLUDING DEVICE

The artificial ileostomy occluding device provides control over fecal discharge in ileostomy patients and eliminates the ileostomy bag.

Rationale and Plan of Use

The rationale of the ileostomy occluding device is to provide a mechanical blockage to the overflow from an ileal pouch or an end ileostomy and so provide control over fecal discharge from the intestinal tract. Moreover, the possibility of valvular malfunction requiring reoperation, as is the case with the Kock pouch, is avoided.

TABLE 1 Outcome of Operations for Ulcerative Colitis and Polyposis Coli

Procedure	Fecal Continence Preserved	Stoma Present	Intubations Required	Disadvantages
Brooke ileostomy	No	Yes	No	Ileostomy bag required
Ileal pouch-anal anastomosis	Yes	No	No	Frequent stools, occasional fecal leakage
Kock pouch	Yes	Yes	Yes	Valve malfunction, diarrhea
Ileostomy obstructing device	Yes	Yes	Yes	Device discomfort, mucus discharge
Ileorectostomy	Yes	No	No	Rectal mucosa remains to cause symptoms and cancer

The device consists of a 28 F catheter that has a soft, inflatable balloon affixed to its internal end. The catheter is inserted into the pouch, the balloon inflated, and the inflated balloon pulled up against the anterior abdominal wall just beneath the stoma. A disk slipped over the external end of the catheter and pushed down to the skin keeps the balloon snugged up against the anterior abdominal wall and occludes fecal outflow from the pouch. To prevent leakage of fecal content through the lumen of the catheter, the catheter is folded over and fixed to the disk.

Type of Patient

The ileostomy occluding device can be used in patients of almost any age or body habitus. For example, it can be employed in elderly patients and in obese patients not ordinarily candidates for ileoanal anastomosis or the continent ileostomy (Kock pouch).

Operative Technique

An ileal pouch is constructed from the terminal 35 cm of ileum, as with a Kock pouch, but the biologic valve of the Kock pouch is not made. The efferent limb from the ileal pouch is simply brought through the anterior abdominal wall and the stoma constructed. The device is then passed through the stoma and positioned in the pouch. The device is connected to straight drainage for the first postoperative month to allow the pouch to heal before it is distended. Intermittent occlusions using the device are begun thereafter, and continence is achieved immediately. At first only short periods of occlusion can be tolerated, but as the distal ileum dilates over a 6-week to 8-week period, 6-hour periods of occlusion can be accomplished.

Outcome

The main advantages of the procedure are its simplicity and its lack of complications. The device can be removed and reinserted at will. Reoperation to change the device is not necessary. The main disadvantage of the procedure is the need to wear the device and the discomfort thereof. The appliance itself, while not large, does produce some bulk on the anterior abdominal wall. In addition, the presence of the appliance stimulates the production of mucus from the terminal ileum, so that absorbent pads must be worn between the appliance and the skin.

ILEORECTOSTOMY

Ileorectostomy has been used infrequently at the Mayo Clinic. The operation does not excise the diseased rectal mucosa, which continues to ulcerate, bleed, and cause pain and diarrhea in patients with ulcerative colitis. In addition, the risk of carcinoma developing in the rectal mucosa remains in patients with colitis or polyposis coli.

Type of Patient

Nonetheless, there are some patients who have such minimal involvement of the rectum that an ileorectostomy is a reasonable choice, especially if these patients are young and anxious to avoid any type of ileostomy or the disabilities and minimal risk to sexual or urinary function occasioned by an ileoanal anastomosis.

Operative Technique

The operation is done with the patient in the supine position through a midline abdominal incision. After excision of the cecum and colon, the ileum is anastomosed end-to-end to the rectum using continuous 3–0 chromic catgut on the mucosal layer and interrupted 4–0 Dacron sutures on the seromuscular layer.

Outcome

Fewer than one-half of patients undergoing this operation will have a satisfactory result over a 5- to 15-year follow-up. Those with a good result experience fewer than eight bowel movements per day, are continent, require no systemic steroids, and maintain a satisfactory style of life. They require yearly proctoscopic examinations to ascertain the presence or absence of continuing inflammation in their rectal mucosa and also to check for dysplasia, polyps, or other signs of malignancy in this mucosa. The other one-half of the patients have more disabling symptoms that require treatment, threaten life, and eventually mandate excision of the remaining rectal mucosa.

CONCLUSIONS

The pros and cons of the various operations for ulcerative colitis and polyposis coli are outlined in Table 1. On balance, I advise and most patients elect ileal pouch-anal anastomosis. Its major advantages, which include total excision of the disease, avoidance of the ileostomy, maintenance of voluntary transanal defecation, and reasonable continence, recommend it over the other options.

RECTAL CARCINOMA: SPHINCTER SPARING PROCEDURES

NORMAN SOHN, M.D., F.A.C.S.

Rectal carcinoma continues to be common. Its treatment presents problems in two areas: first, eradication, so that it no longer represents a threat to the patient, and second, preservation of the normal pathway for defecation following its treatment. In the early part of this century, Miles laid down principles for the surgical treatment of rectal carcinoma. These should represent the standards to which newer therapies can be compared. He recommended excision of the anorectal sphincters, levator ani muscles, and rectum, necessitating a permanent colostomy. Despite the emotional burden which a colostomy can generate, most such patients can be rehabilitated and live normal lives with few modifications in their daily routines.

Two directions can be followed in attempting to preserve the normal defecatory pathway. One is *nonoperative* or *local operative procedures*, which can be performed for selected tumors. The other course is modification of operations resulting in *preservation* of the *anorectal sphincter* mechanism *without compromising potential for cure*.

Techniques for local treatment or local excision are ideal for small lesions in which there are no lymph node metastases. Such therapy would theoretically fail to cure the patient who has lymph node metastases, who might be cured by a more radical operation. Future development of techniques, perhaps utilizing monoclonal antibodies, may better define the patients who could benefit most from local therapy and also those patients who require a radical approach.

There are several surgical techniques, as well as other therapeutic modalities, that can be applied to the patient with rectal carcinoma which may obviate the need for a permanent colostomy. An appreciation of these modalities is important in selecting appropriate therapy. The following will be discussed in this chapter: (1) combined chemotherapy and radiation therapy for squamous and cloacogenic carcinoma, (2) intracavitary radiation therapy, (3) electrocoagulation of rectal tumors, (4) anterior resection, (5) abdominoanal resection, (6) pull-through operations, and (7) abdominosacral resection.

NONOPERATIVE OR LOCALLY DESTRUCTIVE THERAPY

Combined Chemotherapy and Radiation Therapy

Combination chemotherapy and radiation therapy was initially introduced as adjuvant therapy in the treatment of squamous and cloacogenic carcinomas of the anorectum. It was subsequently found that this therapy alone, without further resection, could successfully treat many of these lesions. The treatment protocol involves initial therapy with mitomycin C, 5-fluorouracil (5-FU), and radiation therapy. On the twenty-eighth day following initiation of treatment, the infusion of 5-FU is repeated. Two to 3 weeks later the site of the tumor is biopsied or excised. If no tumor is present, nothing further is done except careful observation. Persistent tumor is considered an indication for abdominoperineal resection with a permanent colostomy. Trials with other chemotherapeutic agents for failures of the initial treatment are under investigation at this time. Utilizing this program, one can expect to cure more than 80 percent of tumors.

Intracavitary Radiation

Intracavitary radiation therapy, introduced and popularized by Papillon, involves the administration of radiation therapy via a modified proctosigmoidoscope. No hospitalization is necessary. The treatment is given in three sessions at intervals of 3 weeks. This technique ideally is applicable to patients with small, mobile lesions located above the anal sphincters and up to the 10 cm level. It can be expected to cure more than 90 percent of cases. This information is supplemented by the chapter *Intraoperative Irradiation*.

Electrocoagulation

Electrocoagulation was introduced many years ago for the treatment of rectal tumors. It was popularized in the mid-1960s and designated the primary preferred treatment of rectal cancer. Original enthusiasm for the technique has waned and at this time it is felt to be applicable only in carefully selected patients with small and mobile lesions. The latter group of patients are usually better managed with intracavitary radiation. Elderly or poor-risk patients or those who refuse a colostomy can be considered for this technique. Laser destruction of tumors has also been used for palliation of rectal cancer.

SURGICAL RESECTION TECHNIQUES

Anterior Resection

There are two important principles involved in the selection of a resection type of operation for rectal cancer. First, the tumor must be excised along with an appropriate margin. There is controversy in the literature as to whether the classic 5-cm level is necessary or whether this margin can be reduced under certain circumstances. In any event it is generally acknowledged that a 5-cm margin represents an adequate margin of resection. Second, the levator muscles and external sphincter must be preserved to ensure continence. An anastomosis at or above the 3-cm level, as measured from the anal verge, is above these important structures. Thus, if a 5-cm margin is to be obtained and the anastomosis is to be above the 3-cm level, tumors that are below the 8-cm level usually have to be treated by means of an abdominoperineal resection with a permanent colostomy.

These measurements are best made with a rigid sigmoidoscope. Measurements with a flexible endoscope often do not give reliable reproducible data. Occasionally the measurements are imprecise. Mobilization of the rectum during the course of the operation may result in the determination that the tumor, along with an adequate margin, can be excised despite preoperative measurements that would have predicted that a sphincter-saving procedure would be unlikely. In general, low anastomoses can be performed more easily in women or in nonobese patients than in obese patients or men.

The most important part of the operation should be the adequate excision of the primary lesion. The surgeon usually has no difficulty satisfactorily resecting the bowel with the tumor via the abdomen; however, reconstruction with the establishment of an anastomosis can be difficult and trying and may even be impossible via the abdominal route. Reconstruction via coloanal or colorectal anastomosis has to be of secondary importance. The techniques to be described can accomplish an anastomosis at any level of the rectum. Therefore, the primary efforts have to be directed toward excision of the rectum with the primary tumor. Reconstruction must have a secondary role.

In the anterior resection an anastomosis is performed via an abdominal approach. Intestinal stapling devices can facilitate, simplify, and expedite this operation if the surgeon is skilled in their use. It is probable that a low anterior resection can be performed with a classic hand suturing technique as well and as low as with the staple technique. A tenuous anastomosis may, in the judgment of the surgeon, require the addition of a complementary transverse colostomy or cecostomy.

Abdominoanal Resection

In abdominoanal resection, in which the anastomosis is too low to be comfortably performed abdominally, the anastomosis is performed transanally. Retractors which are utilized in anorectal surgery can facilitate this anastomosis. A hand-sutured anastomosis can be performed via this route. Alternatively, a purse-string suture can be applied to the upper cut edge of the rectum to utilize the intraluminal intestinal stapling device. Using this technique, an anastomosis can be performed at the 3-cm level.

Pull-Through Procedures

In the pull-through operation, rather than a hand-sutured anastomosis or stapled anastomosis being performed, the proximal end of the colon is drawn out the anus. Union between the upper cut edge of the rectum and the seromuscular coat of the colon occurs. Seven to 10 days postoperatively any residual colon protruding from the anus can be amputated.

When an abdominoanal procedure is performed a complementary transverse colostomy is also constructed. This protects the tenuous coloanal anastomosis from the effects of failure of primary healing of the suture line. The pull-through procedure can be performed without a complementary colostomy. To accomplish a pull-through operation, approximately 3 to 4 inches of additional colon are needed to protrude from the anus. This added length of bowel is frequently not available. In the latter situation the abdominoanal reconstruction can be performed.

Abdominosacral Procedure

In the abdominosacral procedure the colorectal anastomosis is performed transsacrally. The patient is positioned on the operating table in the lateral position with the right side down. A long oblique incision from the right lower quadrant to the left upper quadrant is utilized. The abdominal portion of the operation is performed in this position and is similar to the standard operation. A second incision is made transversely across the sacrococcygeal junction, the coccyx is excised, and the anastomosis performed.

The disadvantage of this operation is that it is performed in the lateral position, a position with which many surgeons are not comfortable or familiar. Furthermore, there is added morbidity from the sacral incision and the possibility of a sacral fistula. This operation offers no advantage over the abdominoanal procedure. The latter is performed in the modified lithotomy position, which is well known to every abdominal surgeon.

Ileal Pouch

In the rare situation in which a near total colectomy along with a low anterior resection has to be performed for multiple carcinomas of the rectum, an ileal pouch can be constructed and anastomosed to the anus. This operation is similar to that performed for ulcerative colitis or familial polyposis. The patient can then be provided with a reservoir and maintain normal rectal sphincter function. The purpose of the reservoir is to minimize the potential for diarrhea. A temporary ileostomy is utilized for 2 months.

In some cases of abdominoanal resection where the anastomosis is performed at the 6- or 7-cm level, it may be difficult to perform it transanally. Under these circumstances it may be advantageous to excise the rectal mucosa from the dentate line to the cut edge of the rectum and perform the anastomosis at the level of the dentate line. At this level an anastomosis is technically easier to perform.

The physician embarking on the care of the patient with a rectal neoplasm has to decide between resection or nonresection. Squamous and cloacogenic carcinomas should be treated with combination chemotherapy and radiation therapy. Small, mobile lesions can often be efficiently and effectively managed with intracavitary radiotherapy. Poor risk patients, those who refuse an inevitable colostomy and those deemed to require only palliative therapy should be considered for electrocoagulation. Lesions considered ideal for intracavitary radiation may alternatively be treated by electrocoagulation if the former modality is not available. The role of laser destruction in these patients remains to be defined.

The surgeon embarking on a resection must have available the knowledge to perform the anterior resection and the abdominoanal and pull-through procedures as well. There is little place for the abdominosacral operation. With these options available the surgeon can then totally excise the tumor and yet be capable of restoring anal continence if possible. In most situations an anterior resection, with an anastomosis constructed via the abdomen, either by hand or with a stapler, can be performed. A pull-through procedure requires more length on the proximal end of bowel than may be available, but can be performed without a protective colostomy. The abdominoanal resection is applicable in most clinical situations but should be performed with a protective colostomy. There should be few cases in which an abdominoperineal resection is performed for the sole reason that it is technically impossible to accomplish an anastomosis.

COLORECTAL CARCINOMA: ADJUVANT THERAPY

ANTHONY N. BRANNAN, M.D.
ROBERT W. BEART, Jr., M.D.

Currently, colorectal carcinoma is the second most common malignancy in the United States. In 1984, approximately 130,000 new cases of colorectal carcinoma were diagnosed, and approximately 59,000 persons died from this disease. "Curative" surgical resection has been the most effective primary treatment for colorectal carcinoma. In spite of improved diagnostic and surgical techniques, however, the overall 5-year survival rate of approximately 50 percent has not improved significantly during the last 30 years. In this chapter we review the adjuvant modalities which, during the last two decades, have been developed in an attempt to decrease the recurrence rate of the tumor and to increase the survival.

NEED FOR SURGICAL ADJUVANT TREATMENT

The Dukes staging system has been useful in determining which subpopulations of patients are most likely to benefit from adjuvant treatment. For tumors confined to the bowel wall (Dukes A and B1), the surgical cure rate is 70 to 80 percent; however, with tumor penetration through the bowel wall and/or metastasis to regional lymph nodes (Dukes B2 and C), the cure rates drop markedly, ranging from 40 to 70 percent.

A modification of the Astler-Coller staging system has been developed by Gunderson and Sosin to distinguish subpopulations of patients who are at greatest risk for local tumor recurrence (Table 1). This staging system differentiates the degrees of extracolonic or extrarectal involvement and indicates that subgroups of patients within each Dukes stage B and C classification have significantly different risks of local tumor recurrence.

Local recurrence is more frequent for rectal than for colon carcinomas. Various autopsy, clinical, and reoperative series indicate that for rectal cancer the incidence of local recurrence is 20 to 25 percent for stage C1, 30 to 35 percent for stage B2 or B3, and 50 to 65 percent for stage C2 or C3. Stage A or B1 tumors have a recurrence rate of less than 10 percent. After local recurrence, significant palliation can be obtained in 75 to 85 percent of the patients by means of radiation alone or by a combination of radiation and chemotherapy; however, the duration of palliation is often limited, and the chance for cure is only 5 percent or less. Therefore, it is imperative that local recurrence be prevented. The patients who could potentially benefit from effective adjuvant therapy are

TABLE 1 Dukes and Modified Astler-Coller Staging of Rectal Cancer by Gunderson and Sosin

Dukes Stage	Modified Astler-Coller Stage	Description
A	A	Nodes negative; lesion limited to mucosa
	B1	Nodes negative; extension of lesion through mucosa but still within bowel wall
B	$B2_m$	Nodes negative; microscopic extension through the entire bowel wall (including serosa if present)
	$B2_{m+g}$	Nodes negative; gross extension through the entire bowel wall (including serosa if present) with microscopic confirmation
	B3	Nodes negative; adherence to or invasion of surrounding organs or structures
C	C1	Nodes positive; lesion limited to bowel wall
	$C2_m$	Nodes positive; extension of lesions through the entire bowel wall (including serosa if present)
	$C2_{m+g}$	Nodes positive; gross extension through the entire bowel wall (including serosa if present) with microscopic confirmation
	C3	Nodes positive; adherence to or invasion of surrounding organs or structures

those with tumor penetration through the bowel wall and/or metastasis to regional lymph nodes (Dukes B2 and C).

COLON CARCINOMA

For the last 25 to 30 years, clinical trials have been performed in hopes of identifying a chemotherapeutic agent capable of improving the survival rates for patients undergoing resection of Dukes B2 and C colon carcinomas. The control groups (surgery alone) in current adjuvant trials remain appropriate because surgical survival rates have improved. One of the earliest adjuvant chemotherapy trials was conducted by the Veterans Administration Surgical Oncology Group (VASOG), employing thiotepa, an alkylating agent (Table 2). Thiotepa was administered intraoperatively and on the first two postoperative days, but there was no change in survival from that of untreated controls.

Subsequent trials involved the use of the fluorinated pyrimidines, 5-fluorouracil (5-FU) or fluorodeoxyuridine (FUDR), on the basis of their ability to produce partial remissions in 10 to 20 percent of patients with advanced colorectal cancer. The VASOG study using FUDR showed no treatment benefit.

The VASOG conducted its third adjuvant study between 1965 and 1969, studying the effect of 5-FU. Therapy with 5-fluorouracil was started 2 weeks after operation and was continued for 5 successive days, and this 5-day course was repeated 6 weeks later. The 5-year survival rate among 338 patients having "curative" resection was 58 percent for those patients treated with 5-FU and 48 percent for the control group. This improvement in survival was not statistically significant.

As years passed, a better understanding of tumor cell kinetics and the action of chemotherapeutic agents influenced the design of clinical trials. It was believed that recurrent disease after "curative" resection probably was caused not by tumor cells dislodged at the time of surgical manipulations but by microscopic metastatic cells that had become established long before the operation.

The importance of administering chemotherapeutic agents in the appropriate dose, route, and schedule was realized, and agents were administered repeatedly during a longer period, usually at least a year. Agents were administered only to patients at high risk for micrometastases, therefore sparing those patients who were likely to be cured by surgery alone from the potential toxic effects of chemotherapy.

The next VASOG study, the so-called prolonged intermittent therapy trial, reflected some of these changes in philosophy. Between 1969 and 1973, 5-FU was given to patients with Dukes B2 and C lesions. Five-day cycles of 5-FU were given postoperatively for 18 months at 6- to 8-week intervals. The 5-year survival rate among the 518 patients having "curative" resection was 49.1 percent for treated patients and 44.7 percent for control patients. Again, a small, statistically insignificant benefit was seen in the patients treated with 5-FU.

The final study of adjuvant 5-FU was conducted between 1971 and 1976 by the Central Oncology Group on 233 patients with Dukes B2 and C lesions. The treatment began within four weeks after operation and was given daily for 4 days, followed by an alternate-day schedule for an additional five doses. After a 1- to 2-week rest, patients were given weekly treatments for 1 year. The 4-year survival rate was 62 percent for the treated patients and 60 percent for the control patients; once again, the difference was not statistically significant. The patients with Dukes C lesions who were treated with 5-FU had a statistically significant prolongation of disease-free interval; the median disease-free interval was 30 months for treated patients and 18 months for control patients ($P = 0.04$).

All of these trials showed that 5-FU improved survival approximately 5 to 10 percent. Because this small benefit was statistically insignificant and because there were risks associated with 5-FU, the routine use of 5-FU in the adjuvant setting has not been universally supported. However, the slight beneficial effect of 5-FU supported the continuation of clinical trials that examined the effect of 5-FU in combination with other chemotherapeutic agents.

Between 1975 and 1979, the Gastrointestinal Tumor Study Group (GITSG) randomized 621 patients who had Dukes B2 and C lesions into a four-arm study to evaluate combination chemotherapy using 5-FU, methyl CCNU, and immunotherapy using a methanol-extraction residue of bacillus Calmette-Guérin (MER). In prior clinical trials, the combination of 5-FU and methyl CCNU had been reported to have produced substantial response rates in patients with advanced large bowel cancer. MER, a nonspecific immunostimulant, was chosen on the basis of reports of its antitumor activity in animal tumor systems and reports of the temporary regression of tumor in patients with advanced gastrointestinal cancer. The four treatment arms were (1) control, (2) 5-FU and methyl CCNU, (3) MER, and (4) 5-FU, methyl CCNU, and MER. At a median postoperative follow-up time of 65 months, there was no statistically significant difference in survival or recurrence rates. One patient died of sepsis associated with bone marrow depression, and six patients from the group receiving 5-FU and methyl CCNU developed leukemia. The importance of a *concurrent* control population was demonstrated because the survival for all four treatment groups was better than that of historic controls. Therefore, comparison with historic controls would have erroneously shown a beneficial effect of adjuvant therapy.

A GITSG trial that has been in progress since 1979 is comparing surgery alone with the combination of 5-FU and whole-liver radiation using 2,100 rads. Results are not available at this time.

Currently, trials examining the immunotherapeutic effect of levamisole are in progress. Levamisole, a proven antihelminthic, stimulates the human immune system by enhancing both the lymphocytic and the macrophage activity. It is administered orally and has only minimal side effects. Studies have reported significant increases in survival rates for patients with various malignancies after treatment with levamisole. Two randomized studies, one by Verhaegen and another by Borden at the University of Wisconsin, indicate that levamisole significantly improves survival rates for patients with colorectal carcinoma. From 1978 to 1984, the North Central Cancer Treatment Group randomized 408 patients with Dukes B2 and C carcinoma to one of three arms: (1) control, (2) levamisole, and (3) levamisole and 5-FU. A confirmatory intergroup study is in progress at this time.

In 1975, Taylor initiated a study to examine the effect of adjuvant liver perfusion with 5-FU by way of the portal venous system in patients with resected Dukes B2 and C lesions. It is hoped that this treatment will decrease the incidence of hepatic metastases by eradicating hepatic micrometastases or any tumor cells that may have seeded the liver via the portal vein. At operation, patients are randomized to either the control or the portal vein infusion group. Portal venous infusion of 5-FU is performed for 7 days during the immediate postoperative period. The results so far are promising. In 1981, Taylor reported that 38 patients (39%) from the control group of 97 patients died and 17 patients (18%) had liver metastases.[1] This compared with the 90 patients in the treated group, of whom 19 (21%) died and 5 (6%) had liver metastases. The median follow-up was 34 months. These data provide suggestive evidence that this treatment may decrease the incidence of liver metastases. Unfortunately, the incidence of local or peritoneal (or both) recurrences remains unchanged. Patients with Dukes B tumors seem to

TABLE 2 Prospective, Randomized, Controlled Trials for adjuvant Therapy in Colon Carcinoma

Date	Group*	Agent†	Result
1957–1961	VASOG	Thiotepa: intraoperatively on postoperative days 1 and 2	No improvement in survival
1960s	VASOG	FUDR: postoperative days 1, 2, and 3, repeat in 6 wk	No improvement in survival
1965–1969	VASOG	5-FU: began 2 wk postoperatively for 5 days and repeated in 6 wk	5-year survival: treated 58%, control 48%; not statistically significant
1969–1973	VASOG PIT	5-FU: began 2 wk postoperatively, 5-day cycles given every 6–8 wk for 18 mo	5-year survival: treated 49%, control 45%; not statistically significant
1971–1976	COG	5-FU: began within 4 wk, daily for 4 days, every other day for 5 doses, 1–2 wk rest, weekly for 1 yr	4-year survival: treated 62%, control 60%; not statistically significant; Dukes C patients, median disease-free interval: treated 30 mo, control 18 mo (p=0.04)
1975–1979	GITSG	1) Control 2) 5-FU and methyl CCNU 3) MER 4) 5-FU, methyl CCNU, and MER Began within 7 wk and continued for 70 wk	No difference in survival and recurrence with median postoperative follow-up of 65 mo
1979–present	GITSG	1) Control 2) 5-FU and external whole-liver radiation (2,100 rads)	Results unavailable at this time
1978–1984	NCCTG	1) Control 2) Levamisole 3) Levamisole and 5-FU	Results unavailable at this time

* VASOG = Veterans Administration Surgical Oncology Group, VASOG PIT = VASOG prolonged intermittent therapy trial, COG = Central Oncology Group, GITSG = Gastrointestinal Tumor Study Group, NCCTG = North Central Cancer Treatment Group.
† FUDR = fluorodeoxyuridine, 5-FU = 5-fluorouracil, CCNU = lomustine, MER = bacillus Calmette-Guérin.

benefit most. These results warrant confirmation, so currently the Mayo Clinic, the Australia and New Zealand Bowel Cancer Trials Group, and the Swiss Group for Clinical Cancer Research are conducting adjuvant liver perfusion trials.

RECTAL CARCINOMA

Approximately 40,000 of the 130,000 new cases of colorectal carcinoma in 1984 were rectal carcinomas. The most ominous long-term complication after "curative" resection of rectal carcinoma is local recurrence. Because radiation therapy for unresectable or recurrent rectal carcinoma in the past has demonstrated significant palliation and occasional cures, strong consideration has been given to the use of radiation therapy as an adjuvant to surgery in hopes of decreasing the recurrence rates.

In 1974, Gunderson and Sosin determined the location of tumor recurrence in a unique series of 75 high-risk patients at the University of Minnesota who underwent reoperation (second or symptomatic look) after "curative" resection of rectal carcinoma. They found 52 patients with recurrent carcinoma. Local recurrence in the tumor bed or regional nodes was noted in 25 patients (48%) and distant metastases alone were found in four patients (8%). Twenty-three other patients had local recurrence in combination with distant metastases. Therefore, 48 patients (92%) had local recurrence as a part of their recurrence. Because a significant number of patients have local recurrence in a well-defined anatomic area (i.e., pelvis), rectal cancer is very amenable to local adjuvant treatment, such as radiotherapy.

Because there are risks to radiation therapy, such as obstructive radiation enteritis, only those patients with a significant risk of recurrence should be treated. Patients with Dukes B2 and C rectal cancers—those who are at highest risk for local recurrence, with rates ranging from 20 to 65 percent—need an effective surgical adjuvant treatment.

Both preoperative and postoperative adjuvant radiation therapies for rectal carcinoma have been investigated, and there are advantages to each. The major advantage of preoperative radiation therapy is the potential damaging effect on cells that may spread locally or distantly at operation. Perhaps a well-designed combination of preoperative and postoperative radiation therapy ("sandwich" technique) could combine the theoretical advantages of each.

PREOPERATIVE RADIATION THERAPY

The rationale for preoperative radiation therapy is to decrease tumor size, increase resectability, prevent tumor seeding during operation, and destroy microscopic foci of tumor that are outside the margins of surgical resection in order to decrease local recurrence. Interest in the use of preoperative radiation therapy was stimulated by a retrospective, nonrandomized study from Memorial Hospital using various radiation techniques and doses from 1,500 to 2,000 rads in patients with rectal carcinoma between 1939 and 1951. When compared with "matched" controls, patients with Dukes C lesions had a significant improvement in 5-year survival rate (37% compared with 23% for patients undergoing surgery alone).

Since that study, numerous prospective trials have evaluated the effectiveness of adjuvant preoperative radiation therapy for rectal cancer (Table 3). Between 1957 and 1967, the Memorial Hospital group randomized 790 patients with rectal cancer to receive surgery alone or 2,000 rads preoperatively. The group found no difference in survival rates but noted a decrease in local recurrence in patients with Dukes C lesions who were receiving preoperative radiation therapy. That study has been criticized because the patients were not randomized during the first 2 years.

From 1964 to 1969, the VASOG conducted a prospective study using 2,000 to 2,500 rads preoperatively in 700 patients. The patients who had preoperative radiation followed by "curative" resection had an improved five-year survival rate (49% compared with 39% for those undergoing surgery alone); however, the difference was not statistically significant. The local recurrence rate was improved in the irradiated group, but the difference also was not statistically significant.

A prospective study initiated in 1965 at Princess Margaret Hospital in Toronto, comparing preoperative treatment using 500 rads with surgery alone, found a statistically significant improved 5-year survival rate (35% compared with 17% for surgery alone) in patients with Dukes C lesions only. The 5-year survival rate for the overall patient population remained unchanged at 35 percent for both treatment groups.

The second VASOG trial was performed between 1973 and 1980, when 357 patients were randomized to one group receiving 3,150 rads preoperatively and another undergoing surgery alone. Preliminary results show that the 5-year survival rate for 97 patients was improved in the group receiving radiotherapy (58% compared with 52% for surgery alone). Final follow-up and determination of statistical significance is not complete.

The European Organization for Research on Treatment of Cancer is currently comparing high-dose preoperative radiotherapy using 3,450 rads with surgery alone. Preliminary reports reveal a significant decrease in pelvic recurrence rates; however, the final results are not available at this time.

All of these studies provide suggestive evidence that radiation therapy given in moderate to low doses before operation reduces the incidence of lymph node involvement and the rate of local recurrence. These prospective, randomized, controlled studies, however, do not show a statistically significant overall survival benefit from preoperative radiation therapy. Because most of the trials used radiation doses only up to 2,500 rads, perhaps further preoperative radiotherapy trials using higher doses (in the range of 4,500 rads) are warranted. Intraoperative radiation is described in a separate chapter in this volume.

TABLE 3 Prospective, Randomized, Controlled Trials for Preoperative Radiation Therapy in Rectal Carcinoma

Date	Group*	Rads	Result
1957–1967	Memorial Hospital	2,000	No survival benefit; decrease in local recurrence in Dukes C patients
1964–1969	VASOG I	2,000–2,500	Improved local recurrence and 5-year survival rate (49% vs. 39%) but not statistically significant
1965	Toronto, Princess Margaret Hospital	500	No survival benefit for overall population (35%); improved 5-year survival for Dukes C patients only (35% vs. 17% surgery alone); statistically significant
1973–1980	VASOG II	3,150	Preliminary results show improved 5-year survival (58% vs. 52%) but final follow-up incomplete
Currently	EORTC	3,450	Final results not available at this time

* VASOG = Veterans Administration Surgical Oncology Group, EORTC = European Organization for Research on Treatment of Cancer.

POSTOPERATIVE RADIATION THERAPY

Hoskins and Gunderson from Massachusetts General Hospital and Withers and Romsdal from M.D. Anderson have reported two prospective but nonrandomized postoperative radiation therapy trials. Patients who had Dukes B2, B3, C1, C2, and C3 lesions were treated postoperatively with 4,500 to 5,500 rads during a 5- to 6½-week period. These patients were compared with historical controls who received operation alone. The local recurrence rate decreased from between 37 and 48 percent for patients with operation alone to between 6 and 8 percent for patients who received postoperative radiation therapy. In spite of the improvement in local control, distant metastases in these two series continued to be a problem in 25 to 30 percent of patients.

In a prospective, randomized trial conducted by the GITSG, 227 patients with Dukes B2 and C rectal cancers gathered between 1975 and 1980 were randomized postoperatively to receive (1) no adjuvant therapy (concurrent controls), (2) radiation therapy (4,000 to 4,800 rads for 4½ to 5½ weeks), (3) chemotherapy (5-FU and methyl CCNU for 18 months), or (4) a combination of radiation and chemotherapy. In February 1980, the "surgery alone" control group was found to have results that were significantly inferior to those of the other three treatment arms. Thus, the study was terminated, and 202 of the 227 patients were evaluable. Fifty-eight patients had no adjuvant treatment, 48 had chemotherapy, 50 had radiotherapy, and 46 had combination chemotherapy and radiation therapy. In 1981, a GITSG interim report indicated that recurrence rates were 49 percent for the control group, 39 percent for the chemotherapy group, 36 percent for the radiotherapy group, and 28 percent for the combination therapy group. There was a statistically significant improvement in disease-free survival for patients receiving combination treatment compared with patients receiving no adjuvant treatment. There was no significant difference in disease-free survival when the other treatment arms were compared with one another. This is the first prospective study with a concurrent control population which provides evidence that postoperative adjuvant treatment with radiation and chemotherapy has a significant advantage as an adjuvant treatment. Unfortunately, these treatment modalities can have associated toxicity. In two of the patients receiving combination therapy, infections developed secondary to hematologic toxicity. In five of the 96 patients receiving radiation, radiation enteritis developed. The symptoms resolved in three of these patients, but the other two died from radiation enteritis. One patient from the chemotherapy group developed acute myelogenous leukemia and died.

Currently, at least two prospective postoperative adjuvant trials are in progress. A GITSG study randomizes patients to receive (1) radiation, 5-FU, and methyl CCNU or (2) radiation and 5-FU alone. This study potentially could answer questions regarding the toxicity and necessity of methyl CCNU. The members of the Gastrointestinal Oncology Group at the Mayo Clinic are randomizing patients to receive (1) radiation therapy alone (5,040 rads) or (2) initial chemotherapy (5-FU and methyl CCNU) followed by delayed radiation therapy (5,040 rads).

RECOMMENDATIONS

There is no proven effective adjuvant treatment for colon carcinoma. After "curative" surgical resection, patients should be followed up with careful periodic observation. Patients with Dukes B2 and C lesions should receive adjuvant treatment only in the setting of well-designed, prospective, randomized studies, with concurrent controls receiving no adjuvant treatment.

The prospective preoperative radiotherapy trials for rectal cancer show no significant decrease in local recurrence or increase in survival, except for the Toronto group, which found a significantly improved 5-year survival rate for patients with Dukes C lesions only. Currently, we cannot recommend preoperative radiotherapy as an adjuvant therapy unless physical examination reveals a large rectal tumor fixed within the pelvis in the absence of apparent metastatic disease. Even though there is no statistically significant evidence, there is suggestive evidence that preoperative radiotherapy for these patients decreases tumor size, tumor adherence, and nodal metastasis to make "curative" resection possible.

Nonrandomized trials show a significant decrease in local recurrence when high-dose postoperative radiation is used for Dukes B2 and C rectal lesions. A recent randomized GITSG study shows a significant prolongation of disease-free survival when a combination of radiation and chemotherapy is used postoperatively, compared with controls receiving no adjuvant treatment. All patients with Dukes B2 and C lesions should at least receive postoperative radiation from a qualified radiotherapist using modern techniques to spare the radiation effects on the small bowel. The "no adjuvant treatment" arm is not present in the randomized trials that are now in progress comparing radiation, chemotherapy, and combination treatment. The results of these studies must be evaluated before any recommendations can be made regarding the use of combined chemotherapy and radiotherapy outside of controlled trials.

The use of low-dose preoperative and high-dose postoperative adjuvant radiation ("sandwich" technique) has not been examined with prospective, randomized, controlled trials. This needs to be done before recommendations can be made regarding this technique.

REFERENCE

1. Taylor I. Studies on the treatment and prevention of colorectal liver metastases. Ann R Coll Surg Engl 1981; 63:270–276.

POLYPS OF THE COLON

JEROME D. WAYE, M.D.

A colon polyp is any tissue protuberance above the surface mucosa. Polyps may be neoplastic or nonneoplastic (Fig. 1); the majority of neoplastic polyps are adenomas, which are premalignant lesions. Most polyps larger than 1 cm in diameter are adenomas, but it is usually impossible for the radiologist, internist, endoscopist, or surgeon to predict the histologic type of adenoma, i.e., tubular, villous, or mixed, from the gross appearance of the polyp. Small polyps, less than 6 mm in diameter, are more often adenomas than not, but the differentiation can only be made histologically. Five to 10 percent of adenomas will become malignant, but it is not possible to predict accurately which adenomas will develop cancer. The incidence of cancer in adenomas correlates directly with their size and with the proportion of villous architecture present. Prior to the advent of colonoscopy, polyps at risk of malignancy or those that contained cancer were pooorly identified because, although polyp size could be estimated by a barium enema x-ray examintion, it was not possible to assess polyp histology. In the precolonoscopy era, polyps within reach of the sigmoidoscope were removed and those more proximal were evaluated by interval colon roentgenograms. The polyp with smooth contours and no growth tendency from one x-ray film to the next was followed periodically by repeat colon roentgenograms; removal of a proximal colon polyp required surgical laparotomy for the indications of surface irregularity, size, or a change in the polyp's shape or diameter on successive roentgenograms.

The ease and safety with which polyps can be removed colonoscopically has markedly altered the treatment of colon polyps. Since a nonsurgical approach is feasible and generally available, it is inappropriate to follow outmoded practice and observe polyps with serial roentgenograms. If a barium enema x-ray film demonstrates a polyp of 1 cm in diameter, it should be removed because of the 1 percent incidence of carcinoma in adenomas of this size. Malignancy in small polyps is extremely difficult to diagnose by gross visual inspection, a factor that mandates their resection for microscopic examination. Removal of the early carcinoma confined to a polyp is curative. The resection of polyps at high risk for cancer will undoubtedly interrupt the adenoma-carcinoma sequence. The small polyp with a high malignant potential can only be identified when the amount of villous component is seen histologically.

DIMINUTIVE POLYPS DISCOVERED ON BARIUM ENEMA X-RAY FILM

The occurrence of carcinoma in a polyp less than 0.5 cm in diameter is so rare that such a finding on a barium enema x-ray film may not, in itself, be sufficient indication for the performance of colonoscopic polypectomy. The clinician must be alert, however, to the probability that the symptoms that prompted the x-ray examination are not explained by a diminutive polyp and that occult or overt bleeding requires investigation by total colonoscopic examination, since blood loss is uncommon with these small polyps. The management of patients with polyps 0.5 to 1.0 cm in diameter is controversial; decisions should be based on the patient's symptoms, age, past history, family history, presence of other illnesses, and the physician's judgment. If a small polyp is detected on barium enema, and there are no symptoms or signs that require urgent colonoscopy, the patient may properly be scheduled for an interval follow-up surveillance examination by colonoscopy rather than by barium enema with the purpose of reevaluating the entire colon and removing the previously identified polyp.

SYNCHRONOUS ADENOMA

Whenever one polyp is discovered in the colon, total colonoscopy is mandated, since there is a 50 percent probability of discovering a synchronous adenoma. Whenever polyps are encountered during colonoscopy, they should be removed and biopsied. Even small polyps are now

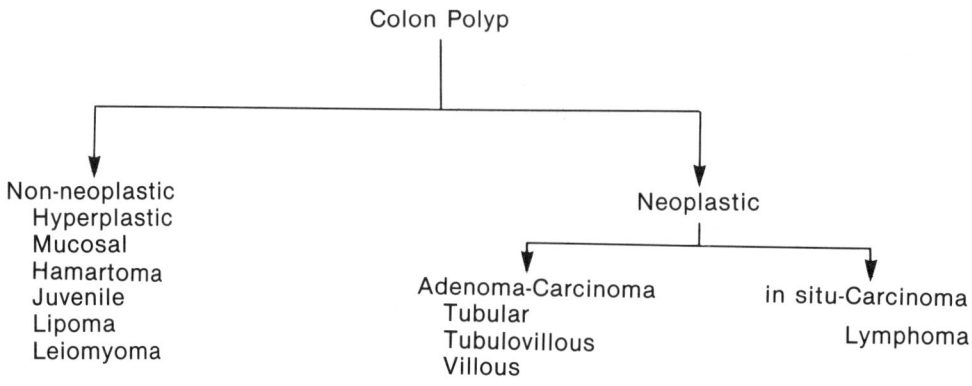

Figure 1 Nomenclature of colon polyps.

known to often contain adenomatous tissue, and if discovered during colonoscopy they should be sampled and ablated with the hot biopsy forceps. The majority of polyps are less than 2 cm in diameter, and experience has shown that most polyps seen during colonoscopy can be completely removed by simultaneous biopsy and fulguration or by cautery snare. In view of the current expertise in the field of colonoscopy, there are few occasions when a patient should be requested to return at some future time for removal of a polyp discovered during the endoscopic examination.

POLYPECTOMY

Complications

Serious complications, such as hemorrhage or perforation, occur in 1.8 percent of all colonoscopic polypectomies, with bleeding being the most frequent. Thermal injury to the bowel wall can occur during polypectomy and may result in a syndrome of peritoneal irritation characterized by abdominal pain, fever, and leukocytosis in the absence of free air on plain x-ray films of the abdomen. Symptoms of this "colon coagulation syndrome" usually subside with symptomatic therapy in 24 to 48 hours.

Surgical Polypectomy

The morbidity, mortality, and cost of colonoscopic polypectomy are significantly less than when polypectomy is performed surgically. The decision to remove a polyp surgically should be made by an experienced endoscopist who can directly assess the feasibility of endoscopic polypectomy by observing size of the polyp base, its position in the colon, and its accessibility for snare placement. The obviously malignant polyp with a waxy, irregular, ulcerated surface should properly be resected surgically. Some adenomas with a wide base or those that straddle an interhaustral fold may require several separate polypectomy sessions with only a small chance of total endoscopic removal; the endoscopist must weigh the risks and benefits of the endoscopic versus surgical approach for each patient before reaching a decision as to which route should be recommended.

Preparation for Colonoscopic Polypectomy

Preparation for a polypectomy should be a routine part of any diagnostic colonoscopic examination in order to avoid repetitive procedures and to control endoscopic costs. These preparations should encompass many areas, the most important of which is the preparation of the endoscopist.

Preparation of the Physician. The physician who performs colonoscopy must be trained in (not just familiar with) the techniques of colonoscopic polypectomy. This cannot be undertaken lightly, and adequate polypectomy experience will ensure the lowest possible rate of complications. The technique of polypectomy should be learned in a preceptor-type of relationship, during a specified training program only after the physician is completely capable of handling the colonoscope well. Initially, small pedunculated polyps can be removed, and with further experience, the physician can resect sessile polyps endoscopically, either with single snare application or in piecemeal fashion. Every endoscopist must be thoroughly knowledgeable with principles of electrosurgery and be familiar with the specific cautery unit available in the endoscopy suite.

Preparation of the Patient. Prior to any colonoscopic examination, the patient should be informed that polyps identified during the procedure will be removed at that time. Informed consent to include the polypectomy should be obtained from the patient before embarking upon any colonoscopic examination. The patient should be made aware of the risks involved in polypectomy, namely, perforation and bleeding. When colonoscopy is being performed specifically to remove a colon polyp, the patient should know that surgery is an alternative method of polyp removal. It is the responsibility of the physicians or an interested staff member to give instructions on the importance of bowel cleansing and to explain the possibility of not performing the procedure if the large bowel is poorly prepared.

Preparation of the Colon. Gases within the lumen of the unprepared bowel may be present in explosive proportions. Placing patients on a liquid diet for 48 hours has been shown to be effective in markedly decreasing the concentration of combustible gases. When this diet is coupled with a purgative, the level of explosive gas further decreases to where it is safe for electrocautery to be performed without the need for carbon dioxide insufflation. A colonic explosion related to the use of mannitol as an osmotic cathartic has been reported, and the use of this cathartic cannot be condoned for bowel preparation if electrocautery current is to be used. Adequate cleansing of the colon may be accomplished by giving the patient a low-residue diet, cathartic, and enemas. Castor oil (2 oz) or citrate of magnesia (10 oz) may be taken in the evening prior to the procedure. A full liquid diet for 24 or 48 hours prior to endoscopy is recommended, as are cleansing enemas on the day of the examination to be completed 2 hours prior to colonoscopy, allowing evacuation of excess water. Balanced electrolyte preparations are excellent cathartics but may leave a considerable amount of fluid within the bowel. Approximately one out of every 20 patients using the electrolyte preparation has a poorly prepared colon that may interfere with the ability to complete the examination. Two major factors account for this problem; a distaste for the solution and a reluctance to ingest the large volume of fluid required.

The patient should receive two instructions approximately 1 week prior to any colonoscopic examination, especially if polypectomy might possibly be performed. These are: (1) discontinue iron-containing medications (because they cause a dark residue in the colon); and (2) discontinue the use of aspirin-containing drugs (to decrease the risk of bleeding in the postpolypectomy period). The patient's coagulation status should be ascertained historically, by specifically inquiring as to previous bleeding episodes, especially with prior operations or tooth extractions. There is no need to obtain a "coagulation work-up" before polypectomy, unless a particular reason exists. In general, the use of carbon dioxide is not necessary for the performance of polypectomy. Adequate preparation of the colon is sufficient to prevent an explosive mixture of gases.

Preparation of the Equipment. For the performance of polypectomy, the following equipment must be available: hot biopsy forceps, two snares, and an electrosurgical unit. Each piece of apparatus should be individually inspected daily to ensure proper function. Since a number of incompatible items are commonly purchased from individual manufacturers, all connections should be checked and appropriate adapters employed.

Preparation of the Gastrointestinal Assistant. A trained gastrointestinal assistant should be available for the performance of colonoscopy and polypectomy. The assistant must be familiar with the principles of polypectomy and with the electrosurgical unit, its dial settings, the need for a ground-plate return, and so on. It is the assistant's role to identify the polypectomy site on the resected specimen with a pin or thread and to label each specimen in the order of its removal, permitting precise site location when the pathologist's report is received. It is customary for the assistant to close the snare around the polyp pedicle or base upon the physician's request. However, the force with which the wire loop guillotines the polyp while electric current is applied mandates training, practice, and experience to prevent complications. The use of an untrained assistant may be detrimental to the patient's safety.

The Site of Polypectomy

There is no contraindication to removal of colon polyps in whatever setting colonoscopy is performed. Most polyps may be removed in an ambulatory facility, either in a hospital endoscopy suite or in a physician's specially equipped office.

The *indications for hospitalizing* patients for polypectomy are as follows: (1) Age or infirmity may make it difficult for patients to ambulate, and they may not tolerate an in-home preparation requiring enemas and frequent trips to the bathroom; (2) the presence of known coagulopathy; (3) the need for prophylactic antibiotics; and (4) multiple polyps, large polyps, or suspected complications may justify hospitalization for observation following the polypectomy procedure.

The low frequency of complications that require hospitalization after polypectomy means that polyps may be removed in a physician's office as well as in the hospital outpatient department. Whenever polypectomy is to be performed on an ambulatory basis, emergency resuscitation equipment must be available for the treatment of the rare but potentially disastrous complications of medication administration. An endotracheal tube should be available with an Ambu-bag, along with various drugs for resuscitation. Narcan should be available to reverse the effect of narcotics. Many physicians administer Narcan routinely to ambulatory patients who have received meperidine for the procedure. Whenever endoscopy is to be performed on an ambulatory basis, it is imperative that the patient bring a companion to assist the partially sedated patient in traveling home.

THE MALIGNANT POLYP

Lymphatic channels are not present superficial to the muscularis mucosa in the polyp head. Because of the lymphatic distribution, malignant cells that do not penetrate the muscularis mucosa have no potential for metastatic spread. The adenoma with carcinoma-in-situ or noninvasive carcinoma may, once resected, be subsequently followed as any other benign adenoma. The three absolute criteria for surgically operating on the malignant polyp are: (1) invasion of lymphatic or vascular channels, (2) the presence of poorly differentiated carcinoma, and (3) malignancy at the resection margin of a sessile adenoma. Any sessile adenoma with malignancy invading beyond the muscularis mucosa is at risk for metastasis, and the patient may properly be advised to have a surgical resection of the colon to remove this site and adjoining lymph nodes. There is controversy concerning the need for such surgery, and the decision may be altered by the condition of the patient (elderly or infirm), the location of the malignant polyp (whether it requires an abdominoperineal resection), and the histopathologic findings in the polyp (only a small amount of malignancy at a distance from the resection margin).

Pedunculated adenomas with cancer invading the polyp head need not be surgically resected unless the malignancy satisfies the above-mentioned absolute criteria for surgery. When the pedicle contains carcinoma, even though the resection margin is not involved, surgery (with the above caveats) should be recommended. The pedicles of some polyps are broad-based and represent a portion of the colon wall pulled upon by peristalsis; these are pseudo-pedicles and should be treated as sessile polyps.

FOLLOW-UP AFTER ENDOSCOPIC POLYPECTOMY

Polyps recur in 30 to 50 percent of patients in whom adenomas are resected. Patients who have multiple adenomas are at greater risk of recurrence than those with a single adenoma resected. If no polyps were missed during the index polypectomy, then the follow-up interval to seek and remove metachronous adenomas should properly be at a time just prior to the development of cancer; more frequent examinations will permit the removal of adenomas but the risk of cancer in small adenomas is extremely slight. Since adenomas may, however, be missed at the time of the index examination, the first surveillance colonoscopy should be scheduled one year following the index polypectomy, and residual polyps removed. Because the growth rate of adenomas is unknown, as is the duration of time required for the development of carcinoma in an adenoma, no exact time period can be suggested for follow-up examinations. It does, however, take a few years for an adenoma to grow to 1 cm in size, when the realistic risk of cancer begins. A suggested surveillance plan would be to perform total colonoscopy every 2 or 3 years after the initial follow-up examination when patients have had multiple polyps removed, and every 3 years when one adenoma was originally resected.

FAMILIAL POLYPOSIS COLI AND HEREDITARY CANCER OF THE COLON

DAVID G. JAGELMAN, M.S.(Lond), F.R.C.S.(Eng), F.A.C.S.

There has been an annual increase in the number of reported cases of carcinoma of the large bowel in the past 20 years. The number of those cancers that arise and are influenced by a genetic component in their development is small; however, the realization that a genetic defect may be responsible for a significant, albeit small, group of patients who develop colorectal cancer is more clear now than previously. It has been estimated that 25 percent of patients who develop colorectal cancer will have a family history of a similar malignancy in a close relative. Within this group will be families who have a very strong family history of colorectal cancer at a particularly young age. This group has been identified as suffering from familial colon cancer syndrome (FCCS) and seems to differ from patients who develop or inherit familial polyposis coli (FPC). The latter condition is the ultimate genetic expression of malignant disease, as there seems to be a 100 percent incidence of large bowel malignancy in affected individuals. This genetically induced malignant transformation is not limited to the large intestine, and indeed in recent years a large number of extracolonic lesions, both benign and malignant, have been identified. These observations lead to the conclusion that FPC is indeed a generalized growth disorder rather than a condition affecting the large intestine alone.

FAMILIAL COLON CANCER SYNDROME

Kindreds in which there seems to be an inordinately high incidence of colon cancer have been investigated and a genetic component to their risk has been defined. In these colon cancer-prone families a number of features have been observed. In FCCS, or hereditary site-specific colon cancer as it is alternatively called, an early age of onset is usual. Colon cancer developing below the age of 40 years is common in these families, and it often may occur below the age of 30 years. A multitude of adenomatous polyps, as is seen in FPC, is uncommon. There is a predominance of right-sided colonic neoplasms and the chance of multiple primary tumors, either synchronous or metachronous, is high. The genetic influence may be autosomal dominant giving rise to ventrical transmission. Remarkably, tolerance to the cancer seems to be unusually favorable in many cases, in spite of advanced staging or poorly differentiated histologic findings. Some families also show cutaneous manifestations, e.g., sebaceous cysts, in association with FCCS, the so-called Torres syndrome.

Further studies of FCCS kindreds have shown a higher than expected incidence of uterine cancer, sometimes in conjunction with colon cancer, and again at an unusually young age. A few female members of the kindreds have also developed breast carcinoma. These ob-

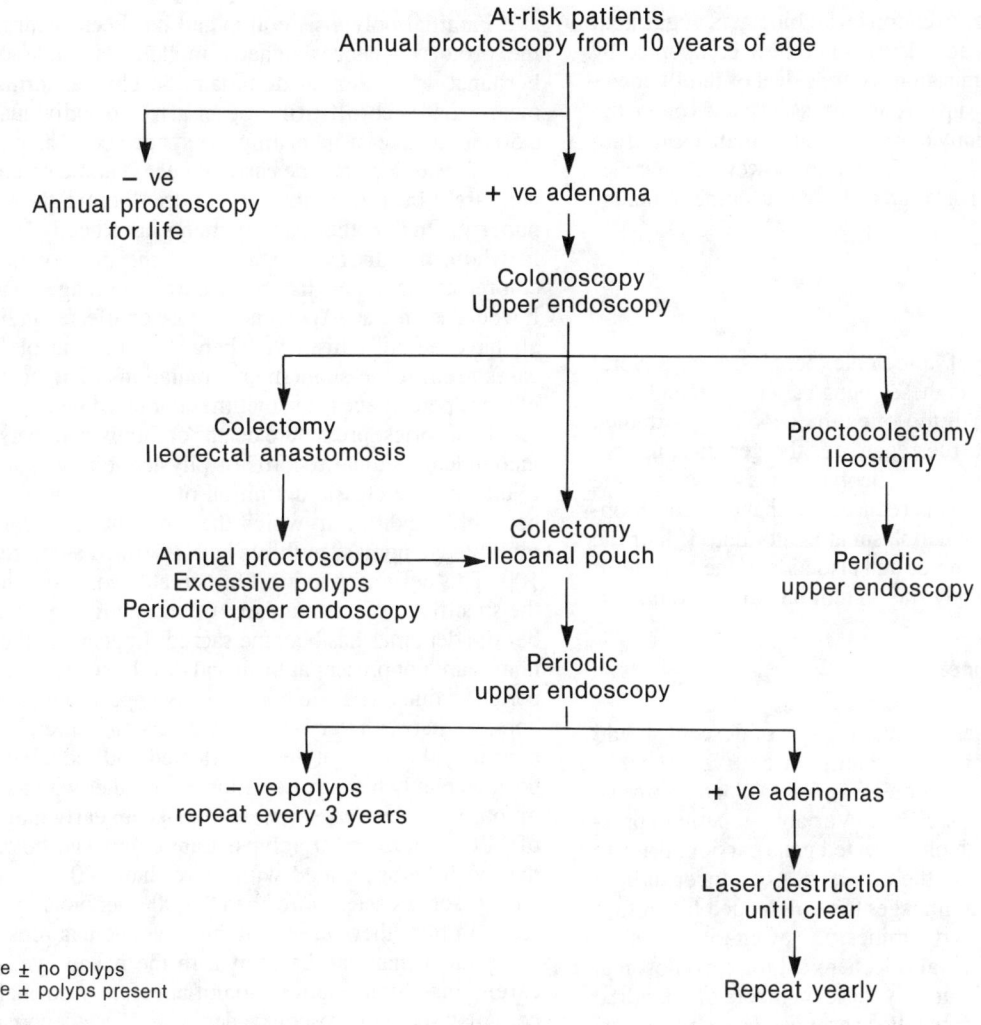

Figure 1 Surveillance program for familial polyposis coli.

servations in a comparatively few well-investigated families have confirmed the suspicion that there is a genetic component other than that seen in FPC in the development of large bowel cancer. This genetic defect may override or be supplemented by the environmental factor that obviously plays a major role in the development of colorectal cancer in the more typical older age groups. The detection of coloretal cancer in a patient younger than 40 should raise the suspicion of FCCS. Once the question has been raised regarding a genetic determination, the treatment becomes that of the family rather than the individual alone. Unfortunately, owing to lack of awareness or time constraints, the treatment of the whole family is not often completed.

Family History

A full history of the patient and his relatives should be taken, with particular emphasis on other family members with colorectal, uterine, or breast cancer. Special attention to the presence of young age of onset and multiple malignancy will add further credibility to the diagnosis of FCCS. Once having developed the family tree or kindred, and having determined the vertical transmission patterns, the physician should recommend particular surveillance programs.

Surveillance Program

Those relatives in a high-risk lineage, i.e., the children of affected individuals, should be screened from the age of 20 years. This seems to be somewhat young, but the risk factors seem high even at this age, especially when one considers the autosomal dominant pattern of inheritance. Presumably these large bowel cancers arise in previously benign adenomatous polyps. Because of the right-sided predominance of colon cancer in these patients, a colonoscopy at 20 years is necessary to establish a baseline surveillance of the large bowel. This should be repeated every 3 years, probably forever. Between colonoscopies annual proctosigmoidoscopic examination with hemoccult testing seems advisable. In women annual

Pap smear and specific endometrial biopsy is suggested, again from a young age. This should be accompanied by thorough breast examination. A great deal of family member education and support is necessary to explain the need for this apparently aggressive surveillance program (Fig. 1). Without this type of program, however, a number of young people will develop and even succumb to malignancy.

Colectomy

The detection of a colonic neoplasm or several adenomatous polyps in these young patients demands surgical intervention. All too often the neoplasm is treated in isolation without true regard for the genetic implications. Total colectomy with ileorectal anastomosis is the procedure of choice. This reduces the chance of developing a second primary neoplasm at a later date if half the large bowel is left behind, and also aids in the long-term surveillance, since only the rectum has to be examined.

Continued Surveillance

Women in the family in direct line of descent should continue to undergo uterine and breast surveillance. A great deal more information is needed to clarify some of the clinical features of FCCS. Variable genetic expression, premature death of suspected gene carriers prior to cancer expression, and the occurrence of cancer in both paternal and maternal lineages have all tended to confuse true analysis of affected families. We await the availability of an accurate clinical, biochemical, or chromosomal marker to identify accurately those members of a kindred at ultimate risk of genetically determined large bowel carcinoma.

FAMILIAL POLYPOSIS COLI

The study and evaluation of FPC over the years by clinicians and geneticists has led to confusion about the accurate name for this condition. The knowledge that a genetic component is present in the disease and that this genetic defect can be expressed in a variable way in various organs throughout the body, in either a benign or malignant manner, has led some to abandon the term familial polyposis coli. Alternatively, the term *hereditary adenomatosis* has been coined, but this also fails to describe the completeness of what appears to be a generalized growth disorder. This is because the defect can be manifested primarily and often fatally in the large bowel, but with extracolonic lesions commonly associated in other organs. *Heritable colorectal cancer syndrome, adenomatosis coli, familial adenomatosis coli,* and *Gardner's syndrome* are alternative terms used. Until a specific genetic defect has been defined it seems reasonable to retain the original term of familial polyposis coli, and this is what I use in this chapter.

Familial polyposis coli is and has been regarded as the prototype cancer genetic model. Its mode of inheritance is autosomal dominant. In clinical terms this means that each offspring of an affected individual has a 50–50 chance of inheriting the syndrome. The expression of the defect may be early or late. Colonic carcinoma has rarely been described in children before the age of puberty. On the other hand, patients have been described in whom the disease, in terms of the development of colorectal adenomas, has not occurred until age 40 to 50. It would seem that 80 percent or more of affected individuals have a family history, whereas 20 percent or fewer cases seem to be spontaneous mutations. The accuracy of these percentages is sometimes confused by inaccurate family histories, premature deaths of family members, and incomplete medical records or physical examinations in relatives. The classic definition of FPC is that of an inheritable condition in which the large intestine contains multiple adenomas, multiple being defined as more than 100. This definition in itself has created confusion in that the specificity of the number 100 in relation to the number of adenomas has become sacred. In general, the adenomas are not present at birth and develop over a variable period of time. They do not suddenly appear in mass numbers, so that with very early diagnosis only a few adenomas may be present in an affected individual with a positive family history, i.e., mother or father with the condition. It is therefore possible to make an early diagnosis of FPC with even 20 polyps. Late diagnosis, however, may well be associated with more than 100 adenomas, and in some cases more than 1,000 adenomas may be seen. In fact, there are many more adenomas present in any patient than can be seen with the naked eye. Very careful histologic examination of apparently normal mucosa may show microscopic adenomas. The adenomas are identical to colonic adenomas seen in the general population without FPC.

Extracolonic Manifestations

Elton Gardner, in the early 1950s, described a kindred with apparent FPC in which family members had extracolonic manifestations. Specifically, these lesions were epidermoid cysts and benign osteomas of bone. This syndrome now bears his name. For a long time it was thought that FPC and Gardner's syndrome (GS) were different conditions. Further investigations of multiple kindreds now suggest that they are indeed the same condition and that the differences can be explained by variable penetrance of the genetic defect. We have examined many kindreds under surveillance at the FPC registry at the Cleveland Clinic Foundation and found that, within families, there are some members with and some without the epidermoid cysts and osteomas. The epidermoid cysts can be located anywhere on the body and do not seem to grow very large or cause any clinical problems. They may be seen in children affected with FPC before the onset of colorectal adenomas. Osteomas can occur in any bone but most commonly are detected on the skull and jaw bones. They rarely cause problems, but there have been two cases of osteogenic sarcoma arising in patients with FPC (who were blood relatives). Panorex x-ray film of the jaw bones will detect a higher percentage of occult osteomas and this technique may have some benefit as a screening tool in children at risk. Again, the osteomas may arise before the onset of colorectal polyps.

Other benign extracolonic manifestations include abnormal retinal pigmentation, and adenomas of adrenal gland, pancreas, and pituitary (Table 1). The recent studies investigating the incidence of upper gastrointestinal polyps have shown them to be much more common than previously thought. Gastroduodenal polyps are often small and not seen on radiologic examination. Gastroduodenoscopy is required for their detection. We have recently analyzed the results of 100 patients undergoing upper endoscopy for FPC and GS. Polyps may arise in the stomach or duodenum. Fifty percent of the patients had polyps and 30 percent had duodenal adenomas. The gastric polyps were all nonadenomatous and usually present in the fundus. Histologically they were hyperplastic or glandular hyperplasia. All the duodenal polyps were adenomatous, mostly tubular adenomas and on a few occasions villous in nature. Adenomas can occur at any age, even in children, in patients with FPC and GS, without any male-female difference. These findings are significant, and, with the apparent increase in reporting of duodenal carcinoma in patients with FPC, suggest strongly the need for routine surveillance of the stomach and duodenum in these patients. Techniques of treatment of such lesions and their success in control have yet to be defined, but options include electrocautery or laser endoscopy. Adenomatous polyps may also be detected in the jejunum and more commonly in the ileum. Adenomatous polyps, both tubular adenoma and villous adenoma, have been seen on ileostomies and in the ileum above an ileorectal anastomosis. Recent reports have documented their presence in continent ileostomy pouches and ileoanal pouches. The malignant potential of these adenomas has yet to be defined.

Malignant extracolonic lesions in association with FPC seem to be reported with increasing frequency (Table 2). With a greater awareness of FPC and with more patients living longer after prophylactic colectomy, thereby avoiding death from colorectal cancer, these cancers in other organs are being detected more commonly. After death from colorectal cancer in patients with FPC, the next most common cause of death is periampullary carcinoma. Duodenal cancer no doubt relates to the presence of adenomas in the duodenum in 30 percent of patients, as seen in our study. Carcinomas of the pancreas and bile duct have also been seen in patients in our study population of 145 kindreds. The exact incidence and its relationship to age and other factors remains to be defined. These malignancies are certainly not restricted to those patients who have the GS variant. The role of bile in periampullary carcinoma is not known.

Desmoid tumors are particularly troublesome lesions that seem to develop in approximately 12 to 15 percent of patients. Isolated cases can be seen within families with or without other extracolonic lesions. Some families seem to be particularly prone to these lesions, and we have seen such a family with six members being affected. Desmoid tumors can occur in the rectus abdominis muscle, on the back, and around the scapula and hip. Most commonly, however, they occur within the abdomen in the retroperitoneal area and specifically in the small bowel mesentery, often wrapped around the origin of the superior mesenteric artery. The intra-abdominal lesions seem to be more aggressive and less easily treated than the extra-abdominal desmoids. Indeed, there is some evidence that they may have a different histologic pattern, which may account for their behavior. The majority of abdominal desmoids occur after some kind of abdominal operative procedure, usually colectomy. Surgical excision, even with massive small bowel resection, has been particularly disappointing in my experience, with most patients developing an early often massive recurrence. The growth pattern seems to vary tremendously from patient to patient, some desmoids remaining dormant for years, others growing rapidly in spite of all therapy. Women seem to develop them more frequently than men. No therapeutic modalities have been proved effective.

In my experience radiotherapy has not been beneficial. One patient in our series of 30 patients with desmoids responded to quadruple chemotherapy. Other somewhat unusual medications have been reported to produce a remission in some patients, including theophylline, in-

TABLE 1 Benign Extracolonic Manifestations of Familial Polyposis Coli

Epidermoid cyst
Osteoma
Gastric polyp
Duodenal adenoma
Small bowel adenoma
Adrenal adenoma
Pituitary adenoma
Retinal pigmentation

TABLE 2 Malignant Extracolonic Manifestations of Familial Polyposis Coli

Carcinoma of the duodenum
Carcinoma of the pancreas
Common bile duct
Hepatoblastoma
Thyroid carcinoma
Myeloid leukemia
Desmoid tumor
Medulloblastoma
Glioma
Adrenal carcinoma
Testicular tumor
Osteogenic sarcoma

domethacin, Clinoril, sulindac, tamoxifen, and progesterone. Their effectiveness alone or in combination is being investigated. Desmoid tumors do not metastasize but create problems from a pressure effect on the intestine and ureters, causing obstruction or necrosis.

Turcot described a family with FPC in which two members developed brain tumors, specifically a glioma and medulloblastoma. Investigation of 12 patients documented in our study population with medulloblastomas suggests that this is another extracolonic manifestation of FPC. Medulloblastomas tend to arise in young children usually before FPC is diagnosed. Indeed, even if the colon is examined there may be only a few adenomas present, as the patients are usually at or near the age of puberty. Gliomas have also been documented but seem to be less common.

Other malignant lesions detected in patients with FPC include hepatoblastoma, testicular tumors, thyroid and adrenal carcinoma, ovarian and breast cancer, and leukemia.

The knowledge of the extensiveness of these extracolonic lesions, both benign and malignant, adds weight to the hypothesis that FPC is truly a generalized growth disorder.

Treatment

The treatment of the individual patient must be combined with the treatment of the whole family. The patient's kindred must be ascertained and all information on relatives obtained from local physicians, hospitals, and autopsy reports. It is only in this way that the pattern of inheritance can be mapped out. The condition does not seem to skip a generation. All remaining relatives in direct line of descent, irrespective of age, should be encouraged to undergo proctosigmoidoscopic examination for the detection of colorectal adenomas. I recommend commencing the examinations at the age of 10 years and yearly thereafter. It is uncertain when to stop the examinations if no polyps appear, since cases have been reported in which polyps have first appeared at or about 40 years of age. After 40 years it is generally recommended that anyone with a family history of colon cancer irrespective of FPC should have annual proctoscopic examination with occult blood testing. The examinations should probably continue for life. Annual examinations starting at 10 years may seem premature, but they do tend to generate an early recognition of the need for check-ups, and I believe they help in the long term to maintain patient compliance with the surveillance program. In discussions with the patients it is important to stress the need for check-ups before symptoms occur. All too often in FPC symptoms come late, with the inevitable development of cancer. Even though it is possible, although rare, to have FPC without at least one adenoma in the rectum, I do not use barium enema or colonoscopy in the absence of rectal polyps. Radiologic examination of the colon will miss the early small adenomas and add to the expense of the surveillance program. If adenomas confirmed on biopsy are detected in the rectum, colonoscopy is required to assess the total number of polyps and, it is hoped, to confirm the absence of colorectal cancer. Histologic confirmation is essential to diagnose adenomatous polyps rather than juvenile polyps or hyperplastic polyps. The latter two types of polyps may also have a familial incidence of an autosomal dominant pattern but without the malignant potential.

To my mind, the diagnosis of FPC demands early prophylactic colectomy. There seems no point in waiting to observe the formation of more and more adenomas, as there is a 100 percent chance of colorectal cancer. Malignant degeneration has been reported before puberty, often in teenage years, and commonly in the 20- to 30-year age group. It has been estimated that 75 percent of patients will develop cancer before the age of 40 years. Prior to operation an upper endoscopy is performed to document the presence of upper gastrointestinal polyps, as we have found that a high percentage of patients have adenomas in the duodenum. It is uncertain whether surveillance and endoscopic destruction of such adenomas will alter the natural history of the adenoma-cancer sequence in the duodenum. Although many other extracolonic malignancies have been noted in FPC patients, their true incidence remains unclear. It is not thought necessary at this time to schedule other tests regularly, e.g., abdominal computed tomographic scans. Ideally, as we gain more information on FPC patients, we will be able to define certain groups who have particular risks for desmoid tumors, adrenal or thyroid cancers, and so on.

Apart from the definition of a clinical surveillance program for these patients and its institution, a great deal of general support is required. We have seen that, in general, the task of truly treating the family rather than the individual patient is beyond the scope of practicing physicians. They really do not have the time to complete the task. As a result, many family members are either not knowledgeable concerning the disease or fail to undergo surveillance. A registry format certainly improves the family care. Designating one or more persons in the registry to spend the time building the family tree, answering questions, and trying to make some family members adhere to a surveillance program are essential. The registry personnel can also give uniform medical advice which might have confused patients previously. Greater knowledge of their disease and risks and those of their children has certainly improved the follow-up program in our institution.

Surgical Options

The three surgical options available for patients with FPC are proctocolectomy and ileostomy, colectomy and ileorectal anastomosis, and colectomy with rectal mucosectomy and ileoanal J pouch.

Proctocolectomy and Ileostomy. This procedure removes the whole of the large intestine and prevents death from colorectal cancer. It does not, however, necessarily cure the disease, owing to the possibility of developing one or more of the extracolonic malignancies that have been documented. Most of these patients are young and often asymptomatic and it is difficult for them to accept an ileostomy. Indeed, it seems to act as a deterrent to other family members ever getting involved in the surveillance program. If this is true, they will of course go on to develop colorectal cancer, the risk being 100 percent. Because of this, and because of the availability of other options, this procedure is less often required. Suitable candidates currently would be a patient who already has a rectal cancer or an older patient who has an excessive number of polyps in the rectal segment.

Colectomy and Ileorectal Anastomosis. Colectomy and ileorectal anastomosis is a more acceptable procedure. It reduces the risk of colorectal cancer tremendously but does not abolish it, as approximately 10 to 15 cm of rectum remains behind. This rectal segment can develop new adenomas or cancer in the future. The follow-up results of previously operated upon patients at the Cleveland Clinic suggest that 80 percent of patients who have had ileorectal anastomosis will be free of rectal cancer 25 years after colectomy. They also suggest that adherence to a follow-up program will not necessarily eliminate rectal cancer risk, but if it does occur it is likely to be detected at an earlier stage. I tend to use ileorectal anastomosis as my main operative procedure, combined with long-term surveillance of the rectal segment. It seems particularly appropriate in younger patients detected through the registry who have only a few polyps in the rectal segment. The relatively normal bowel function and avoidance of a permanent ileostomy make it acceptable to other family members, thereby enhancing overall compliance with the surveillance program.

Colectomy and Ileoanal Pouch. Removal of the whole of the large bowel mucosa, thereby removing the risk of colorectal cancer and at the same time maintaining defecation through the anus, is certainly an attractive option. The operation, however, is much more complex and potentially complicated. It is a two-stage procedure, with most if not all patients requiring a temporary loop ileostomy. There is no doubt in my mind from our own clinical experience that the functional results and overall satisfaction are *less* and the period of recovery is more prolonged than with a one-stage colectomy and ileorectal anastomosis. There has been a tendency to suggest that this operation is the procedure of choice; however, I would tend to reserve it for younger patients with many rectal polyps or for patients who had previously had an ileorectal anastomosis in whom the number of recurring rectal polyps seems to be getting out of control.

These three operative procedures, together with conversion to a continent ileostomy in those patients already committed to a proctocolectomy, all have a place. The type of procedure is chosen by individualizing patients, taking into account their personal attitude, life style and age. The surgical management of FPC is only part of treating these patients. Continuing support, education, and genetic counseling play a major and ongoing role in their care. I believe this is best achieved via a formalized clinical registry for this disease.

LOWER GASTROINTESTINAL BLEEDING

JAMES H. JOHNSTON, M.D.

Lower gastrointestinal (GI) bleeding is a challenging problem in terms of both diagnosis and treatment, often requiring the coordinated efforts of the gastroenterologist, radiologist, surgeon, and nursing staff. In contrast to upper GI bleeding, in which endoscopy has assumed an important role with rapid accurate diagnosis as well as definitive hemostatic therapy, there is often no single approach to lower GI hemorrhage.

The management of major acute lower GI hemorrhage is quite different from minor hematochezia or occult bleeding. These topics will be discussed separately, while the primary focus of the chapter will be on management of the patient with acute bleeding.

MAJOR ACUTE HEMORRHAGE

Massive bleeding is a true medical emergency that must be handled in an expedient manner. After initial passage of a formed stool with blood, further bowel movements typically consist of frank blood and clots. In contrast to the common delay in recognition of the significance of melena, the patient with hematochezia usually seeks medical attention urgently. Resuscitative measures should begin immediately with correction of hypovolemia by rapid infusion of intravenous fluid via large-bore catheter. Blood is typed and crossmatched for transfusion as needed. Relatively minor changes in blood pressure and pulse may reflect significant deficits in blood volume. Coagulopathies should be corrected if present.

Diagnostic Approach

History and Physical Examination

Initial evaluation includes general medical assessment with a concise but thorough history and physical examination. With major hemorrhage of suspected lower GI origin, it is important to search for clues suggesting a possible upper GI source of bleeding (history of peptic ulcer or dyspepsia, liver disease, alcoholism, anti-inflammatory drugs, and so on). Abdominal pain precedes rectal bleeding in ischemic bowel disease, whereas a history of diarrhea and anal fistulas suggests inflammatory bowel disease. Prior radiation therapy is an important clue. Acute major lower GI bleeding is most often due to either a colonic diverticulum or a vascular ectasia in patients over 45 years of age, but other lesions, such as a Meckel's diverticulum, inflammatory bowel disease, and colonic polyps, are more important causes in young patients. Causes of lower GI bleeding are listed in Table 1.

After the patient is stabilized in an intensive care unit, the search for a specific diagnosis continues (Fig. 1).

Anorectal Examination

Careful digital, anoscopic, and proctosigmoidoscopic examination is the next step. This usually reveals copious blood and clots coming from above the proctoscopic level. It is important, however, not to overlook a hemorrhoidal source of massive bleeding, especially in a cirrhotic patient with portal hypertension. Similarly, a minute rectal ulcer with arterial bleeding should be carefully excluded, as well as signs of inflammatory bowel disease. The rigid proctoscope permits much better suctioning, but the flexible fiberoptic instrument provides a superior image if large rectal clots are removed manually or rendered dependent by changing the patient's position and examining the exposed mucosa. Retroflexion of the flexible instrument may aid in inspection of the anorectal junction. Careful exclusion of the uncommon anorectal source of major hemorrhage is an important but often underemphasized task. Its significance can be stressed by considering the implications of a subtotal colectomy done for uncontrolled hemorrhage, only to discover postoperatively an anorectal cause for the persistent bleeding.

Exclude Upper Gastrointestinal Source of Bleeding

Traditionally, the next diagnostic step is passage of a nasogastric tube in search of gross blood. If there was syncope or orthostatic hypotension, however, or if dark stools preceded passage of red blood, then a negative nasogastric aspirate is not sufficient to rule out a bleeding duodenal ulcer with competent pyloric sphincter, and upper endoscopy should be performed.

After exclusion of anorectal and upper GI sources of hemorrhage, the evaluation becomes considerably more difficult. Further diagnostic studies include radionuclide scanning, arteriography, and/or colonoscopy. There is no longer a place for barium x-ray studies in the setting of acute GI hemorrhage.

Bleeding Scan

The radionuclide scan frequently receives mixed reviews regarding its usefulness in the evaluation of a patient with GI bleeding. Many clinicians have been disappointed with its low sensitivity and specificity. It is true that the yield is low, but this is primarily because active bleeding has stopped by the time the test is performed. When positive, the bleeding scan provides valuable localization of the source of hemorrhage with little discomfort, risk, or expense to the patient (especially as compared with the alternatives of arteriography, colonoscopy, and surgery).

I order the bleeding scan only if I believe the patient is continuing to bleed actively at that moment. A nuclear medicine technician is on call 24 hours a day for emergency scanning. Nocturnal participation by the radiologist is required only when there is immediate diagnostic confusion; most scans can be fully interpreted later and do not have urgent therapeutic implications. An unequivocal hot spot on scan that appears in the first few minutes after injection is considered to be useful; overinterpretation of subtle findings is fraught with error. The diagnostic accuracy of the technetium sulfur colloid scan is claimed to exceed that of the technetium-labeled red blood scan, although the latter technique allows delayed scanning to detect intermittent hemorrhage. In my experience, however, delayed scans are of limited benefit for specific localization because the isotope migrates substantially by the time the scan is done. If the bleeding scan is negative, this implies that active bleeding has stopped at least temporarily and the urgency for specific diagnosis and therapy may be reduced.

Arteriography

If major lower GI bleeding persists or recurs, requiring therapeutic intervention, then emergency arteriography may offer specific localization of the bleeding site as well as definitive therapy by selective vasoconstrictor infusion. This procedure requires an interested, readily available and experienced radiography team, and, in practical terms, this service is not universally available. It is important to maintain the intensive care unit environment

TABLE 1 Causes of Lower Gastrointestinal Bleeding

Disorder	Major Acute Hemorrhage	Minor Chronic Hemorrhage
Hemorrhoids		*
Anal fissure		*
Colonic diverticulum	*	
Vascular ectasia	*	*
Polyp		*
Cancer		*
Solitary colonic ulcer	*	
Colonic varices	*	
Post-polypectomy	*	
Ischemic colitis		*
Inflammatory bowel disease		*
Radiation colitis		*
Small bowel lesion		
Meckel's diverticulum	*	
Tumor		*
Upper gastrointestinal lesion	*	

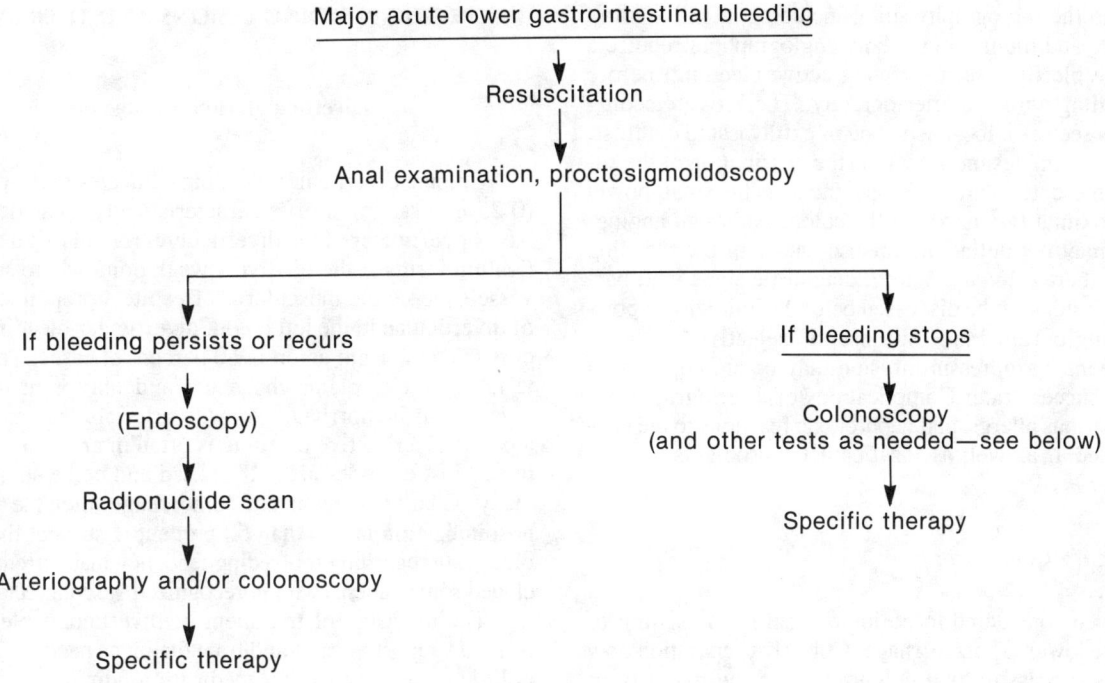
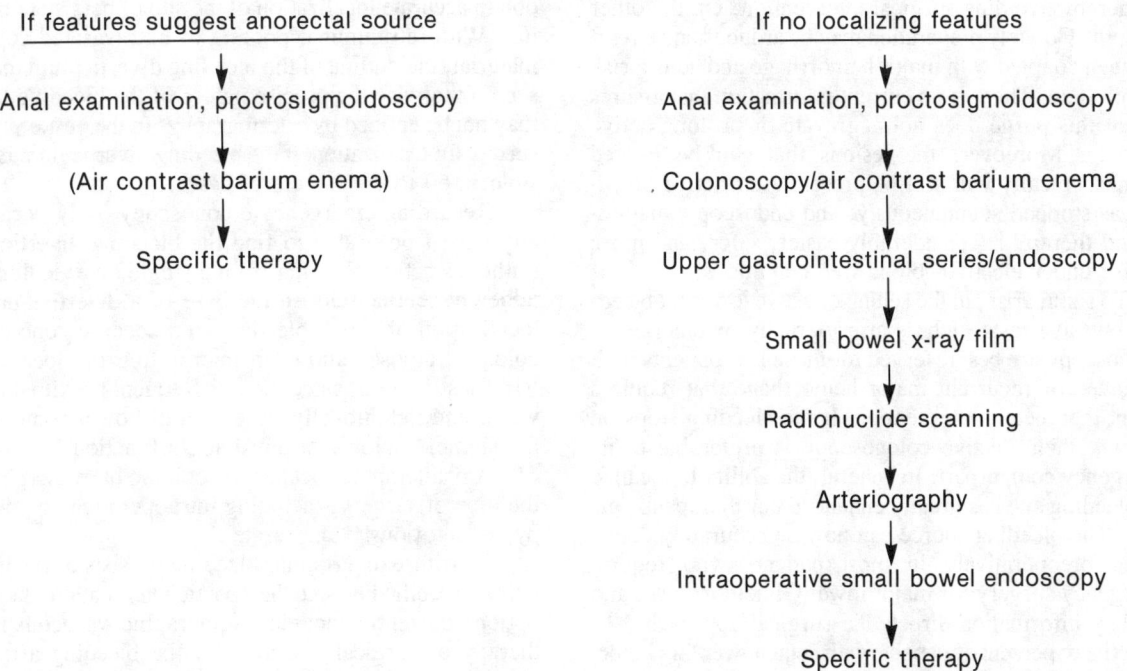

Figure 1 Algorithms for management of lower gastrointestinal bleeding.

while in the radiography suite, including attentive nursing care and monitoring. Many angiographers require a positive bleeding scan (proving active bleeding) before proceeding with full arteriography. The active bleeding point is seen as a localized zone of extravasated contrast. Most bleeding lesions lie within the distribution of the superior mesenteric artery, which includes the small bowel and proximal two-thirds of the colon. Although angiography may not define the precise nature of the bleeding lesion, there often are helpful diagnostic signs with particular lesions (to be discussed below). Following a positive angiogram and successful selective catheter placement, vasopressin infusion may be employed with a high success rate. Complications of arteriography include serious allergic and nephrotoxic reactions to the contrast media, as well as local catheter problems.

Emergency Colonoscopy

Once considered to be impractical in the setting of massive lower GI hemorrhage, Golytely preparation now permits successful total colonoscopy in the majority of cases. Within several hours of Golytely administration by mouth or by nasogastric tube, colonoscopy can usually be performed.

Although the technical feat of colonoscopy is usually possible during active major hemorrhage, I have mixed feelings about its usefulness as an emergency procedure. On one hand, valuable information is gained when the site and nature of the bleeding lesion are accurately determined. Additionally, there are certain bleeding lesions which can be effectively and safely treated endoscopically, thereby avoiding surgical intervention. On the other hand, the Golytely preparation may be arduous and stressful when coupled with major hemorrhage and adds a risk of aspiration. There is no current information that assures us that this purge does not aggravate or prolong active bleeding. Moreover, the lesions that can be treated colonoscopically will still be present after active bleeding has stopped spontaneously, and endoscopic diagnosis and therapy is considerably easier, safer, and more precise under elective, blood-free conditions.

To summarize, in the setting of active lower GI bleeding, invasive tests such as arteriography or emergency colonoscopy are best reserved for those few patients with continued or recurrent major hemorrhage that requires urgent therapeutic intervention. If the bleeding stops on its own, then elective colonoscopy is preferable to its emergency counterpart. In general, the ability to localize the bleeding site has greatly enhanced our therapeutic efforts. The bleeding source can now be accurately determined preoperatively in most patients who require emergency surgery for major lower GI hemorrhage, and this key information directs the surgical approach. Ninety percent of patients with acute lower GI hemorrhage are bleeding from a colonic diverticulum or a vascular ectasia. Common as well as uncommon causes of acute lower GI bleeding will now be discussed.

SPECIFIC BLEEDING LESIONS AND THERAPY

Diverticular Hemorrhage

Colonic diverticular bleeding emanates from a small (0.25-mm range) artery characteristically located in the base or perimeter of the diverticulum (recall that a diverticulum forms at the relatively weak point where serosal vessels pierce the muscularis). Despite a preponderance of diverticulae in the left colon, diverticular bleeding occurs from the right colon in 60 percent of cases. This arterial source explains the acute and abrupt nature of diverticular hemorrhage. As with arterial bleeding from a peptic ulcer, active bleeding is often intermittent in nature. Most episodes are self-limited and cease spontaneously. Chance of recurrent hemorrhage after the initial hospitalization is less than 50 percent (I suspect that the older data regarding rebleeding tendency inadvertently included some patients with unrecognized vascular ectasias).

The mainstay of treatment of diverticular bleeding is good supportive care and transfusion as needed. There is little evidence that any medication administered systemically (e.g., intravenous vasopressin) is effective in halting diverticular hemorrhage; this therapy cannot be recommended because of dangerous problems with myocardial and mesenteric ischemia in this elderly population.

If *specific* therapy is needed because of persistent hemorrhage, then it depends upon accurate localization of the bleeding point. Localization may occasionally be accomplished by bleeding scan. If good emergency arteriography is available, this generally is the best way to obtain accurate localization of the site of persistent bleeding. With intraluminal pooling of extravasated contrast material, the outline of the bleeding diverticulum may be seen, otherwise the precise nature of the bleeding lesion may not be defined by arteriography. In the best of hands, successful localization of the bleeding diverticulum is possible in 60 to 70 percent of cases.

Regarding emergency colonoscopy, only occasionally have I been able to find the bleeding diverticulum (either as active bleeding from a single diverticulum, an adherent sentinel clot in the base of a diverticulum, or localization of active bleeding to a specific zone of the colon). I advise caution in interpreting the location of "freshest" blood, since there is frequent proximal backwash, and, additionally, retention of bowel contents by the sigmoid colon is a physiologic function.

Any attempt to localize the colonic bleeding point at the time of surgery, including intraoperative colonoscopy, is notoriously inaccurate.

If profuse diverticular bleeding persists or recurs requiring specific invasive therapeutic intervention, the main options currently include angiographic vasoconstrictor therapy or surgical resection. If the bleeding artery is selectively catheterized, *intra-arterial vasopressin* can be infused locally. If successful in halting bleeding, vasopressin infusion is usually continued for 24 hours, then gradually tapered. If rebleeding occurs, repeat vasopressin infusion can be performed, but surgical treatment is usually recommended. Most angiographers are reluctant to consider embolic therapy in the superior mesenteric artery circulation.

Surgical resection is required as definitive therapy if profuse bleeding persists or recurs repeatedly and if nonoperative measures are not successful or available. In general, surgery is required sooner in an elderly patient with other serious medical problems than in a younger healthy patient. There may be less enthusiasm for early operation if subtotal colectomy will be required as opposed to segmental resection. Surgical resection is not generally recommended following a single self-limited hemorrhage from a colonic diverticulum. I agree with most authorities who currently recommend segmental resection if the bleeding point has been accurately localized preoperatively. Although there apparently have been rare instances of simultaneous hemorrhage from two different diverticulae, it is generally considered that diverticular hemorrhage is solitary and can be treated effectively by segmental resection if preoperative localization is truly accurate. Attempts to find the bleeding diverticulum at surgery are typically frustrating, often misleading, and generally have been abandoned by most surgeons. If accurate preoperative localization has not been possible, then subtotal colectomy is the procedure of choice. Before this operation is performed, it is important to take a second careful look at the anorectal zone to exclude a distal bleeding source.

In passing, I note a couple of instances in which high-risk patients have been found at colonoscopy to have active arterial bleeding from a single diverticulum, and I employed the heater probe to halt bleeding effectively. In each case, the probe was gently inserted into the diverticulum with just enough pressure to tamponade active bleeding, at which point heat was delivered and coaptive coagulation was achieved. This new and unorthodox therapy was considered reasonable in view of the absence of any acute erosive potential with the heater probe, our large experience with this device, and the high-risk status of each of these patients. Further experimental study of this technique is in progress.

Bleeding Vascular Ectasia

Vascular abnormalities of the colon have been increasingly recognized as a frequent cause of gastrointestinal hemorrhage. Although a variety of terms have been used to describe these lesions (angiodysplasia, vascular ectasia, arteriovenous malformation, telangiectasia, and so on), for the purpose of this chapter our attention will be directed to the vascular ectasia[1]. The vascular ectasia, occurring predominantly in the right colon, may be viewed endoscopically as a discrete mucosal red spot, often intensely red in color and sharply demarcated with a fern-like perimeter. Lesions may be single or multiple, and size may vary from less than 1 mm to larger than 1 cm. Three-dimensional morphologic study has revealed these lesions to be similar to an oak tree, with a mucosal canopy of dilated venules and capillaries that converge into a large draining submucosal vein. The vascular ectasia is confined to the submucosa and mucosa, in contrast to a hemangioma, which may be transmural in location. Angiographically, the vascular ectasia may be seen as a vascular tuft on the tip of the feeding artery. There may be early filling of a draining vein, indicating a significant arteriovenous connection. Histologically, the elderly patient with a vascular ectasia in the right colon typically has a preponderance of dilated submucosal veins. Vascular ectasias are occasionally found incidentally at colonoscopy, without history of overt bleeding or anemia, and these lesions do not require treatment.

The patient with a vascular ectasia may present with chronic anemia from intermittent low-pressure oozing. The same lesion may also mimic diverticular arterial bleeding when a direct arteriovenous communication is present. Endoscopically, a white spot or erosion in the center of a vascular ectasia may represent a stigma of recent hemorrhage and is helpful in deciding which of several lesions may have been the true bleeding culprit. Histologically, there may be only a thin layer of epithelial cells overlying the vascular channels, and it is common for endoscopic trauma to induce transient bleeding. Induced hemorrhage is usually an ooze, although in rare instances we have observed pulsatile arterial bleeding from these lesions.

Treatment options include angiographic, endoscopic or surgical therapy. At *angiography* selective vasopressin infusion might be used to halt active bleeding, but this would not represent definitive therapy because of the high rebleeding rate with these lesions. Embolic therapy is considered unwise in the right colon by most angiographers.

There has been increasing interest and experience with *endoscopic* methods for coagulation and destruction of vascular ectasias. Thermal modalities include monopolar electrocoagulation (e.g., ''hot biopsy'' forceps), bipolar electrocoagulation (BICAP unit, American ACMI, Stamford, CT), thermal cautery (Heat Probe, Olympus Corp., Lake Success, NY), and laser photocoagulation (Neodymium: YAG and argon lasers). The most promising nonthermal method is injection sclerotherapy. These hemostatic modalities were recently comprehensively reviewed.[2] There is a separate chapter in this volume on *Laser Treatment in Gastrointestinal Disease*.

In general, the vascular ectasia is an easy lesion to treat with any of these endoscopic hemostatic methods. I currently prefer the nonerosive contact probes (Heat Probe or BICAP) because of low cost, portability, precise control of tissue heating, no potential for tissue erosion, adjustable depth of coagulation, and potential for coaptive coagulation.

Regarding treatment technique, I recommend applying thermal treatment directly at the vascular lesion to produce tissue coagulation or whitening. Suggested initial instrumental settings include the following: heat probe, 10 joule pulses, light touch; BICAP (25 watt unit), 1- to 2-second pulses of power 5, light touch; ''hot biopsy'' forceps, grasp and ''tent'' the lesion, then apply short pulses with a low power coagulation setting; YAG laser, 40 to 60 watts, 2-cm treatment distance, 0.5-second pulses; argon laser, 5 watts, 2-cm treatment distance, 1- to 2-second pulses. Induced bleeding is common in treatment of the vascular ectasia regardless of which modality is used. It is important to deliver only enough thermal energy to ultimately destroy the lesion, but it is unwise to overtreat just to control "cosmetic" induced bleeding. Unfortunately, precise guidelines for "safe and effective" energy limits cannot be defined, but in general, it is better to undertreat initially than to overtreat.

"Ideal" therapy for the vascular ectasia involves coagulation down to the submucosa but avoids a full-thickness burn. It is not necessary to treat the normal mucosa surrounding a vascular ectasia. The peripheral parts of a large lesion may be treated quite superficially, whereas the deeper central vessels may require deeper coagulation (increased energy setting and appositional force with the contact probes). Because of endoscopic problems with accurate lesion identification and traumatic artifacts, I recommend searching for and treating vascular lesions as the colonoscope is introduced, rather than on withdrawal. I see no reason to take the risk of biopsying a typical appearing vascular ectasia.

The main risks of endoscopic treatment of the vascular ectasia include perforation of the thin-walled cecum and delayed hemorrhage. Acute perforation can be prevented by using a nonerosive contact probe or by avoiding high power density with the lasers or electrical sparking with the monopolar probe. Delayed perforation one to seven days after treatment is possible after any full-thickness bowel injury but is prevented by keeping intraluminal pressure low (liquid diet and avoiding repeat endoscopy) and by the body's effective response in sealing the injured bowel with adjacent bowel loops and omentum. Delayed hemorrhage, an uncommon but potentially serious complication, may be caused by thermal-induced ulceration of a normal underlying submucosal artery. It is unwise to assume that rebleeding during the week following thermal treatment is due to inadequate coagulation of the vascular ectasia and attempt repeat endoscopic treatment. If the patient is supported and hemorrhage ceases spontaneously, then repeat colonoscopy 1 month later will usually reveal complete tissue healing with no residual vascular ectasia.

Although *surgical* resection has traditionally played a major role in definitive treatment of colonic vascular ectasia, I now reserve surgery (usually right hemicolectomy) for patients with widespread or particularly large vascular lesions, or when poor endoscopic orientation prevents effective endoscopic therapy. Typically, vascular ectasias are difficult or impossible to see at surgery or in the resected specimen, and special techniques with silicone rubber injection followed by tissue clearing are required.

Upper Gastrointestinal Bleeding

In the setting of major hemorrhage manifest as hematochezia and hypotension, endoscopy is indicated to exclude a bleeding lesion in the upper gastrointestinal tract, most of which are now amenable to endoscopic therapy. In the absence of hypotension or significant transfusion requirement, it is unlikely that an upper GI source explains passage of red blood from the rectum.

Colonic Ulcer

A solitary ulcer of the colon with arterial bleeding is an uncommon but important cause of major lower GI hemorrhage (cecum and rectum are the most frequent sites in our experience). Size of the bleeding artery is typically small, and direct endoscopic coagulation can usually be easily accomplished. Surgical oversewing of the ulcer or limited resection may be employed if effective endoscopic therapy is not possible.

Colonic Varices

In the setting of portal hypertension, colonic varices are an uncommon but potentially treatable cause of lower GI bleeding. As with their esophageal counterpart, injection sclerotherapy can be tried if the specific point of bleeding can be found, although portocaval shunt surgery is usually required.

Meckel's Diverticulum

An ulcerated Meckel's diverticulum should be considered as a cause of major hemorrhage in a young patient. Technetium sulfur colloid or technetium-labeled red blood cell scan may be helpful during active bleeding, whereas a technetium pertechnetate scan or small bowel x-ray film may show the diverticulum after bleeding has ceased. Lateral films or delayed films after barium enema or small bowel series may help demonstrate a Meckel's diverticulum. Surgical resection is required.

Postpolypectomy Bleeding

Delayed major hemorrhage during the week following colonic polypectomy occurs infrequently and usually subsides spontaneously with observation. Whereas the acutely bleeding stalk can be resnared and tamponaded by pressure, with delayed hemorrhage the polypectomy site is ulcerated and the bleeding artery may be retracted deeply into the submucosa. Spontaneous hemostasis is most desirable, but if therapeutic intervention is required, either injection sclerotherapy or coaptive coagulation with a nonerosive contact probe is optimal for this deep arterial bleeding site; caution must be exercised regarding the weakened wall.

Hemorrhoids

Hemorrhoids are a rare cause of major lower GI bleeding, most often associated with obstructed venous return from the superior hemorrhoidal veins (cirrhosis, cancer, and so on). Injection sclerotherapy with a variety of agents is typically effective in the control of acute bleeding. Other definitive therapy, such as rubber band ligation or possibly operative hemorrhoidectomy, may subsequently be required for third-degree hemorrhoids.

Radiation Colitis

Major hemorrhage from radiation colitis is distinctly uncommon. Whereas minor bleeding may be due to diffuse proctitis with granular, friable mucosa and characteristic telangiectasias, major bleeding usually implies an arterial source within the base of a radiation-induced ulcer. Although minor bleeding may respond to steroid enemas, persistent major hemorrhage requires definitive endoscopic or surgical therapy. If the bleeding point is found endoscopically, my treatment technique is similar treatment of a bleeding peptic ulcer (namely tamponade of bleeding with a nonerosive contact probe, followed by coaptive coagulation). If massive bleeding cannot be controlled endoscopically, surgery is needed to oversew or resect the bleeding ulcer. Unfortunately, diverting colostomy alone is not usually sufficient to control major hemorrhage.

Inflammatory Bowel Disease

Crohn's disease will rarely cause major bleeding from a deep ulcer which has eroded into an artery. This may require surgical intervention if the hemorrhage does not cease spontaneously. In contrast, the superficial ulceration of chronic ulcerative colitis characteristically produces only minor intermittent bleeding.

MINOR CHRONIC OR OCCULT BLEEDING

Small volume intermittent hematochezia typically implies a bleeding source in the left colon, rectum or anus, with benign anal causes predominating (see Table 1). Clues obtained from a careful history may be helpful. Passage of fresh blood after normal stool suggests an anal lesion, especially if there is dripping of bright red blood into the toilet. Hematochezia associated with painful defecation suggests an anal fissure. Streaks of blood on the stool or blood mixed in the stool suggests a lesion higher in the rectum or colon.

When historical features strongly suggest an anorectal cause of bleeding, and if careful digital, anoscopic and proctosigmoidoscopic examinations confirm a likely source of bleeding, then full colonic examination may not be required. There is additional support for this approach if a stool specimen, obtained from the sigmoid colon at the time of endoscopy, is negative for occult blood. However, if the patient is over age 40, or if a convincing distal source of bleeding is not found, or if features of bleeding suggest a higher bleeding site, then full colonic examination by good quality air contrast barium enema and colonoscopy or both should be performed.

Occult GI bleeding does not have any inherent localizing features and therefore requires examination of the entire GI tract. The main worry with occult bleeding is neoplasia, especially of the colon. Evaluation includes anorectal examination, proctosigmoidoscopy, and air contrast barium enema or colonoscopy. If the barium enema is negative except for diverticulae, colonoscopy is indicated and will reveal a missed colonic lesion in approximately 40 percent of cases. Conversely, if the colonoscopy is technically suboptimal or if the entire colon is not carefully examined, then air contrast barium enema is needed. Examination of the upper GI tract is accomplished either by air contrast x-ray film or endoscopy, depending upon clinical suspicions. With occult or recurrent overt GI bleeding and negative examination of the colon and upper GI tract, further possible diagnostic tests include small bowel x-ray films (enteroclysis is preferred), radionuclide scans, arteriography and use of a bleeder tube. A peroral attempt to endoscope the small bowel beyond the ligament of Treitz is usually not very rewarding, and the length of ileum that can be inspected at the time of colonoscopy is limited. As a last resort, if the clinical situation warrants, laparotomy with intraoperative small bowel endoscopy can be performed. Although a variety of techniques have been suggested, I have found that it is best to make a single small enterotomy in the mid small bowel, then pass the gas-sterilized colonoscope proximally and distally to inspect the entire small bowel. This is accomplished by a patient surgeon gently passing the endoscope as the endoscopist carefully observes the mucosa. Telescoping over the endoscope can be very traumatic to mucosal as well as serosal surfaces of the bowel, and it is therefore important to inspect adequately on insertion, since artifacts may preclude a satisfactory examination as the endoscope is withdrawn.

Evaluation of intermittent melena is similar to the approach outlined for occult bleeding except that suspicion of an upper GI source is greater and upper endoscopy should be considered earlier.

Once a precise diagnosis has been established, specific treatment options depend upon the particular lesion (see other chapters for full discussion). For example, medical therapy may include steroids for inflammatory bowel disease or stool softeners for anal fissure. Endoscopic therapy may be effective for removal of a bleeding polyp, for coagulation of bleeding telangiectatic vessels with localized radiation colitis, or for palliative treatment of a bleeding rectal malignancy. Surgery may offer definitive treatment of colon cancer, an intractable anal fissure, third-degree hemorrhoids, a Meckel's diverticulum, or ischemic colitis with peritoneal signs.

REFERENCES

1. Boley SJ. On the nature and etiology of vascular ectasias of the colon: degenerative of aging. Gastroenterology 1977; 72:650.
2. Johnston J. Endoscopic thermal treatment of upper gastrointestinal bleeding: overview and guidelines. Endoscopy Rev 1982; 2:12–33.

INTESTINAL GAS

JACK D. WELSH, M.D.

Increased intestinal gas is a common primary or secondary complaint. The patient's symptoms usually take the form of abdominal discomfort and bloating, or less frequently, increased belching or the passage of flatus via the rectum. A careful history concerning the timing of the symptoms and the patient's dietary intake is more important in determining therapy than a series of diagnostic tests. Patients should be questioned concerning any relationship of their symptoms to alterations in bowel habits or eating patterns. In some instances there may be obvious contributory dietary factors, whereas a few patients complain that "everything I take turns to gas." For the difficult patient a dietary diary for a week or 2, along with a record of the time and severity of symptoms, is frequently helpful. Not only will this occasionally document unusual dietary habits, but it also may uncover contributing situational factors.

EXCESSIVE BELCHING

Belching can be of recent onset, occur only occasionally, and come on at certain times of the day, or it can be a chronic daily occurrence. As a symptom, belching is of little concern to many patients and only an irritation to the family. In these instances the patient may say the belching relieves abdominal discomfort and fullness. In some cases it may represent a conscious or unconscious effort to produce social embarrassment to family members.

To other patients, chronic daily belching may be a matter of concern in that they feel it represents a serious underlying problem. Informing the patient of the cause and providing reassurance as to its benign nature are helpful. The physician should explain that the expelled gas is not formed in the stomach or intestine from "poor digestion," but is mainly air that has been swallowed or aspirated into the esophagus. The patient should be instructed on how to palpate his larynx to demonstrate that every belch is preceded by elevation of the larynx during the aspiration of air. This is best done initially under the physician's supervision. The demonstration is not only useful in explaining to the patient what is happening, but is helpful for therapy. Patients should be told that the sequence of aspirating air and belching is a learned response, and therefore can be "unlearned." Many patients will understand and accept that it is a habit. When belching episodes occur the patient should place a hand on his larynx and consciously try to prevent the aspirations. Practicing the "no-aspiration, no-belch" exercise cures many patients. Further reinforcement through documentation by family members that belching does not occur while the patient is asleep may be helpful in the overly concerned and anxious patient. Operant conditioning may help the patient to "break" the habit of belching.

Dietary factors should be considered by the physician if eructation occurs during or soon after a meal. Occasionally this is the only symptom in lactose malabsorption. In other cases the patient may be ingesting large amounts of gas-containing foods or beverages. Obvious examples are carbonated beverages and foods with air added during preparation. Less obvious examples are apples and other foods that contain a lot of air as part of their natural structure.

The patient or his family usually does not mention any particular odor of the belched gas. Since the patient may not volunteer such information it should be sought. "Sulphur" smelling or tasting belches of either acute or chronic nature should alert the physician to the possibility of giardiasis. Eradication of the parasite eliminates the odoriferous belches. The chapter *Parasites of the Small Intestine* provides information on treatment of giardiasis.

Most teaching in the past emphasized poor eating habits, bad dentures, gum chewing, and the use of drinking straws as causes of excessive swallowed air. Little evidence supports these as important contributors. Concentration on correcting these factors is usually of little therapeutic help and detracts from more primary causes.

ABDOMINAL PAIN AND BLOATING

Patients with functional abdominal pain and bloating are usually convinced that their symptoms are due to excessive intestinal gas. It has been demonstrated that the volume of intestinal gas in such patients before or after a meal is not excessive. The symptoms appear to be the result of altered motility and an increased awareness of discomfort and pain with volumes of intestinal gas tolerated by most individuals. In contrast, an occasional patient with lactase deficiency will demonstrate rather dramatic abdominal swelling, not always accompanied by diarrhea. The time sequence following ingestion of milk or lactose-containing foods is easy to identify through questioning. A positive response to a low-lactose diet is both diagnostic and therapeutic.

Once organic causes for the abdominal pain have been eliminated, it should be explained to the patient that he has an increased awareness of visceral responses to normal volumes of gas. If the episodes are related to periods of stress or depression, this should be pointed out to the patient.

Reduction of any intestinal gas or prevention of sudden increases in gas volumes is beneficial, since these individuals appear particularly sensitive to even normal amounts of gas. If belching is an additional part of the patient's symptom complex, measures to decrease this as outlined above should be instituted. When the patient is purposefully taking gas-producing agents such as sodium bicarbonate to induce belching to relieve symptoms, this practice should be discouraged. Individuals who have a history of a high-fat diet should be encouraged to reduce their fat intake. Large amounts of carbon dioxide are produced when fatty acids or hydrochloric acid are neu-

TABLE 1 Gas-Forming Potential of Common Foods

High Gas Producers	Low Gas Producers
Beans, cabbage, Brussels sprouts	Rice (white)
Bread, pasta, other wheat products	Bananas, citrus fruits, grapes
	Hard cheese
Apples, pears, peaches	Meats, eggs, peanut butter
Prunes	Noncarbonated, sugar-containing beverages
Corn, oats, potatoes	Saccharine
Processed bran	Unprocessed bran

tralized by bicarbonate. A hydroxide-containing antactid taken 15 to 30 minutes after a meal therefore may be helpful.

Nonabsorbable dietary carbohydrates provide the major exogenous fermentable substrate for bacteria to form gas in the colon. Elimination of gas-producing foods from the diet may thus be a major factor in decreasing the patients' symptoms (Table 1). Fruit juices are a contributing factor in some patients, while large amounts of diet drinks containing fructose or sorbitol may be a source of the problem in other patients. Those who drink large amounts of diet drinks should check the labels to determine their content. Even in the patient who has normal amounts of intestinal lactase, a decrease in the daily intake of lactose-containing foods, for those who ingest excessive quantities, may be helpful. The chapter *Carbohydrate Absorption*, should be reviewed for low-lactose diets.

Simethicone, a defoaming agent, has been used rather extensively alone or in combination with various antacids in the treatment of gas-related distress. As any endoscopist knows, the liquid form readily breaks up foam in the stomach, but relief of symptoms in the patient with gaseous distress is variable. This may be due to the fact that the symptoms are not related as much to the volume of gas present as to an increased awareness of its presence. Simethicone may be tried for a short period when dietary modifications or other treatment modalities have failed. In some patients it may provide a degree of benefit, particularly after ingestion of gas-forming foods.

Acute episodes of pain are frequently best relieved by a heating pad to the abdomen and having the patient recline and relax. The sooner after the onset of symptoms the patient can start this therapy, the more likely it is to help. The reclining position may bring about a more uniform distribution of any gas in the intestine.

On the whole, pharmacologic agents directed at the underlying motor disorder are often unsatisfactory. They should be tried only for acute episodes or when other measures have failed. Metoclopramide, which increases intestinal transit, may be given in doses of 10 mg orally 15 to 30 minutes before meals. It should not be combined with anticholinergic agents, since its action is antagonized by these drugs. It has a decreasing action from the proximal to distal intestine, but may increase the passage of gas through the intestinal tract. Any of the various anticholinergic agents may occasionally help. Some evidence supports the use of dicyclomine hydrochloride (Bentyl) in doses of 10 to 20 mg 3 or 4 times a day in these patients.

Increased intestinal gas in the patient with prior gastric surgery or inflammatory bowel disease may be a real factor in their abdominal pain. It may be a part of the dumping syndrome in the patient who has undergone gastric surgery or a daily feature of the patient with inflammatory bowel disease. The basic therapy for these conditions are outlined in the chapter *Idiopathic Inflammatory Bowel Disease and Neoplasia*, but many patients still benefit from the measures described above to decrease intestinal gas.

EXCESSIVE FLATUS

Excessive or foul smelling flatus can be a source of social embarrassment or cause a patient to think that it is an indication of a serious gastrointestinal problem. The increased passage of rectal gas and its odor are usually the result of the composition of the diet rather than a symptom of underlying disease. Except for some patients with prior gastrointestinal surgery who may pass swallowed air, rectal gas is produced in the intestinal tract. The patient with inflammatory bowel disease frequently has increased rectal gas and particularly foul smelling flatus. Treatment of the basic disease and following the suggestions listed below can be of value.

Large amounts of lactose-containing foods may be the offending agents in those with a lactase deficiency, prior gastric surgery, and in some otherwise normal individuals. The person with normal intestinal lactase may still malabsorb substantial amounts of lactose, particularly when drinking milk. A trial of a low-lactose diet for a week or two followed by reintroduction of lactose into the diet is often a helpful test. If symptoms disappear and then come back it is not only diagnostic, but reinforces the importance of the diet to the patient.

Reassurance that the increased gas does not represent a serious problem or disordered digestion alleviates the anxiety of most patients. In the rare individual in whom concern seems excessive and disproportionate, a deeper psychologic dysfunction must be considered.

In the otherwise healthy person when lactose does not seem to be a contributing factor, the role of other foods should be investigated. The 1- or 2-week diet diary can be very helpful and frequently saves time in the difficult patient. Some high gas forming foods are usually well recognized by the patient but others may not be as obvious. Fruits (raisins, bananas, apples, pears, and peaches) and fruit juices (apple, grape, and prune) may be gas producers in some individuals. Although undigested fiber plays a role in these cases, probably other, as yet unstudied, fermentable materials also contribute to the gas formation. Orange juice and apricot nectar are usually well tolerated without increased gas production. Red wines and tap beer in particular are major gas producers in some individuals. Added dietary fiber and roughage may be the cause of an acute increase of flatus. Processed bran is fermentable and can cause increased gas production in the colon. To a lesser degree this is also true in some individuals taking unprocessed bran. Therefore any increase in bran intake that correlates with increased gas formation is suspect. Ingestion of "sugar-free" products that contain sorbitol or fructose must also be considered.

Most patients gain relief from their symptoms by eliminating or reducing foods that they recognize as causing their increased gas. Those who continue to have symptoms should keep a record of their diet and symptoms until they can identify the foods that are causing their problem through systematic deletion. The emphasis on diet as the causative factor of their symptoms also helps to take their minds off any possible underlying disorder, and frequently relieves anxiety. Occasionally elimination of foods has to be monitored, as the patient's omissions may be too excessive.

Treatment of excessive or odorous flatus through pharmacologic agents is not beneficial, except possibly for the use of activated charcoal. Although the physician has only the patient's word that the charcoal decreases the embarrassing odor, that is what is important. Charcoal tablets of 325 mg or more are available but may have to be obtained from local health food stores. The required dosage, 1 to 2 tablets 2 or 3 times a day, seems to vary among individuals. Pancreatic enzymes with bile salts alone or combined with the activated charcoal to provide "better digestion" are of little value. There is no evidence that any reported improvement is not due to a placebo effect. Although the increased flatus in some instances seems to be due to a colonic bacterial flora particularly efficient in fermenting carbohydrates, or follows some episode of gstroenteritis or foreign travel, the use of antibiotics is not advised. Results are unpredictable, and occasionally patients will even recall that flatus increased following antibiotic treatment for some other condition.

IRRITABLE BOWEL SYNDROME

MARVIN M. SCHUSTER, M.D.

Although irritable bowel syndrome is the most common gastrointestinal condition, little is known concerning its etiology. Recently acquired knowledge concerning pathophysiology and precipitating factors permits a rational approach to treatment based on these factors as well as empiric observation. Irritable bowel syndrome is characterized by abdominal pain and altered bowel habits, usually alternating constipation and diarrhea with one of the two symptoms predominating. The syndrome is recognized as a motor disorder which is strongly influenced by emotional stress and by food intake, and occasionally by specific food intolerances.

GENERAL PRINCIPLES OF TREATMENT

Since the etiologic determinants of irritable bowel syndrome are unknown, treatment focuses on correcting the underlying motor disorder and modifying those factors which are known to precipitate or aggravate the motor disorder and associated symptoms (Table 1). Treatment is therefore multidimensional and predominantly symptomatic. A consistent approach with persistent attention to details and a sensitive understanding of the individual patient can lead to significant improvement with time.

Establishing Confidence

The initial visit sets the stage and begins the ongoing process of the developing doctor-patient relationship. The interest and compassion shown by the physician at this time serves not only to inspire confidence but also to assist in the diagnostic pursuit of relevant information concerning the patient and the factors affecting his illness.

TABLE 1 Treatment of Irritable Bowel Syndrome

General Principles of Treatment
  Establish confidence
  Educate and reassure
  Dispel fears and misconceptions
  Schedule return visits

Dietary Management
  Investigate and treat lactose intolerance
  Eliminate offending foods
  High-fiber diet
  Hydrophilic colloids

Medications (as appropriate)
  Antispasmodics
  Antidiarrheals
  Intestinal stimulants
  Analgesics
  Antiflatulents

Psychological Management
  Anxiety
    Manage situational stressors
    Improve coping techniques
    Relaxation training
    Mild tranquilizers as needed
  Depression
    Manage situation stressors
    Support
    Tricyclic antidepressants
  Illness Behavior
    Avoid reinforcement of illness behavior
    Reward healthy behavior
    Push toward maximal performance

Adapted from Schuster MM. Irritable bowel syndrome. a coordinated approach to therapy. Drug Therapy 1962; August.

A dogged pursuit of details can produce helpful and rewarding results.

Education and Reassurance

It is important that the patient understand that irritable bowel syndrome is an intestinal motor disorder, that it is chronic and recurrent, and that it is influenced by a number of factors, including emotional stress, food intake, and drugs. The patient will then be more likely to accept recurrence as part of the disease process rather than as an indication of inappropriate diagnosis or inadequate treatment. This will alleviate one of the stresses that every person with irritable bowel syndrome undergoes, namely, concern about the significance of persistent, recurrent, or intensified symptoms. It is often helpful to utilize as an analogy chronic disorders, such as hypertension or diabetes, which, like irritable bowel syndrome, are not cured but can be controlled.

Managing Fears and Misconceptions

A frank and open invitation to discuss concepts and concerns is perhaps the best way to elicit information which may be highly specific to the individual. This invitation may have to be repeated in subsequent sessions as the patient develops confidence and as the physician develops knowledge of the patient. Relatives may also be quite helpful in providing useful information in this regard. Patients also should understand that, although bothersome, irritable bowel syndrome does not lead to any serious disorder such as ulcerative colitis or cancer, nor does it in any way influence life expectancy.

Scheduling Return Appointments

A scheduled return visit will provide reassurance of continued interest, will avoid a sense of abandonment, will provide support, and will permit the continued gathering of information that can help to fine-tune the treatment program. During subsequent visits the patient's response to the therapeutic regimen can be ascertained and modifications can be made in the program as indicated. The support provided by this expression of ongoing interest, while not tangible, may be extremely meaningful and useful. Subsequent visits may be more brief and less frequent as improvement occurs and the patient is encouraged to assume a more active and independent role in the management of his disorder.

DIETARY MANAGEMENT

Investigate and Treat Lactose Intolerance

Symptoms of lactose intolerance can mimic in every way the symptoms of irritable bowel syndrome. In addition, lactose intolerance can aggravate the symptoms of irritable bowel syndrome. For these reasons lactose intolerance should be ruled out in every patient presenting with symptoms of irritable bowel syndrome. This can be achieved by performing a lactose tolerance test, or more simply by placing the patient on a lactose-free diet for a trial period of 2 weeks. Initially this diet should be quite strict, eliminating all milk and milk products. At a later stage, if lactose intolerance is demonstrated, the level of intolerance can be tested by gradually adding small quantities of the milk-containing products which the patient misses most until a threshold is reached at which symptoms recur. Only about 2 percent of patients who present with symptoms of irritable bowel syndrome will have lactose intolerance as the sole basis for their symptoms. Though small in number, this will be a very grateful group of patients who are cured by control of the quantity of lactose in their diets. In a larger number, about 40 percent, lactose intolerance is superimposed upon irritable bowel syndrome. Elimination of lactose in this group will improve but not alleviate symptoms completely. I generally reserve lactose tolerance tests for patients who appear to have lactose intolerance but refuse to accept the concept that small quantities of milk can be deleterious. Intolerance of other foodstuffs is a highly individual phenomenon and best demonstrated by the keeping of a careful dietary diary.

High-Fiber Diet

Diets high in bran (and perhaps other fibrous foods) may be helpful especially when constipation is a dominant feature of irritable bowel syndrome. One may begin by prescribing bran cereals, whole wheat or rye bread, and progress as needed to unprocessed bran which can be sprinkled on foods. It is perhaps best to start with small doses, increasing as needed and as tolerated to 16 g per day (2 tablespoons 3 times daily). More palatable forms of brans such as crackers (Fibermed) are also available. A transient increase in gas and bloating occurs not infrequently for the first several weeks but often disappears. Patients should therefore be encouraged to continue with the diet for about 3 weeks unless symptoms are extremely disturbing. Only about 15 to 20 percent cannot tolerate bran because of the intensity of the symptoms or because they persist for longer than 3 weeks.

Hydrophilic Colloids

Bulk agents containing psyllium seeds are particularly helpful when alternating constipation and diarrhea exist, since these agents are hydrophilic and tend to solidify diarrheal stools and also soften hard stools. They are therefore safer than antidiarrheal agents to treat the diarrheal phase and safer than laxative agents to treat the constipated phase. Dosage requirements are highly individual; one should begin at small doses, increasing as required until an effective dose is reached. The preference for one hydrophilic colloid over another is based predominantly on palatability, and in some specific instances on salt and sugar content for patients who require restriction of these ingredients. Some of the more popular agents are Metamucil, Perdiem plain, LA formula, Hydrocil, Konsyl, and Mitrolan. These agents may be more effective when administered with meals rather than at bedtime, because then they mix with the stool as it is being formed. Because of taste factors and because some swelling of the psyllium seeds takes place in the stomach, there may be some appetite suppression if administered before meals. Therefore these agents should be taken by obese people before meals and by thin people after meals.

DRUG THERAPY

Antispasmodic Agents

Although they are the most physiologically reasonable drugs for treatment of the intestinal motor disorder of irritable bowel syndrome, antispasmodics have been less than dramatic in their success. Still, they do play a role and provide varying degrees of relief for many sufferers of irritable bowel syndrome. Antispasmodics may be particularly useful in patients who have postprandial symptoms induced by increased intestinal motor activity. Anticholinergic drugs that have more spasmolytic than antisecretory activity are the logical choice for the treatment of the majority of patients with irritable bowel syndrome who do not have dyspepsia. In the United States, dicyclomine hydrochloride (Bentyl) is used; it has a high ratio of spasmolytic to antisecretory action. Therefore, side effects of dry mouth and decreased gastric secretion are less prominent. While it is generally prescribed in dosages of 20 mg 4 times daily, a recent study indicates that as much as 40 mg 4 times daily may be required. It is probably wise to start with doses of 10 mg 4 times daily for elderly patients, who are often not able to tolerate higher doses. At least 3 weeks should be allowed to judge clinical efficacy. Spasmolytic agents are generally best administered half an hour to an hour before meals and at bedtime (particularly in those patients with meal-aggravated symptoms). This allows time for peak blood levels to be reached during the postprandial period. Blurred vision, urinary retentin, and aggravation of glaucoma are possible side effects with any anticholinergics.

When dyspeptic symptoms suggest hyperacidity, anticholinergics with more antisecretory activity may be preferred. Tincture of belladonna has the advantage of permitting graded dosage, starting with 10 drops and increasing until side effects of dry mouth or blurred vision appear, then dropping back to the dosage immediately preceding the one that caused the side effects. The liquid form may, however, be inconvenient outside the home. Other anticholinergics, such as propantheline, Levsin, and Cantil, are often used.

Antidiarrheal Drugs

Although mild diarrhea usually responds to hydrophilic colloids or dietary manipulations, severe diarrhea may require drugs such as diphenoxylate and atropine (Lomotil), one or two 2.5-mg tablets every 4 to 6 hours as long as diarrhea persists, or loperamide (Imodium), which has a rapid but longer duration of action and generally need be given as 2 or 4 mg only every 8 hours. When diarrhea is unremitting or accompanied by severe disabling pain, codeine, 30 to 60 mg every 4 to 6 hours, may be helpful but carries the danger of addiction. Since the effective antidiarrheal dose of codeine remains constant over time, increased dose requirements should suggest problems with addiction and possible need for withdrawal from the medication. Another problem associated with antidiarrheal agents of this type is induction of constipation, especially in patients with alternating diarrhea and constipation.

Stimulant Laxatives

As with antidiarrheal agents, stimulant laxatives should be used only when absolutely necessary, because they may induce diarrhea in patients with alternating constipation and diarrhea. They are also habit forming and should be prescribed only in the smallest possible effective doses and for the briefest period of time. Stimulants such as milk of magnesia, cascara, Senokot, and Dulcolax may aggravate a painful condition by stimulating intestinal spasm.

Analgesic Medication

The pain of irritable bowel syndrome can often be relieved by antispasmodic medications. When pain is severe and unresponsive to anticholinergics, analgesics may be required, but they should be reserved only for acute stages of severe pain. A heating pad applied to the abdomen or warm baths may also be helpful. When a chronic pain syndrome is present, referral to a pain treatment center may be appropriate. Such a clinic is described in the chapter *Chronic Intractable Abdominal Pain*. Nonsteroidal anti-inflammatory agents, including aspirin, 2 tablets every 6 hours, may alleviate acute exacerbations of pain. Pentazocine (Talwin), 50 to 100 mg every 6 hours, should be used in preference to opiates for severe, acute, limited situations. Morphine particularly is to be avoided because of its addiction potential as well as the fact that it aggravates spasm even though its central action may diminish perceived pain.

Antiflatulents

The effective antiflatulent is yet to be discovered. Trial and error seems to be the most useful way of finding drugs that provide some relief. Simethicone (Mylicon), two to four tablets, or activated charcoal (4 tablets), may be prescribed with meals and at bedtime. Pancreatic supplements, Phazyme 95, Ilozyme, Pancrease, Viokase, Cotazyme, and so on, 1 to 2 tablets before meals and at bedtime, are helpful for some.

MANAGEMENT OF PSYCHOLOGIC FACTORS

Since emotional stress is one of the most commonly recognized factors aggravating irritable bowel syndrome, and since 70 to 80 percent of patients with irritable bowel syndrome demonstrate psychopathologic factors on psychological tests, psychological management is an important aspect of treatment. In the vast majority of instances this can be effectively handled by the primary physician or consulting gastroenterologist. Psychiatric referral is appropriate only for those conditions that would require psychiatric referral whether or not irritable bowel syndrome were present. A life history chart compiled by the patient can be quite helpful in detecting stressful factors that are associated with exacerbation of symptoms. This information is best obtained simply by probing into life events that surround periods of exacerbation and remission.

Anxiety

Although anxiety is easily recognized by patients, somatization (which represents an internalization of anxiety) is less readily detected. Correlation of life events with anxious periods provides useful clues. In some instances direct environmental manipulation may successfully remove the stressful stimulus. For example, with the physician's questions acting as a catalyst, a patient may arrive at the conclusion that his interest would be better served by changing jobs or locations. This type of milieu therapy can produce dramatic improvement. Often, however, these changes are either impossible or inadvisable, and the patient must be helped to learn appropriate coping techniques for dealing with stresses that cannot be removed. A number of audiotapes are available for relaxation training e.g., Budzynski narration MV 3–B (BMA Audiocassettes Department C1, 200 Park Avenue South, New York, NY 10003). Infrequently tranquilizers may be required for brief periods of intensive anxiety, but long-term use should be avoided if possible.

Depression

Depression is less readily recognized than anxiety, since it is often masked and expressed as somatic symptoms. As with anxiety, precipitating factors can sometimes be altered but more commonly they cannot. Supportive therapy is often helpful. Tricyclic antidepressants may be useful when given in a single night-time dose, e.g., 25 to 50 mg of amitriptyline (Elavil), or 50 to 100 mg of maprotiline (Ludiomil).

There is some evidence that symptoms of irritable bowel syndrome represent illness behavior learned in early childhood and perpetuated by social reinforcement (secondary gain). A behavioral approach to this aspect is the most direct, and often the most successful. Patients and relatives are instructed to avoid disscussion of illness and by all means to avoid rewarding illness by attention, while focusing on and rewarding healthy behavior. Patients are asked to distract themselves from thinking about their symptoms whenever they become more aware that they are doing so. They are told to avoid discussion of symptoms except during their routine visits with their physicians. Patients are instructed to view their irritable bowel syndrome as they would view a physical disability which they would try to overcome. Rather than give in to the illness, they are encouraged to push themselves to maximal performances as they would if they had visual impairment, hearing deficit, or other physical disability.

While no single drug or therapeutic maneuver may be curative, gratifying relief can result for a coordinated program based on sound physiological principles and empiric observations.

DIVERTICULAR DISEASE OF THE COLON

ADAM NEIL SMITH, M.D., F.R.C.S.

A recent Scottish survey has shown that there was no decrease in the number of operations performed for uncomplicated or complicated diverticular disease in the first 5 years of the "bran era." Yet there is little doubt that nowadays the majority of patients with diverticular disease of the colon are initially treated with high-fiber diets, usually including the combination of fiber, hydrophilic colloid compounds, and antispasmodics.

MEDICAL THERAPY

Good initial treatment ought to include the following: A precise diagnosis should be made before putting the patient on a high-fiber intake. This requires sigmoidoscopy and barium enema examination which should exclude carcinoma of the colon. Fiber is taken as 20 g per day and should be increased in stages over a 2- to 3-week period to diminish the risk of bloating or other abdominal discomfort associated with the change in intestinal filling. The patient should be informed, and should note, that the daily fecal output will increase. An antispasmodic agent, such as propantheline bromide, 15 mg 3 times daily, or mebeverine hydrochloride, 100 to 400 mg per day, is often added for the first month. Rarely, diarrhea dominates the picture and codeine phosphate or sulfate, 20 to 60 mg, usually controls these symptoms; like morphine, however, it can increase the intraluminal pressure and it is therefore preferable to use diphenoxylate hydrochloride, 5 mg 3 times a day.

Seventy-eight percent of patients with painful uncomplicated diverticular disease can expect to get relief of symptoms with bran and a high-fiber diet, and this has become the basis of present day initial management. Bran is denatured by cooking, so the advice of a dietician may have to be sought to achieve the most advantageous means of consumption. Most patients consume it as breakfast cereal or mix it into soup. Like other hydrophilic compounds which act mainly as fecal bulking agents, bran acts by providing unabsorbed fiber residues which bind salt and water to them in the gut.

SURGICAL MANAGEMENT OF UNCOMPLICATED DIVERTICULAR DISEASE

Few patients require elective surgery, since most respond to the measures outlined above. Yet perhaps because fiber is at first so outstandingly successful, patients who fail to improve all the more readily come to surgery. The main indication for resection thus becomes either failure on a high-fiber diet or an inability to adhere in someone having constantly painful attacks of diverticular disease. Such patients usually have left-sided pain with varying local tenderness; the absence of fever and rigidity of the overlying muscles and a marginally higher than normal white blood count at this stage indicate that the condition is basically noninflammatory. Many observers have advanced the view that this phase of the disease is the result of the thickened circular muscle of the colon producing luminal obstruction of the sigmoid colon. Resection of the sigmoid colon, especially of the rectosigmoid part where the obstructive process commonly begins, combined with end-to-end anastomosis brings immediate relief.

This "localized" resection may occasionally be accompanied by painful recurrence of the disease with further high intraluminal pressure inducing further episodes of diverticular disease. It has been shown that the muscle dysfunction of the colon is more widely distributed along the colon wall than at first thought. Most patients therefore benefit from maintaining a high-fiber or bulk additive diet postoperatively to ward off further pain and as a prophylaxis against the risk of intraluminal pressure rises which extrude the mucosa through the wall of the colon. This is a basic factor in the origin of the condition and predominantly affects the left or sigmoid colon, at least initially. An anomalous feature of some patients is that they may refer some of the problem to the right side of the colon—perhaps because the thick circular muscle of the left colon shuts down so completely that it produces obstructive distention of the cecum and ascending colon. These patients can expect to become free of right iliac fossa features of the disease only if the primary troublesome area in the left iliac fossa is detected and treated correctly.

Parks, in the article on this subject in the first edition of this work (Current Therapy in Gastroenterology and Liver Disease, 1984–1985) reviewed the position of *myotomy*. Whatever the pros and cons of this operation, the need for it has diminished greatly since. Whatever its applicability, it has been superseded largely by the use of fiber.

SURGICAL MANAGEMENT OF COMPLICATED DIVERTICULAR DISEASE

Most patients with more severe disease require surgery. The largest group is those with *inflammatory* disease. The inflammation may be local but may increase in severity by spreading transmurally from a stage of peridiverticulitis to one of pericolic abscess or to a local or generalized peritonitis. Inflammation may be dramatically precipitated by rupture of a diverticulum, and it may also lead to fistula into other parts of the intestinal tract or adjacent viscera. Other important complications are bleeding, pseudotumor formation, and obstruction.

Inflammation

The clinical severity of already known diverticular disease have recently increased. Many patients have had prior mild temporary attacks of fever and tenderness in the left iliac fossa, often subsiding on a course of antibiotic directed at alimentary tract organism, such as *Escherichia coli* and *Bacteroides*. Many of these patients have had earlier hospital admissions and have been managed by measures such as gastric suction to rest the alimentary tract and intravenous glucose and saline infusion to correct fluid and electrolyte imbalance. They normally settle down and may not require surgery—indeed this is rare in "first attacks."

Should the temperature become significantly elevated to 39 °C, however, or fail to resolve with effective antibiotic management or become subnormal, accompanied by tenderness or guarding in the left iliac fossa and a white count elevated above $15 \times 10^9/L$, then such patients must be considered to have peritonitis becoming a pericolic abscess and preparation has to be made for surgical drainage and/or resection.

I believe ideally in letting such sepsis localize if possible and in draining a resultant abscess with resection of the colon postponed to a later date. This course is favored particularly because many are elderly and often poor-risk patients.

The majority of patients, however, do eventually undergo surgical drainage combined with resection of the pelvic colon, for the following reason: It is necessary when draining a pericolic abscess to evacuate all the thick, purulent content from what has been a cavity of phlegmonous inflammation in and around one or several diverticula. This may have advanced to the stage of necrosis of the bowel wall, with the implication that in the depth of the abscess cavity there is a direct fistulous connection into the lumen of the colon. The use of the surgical suction apparatus is important: If the evacuation of pus is followed by the recognition of a fecal leak, then the diverticular abscess is of the so-called communicating type and must be treated by resection. The results of a Hartmann's resection, i.e., resection without anastomosis plus proximal colostomy, have been shown to be preferable to those of proximal colostomy. Attempts to close or patch the hole in the colon are much less satisfactory and have a higher mortality. Performing a Hartmann's resection also means that if staged resections are required, fewer stages are necessary. The introduction of the "stapling gun" has greatly simplified the reanastomosis of the bowel in the pelvis and makes the procedure of closure easy for most surgeons.

Should the sepsis fail to localize, more urgent measures are necessary. This may also happen if a localizing collection ruptures. Roentgenograms taken of the abdomen may show localized intestinal gas collections in the left iliac fossa or even free gas there or underneath the diaphragm. Such patients need maximum resuscitation in an intensive care unit with intravenous fluid, including blood and colloid administration, and intravenous antibiotics aimed at *E. coli, Streptococcus faecalis*, and *Bacteroides*. A central venous line is necessary to monitor hypovolemic shock and an indwelling catheter is mandatory to estimate hourly urine flow. The surgeon's judgment must be brought to bear in the timing of surgical intervention. This is usually done when the "infective storm" is passing, when the blood pressure is returning to normal levels, and the associated tachycardia is settling. Such patients almost always benefit from antibiotic lavage of the peritoneal cavity after resection of the pelvic or left colon. There is often an associated ischemia of the left colon in such patients, so a careful appraisal should be made at laparotomy not only of the extent of the diverticular disease present, but also of the possible associated ischemia in elderly patients affecting the bowel from the splenic flexure downward to the pelvic brim.

Occasionally this dramatic clinical picture is arrived at almost immediately. Patients with or without known diverticular disease may collapse with varying degrees of tenderness in the left iliac fossa; they may be febrile but more often suffer from a subnormal temperature (36 °C), and blood cultures taken at this time show a coliform bacteremia. Admitted to the hospital often grievously ill, they require urgent resuscitation as already outlined. Roentgenography of the diaphragmatic area commonly shows copious gas underneath the diaphragm (if done in the left lateral position the film shows a 2- to 4-cm gaseous space above intestinal loops which may or may not be dilated).

If there is any remaining doubt of a fecal leak, *abdominal paracentesis* with syringe, needle, and saline shows gas and fecal fluid on aspiration in the left iliac fossa. At subsequent laparotomy after resuscitation these patients are found to have a ruptured diverticulum with resultant varying degrees of fecal contamination of the abdomen. Some elderly patients become so ill and toxic that they are not ever fit for a full laparotomy and are treated as a last resort by intraperitoneal dialysis catheter perfusion of the peritoneal cavity. The main objective, however, must be to resect the affected colon. In most circumstances this again leads to a Hartmann's resection.

There is a subgroup in which this problem presents in a lesser manner, in which the fecal contamination is less and the systemic reaction is minimal. In such patients the colon may be resected, the peritoneal cavity washed clean, and a restorative anastomosis performed. It is my practice, however, to protect a primary anastomosis in these cases by a proximal colostomy. Occasionally elderly patients are seen in whom the entire process has been missed in the first few days. Presumably the elderly do not always react systemically to the infective process to the same extent. The fecally contaminated abdomen responds with a layer of granulation tissue in and around loops of bowel, matting them together. It may be impossible to find the point of fecal leakage. In such patients extensive lavage of the peritoneal cavity is imperative and a blind transverse colostomy may be required.

Fistula

Fistula may follow a possibly unrecognized abscess and is really an affirmation of this. The most common fistula developing in diverticula is *colovesical fistula* and it is an exception to the above rule in that it nowadays almost always is de novo without abscess as its forerunner. The type of patient affected by this fistula has also changed. Most patients are male, and in the unlikely event of it arising in a female it can be predicted that a hysterectomy has been performed previously.

Those affected do not necessarily have a lengthy or complicated preceding history of the diverticular process. Examination of hospital records shows that more and more patients present with a short history because there is a relatively mobile pelvic colon, often minimally affected by diverticular disease, able to adhere to the bladder and able to penetrate the relatively thin bladder wall. Thus, fewer patients require staged operations than was formerly necessary when the fistula was a passage from the bowel to the bladder through a complex abscess cavity which resulted from years of diverticular disease. Indeed, at operation the two structures are usually readily separated surgically, the bladder is closed by local suture (protected from dehiscence by an indwelling catheter, e.g., draining via a Foley catheter), and a resection of sigmoid colon is performed at the same time.

The more demanding aspect of the problem lies in the recognition that a colovesical fistula exists, because it is often an elusive diagnosis. First, the patient's symptoms may be bizarre and vary from a persistent cystitis unremitting after courses of antibiotics to pneumaturia and fecaluria. The former may become clinically confirmed when the patient reports a bubbling urinary stream or the latter by the passage of fecal pellets. Cystoscopic examination of the bladder commonly fails to show any lesion other than an occasional localized bullous cystitis in the vault of the bladder. These factors are all inherent to the dynamics of the situation: The intraluminal pressure in the bowel is mostly higher than in the bladder and the passage of gas, fluid, and solids is from the bowel to the bladder. The fistula may be identified by making use of this very principle—if the patient is sigmoidoscoped and has the bladder filled with contrast medium, air will be seen to pass according to the gradient from the bowel to the upper part of the contrast-filled bladder and rise to set up a fluid level in the region of the vault of the bladder outlined in this way in an x-ray film. Computed tomographic scans are proving very useful in some centers as a method of demonstrating air in the bladder. A thickened, adherent bowel loop completes the computed tomographic picture of a colovesical fistula.

Fistulas formed in other areas, such as the vaginal vault, to another intestinal loop, and sometimes to the skin surface, require resection of the affected diverticular sigmoid colon. The fistula tract proper thereafter heals spontaneously.

Bleeding

Serious bleeding arises when a fecalith erodes into the major vessels which are arranged around the neck of a diverticulum. Rarely, the amount of blood expelled per rectum is copious and red and the patient runs the risk of rapidly becoming exsanguinated. Left hemicolectomy is urgently indicated for the control of such serious hemorrhage.

The majority of incidents of bleeding are less dramatic and the site is less apparent. These patients are usually transfused and the majority stop bleeding. The problem then becomes one of prevention of the risk of recurrent episodes and identifying the source of hemorrhage, which is done in one of two ways:

First, in recurrent bleeding *colonoscopy* is done between episodes to identify not only the location of the diverticular disease but also the site of the mucosal lesion. The chance of bleeding from the right side of the colon in diverticular disease was considered high a few years ago. It is now known that the explanation lies in the overlap between two conditions, both of which affect patients of mature years. *Angiodysplasia* commonly coexists with and was the cause of the erroneous attribution of right-sided bleeding to diverticular disease. It affects the right colon, is commoner in women, and produces mucosal microvascular lesions (aneurysmal vascular ectasia or arteriovenous fistulas of small vessels). These vascular malformations appear as vascular "floral-like" mucosal patches at colonoscopy and may be seen actively bleeding. After excision by right hemicolectomy, microperfusion of the vessels and radiography performed on the specimen in vitro confirm the lesion.

Second, in the more urgent recurrent bleeding episode *arteriography* produces the higher diagnostic yield. The vessel usually cannulated is the superior mesenteric artery; the detail is not good in the inferior mesenteric and many radiologists consider it not worth doing. Blood loss of the order of 1 to 2 ml per minute can also be identified using technetium hydrochloride. To many this is easier than colonoscopy, since the colon can rarely be made clean enough for urgent endoscopy. Additionally, colonoscopy in diverticular disease is often technically demanding because the hypertrophied circular muscle impedes and distorts the passage of the instrument. The chapter *Lower Gastrointestinal Bleeding* contains details on the management of such bleeding.

Most surgeons now proceed by "consecutive colectomy" and mobilize and free the left colon. The specimen is then examined to see if it confirms a bleeding lesion. If not, one proceeds to the right colon looking for a further area of diverticular disease or angiodysplasia. The patient is given a temporary ileostomy on the right abdominal wall and a mucous fistula on the left and 3 months later has a restorative procedure.

Pseudotumor

A mass may be palpable in patients known to have diverticular disease, and if there is an absence of inflammatory features the differential diagnosis includes colon carcinoma. A computed tomographic scan may be helpful in such circumstances and may demonstrate the infiltration of a tumor or the more circumscribed outline of a pseudotumor in diverticular disease. The two lesions occasionally coexist and a relatively small tumor may, by obstructive effects, have precipitated diverticular disease and intensified its features. The management is the same, however. If otherwise operable, resection of the left colon with end-to-end anastomosis is performed, with removal of involved lymph nodes and an assessment of the presence or absence of metastases in the liver. The overall pathologic confirmation of the extent of the disease and the staging of any tumor present are ascertained from the specimen.

Obstruction

After repeated attacks of inflammation, the sigmoid colon may become embedded in *fibro-fatty degenerative tissue*. This, plus the thick bars of obstructing circular muscle of the colon wall encroaching on the lumen, add to distortion and fixation of the pelvic colon. This commonly leads to mildly obstructive features but may also provoke a true obstructive attack. When true obstruction develops, however, it is more often related to the presence of *peridiverticulitis* or a *pericolic abscess*. This obstruction can also affect the small intestine and both are of the *ileus* type. They follow a local toxic paralysis induced by infection developing in or around the colonic diverticulum. The latter responds to conservative management (nasogastric suction and intravenous fluids) as the infection is controlled. If there is a truly mechanical obstruction precipitated by colonic fibrosis and distortion, this is another indication for sigmoid resection, and since the bowel may be inadequately prepared in most of these patients it must be washed out "on the table" in the operating room. The patient is also protected intraoperatively and postoperatively by full antibiotic regimens, such as metronidazole and cefotaxime given intravenously.

RELATED CONDITIONS

The chances of finding diverticular disease in the right colon are notably higher among the Japanese in Hawaii. This is an as yet unexplained local variant of the disease in Southeast Asia.

Diverticular disease is commonly associated throughout the Western world with gallstones and hiatus hernia. Since patients may have complications relating to these diseases, relevant investigation should be directed toward elucidating the function of the gallbladder and esophagogastric junction by cholecystography and upper endoscopy.

Overlap with idiopathic inflammatory bowel disease occurs and may affect the clinical management in two ways. Patients with inflammatory bowel disease of the ulcerative colitis and Crohn's disease type combined with diverticular disease fare less well surgically; they tend to have more inflammatory problems (peritonitis, intraperitoneal abscess, wound healing problems). It has also been noted that a proportion of patients with recurrences of so-called diverticular disease have actually developed other inflammatory bowel diseases.

Surveys have been undertaken recently to demonstrate groups at special risk in diverticular disease. Patients with rheumatoid arthritis, asthma, renal transplantation, and collagen disease were found to have more complications, but this can be related to the added risk of being on steroids, chemotherapy, radiotherapy, and immunosuppressants. Some of their lesions may have started as vasculitis.

Overall, the management of diverticular disease is colored by the fact that it affects patients of a significantly older age group. For a benign condition such as this it is necessary that surgical resection be associated with consistently low mortality. For this reason there should be wise selection of the time and need for operation. Attention should first be directed toward avoiding the need for operation. If the dietary fiber theory is proven, then all surgeons should join in schemes of avoidance, all the more so as the number of elderly people who are specially at risk is continually rising in all Western countries. The figures establishing this come from an impeccable source: The Queen of England sends a congratulatory telegram to every citizen who reaches 100 years and has kept a record over the years of her reign. In 1952, there were just over 200 who attained their 100th birthday in the United Kingdom, but by 1984 this had risen to 1,750 centenarians who were congratulated in this way. It is a fair assumption that most of them would have diverticular disease of the colon.

RECURRENT ABDOMINAL PAIN IN CHILDHOOD AND ADOLESCENCE

RONALD G. BARR, M.A., M.D.C.M., F.R.C.P.(C)

Recurrent abdominal pain (RAP) syndrome presents both a diagnostic and therapeutic dilemma for physicians. The cardinal presenting symptom is intermittent, paroxysmal episodes of abdominal pain occurring during the school years. They are usually unrelated to other symptoms of organic disease. Traditionally, the approach to this symptom has been to determine whether the pain is "organic" or "psychogenic" ("functional") in nature and to base therapy on this determination. Since organic disease is rare as a cause (usually less than 5%), physicians tend either to overuse diagnostic tests which are invasive, expensive, and often painful (to rule out organic causes) or to underuse these tests (since they are so seldom positive) and assume that the cause is psychogenic. The usual result is that the symptom itself is treated as the manifestation of emotional problems in the child or an interactional problem in the family even in the absence of independent evidence confirming this assessment.

In my experience, this somewhat oversimplified classification and the diagnostic and clinical strategies which are entailed are misleading. As an alternative, I prefer to base the approach on a classification that does *not* assume that the pain represents a symptom of either organic or psychologic disease, and on a clinical strategy that aims to minimize the dysfunction when the symptom persists. In general, this approach acknowledges the possibility that nonspecific abdominal pain in the absence of disease may occur as a result of normal physiologic processes. Consequently, for most children and adolescents with the syndrome, prevention of secondary dysfunctional consequences is an appropriate and achievable therapeutic goal.

RATIONALE FOR CLINICAL STRATEGY

This approach assumes that a patient who complains of recurrent abdominal pain presents with a problem which includes the pain symptom itself, secondary anxiety associated with the pain symptom, and the secondary dysfunctional consequences of being a child with abdominal pain. The most significant feature of recurrent pain is its paroxysmal nature, such that its time of both occurrence and remission is unpredictable and usually unexpected. The anxiety stems primarily from not knowing the cause of the pain and is usually exacerbated by knowledge of a relative whose serious disease presented in a similar manner. Commonly, this anxiety is more pronounced in the child's parent(s) than in the patient. Typical examples of secondary dysfunction for the child include alternating support and anger from the parents who are uncertain about whether the pain is "real," accusations of malingering from schoolteachers, and overinvestigation by physicians. These aspects of the problem are usually present regardless of the origin of the symptom. Consequently, the clinical strategy requires attention not only to symptom resolution but also to secondary anxiety and dysfunction.

The clinical classification refers to the presumed cause of the pain symptom itself, regardless of the secondary consequences. In our alternative classification, a third major diagnostic category—dysfunctional pain—is added to organic and psychogenic possibilities, and a number of subcategories are recognized (Table 1).

Organic Pain

Organic pain refers to cases in which the pain sensations are presumed to originate intra-abdominally, a specific disease process in an organ system(s) is recognized, and treatment of that disease results in amelioration of the symptoms. As subcategories, one would include diseases referable to the gastrointestinal tract, the genitourinary tract, and others. While it is commonly stated that organic causes are approximately half gastrointestinal and half genitourinary, available studies are insufficient to establish diagnostic guidelines based on relative prevalence. The symptom presentation of many disease entities is not typical of that seen in adults and may vary with age. For example, only about 30 percent of children with ulcers show the typical pattern of pain related to meals, which is relieved by food, and night or early morning awakening. Vomiting is a more common primary complaint in children than it is in adolescents. Finally, the spectrum of relevant organic entities changes as patients get older, especially concerning entities referable to the genitourinary tract in adolescent females (e.g., pelvic inflammatory disease, secondary dysmenorrhea). In this classification, recognizable symptom patterns related to nonpathologic physiologic mechanisms are not considered "organic" (e.g., lactose intolerance, primary dysmenorrhea).

Psychogenic Pain

The diagnosis of psychogenic pain is reserved for situations in which the subject experiences pain in the absence of disordered patterns originating in intra-abdominal sensory nerve endings, and it always relies on clinical judgment, since it is impossible to determine with certainty whether these criteria are met in the clinical setting. Subcategories include stress-related exacerbations of otherwise tolerable pain in response to severe acute or chronic stress, behavioral pain complaints, pain occurring as part of a broader psychiatric syndrome, and other recognizable behavioral syndromes (.e.g, school phobia). In general, pain is the presenting complaint because of the meaning of the pain experience to the child or relevant adults in the child's environment. Self-conscious "malingering," as we use that term with adults, is rare in children. Its use as a complaint usually stems from the fact that it is "legitimate" to complain about

TABLE 1 Clinical Classification of Recurrent Abdominal Pain Syndrome

Category	Subcategory	Examples
Organic	Gastrointestinal	Inflammatory bowel disease Ulcer disease
	Genitourinary	Pelvic inflammatory disease Secondary dysmenorrhea
	Other	Acute intermittent porphyria Familial Mediterranean fever
Psychogenic	Major stress reaction	Loss of relative
	Behavioral pain complaint	Complaint modeling Complaint maintenance by secondary gain
	Psychiatric	Depression Conversion hysteria
	Behavioral syndromes	School phobia
Dysfunctinal	Nonspecific	"Spontaneous" resolution Persistent
	Specific	Chronic stool retention Lactose intolerance Normal motility changes Primary dysmenorrhea

pain, whereas other complaints (whining, sexual abuse) are not acceptable within the child's social network. Therapeutically, recognition by the patient of the relationship between the pain episode, relevant psychologic events, and its meaning for the patient strengthens the classification and the prognosis. Unfortunately, psychogenic pain may present nonspecifically. Assessment may be complicated by the fact that complaints such as eating, sleeping, or weight disturbances occur in both organic and psychogenic cases. They also occur normally as part of the developmental transition to adolescence. Abdominal pain is seldom the only manifestation of truly disturbed personal relationships, however, and absence of other evidence of problem relationships makes a psychogenic origin considerably less likely.

Dysfunctional Pain

The dysfunctional pain category includes cases in which the pain sensations are assumed to originate intra-abdominally and result from normal rather than disordered physiologic processes. There are two main subcategories. Specific syndromes are those in which the physiological mechanism of pain production is identifiable, as in lactose intolerance and primary dysmenorrhea. Nonspecific pain syndromes are those in which no mechanism is apparent. I typically distinguish further between nonspecific dysfunctional pain that subsides without specific treatment ("spontaneous resolution") and that in which it continues ("persistent"). In my experience, adolescents appear to have persistent nonspecific pain more often than younger children.

CLINICAL STRATEGY

Whatever the etiologic classification, the therapeutic goals include reduction of secondary parental and patient anxiety and reduction of dysfunction for the patient. In organic cases, additional disease-specific therapy will be indicated; for psyhogenic pain, referral to an appropriate mental health specialist is indicated. The psychogenic nature of the complaint may not become apparent in early visits, however, since it is often possible only to "discover" emotionally significant feelings rather than to elicit them in response to direct questioning. Consequently, the clinical strategy aims to (1) provide a basis for management of persistent nonspecific pain, (2) reduce secondary consequences of being a child with pain, and (3) identify psychogenic etiologic agents, especially those which may only become evident after initial visits.

Assessment Phase

Traditionally, medical investigation consists of a sequential progression through diagnosis, treatment, and patient education stages. I reverse this procedure and begin with a description of the syndrome, what I expect to find, possible mechanisms and their probabilities, a "contract" for following the patient at regular intervals, and the kind of information the patient/parent can help obtain. The purpose is to focus the secondary anxiety at the beginning of the assessment, recruit (rather than neutralize) the patient and his family as coinvestigators, and decide mutually on a program that deals with both the symptom and the secondary anxiety concerning its significance.

The history includes classic questions designed to describe the pain phenomenon and the associated symptomatology, and to narrow down etiologic possibilities. With a few notable exceptions, I have not found the pain description to be exceedingly helpful diagnostically, but it is helpful in defining the individual's particular pain pattern and in evaluating therapeutic trials. Adolescents are more likely than younger children to describe nonperiumbilical pain, even though no organic pathologic factor is found. Parents often have little or no idea of their children's bowel patterns, and this information is usually more accurate from children. The family history may indicate an extended history of pain complaints, but it is also helpful in finding out about serious illnesses in other family members which provoke anxiety about the child's pain. Questions directed at determining the psychological significance of the pain must be highly individualized; they aim at understanding how the pain is experienced, how it is responded to by those around the child, and whether it is being used as a substitute complaint.

A thorough physical examination is important but the results will usually be normal, although abdominal tenderness is not uncommon. I always perform a rectal examination but may defer it until the second visit. The absence of hard stool does not rule out chronic stool retention, since the stool may be soft rather than hard in chronic retention, and the rectum may be empty after a recent bowel movement. A sensitive and carefully done pelvic examination is indicated in adolescent females.

In the patient with other historical or physical evidence of disease, the laboratory work-up will be determined by the findings. In the typical patient with no other symptoms but the pain itself, I perform tests selectively. Baseline tests include complete blood count, erythrocyte sedimentation rate, reticulocyte count, urinalysis and urine culture, and tests of stool for occult blood and ova and parasites. The carmine marker dye transit time is used as an index of occult stool retention. I add a supine abdominal roentgenogram carefully evaluated for colonic and rectal stool if stool retention is suspected but not certain. If these tests are not contributory, a lactose breath hyrogen test (LBHT) is used to define whether the patient is *predisposed* to lactose intolerance. Confirmation of intolerance in LBHT-positive subjects requires a carefully monitored elimination and rechallenge diet trial. In adolescent females, I would add a pregnancy test in the absence of a clear history of a recent and normal period and pelvic examination. In my experience, other evaluations (blood chemistries, sonogram, contrast radiography, endoscopy, computed tomography scan, laparoscopy) are not indicated in the absence of specific indications, and diagnostic laparotomy is never indicated.

Management Phase

In the absence of organic and emotional disease states, the therapeutic goals are aimed at reducing secondary anxiety and preventing the negative consequences of being a child with a symptom of disease. The general strategy is applicable to all patients. Most of those with dysfunctional pain will need to live with its persistence or likely recurrence. Additional strategies related to symptom reduction may be available in those with dysfunctional pain due to an identifiable mechanism.

General Strategies

While each case must be individualized, additional components of the management strategy include the following:

1. Keeping a *diary* of pain episodes. The diary includes space to record time of pain onset and cessation, severity when it was "at its worst" on a visual analogue scale, and recording of number of bowel movements. It can also be modified to collect information on any other particular hypothesis under study, such as milk and ice cream ingestion in lactose intolerance, stress events, and so on. Children over 8 years can often keep accurate diaries themselves, and they (and their parents) become cognizant of the child's own particular pain pattern. The diary record is especially valuable as a baseline in evaluating subsequent therapeutic trials.
2. *Monitoring* for organic disease. Contrary to usual

practice, I do not claim to rule out organic disease. As an alternative, I propose to monitor for that possibility at regular intervals. This includes repeat visits at three-month intervals for physical examination and blood, urine, and stool examinations.

3. *Enrolling* the patient and parent as *coinvestigators*. In addition to the diaries, the parent is asked to take regular weight measurements and sometimes temperature measurements during pain episodes.

4. *Demythologizing* the pain symptom. The children are encouraged to express their own ideas about bowel function and what occurs in their tummies. I attempt to give them a usable and accurate description of what is happening with the help of drawings, showing and discussing their radiographs, and so on.

5. *Agreeing on a plan of action.* A clear decision tree is worked out as to how to deal with each pain episode and what to do if changes in the patient's personal symptom pattern occur (for example, "If the pain remains the same we would like to see you in one month, but if it is accompanied by fever, vomiting, or blood in the stools, we would like to see you earlier").

6. *Pursuing etiologic hypotheses.* Specific hypotheses of concern to the parent (such as "too much sugar") are evaluated using the diary recordings as a baseline. To prevent misinterpreting a spontaneous remission as a diet response, a rechallenge period is included as part of the trial. Being able to pursue suspected hypotheses helps relieve parental anxiety as well as remove unnecessary parental pressure on the children for dietary restrictions.

7. *Involving other family members.* All family members having an interest in the symptom are encouraged to make explicit their concerns and hypotheses. This is especially important if parents have different, or even antagonistic, opinions concerning etiologic agents.

8. *Prognostic* advice. The parents are never told that the patient will grow out of it. The aim is to arrange ways of dealing with the pain which may persist for months or years.

9. *Anxiety* about underlying disease. Contrary to usual practice, I ask directly about concern for underlying disease, and specifically bring up cancer if the parents do not. In my experience, more anxiety is allayed by discussing these entities than "induced" by bringing it up.

10. Establishing a "*contract*" with the patient. The "contract" for evaluating and monitoring the symptom is usually directed as much as possible at the child, with the parent cast in the role of facilitator. In addition, time is reserved each visit for the child alone. Individual time with the parent is usually over the phone or during a separate visit, since considerable trust may be lost if the child is excluded from the examining room.

11. *Telephone follow-up.* I routinely do a physician-generated telephone follow-up at predetermined intervals known to the patient/parents. This effectively lessens secondary parental anxiety about the symptom.

Specific Strategies

In patients in whom a nondisease mechanism is probable, additional maneuvers aimed at symptom reduction are included.

Stool Retention. If stool retention is certain or probable, a therapeutic trial of laxative therapy is indicated. Since the stool retention will be chronic rather than acute in this syndrome, management consists of both a "clean-out" phase and a "maintenance" phase. During the clean-out phase, any combination of stimulant and hydrophilic agents which are acceptable to the patient are used. Mineral oil is effective, but compliance is poor. It may be improved by using light mineral oil, keeping it in the refrigerator, and serving it with carbonated beverages ("light, cool, and fizzy"). During the maintenance phase, mild laxatives are recommended in addition to dietary advice to increase roughage. Oral laxatives are much preferred in children, but rectally administered enemas may occasionally be required.

Lactose Intolerance. In a patient whose LBHT indicates inability to handle a standard lactose load (usually 2 g per kilogram, maximum 50 g), a diet trial including baseline, lactose elimination, and rechallenge periods is recommended. The duration of each of the trial periods should be at least two weeks but may be longer depending on the frequency of pain episodes. A positive trial usually requires a large reduction in frequency (at least 50%). Patients in whom other factors coexist (such as intermittent constipation) may be difficult to evaluate. In children positive for both incomplete lactose absorption (by LBHT) and lactose intolerance (by diet trial), complete elimination of dietary lactose is seldom necessary for long-term management, and the tolerable limit of lactose ingestion can be worked out by trial and error. Avoidance of milk and ice cream is sufficient for most children. Use of prehydrolyzed milks or addition of Lactaid to milk is also effective. The chapter *Carbohydrate Absorption* provides additional details.

High Fiber Diets. High fiber diets provided in the form of biscuits seem to be effective in some children with nonspecific RAP syndrome, although the mechanism is unclear. In persistent cases a therapeutic trial may be effective.

Medications. Analgesics, anxiolytics, antispasmodics, and anti-gas medications have never been demonstrated to be successful and have been singularly unhelpful in my experience. Anticonvulsants are not indicated in nonspecific RAP syndrome unless a seizure disorder is independently documented.

Normal Motility Changes. Sometimes pain calendars will indicate that pain episodes most often take place at times when motility changes are known to occur (asleep to awake, preceding bowel movements, in response to meals). In such cases, the predictability of the pain makes it easier to understand, and watchful expectancy rather than secondary anxiety often follows.

Psychosocial Strategies

In the course of evaluation and management of RAP syndrome, other health or psychosocial concerns may become apparent. Unless they are shown to be directly related to the pain episodes, they are treated as separate problems, and the pain symptom continues to be managed as described. If these concerns are found to be related, specialized behavioral techniques, or play, family, or psychotherapy may be indicated. To date, there is no evidence that general stress or anxiety reduction techniques have been helpful for nonspecific RAP syndrome in childhood and adolescence. Some approaches to chronic abdominal pain in adults are discussed in the chapters *Chronic Intractable Abdominal Pain* and *Chronic Abdominal Pain: A Cognitive Behavioral Treatment Approach*.

PROGNOSIS

The extent to which children with RAP syndrome are classified as having organic, psychogenic, or dysfunctional disease will depend on the population served and the selectivity of the practice. In my experience, organic and psychogenic cases account for 5 to 10 percent each, specific dysfunctional pain occurs in 30 percent, and the remainder of cases are nonspecific. Of those, three of five will have had a "spontaneous" remission by 6 weeks after presentation without specific therapy. The long-term outlook for children with persistent nonspecific RAP is unclear, and it is unknown for adolescents. The possibility of a relationship with adult irritable bowel syndrome has been suggested but not consistently demonstrated. In the absence of a clearly demonstrable mechanism of pain production, however, the prevention of unnecessary concurrent secondary anxiety and dysfunction is both feasible and achievable in the majority of patients and their families. When that is not achieved, consideration of additional forms of psychosocial intervention by relevant health care professionals may be warranted.

FUNCTIONAL DIARRHEA

GUENTER J. KREJS, M.D.

In the United States up to 50 percent of all patients seen by primary care physicians for digestive tract problems have irritable bowel syndrome. In these patients abdominal pain and discomfort are typically associated with either constipation or diarrhea. Such diarrhea is usually referred to as functional diarrhea, since no obvious cause can be found with extensive routine clinical testing. Special investigations have revealed altered myoelectric activity in the large bowel. Forty percent of colonic slow-wave activity occurs at a frequency of 3 cycles per minute instead of 6 cycles per minute (only 10% of normal subjects test at 3 cycles per minute). In addition, a significant acceleration in small bowel transit has been demonstrated in patients with irritable bowel syndrome and diarrhea. At the present time, however, it is unclear what clinical relevance these findings may have in the diagnostic and therapeutic management of such patients. Functional diarrhea is a form of chronic diarrhea which is arbitrarily defined as lasting more than four weeks, to distinguish it from shorter lasting, self-limited diarrheal states that remain likewise unexplained by routine clinical testing.

DIAGNOSIS

Although functional diarrhea as part of the irritable bowel syndrome is generally considered a diagnosis of exclusion, this does not mean that extensive testing is necessary when one is initially confronted with such a patient. Rather, some experienced gastroenterologists emphasize that irritable bowel syndrome is a positive diagnosis which often can be made at the first interview, at which time treatment should commence. This positive diagnosis is mainly based on a typical history: abdominal pain of long duration (often for several years), discomfort and pain in different areas of the abdomen, bloating associated with various so-called food intolerances, alternating diarrhea and constipation, or one or the other on "bad days" alternating with "good days" of normal bowel function. Functional diarrhea may show a temporal relation to meal intake, and nocturnal diarrhea is typically absent. Furthermore, signs of systemic disease such as weight loss are usually absent. Classically, patients are female, in their twenties and thirties, and a history of emotional conflict, stress, or anxiety is common.

With such a typical history and a normal physical examination, complete blood screen, and urinalysis, only routine examination of stool appears necessary. This should include a stain for pus, search for occult blood, Sudan stain for excess fat, and alkalinization to test for phenolphthalein (laxative abuse). If the patient is more than 40 years of age, however, a proctosigmoidoscopy and barium enema should be performed to rule out colorectal cancer. Although it is not a routine test, measurement of stool weight is often performed and may be very helpful. In patients with functional diarrhea this weight rarely exceeds 500 g per 24 hours (N <200 g or >200 g) and in a patient who complains of an increased frequency of defecation a normal or near normal 24-hour stool weight may be the first clue to fecal incontinence, a diagnosis often confused with functional diarrhea.

TREATMENT

Since, by definition, functional diarrhea is not a specific diagnosis, treatment is necessarily nonspecific. The goals are to decrease both stool volume and frequency, improve incontinence, and prevent dehydration.

Fluid and Salt Repletion

Fluid and salt repletion is rarely a problem in functional diarrhea; however, if rehydration is deemed necessary, oral salt-sugar solution should be used as described in the chapter *Secretory Diarrhea*.

Opiates

Opiates are very effective antidiarrheal agents that have been used for many centuries. While in vitro opiates enhance intestinal ion absorption, their major mode of action in man appears to be a decrease in intestinal motility. Most of the conventional opiates are thought to act primarily through intestinal μ receptors. Available for treatment are the naturally occurring opiates codeine and deodorized tincture of opium (DTO), which is 1 percent morphine, and also the synthetic opiates loperamide and diphenoxylate. To start therapy I use either loperamide or diphenoxylate.

Loperamide hydrochloride (Imodium) was designed to have antidiarrheal action but not cross the blood-brain barrier. Thus it has no effect on the central nervous system and does not cause physical addiction. Loperamide decreases intestinal motility, enhances intestinal water and ion absorption, and may strengthen the rectal sphincter to improve incontinence. Loperamide is usually given as 2 mg 3 or 4 times a day but can be increased to 16 mg per day.

Diphenoxylate hydrochloride can either be prescribed alone (2.5 mg 3 or 4 times a day) or in combination with atropine (Lomotil). Each tablet contains 2.5 mg of diphenoxylate plus 25 μg of atropine. Atropine is added to cause nausea and vomiting when the drug is abused in larger amounts to achieve opiate effects on the central nervous system. Diphenoxylate can be increased to 20 mg per day if necessary. In the United States the drug is a Schedule V controlled substance. Because of its lack of solubility in aqueous solutions, parenteral abuse is not a problem.

Some patients' functional diarrhea will respond to loperamide and not to Lomotil, and vice versa. Those who do not respond to either one receive codeine (codeine phosphate, 30 mg 3 times daily, can be increased to 60 mg 3 times daily) or DTO (5 drops 3 times a day, can be titrated and increased to 15 drops 3 times per day).

The side effects of opiates are similar and (except for loperamide) include addiction, tolerance, sedation, and worsening of hepatic coma. Other common side effects include abdominal cramps, constipation, nausea, vomiting, dry mouth, and drowsiness. In addition, administration of these agents may predispose a patient to develop toxic megacolon when ulcerative colitis, infectious colitis due to invasive organisms, or pseudomembranous colitis is the underlying disease. Acute side effects due to overdose of all three agents respond to naloxone.

Other Therapies

High-fiber Diet, Fiber Supplements and Mucilaginous Agents. These are used for the treatment of both constipation and diarrhea. Their success must be judged on an individual basis, as clinical trials have produced conflicting data. It appears that these treatments may reduce liquidity of stool in patients with functional diarrhea but have little effect on stool volume. The two common agents are bran or psyllium hydrophilic mucilloid. The former is usually given as 10 to 30 g of either corn or wheat bran, the latter as 1 tablespoon 3 times a day (11 g). Both should be supplemented with fluids. One teaspoon of psyllium may be sufficient in some patients.

Anticholinergic Agents. Since abnormalities in the contractile response of the intestine are assumed to be a cause of functional diarrhea, anticholinergics have been used. Several preparations are on the market in the United States, such as Bentyl, ProBanthine, and Donnatal. The efficacy of these agents is not convincing and clinical trials have not been rigorously controlled; however, they may be tried on an empiric basis.

Cholestyramine. This anion exchange resin is believed to act by binding intraluminal anions—including bile salts, fatty acids, hydroxy fatty acids, and several drugs—and constipates normal volunteers. While this agent is useful for bile acid-induced diarrhea, there is no proof that it is useful in functional diarrhea. A therapeutic trial may be attempted, however. Cholestyramine is given as 4 g before meals and at bedtime stirred in 250 ml of water or juice. Some patients with postcholecystectomy diarrhea have responded to cholestyramine and loperamide.

Anxiolytic Agents. The prevalence of anxiety and depression is high in patients with irritable bowel syndrome, approaching 50 percent. Thus antidepressant agents are frequently used. In one study desipramine (150 mg at bedtime) improved (self-rated) diarrhea and (self-rated) anxiety in the diarrhea-predominant group of patients with irritable bowel syndrome but not in constipation-predominant patients. Other agents that have been used successfully are mepiprazole and Librax (a combination of chlordiazepoxide and clidinium bromide).

Psychotherapy. Owing to the psychological background of many patients with functional diarrhea (stress, anxiety, frustration), psychological management and guidance appear very reasonable. To a certain degree this is accomplished by the primary care physician who provides guidance and reassurance (explanation of absence of organic disease). Formal psychotherapy with discussion of symptoms and exploration of possible contributory emotional problems and life events has been shown to improve symptoms in irritable bowel syndrome. This improvement, however, refers mainly to abdominal pain. A significant improvement of diarrhea per se has not been demonstrated in controlled trials.

Hypnotherapy. Since psychological factors are thought to contribute to functional diarrhea and hypnosis may influence physiologic mechanisms not readily amenable to conscious control, hypnotherapy has been used for treatment. When seven half-hour sessions of decreasing frequency were given over a 3-month period (plus daily autohypnosis after the third month by using a tape), a significant decrease in frequency of bowel activity was observed when compared to a control group.[1] In the same study psychotherapy plus placebo medication had no effect on bowel frequency, although it slightly improved abdominal pain. Thus, hypnotherapy with emphasis on control of intestinal motility appears a promising therapeutic modality and wider use is recommended.

Biofeedback. Biofeedback provides instant information concerning unconscious bodily functions so that the patient may gain control over these functions. This has become an important technique to control fecal incontinence. In irritable bowel syndrome with functional diarrhea, attempts have been made to decrease the frequency, amplitude, and contractions in the rectosigmoid by use of a rectosigmoid balloon and manometer. In another study an electronic stethoscope taught patients to decrease borborygmi. Since controlled studies are hard to conduct with these techniques, no conclusions about the efficacy of biofeedback in functional diarrhea can be made at this time.

Additional Drugs

Mebeverine hydrochloride. Mebeverine hydrochloride (Colofac in England, Duspatal in West Germany) is a musculotropic spasmolytic drug without anticholinergic side effects. It improves symptoms (abdominal pain, gaseous distention, pain on moving bowels) in irritable bowel syndrome, but any effect on diarrhea per se has been poorly documented.

Lidamidine. Lidamidine increases intestinal water and ion absorption and is effective in several diarrheal diseases. It is on the market in Mexico (Lidral), but United States trials on its efficacy are still being conducted.

Peppermint Oil. Peppermint oil in enteric coated capsules was shown to relieve symptoms in irritable bowel syndrome, but again, any effect on diarrhea remains unclear.

Miscellaneous Agents. A number of pharmacologic agents have been shown in experimental animals either to enhance absorption or to decrease intestinal secretion of water and electrolytes. While such agents are mainly used on an empiric basis in chronic idiopathic secretory diarrhea, they may occasionally be considered for treatment of functional diarrhea. These include adrenergic receptor agonists (Clonidin), lithium carbonate and inhibitors of arachidonic acid metabolism (indomethacin, aspirin), glucocorticoids, and calmodulin antagonists (trifluoperazine, chlorpromazine).

REFERENCE

1. Whorwell PJ, Prior A, Faragher EB. Controlled trial of hypnotherapy in the treatment of severe refractory irritable-bowel syndrome. Lancet 1984; 1232–1234.

LIVER, BILIARY TRACT, AND PANCREAS

DRUG USE IN PATIENTS WITH HEPATIC DISEASE

GILBERT DERAY, M.D.
ROBERT A. BRANCH, M.D.

The liver occupies a key position in the metabolism of many drugs: Its function is to change lipid-soluble agents to water-soluble ones for biliary and urinary excretion. Intuitively, the disposition of drugs that undergo metabolism in the liver should be altered in hepatic disease. In fact, patients with liver disease develop a higher frequency of adverse drug reactions (ADRs) when compared with patients without liver disease. This increased frequency of ADR is related to the degree of hepatic biotransformation of a given drug as well as to clinical characteristics indicative of severe hepatic dysfunction. Altered drug metabolism can be an important clinical problem in patients with liver disease. There are few guidelines, however, to help the physician predict which individual patient will have impaired hepatic drug metabolism and to what extent drug metabolism will be altered.

Pharmacokinetics, the study of the time course of drugs and their metabolites in the body, assists the physician developing rational dosing regimens in many situations and should be able to provide practical help in patients with liver disease. Classic pharmacokinetic teaching has considered drug elimination in terms of compartmental models which, despite their descriptive accuracy, tell us little of the biologic determinants of drug disposition. In the last decade, interest in purely descriptive studies of drug pharmacokinetics in healthy individuals, or in specific patient populations, has expanded to include an interpretation of how physiologic variables, such as blood flow, intrinsic metabolic activity of an eliminating organ, and plasma and tissue protein binding can influence drug pharmacokinetic parameters.

This discussion is focused first on a physiologic approach to understanding pharmacokinetics; second, on how liver disorders influence physiologic determinants of drug disposition; and third, on how this information can be used to modify therapy.

PHARMACOKINETIC CONCEPTS

Because of the complexity of the influence of hepatic disease on various aspects of drug disposition, physiologic models of hepatic drug elimination have been especially useful in advancing our understanding of drug disposition in this disease state. A key feature of this approach has been the quantitation of the efficiency of drug elimination as drug clearance and then assessment of the contribution that hepatic blood flow, intrinsic hepatic clearance, and protein binding have on overall hepatic clearance. A physiologic approach to developing a model of drug disposition defines the action of the body on a drug in terms of variables that are of clinical relevance.

The efficiency of the liver in irreversibly removing a drug from the blood is referred to as the hepatic clearance (Cl_H). This clearance is the volume of blood from which a drug is completely removed per unit time and is equal to the product of blood flow to the liver (Q) and extraction ratio (E).

$$Cl_H = Q \cdot E$$

Under steady state conditions, E can be defined as:

$$E = \frac{Ca - Cv}{Ca}$$

where Ca and Cv are the mixed portal venous and hepatic arterial and hepatic venous total blood drug concentrations, respectively. Thus hepatic clearance is a function of organ flow and the ability of the organ to extract the drug as it perfuses hepatic capillaries.

The intrinsic clearance (Cl'_{int}) of unbound drug may be defined as the volume of liver water cleared of drug in unit time. For drugs that are eliminated by metabolism, Cl'_{int} can be defined in terms of enzyme kinetics as:

$$Cl'_{int} = \frac{Vmax}{Km + C}$$

where Vmax is the maximum rate of metabolism by the whole organ and Km is the apparent dissociation constant and C the drug concentration. Under first-order conditions, this reduces to:

$$Cl'_{int} = \frac{Vmax}{Km}$$

From this relationship, it is evident that the intrinsic clearance depends on the affinity of the enzyme, its concentration in the liver, and the mass of the liver. The efficiency of the liver in removing the drug will also depend on the fraction of unbound drug in blood (f_B) and hepatic blood flow.

The relationship that describes the extraction ratio of a drug by the liver with its free intrinsic clearance, free fraction in the blood, and the total effective liver blood flow is given by:

$$Cl_H = Q\,E = Q\,\frac{f_B\,Cl'_{int}}{Q + f_B\,Cl'_{int}}$$

It is apparent that hepatic clearance is influenced by (1) the blood flow to the organ of elimination; (2) the intrinsic clearance, which is the maximal ability of the liver to remove a drug irreversibly by all pathways in the absence of flow limitations; and (3) the percentage of drug bound to plasma proteins and cellular components of blood.

If the liver is highly efficient in removing a drug from the blood (highly extracted drugs), $f_B\,Cl'_{int} >> Q$ and equation 2 reduces to:

$$Cl_H = Q$$

Equation 5 indicates that *hepatic clearance of a drug that is highly extracted by the liver is sensitive to hepatic blood flow* (Fig. 1) and not to either the unbound fraction of drug in blood or the intrinsic ability of the liver to clear a drug. Changes in hepatic blood flow should be reflected directly in changes in hepatic clearance. It should be noted, however, that severe liver disease can be associated with such a marked reduction in drug metabolizing activity that drugs that are normally considered to have a high intrinsic clearance can be handled as a low clearance drug.

For drugs that are poorly extracted by the liver, $f_B\,Cl'_{int} << Cl_H$ and equation 2 reduces to:

$$Cl_H = f_B\,Cl'_{int}$$

The disposition of these drugs will be sensitive to changes in Cl'_{int} and f_B rather than to changes in hepatic blood flow (see Fig. 1). Therefore, in discussing the therapeutic recommendations in patients with liver disease it is useful to distinguish highly from poorly extracted drugs.

DRUG CLASSES

Drugs can be divided into two broad categories based on their extraction ratio and clearance rates in normal subjects (Table 1).

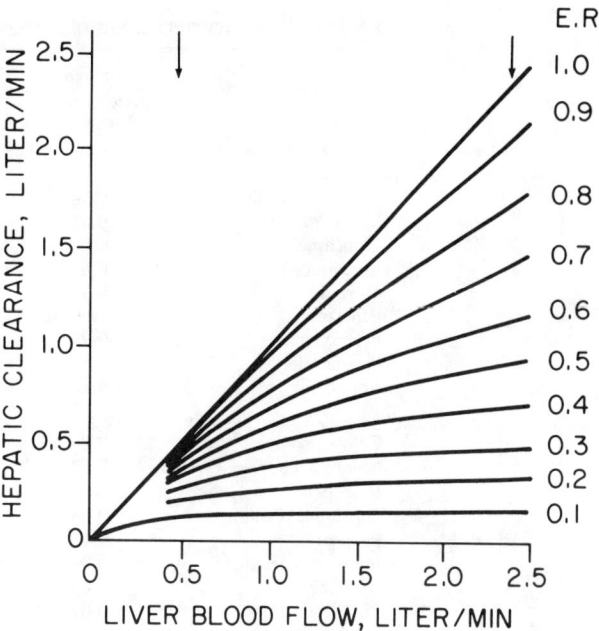

Figure 1 The relationship between liver blood flow and total hepatic clearance for drugs with varying extraction ratios (ER). The arrows indicate the normal physiologic range of liver blood flow and the extraction values refer to a normal flow of 1.5 L per minute. (From Wilkinson et al. Clin Pharmacol Ther 1975; 18:377.)

Highly Extracted Drugs

For a high clearance drug (i.e., $E > 0.6$), the rate of hepatic metabolism is limited by the amount of drug presented to the liver. This in turn is proportional to hepatic blood flow. Thus, an alteration of hepatic blood flow will result in a nearly equal change of the extraction ratio in the opposite direction.

The disposition of highly extracted drugs is relatively insensitive to changes in protein binding, as both free and bound drug are available to extraction on a single pass through the liver. However, only the unbound drug determines the concentration at the site of pharmacologic effect. If protein binding is decreased in the presence of liver disease, the net effect will be an increase in unbound drug concentration, and therefore an alteration in pharmacologic effect.

Poorly Extracted Drugs

The rate of metabolism of drugs in this class is low enough that hepatic clearance is not limited by the amount of drug brought to the liver. These drugs therefore have low hepatic extraction ratios ($E < 0.2$). A change in the intrinsic clearance and extraction will considerably affect the elimination half-life of these drugs. The rate of metabolism of these drugs depends on the concentrations of drug at the hepatic enzyme receptor site, which is proportional to the free concentration of drug in plasma. Consequently, poorly extracted drugs are further divided

TABLE 1 Characterization of Drugs Eliminated Primarily by the Liver

	Approximate Extraction (E)	Protein Binding (%)	Comments on Effects of Liver Disease
Highly Extracted Drugs			
Chlormethiazole	0.70	99	Changes in liver blood flow and
Labetalol	0.85	40	intrinsic clearance associated
Lidocaine	0.60	65	with liver disease will affect
Lorcainide	0.65	70	these drugs. The shunting of
Morphine	0.75	35	blood around the liver will
Pentazocine	0.60	65	have important effects on the
Propoxyphene	>0.90	75	bioavailability of these drugs.
Propranolol	0.65	95	
Verapamil	0.80	92	
Poorly Extracted Binding Sensitive			
Cefoperazone	0.04	90	This class of drugs will be
Chlordiazepoxide	0.02	96	influenced by changes in both
Diazepam	0.02	97	free fraction of drug in blood
Diphenylhydantoin	0.03	92	and free intrinsic drug clear-
Fenprofen	0.13	>99	ance. The overall change in
Indomethacin	0.08	90	drug clearance will be
Naproxen	0.005	>99	governed by which one of
Phenylbutazone	0.01	99	these factors changes the most
Rifampin	0.11	85	as a result of the disease
Tolbutamide	0.02	98	process.
Valproic acid	0.02	89	
Warfarin	0.005	99	
Poorly Extracted Binding Insensitive			
Antipyrine	0.05	10	This class of drugs is most
Amobarbital	0.03	60	sensitive to changes occurring
Caffeine	0.04	31	in the free intrinsic drug
Cyclophosphamide	0.08	14	clearance with liver disease.
Hexobarbital	0.15	47	
Theophylline	0.05	62	
Flow-Enzyme Sensitive Drugs			
Acetaminophen	0.30	20	Changes in liver blood flow,
Chloramphenicol	0.28	70	free intrinsic clearance, and
Chlorpromazine	0.30	95	free fraction of drug in blood
Erythromycin	0.30	80	may be important for this
Isoniazid	0.27	10	class of drugs.
Meperidine	0.50	70	
Methohexital	0.53	—	
Metoprolol	0.56	10	
Nafcillin	0.27	90	
Nortriptyline	0.50	95	
Quinidine	0.27	85	
Rantidine	0.28	15	
Zimelidine	0.34	91	

Adapted from Wedlund, Branch RA. Adjustment of medications in liver failure. In: Chernow B, Lake CR, eds. The pharmacologic approach to the critically ill patient. Baltimore: Williams & Wilkins, 1983:84.

according to the extent of their binding to plasma proteins.

Poorly Extracted, Binding Sensitive Drugs. At therapeutic concentrations these drugs are more than 85 percent bound to plasma proteins. Their hepatic clearance is sensitive to changes in protein binding within the blood and/or liver enzyme activity. Conditions that can affect plasma protein binding or liver enzyme activity or both can have a significant effect on the hepatic clearance of such drugs. In addition to an effect on drug clearance, changes in drug binding to plasma can also enhance the drug effect, as more unbound drug becomes available to receptor sites.

Poorly Extracted, Binding Insensitive Drugs. These drugs have a low affinity for plasma proteins and are less than 30 percent bound to plasma proteins. At therapeutic concentrations, the clearance of drugs in this class is unaffected by conditions that produce changes in protein binding alone. This drug class will be affected only by factors that change the level or activity of liver enzyme responsible for their elimination (see Table 1).

In addition to drugs that can be categorized as having high and low intrinsic clearance, there is a mid-zone where normal hepatic extraction ratios vary between 0.2 and 0.6. In this intermediate group changes in intrinsic clearance, liver blood flow, and protein binding can all contribute to changes in hepatic clearance. The extent will depend on the precise characteristic of the drug and the extent of change in the physiologic variable.

INFLUENCE OF ROUTE OF ADMINISTRATION

The level of drug in the plasma depends on the route of administration, intestinal absorption (if given orally), systemic availability, distribution, protein binding, and clearance.

Intravenous Administration

If a drug is given intravenously, it is considered to be completely available systemically. Changes in the hepatic clearance of a drug with dose-independent kinetics will be reflected by inversely proportional changes in the area under the plasma concentration versus time curve, and half-life will be prolonged.

As indicated in the previous section, reductions in liver blood flow will reduce hepatic clearance of high clearance drugs, and changes in intrinsic clearance and binding will influence hepatic clearance of low clearance drugs. The net effect in both instances is that liver disease usually results in a reduced hepatic clearance.

Oral Administration

When a drug is administered orally, it may not completely reach the general circulation. After an orally administered drug is absorbed from the intestine, it is carried by the mesenteric and portal circulation to the liver before it gains access to the systemic circulation. If a drug is completely absorbed from the gastrointestinal tract and is metabolized only by the liver, then the fraction of the oral dose (Do) reaching the systemic circulation (F) is the fraction removed by the liver during transit to the systemic circulation. Under these circumstances, systemic clearance (Cl_s):

$$\frac{FDo}{AUC_o}$$

where AUC_o is the area under the curve of drug concentrations in blood against time. Since $F = 1-E$:

$$\frac{D_o}{AUC_o} = \frac{QE}{1-E} = Cl_{int}$$

This equation indicates that the area under the concentration time curve after an oral dose (AUC_o) is independent of flow and depends only on the dose and the Cl_{int}.

For drugs with a high hepatic clearance, the fraction of drug removed from the blood during a single transit through the liver is high. For these drugs, a change in Cl_{int} will result in large changes in F, and consequently a large change in peak concentration with little change in half-life (Fig. 2). In contrast, poorly extracted compounds undergo little presystemic removal. The fraction of an oral dose (F) reaching the systemic circulation is high. Changes in intrinsic clearance will not affect peak concentration, but AUC will change because of an altered half-life (see Fig. 2).

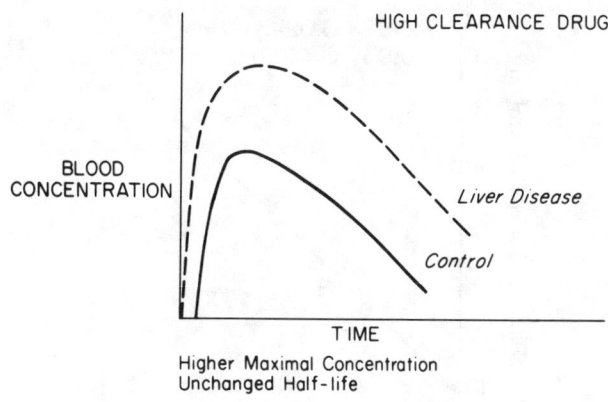

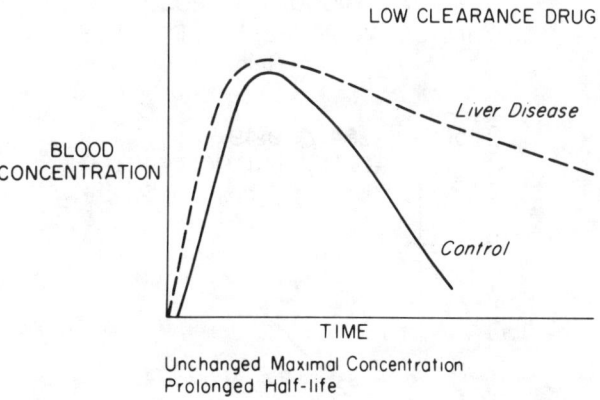

Figure 2 Modifications of blood concentration time curves in liver disease after oral administration, according to the type of drug.

In addition to alteration of intrinsic clearance, intrahepatic and extrahepatic shunts also may profoundly change drug availability. In cirrhotic patients with extensive disease, this shunting may involve 60 percent or more of the total portal vein blood flow. For a highly extracted drug, this can allow a large amount of an orally administered drug that would normally not reach the systemic circulation to bypass the liver. As a result of an increase in bioavailability, blood levels following oral dose administration will be higher in these subjects. This implies that single dose administration of a high clearance drug with a low therapeutic ratio could be hazardous in such a patient almost immediately following drug administration.

INFLUENCE OF HEPATIC DISEASE ON DRUG DISPOSITION

Injury to the liver is expressed in different ways, depending on the cause, type, extent, and duration of the lesion, as well as the magnitude of the reparative processes. Furthermore, there are indirect and associated manifestations of liver injury. Despite these many variables, chronic liver disease tends to present a similar pathophysiologic and clinical picture irrespective of etiology. The initial pathologic process is hepatic parenchymal

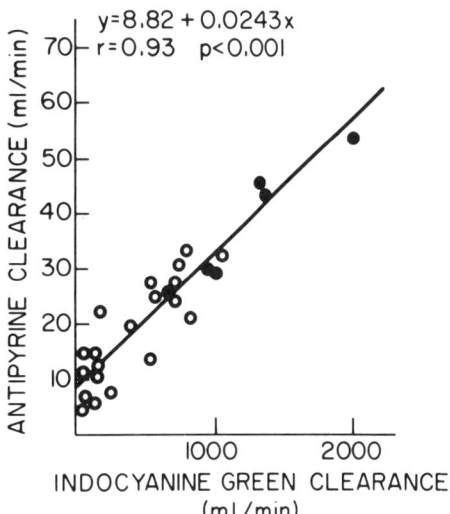

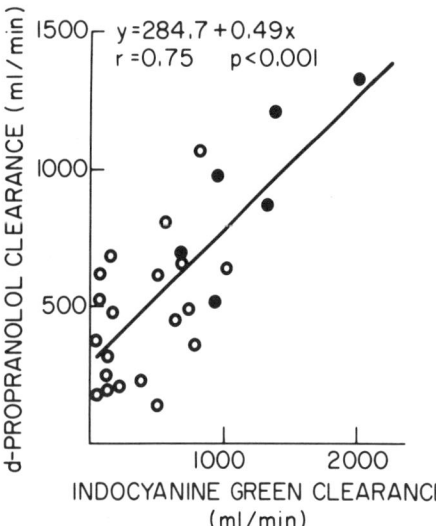

Figure 3 Relationship between the clearance of indocyanine green, d-propranolol, and antipyrine in 6 normal subjects (o) and 20 patients with chronic liver disease (o). (From Branch et al. Clin Pharmacokin 1976; 1:264.)

cell damage which produces an acute inflammatory response. Then a chronic inflammatory response develops with a cellular infiltrate at the site of cellular injury, new blood vessel proliferation, and the activation of resting fibroblasts to form collagen. A further response to hepatocyte damage is for the remaining viable hepatocytes to regenerate.

Regardless of etiology, the combination of cell injury, fibrosis, and hepatocyte regeneration results in a marked and relatively similar derangement of normal hepatic architecture, including (1) parenchymal damage of varying degrees; (2) a grossly distorted architecture in which islands of regenerative tissue develop; (3) the development of portal systemic vascular shunts, both within the liver and outside of it; and (4) failure of hepatic metabolic function. All of these factors can potentially affect drug metabolism.

Measurement of hepatic blood flow is difficult in the presence of liver disease. A comprehensive assessment of flow should include identification of portal flow, hepatic arterial flow, flow through intra- and extrahepatic portasystemic shunts, as well as flow to functioning hepatic parenchyma. In practice, the usual methods for estimation of liver blood flow are based on the simultaneous measurement of the clearance of a compound with high intrinsic clearance where hepatic clearance is dependent on liver blood flow using arterial and hepatic venous blood sampling, a method that measures only total intrahepatic flow.

In a number of studies, investigators have compared clearances of a high clearance drug with clearances of a low clearance drug. In many instances there has been a positive correlation between the clearance of high and low clearance drugs (Fig. 3). In theory, the positive correlation between high and low clearance drugs could arise if flow and Cl_{int} fall in parallel. Where this is the case, however, hepatic extraction should not fall. Direct measurement of the hepatic extraction of several drugs with high intrinsic clearance has demonstrated reductions in the hepatic extraction ratios of patients with liver disease. One explanation for this discrepancy has been explained by the "intact hepatocyte hypothesis." This hypothesis states that hepatic disease reduces the total mass of functioning hepatocytes but that these hepatocytes are normally perfused and function normally. According to this hypothesis, the reduction in clearance of highly extracted drugs may be attributed to blood that is shunted past normally functioning hepatocytes, while the reduction in clearance of poorly extracted drugs is attributable to the reduced mass of functioning hepatocytes. This model, which is analogous to the "intact nephron hypothesis" widely used in renal disease, provides a useful operational model describing the effects of cirrhosis on hepatic drug elimination.

INFLUENCE OF LIVER DISEASE ON PROTEIN BINDING

As chronic liver disease progresses, hepatic synthetic function deteriorates and results in a decrease in the synthesis of albumin. This would be expected to reduce the total number of albumin binding sites. Furthermore, even in the absence of measurable changes in albumin concentration, the binding of drugs to plasma protein may be decreased in patients with liver disease. The relative importance of qualitative changes in the albumin molecule or of increased concentrations of endogenous substances such as bilirubin remains unknown. A further factor that can influence distribution is the total size of the plasma protein pool. For instance, the development of ascites is associated with a twofold increase in the volume of distribution of propranolol in patients with a similar degree of protein binding.

A decrease in the binding of highly extracted (flow limited) drugs will not cause substantial changes in their hepatic clearance. On the other hand, drug binding alteration should influence the Cl_H of the poorly extracted drugs. Decreases in protein binding, however, produce an increase in free drug concentration, which in turn would be expected to increase the rate of metabolism of the drug. An example of this phenomenon has been shown with tolbutamide when a decreased half-life has been observed in patients with viral hepatitis due to changes in binding rather than free intrinsic clearance. Thus, the effect of liver disease on the disposition of these drugs can be difficult to predict. Furthermore, a change in binding increases the pharmacologic response to drug, since response depends on the free concentration of the drug.

SAFE PRESCRIPTION OF DRUGS TO PATIENTS WITH LIVER DISEASE

The rational administration of a drug to a patient requires knowledge of the anticipated toxicity and efficacy of the drug dose administered. Because hepatic disease states may alter hepatic blood flow, enterohepatic cycling, drug protein binding, or intrahepatic functional processes, the influence of a particular disease on the elimination of a drug is highly variable and frequently unpredictable.

If a drug whose disposition may be affected by the liver disease is to be prescribed to a patient with liver disease, then a number of factors need to be considered, including (1) the type and extent of the disease and its influence on the fundamental biologic parameters of drug disposition, (2) the category (highly or poorly extracted) of the drugs, and (3) the route of administration.

It is still not possible to predict changes in drug kinetics in patients with hepatic disease with the same degree of precision as in renal failure. However, the concepts presented previously permit a reasonable "a priori" prediction of dosage requirement. One can predict that for highly extracted drugs, the risk of toxicity on first dose of oral therapy is increased due to an increase in systemic availability (see Fig. 2). Furthermore, these drugs will accumulate during chronic treatment. Consequently, both the loading and the maintenance dose should be decreased in patients with hepatic disease. For those drugs with a low extraction dose, the major risk is accumulation during chronic therapy due to delayed elimination and a prolonged half-life (see Fig. 2). Accordingly, the loading dose should not be changed, but the maintenance dose of these drugs will have to be decreased in hepatic disease.

The extent of these modifications is difficult to anticipate in hepatic disease. In managing patients with renal failure, it is possible to arrive at a reasonable drug dose based on the assessment of renal function by creatinine clearance. The same approach in hepatic disease, using the intact hepatic hypothesis, has three major limitations. First, this hypothesis assumes a linear relationship between the extent of the disease state and hepatic function. For this, a reliable measure of the extent of impairment of hepatic function is required. Unfortunately, such a means is not routinely available. The second limitation is that the intact cell hypothesis assumes a change from a constant baseline. Intersubject variation in renal function in normal subjects is minor. Studies of drugs that are metabolized by the liver, however, have shown considerable intersubject variability in normal subjects. Thus, estimates derived from change from a mean of normal values will not be precise, since the initial baseline starting point for an individual subject is unknown. The third limitation of this approach is that even if hepatic function is known, the extent and nature of portasystemic shunts remains unknown.

Faced with such a wide array of variables influencing drug disposition, the best advice is still: (1) Do not use drugs in patients with hepatic disease unless a specific indication exists; (2) be familiar with the pharmacologic and potential toxic effects of drugs used in patients with hepatic disease; (3) use caution when dosing and, when possible, modify drug dosage regimens by using dosage schedules previously evaluated in patients with hepatic disease; (4) be alert for signs of drug toxicity; (5) when possible, monitor the drug level, (6) where feasible, use drugs that are predominantly eliminated by the kidney; and (7) reduce the drug dosage in parallel with the perceived severity of the liver disease.

This work was supported in part by USPHS Grant GM31304.

The authors wish to express their appreciation for the secretarial assistance of Susan Britt. Dr. Deray was a Merck Sharp & Dohme International Fellow.

HEPATORENAL SYNDROME AND ASCITES

H. FRANKLIN HERLONG, M.D.

ASCITES

Ascites, the accumulation of fluid within the abdominal cavity, may develop because of hepatic, cardiogenic, neoplastic, or inflammatory disorders. Modest amounts of ascites are not reliably detectable on physical examination. In one study the overall accuracy of detection was only 58 percent when the presence of ascites was questionable, with many false-positive assessments. If there is any doubt as to the presence of ascites, a blind paracentesis should not be performed. Since ultrasonographic examination of the abdomen can reliably detect even small amounts (100 ml) of ascites, this procedure should be used to confirm its presence. The sonogram can not only locate a site at which a paracentesis can safely be performed but also can detect abdominal or pelvic masses or organomegaly.

When a patient develops ascites for the first time, or when a patient with chronic ascites develops unexplained fever, encephalopathy, or other significant changes, he should be hospitalized and should undergo a diagnostic paracentesis. A Z-track technique is employed to avoid a post-paracentesis leak. Under aseptic conditions, 100 ml of ascitic fluid is removed and the syringe is immediately capped. A portion of the fluid is sent for routine studies, including protein and glucose determinations, cell counts with differential, and bacteriologic cultures. The rest of the specimen should be transported to the laboratory anaerobically and on ice for a pH determination. If cancer is suspected an additional 100 ml of fluid should be obtained for cytopathologic examination. Appropriate analysis of these tests should allow a correct diagnosis to be made and institution of appropriate therapy.

The most common cause of ascites is cirrhosis, which accounts for approximately 70 percent of all cases. Extrahepatic disorders also produce ascites. Table 1 summarizes the laboratory and clinical features of some diseases associated with ascites. When possible, therapy is directed toward underlying conditions; this often leads to resolution of the ascites. There is no effective treatment for some of the conditions, however, and the ascites can only be palliated.

Treatment of Ascites in Patients with Underlying Liver Disease

In most patients with underlying liver disease, ascites develops as a complication of the cirrhosis itself; however, patients with cirrhosis may have coexistent disorders that contribute to the production of ascites. For instance, alcoholic cirrhotics are predisposed to tuberculous peritonitis, and patients with chronic hepatitis B infection may develop hepatocellular carcinoma with peritoneal metastases.

Spontaneous Bacterial Peritonitis

Patients with cirrhosis are also predisposed to developing spontaneous bacterial peritonitis. Early recognition and prompt institution of therapy for this disorder dramatically reduce mortality. If the condition is diagnosed before patients become febrile or develop peritoneal signs, the mortality can be reduced by 50 percent.

The presence of more than 500 polymorphonuclear (PMN) leukocytes per cubic millimeter in ascitic fluid is evidence of bacterial peritonitis even if the patient is asymptomatic. Immediate antibiotic therapy should be instituted in such cases or for patients who have evidence of systemic infection, even if the fluid PMN cell count is less than 500 per cubic millimeter.

Antibiotic therapy should be appropriate for gram-positive organisms, including streptococci and staphylococci, and gram-negative bacilli until culture results are available. Anaerobic infections are uncommon except in patients who have recently undergone abdominal surgery. I recommend either *cefamandole* or a combination of *ampicillin* and *gentamicin*. When possible I avoid aminoglycosides, since patients with cirrhosis are at increased risk of aminoglycoside-induced nephrotoxicity. The choice of antibiotics should be adjusted once the results of the ascitic fluid culture are known.

Potential Aggravating Factors

Some medications may precipitate ascites formation in patients with cirrhosis. Nonsteroidal anti-inflammatory agents which inhibit prostaglandin synthetase cause retention of sodium by the kidneys. This increased renal sodium retention may expand the plasma volume sufficiently to cause ascites. Discontinuation of these medications results in mobilization of the ascitic fluid.

Perhaps one of the most important management steps is to look for reversible components of the underlying liver disease. Treating these components may make it unnecessary to prescribe specific therapy for the ascites. For instance, when patients with severe alcoholic hepatitis are forced to abstain from drinking alcohol over several weeks, they may have enough improvement in their liver function that they may not need diuretic therapy. Restoration of blood volume after a gastrointestinal hemorrhage may also promote ascites reabsorption (Table 2).

Primary Treatment of Ascites

Once complicating extrahepatic conditions have been excluded or treated, therapy may be directed specifically toward mobilization of ascites. Patients with only mild ascites do not need therapy. Use of diuretics should be restricted to those patients in whom ascites has become uncomfortable or causes specific complications, since injudicious use of diuretics may lead to serious complications.

While a mild to moderate amount of ascites may be cosmetically unattractive, it rarely harms the patient. Specific therapy is indicated when the ascites becomes extensive enough potentially to cause complications. For example, respiratory compromise due to decreased diaphragmatic excursion may predispose to pneumonia. Associated pleural effusions can exacerbate the respiratory compromise. In addition, ascites may increase risk of variceal bleeding by increasing portal pressure. Other important complications are anorexia and development of inguinal and umbilical hernias.

The mainstays of therapy for ascites caused by cirrhosis are *sodium restriction* and/or *diuretics*. The rationale for this approach is based on the three factors that produce ascites in patients with cirrhosis. Ascites develops in patients with cirrhosis because of increased renal retention of sodium in combination with portal hypertension and decreased plasma colloid oncotic pressure. All three factors favor the transudation of fluid from the liver into the abdominal cavity. When the production of fluid overcomes the removal of fluid by the lymphatic system, ascites accumulates.

TABLE 1 Causes of Ascites

Associated Diseases	Fluid Analysis			Other Laboratory Features	Clinical Features
	WBC (/mm³)	RBC	Protein (g/dl)		
COMMON					
Cirrhosis	< 250 (mono)	Few	< 2.5	pH > 7.4	Signs of portal hypertension frequently present
Infection					
Bacterial	> 500 (poly)	Few	> 2.5	pH < 7.35	Fever, rebound tenderness; some patients are asymptomatic
Tuberculous	> 500 (mono)	Few	> 2.5	pH < 7.35	Low-grade fever, cachexia, alcoholic liver disease
Tumor	Few	Many	> 2.5	pH < 7.35 (tumor cells present)	Cachexia, abdominal pain, primary site may be occult
Pancreatitis	> 500 (poly)	Many	> 2.5	Fluid amylase > 1,000 IU/L	Severe abdominal pain, leukocytosis
Congestive heart failure	Few	Few	< 2.5		
RARE					
Nephrotic syndrome	Few	Few	< 2.5		Urinary protein > 2 g/24 hr
Pseudomyxoma peritonei	Few	Few	< 2.5	Gelatinous fluid, occasionally with tumor cells	Marked abdominal distention, pain, cachexia
Chylous ascites	Few	Few	Variable	Fluid triglycerides elevated > 400 mg/dl	Results from lymphatic obstruction; may be due to tumor, trauma, tuberculosis

The limited capacity to reabsorb ascites must be taken into consideration in designing therapy. When patients have peripheral edema in addition to ascites, a maximum of 3 L of fluid can be mobilized within a 24-hour period. In the absence of edema, a maximum of only 900 ml of ascitic fluid can be removed in 24 hours.

If diuresis exceeds these amounts, the extra fluid is removed at the expense of the intravascular space and hypoperfusion may ensue. Therefore, in treating ascites the goal is to use the simplest regimen that will produce a diuresis of about 900 ml (1 to 1½ lb) a day in patients without peripheral edema, and 2 L (3 to 4 lb) a day in patients with edema. Once edema has resolved, the diuretic regimen may have to be adjusted to ensure continued safety.

Since renal retention of sodium is one of the most important factors responsible for the development of ascites, assessing quantitative renal sodium excretion is of value in planning a quantitative therapeutic regimen. Before beginning diuretic therapy, 24-hour urinary sodium excretion should be measured while the patient is on a 1-g sodium diet. This allows accurate prediction of diuretic effectiveness at the start of therapy, rather than using the trial-and-error method of adding various agents depending on patient response. Table 2 outlines various dietary and diuretic regimens based on renal excretion of sodium. Fluid restriction is not necessary unless the patient develops hyponatremia.

In most patients, ascites will resolve with a combination of salt restriction and diuretics. If patients fail to lose weight on an appropriate diuretic regimen, however, it is useful to remeasure their urinary sodium excretion. Excretion of an adequate amount of sodium without the mobilization of ascites suggests surreptitious ingestion of extra salt. Refractory ascites is defined as excretion of less than 10 mEq of sodium in 24 hours while taking less

TABLE 2 Treatment for Ascites in Patients with Cirrhosis

1. Hospitalize patients with new onset of ascites.
2. Perform diagnostic paracentesis
   If > 500 PMNs/mm³ in ascitic fluid, treat empirically for bacterial peritonitis with either cefamandole or ampicillin/gentamicin. Adjust antibiotics depending on culture results.
3. Discontinue drugs that increase sodium retention.
4. If ascites is uncomplicated, collect 24-hour urine to measure sodium excretion.
5. Base diuretic therapy on urinary sodium excretion.

Urinary Na+ Excretion (mEq/24 hr)	Dietary Sodium (g/day)	Therapy
> 50 (= 1 g Na+)	2.0	None
25–50 (0.5–1.0 g)	1.5	Spironolactone (100–300 mg/day)
10–25 (250–5 mg)	1.0	Spironolactone (100–300 mg/day) and furosemide (40–160 mg/day) or bumetanide (2–8 mg/day)
< 10 (<250 mg)	0.5	Maximal diuretic dose Therapeutic paracentesis (?) Peritoneovenous shunt (?)

than 500 mg of sodium in the diet and maximum doses of diuretics. In these patients the tendency to form ascites is so severe that ascites accumulates at a rate exceeding reabsorption despite intravascular volume depletion sufficient to cause prerenal azotemia. Patients with intractable ascites may, if they are suitable candidates, require surgical therapy to mobilize their ascites.

Alternative Treatment

Alternatives for removing ascites include *portosystemic shunting, therapeutic paracentesis,* and *ascites reinfusion* via *peritoneovenous shunt*. Portosystemic shunts will reduce portal hypertension and mobilize ascites, but surgical morbidity and/or subsequent encephalopathy makes shunting unacceptable therapy for ascites.

Therapeutic Paracenteses

Several recent studies have demonstrated the efficacy and safety of therapeutic paracenteses for patients with resistant ascites. In these patients, paracenteses of up to 6 L per day led to effective ascites control, with no more complications than diuretic therapy. These large-volume paracenteses did not cause a higher incidence of renal insufficiency, systemic hypotension, or plasma protein depletion compared with diuretic therapy. I have used this technique successfully in a number of patients whose ascites was refractory to a potent diuretic regimen.

An 18-gauge plastic catheter is placed in the linea alba inferior to the umbilicus and attached via plastic tubing to evacuated bottles to facilitate large-volume fluid removal. Continuous removal of ascites at a fixed rate may be accomplished by attaching the plastic tubing to a continuous infusion pump (I-Med).

Ascites Reinfusion

Ascites may be reinfused into the intravascular space through *peritoneovenous shunts*. These shunts allow ascitic fluid to flow unidirectionally from the peritoneal cavity into the superior vena cava. Several pressure-sensitive valves have been developed which allow fluid to flow up the shunt when the intraperitoneal pressure exceeds the intrathoracic pressure. The LeVeen shunt is the most popular. It consists of a silicone valve that remains open and permits ascites flow when a pressure gradient between the intraperitoneal limb and intrathoracic limb exceeds 5 cm H_2O. Two modifications of the LeVeen shunt have been developed and are commercially available: the Cordis-Hadin shunt and the Denver shunt. These newer shunts include pumping mechanisms which create turbulence within the valves and reduce the chances of mechanical shunt failure because of valve occlusion.

Soon after the peritoneovenous shunt is implanted, diuresis and natriuresis produce significant decreases in abdominal girth and body weight. Some patients have an increase in creatinine clearance accompanied by a fall in renin and aldosterone secretion.

Unfortunately, a number of potential complications limit the usefulness of peritoneovenous shunts. In about 30 percent of patients, the shunt fails for mechanical reasons. In some of these patients, repositioning the distal end of the shunt may restore function. In others the valve becomes clogged and needs to be replaced. Some patients with underlying heart disease fail to increase their cardiac outputs in response to the increased delivery of fluid into the right heart. Unless left ventricular function improves, the shunt will fail.

The most serious complication of peritoneovenous shunts is associated *coagulopathy*. Patients with acute liver disease such as alcoholic hepatitis seem particularly predisposed. Although the etiologic agent of this coagulopathy has not been clearly established, the problem seems to result from introduction of thromboplastic substances from the peritoneal fluid into the intravascular space. Complete removal of ascites with partial replacement by normal saline at the time of surgery has been reported to reduce the risk of severe coagulopathy.

When disseminated intravascular coagulation is accompanied by significant bleeding, heparin and/or epsilon-aminocaproic acid may be necessary to control the hemorrhage. Some patients require shunt removal. Low-grade fever is common during the first week after the peritoneovenous shunt is placed. Most patients have negative cultures and the fever resolves without therapy.

Expansion of intravascular volume in some patients may increase portal pressure and flow, precipitating variceal hemorrhage. Therefore, peritoneovenous shunts should not be used in patients who have recently bled from esophageal varices. Another absolute contraindication to peritoneovenous shunting is intrinsic renal disease, such as acute tubular necrosis, which prevents the kidneys from excreting the additional salt load. Since patients with active hepatocellular injury are predisposed to severe bleeding, the shunt is also contraindicated in patients with active hepatocellular disease such as alcoholic hepatitis.

HEPATORENAL SYNDROME

Progressive oliguria and renal insufficiency may complicate both acute and chronic liver disease. Patients with liver disease may develop renal insufficiency from hypoperfusion caused by intravascular volume depletion or a reduced cardiac output, from acute tubular necrosis because of ischemia or nephrotoxic agents, and from obstructive uropathy.

The initial approach to oliguria in patients with liver disease should include a vigorous search for reversible precipitating factors. Insertion of a urinary catheter will promptly relieve prostatic obstruction in men. An ultrasonogram may reveal ureteral dilatation in patients who have obstruction at the level of the urinary bladder. Patients should be examined carefully to assess intravascular volume status. When doubt exists as to whether they are volume depleted, measurement of central venous pres-

TABLE 3. Treatment for Acute Renal Insufficiency in Patients with Liver Disease

1. Rule out obstruction, urinary tract infection.
2. Obtain 24-hour urine collection to measure sodium and creatinine for differential diagnosis.

	Urinary Sodium (mEq/L)	Urinary/Plasma Creatinine Ratio
Prerenal azotemia	< 10	> 30
Acute tubular necrosis	> 30	< 20
Hepatorenal syndrome	< 10	> 30

3. If urine Na$^+$ < 10 mEq/L, carefully assess intravascular volume.
4. If central venous pressure < 6 cm H$_2$O, try volume expansion with albumin or blood.
5. Therapy for hepatorenal syndrome
   Diet: 3,000 calories, 40 g protein, 40 mg potassium, 1 g sodium.
   Avoid *indwelling* catheter to prevent infection.
   Avoid drugs that adversely affect renal function: nonsteroidal anti-inflammatory agents, demeclocycline
   No specific therapy (i.e., vasodilator drugs, diuretics, ascites reinfusion) is of proven efficacy.
   Dialysis depends on reversibility of underlying liver disease.
   Liver transplantation (?)

---

sure is necessary. In addition, all potentially nephrotoxic drugs should be discontinued.

In some patients with advanced liver disease, no specific cause is found for the renal insufficiency and the disorder is termed the "hepatorenal syndrome." The hepatorenal syndrome is a disorder of unknown origin that develops in patients with severe acute or chronic liver disease and is characterized by progressive oliguria and azotemia. It may develop insidiously, with a gradual decrease in urine volume over days to weeks, or it may develop suddenly, with profound oliguria or even anuria developing within a few days. Most patients have cirrhosis and portal hypertension with ascites; however, there are reports of the hepatorenal syndrome developing in the absence of ascites. The hepatorenal syndrome may also complicate acute liver failure.

In patients with the hepatorenal syndrome, the kidneys are anatomically and morphologically normal. There is, however, a profound shift in intrarenal blood flow, from the cortical nephrons to the medullary nephrons. This shift may be produced by afferent vasomotor constriction of vessels supplying the cortical nephrons, perhaps mediated by prostaglandins. This shift in blood flow results in avid reabsorption of sodium, with preservation of the kidneys' capacity to concentrate the urine.

Using urinary electrolyte measurements and urinalysis, one can often differentiate between the hepatorenal syndrome and oliguria produced by acute tubular necrosis. The urine osmolarity in the hepatorenal syndrome is normal but contains virtually no sodium (<3 mEq per 24 hours). The urinary/plasma creatinine ratio is often greater than 30. In contrast, in acute tubular necrosis the urinary/plasma creatinine concentration is approximately 1, and significant quantities of sodium are found in the urine (Table 3).

Many patients with the hepatorenal syndrome are hyponatremic and have a compensated respiratory alkalosis. Most patients have modest systemic hypotension. Despite prolonged oliguria the serum creatinine and urea concentration may remain minimally elevated because of reduced muscle mass and impaired hepatic urea synthesis. The urine sediment is unremarkable in patients with the hepatorenal syndrome, but in patients with acute tubular necrosis it contains cellular debris and casts.

Urinary biochemical tests and urinalysis results in patients with the hepatorenal syndrome are indistinguishable from those seen in patients with prerenal azotemia in the absence of acute tubular necrosis. Careful assessment of intravascular volume is essential in all patients with liver disease and renal insufficiency. This may be difficult from the physical examination alone. Frequently it is necessary to measure the central venous pressure. If the central venous pressure is less than 6 cm H$_2$O, patients should receive a trial of volume expansion, preferably with 50 g of albumin, or with blood if patients are anemic. Overexpansion of the intravascular volume should be avoided (central venous pressure >12 cm H$_2$O), as the excess volume may increase portal flow and/or pressure, precipitating variceal hemorrhage. If initial volume expansion does not increase urine output and sodium excretion, volume expansion with intravenous fluid should be discontinued.

Management of patients with the hepatorenal syndrome is similar to that of patients with other forms of acute renal failure (see Table 3). Dietary protein should be restricted and electrolyte disturbances corrected. If oliguria persists, complications of renal insufficiency and azotemia will develop.

Dialysis

Although peritoneal or hemodialysis may improve metabolic acidosis and associated complications of azotemia (platelet dysfunction with bleeding, altered mental status, and pericarditis), these benefits are usually transient without improvement in survival. I make the decision to dialyze patients with renal insufficiency and advanced liver disease based primarily on the potential reversibility of their underlying liver disease. I dialyze patients with advanced cirrhosis and portal hypertension only if they have treatable complicating factors and/or reversible components of their liver disease.

Vasodilating drugs and peritoneovenous shunting have been used in attempts to reverse the hepatorenal syndrome. Unfortunately, none of these has been consistently effective. Orthotopic liver transplantation cures the hepatorenal syndrome but can be considered only if the patients are appropriate candidates for this procedure.

PORTOSYSTEMIC ENCEPHALOPATHY

LAURENCE M. BLENDIS, M.D., F.R.C.P., F.R.C.P.(C)

Portosystemic encephalopathy (PSE) is a potentially reversible neuropsychiatric syndrome occurring in patients with chronic liver disease. It can occur at any age but is more common in older patients. Its pathogenesis is unknown but there are several theories. Portosystemic encephalopathy may be due to a number of factors including; toxic nitrogenous substances, false neurotransmitters, and decreased physiologic neural excitation (Table 1).

Toxic nitrogenous substances, e.g., ammonia, are produced by and absorbed from the right side of the colon and normally detoxified by the liver. In cases of severely decompensated liver disease, with or without shunting, these substances pass to the brain with toxic effects. This is an old theory and has stood the test of time despite many imperfections.

The theory of *false neurotransmitters* as a cause of PSE is based on the observation of increased circulating levels of aromatic amino acids, e.g., phenylalanine, and decreased levels of branched chain amino acids competing for the same amino acid transport system across the blood-brain barrier. The possible result is increased phenylalanine concentrations in the brain, with saturation of the normal neurotransmitter metabolic pathway to form dopamine and norepinephrine. This results, via alternate pathways, in the production of weak or false neurotransmiters such as octopamine, which block normal neurotransmission. The problem with this theory is that the altered amino acid ratios in patients with PSE compared to those with uncomplicated cirrhosis are not different and are probably a manifestation of liver dysfunction rather than encephalopathy. Thus the development of PSE by this theory remains controversial.

Another theory is that involving *decreased physiologic neural excitation*, e.g., due to glutamate or increased physiologic neural inhibition due to gamma-aminobutyric acid (GABA), in which GABA synthesized from glutamate in presynaptic neurons interacts with specific receptors or postsynaptic neurons to exert its inhibitory effect. This appears to result from increased chloride ion conductance across the postsynaptic neural membrane with generation of an inhibitory postsynaptic potential. Support for this hypothesis includes evidence that GABA is generated by gut bacteria and that serum levels of GABA-like activity are increased in patients with PSE and in cirrhotic patients following gastrointestinal hemorrhage. Other precipitating factors, however, do not closely relate to nitrogen metabolism (see Table 1), thus supporting the concept that PSE is multifactorial.

Whatever the pathogenesis of PSE, it is clear that it can be induced by a number of clearly defined precipitating factors, most of which are treatable or reversible (see Table 1).

ACUTE PORTOSYSTEMIC ENCEPHALOPATHY

Diagnosis

Diagnosis of acute PSE requires a clinical suspicion of chronic liver disease aroused by clues in the history, if available, or by signs of hepatic dysfunction on physical examination. In addition, there may be neuropsychiatric signs of a metabolic encephalopathy, e.g., fetor, asterixis, cogwheel rigidity, hyperreflexia, ankle clonus, and so on. Frequently the patient will come to the emergency department at a time of day when confirmatory diagnostic tests such as arterial ammonia measurement or electroencephalogram may be difficult to obtain. Therefore the diagnosis may have to be entirely clinical.

Once the diagnosis is made, the next problem, management of the disease, requires the detection and treatment of the precipitating cause(s) (see Table 1) as well as specific treatment of PSE. Once again a history of recent excessive protein load to the gastrointestinal tract, either exogenous, such as a large steak, or endogenous; melena or constipation; or diuretic or sedative therapy may provide a clue to the precipitating cause. A full clinical examination is essential and may reveal melena or severe constipation. Intravascular volume depletion is diagnosed by a postural drop in blood pressure and absent jugular veins. The presence of a fever may indicate infection. Pneumonia can be diagnosed clinically, whereas spontaneous peritonitis in the presence of ascites may produce little in the way of physical signs and can be very difficult to diagnose.

Tests at the bedside, such as that for fecal occult blood, are important. In addition, routine laboratory investigations, e.g., blood count, serum electrolytes, BUN and creatinine, and urine for microscopy, culture, and sensitivity, may reveal the precipitating cause. Other tests, such as blood gas measurements, indicate the consequence, and not the cause of the disorder. In the presence of ascites with negative preliminary results, a diagnostic peritoneal tap is indicated to exclude peritonitis. A chest roentgenogram for evidence of pneumonia is essential, and an abdominal roentgenogram to assess colonic fecal content is useful.

General Therapeutic Measures

Management initially requires securing the patient's airway if necessary and maintaining the vital signs. In patients who have had a gastrointestinal bleed, glucose and colloid infusions prior to blood replacement are preferable to saline, which is likely to be "third spaced." In patients with nonhemorrhagic intravascular depletion, colloid is preferred if possible. Electrolyte disturbances, such as hyponatremia due to excessive diuretic therapy, are best managed by complete cessation of diuretic therapy and strict fluid restriction to about 1,200 ml per day in patients who can drink, or 50 ml per hour of intravenous fluid in the comatose patient. When infection is diagnosed,

TABLE 1 The Precipitating Causes of Portosystemic Encephalopathy

Precipitating Cause	Diagnosis
Increased Colonic Nitrogen Load	
Excessive protein intake	History
Upper gastrointestinal hemorrhage	Rectal examination—melena, occult blood
Constipation	Abdominal examination
	Rectal examination
	Abdominal x-ray films
Metabolic Disturbance	
Excess sedation	History
Infection	White blood cell—total and differential
Pneumonia	Chest x-ray films
Urinary tract infection	Urinalysis—microscopy, culture, and sensitivity
Peritonitis (ascites)	Peritoneal tap—polymorph count
Acid-Base disturbance	Blood gases
Electrolyte abnormality	Serum electrolytes
Intravascular Volume Depletion	Clinical—postural drop in blood pressure, absent jugular vein, elevated BUN, creatinine

a broad-spectrum antibiotic regimen is begun until culture results are available. For pneumonia, ampicillin is used; for peritonitis a cephalosporin and an aminoglycoside are chosen.

Specific Therapeutic Measures

In patients with acute PSE, with or without coma, oral protein intake can be withheld completely for two to three days with the patient receiving intravenous fluids only. Colonic washout with tap water enemas until the returns are clear should be started immediately and continued every 6 to 12 hours. At the same time lactulose, the specific treatment of choice (Table 2), in a dosage of 30 ml (20 g lactulose) by mouth every 2 to 4 hours should be instituted to produce at least two or three loose watery stools. If the patient cannot cooperate, a thin nasogastric feeding tube should be passed and, after one is certain that it is indeed in the stomach, lactulose can be administered via this route. In the comatose patient it is preferable to give lactulose per rectum as an enema, e.g., 300 ml lactulose made up to 1 L with water, but only after the tap water enema has been completed. When lactulose enemas are given from the first, the importance of colonic cleansing is forgotten by both nursing and medical staff. The result is that the lactulose remains in the sigmoid or descending colon while the right side of the colon remains full of feces.

Most patients will respond within 3 to 5 days to this combined treatment of the precipitating cause and the encephalopathy. In any event, by the third day, as the patient recovers, oral protein intake should be reinstituted at 20 g per day, often in the form of enteral feedings. At the same time the dose of lactulose should be reduced to not more than 30 ml 4 times per day. With further improvement the lactulose dose should be reduced again, provided the patient continues to have one to two loose bowel movements daily. It is most important to reduce the dose of lactulose as soon as possible, otherwise the patient may become severely dehydrated and in addition develop an anion gap metabolic acidosis.

Resistant Comatose Patients

Differential Diagnosis

In some cases the patient does not appear to respond to standard medical therapy, i.e., resistant coma. First it is essential to exclude the possibility of a missed precipitating cause perpetuating the hepatic coma, such as a masked spontaneous peritonitis, other cerebral disease, and so on. We would, however, repeat or perform for the first time an electroencephalogram to confirm the diagnosis and to assess the severity of PSE. A decrease rather than an increase in wave amplitude or an absence of recognizable wave forms would indicate a poor prognosis and the necessity of additional measures.

Management

In my experience, the majority of these patients will eventually respond to continued standard therapy (5 to 7 days) without altering the management. Theoretically, the addition of neomycin to lactulose does not make sense, since the therapeutic effect of lactulose is thought to result from the alteration of the colonic flora by creating an acidic pH with the suppression of urease-containing bacteria (see Table 2). Thus, at that stage the antibacterial effect of neomycin should not be beneficial. Nonetheless, there is some evidence that the combination of neomycin and lactulose may result in an additional therapeutic effect.

TABLE 2 Specific Therapy for Portosystemic Encephalopathy

Medication	Mode of Action
Proven	
Lactulose	Laxative
	Acidification of colon:
	Converts ammonia to ammonium, decreases faster nonionic diffusion across colonic mucosa
	Suppresses bacterial reproduction or metabolism
	Increases fecal bacterial ammonia excretion
Neomycin	Antibacterial action in colon
Metronidazole	
Unproven	
L-dopa	Increased cerebral dopamine production
Bromocriptine	Dopamine agonist
Branched chain amino acid	Promotes cerebral neurotransmission production

Nonproven Treatment of Acute Portosystemic Encephalopathy

L-Dopa

The suggestion that PSE might be due to a relative deficiency of the neurotransmitters led to the use of L-dopa. Although initial anecdotal reports indicated that it might be beneficial, carefully controlled trials failed to show any significant improvement in patients so treated.

Bromocriptine

Similarly, it was suggested that the dopamine agonist bromocriptine might be helpful. Again, although initial studies were optimistic, a controlled trial showed no beneficial effects.

Branched Chain Amino Acids

The controversy still rages as to whether branched chain amino acids (BCAAs) are beneficial either intravenously or orally in PSE. In comatose patients there are few controlled data in favor of their use and a considerable number of controlled trials showing no obvious improvement in the level of PSE with amino acid infusions rich in BCAAs. The longer the patients remain in coma, however, the more they are at risk of developing serious effects of protein malnutrition. Thus an argument can be made that in this regard there is an indication to use amino acid solutions that do not use hepatic metabolic pathways, such as BCAAs. The benefits may be marginal, however, and insufficient to compensate for the high costs even if the solutions are available. Therefore I do not use them in this situation.

Finally, it is important to emphasize that cirrhotic patients who are in coma with resistant PSE often have severely decompensated or end-stage liver disease and may have entered the final, irreversible stage of their disease. Thus it is important to resist heroic measures, particularly if the electroencephalogram shows marked flattening of the wave forms.

CHRONIC PORTOSYSTEMIC ENCEPHALOPATHY

Cirrhotic patients with chronic PSE present a different group of problems. First there is the question of diagnosis. It is well recognized that stage I PSE may be difficult to diagnose. The patients can present with myriad symptoms, e.g., changes in personality, such as becoming more irritable or being depressed, possibly associated with a failure to recognize a deterioration in mental function or absent-mindedness. Deterioration of mental function is an important symptom because, if the cause goes unrecognized, it can lead to loss of employment. These presentations are much more common than the classic reversal of sleep pattern with a tendency to sleep during the day and for which sedatives at night can have disastrous consequences.

Diagnosis

In the treatment of chronic PSE the first prerequisite is to make the diagnosis and then treat. In the absence of clear-cut history or neurologic signs, such as asterixis, hypertonicity with cogwheel rigidity, and hyperreflexia, the diagnosis may be difficult. In such patients the use of a simple psychometric test, such as the number connection test, is invaluable. It can be performed immediately in the office and, particularly if there is a previously normal test (i.e., less than 40 seconds), an increase in the time taken to complete the test to more than 90 seconds is highly suggestive of PSE. Other tests, such as a fasting arterial ammonia level or an electroencephalogram, are much more difficult to obtain.

Treatment

There are several proven therapeutic regimens for the treatment of chronic PSE.

Lactulose to Prevent Constipation. This in itself may be sufficient to treat very mild cases of PSE. Lactulose is still the drug of choice but is expensive. I usually start treatment with a dose of 30 ml four times a day to produce two loose bowel movements daily before decreasing to a maintenance dose of 30 ml twice a day. Similar laxative effects may be achieved by other cheaper combinations, including a fiber substitute (Metamucil), or stool softener (Colace), as well as an osmotic laxative (sorbitol). Alternatively, a high-fiber diet is a more natural way of preventing constipation. As previously stated, however, the benefit of lactulose is not simply due to its laxative effect but is multifactorial (see Table 2).

Reduction in Animal Protein. There is no doubt that a reduction in protein intake is an effective treatment of PSE. Yet many of these patients are already suffering from protein malnutrition. It is therefore often necessary to decrease the protein from the normal amount of about 70 g per day to 40 g, which is usually the reduction required to achieve a therapeutic effect. Vegetarian diets, which are higher in fiber, appear to be less encephalopathogenic than animal protein diets. It is extremely difficult, however, to convert a life-long meat eater to vegetarianism but relatively easy to encourage someone to increase the fiber content of his diet.

Antibiotics. A small group of patients either cannot tolerate lactulose or are resistant to it, the alternative medication for many years has been neomycin. Because of its side effects of ototoxicity and nephrotoxicity which occur in about 5 percent of the patients, alternatives have been sought. Recently metronidazole, in a dosage of 250 mg 3 times daily, has been shown to be as effective as neomycin and therefore it is now the alternative drug of choice.

Subclinical Portosystemic Encephalopathy

It has become clear in the past few years that many cirrhotic patients who appear totally asymptomatic may have a subclinical form of PSE. More sophisticated techniques, such as a battery of psychometric tests, can show a classic pattern of abnormalities in patients with clinical PSE. Similar abnormalities have also been found in asymptomatic patients, even with apparently normal electroencephalograms.

In the future we will be faced with the necessity of developing even more sensitive diagnostic tools, such as visually evoked potentials, and better therapeutic regimens that will not necessitate the reduction in dietary protein with its possible drastic nutritional and metabolic consequences.

ALCOHOLISM

ENOCH GORDIS, M.D.

Alcoholism is recognized by its consequences, but the treatment of its consequences is not the treatment of alcoholism (Table 1). Gastroenterologists are familiar with many of the toxic consequences of alcohol abuse. In fact, medical complications of alcoholism account for more than 25 percent of all general hospital admissions. The management of these complications is certainly important; however, the treatment of alcoholism means the modification of the *alcohol-seeking and alcohol-abusing behavior*. If this behavior is not arrested, the patient goes on to repeated problems from his drinking or dies. To treat the hemorrhage or the pancreatitis and not to treat the alcoholism is bad medicine, akin to treating iron-deficiency anemia without treating the colon cancer that is causing it.

Physicians, because of their authority and knowledge, are in a highly advantageous position to begin the management of alcoholism. Nevertheless, many physicians are reluctant to address the question. There are several reasons for this reluctance. They may believe that alcoholism is simply a symptom of some underlying psychological problem and that alcoholism itself cannot be addressed directly. They may see alcoholism as a moral, not a medical, issue. They may consider the condition hopeless. These views are almost certainly incorrect. Physicians also may fear that by discussing drinking behavior with a patient, the patient will be offended and find another doctor. This argument has some merit, but obviously that cannot be justification for not practicing good medicine. Furthermore, if all physicians behaved properly, they might gain patients, because some who had walked out angrily on other physicians might now be ready for help. Finally, a minority of physicians have problems with alcohol themselves, and find it impossible to examine someone else's drinking objectively.

I have written this chapter with the following assumptions: The physician reading it is busy, and his or her primary interest is in clinical gastroenterology and its scientific basis. Yet he or she has a conscience and is willing to take a certain amount of time to address the problem of alcoholism, but then will probably refer the patient to long-range treatment by others. That first step, however, is critical, and the reward is the saving of many more lives than can be saved currently by intimate knowledge of hepatic cytoarchitecture or liberal application of sclerotherapy.

Alcoholism is a chronic relapsing disease characterized by four main clinical features: *tolerance*, a state of adaptation in which more and more alcohol is needed to produce desired effects; *physical dependence*, which means that upon interruption of drinking, a characteristic withdrawal syndrome appears which is relieved by alcohol itself (e.g., morning drinking) or by other drugs in the alcohol-sedative group; *loss of control*, which means that the alcoholic person cannot invariably regulate his total alcohol intake at any drinking occasion once drinking has begun; and finally, the *dysphoria of abstinence*,

TABLE 1 Alcoholism Vs. Complications of Alcoholism

Alcoholism →	Toxic → Consequences	Medical, surgical, and psychiatric Social Financial Spiritual Legal
Behavior: (Alcohol-seeking) (Alcohol-abusing)		

or "craving," which is the most elusive feature of alcoholism and which leads to relapse.

TREATMENT OF ALCOHOLISM

Treatment of alcoholism consists of (1) recognition of alcoholism, (2) confrontation of a patient with the problem, (3) safe conduct through withdrawal, and (4) long-term management in the abstinent state.

Recognition of Alcoholism

Recognition is no problem in the acutely ill hospitalized patient who has one of the major alcohol-related medical complications, but in the office things are more difficult. The patient is not acutely ill, will choose to hide or deny the problem, and will prefer that the medical complication be addressed and the drinking overlooked. The denial of the problem is not simply deliberate lying; much of the denial is unconscious because the thought of living without alcohol can be terrifying to one addicted to it. Here the physician must use a combination of clinical clues, laboratory clues (well-known abnormalities of bone marrow, liver, and urate metabolism), and social clues (especially job, marital, and legal problems) to make the diagnosis likely. Alcoholics are tolerant of large concentrations of alcohol: They may be vertical and coherent at a time when their blood alcohol level would be lethal to a nondrinker. The small, commercially available breath alcohol meters, no larger than a paperback, are very convenient and settle doubts and disagreements in a few seconds. When a drinking bout has ended more than 12 hours or so before the consultation, and the blood level is zero, clues to alcoholism may be provided by tremor, tachycardia, and hypertension in a usually normotensive patient. These are early signs of withdrawal.

Confrontation of Patient with Problem

Confrontation must be handled in a firm but tactful way. It can be managed as a mutual exploration of the possibility that alcohol is causing many of the patient's troubles. Standardized questionnaires (MAST,[1] Short MAST,[2] CAGE,[3] and REICH[4]) are helpful, because the patient sees that his situation is not unique and that he has not been singled out for harassment. If the patient consents to have the physician contact a family member or close friend, or if a family member comes on his or her own to see the doctor about the patient, the physician can enlist the help of these relatives or friends to join in a meeting with the patient. At this meeting, the others can quietly describe to the patient the impact of the patient's drinking on their lives and urge the patient to enter treatment. The impact of such a meeting is stronger if family or friends are prepared to threaten the patient with termination of contact until he enters treatment.

If the confrontation is successful, and if the physician chooses not to manage the alcoholism any further, the patient should be referred immediately to another therapist or agency for help, as well as to Alcoholics Anonymous.

Safe Conduct Through Withdrawal

Many patients will be alcohol free at the time of the confrontation, and in no discomfort from withdrawal. For these patients, the approaches described in the section Long-Term Management of Alcoholism (below) may be begun promptly. Patients who still have alcohol in their system or who are uncomfortable with symptoms of withdrawal may need treatment for withdrawal.

For clarity, I have divided this discussion into two parts: first, description of the withdrawal syndrome and practical details about its treatment, and second, a guide to modifications appropriate for the several ways the situation may present itself to the physician.

Withdrawal Syndrome

Upon interruption of drinking, even before the blood alcohol has reached zero concentration, the patient may experience a group of adrenergic symptoms: agitation, sweating, systolic and diastolic hypertension, tachycardia, and tremor. These vary in intensity and subside within several days or, rarely, 1 or 2 weeks. The diastolic pressure may be as high as 115. I do not treat hypertension below this level, since it usually disappears within a few days as the withdrawal itself subsides. Some patients, of course, are hypertensive as well as alcoholic, and will need treatment while sober, but there is no way of knowing this beforehand unless a physician had to treat the patient for hypertension in a previous period of abstinence. The tremor is a postural tremor at about 6 per second; sometimes it is hard to distinguish it from anxiety, but if the fingers continue to shake when the examiner immobilizes the wrist and elbow it is probably alcohol withdrawal. A tongue tremor, if present, is virtually pathognomonic. The patient may be nauseated and unable to hold food at the beginning of withdrawal. Some patients hallucinate during the first 1 or 2 days: hallucinations may be visual or auditory, are recognized by the patient as abnormal, are not associated with persistent belief (as in delusion), and are *not* a sign of psychosis.

Patients may experience seizures, usually 2 or 3 days into withdrawal. They are epileptiform, characteristically are not preceded by an aura, are temporally related to the cessation of drinking, and of course are accompanied by a brief period of unconsciousness. Electroencephalograms and brain scans are normal. I order these only once in any patient. Competing causes of seizures (childhood epilepsy, hypoglycemia, old head injury with organized seizure focus) must be considered but are rarely found. Whether withdrawal seizures are an indication for Dilantin therapy is controversial. I do not use Dilantin, since I believe that the seizures are controlled with adequate sedative therapy for the whole period of withdrawal. (There is no controversy about the fact that anticonvulsants have *no* role in long-term management in the abstinent state. The long-term treatment for withdrawal seizures is abstinence.) A minority of patients enter a severe form of withdrawal on about the third day: delirium tremens (DT). During this state of disorientation, agitation, fever, fluid loss, and tremulousness, the essential part of treatment is support of the airway and maintenance of fluid and electrolyte balance. Most of us sedate patients in DT, but probably this adds very little, since DT seems to have a distinct physiology. It usually subsides in 18 to 36 hours, with a period of terminal sleep from which the patient awakes tired but oriented. Currently, DT seems to occur mainly in patients who are sick with another condition as well, such as pneumonia. It is quite rare to see DT in patients with severe liver disease.

Hyperglycemia in nondiabetics is often seen in early withdrawal. It is probably more common in malnourished patients since normal glucose tolerance depends on adequate nourishment. In addition, alcohol is known to blunt the insulin response of the pancreas to a glucose load. With abstinence and eating, this condition rapidly clears and a diagnosis of diabetes should not be made.

For mild withdrawal, drugs may not be needed at all. For the more uncomfortable patients, I use *chlordiazepoxide*, 50 mg orally twice a day for an average size man, larger or smaller doses when appropriate. Heavy drinkers are tolerant of this drug, and for severe withdrawal even 100 mg twice a day is easily tolerated. I avoid orders on an "as needed" basis. This spares the nurses endless confrontations with the patient who often prefers to think about drugs rather than his plans for sobriety. Oversedation should be avoided, so the patient may begin to reflect on his problem and benefit from the counseling and Alcoholics Anonymous meetings that may be available in an inpatient setting. Chlordiazepoxide has a half-life of close to 1 day, and that has three implications. First, more than twice-a-day dosing is unnecessary. Second, if the same dose is used daily, it will accumulate, so it should be tapered. Third, even if the order is written to stop it, its effects will persist for several days. Paraldehyde works but I do not use it. It has a bad odor, it deteriorates upon standing and must be replaced, and since it is a trimer of acetaldehyde, disulfiram treatment cannot be started while it is in use. Propranolol and clonidine can control many of the adrenergic manifestations of withdrawal, but I see no advantage in their use, unless the early hypertension is severe. One drug then might control both withdrawal and blood pressure.

Although safe and comfortable withdrawal can be accomplished by giving tapering doses of alcohol over several days, I do not do this. True, this is the substance the patient is addicted to, and one does not have to rely on other drugs which do not have identical pharmacology; however, the arguments against using alcohol make sense. First, nurses would be kept busy giving alcohol around the clock. Second, it is hard to maintain an ambience conducive to serious counseling about sobriety when patients reek of alcohol. Third, there is an ethical question in prescribing a known liver and marrow toxin to patients already sick with these complications. Finally, disulfiram therapy cannot be started while ethanol is used for detoxification.

Sometimes it is safer to let the patient shake rather than to risk drug toxicity. I avoid sedation if possible in patients with chronic obstructive pulmonary disease. With advanced liver disease, I use very little sedative or none, since the metabolism of benzodiazepines is retarded in this state. Alcohol and benzodiazepines make depression worse, and in a severely depressed patient, I avoid sedatives. Note that a mild depression is expected and appropriate, and is almost always self-limited.

The physician should be concerned with *nutrition*. Middle-class alcoholics are generally not particularly malnourished. Among patients who are, the commonest deficiencies are folate, thiamine, and magnesium. Many therapists routinely administer all three, and this can do no harm. Magnesium deficiency manifested by low serum magnesium levels must be corrected promptly, since magnesium depletion lowers the threshold for withdrawal seizures. Claims that magnesium alone is a suitable regimen for withdrawal have not been validated. Thiamine must be administered to malnourished patients before glucose; if this is not done, Wernicke's syndrome may be precipitated.

The following management choices are based on the condition of the patient *when seen in the office* (Table 2). (Patients hospitalized for complications of alcohol may undergo withdrawal at the same time and may need treatment for it.)

TABLE 2 Office Management of the Alcoholic Patient

Sober (no alcohol aboard). Verify with breath meter.
  Comfortable, can listen:
    Confrontation; then *long-term management* (see text), including immediate offer to disulfiram.
  Uncomfortable, in withdrawal:
    Withdrawal troublesome (or patient has had seizures or DT during a prior withdrawal): admit for detoxification.
    Withdrawal mild: prescribe one day's sedative dosage, return to physician next day, then proceed with confrontation and long-term management. The mistake here is to prescribe a whole bottle of sedative: this accomplishes nothing, and the patient is likely to drink and use the pills together.

Has alcohol aboard
  Can stop drinking: Return sober next day, continue as under "Sober." It is safer not to offer sedatives to a drinking patient.
  Cannot stop drinking: admit for detoxification. The gastroenterologist may choose to manage the inpatient withdrawal him- or herself on a general service, or may admit the patient to a specialized unit. Insurance coverage for alcoholism detoxification is now provided in many if not most policies. Do not admit the patient under a false diagnosis such as "gastritis." That fuels the patient's denial and impedes recovery. The advantage of a specialized detoxification unit is that nonmedical services, such as AA, counseling, and group therapy, are generally available.

Long-Term Management of Alcoholism

The goal of long-term management is the maximum restoration of physical and social functioning. Complete abstinence is the only recommendation that can ethically be made at present. The commonly offered advice, "You should try to cut down on your drinking" is not worth the breath it takes to give it. Nor can the memory of past pains alone be relied upon to turn things around. If it could, we would not see relapsing pancreatitis or repeat episodes of hemorrhagic gastritis. The outlook for recovery from alcoholism may be seen to hinge on the outcome of a struggle between two functional parts of the brain: that which determines appetite, and that which can understand the consequences of surrendering to that appetite and can decide not to. At present, we have no therapy to modify the pathologic appetite for alcohol. Instead, we can appeal only to the cognitive function of the brain with teaching, persuasion, and coercion.

The physician is the most competent person to describe the health consequences of alcoholism, and this should be done in detail. The physician can also counsel; he or she can indicate to the patient those other areas in life which are being damaged by alcohol. For the patient, merely to know all this is not enough. He must also be *persuaded* that the struggle for a better life is worthwhile, despite the fluctuating discomfort of abstinence. The fellowship of Alcoholics Anonymous (AA) can be a potent force. Alcoholics Anonymous is neither an encounter group nor a religious denomination. Its sole aim is to help other drinkers to stay sober. Patients benefit from the sense of dignity and personal worth that AA imparts. All alcoholics should be encouraged to attend, although they will not all respond to AA's style and message. The generosity of AA members knows few bounds, and every physician should have available the names and telephone numbers of several AA members of diverse backgrounds who, with the patient's consent, can be called while the patient is in the office. The patient can often be taken to his first meeting that evening. There are several AA meetings each day, in different locales, in most medium and large sized cities. A list of these sites and meeting times is generally available upon inquiry.

Disulfiram

Disulfiram (Antabuse) is a valuable adjunct to therapy and should be offered to all patients in whom there is no contraindication. Whatever its long-term value, it buys time initially by putting up a "chemical fence" so the patient knows he cannot drink that day, and even for 3 or 4 days after stopping it. It can be given as soon as 12 hours after the last drink. Nowadays, the dosage is designed first for safety and then for efficacy. A common routine, for which there is more tradition than pharmacokinetic evidence, is 0.5 g daily for 5 days, then 0.25 g. A full-blown alcohol-Antabuse reaction includes immediate flushing of the face and neck (sometimes the rest of the body as well), an initial hypertension, tachycardia, and conjunctival injection. Within minutes the flush resolves, the blood pressure falls, and the patient feels faint, and often nauseated, chilled, and generally sick. Convulsions are not part of the usual reaction. Finally, after a variable amount of time, but not more than 2 hours, the patient becomes sleepy, and may sleep for several hours. On awakening, he is well. Compensated liver disease and diabetes are *not* contraindications to therapy. Antabuse is a very safe drug; the most common side effect is sedation, which wears off usually in the first two weeks. Other side effects, including a rare but well-documented drug-induced hepatitis, are infrequently seen. Ambivalence about taking it is common, and the physician can point out to the patient that this indicates a less-than-total commitment to sobriety. Patients may reflect on this and change their minds about disulfiram.

Absolute *contraindications* to disulfiram are pregnancy, severe depression, organic brain syndrome, severe active liver disease, and cardio- or cerebrovascular disease. The last two are contraindications not because Antabuse is in itself toxic to the heart or the brain, but because the rare patient who drinks while taking Antabuse (most stop it several days before drinking) will un-

TABLE 3 Checklist: What the Concerned Physician Should Know and Have Available in his Practice to Manage Alcoholism

To Know:	1.	The pharmacology of alcohol: its distribution, metabolism, tolerance, physical dependence
	2.	The pharmacology of disulfiram and how to use it
	3.	The pharmacology of one sedative, for example, chlordiazepoxide
To Have Available:	1.	A supply of disulfiram in the office so it can be started immediately on acceptance. The remainder of the patient's supply is prescribed in the usual way.
	2.	A small alcohol breath analyzer. Test for heavy drinking and tolerance. We have been satisfied with the Alco-Sensor, manufactured by Intoximeters, Inc., 1901 Locust Street, St. Louis, MO 63103.
	3.	Photocopies of one standard questionnaire (MAST, short MAST, etc.) so patient can be engaged in a neutral way.
	4.	The following telephone numbers: • Several willing members of AA of both sexes and various ethnic and occupational backgrounds who will respond to a telephone call, if possible while the patient is in the office. • The local AA Intergroup Office (see telephone directory) for help in finding AA members as above, and also for other members if those known are unavailable. The AA Intergroup Office often knows which detoxification units have available beds. • The local Affiliate of the National Council on Alcoholism for further screening and referral, especially to outpatient services. • Three or four of the available public or private inpatient detoxification units. • Three or four of the available public or private outpatient multidisciplinary programs.

dergo a hypotensive episode. I must emphasize again, however, that the vast majority of alcoholic patients can benefit from Antabuse, and that it is easy and safe to prescribe.

I see little evidence to suggest that relapses result from life's stresses and problems. Patients taking Antabuse who relapse have almost all stopped Antabuse several days before the alleged drink-provoking stress occurred. Counseling and social work are valuable because they help the patient undo the damage that drinking has done and help the patient adjust to a sober routine. When life has some rewards, the patient is more likely to view the struggle for sobriety as worthwhile.

In general, no psychiatric diagnosis can be made while the patient is either drinking or in early withdrawal. Most alcoholics do not need a psychiatrist; they are drunk, but not mentally disturbed. Once sober, however, a minority will need treatment by a psychiatrist for an affective disorder, manic-depressive disorder, or panic attacks. In the sober state, they can respond to competent psychiatry as do nonalcoholics.

There is no role for sedation in the long-term management of alcoholism. It does not control the drinking, and sets the patient up for a possible second drug habit. *Insomnia* may persist many months after withdrawal; the sleep electroencephalogram may not become normal in a year's time. Sleeping pills should not be prescribed. The patient should be told that the condition will improve if he doesn't take pills. The commonest cause of insomnia, however, is caffeine. Alcoholics are inveterate coffee drinkers, and most insomnia will respond to the cessation of all caffeine, including coffee, tea, and cola beverages.

I know physicians who genuinely enjoy the long-term management of alcoholism, including nonmedical counseling (Table 3). Most physicians, however, cannot or prefer not to do this, and will choose to refer their patients to a competently run outpatient alcoholism program. There, a variety of counseling and social work services are frequently available, and many of these programs will also handle the prescription of Antabuse and have AA meetings on their premises.

There are now many inpatient rehabilitation units which offer programs of several weeks' duration. Most patients do not need them. Whether the extensive group therapy, didactic sessions, and educational movies really add much has not been carefully evaluated, but one can argue that the chance to heal liver and brain, eat well, "get away for a while," and restore cognitive function and optimism is occasionally valuable.

When voluntary approaches fail, *coercion* may become necessary. Sometimes it has already been applied by others. The spouse may be contemplating divorce. The job may be in danger. There may be court pressure after driving while intoxicated or family violence. In many states, recent legislation has tightened the requirement for prompt reporting to medical licensing agencies of alcoholic physicians. In these situations, the added use of mandatory Antabuse can be very helpful. Finally, a trusted physician confronted with a patient's repeated alcoholic hemorrhage or pancreatitis may tell the patient that after the acute episode is over, he or she will no longer be responsible for the patient's care if the patient does not immediately begin Antabuse under supervision and enter treatment for alcoholism. Coercive measures may seem harsh but the stakes are very high: Alcoholism is a malignant disease.

(The MAST and short MAST are the most widely used. None is a perfect screener; patients do lie.)

REFERENCES

1. Selzer ML. The Michigan Alcoholism Screening Test: The quest for a new diagnostic instrument. Am J Psych 1971; 127:89.
3. Mayfield D, Mcleod G, Hall P. The CAGE questionnaire: Validation of a new alcoholism screening instrument. Am J Psych 1974; 131:1121.
2. Pokorny A, Miller BA, Kaplan H. The Brief MAST: A shortened version of the Michigan Alcoholism Screening Test. Am J Psych 1972; 129:118.
4. Reich T, Robins LN, Woodruff RA Jr, et al. Computer-assisted derivation of a screening interview for alcoholism. Arch Gen Psych 1975; 32:847.

SUGGESTED READING

Bieder L, O'Hagan J, Whiteside E. In: Paton A, ed. Handbook on alcoholism for health professionals. London: William Heinemann Medical Books Ltd, 1985. (This book, written in New Zealand and re-edited in Great Britain, is the best single book on alcoholism for the practicing physician that I know. Short, crisp, stylish, gets to the point. A few details pertaining to Commonwealth practice need revision for Americans, but no matter. Get it.)

Fox R. Treatment of the problem drinker by the private practitioner. In: Bourne PG, Fox R, eds. Alcoholism, progress in research and treatment. New York: Academic Press, 1973. (Dr. Ruth Fox was a master clinician and stylist. Much of this book remains among the best writing on alcoholism.)

Hurt RD, Morse R, Swenson WM. Diagnosis of alcoholism with a self-administered alcoholism screening test (SAAST). Mayo Clin Proc 1980; 55:365.

Lieber C. Medical disorders of alcoholism. Philadelphia: WB Saunders, 1982. (A tour-de-force. Comprehensive, detailed, well-referenced one volume on the impact of alcohol on major organ systems. Excellent on alcohol metabolism also.)

Lisansky E. Alcoholism—the avoided diagnosis. Bull Am Coll Phys March 1974; 18.

ALCOHOLIC LIVER DISEASE

ESTEBAN MEZEY, M.D.

Chronic alcoholism is a leading cause of liver disease. Both alcoholism and the mortality from cirrhosis have been increasing in the United States and in other industrialized countries. In the United States, cirrhosis is now the fifth leading cause of death. The types of histologically demonstrable liver injury in alcoholics which can occur singly or overlap include fatty liver, alcoholic hepatitis, and cirrhosis. Both clinical features and laboratory tests often do not distinguish among these types of liver injury. In addition, approximately 20 percent of patients suspected of having alcoholic liver disease are found to have other lesions. Therefore, whenever feasible, a liver biopsy should be done to ascertain the type of liver injury and its activity and chronicity. A direct toxic effect of alcohol is the principal cause of the development of alcoholic liver disease, and the development of cirrhosis correlates with the daily dose and duration of alcoholic abuse. Women are more susceptible than men to hepatic damage. Intakes of ethanol as low as 40 g for men and 20 g for women result in an increased risk of development of cirrhosis. Only 10 to 20 percent of alcoholics develop cirrhosis, however, indicating that other factors, either genetic, environmental, or nutritional, may contribute to the pathogenesis.

FATTY LIVER

Fatty liver occurs in all individuals after the ingestion of moderate to large amounts of alcohol for even a short period of time, i.e., even after a weekend binge. It is a direct result of an increased synthesis and decreased degradation of fatty acids, which is a consequence of the increased redox state occurring during alcohol metabolism. The increased amount of fatty acids accumulated results in an increased formation of triglycerides. The accumulation of fat is particularly enhanced when alcohol is ingested with a high-fat diet.

Severe fatty infiltration of the liver is associated with malaise, weakness, anorexia, nausea, abdominal discomfort, and tender hepatomegaly. Jaundice is present in about 15 percent of patients admitted to the hospital because of their symptoms. Fluid retention, portal hypertension with splenomegaly, and occasionally bleeding esophageal varices may occur in the most severe cases. Mild elevation of serum aspartate aminotransferase (AST) and serum alkaline phosphatase are common, while reduced serum albumin and elevated serum globulins are found in about 25 percent of patients. Liver biopsy, as mentioned previously, is necessary to differentiate fatty liver from other types of alcoholic liver disease. Fatty liver is generally considered to be a benign condition; however, the presence of fibrosis around the central vein and in Disse's space in association with fatty liver indicates a propensity toward cirrhosis if alcohol ingestion is continued.

The treatment of fatty liver consists of abstinence from alcohol and an adequate diet. Under this regimen, the abnormal accumulation of fat disappears from the liver in one to four weeks. Bed rest has no proven benefit. Androgenic steroids, which are found to increase the rate of hepatic lipid removal in some studies but not in others, may be detrimental by producing cholestasis and are not indicated. Recurrent episodes of symptomatic fatty liver are common but there is no evidence that they lead to cirrhosis.

ALCOHOLIC HEPATITIS

Patients with alcoholic hepatitis often have symptoms of fatigue, anorexia, weight loss, jaundice, fever, and tender hepatomegaly. Serum aminotransferase levels are rarely elevated to more than ten times above normal, and characteristically that of AST is higher than that of alanine aminotransferase (ALT). This finding may be related to pyridoxine deficiency, since aminotransferases require, as a cofactor, pyridoxal phosphate, which is often deficient in alcoholics. Pyridoxine deficiency in rats results in a greater decrease in liver and serum ALT than AST. Low liver ALT, but not AST, correlates with decreased circulating levels of pyridoxal phosphate, and can be increased in vitro by incubation with pyridoxal phosphate. The serum albumin is frequently depressed and the prothrombin time prolonged. Cholestasis with striking elevation of serum alkaline phosphatase may occur, and when associated with right upper abdominal pain, fever, and leukocytosis, may be mistaken for extrahepatic biliary obstruction. The typical histologic picture of alcoholic hepatitis includes hepatocellular necrosis and ballooning degeneration, alcoholic hyalin, and an inflammatory reaction with many polymorphonuclear leukocytes.

Deterioration of clinical state and laboratory test results often occurs following admission to the hospital despite abstinence from alcohol, bed rest, and intake of an adequate diet. The mortality rate in hospitalized patients with alcoholic hepatitis has been estimated to be 15 to 20 percent. Findings that correlate with a poor prognosis are encephalopathy, a low serum albumin, a serum bilirubin over 20 mg per deciliter, and a very prolonged prothrombin time (more than 8 seconds above control) unresponsive to vitamin K administration. Long-term follow-up in one study revealed that 38 percent of the patients who had no evidence of fibrous septum formation or cirrhosis on initial liver biopsy developed cirrhosis after a mean of 3.3 years. Only 10 percent had complete resolution to normal, while the remainder continued to have evidence of alcoholic hepatitis.

The treatment of alcoholic hepatitis consists of abstinence from alcohol, bed rest, and intake of a normal or high-protein diet, provided that there is no encephalopathy. Replacement of nutrients and vitamins appears to be indicated because of the poor dietary intake, disturbed absorption and metabolism, and greater nutritional requirements induced by alcohol. In one study, parenteral administration of 70 to 85 g of amino acids per day, as either 7 percent Aminosyn or 8.5 percent Travasol, for 4 weeks to patients with alcoholic hepatitis resulted in greater clinical and laboratory improvement and in fewer deaths than in a control group.

Adrenal Corticosteroid Therapy

Because alcoholic hepatitis may have a prolonged clinical course, high mortality rate, and frequent progression to cirrhosis, the potential benefits of more specific anti-inflammatory, immunosuppressive, and antifibrotic therapies have been evaluated. The usefulness of corticosteroid therapy remains controversial despite numerous controlled studies assessing their effect on mortality. Prednisone, prednisolone, or 5-methylprednisolone was given in doses ranging from 35 to 80 mg per day for either 4 or 6 weeks. All studies showed that corticosteroids do not alter survival when patients with alcoholic hepatitis in each study are considered as a group. Corticosteroids did increase survival in a subgroup of patients with more severe illness manifested by encephalopathy or by very abnormal prothrombin time and bilirubin level. In one study, a discriminant function, 4.6 × prothrombin time (seconds) + bilirubin (milligrams per deciliter) >93, predicted a very high mortality, which was reduced in patients receiving corticosteroids.[1] Decrease in serum bilirubin and prothrombin time and improvement in serum albumin occur after corticosteroid therapy; however, the histologic findings remain unchanged. My present recommendation is to consider the use of corticosteroids only as a last resort in patients who are seriously ill with alcoholic hepatitis.

D-Penicillamine

Treatment with D-penicillamine, an inhibitor of collagen synthesis, for one month did not result in any significant improvement in the histologic appearance of the liver. Whether or not therapy with D-penicillamine for a longer period of time will reduce hepatic fibrosis is unknown.

Propylthiouracil

Propylthiouracil was also suggested as treatment for alcoholic hepatitis because it decreases an alcohol induced hypermetabolic state and prevents hepatocellular necrosis in animals exposed to low oxygen tensions. One trial with propylthiouracil in a dose of 300 mg per day for up to 46 days showed a more rapid improvement in clinical symptoms and laboratory tests than treatment with placebo. In another study, however, propylthiouracil was found to be ineffective in a group of more severely ill patients with alcoholic hepatitis. A tentative conclusion would be that propylthiouracil may be beneficial in moderately ill patients but not beneficial in severely ill patients with a high mortality. Clearly this drug requires additional evaluation in treatment of alcoholic hepatitis.

Abstinence

The principal long-term goal in the treatment of alcoholic hepatitis is to obtain permanent abstinence from alcohol, since this markedly increases survival. This goal is more likely to be accomplished in patients who were socially stable before their illness and frequently attend Alcoholics Anonymous or group alcoholism treatment programs. The monitoring of abstinence is difficult because the history of alcohol intake is often inaccurate. Approximately one-half of the patients with alcoholic liver disease in whom alcohol is detected in the urine deny ingestion. Laboratory abnormalities that have been useful in detecting alcohol abuse are elevated mean red cell volume (macrocytosis) and elevated serum gamma glutamyl transpeptidase. Macrocytosis, which is not related to folate deficiency, is more common in female than male alcohol abusers and is probably caused by changes in red cell membrane structure and fluidity. Elevated serum gamma glutamyl transpeptidase is caused by alcohol-induced microsomal enzyme induction, liver injury, or a combination of both.

CIRRHOSIS

Cirrhosis is the irreversible stage of liver disease. The onset of cirrhosis is often insidious and associated with nonspecific symptoms such as fatigue, anorexia, weight loss, nausea, and abdominal discomfort. As the disease progresses, signs of hepatocellular failure become prominent. The most severe complications of cirrhosis are hepatic encephalopathy, bleeding from esophageal varices, and infection. Rapid deterioration should raise the suspicion of a complicating hepatocellular carcinoma.

The treatment of uncomplicated cirrhosis consists of voluntary restriction of activity, if the patient has weakness or fatigue, a diet high in protein but low in salt, and abstinence from alcohol. Multivitamins and folic acid, 1 mg per day, are given if the patient has evidence of vitamin deficiencies or is unable to achieve an adequate dietary intake. This regimen almost invariably results in improvement in hepatocellular function. Tranquilizers and sedatives should be avoided. Infection and gastrointestinal bleeding, which in addition to alcohol ingestion are frequent precipitating factors of decompensation, should be searched for and treated. Common sites of infection are the urinary tract and ascitic fluid. Gastrointestinal bleeding can be due to esophageal varices or other causes. Vitamin K, 15 mg parenterally, may improve abnormal prolongation of the prothrombin time. Potassium deficiency is frequent and may contribute to the precipitation of hepatic encephalopathy, but its extent is difficult to assess because serum potassium concentration is a poor reflection of the total body potassium. When serum potassium falls below 3.5 mEq per liter however, the deficit to body potassium is approximately 300 to 500 mEq. This can be replaced over a period of a few days with oral solutions of 10 percent potassium chloride, which provides 40 mEq of potassium per ounce. Fluid retention is treated with sodium restriction (1.0 g of sodium chloride per day) and diuretics. The induced diuresis should be slow and should result in a loss of no more than 2.27 kg (5 lb) of weight per week because of the danger of precipitating electrolyte abnormalities, including hypokalemia. Diuresis can be initiated by Aldactone, 25 mg orally three times a day. If this is not successful, Laxis can be added in a dosage of 40 mg a day, with an increase in the dose in increments of 40 mg every 3 to 5 days, until diuresis is achieved. Hepatic encephalopathy manifested by asterixis or changes in mental status can be treated with protein restriction and lactulose in a total daily dose of 60 to 120 g a day in divided doses. Lactulose usually is not effective unless it also increases the frequency of bowel movements. Abstinence from alcohol improves long-term survival of patients with cirrhosis, with the exception of patients with advanced cirrhosis and severe portal hypertension. Treatment with corticosteroids is not indicated. Steroids do not improve the clinical manifestations of the disease and may result in an increased susceptibility to infection and other complications. Long-term prednisone therapy does not alter the survival of patients with cirrhosis, with or without superimposed alcoholic hepatitis.

Therapy with colchicine, which interferes with collagen metabolism, in a dose of 1 mg a day for 5 days of each week, was found in one study to result in greater clinical improvement—manifested by diminution of ascites, encephalopathy, and splenomegaly—than in control patients. In addition, serum albumin remained constant in patients taking colchicine, while it decreased in the control groups. In some instances, a decrease in fibrosis was noted on repeat liver biopsy in patients receiving colchicine. Ten-year survival was significantly increased in patients taking colchicine as compared with controls. This preliminary trial of colchicine therapy is encouraging and has stimulated further controlled trials.

REFERENCE

1. Maddrey WC, et al. Corticosteroid therapy of alcoholic hepatitis. Gastroenterology 1978; 75:193–199.

PORTAL HYPERTENSION

FRANK LYNN IBER, M.D.

Portal pressure is not frequently measured in the routine management of patients except when the diagnosis is in doubt or when the measurement is utilized to make management decisions. It may be measured at operation, or may be indirectly measured via a cardiac catheter wedged into a large hepatic vein or by measuring the intraparenchymal pressure in the substance of the liver or splenic pulp. The direct portal measurement as well as splenic pulp pressures are elevated more than 12 cm H_2O in all patients with portal hypertension. The wedged hepatic venous pressure or the liver parenchymal pressure is elevated only in patients with sinusoidal or postsinusoidal blockage.

Clinically, portal hypertension is assumed to be present when esophageal varices are present, when there is impressive abdominal collateral circulation, and when there is transudative ascites without edema. Its presence is seriously considered in any case of cirrhosis, hepatomegaly, or splenomegaly. Varices are most reliably detected by esophagoscopy, but they also may be detected by barium esophagogram or sonography of the gastroesophageal juncture. Sonography and computed tomographic scans also identify enlargement of the portal vein and tortuosity of its course. Angiography of the venous phase after celiac artery injection is reliable only when varices are extensive.

The common causes of portal hypertension are cirrhosis of the liver; infiltration of the liver with malignant tumor, inflammation, or fat; or thrombosis of the portal vein outside the liver. Idiopathic fibrosis and schistosomiasis occur frequently in certain developing countries. The consequences of portal hypertension are bleeding varices, mesenteric or splenic vein thrombosis, splenomegaly with hypersplenism, ascites, and shunting of intestinal blood around the liver through collateral veins. Of these, bleeding varices are by far the most important.

CONFIRMATION OF PORTAL HYPERTENSION

If the patient has varices and cirrhosis as established by biopsy, or typical cirrhosis patterns on scintiscan or sonogram of the liver, diagnosis is considered established. Portal pressure measurement is of clinical value only when the liver seems normal, or when there are less common features, such as obscure ascites without varices, splenomegaly, or peculiar intestinal pain consistent with venous thrombosis. In such cases, the radiologist or cardiologist can usually directly pass a catheter into the wedged hepatic venous pressure position and compare that measurement with the inferior vena cava or right auricle pressure. If serious consideration is given to extrahepatic portal obstruction, then direct visualization of the portal vein or its collaterals by angiography is undertaken.

Esophageal varices bleed into the wall of the esophagus, which then ruptures into the lumen. Bleeding is more prone to occur when the varices are extensive, have been present a long time, and when the portal pressure is quite elevated. Direct observation of the bleeding at endoscopy is the most convincing means of diagnosis but is seldom seen. Angiography occasionally demonstrates such hemorrhage. However, the plasma volume depletion associated with hemorrhage usually lowers portal pressure, causing temporary cessation of variceal bleeding. Direct observation of bleeding is seen about 25 percent of the time, topical erosion or clot is seen in an additional 10 to 20 percent of patients, and at least half of the patients reveal no diagnostic bleeding lesion, even though varices are subsequently believed to be the basis of hemorrhage. Other gastrointestinal lesions are the cause of hemorrhage in a third of patients with known varices. Approximately 10 percent of known varices bleed for the first time each year after recognition, but the risk of subsequent hemorrhage is 65 to 81 percent per year with more bleeds in the first 90 days. Although 75 percent of diagnosed variceal bleeds are clearly upper gastrointestinal hemorrhage, occult bleeding and anemia are known consequences of variceal bleeding.

TREATMENT OF ACTIVE VARICEAL HEMORRHAGE

Treatment is, first, resuscitative to preserve the life of the patient (with consideration that the patient has liver disease), second, directed to those unique aspects of therapy that stop variceal bleeding, and third, aimed at preventing the progression of liver disease (Table 1).

Resuscitative Measures

General resuscitative measures must be applied rapidly in the active bleeder who has lowered blood pressure. Patients who have less severe bleeding need fewer urgent measures, but hospitalization is needed in all. The initial measures consist of assessment of the blood volume deficit and appropriate replacement with whole blood. Adequate access lines should be established and maintained. Baseline information on mental status, blood gases, liver chemistries, and urine output should be obtained. Combined surgical and medical management is usually essential for all of these patients. Once initial resuscitation to control pulse and maintain blood pressure is complete, endoscopy may be undertaken. A central venous line is of great value in the management of portal hypertension; the central venous pressure should be maintained at 5 to 10 cm H_2O to perfuse the brain, liver, heart, and kidneys adequately while preventing rises in the portal pressure which may be sufficient to restart bleeding. All acute cases of gastrointestinal bleeding need hematocrit, electrolytes, and blood gases monitored. All patients should be given synthetic vitamin K (5 mg menadione) and should receive parenteral ranitidine for the next 3 days. If there is massive ascites, a 2- to 3-L paracentesis will lower the portal pressure for about 24 hours as the ascites re-forms. Monitored central pressure and volume control will usually control bleeding in at least 75 percent of the patients.

A nasogastric tube should not remain in place but can be inserted every 6 to 12 hours if information on continued bleeding is needed. The history may indicate recent alcoholism or poor nutrition, which would dictate the need for vitamin and mineral supplements. A history of previous encephalopathy or ascites would dictate actions restricting the free use of salt or protein or both. If there is cirrhosis, salt and water will usually be handled poorly, so some restriction should be instituted once blood pressure is maintained. A tendency to encephalopathy is common and can often be avoided by limiting the protein in the diet to 40 g total, purging the gastrointestinal tract of unabsorbed blood, and administering antibiotics. Ampicillin or tetracycline is often used in the very ill patient to avoid nephrotoxicity. Assessment of continued bleeding should be made (continued fall in hematocrit, passage of blood into the stomach, observation at endoscopy), and the patient should receive histamine$_2$ blocking agents, antibiotics, and vitamin K. If the patient is agitated, sedation with diazepam in small doses is appropriate. Nutritional needs should be determined based upon the history and examination. If the patient can eat, frequent feedings of normal food limited to 40 g of protein should be given.

Specific Measures to Control Bleeding

A variety of specific measures to control variceal bleeding are available and each has potential for harm. More than half the hospitalized patients will stop variceal bleeding if care is taken to avoid too great an increase in plasma volume. If ascites is present, a 2-L paracentesis may help. If these fail, additional measures are employed in this sequence: (1) vasopressin given intravenously, (2) vigorous volume depletion, (3) endoscopic sclerotherapy, (4) esophageal balloon tamponade, and (5) surgery.

Vasopressin Infusion

A bolus of 20 units of vasopressin is infused intravenously at the rate of 1 to 1.5 units per minute and should be associated with severe abdominal cramps, one or two spontaneous bowel movements, and tachycardia. After 20 units are given, the infusion rate is slowed to

TABLE 1 Measures for Treatment of Variceal Bleeding

Resuscitative:
 Restore blood volume with blood. Follow loss with serial hematocrits and occasional gastric intubation. Evaluate the effect on the body by blood gases, electrolytes, and urine output. Massive bleeding may require Swan-Ganz catheter to monitor replacement.

For liver disease:
 Give all patients intramuscular menadione (vitamin K) IM. Measure liver tests and cleanse the bowel of blood with purgatives or enemas. Limit salt and water intake when possible, treat or prevent encephalopathy by administering antibiotics that are safe for the kidneys and a low-protein diet. Provide glucose calories each day.

Specific measures to arrest variceal bleeding:
 Restore plasma volume slowly and carefully (central venous pressure under 10 cm H_2O). Consider 2-L paracentesis and furosemide to lower portal pressure. Use intravenous vasopressin (20 units in 15 to 20 minutes), balloon tamponade, sclerotherapy of varices, and surgical procedures to interrupt bleeding or lower portal pressure.

0.5 unit per minute. Nearly all patients will stop bleeding with this treatment, but the bleeding may recur as the infusion continues and subsequent treatments are progressively less effective. If the patient rebleeds or if the bleeding did not stop, endoscopic sclerotherapy is indicated. The chapter Acute Upper Gastrointestinal Bleeding provides additional details.

Endoscopic Sclerotherapy

If the team is experienced, sclerotherapy may be employed before and during vasopressin infusion. The experienced endoscopist should inject four to seven sites, selecting those in the most distal esophagus. Although gastric varices hemorrhage, the massive recurrent bleeding more characteristic of esophageal varices is not seen.

Esophageal Balloon Tamponade

The Blakemore-Sengstaken or the Nachlas tube is an effective means of stopping variceal hemorrhage for up to 24 hours. Both of these devices have a large gastric balloon that is inflated in the stomach. The balloon is then pulled up tightly against the diaphragm, which constricts the flow of portal blood into the varices and causes immediate cessation of bleeding. There is a stomach aspiration port that permits bleeding to be monitored. The tube should be inserted into the stomach and 300 ml of air carefully measured into the gastric balloon. This should produce no discomfort. The balloon is then snugged up against the diaphragm, pulled by hand until resistance is felt, and held there firmly while an assistant aspirates from the stomach until fresh bleeding stops. The pressure on the balloon rarely need exceed 500 g (some sort of gravity and pulley arrangement is needed to sustain this pressure) when it is successfully in position. As soon as possible (in the next hour or two) the position of the gastric balloon should be verified by an x-ray film of the upper portion of the stomach. The esophageal balloon is rarely needed and emergency scissors should be available nearby to cut through all channels of the device should the patient develop chest or respiratory distress. Patients should be in an intensive care unit as long as tamponade is taking place. After 12 to 24 hours, the patient should have the tension relieved and the gastric balloon deflated. Before withdrawal, a swallow of 1 oz of mineral oil will facilitate nontraumatic removal. The Blakemore-Sengstaken or Nachlas balloon tamponade and vasopressin therapy are temporary measures, and there is a tendency toward recurrent hemorrhage when therapy is stopped.

Volume control and sclerotherapy provide much longer benefit. Fluid and electrolyte intake sufficient to maintain urine flow is essential, but keeping the central venous pressure at 10 cm H_2O or less using limited saline replacement, paracentesis, and furosemide doses or osmotic diarrhea to deplete the body often will control hemorrhage when other measures fail. The hemorrhage remains the patient's primary problem for the first 3 to 4 days, and limited urine output or rising creatinine should not be designated the primary problem, because excessive volume overload as part of a nonmonitored fluid challenge may lead to recurrent hemorrhage.

Emergency Surgery

Propranolol should not be used to control acute hemorrhage. Emergency surgical procedures to control acute variceal hemorrhage are occasionally needed, and the choice is dictated by the training and experience of the surgeon and the degree of urgency. A portacaval shunt utilizing the H graft between the superior mesenteric vein and the inferior vena cava is the quickest to perform and probably should take precedence over the selective splenorenal shunt in the emergency situation. A complete transection of the stomach and its blood vessels from the esophagus can be carried out by nearly all general surgeons, utilizes an abdominal incision, and controls the hemorrhage for a number of months.

PREVENTION OF SUBSEQUENT HEMORRHAGE

Many patients recover adequately from the bleeding episode. Most of these patients have varices but, although no other lesion is found to account for the hemorrhage, the varices were not actually demonstrated to be bleeding. The high recurrence of bleeding requires that a plan of action be undertaken and appropriate assessment made to ensure that the goals of the plan are met.

If the liver condition seems reversible by treatment (such as disappearance of fat with abstinence or diabetes management), then it is likely that the portal pressure will fall and the varices diminish. Such patients may be monitored under treatment with portal pressures or esophagoscopy repeated at 3-month intervals. Failure of the portal pressure to fall or the varices to diminish is the basis for more direct treatment. In the majority of patients with cirrhosis, portal pressure increases with the passage of time and other measures are indicated.

Minimizing Sodium Retention and Esophagitis

The size of varices and the portal pressure increase with sodium overload and decrease with diuresis. Esophagitis and gastritis may facilitate hemorrhage. All patients who have bled from varices, proven or possible, are placed on a sodium-restricted diet, encouraged to weigh themselves daily, encouraged to avoid salt splurges in the diet, and usually are given hydrochlorothiazide or furosemide to use when indiscretions occur in sodium intake or there is weight gain. Aspirin and nonsteroidal anti-inflammatory agents are to be avoided and a liquid antacid can be used postprandially and at bedtime if there are episodes of regurgitation. These measures of unproven value seem innocuous and remind the person of the importance of the disease.

Beta-Adrenergic Blockade

Propranolol diminishes the size of varices and the blood flow in them as well as the portal pressure in many patients. It is administered four times daily in a dose sufficient to lower the heart rate by one-fourth. Available controlled trials differ as to the benefit of this treatment, but the medication is well tolerated by patients and seems a minimal undertaking for a potentially large benefit. Patients whose portal pressure lowers during an acute trial of the drug are much more likely to benefit than those who have no change in the pressure, but not enough patients have been tested in this manner to advise generally about its use. Sufficient trials have been completed to indicate that there are a few serious adverse effects particularly if the patient rebleeds, that about equal the benefit.

Sclerotherapy

Endoscopic sclerotherapy and shunt surgery are proven measures to diminish variceal bleeding and lessen days spent in hospital for bleeding. The long-term adverse effects of sclerotherapy are less clearly known than those from shunt surgery and this is the basis for its current favor. There have been more than 500 articles on sclerotherapy of varices in the past 5 years. Sclerotherapy destroys the larger varices near the gastroesophageal junction in a series of treatments. As varices are thrombosed and fibrosed by this process, additional collaterals develop, some as new varices but others in the mediastinum which are much less prone to hemorrhage. Various trials indicate that even a few treatments lessen the likelihood of hemorrhage; that complete eradication eliminates the hazard of variceal hemorrhage as long as they do not recur, but that recurrence of the varices is increasingly likely in the months following sclerosis. Efforts to predict, via endoscopic appearance, which varices are more likely to bleed are under way. Reportedly, varices *on* large varices, seen as "black spots," "cherry red spots," and "red whales" may indicate a propensity to hemorrhage.

In our unit, we undertake sclerotherapy as soon as the patient is stable after variceal bleeding—usually the first to fifth day. We inject three to five veins with sodium morrhuate (5%), using about 2 ml per varix and a total of no more than 10 ml per session attempting to inject into the varix. The injection needle is ⅝ inch long. Patients are usually hospitalized for one day following the first treatment, but subsequent treatments are conducted on an outpatient basis. Varices are injected weekly for three sessions, then monthly until eradicated; approximately six treatments are required. After eradication, endoscopy is repeated every 3 to 6 months and further treatment utilized if there is recurrence. The chapters *Sclerotherapy of Esophageal Varices* and *Acute Upper Gastrointestinal Bleeding* provide additional opinions and details on this procedure.

Shunt Surgery

Portacaval shunt is utilized in patients who continue to bleed despite other treatment. Patients who are over age 60, patients who have had prominent encephalopathy other than with an acute bleed, or patients who are expected to live more than 10 years based on the prognosis of their primary liver condition are less favored for a shunt because of the occurrence of incapacitating encephalopathy. If transplantation is contemplated a shunt may interfere. On the other hand, patients with cirrhosis and varices who are not expected to live more than 10 years, patients under age 60, and those who have not had encephalopathy undergo elective shunt after two certain bleeds or three probable bleeds uncontrolled by less definitive methods. The choice of shunt depends heavily upon the surgeon's experience; most surgeons perform only one operation well. When longer survival is anticipated (5 to 10 years), we refer the patient to those doing distal splenorenal shunts; for shorter anticipated survival, the technically less demanding H graft is recommended.

Operative Risk: Criteria

The criteria developed by Childs to predict operative and perioperative mortality following portacaval shunt surgery are useful. Patients with jaundice (bilirubin over 3.0 mg per deciliter), clinical ascites, prominent encephalopathy, or hypoalbuminemia (albumin < 3.0 g per deciliter) are rated Childs C if three or more of these findings are present. Childs B if one or two are present. If none of these findings is present they are Childs A. Childs A patients have operative mortality of under 3 percent, rarely die with variceal hemorrhage, and have long-term survival with their disease. Childs C patients have 20 to 50 percent operative mortality, nearly one-third die with variceal bleeding, and most are dead in 1 year[1]. The Childs B patients are intermediate. This clinical estimate of prognosis is useful in making decisions in management. Alcoholic patients may improve their Childs classification with several months of alcohol abstinence.

OTHER COMPLICATIONS OF PORTAL HYPERTENSION

Ascites is discussed in the chapter *Hepatorenal Syndrome and Ascites*. Patients with symptomatic low platelet counts or severe leukopenia accompanying splenomegaly of portal hypertension are seldom clinically benefited by splenectomy. Emergency cases can best be handled by the injection of an autologous clot into the splenic artery by angiography, and if this is beneficial a surgical splenectomy is performed. In my experience, the most severe leukopenia and lowered platelet counts attributed to hypersplenism have not been corrected by surgical or angiographic splenectomy.

Other complications of portal hypertension are less frequently subjected to specific treatment. Splenic or mesenteric infarctions are difficult to diagnose and there is no extensive experience with portacaval shunts to lessen their recurrence. Hepatic encephalopathy requires the shunting of large amounts of blood from the intestine around or through the liver. Rarely, a single large collateral is responsible for medically refractory encephalopathy and control has been gained by ligation of this collateral. Angiographic demonstration of such collaterals is readily possible. Other measures of treatment for hepatic encephalopathy are discussed in the chapter *Portosystemic Encephalopathy*.

REFERENCE

1. Cello et al. Endoscopic sclerotherapy versus portacaval shunt in patients with severe cirrhosis and variceal hemorrhage. N Engl J Med 1984; 311:1589.

ACUTE VIRAL HEPATITIS

LEONARD B. SEEFF, M.D.

The remarkable advances of the past two decades in diagnostic serology and molecular virology of viral hepatitis have, unfortunately, not been paralleled by improved techniques for treatment of the disease. On the contrary, current management of the acute illness is characterized by the omission of certain approaches that were common a decade ago, items such as mandatory hospitalization, mandatory bed rest, the use of special diets, and treatment with glucocorticoids in certain circumstances. Prevention of the disease, however, or at least some of its forms, has made dramatic progress, testimony to the persistent and innovative research of the clinical epidemiologist, virologist, and molecular biologist.

DIAGNOSTIC CONSIDERATIONS

A prerequisite for specific and effective treatment of any disease is the ability to establish a definitive diagnosis. In the case of acute hepatitis that has no pathognomonic features, diagnosis depends on the accumulation of historical facts, clinical findings, and biochemical alterations that, taken together, suggest the presence of acute hepatocellular necrosis. Attention must then be directed toward finding a specific etiology, since the liver responds in only a limited number of ways to numerous, diverse noxious stimuli. For example, it is now recognized that viruses other than those of hepatitis A and B can induce identical acute liver disease, namely, those causing delta hepatitis, non-A, non-B hepatitis (of which there are almost certainly two), and epidemic non-A, non-B hepatitis. The illness can be mimicked also by adverse reactions to certain drugs, by congestive cardiac failure, and by severe hypotension. Finally, a similar although generally distinguishable liver disease can result from other infectious agents (e.g., cytomegalovirus, Epstein-Barr virus, herpes simplex virus, coxsackievirus, rubella, and so on), in association with acute choledocholithiasis, from alcohol excess (alcoholic hepatitis), and occasionally in connection with certain metabolic disorders (Wilson's disease, alpha$_1$-antitrypsin deficiency). Thus, etiologic identification is imperative not only as a guide to specific therapy but also as an aid in the institution of appropriate preventive measures.

PRELIMINARY EVALUATION

In persons with apparent acute liver disease, a presumptive etiologic diagnosis can generally be achieved through the combination of a detailed historical interview (with special emphasis on the circumstances that favor exposure to viral hepatitis), extensive questioning regarding the use of all drugs (prescription and over-the-counter), a carefully administered physical examination, and the use of appropriate biochemical and serologic tests. If the diagnosis remains unclear, additional evaluation is necessary, as dictated by clinical circumstances. This may include ultrasound and computed tomographic scanning of the abdomen, immunologic tests, screening procedures for Wilson's disease, and so on. A liver biopsy is no longer considered a routine procedure when acute viral hepatitis is strongly suspected. The biopsy is now reserved for instances in which there is a diagnostic dilemma that is likely to be resolved by the finding of characteristic morphologic changes, or for the further evaluation of a bout of acute viral hepatitis that follows a disturbing course or persists for an unusual period of time (more than 4 to 6 months).

Once a diagnosis of acute viral hepatitis is established, the next step is definition of the severity of the disease and of the responsible virus. The basis for the latter exercise is to permit the adoption of the appropriate preventive and prophylactic measures for contacts of the patients.

Biochemical Tests

Routine biochemical tests should include measuring the activities of the aminotransferases (SGOT or AST; SGPT or ALT) and alkaline phosphatase, the levels of serum bilirubin and the serum proteins, and the prothrombin time. Of these, the tests that best define severity and prognosis are the prothrombin time and the serum bilirubin value. A prothrombin time in a patient which exceeds that of the control by 3 to 4 seconds is a disturbing finding, as is deep jaundice (> 25 mg/dl, unless superimposed hemolysis is the basis for the increased value). There is little correlation between the height of the aminotransferase values and the severity of the disease.

Serologic Tests

The most useful panel of serologic tests are HBsAg, IgM anti-HBc, and IgM anti-HAV, with the addition of HBeAg and IgM anti-delta (anti-HD) as needed. Thus, acute liver disease associated with a positive test for IgM anti-HAV establishes a diagnosis of acute hepatitis A. It must be noted, however, that in about 15 percent of instances, this antibody persists for 200 days or longer. Hepatitis B is diagnosed by the presence of HBsAg and/or IgM anti-HBc. If, instead, IgG anti-HBc is present together with HBsAg, the diagnostic consideration is a superimposed bout of acute hepatitis A, non-A, non-B hepatitis, or delta hepatitis, or a flare of hepatitis B (which sometimes occurs when HBeAg spontaneously seroconverts to anti-HBe) in an HBsAg carrier. Acute non-A, non-B hepatitis requires the exclusion of all known causes of acute hepatitis and the absence of IgM anti-HAV and of IgM anti-HBc.

MANAGEMENT OF ESTABLISHED ACUTE VIRAL HEPATITIS

There are two aspects to management when the precise diagnosis is finally made, namely, active treatment and prevention and prophylaxis.

Active Treatment

Site

The site of treatment is dictated by the severity of the disease and the adequacy of home support. If the disease is not classified as severe (bilirubin <25 mg per deciliter, prothrombin time <4 seconds prolonged), and there is an acceptable level of home care available, hospitalization is not needed. Adequate care implies that there is a household member willing to observe the patient daily for any signs of unusual physical or mental change, and to supply the necessary nursing and subsistence support. Such patients need not be seen by the physician any more frequently than is necessary for appropriate blood testing (see below).

Hospitalization will, however, need to be considered at the outset of the illness or during its course if the patient has persistent vomiting with the threat of dehydration, has a serum bilirubin value that is greater than 25 mg per deciliter or a prothrombin time that is greater than 4 seconds prolonged, has clinical evidence of encephalopathy, shows rapidly declining aminotransferase activity in the face of a rising bilirubin level, or develops other evidence of hepatic failure (falling albumin level, ascites, and so on).

Evaluation

Ideally, biochemical evaluation should be performed twice weekly while values continue to rise, once a week after they have reached a plateau and begin to decline, and at 1- to 2-week intervals when a slow but inexorable reduction toward normal becomes apparent. It is worth recording normalization of all values even though this may require a prolonged period of observation. It is also important in persons with proven hepatitis B to establish the loss of HBsAg and, if possible, the appearance of anti-HBs (although this may take many months).

Bed Rest

There is now general agreement that complete bed rest is not essential. Indeed, physical activity within the bounds of fatiguability can be permitted without fear of permanent damage. The exception to this rule is evidence of persistent biochemical or neurologic worsening, particularly in an older person (>40 years of age), even though there are no scientific data that demonstrate a beneficial effect of bed rest.

Diet

Contrary to earlier practice, it is no longer believed necessary to restrict fats. A nutritious diet should be encouraged which need not include vitamin supplementation unless there is evidence of a specific deficiency. If there is persistent nausea and vomiting, repeated small feedings of caloric liquid formulas may be helpful. Occasionally nausea and vomiting may be severe enough to culminate in dehydration, which would require appropriate intravenous fluid and electrolyte replacement. Protein restriction is required only if overt encephalopathy develops.

Drugs

There are no drugs available for the treatment of acute hepatitis. Because corticosteroids accelerate the reduction in bilirubin levels and aminotransferase activity, they have been used in the past therapeutically in different stages of the disease, (e.g., during the early acute phase, for fulminant hepatitis, in suspected subacute hepatic necrosis, for chronic viral hepatitis). Available data suggest that they are not only unhelpful, but they may well be harmful by increasing viral replication. Certain experimental drugs (e.g., cyanidanol, isoprinosine, ribavirin, levamisole, high-titer anti-HBs) have also been evaluated in patients with acute viral hepatitis but without demonstrable benefit.

Because the liver is the major site of metabolism of many drugs, all medications, particularly narcotics, analgesics, and tranquilizers, should be strictly avoided during the acute illness. The reduction in drug clearance when there is widespread necrosis may promote hepatic encephalopathy or even respiratory depression. If sedation is essential, reduced doses of benzodiazepines can be employed, or preferably oxazepam, a drug whose metabolism is not impaired in the presence of acute liver damage. (See chapter, *Drug Use in Patients with Hepatic Disease*). Protracted nausea and vomiting may require the judicious use of phenothiazines or antihistamines. Rarely, pruritus may be sufficiently severe and persistent as to warrant the use of medication, such as the exchange resin cholestyramine. Vitamin K_1 is often administered in the hope of preventing or improving coagulation abnormalities; however, no benefit derives from its use in acute hepatocellular disease, although it may be effective in cholestatic liver disease.

A question that sometimes arises is whether or not alcohol can be used. Generally this is in reference to the period after recovery but occasionally it relates to the taking of alcohol during the acute illness as symptoms begin to wane. It has been traditional to proscribe its use during the acute illness and for a period of 6 to 12 months after recovery based on early data which suggested that fulminant hepatitis could be provoked or that relapse of acute hepatitis could result. Despite the lack of firm data to support these observations, it seems prudent to continue this approach, if for no other reason than to reduce confusion regarding the meaning of subsequent enzyme abnormalities (alcohol effect versus disease exacerbation). If, on the other hand, enzyme abnormalities persist for more than 12 months, suggesting transition to chronic hepatitis, it is wise to recommend to the person who strongly desires alcohol to use it in moderation and infrequently.

Finally, while the use of oral contraceptives can be continued during acute hepatitis without fear of harm, sexual activity during the early acute phases of hepatitis should be discouraged so as to avoid transmission of the virus to the partner.

Preventive Measures and Prophylaxis

Prevention

The institution of appropriate preventive public health measures is predicated on a thorough knowledge of the modes of spread of hepatitis. The *hepatitis A virus* is excreted in stool from the latter half of the incubation period to approximately the time of peak illness, generally within a week of onset of overt disease. Transmission from person to person is via fecal-oral contact; accordingly, those at risk are susceptible household or institutional contacts. Because of this pattern of viral excretion, many of these contacts are likely to have been exposed by the time the index case is brought to medical attention. Nevertheless, to curtail further spread, the modes of disease transmission should be discussed with the patient, and strict standards of personal hygiene should be imposed. This includes regular hand washing, particularly after using the toilet (separate facilities are not required), a warning against intimate contact, and a prohibition of the sharing of food and drink. With regard to eating utensils, either disposable or regular crockery can be used as long as a hot-water dishwasher is available, which provides adequate sterilization. If hospitalization is required, there is no need to impose reverse isolation procedures or require the use of separate bathroom facilities. Needle precautions continue to be advised even though there is no carrier state for hepatitis A and percutaneous transmission of hepatitis A is uncommon (but by no means unheard of).

The *hepatitis B virus* is present in blood and in all physiologic and pathologic body fluids, with the exception of stool; presumably the same holds true for the viruses of *non-A, non-B hepatitis* and the *delta agent*. Thus, blood and body secretions are the source of transmission, and high-risk individuals are those who are likely to come into contact with blood or its products or who have close intimate contact with the index case. Nonpercutaneous transmission other than through sexual contact also occurs but the precise mechanism often cannot be established. Consequently, preventive measures that can be adopted include efforts to reduce the number of blood transfusions; the development and maintenance of hospital surveillance to identify HBsAg carriers; the requirement that gloves be worn by personnel who are in regular contact with blood, followed by careful hand washing; the requirement that needles be appropriately disposed of and that instruments in contact with blood and secretions be adequately cleaned (with soap and water), disinfected (sodium hypochlorite, formalin, glutaraldehyde), and sterilized (autoclaving, ethylene oxide); and the recommendation that sexual abstinence be followed during the acute disease and that sexual contact be limited by the carrier. Finally, as will be discussed, if immune prophylaxis is provided for all susceptible high-risk individuals, many of these problems would be avoided.

Prophylaxis

Prophylaxis is the area of most impressive gains. For *hepatitis A*, passive protection with immune globulin (IG, formerly ISG) remains the backbone of prophylaxis, and, provided IG is administered to susceptible contacts within 2 to 4 weeks of exposure, complete inhibition or modification of the disease can be anticipated. A practical dose formulation is the administration intramuscularly of 0.5 ml of IG to children weighing less than 50 lb, 1.0 ml to persons weighing 50 to 100 lb, and 2.0 ml to those who weigh more than 100 lb (based on a dose of 0.02 ml per kilogram of body weight). Now that the hepatitis A virus has been cultured, an attenuated, live hepatitis A vaccine has been developed. Recombinant vaccine, made possible by the cloning of hepatitis A, is also in the process of development. Early studies with the live vaccine indicate that it is immunogenic, and human studies are now in progress to determine its efficacy.

Hepatitis B prophylaxis is more complex because of the carrier state of this virus, often in totally asymptomatic individuals. Therefore, prevention has to be considered in two contexts, namely, postexposure prophylaxis that follows an episode of known contact (e.g., percutaneous exposure to a contaminated needle, sexual contact with a partner incubating the disease or carrying the virus, the birth of an infant to a mother with acute disease or who is a carrier), or preexposure prophylaxis (e.g., high-risk individuals in whom contact can be anticipated in the future). In the former situation, hepatitis B immune globulin should be administered intramuscularly to contacts as soon as possible after exposure (5 ml on two occasions to an adult, 0.5 ml once to a newborn). Adults who already have adequate titers of anti-HB^s (10 sample ratio units or more by radioimmunoassay or positive by enzyme immunoassay) do not require prophylaxis; pre-screening of exposed neonates is unnecessary. The "needlestick" and neonatal contacts should also receive hepatitis B vaccine (20 μg for adults, injected into the deltoid; 10 μg for neonates, injected into the thigh immediately and 1 and 6 months after exposure). Postexposure prophylaxis for sexual contact is controversial; the current official recommendation is that either IG or HBIG be administered once only, with the addition of the vaccine reserved for contacts of a carrier but not of a person with acute hepatitis B. Preexposure prophylaxis with hepatitis B vaccine is strongly recommended for all susceptible high-risk contacts. There is overwhelming evidence that it provides a high rate of immunogenicity, protection, and safety. Deltoid injection may induce a more consistent response than buttocks injection. The current plasma-derived vaccine may be replaced in the future by vaccines that are genetically engineered or synthesized from defined immunogenic HBsAg peptide sequences. In a population with a high prevalence of hepatitis B, such as homosexually-active men or nurses in a dialysis unit, screening for hepatitis B antibody is cost-effective.

No specific prophylactic measures are available for the delta agent or non-A, non-B hepatitis. None is needed for delta hepatitis; this agent is entirely dependent for its expression on the coexistence in the human host of hepatitis B, and hence prevention and prophylaxis of the latter affords equal protection for the former. The development of passive or active immunizing products against non-A, non-B hepatitis obviously awaits the identification of the responsible viral agents. In the interim, since this disease has many epidemiologic similarities to hepatitis B, the same general preventive measures should be instituted as those described for hepatitis B. Indeed, the use of IG as postexposure prophylaxis for the same circumstances as it is used in hepatitis B has become common practice. This should probably continue even though it is impossible to determine whether a specific lot of IG contains any or sufficient concentrations of specific antibody. Research in this area continues.

FULMINANT HEPATIC FAILURE

S. CHRIS PAPPAS, M.D., F.R.C.P.(C)

Fulminant hepatic failure (FHF) is the syndrome that arises as a result of the acute failure of the liver in an individual in whom there is no antecedent hepatic dysfunction. By definition, FHF includes the occurrence of hepatic encephalopathy within 8 weeks of the onset of clinical illness. This distinguishes FHF from subacute hepatic failure or decompensation of chronic liver disease, although all the entities may share many clinical and pathophysiologic features. Fulminant hepatic failure is not common; some 2,000 cases occur annually in the United States. Since FHF can, and often does, occur in young patients and is associated with a 65 to 85 percent mortality rate, it remains one of the most challenging and dramatic clinical problems. The major problems in the treatment of FHF include the diverse etiologic processes of the disorder, the often rapid evolution of the syndrome culminating in death before important biochemical, histologic, or serologic data are available, and the lack of good, controlled clinical trials assessing recent treatment modalities.

Unfortunately, there is little that is truly new in the area of treatment of FHF. This, plus the high mortality of the syndrome, often combine to discourage physicians from aggressively supporting these patients in an optimal, intensive care setting. Data exist which support the concept that the application of standard intensive care surveillance and nursing is the major factor responsible for the improved survival of patients with FHF noted over the past two to three decades. It is reasonable to expect that about one-third of patients with FHF will survive with aggressive intensive care. Accordingly, the major principle of the treatment of FHF is that such treatment should take place in specialized intensive care units, and preferably units experienced and interested in the management of patients with severe liver disease. The Acute Care Liver Unit, a concept that is popular in Europe and seeing increasing development in North America, is probably the ideal setting in which to manage the patient with FHF.

SUPPORTIVE CARE

Table 1 summarizes the major complications of FHF and their treatment. In general, initially the patient should be admitted to the intensive care unit as soon as the diagnosis is made (i.e., with the onset of hepatic encephalopathy). The laboratory, blood bank, and other medical specialists (i.e., nephrologist, infectious disease specialist)

TABLE 1 Complications of Fulminant Hepatic Failure and Their Treatment

Complication	Treatment
Hypoglycemia	IV glucose
Hypokalemia	IV potassium chloride
Hyponatremia	Sodium chloride not usually needed
Renal failure / Metabolic acidosis / Fluid overload	Dialysis
Hypoxemia / Pulmonary edema	Assisted ventilation
Infection	Antibiotics
Increased intracranial pressure	Mannitol (1 g/kg of body weight)
Hypotension	IV fluids, vasopressors
Gastrointestinal bleeding	Cimetidine, 200 mg IV TID
Coagulopathy with bleeding	Fresh frozen plasma, platelets, whole blood
Disseminated intravascular coagulation	Heparin not usually indicated
Pancreatitis	Nasogastric suction, IV fluids, nothing by mouth

should be notified. The laboratory should be advised that the results of blood tests may be required on a "stat" basis, including tests not normally ordered as such (e.g., serum copper, hepatitis serology). Blood should be obtained for serum liver biochemical and other appropriate tests; if indicated, acetaminophen levels should be determined. Orders should then be written to ensure regular monitoring for the complications of FHF, with particular attention paid to frequent neurologic assessment, blood glucose levels, and renal function.

As can be appreciated from Table 1, the treatment of the complications of FHF are individually not exotic but actually quite simple; the complexity arises from the tendency for multiple problems to occur simultaneously. A few specific comments should be made. Large amounts of glucose and potassium may be required during the course of therapy; up to 400 to 600 mEq of potassium per day is necessary in some patients. In general, it is best to provide at least 300 g of glucose per day (for its protein-sparing effect) in the form of intravenous fluid; this will require modification if electrolyte or fluid imbalances are present. Treatment for hyponatremia is not usually indicated unless the problem is particularly severe and there are neurologic disturbances which are felt to be related to hyponatremia. Dialysis may be very useful to correct fluid overload, hyperkalemia, acidosis, and so on. The usual indications for dialysis prevail in patients with FHF, since it must be understood that this treatment is undertaken as part of the *supportive*, as opposed to specific, therapy for FHF. Either peritoneal or hemodialysis (HD) may be employed, with the former preferred because it obviates the need for anticoagulation. Experience with HD and other extracorporeal circulation devices has suggested that, despite the presence of severe coagulopathy, patients with FHF still require anticoagulation, and in fact, heparin requirements may be increased due to antithrombin III deficiency. The unpredictable response of individual patients with FHF to anticoagulant or antiplatelet active agents (e.g., prostacyclin) makes systemic or regional anticoagulation difficult, but not impossible or excessively dangerous.

As with dialysis in FHF, the usual indications for assisted ventilation and endotracheal intubation apply. Hypocapnia, a common finding in FHF, should not be treated, since it is often not severe and may be beneficial as regards cerebral edema. Sepsis must be vigorously watched for with daily cultures of biologic fluids, since the usual signs of sepsis may be absent in the patient with FHF. There is no role, however, for prophylactic antibiotics. Systemic fungal infections, perhaps related to cimetidine therapy (see below), occur not infrequently and should be aggressively treated.

Increased intracranial pressure (ICP) as a result of cerebral edema remains the most difficult complication of FHF and is now the most common cause of death in these patients. In specialized units where the facility exists, direct ICP monitoring with an extradural pressure transducer should be employed because it allows moment-by-moment measurement of ICP and thus permits prompt institution and assessment of treatment for the precipitous rises in ICP which patients with FHF may exhibit. Such extradural pressure monitors can be safely placed in patients with FHF despite the presence of coagulopathy. The procedure can be performed in the intensive care unit. Steroids are of no value in the treatment of cerebral edema in FHF. For sustained increases in the ICP above 25 to 30 mm Hg for more than 5 minutes, *mannitol*, 1 g per kilogram body weight (up to a maximum of 100 g) should be given in a 20 percent solution as an intravenous bolus. This may be repeated as necessary if urine output is sustained but should not be continued if renal failure is present or ICP monitoring demonstrates a lack of response or a paradoxic increase in ICP, as occasionally occurs in patients with FHF, especially when ICP is initially high. This latter observation underscores the value of direct ICP measurement, although it is admitted that the value of the routine use of such monitoring has not been rigorously assessed. In the absence of direct ICP measurements, continuous electroencephalogram monitoring (which may also be useful in detecting seizure activity or hypoglycemia) and careful, repeated neurologic examination can be used to detect increased ICP. The main neurologic signs which may indicate raised ICP are listed in Table 2. Treatment

TABLE 2 Findings Suggesting Raised Intracranial Pressure in Patients with Fulminant Hepatic Failure

Decreasing level of consciousness
Abnormal, unequal, or absent pupillary light reflexes
Absent or abnormal oculovestibular reflexes
Decerebrate posturing
Focal or generalized seizures, myoclonus
Hypertension, bradycardia
Electroencephalogram changes—marked slowing, asymmetry

with mannitol, as described above, should be instituted should these signs appear or the electroencephalogram deteriorate with hypoglycemia having been ruled out. In certain patients, particularly children and young adults, in whom cerebral edema has become a major problem unresponsive to usual therapy, consideration should be given to decompressive craniotomy if an aggressive therapeutic approach is felt to be indicated. Experience with this form of treatment in children with Reye's syndrome and a patient with FHF suggests that it may be useful in selected cases. Finally, drugs that are known to increase ICP (e.g., fentanyl, ketamine, halothane) should be used with extreme caution in patients with FHF; fortunately, they are rarely indicated.

The treatment of hepatic encephalopathy complicating FHF is, in general, not different from that in chronic liver disease. Identification and treatment of exacerbating factors remain an important principle of therapy. Most patients are protein restricted by necessity. It is suggested that lactulose or neomycin be employed, although the hepatic encephalopathy of acute liver failure may not respond to any of the usual measures. Lactulose therapy is probably preferable since it is easy to administer and, in general, safer in patients with renal dysfunction when compared with neomycin. Lactulose treatment should be promptly discontinued, however, if problems arise, such as excessive diarrhea, volume contraction, or hypokalemia. Although patients with early hepatic encephalopathy, especially children, may exhibit hypomania or delirium, the temptation to use sedative/hypnotic drugs should clearly be avoided. If seizures occur, however, treatment must be undertaken despite the sedative properties of the anticonvulsant drugs. Diazepam appears to be the most effective drug; the doses required are generally small and in the range of 2 to 10 mg IV. The principles of treatment dictate that the smallest doses necessary for seizure control be used, increased ICP be aggressively treated, and that a search for alternate causes of seizures (e.g., electrolyte imbalance or intracranial hemorrhage) be undertaken. When seizures become a major problem, treatment should be along conventional lines, with the dosage of drugs adjusted for the presence of severe liver disease; neurologic consultation should be sought. Barbiturate coma is used in the treatment of status epilepticus and, despite seemingly major contraindications, may be useful in the rare patient with FHF and continuous seizure activity; unfortunately, no published clinical information exists with reference to this.

Hypotension not related to obvious volume depletion is a common accompaniment of FHF but should be treated only if the systolic blood pressure is sustained below 90 mm Hg in association with a falling urine output and/or neurologic deterioration. A decreased mean arterial pressure with a low systemic vascular resistance and increased cardiac output is typical of FHF and treatments to arbitrarily increase the blood pressure to the normal range are not appropriate. When treatment is indicated, however, low-dose dopamine or other vasoactive agents may be used.

The coagulopathy of FHF may be severe and is often complex. A general principle is that treatment is indicated only if active and dangerous bleeding is occurring. There is no role for the prophylactic treatment of the coagulopathy with fresh frozen plasma, platelets, and so on. The sole exception would be the use of fresh frozen plasma and platelets at the time of any invasive procedure, such as the placement of extradural pressure transducers or arterial and central venous catheters. Vitamin K, 10 mg given by slow intravenous infusion, should be administered once on admission and weekly thereafter. While disseminated intravascular coagulation may occur in patients with FHF, this is not usually a major problem and does not appear to resemble disseminated intravascular coagulation occurring in other settings. Accordingly, the use of heparin and large amounts of factor concentrates is not indicated, and in fact the latter may pose a danger by accelerating microthrombus formation. Prophylaxis for gastrointestinal bleeding should be employed, as dictated by guidelines for the management of any critically ill patient. Cimetidine, 200 mg IV three times a day, is a suggested treatment; unfortunately, there is no good information on appropriate doses of other gastric acid-lowering agents in FHF, and gastric pH should be closely monitored whatever treatment is employed. While the central nervous system side effects of histamine$_2$ receptor blockers are of theoretical concern, this is not usually a practical problem and may be avoided by the use of antacids to increase gastric pH. In addition, while systemic fungal infection related to gastric hypochlorhydria and a subsequent lack of resistance to gut colonization and invasion by pathogenic fungi are concerns, the risk of gastrointestinal bleeding is too great to consider avoiding prophylactic treatment for it. Hemorrhagic pancreatitis complicating FHF is treated in the usual manner.

SPECIFIC THERAPY

In contrast to supportive care, the specific treatment of FHF is an area of much controversy, and there is little in the way of good, controlled data. Aside from accumulated evidence demonstrating the lack of value of steroids (with some exceptions; see below) and exchange transfusions, there is little to guide the physician in the choice of specific therapy (if any) to be employed in FHF. Accordingly, since some of these treatments may be dangerous, and all are time-consuming and expensive, for the present, any specific treatment of FHF should be undertaken only in the setting of careful pilot studies in experienced liver failure units or as part of large randomized and controlled clinical trials conducted by experienced and interested investigators. While there is little doubt that certain specific treatments involving temporary hepatic assist, in particular, *charcoal hemoperfusion with prostacyclin infusion*, appear to offer hope for more successful management of patients with FHF, this type of treatment cannot be routinely advocated despite claims of ethical justification. Clearly, more controlled data are badly needed and ongoing research is imperative. The early identification of those patients unlikely to survive with

TABLE 3 Clinical Coma Profile

1. Verbal ability 　None 　Incomprehensible	6. Oculocephalic-oculovestibular response 　Absent 　Present but abnormal 　　(describe) 　Normal
2. Eye opening 　None 　To painful stimuli only 　To noise 　Spontaneous	7. Motor response (best limb) 　None 　Abnormal extensor 　Abnormal flexor 　Withdrawal
3. Pupillary light reflex 　Absent 　Present	8. Pattern of respiration 　None (apnea) 　Irregular (or abnormal) 　Regular >22/min 　Regular <22/min
4. Corneal reflex 　Absent 　Present	9. Deep tendon reflexes 　Absent 　Increased 　Normal or decreased
5. Spontaneous eye movements 　None 　Roving dysconjugate 　Roving conjugate 　Orienting	10. Skeletal muscle tone 　None (flaccid) 　Abnormal 　Normal

From Pappas SC, Jones EA. Methods for assessing hepatic encephalopathy. Sem. Liver Disease 1983; 3:298.

supportive care alone would greatly aid in the selection of patients to receive newer therapies, including liver transplantation if it is indicated (see below). Exciting potential therapies, in addition to charcoal hemoperfusion and prostacyclin, include such alternatives as the use of auxiliary liver transplantation (heterotopic transplantation of part of a donor liver to simultaneously provide hepatic assist and stimulate hepatic regeneration) and interferon treatment in FHF due to viral hepatitis.

With regard to orthotopic liver transplantation, this formidable procedure can be carried out in patients with FHF with occasional dramatic results and survival reported. However, except in patients with *Wilson's disease* presenting as FHF and possibly patients with *Budd-Chiari* syndrome and FHF (see below), it is unlikely that orthotopic liver transplantation will ever play a major role in the treatment of FHF. For the present, this procedure should be considered only in the specific instances noted above and possibly in patients with so-called *subacute hepatic failure*, an as yet poorly characterized clinical syndrome with diverse etiologic factors in which the clinical course tends to be slower and the development of hepatic encephalopathy delayed (i.e., from 8 to 26 weeks after the onset of the initial illness). The rationale for liver transplantation in these patients is the apparent similarly high mortality with this syndrome and, in contrast to patients with FHF, frequent progression to severe chronic liver disease in the few survivors.

ASSESSING RESPONSE TO TREATMENT

Unless a specific treatment for FHF is being used, assessing the response to therapy in patients with FHF involves, more than anything else, the assessment of spontaneous hepatic recovery while the patient is being supported. The main aspect of assessment involves careful neurologic review, since the sustained improvement of hepatic encephalopathy accompanying FHF is associated with a much improved prognosis. A clinical coma profile, such as that shown in Table 3, should be employed. The meticulous repeated application of such a coma profile, especially in combination with continuous electroencephalogram monitoring, may well facilitate the detection of early recovery or the earliest response to therapeutic measures. Similarly, neurologic deterioration, especially loss of the oculovestibular reflexes, portends a poor prognosis and survival is unlikely. Serum biochemical assessment includes the usual tests reflecting hepatic function, and with regard to assessing recovery from FHF, particular attention should be paid to the prothrombin time, and serum bilirubin, and glucose measurements. If more sophisticated testing is available, monitoring factor VII levels is useful if serial values can be obtained. The precise role of routine use of true liver function tests, such as the galactose elimination capacity or aminopyrine clearance test, is unclear, but if they are available, these tests should be done.

SPECIFIC CONSIDERATIONS

Certain causes of FHF merit special consideration. As alluded to above, the rare presentation of Wilson's disease with FHF is a situation in which liver transplantation should be considered, since it offers the best hope for these patients. This diagnosis must be suspected in any young person with FHF, especially if it is accompanied by hemolytic anemia and the impression of lower than expected serum transaminase and alkaline phosphatase levels. Rapid diagnosis of Wilson's disease in this setting may be difficult; serum copper is markedly elevated in patients with FHF and Wilson's disease but low or low-normal in other patients with FHF. Similarly, patients with acute Budd-Chiari syndrome and FHF may benefit from liver transplantation or such surgical procedures as mesocaval or mesoatrial shunts; the diagnosis must be considered in patients with the usual etiologic predispositions and prompt surgical therapy undertaken. Once the disorder develops, there is little that medical therapy can offer.

Other instances in which specific therapies may be of use include the rare occurrence of FHF due to herpes simplex infection, for which intravenous acyclovir may be of value; acute fatty liver of pregnancy, for which, in contrast to other causes of FHF, antithrombin III infusions may be useful in the management of the accompanying coagulopathy; and drug-induced FHF accompanied by a hypersensitivity syndrome (e.g., halothane, phenytoin), in which the use of corticosteroids is reasonable and may be useful. Acetaminophen-induced FHF is a difficult problem, since most patients with this form of FHF present more than 24 hours after ingestion, beyond the time when the treatment with acetylcysteine is of value. Rarely, however, patients will have "acute on chronic" or "repeated" overdoses such that they may present with FHF within 24 hours of the last major ingestion. It would seem reasonable to treat these patients with acetylcysteine in the usual doses, although experience in this setting is limited. Finally, in children with FHF, the inborn errors of metabolism—galactosemia, tyrosinemia, and fructosemia—must be considered and, if diagnosed, appropriate specific therapy commenced in addition to the general supportive measures described above.

CHRONIC HEPATITIS

RAYMOND S. KOFF, M.D.

Chronic hepatitis refers to a set of necro-inflammatory liver disorders in which clinical, biochemical, and histologic abnormalities persist for more than six months. Chronic hepatitis can be caused by viral hepatitis (persistent hepatitis B virus (HBV) infection, delta agent infection of HBV-positive individuals, persistent non-A, non-B hepatitis virus infections, but not hepatitis A virus infection), adverse hepatic drug reactions, and metabolic disorders such as Wilson's disease, alpha$_1$-antitrypsin deficiency, and iron overload disorders. In a large proportion of patients no etiologic agent can be defined and the term *idiopathic chronic hepatitis* seems appropriate. Some of these may be examples of autoimmune-initiated disease (autoimmune chronic hepatitis), but it is likely that primary defects in immunoregulation are responsible for only a minority of cases. Patients with primary biliary cirrhosis may have features resembling those seen in chronic hepatitis; this disorder is discussed in the chapter on *Primary Biliary Cirrhosis*. Similarly, patients with alcoholic liver disease occasionally may present with features typical of chronic hepatitis (this disorder is also discussed elsewhere in this volume). In this chapter, the treatment of viral and idiopathic chronic hepatitis will be discussed.

Liver biopsy is essential for confirmation of the diagnosis of chronic hepatitis, histological classification of the form of chronic hepatitis present, and identification of severity of the lesion. The presence of sequelae and some clues to etiology may also be provided.

Three major forms of chronic hepatitis have been recognized: chronic persistent hepatitis, chronic lobular hepatitis, and chronic active hepatitis.

CHRONIC PERSISTENT HEPATITIS

Chronic persistent hepatitis is a benign form of chronic hepatitis characterized histologically by the presence of a dense infiltrate of mononuclear cells in the portal tracts, with minimal stromal collapse, slight or no periportal hepatocyte necrosis, and little if any fibrosis. While some authorities have suggested that liver biopsy may be unnecessary because management of this form of hepatitis is not altered by confirmation of the diagnosis, biopsy confirmation provides reassurance that a more serious disorder is not present and seems an appropriate measure. Hepatitis B virus (the hepatitis B surface antigen [HBsAg] is detected in the sera of 10 to 40% of patients) and non-A, non-B viral hepatitis are responsible for most cases. Chronic persistent hepatitis is a nonprogressive disorder which rarely, if ever, evolves into cirrhosis. An identical lesion may be seen, however, following spontaneous or treatment-induced remission in some patients with chronic active hepatitis. In this case, the natural history of the disease is that of chronic active hepatitis, and relapses may occur with clinical, biochemical, and histologic progression. One additional exception to the general benign course of chronic persistent hepatitis is the occurrence of delta agent superinfection of patients with HBsAg-positive chronic persistent hepatitis. In this event, the disease may be progressive and can lead to the development of chronic active hepatitis and cirrhosis.

Most, but not all, patients with chronic persistent hepatitis are asymptomatic and appear healthy. Such patients come to medical attention because of the detection of persistently elevated levels of serum aminotransferases or during the evaluation of the HBsAg carrier state. Nonspecific complaints of mild fatigue, anorexia, and abdominal discomfort or pain may be seen in a few patients, but physical findings are usually absent except for minimal hepatomegaly. Serum bilirubin levels are mildly elevated in about 10 percent of patients, but with the exception of the serum aminotransferases other liver tests are usually within normal limits.

No specific therapy has been shown to alter the natural history of this disorder irrespective of its etiologic agent. Neither immunosuppressive therapy nor antiviral therapy has established a role in the management of affected patients. Treatment of chronic persistent hepatitis is limited to reassurance, simple supportive measures, the avoidance of known hepatotoxins (small amounts of alcohol may be permitted if well tolerated), avoidance of parenteral exposures that might result in delta agent superinfection of HBsAg-positive patients, and annual follow-up to ascertain that the disease remains nonprogressive as determined by physical examination and serial liver chemical tests. Liver biopsy is not repeated unless clinical or biochemical deterioration suggests that the original diagnosis of chronic persistent hepatitis may have been erroneous. This is a rare event. The disease may persist for many years before resolution, which is signaled by normalization of the serum aminotransferase levels and, in some instances of HBV-induced disease, seroconversion from HBeAg-positive to anti-HBe-positive and loss of HBsAg.

CHRONIC LOBULAR HEPATITIS

This uncommon form of chronic hepatitis appears to be a sequel of hepatitis B and non-A, non-B viral hepatitis in which the features of acute hepatitis may persist for a prolonged period, with moderately increased levels of serum aminotransferases typical of those found in acute hepatitis. The course is characterized by multiple biochemical remissions and relapses over many years. During the relapses the hepatic histopathologic lesion is that of acute hepatitis. During remissions the lesion resembles chronic persistent hepatitis. Physical findings are minimal; about one-third of patients have hepatomegaly. Signs of portal hypertension are absent. Neither cirrhosis nor hepatic failure is a sequela of chronic lobular hepatitis. No specific therapy is available. Biochemical and histologic resolution may occur after years of follow-up, as in chronic persistent hepatitis.

CHRONIC ACTIVE HEPATITIS

Chronic active hepatitis is the most serious form of chronic hepatitis because, in its most severe and aggressive form, the disorder may progress to fatal hepatic failure and/or the development of cirrhosis with associated complications of portal hypertension. Liver biopsy reveals enlarged portal tracts which are infiltrated with mononuclear and plasma cells, spilling out into the hepatic parenchyma and eroding and obscuring the limiting plate. Periportal (piecemeal) necrosis is a characteristic feature. In some patients a more aggressive form of confluent, bridging hepatic necrosis is prominent and fibrous septa appear to isolate clusters of hepatocytes into precirrhotic nodules. Cirrhosis may be present upon initial examination in as many as one-third of patients with the severe form of chronic active hepatitis and may develop in a similar proportion during follow-up, whether or not such patients are treated with currently available regimens. In contrast, patients with the less severe forms of chronic active hepatitis (without bridging necrosis) infrequently develop cirrhosis and, in general, have a more favorable prognosis.

Identification of orcein-positive, ground-glass hepatocytes in the biopsy specimen strongly suggests that the patient has persistent HBV infection; similarly, recognition of intracytoplasmic, acidophilic PAS-positive, diastase-resistant alpha$_1$-antitrypsin globules suggests the presence of alpha$_1$-antitrypsin deficiency rather than idiopathic or viral-induced chronic active hepatitis. Identification, by immunohistologic techniques, of delta antigen in the hepatocytes of patients with HBsAg-positive chronic active hepatitis or the presence of IgG anti-delta antibody in such patients indicates that superinfection by this defective, pathogenic RNA virus may have occurred. Because the delta agent requires HBV for its expression and replication, delta infections are limited to HBsAg-positive patients. Although the severity of delta-induced liver disease appears to be variable, a rapidly progressive and fatal form of HBsAg-positive chronic active hepatitis has been described in association with delta infection, and cirrhosis may be a consequence of persistent delta infection.

Because ideal treatment for chronic active hepatitis is predicated on the etiologic agent of the disease, discussion of management will focus on the etiologic factors. All patients with chronic active hepatitis, with or without cirrhosis, should be immunized with the polyvalent pneumococcal vaccine. This may be particularly important for those patients who will receive immunosuppressive therapy.

Chronic Active Hepatitis-HBV

Between 5 and 10 percent of adults with clinically apparent acute hepatitis B will become persistent carriers of HBV and are identified by the prolonged presence (more than 6 months) of HBsAg in sera. Of this group about half are asymptomatic carriers without aminotransferase abnormalities and without histologic evidence of chronic hepatitis. In many of these individuals, markers of viral replication are absent or low, or decrease on follow-up over many years. Available longitudinal studies suggest that these individuals will not develop signs or symptoms of chronic hepatitis in the future unless superinfection with the delta agent occurs. In those in whom HBV-DNA has become integrated into the genome of the host hepatocyte, however, malignant transformation into primary hepatocellular carcinoma may occur after a variable, but generally long, latent period (several decades).

In most of these asymptomatic infections inhibitors of viral replication would appear to have little therapeutic value. Elimination of clones of hepatocytes containing HBV-DNA or which have undergone malignant transformation is the major goal. Monoclonal antibody-toxin conjugates have been studied in experimental models but therapeutic studies in man are not available. Management of HBsAG carriers is currently limited to prevention of contact transmission by vaccination of susceptible household members, prevention of delta agent superinfection by avoidance of parenteral exposure, and periodic screening for early hepatocellular carcinoma by polyclonal or monoclonal assays for alpha-fetoprotein.

In addition to the 50 percent of carriers without evidence of liver disease, about one-third of adults identified as HBsAg carriers after recognized HBV infection will have histologic evidence of chronic active hepatitis (the remaining 20% of carriers have chronic persistent hepatitis or nonspecific minor histologic lesions). Two phases of HBsAg-positive chronic active hepatitis have been identified. The initial phase is characterized by the presence in serum of markers of viral replication, i.e., HBeAg, HBV-DNA polymerase, and HBV-DNA. In the subsequent phase viral replication is dramatically reduced and HBV-DNA may be integrated into the DNA of the infected hepatocyte. Therapeutic trials have focused primarily upon HBsAg-positive patients with active viral replication. As in the case of chronic persistent and chronic lobular hepatitis, therapy of HBsAg-positive chronic active hepatitis is largely supportive.

Recent studies using monoclonal assays for HBsAg and hybridization techniques for the detection of HBV-DNA in serum and liver suggest that some HBsAg-negative patients with chronic active hepatitis also may have persistent HBV infection. Few therapeutic trials have been directed toward the use of immunosuppressive drugs, antiviral chemotherapy, immunostimulant drugs, or other agents in HBV-infected patients without HBsAg.

Immunosuppressive Therapy

Immunosuppressive treatment with prednisone (or prednisolone) with or without azathioprine appears to have little therapeutic value in HBsAg-positive chronic active hepatitis. In HBeAg-positive patients, markers of HBV replication increase in titer and seroconversion to anti-HBe positivity appears to be delayed. In patients with negative tests for both HBeAg and anti-HBe, immunosuppressive therapy may result in the reappearance of HBeAg. Abrupt discontinuation of short-term corticosteroids, resulting in "rebound immune stimulation," also has failed to have a clearly beneficial influence on the course of the disease. Despite the nearly overwhelming evidence that corticosteroid therapy has no value in the treatment of these patients, anecdotal data suggest that a few patients with severe, progressive HBsAg-positive chronic active hepatitis may receive short-term benefit from high-dose steroid therapy. Such therapy should be restricted to those patients in whom the clinical course has been inexorably downhill. Setting a time limit for the trial seems reasonable. At present there are no unequivocal means of identifying HBsAg-positive patients likely to respond. Delta agent superinfection is clearly not such a marker. In fact, because the liver injury associated with persistent delta agent infection is believed to be a consequence of a direct cytopathic effect, it is not surprising that immunosuppressive therapy with corticosteroids and azathioprine appears to have no beneficial influence on the course of the disease.

Antiviral Therapy

The use of antiviral drugs in the management of HBsAg-positive chronic active hepatitis remains experimental. Trials of human leukocyte or fibroblast interferon have revealed that such therapy may transiently reduce HBV replication and aminotransferase elevations in some patients, but that following drug withdrawal no consistent beneficial effect can be recognized. Whether interferons produced by recombinant DNA technology will have greater efficacy when used alone or in combination with other antiviral drugs remains to be determined. Combination therapy with interferon and the aqueous salt of adenine arabinoside (ARA-A), adenine arabinoside 5″ monophosphate (ARA-AMP), is currently in progress in controlled clinical trials. Despite in vitro activity as inhibitors of DNA polymerase, ARA-A and ARA-AMP appear to have a minimal or inconstant favorable influence on markers of HBV replication when used individually. Furthermore, severe neuromuscular toxicity has been reported in several patients treated with these agents. Therapy combining immune stimulation and inhibition of viral replication resulting from discontinuation of a short-course of corticosteroids followed by ARA-AMP may be more effective than either therapy alone and may reduce the frequency and severity of neuromuscular side effects.

Acyclovir appears to reduce markers of HBV replication, but a consistently beneficial effect on disease activity has yet to be described. Other antiviral agents, such as ribavirin, isoprinosine, intercalating agents such as quinacrine, and phosphonoformate analogues also have yet to be shown to have any beneficial effects. Until the results of large-scale controlled trials are available, all treatment with antiviral chemotherapy must be considered experimental.

Other Drugs

Levamisole and other agents with potential immunostimulant activity have been studied but none appears promising. Active immunization with the hepatitis B vaccine and passive immunization by infusion of anti-HBs have no beneficial effect on established HBV infection. The efficacy of transfer infection remains uncertain.

Non-A, Non-B Chronic Active Hepatitis

Chronic active hepatitis is believed to be a common sequela of non-A, non-B viral hepatitis. As many as 33 to 85 percent of patients with transfusion-associated non-

A, non-B hepatitis will have persistent aminotransferase abnormalities 6 months after the recognition of hepatitis, and the majority of these have histologic evidence of chronic active hepatitis. The frequency of progression to chronic active hepatitis appears to be lower in sporadic non-A, non-B hepatitis, and chronic persistent hepatitis may be at least as common as chronic active hepatitis in this setting. Most patients with chronic active hepatitis associated with persistent non-A, non-B viral hepatitis have a generally mild disease and many are entirely asymptomatic. Despite this benign picture as many as 10 to 15 percent may develop cirrhosis after a relatively short follow-up period of 2 to 5 years.

Treatment is supportive. Corticosteroids appear to have little, if any, efficacy, and a limited study of the antiviral agent acyclovir has failed to provide convincing evidence of clinical value.

Idiopathic Chronic Active Hepatitis

The origin of idiopathic chronic active hepatitis is multifactorial. Some patients may have previously unrecognized persistent non-A, non-B hepatitis infection and some may have HBV infection despite the absence of circulating HBsAg. Although an autoimmune-initiated form (autoimmune or lupoid hepatitis) has long been recognized as a serious, progressive disease of young women associated with HLA type B8, DRw3, fewer than 20 percent of patients with severe HBsAg-negative chronic active hepatitis have other associated autoimmune disorders. Furthermore, serologic markers of autoimmunity, such as the LE factor, antinuclear antibody, and smooth muscle antibody, are found in more than 50 percent of patients with idiopathic chronic active hepatitis. Despite the belief that autoimmune hepatitis is a form of chronic active hepatitis that is highly responsive to immunosuppressive therapy with corticosteroids, the rates of remission, treatment failure, progression to cirrhosis, death from hepatic failure, and 5-year survival are similar in HBsAG-negative patients with or without LE cells or antinuclear antibodies and in patients with or without associated autoimmune disorders. These data suggest that a corticosteroid-responsive subset of patients with autoimmune chronic active hepatitis cannot be readily identified with current markers of autoimmunity.

Immunosuppressive Therapy

Although the mortality of severe idiopathic chronic active hepatitis (severity defined by prolonged and progressive symptoms of liver disease associated with jaundice, signs of portal hypertension, and the presence of bridging necrosis or cirrhosis on liver biopsy) is high in the absence of corticosteroid therapy, cirrhosis and complications of portal hypertension may develop despite prolonged treatment with corticosteroids. The course of asymptomatic or mild forms of idiopathic chronic active hepatitis has not been shown to be influenced by such therapy.

In light of this information *corticosteroid* therapy should be reserved for patients with symptomatic disease. Therapy is initiated with a maintenance dose of 20 mg of prednisone. (There are no data supporting increased efficacy resulting from the use of a higher dose tapered to this maintenance dose.) If 20 mg is not sufficient to reduce symptoms and return the serum aminotransferases to near-normal levels within several weeks, 50 mg of *azathioprine* may be added. Azathioprine also may be useful if corticosteroid-induced side effects are prominent, since its addition may permit reduction of the prednisone dose. Whether supplemental oral calcium and vitamin D reduce the frequency of prednisone-induced bone thinning is uncertain.

Most patients require treatment for one or more years before histologic remission is likely. Alternate-day therapy has no value in achieving histologic remission. Cessation of therapy is associated with relapse in about 50 percent of patients. While a number of tests, such as serum bile acid concentration, ^{14}C-aminopyrine breath test, molar ratio of branched chain to aromatic amino acids, and antibodies to liver-specific protein, have been used to assess the probable outcome of corticosteroid withdrawal, all are imperfect prognostic indicators. For those patients who relapse on corticosteroid withdrawal a second course of therapy may reinduce remission. Overall, remission is achieved in 60 percent of patients within 3 years of beginning therapy. The 5-year survival rate of treated patients is about 90 percent. About 30 percent will develop cirrhosis during the treatment period and another 10 percent will develop cirrhosis after cessation of therapy. Despite histologic evidence of cirrhosis, clinically important complications of portal hypertension are infrequent in treated patients.

Treatment failure may be most common in patients with non-A, non-B hepatitis associated disease or in those with HBsAg-negative HBV infection. However, data to support this hypothesis are not yet available. No treatment of patients who have failed to respond to corticosteroid therapy is known to influence the course of the disease.

DRUG-INDUCED LIVER DAMAGE

MACK C. MITCHELL, M.D.

Drug-induced liver damage is becoming an increasingly common cause of both acute and chronic liver diseases. Injury may result from an idiosyncratic reaction to medication or from exposure to known hepatotoxic chemicals. Management of drug-induced liver damage requires prompt recognition of hepatic injury and elimination of exposure to the offending agent. In some instances, administration of specific agents may be useful in preventing injury or reducing its severity. One example, which will be discussed in detail later in this chapter, is acetaminophen overdose. With the majority of drugs, however, therapy for hepatotoxicity is limited to supportive treatment for the complications of resulting hepatic dysfunction.

CLASSIFICATION

Drug-induced liver damage may be classified according to the histologic features of liver injury (Table 1) or the mechanism of injury (Table 2). Both classifications are useful and are by no means mutually exclusive. Classification based on histopathology is valuable in recognition of the offending agent, since the features of injury are often characteristic for a particular hepatotoxin. For example, chlorpromazine typically causes cholestasis and periportal inflammation, whereas isoniazid most often causes centrilobular necrosis and patchy lobular inflammation. Classification by mechanism of injury is likewise helpful because it provides a rational basis for prevention and treatment of the injury.

As shown in Table 1, both acute and chronic liver diseases may result from drug hepatotoxicity. Furthermore, the length of time between exposure to the drug and development of clinical manifestations of liver disease may vary. Acute injury from exposure to intrinsic hepatotoxins, such as carbon tetrachloride, results in rapid elevation of aminotransferases and clinical signs of injury when severe. These abnormalities are usually apparent within several days of exposure.

By contrast, idiosyncratic drug hepatotoxicity almost always requires a longer period of exposure before development of damage. Adverse hepatic reactions to medications and other pharmaceuticals is more often idiosyncratic than due to intrinsic hepatotoxicity, since most drugs known to be hepatotoxic are eliminated during preclinical testing. With few exceptions, intrinsic hepatotoxins cause liver injury in animals similar to that which might occur in man, thereby preventing widespread exposure of patients to these agents. However, idiosyncratic injury may be equally severe and can result from immunologic hypersensitivity or because of metabolic abnormalities that might alter normal drug detoxification within an individual (see Table 2). Hypersensitivity reactions may involve organs other than the liver and frequently produce systemic manifestations such as fever, arthral-

TABLE 1 Classification of Drug-Induced Liver Disease by Histopathology

Type of Injury	Biochemical Abnormalities (× normal)		Examples
	Aminotransferase	Alkaline Phosphatase	
Hepatocellular			
Acute necrosis	10–500	1–2	Acetaminophen, carbon tetrachloride
Acute hepatitis	10–200	1–2	Isoniazid, alpha-methyldopa, aspirin, phenytoin
Chronic hepatitis	5–50	1–2	Isoniazid
Steatosis			
"Steatohepatitis"	5–10	1–3	Tetracycline, valproate, corticosteroids
Cholestasis	5–10	1–3	Ethanol, amiodarone, perhexiline maleate
Inflammatory	1–10	3–10	Chlorpromazine, erythromycin
Noninflammatory	1–5	1–5	Oral contraceptives, rifampicin
Granulomatous inflammation	5–25	2–10	Numerous
Vascular			
Peliosis hepatis	1–2	1–2	Anabolic steroids, oral contraceptives
Hepatic vein thrombosis	2–5	1–2	Oral contraceptives
Veno-occlusive disease	2–5	2–5	Several antineoplastic agents
Tumors			
Hepatic adenomas	Variables	1–3	Oral contraceptives
Hepatocellular carcinoma	Variables	1–3	Anabolic steroids, oral contraceptives
Angiosarcoma	Variables	1–3	Vinyl chloride

TABLE 2 Classification of Drug-Induced Liver Damage by Mechanism of Injury

Mechanism	Example
Intrinsic Toxins	
Direct	Carbon tetrachloride, arsenic
Metabolite-mediated	Acetaminophen, carbon tetrachloride, chlorpromazine
Idiosyncratic Toxins	
Hypersensitivity	Phenytoin, sulfonamides, para-aminosalicylic acid, halothane
Host idiosyncrasy metabolic	Phenytoin?, valproate, isoniazid?, halothane?

gias, and rash. Peripheral eosinophilia and granulomatous inflammation in the liver are common. These reactions usually develop within 2 weeks to 2 months after initiation of therapy but recur promptly upon rechallenge after discontinuation. Reactions due to host metabolic idiosyncrasy may require a longer exposure before clinical signs become manifest. In many instances a minor but potentially toxic metabolite of the drug is responsible for the injury. The dose of drug given, and the rate of formation and elimination of the metabolite(s) will determine the concentration of the metabolite to which the patient is ultimately exposed. For this reason, it is difficult to predict a time for onset of symptoms.

MONITORING

Since most adverse hepatic drug reactions are idiosyncratic, it is often difficult to identify which patients are at risk. However, the incidence of hepatic drug reactions appears to be higher in women, in elderly patients, and in those individuals who have a previous history of drug reactions, including nonhepatic reactions. The incidence of reactions to some agents, although idiosyncratic, may be high enough to justify periodic monitoring of liver enzymes. The anticonvulsants *phenytoin* and *sodium valproate* both may cause hepatitis in susceptible individuals. Although the occurrence of hepatitis is rare, it is serious and potentially fatal. Monitoring serum aminotransferase levels may be helpful in predicting which patients will develop serious liver injury. Not all patients with elevated aminotransferase levels develop serious hepatic necrosis, but these patients are at highest risk and thus require close supervision. A similar situation exists with *isoniazid*, which is associated with a 10 percent incidence of abnormal aminotransferase levels, but only a 1 percent incidence of serious toxicity. *Nonsteroidal antiinflammatory drugs, antidepressants*, and *antiarrhythmics* are other categories of drugs for which periodic monitoring of aminotransferases may be indicated. Patients given medications known to cause hepatotoxicity should be alerted to report any symptoms of hepatitis, such as anorexia, nausea, abdominal pain, jaundice, or dark urine, to their physician immediately.

When confronted with an asymptomatic patient in whom liver enzymes have become abnormal, the physician must decide whether the suspected drug is necessary and whether another compound might be equally effective. If the medication is the only effective therapy for a patient's illness, such as life-threatening arrhythmia, the drug could be continued with careful monitoring of enzymes. In these instances liver biopsy may help to determine the severity of liver damage. If the patient develops symptoms of hepatitis, hypersensitivity, or jaundice, the drug should be stopped. Continuing therapy in a symptomatic patient with hepatitis is hazardous.

A more difficult problem is determining whether abnormal liver enzymes are drug-related or are related to another condition, such as non-A, non-B viral hepatitis. Assuming that no other cause for liver disease is found in a patient with hepatitis, discontinuation of the presumed offending agent usually results in improvement, although not necessarily complete resolution, in symptoms and liver enzymes within 2 weeks. There are exceptions to this general rule, but failure to improve in this time suggests an alternative cause for liver disease. Rechallenge is often carried out in an attempt to determine whether the presumed agent was responsible for the liver disease. There is always a risk involved in rechallenge, and it is probably greatest for those drugs that cause allergic hypersensitivity. For example, fatal hepatic necrosis may occur after only the second administration or "rechallenge" with halothane. Rechallenge does not always produce prompt increases in aminotransferases or recurrence of symptoms. For some drugs that are hepatotoxic because of metabolic idiosyncrasy, several weeks or months may be required before recurrence becomes apparent. Whenever rechallenge is carried out, the physician should be prepared for an exaggerated response to readministration of the drug. Hospitalization is advisable in most instances. For these reasons, I do not believe that rechallenge is necessary in the majority of patients with suspected drug-induced liver damage.

TREATMENT

In cases of suspected drug hepatotoxicity, *discontinuation* of the presumed offending agent is the first step in treatment. Asymptomatic patients do not usually require hospitalization, but careful follow-up must be ensured. Occasionally patients will continue to self-administer medications which they believe to be beneficial for a medical problem other than liver disease. If the patient does not have symptoms of liver disease, he may not recognize the potential danger in continuing therapy. The physician must be alert to such a possibility and instruct the patient carefully. Patients with jaundice or other symptoms of liver injury require more thorough evaluation. Prolongation of the prothrombin time and/or development of hepatic encephalopathy are poor prognostic signs. Liver biopsy, when possible, is helpful in determining the severity of injury as well as the histologic pattern of damage.

In patients with fulminant hepatic failure, supportive care and close monitoring in an intensive care unit is indicated. These patients may require vasopressor therapy for hypotension, administration of intravenous dextrose solutions to prevent hypoglycemia, fresh frozen plasma for active bleeding, and judicious management of fluids and electrolyte balance. The routine use of cimetidine as prophylaxis against gastrointestinal bleeding should be avoided, since cimetidine may interfere with metabolism and elimination of some drugs. Lactulose may be indicated for encephalopathy and mannitol may be helpful in patients with cerebral edema.

Corticosteroid therapy does not directly alter the cause of fulminant hepatic failure and should not be used routinely. In patients with fever, skin rash, or other signs of allergic hypersensitivity, however, steroids may attenuate the exaggerated immune response and further reduce hepatic injury that is immunologic rather than due to direct toxic effects of the drug. For example, steroids may be beneficial in patients with phenytoin or halothane hepatitis, both of which involve allergic hypersensitivity.

Charcoal or *resin hemoperfusion* has been used successfully in some patients to increase the rate of elimination of highly lipid–soluble drugs with a long half-life. Experience with these techniques is limited and both may cause complications, such as thrombocytopenia. Hemodialysis is seldom necessary, except for associated renal failure, since most drugs that can be easily eliminated with this technique have short half-lives.

These recommendations are general measures that apply primarily to management of patients with idiosyncratic drug-induced liver damage. A few drugs and unusual lesions associated with drug injury merit special attention.

Acetaminophen Poisoning

Acetaminophen is becoming the most widely used analgesic in Western countries. In general, the drug has a wide therapeutic index with toxicity occurring at doses more than ten times the usual therapeutic dose of 1 g every 4 hours. In some individuals, particularly alcoholics, this therapeutic index may be narrower for reasons discussed below. Fulminant hepatic failure and death may occur in individuals after massive overdoses of this drug. Acetaminophen hepatotoxicity develops because of excessive formation of a highly reactive electrophilic metabolite which is formed by a minor metabolic pathway of elimination, cytochrome P-450 mediated oxidation. Usually this reactive metabolite is further detoxified by hepatic glutathione; however, after massive overdose, glutathione is depleted, allowing the reactive metabolite to damage cellular macromolecules. Long-term heavy alcohol consumption or use of phenobarbital causes induction of cytochrome P-450 and enhances the formation of the toxic metabolite of acetaminophen.

Symptoms of acetaminophen hepatotoxicity usually appear after 24 hours, often resulting in delay in the patient seeking medical attention. The clinical course of hepatotoxicity is outlined in Table 3. Symptoms of liver failure usually begin after 48 to 72 hours. Patients with bilirubin levels over 4 mg per deciliter and prolongation of prothrombin time more than two and a half times that of controls are at highest risk for serious liver damage.

The key to management of acetaminophen overdose is prompt recognition and initiation of treatment. If the patient is seen 24 or more hours after ingestion, therapy is supportive only. Less than 12 to 18 hours after ingestion, specific treatment with N-acetylcysteine (Mucomyst) can prevent or reduce the severity of liver damage. Treatment may be initiated up to 24 hours after poisoning but is most effective when given early. For oral administration, the recommended dose is 140 mg per kilogram mixed in juice or soft drinks to disguise the unpleasant taste and odor. Repeat doses of 70 mg per kilogram should be given at 4-hour intervals for a total of 72 hours. N-acetylcysteine can also be given by gavage. If the patient vomits within 1 hour the dose should be repeated. In Europe intravenous therapy has been used: 150 mg per kilogram in 200 ml of 5 percent dextrose over 15 minutes, followed by 50 mg per kilogram over the next 4 hours, and 100 mg per kilogram over the following 16 hours. Both routes of administration are effective, although at present an intravenous formulation is not available in the United States. If signs of liver failure develop, additional doses should be withheld to prevent worsening of hepatic encephalopathy.

Liver Disease Associated with Oral Contraceptives

A variety of liver diseases, including intrahepatic cholestasis, hepatic tumors, Budd-Chiari syndrome, and peliosis hepatis (blood-filled "lakes"), have occurred in

TABLE 3 Clinical Course of Acetaminophen Hepatotoxicity

Time After Ingestion	Signs and Symptoms	Laboratory Studies
1–8 hr	Nausea, vomiting, anorexia	Normal
24–48 hr	Nausea, vomiting, anorexia, right upper quadrant pain	Aspartate aminotransferase and prothrombin time
48 hr	Jaundice	Aspartate aminotransferase and prothrombin time, bilirubin
72 hr		Peak of all tests
4–6 days	Encephalopathy, coma, death	

patients taking oral contraceptives. Intrahepatic cholestasis is usually mild and always responds to discontinuation of the pill. There may be a higher frequency of this lesion in women with a history of jaundice during the third trimester of pregnancy. Hepatic adenomas and hepatocellular carcinoma also occur, although the incidence is low. Hepatocellular carcinoma should be resected, if possible, as medical and radiation therapy are mostly palliative. Although hepatic adenomas may regress after withdrawal of the drug, the propensity of this tumor to bleed massively into the peritoneal cavity suggests that surgical resection is advisable.

Budd-Chiari syndrome and peliosis hepatis are both vascular lesions associated with oral contraceptive use. Peliosis may rupture and bleed into the peritoneum. Surgical treatment is recommended only if there is hemoperitoneum. Otherwise, the drug should be withdrawn and the patient followed conservatively. *Budd-Chiari syndrome* is a dramatic illness characterized by abdominal pain, hepatomegaly, and ascites. Although the outlook for these patients is usually poor with only medical management, one recent report suggests the prognosis may be better in those women who develop Budd-Chiari syndrome while taking oral contraceptives. In patients in whom there is complete occlusion of both hepatic veins, either side-to-side portocaval or mesocaval shunting is indicated to relieve the severe outflow obstruction and prevent further loss of hepatocytes. With associated thrombosis of the vena cava, mesoatrial shunting is the preferred operation. In cases in which only one vein is obstructed, a trial of medical therapy is permissible although surgery may ultimately be needed.

Liver Disease Associated with Anabolic Steroids

Anabolic steroids, particularly methyltestosterone, are widely used by weight lifters and some other athletes. Although the incidence of liver disease in these individuals is low, peliosis hepatis, hepatocellular carcinoma, and angiosarcoma have been reported. Treatment for peliosis is withdrawal of the drug. Hepatocellular carcinoma should be resected, if possible. Angiosarcoma has a dismal prognosis and is not amenable to any therapy.

Occupational Liver Disease

Since discontinuation of the widespread open use of carbon tetrachloride in dry cleaning and other industries, the incidence of documented hepatotoxicity through occupational exposure has diminished. Nonetheless, there are still many potentially hepatotoxic organic compounds to which workers are exposed which may cause liver damage. Haloalkanes (tetrachlorethane, trichloroethane, and TNT), arsenic, beryllium, and vinyl chloride all cause liver damage or hepatic tumors or both. Pesticides, particularly chlordecone (Kepone), may cause damage to liver and other organs. The herbicides paraquat and diquat have been reported to cause hepatic necrosis, although pulmonary damage is more commonly seen. Prevention of exposure to these potentially hazardous compounds is vital, since there is no specific treatment for hepatotoxicity once it has occurred.

LIVER TRANSPLANTATION: GASTROENTEROLOGIC CONSIDERATIONS

DAVID H. VAN THIEL, M.D.
MARK APPLER, M.D.
DAVID SCHREIBER, M.D.
JEFFERY GRAY, M.D.
RENE PELEMAN, M.D.
BYRON DeLEMOS, M.D.
WILLIAM PETERSON, M.D.

Orthotopic liver transplantation is a heroic surgical procedure that enables patients with otherwise hopelessly advanced liver disease an opportunity for a meaningful life. Although liver transplantation certainly is an immediate surgical problem, pediatricians, gastroenterologists, and hepatologists must be crucially involved in the decision to perform the procedure (identify candidates) and in confirming the diagnosis in patients selected for the procedure. They must be knowledgeable as to the types of medical problems that occur as a consequence of the transplantation procedure and the putative requirement for lifelong immunosuppression. They must also be aware of and help with the psychosocial adjustments that occur in patients and their parents following successful transplantation. It is the purpose of this chapter to clarify these unique issues for the practicing physician.

WHO ARE CANDIDATES FOR ORTHOTOPIC LIVER TRANSPLANTATION?

As the surgical success achieved with orthotopic liver transplantation increases, the indications for the procedure will be expanded and made progressively less restrictive. Thus, the following discussion can be used only as a guide for future decision-making concerning the candidacy of a given patient for orthotopic liver transplantation and must be viewed in terms of the time frame during which it was prepared. With this important disclaimer in mind, as of mid-1985, candidates for liver transplantation can be classified as having one of three major indications for the procedure. These are, in order of their frequency: (1) advanced chronic liver disease; (2) hepatobiliary malignancy; and (3) fulminant hepatic failure.

Advanced Chronic Liver Disease

Multiple algorithms have been developed to identify those individuals with advanced chronic liver disease who are likely to die in 6 months to a year. Unfortunately, none of these algorithms is foolproof. Moreover, some apply only to a specific type of liver disease while others have not yet been validated. Therefore, we have identified the following easily determined criteria for selecting candidates for orthotopic liver transplantation among those with chronic advanced liver disease. Legitimate transplant candidates should have two of the following four identifying factors: (1) a serum bilirubin greater or equal to 12 mg per deciliter; (2) a serum albumin less than or equal to 2.5 g per deciliter; (3) prothrombin time greater or equal to 5 seconds above control; or (4) hepatic encephalopathy that limits the individual to being home- or hospital-bound and requiring nearly constant care despite the maximal use of available medical treatment.

Legitimate candidates with *cholestatic liver diseases of childhood*, such as biliary atresia, Alagille's syndrome, and other biliary hypoplasia syndromes, and adults with *primary biliary cirrhosis* and *primary sclerosing cholangitis* will have bilirubin levels greater than 12 mg per deciliter and usually serum albumin levels less than or equal to 2.5 g per deciliter. In contrast, patients with primarily *hepatocellular* disease, such as *alpha-1-antitrypsin deficiency, postnecrotic cirrhosis, chronic active hepatitis,* and *cryptogenic cirrhosis,* will usually have a prothrombin time greater or equal to 5 seconds above control and hepatic encephalopathy. Many of the latter patients will also have an albumin level less than or equal to 2.5 g per deciliter.

There are unusual exceptions to these simple guidelines which should suggest that transplantation be offered earlier than otherwise indicated by the above criteria. These are (1) the presence of severe incapacitating bone pain or spontaneous fractures in patients with cholestatic liver disease; (2) pruritus—again in patients with cholestatic liver disease—that is severe enough to cause the individual to have suicidal ideation; (3) indications for consideration of a portocaval shunt procedure; (4) the presence of a small hepatocellular carcinoma in an established chronic liver disease detected on the basis of a positive alpha-fetoprotein determination or other technique, such as computed tomographic (CT) scanning or sonography; and (5) recurring episodes of spontaneous bacterial peritonitis. The presence of any one of these problems should cause the physician to suggest early rather than delayed transplantation for a given patient.

Hepatobiliary Malignancy

Patients with hepatobiliary carcinoma are those who have a neoplastic lesion which is confined solely to the liver but which is not resectable because of coexistent cirrhosis, large size of the lesion, or unique location in or involving the porta hepatitis. All available techniques, including CT scanning, sonography, chest roentgenography, laparoscopy, and tomography, must be used in these patients to detect the presence of occult metastases, as such lesions prohibit successful transplantation and appear to become more aggressive following the immunosuppressive therapy administered to patients after successful transplantation to prevent graft rejection.

Despite its small size, central location, and apparent slow course, cholangiolar carcinoma has been a universally poor indication for liver transplantation. In all our cases to date, recurrent aggressive cholangiolar carcinoma has become apparent within a year of transplantation and has led to the patient's death. Fortunately, such tumors are rare in the pediatric population. In contrast, one-third of the patients with hepatocellular carcinoma who have received transplants appear to be "cured" following successful transplantation, while the remaining two-thirds tend to have one or more years of clinical remission prior to developing recurrent clinical disease. Thus, although the short-term prognosis for such candidates is good as compared with that following other treatment modalities, the long-term prognosis for these patients must continue to be quite guarded.

The patients with hepatocellular carcinoma who have the best prognosis after orthotopic hepatic transplantation are those who have either an incidental carcinoma in an otherwise advanced chronic liver disease or a metabolic liver disease such as alpha$_1$-antitrypsin disease, glycogen storage disease, or tyrosinemia (either of which is the primary indication for the transplant procedure); or a fibrolamellar carcinoma. The latter patients are preferred transplant candidates, since their tumors clinically appear to grow slowly and are frequently cured by surgical removal.

Fulminant Hepatic Failure

Fulminant hepatic failure is an *evolving* indication for orthotopic hepatic transplantation. Fulminant hepatic failure initially would appear to be a superior indication for transplantation because of the uniform poor prognosis (80 to 90% death rate) in patients treated either medically or with operations other than orthotopic liver transplantation. The major problem restricting the more general application of orthotopic liver transplantation for this indication is the late referral of such patients to transplant centers.

Patients with fulminant hepatic failure should be referred early, well before they are in coma. Certainly, many such patients not in coma at the time of referral will not require transplantation, but, if one waits until these critically ill patients are comatose before transferring them, the logistic problems experienced by the transplant team are considerable and usually predict failure. In caring for such patients, particular attention must be given to the prevention of brain stem herniation, hypoglycemia, and bleeding at the sites of the numerous intravenous and endotracheal intubations required by the patient prior to transfer to the transplant center.

In addition, the risk of recurrent disease following transplantation in this group of patients, comprised in large measure of those with fulminant viral hepatitis, is substantial indeed. The single most important factor that limits the application of liver transplantation for this indication, however, is the urgency with which it must be applied once the patient becomes comatose at the transplant center. The speed with which these patients die unless they receive a transplant requires that an appropriate donor be identified rapidly, usually within hours, or within a maximum of 1 or 2 days.

WHO ARE NOT CANDIDATES FOR THE PROCEDURE?

In addition to recognizing the characteristics of good candidates for the procedure, physicians should also be cognizant of the factors that either prohibit consideration or enhance the risks experienced by a candidate subjected to liver transplantation. For example, a prior surgical portal venous shunt procedure or portal venous thrombosis enhances the intraoperative risk of death by approximately 10 to 15 percent. Other prior operations in the right upper quadrant, such as biliary tract reconstruction procedures or a complicated gastric or pancreatic operation also increase the difficulty of the recipient hepatectomy and make the transplant procedure more dangerous and costly in terms of operative blood loss and risk of postoperative abdominal infection.

Medical problems such as primary cardiorespiratory disease (a limited cardiac output or hypoxemia) also increase the risk experienced by the recipient and are relative, if not absolute, contraindications to the procedure.

The presence of extrahepatic biliary sepsis or clinically active cancer is an absolute contraindication to the procedure. Should such sepsis be eliminated, however, the patient can be reconsidered for the procedure. Similarly, the presence of intrinsic hepatic or biliary sepsis is a relative but not absolute contraindication to the procedure, and in fact may be the primary reason for considering transplantation in a given subject. Nonetheless, it increases the risks of postoperative sepsis, abscess formation, and the need for subsequent surgical procedures to control sepsis or anastomosis breakdown.

The presence of HBsAg positivity plus HBe-antigen positivity has been considered to be an absolute contraindication to the procedure, since infection of the donor organ is to be expected in the immediate postoperative period. In our experience, in each such case the donor organ has been infected and an episode of acute type B hepatitis has occurred. In two of five such patients, recurrent chronic liver disease supervened within 1 year. Thus, we do not consider such patients candidates for the procedure except under research protocols attempting to prevent infection of the donor organ. Trials of interferon during and immediately after the transplant operation, use of specific antiviral drugs yet to be developed, and current use of massive doses of HB1G intraoperatively and during the postoperative period would appear to be indicated.

THE PERIOPERATIVE PERIOD FOLLOWING THE TRANSPLANT PROCEDURE

The perioperative period lasts from operation through the sixth postoperative week. During the immediate postoperative period the physician serves primarily as a consultant by providing information to the operating surgeon as to when a given patient should be dialyzed, what diagnostic procedures are most likely to yield a specific diagnosis should an untoward course be followed, and the choice of drugs to be used for a given patient for the treatment of infection, seizures, and hypertension.

Problems occurring in the first 2 to 3 days are usually technical and require immediate surgical attention or early retransplantation. They include hepatic artery or portal vein thrombosis or a biliary tract obstruction, dehiscence, or leak. These problems are best evaluated using ultrasonic methods, xenon-CT scanning techniques, and cholangiography or a HIDA scan, depending upon the type of problem suspected and the type of biliary drainage procedure used at the time of transplant surgery.

After the first postoperative week, the major concerns for transplant recipients are *rejection* and/or increasing *renal dysfunction* due to the antibiotics and cyclosporin they are receiving. The latter problem can be particularly difficult, since it occurs as a consequence of treating rejection and is exacerbated by the antibiotics the patient may be receiving in an effort to control infection. By maintaining hydration and an adequate salt intake during the second to third postoperative weeks, the physician serves both the patient and the surgeon and can either reduce or avoid cyclosporin nephrotoxicity, which is otherwise quite common during this period.

During the late second and early third through fourth postoperative weeks, the major goal is to treat and control the rejection process. This should be accomplished by using the least amount of immunosuppressive drug possible (both cyclosporin and prednisone) and by avoiding the excessive use of bolus steroids or steroid recycling episodes. Keen attention to the latter issue will result in a reduction in the number of viral and fungal infections seen in the transplant patient during this critical period. Should such infections occur, however, the physician should make every attempt to identify the specific pathogens responsible and treat them with the most appropriate therapy (amphotericin or acyclovir). The use of drugs that are of no benefit to the patient (such as acyclovir for cytomegalovirus or Epstein-Barr virus infections) but may react adversely with other drugs or produce their own intrinsic toxicity must be avoided.

Late in the fourth through sixth postoperative weeks, fever is likely to be due either to an abscess in or about the operative site (liver/biliary tree) or to a pancreatic pseudocyst, or to be drug related. Sonographic and CT techniques can be used to identify abscesses (fluid collections) and have been more successful in our hands than have been the various nuclear medicine techniques using either gallium or radiolabeled white blood cells.

During this same time period the patient will require education concerning the need for lifelong monitoring of his cyclosporin levels, recognition of putative rejection episodes, and attention to the many adjustment problems related to returning to a life outside the hospital without hepatic failure: sibling rivalry for parental attention, attending school, and competing with other children on an equal basis or returning to work. The latter problem can be a difficult one for the patients who have had a prolonged, debilitating course prior to their transplant procedure. They and their families will need frequent reassurance and encouragement to accept responsibility and independence for the patient. This transition is best accomplished using a team approach, with the gradual transfer of care from the physicians and surgeons to nurses and nurse practitioners in an outpatient setting, and finally to the family and individual patient.

THE FOLLOW-UP PERIOD

After discharge from the hospital, which usually occurs at 6 weeks, patients are followed for an additional 6 weeks as outpatients while the transfer of responsibility occurs. From this point the physician's responsibility consists primarily of monitoring cyclosporin dosage, compliance, and toxicity, and recognizing rejection or late infection episodes.

The particular problems that occur with cyclosporin use and that must be watched for are tremor and dysesthesias, nephrotoxicity, hypertension, gingival hyperplasia, and the polyglandular hyperplasia syndrome (pseudolymphoma). Each of these problems responds to a reduction in immunotherapy and should be recognized early and managed with a reduction in immunotherapy if at all possible. The goal of immunotherapy during this period is to use the least amount of drug that maintains graft function and prevents graft rejection.

PRIMARY BILIARY CIRRHOSIS

JOHN H. HELZBERG, M.D.
JAMES L. BOYER, M.D.

Primary biliary cirrhosis (PBC) is a chronic cholestatic liver disease of unknown cause. It is characterized histologically by inflammatory destruction of the intrahepatic bile ducts with frequent progression to periportal fibrosis, bridging necrosis, and biliary cirrhosis. Epidemiologic studies in England and Sweden have estimated the point prevalence of the disease to be 54 and 92 per million population, respectively. The classic symptoms of PBC are fatigue, pruritus, and jaundice in a middle-aged woman. The disease is often suspected, however, in an asymptomatic patient with unexplained hepatomegaly or an elevated alkaline phosphatase level. The diagnosis is confirmed by characteristic liver biopsy findings and the presence in the serum of an antimitochondrial antibody.

Long-term follow-up studies in the past have suggested a mean survival time of between 5 and 12 years from the diagnosis of PBC. Patients presenting with asymptomatic PBC, however, have life expectancies that do not differ from age- and sex-matched controls, as determined from epidemiologic studies from the United States, Great Britain, and Sweden (Fig. 1, 2)[1,2,3,4] Therefore, treatment of asymptomatic patients with PBC using anything other than innocuous means is difficult to justify.

EPIDEMIOLOGY AND ETIOLOGY

Primary biliary cirrhosis occurs worldwide and in all races. Approximately 90 percent of cases occur in middle-aged women. Annual incidences of 5.8 and 13.7 cases per million population were reported in recent studies from Britain and Sweden, respectively.[2,3] The etiologic agent of PBC is unknown but several agents have been postulated, including hepatotropic viruses and fungi, hepatotoxic medications, environmental toxins, and toxic bile acids. Genetically determined factors may play a role in the expression of the disease and occasionally more than one family member is affected. Host susceptibility may also be influenced by hormones as demonstrated by the predominance of PBC in women. The disorder is characterized histologically by a nonsuppurative cholangitis and infiltrate of plasma cells and lymphocytes suggesting an immunologic mechanism for its pathogenesis. Many of the clinical and histologic features resemble a graft versus host disorder.

CLINICAL FEATURES

The most frequent presenting symptoms of PBC are malaise and fatigue, pruritus, and jaundice. Hyperpigmentation, xanthomas, portal hypertension, abdominal pain, anorexia, weight loss, amenorrhea, bone pain, easy bruising, and nausea and vomiting occur less commonly. Hepatomegaly is found in three-quarters of symptomatic patients and half of asymptomatic patients on initial presentation.

Virtually all patients with PBC have abnormal biochemical hepatic studies that demonstrate a cholestatic rather than hepatocellular pattern. Serum alkaline phosphatase and bile acids are elevated in more than 95 percent of patients. The alkaline phosphatase is hepatobiliary in origin as shown by simultaneous elevations of serum 5'-nucleotidase and gamma glutamyl transpeptidase.

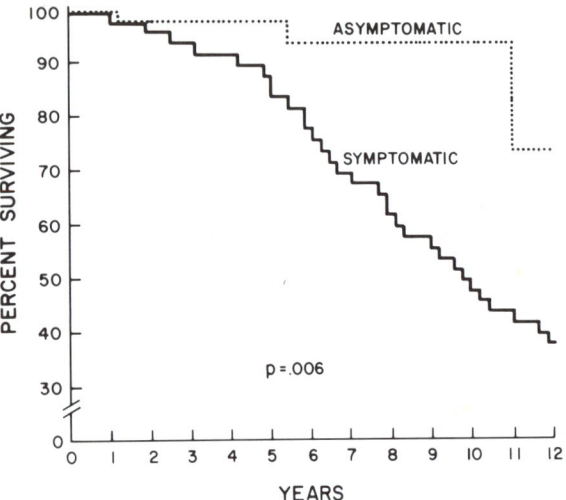

Figure 1 The survival time for 37 asymptomatic patients was significantly longer than for 243 symptomatic patients. Survival was calculated according to the Kaplan-Meier method. Year 0 denotes the date of onset of symptoms of primary biliary cirrhosis.

Transaminase elevations are usually present but are generally less than four times normal levels. Total serum cholesterol is raised in approximately 50 percent of cases and values are higher in symptomatic patients. Serum bilirubin levels vary with the stage of the disease and have prognostic importance. Elevations of serum bilirubin are seen in 50 percent of patients at the time of initial presentation. Elevated serum IgM levels occur in 90 percent of patients with PBC, and this disproportionate increase in IgM distinguishes PBC from the hypergammaglobulinemia seen in most other chronic liver diseases.

DIAGNOSIS

The most important laboratory study in the diagnosis of PBC is the *antimitochondrial antibody*. It does not, however, appear to be related to the pathogenesis of the disease, since the titer of antimitochondrial antibody does not correlate with clinical or histologic disease severity or prognosis and is not tissue- or species-specific. Between 1 and 19 percent of patients with PBC have negative tests for the antimitochondrial antibody. This antibody is not specific for PBC and can be seen in some patients with chronic active hepatitis and collagen vascular diseases. Several types of antimitochondrial antibodies have been described. Most often, patients with PBC have antibodies that react only with antigens from the inner mitochondrial membrane, whereas patients with chronic active hepatitis have antibodies that react with antigens from both the inner and outer mitochondrial membranes.[5] Nonetheless, the absence of antimitochondrial antibody in a patient with cholestasis should alert the physician to consider other diagnoses.

The presence of florid, nonsuppurative, inflammatory destruction of the intrahepatic bile ducts is characteristic of PBC but unfortunately is usually seen only in the early histologic stages (stage 1 or 2). Stage 1 PBC is characterized by a nonsuppurative destructive cholangitis with expansion of the portal tracts with mononuclear cells, lymphocytes, and plasma cells. Stage 2 PBC is defined by proliferation of bile ductules within the portal tracts. Stage 3 disease is characterized by the presence of fibrous septa extending from the portal triads. Stage 4 represents a frank histologic cirrhosis. The presence of granulomas in the liver biopsy is associated with a better clinical prognosis.[4,6] Granulomas are found more frequently in liver biopsy specimens from patients with stage 1 and 2 disease.

In patients in whom PBC is suspected but who do not have a pathognomonic liver biopsy and a positive antimitochondrial antibody, cholangiography is necessary to assess patency of the intrahepatic and extrahepatic biliary ducts. This can be achieved either with endoscopic retrograde cholangiopancreatography or percutaneous transhepatic cholangiography. An adequate cholangiogram will exclude sclerosing cholangitis, choledocholithiasis, and pancreatic or ampullary cancer, which must be considered in the differential diagnosis of PBC and other chronic cholestatic liver diseases.

ASSOCIATED DISEASES

Up to 17 percent of patients with PBC have associated progressive systemic sclerosis. The most frequent in-

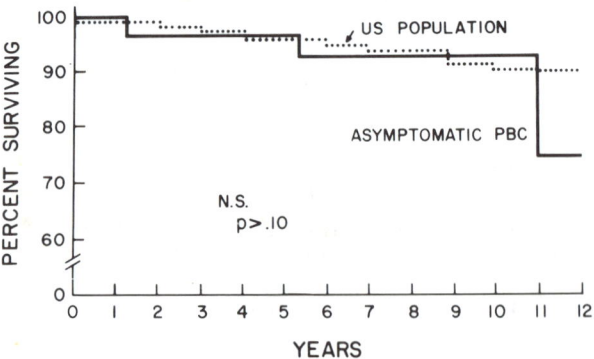

Figure 2 No difference in survival time was found between asymptomatic patients with primary biliary cirrhosis and age-matched and sex-matched controls from the United States population. Year 0 denotes the date of diagnosis of primary biliary cirrhosis in asymptomatic patients. (Reproduced with permission from Roll J, Boyer JL, Barry D, Klatskin G. The prognostic importance of clinical and histologic features in asymptomatic and symptomatic primary biliary cirrhosis. N Engl J Med 1983; 308:1–7.)

volvement includes esophageal dysmotility, decreased carbon monoxide diffusion capacity in the lung, Raynaud's phenomenon, and sclerodactyly. Raynaud's phenomenon, sclerodactyly, and telangiectasia) may be found and is characterized by the presence of anticentromere antinuclear antibodies.[7] Polymyositis and scleroderma can occur simultaneously in patients with PBC, implying an association with mixed connective tissue disease. The association of PBC and systemic sclerosis appears to be related to the presence of PBC, since scleroderma patients do not have an increased prevalence of liver disease over matched controls.

The sicca complex of keratoconjunctivitis sicca and xerostomia is commonly associated with PBC. More than one-quarter of patients with PBC will have Sjögren's syndrome as defined by an abnormal Schirmer's test of lacrimation. Symptomatic disease is less frequent, however. An antinuclear antibody fluorescence pattern of multiple large dots has recently been described in association with the sicca syndrome and PBC and can be demonstrated as a specific antinuclear antibody when using human hepatoma cell (HEP-2) culture line substrates.[8,9]

Other diseases associated with PBC include autoimmune thyroiditis, seronegative arthritis, and renal tubular acidosis, usually type 1. Xanthomatous neuropathy is fortunately rare and only seen in patients with severe hypercholesterolemia. Plasmapheresis is usually indicated for this often incapacitating disorder, as therapy with cholestyramine is generally ineffective.

PROGNOSIS

The mean survival for patients presenting with symptomatic pruritus and jaundice is generally less than eight years but has ranged from 5.5 to 11.9 years in various studies. In contrast to this dismal outcome in symptomatic patients, the prognosis of patients with asymptomatic PBC is excellent and does not differ from that of age- and sex-matched controls in follow-up periods of 10 to 13 years (Figs. 1 and 2). In addition, only 40 percent of asymptomatic patients appear to develop symptomatic PBC. Multivariate analysis of clinical and histologic features has revealed that at the onset of disease, age, hepatomegaly, elevated serum bilirubin, and bridging fibrosis or cirrhosis on liver biopsy are independent risk factors of a poor prognosis. Early detection of disease cannot be invoked to explain the benign course in asymptomatic patients, as the average age at diagnosis of symptom-free patients is the same or higher than that of symptomatic patients.[1]

TREATMENT

There is no specific treatment for PBC that alters morbidity or improves survival. Consequently, therapy is generally directed toward the symptoms of pruritus, osteodystrophy, fat malabsorption, hypercholesterolemia, and portal hypertension. Corticosteroids, azathioprine, chlorambucil, cyclosporin, colchicine, and D-penicillamine have been used in an attempt to halt disease progression but are without proven benefit. D-Penicillamine has been extensively studied at the Royal Free Hospital, the Mayo Clinic, and the New England Medical Center. The rationale for its use includes reduction of the extensive hepatic copper accumulation seen in PBC, depression of the inflammatory response, and prevention of cross-linkage of collagen. Although preliminary reports suggested biochemical improvement and possible impedance of histologic disease progression, no increase in mean survival has been demonstrated in later studies. D-Penicillamine has potential severe side effects, including dermatitis, proteinuria, and bone marrow suppression, and its use cannot be advocated except in randomized trials.[10] Unfortunately, orthotopic liver transplantation remains the only definitive treatment for PBC. It is recommended, however, only for end-stage disease, as the mortality one year after transplantation is approximately 50 percent. Therapy for asymptomatic patients with PBC is not indicated because of their excellent overall prognosis.[1,4]

Pruritus in PBC is common and can be disabling. It is usually generalized, though most severe on the palms and soles. The cause of pruritus is not known, but it has been attributed by some to the accumulation of bile salts in the skin. *Cholestyramine* is the most effective agent to control pruritus and is usually administered in doses of 4 g, or one packet, three to four times a day, 20 minutes before meals and on awakening in the morning. This takes advantage of meal-stimulated gallbladder discharge of bile. Cholestyramine is an ionic resin that nonspecifically binds bile acids and other potential pruritogens in the small intestine. Unfortunately, cholestyramine is expensive, can interfere with the absorption of other medications, and often causes constipation, abdominal discomfort, nausea, and flatulence. Its unpleasant taste and consistency can be minimized by mixing the drug with applesauce or fruit juice. Fat malabsorption can be worsened by cholestyramine and necessitates supplementation of the fat-soluble vitamins in patients with PBC.

For patients who continue to itch with cholestyramine or are intolerant of the side effects, *phenobarbital*, in divided doses of 2 to 4 mg per kilogram per day in the morning and at bedtime, may be beneficial. Phenobarbital increases hepatic bile secretion but has disturbing addictive and sedative effects. Antihistaminic drugs such as hydroxyzine are usually of limited usefulness.

Severe hypercholesterolemia, xanthomatous neuropathy, and cosmetically unattractive xanthomas can also be treated with 12 to 16 g per day of cholestyramine. Plasmapheresis is occasionally used for refractory cases.

Hepatic osteodystrophy is a severe complication of longstanding cholestasis from PBC. Its origin is multifactorial and related to malabsorption of calcium and vitamin D as a consequence of steatorrhea. Moreover, many patients with PBC are postmenopausal. Bone pain and spontaneous fractures from osteoporosis or osteomalacia are unfortunately common. Patients with PBC should be encouraged to ingest 1 g of elemental *calcium* daily, usually through oral calcium supplements. *Vitamin D sup-*

plementation is also indicated with 50,000 units per day of water-soluble vitamin D_2 (ergocalciferol) or 50 μg per day of 25-hydroxyvitamin D_3 (calcifediol). Blood and urine calcium levels should be monitored frequently to prevent toxicity. The efficacy of vitamin D supplementation can be assesed by measuring serum 25-hydroxyvitamin D_3 or 1,25-hydroxyvitamin D_3 levels.

Ineffective micelle formation from impaired hepatic secretion of bile acids can lead to fat malabsorption in patients with PBC. If clinically significant steatorrhea develops with abdominal bloating and diarrhea, fat ingestion can be restricted to approximately 40 g per day. Caloric supplementation can then be added if indicated with medium-chain triglyceride oil.

Deficiencies of the fat-soluble vitamins A, D, E, and K can develop. Water-miscible vitamin A in doses of 25,000 units per day is generally administered to patients with symptomatic PBC to prevent vitamin A deficiency. Unfortunately, oral vitamin K supplementation is usually ineffective, and it is therefore recommended that 10 mg of *vitamin K* (phytonadione) be given subcutaneously or intramuscularly at monthly intervals. Supplementation with vitamin E is controversial, as no clinical syndromes are known to result in adults, as opposed to children, from vitamin E deficiency.

REFERENCES

1. Roll J, Boyer JL, Barry P, Klatskin G. The prognostic importance of clinical and histologic features in asymptomatic and symptomatic primary biliary cirrhosis. N Engl J Med 1983; 308:1–7.
2. James O, Macklon AF, Watson AJ. Primary biliary cirrhosis—a revised clinical spectrum. Lancet 1981; 1:1278–1281
3. Eriksson S, Lindgren S. The prevalence and clinical spectrum of primary biliary cirrhosis in a defined population. Scand J Gastroenterol 1984; 19:971–976.
4. Beswick DR, Klatskin G, Boyer JL. Asymptomatic primary biliary cirrhosis: a progress report on long-term follow-up and natural history. Gastroenterology 1985; 89:267–271.
5. Berg PA, Baum H. Serology of primary biliary cirrhosis. Semin Immunopath 1980; 3:355–373.
6. Lee RG, Epstein O, Jauregui H, et al. Granulomas in primary biliary cirrhosis: a prognostic feature. Gastroenterol 1981; 81:983–986.
7. Powell F, Winkelman RK, Venencie-Lemarchand F, et al. The anticentromere antibody: disease specificity and clinical significance. Mayo Clin Proc 1984; 59:700–706.
8. Bernstein RM. Antinuclear antibodies in primary biliary cirrhosis. Lancet 1984; 1:508.
9. Powell F, Schroetter AL, Dickson ER. Antinuclear antibodies in primary biliary cirrhosis. Lancet 1984; 1:288–289.
10. Dickson ER, Fleming CR, Ludwig J. Primary biliary cirrhosis. In: Popper H, Schaffner F, eds. Progress in liver diseases. Vol VI. New York: Grune and Stratton, 1979; 487.

CHOLESTASIS AND SCLEROSING CHOLANGITIS

JOHN GREGORY FITZ, M.D.
JOHN RICHARD LAKE, M.D.
BRUCE F. SCHARSCHMIDT, M.D.

This chapter deals with the treatment of cholestasis. Because the management of specific types of biliary obstruction is covered in detail in subsequent chapters, our focus will be on the medical management of the complications of cholestasis. Biliary obstruction will be addressed only briefly and with respect to how therapeutic considerations enter into the initial approach to the patient. Sclerosing cholangitis is the only disease entity that will be discussed in detail.

CHOLESTATIC SYNDROME

The term cholestasis, as used in this chapter, refers to a constellation of clinical and biochemical abnormalities that can accompany a variety of hepatobiliary disorders (Table 1). Elevations in serum alkaline phosphatase activity and bile acid concentration are nearly always present, and pruritus is the most frequent clinical manifestation. Hyperbilirubinemia is also typically present; however, cholestasis severe enough to produce secondary biliary cirrhosis is known to occur in the absence of hyperbilirubinemia. Also, conjugated hyperbilirubinemia (as in the Dubin-Johnson or Rotor's syndrome) does not necessarily signify cholestasis. Hypercholesterolemia and hypoprothrombinemia (correctable by parenteral vitamin K administration) are variable biochemical findings, as are the clinical features of jaundice and fat malabsorption. Finally, chronic cholestasis, which occurs with biliary atresia, primary biliary cirrhosis, or sclerosing cholangitis, may occasionally be associated with elevated levels of copper in the liver comparable to those seen with Wilson's disease. Additional clinical and biochemical features of the cholestatic syndrome will be discussed below in conjunction with treatment.

Certain additional points merit emphasis. First, the hepatic origin of an elevated alkaline phosphatase level must be confirmed by more specific tests, such as 5'-nucleotidase. Second, direct- and indirect-reacting bilirubin levels are inaccurate measures of conjugated and unconjugated bilirubin, respectively. Moreover, a substantial proportion (up to 80%) of the total direct-reacting fraction in patients with cholestasis may represent conjugated bilirubin bound covalently to albumin. This pigment fraction cannot be excreted in urine, is not taken up by the liver, and therefore disappears slowly following resolution of hepatobiliary disease. Third, while serum bile acids are perhaps the most sensitive indicator of cholestasis, measurement of serum bile acids adds relatively little to the conventional battery of liver function tests. Finally, because most drugs are capable of producing liver damage in few patients, potentially hepatotoxic drugs or other agents known to cause cholestasis (e.g., hormones, see Table 1) should be eliminated.

TABLE 1 Causes of Cholestasis

Adults	Children
Hepatic Disorders	Hepatic Disorders
Alcoholic hepatitis	Inherited Disorders
Amyloidosis	Alpha$_1$-antitrypsin deficiency
Benign recurrent cholestasis	Arteriohepatic dysplasia
Cholestasis of pregnancy	Byler's syndrome
Chronic active hepatitis	Cystic fibrosis
Drug- and hormone-induced cholestasis (phenothiazines, estrogens)	Galactosemia
Graft-versus-host disease	Zellweger's syndrome
Hodgkin's disease	Infectious Disorders
Infiltrating neoplasm (leukemia, lymphoma)	Coxsackievirus
Parenteral nutrition	Cytomegalovirus
Primary biliary cirrhosis	Hepatitis B virus
Sarcoidosis	Herpesvirus
Viral hepatitis	Syphilis
Wilson's disease	Toxoplasmosis
Biliary Disorders	Biliary Disorders
Gallstones	Biliary atresia
Malignancy	Choledochal cyst
Sclerosing cholangitis	Malignancy

TREATMENT OF BILIARY OBSTRUCTION

Virtually every patient with prolonged cholestasis should undergo visualization of the biliary tree to exclude the possibility of biliary obstruction. If obstruction is present, every effort should be made to relieve it. The management of specific types of obstruction (e.g., gallstone disease, periampullary neoplasm, high obstruction) is discussed in other chapters and the focus of this chapter is on therapy, not diagnosis. It is important, however, to appreciate that the approach to a patient with suspected obstruction depends upon the clinician's educated guess as to the probable nature of the obstruction and most appropriate therapy.

The early establishment of a "game plan" is thus important. Since this process must be highly individualized, it is best illustrated by example. First, given a patient with a recent cholecystectomy for stones who now presents with right upper quadrant pain, fever, and biochemical evidence of cholestasis, retrograde cholangiography with anticipated sphincterotomy would be an appropriate first procedure, the presumptive diagnosis being a retained stone(s). Second, given a patient with similar symptoms but without prior cholecystectomy in whom an ultrasound examination demonstrates gallbladder stones and ductal dilatation (with or without stones) and no other abnormalities, laparotomy with anticipated cholecystectomy and common duct exploration would be an appropriate next step, the presumptive diagnosis being cholecysto- and choledocholithiasis. Third, given an elderly patient with severe symptomatic cholestasis in whom an ultrasound examination demonstrates dilatation of the intrahepatic biliary tree without dilatation of the extrahepatic biliary tree or gallbladder, percutaneous cholangiography with anticipated drainage would be a reasonable next step, with proximal obstruction being the most likely diagnosis. Other examples could, of course, be given; however, these adequately illustrate the point that considerations regarding therapy enter into the decision-making process early in patients with suspected obstruction. A complete coverage of a number of specific entities is provided in separate chapters.

PRURITUS

Pruritus is the most frequent and perhaps most distressing manifestation of cholestasis. It occurs in 20 to 25 percent of jaundiced patients and in nearly all patients with advanced primary biliary cirrhosis. It may occur with either intra- or extrahepatic cholestasis and is commonly the presenting symptom. The cause of this type of pruritus remains obscure and may be difficult to treat.

Initially it was believed that cholestasis-associated pruritus resulted from the deposition of circulating bile salts in the skin. Evidence supporting this hypothesis included (1) increased concentrations of bile acids in the skin of patients with cholestasis and itching; (2) the production of pruritus by the injection of bile acids at the base of preexisting blisters, and (3) relief of pruritus with nonabsorbable, orally administered, anion exchange resins (cholestyramine) which bind bile acids in the intestine. A causative role for bile acids is not established, however, because (1) no consistent relationship has been found between cutaneous levels of bile acids and the presence of pruritus; (2) cholestyramine relieves pruritus associated with other systemic diseases (e.g., polycythemia vera) in which serum bile acid levels are not elevated; and (3) androgens, which occasionally relieve cholestasis-associated pruritus, actually increase the level of circulating bile acids. Therefore, bile acids may not be the sole or even primary cause of cholestasis-associated pruritus. They may, however, serve as a marker for the putative pruritogen(s), which is also presumably excreted in bile and reabsorbed by the gut.

A wide range of therapeutic agents (e.g., anion exchange resins such as cholestyramine, phenobarbital, antihistamines, androgens, choleretic agents) as well as therapeutic procedures (e.g., ultraviolet light, plasmapheresis, and plasma perfusion) have been tried in the treatment of pruritus (Table 2). Treatment should begin first with simple skin care followed by other measures as required.

General Measures and Topical Agents

Simple *skin care* alone often provides some relief from the itching. General skin care should include frequent cutting of fingernails and wearing of light clothing

TABLE 2 Therapeutic Measures Used in Treatment of Cholestasis-Associated Pruritus

Treatment	Regimen	Efficacy	Adverse Effects
Antihistamines			
Diphenhydramine	25–50 mg q.i.d.	Rarely provides significant relief apart from sedation	Drowsiness
Hydroxyzine	25 mg t.i.d.		
Cimetidine	200 mg q.i.d.	None established	Antiandrogen effects, mental confusion, hypersensitivity reactions
Cholestyramine	12–20 g/day: 4-g dose 30 min before meals; double dose at breakfast; evening dose may be skipped to facilitate taking other medications	Beneficial in most patients, but may require up to 2 weeks for an effect	Fat malabsorption; decreased absorption of other medications, constipation, hypercholeremic acidosis
Phenobarbital	Starting dose: 120 mg/day in adult, 3–5 mg/day in child; dosage subsequently altered to maintain therapeutic response and plasma concentration of drug between 10–40 µg/ml	Variable, typically incomplete relief	Drowsiness; potent inducer of hepatic enzymes involved in drug metabolism
Plasma perfusion or exchange	2–3 procedures on consecutive days, then p.r.n. Each procedure lasts approx. 4 hr and 1–6 L of plasma is perfused	Good in the few patients tested, but limited by availability of equipment/personnel	None reported
Ultraviolet-B light	2–3 treatments/week at a dose slightly below minimal erythemal dose	Good in the few patients tested, but no controlled trials to date	None reported

and few bedclothes. A lukewarm bath or shower before retiring may provide temporary relief; however, excessive bathing and the use of soaps or detergents have a drying effect on the skin which may aggravate the problem and should be avoided. Topical application of emollients should be tried even in the absence of xerosis, and lotions containing menthol or phenol may provide some additional relief by soothing the skin. Topical anesthetic agents or topical antihistamines should not be used, as they may cause sensitization.

Antihistamines

Oral antihistamines, both the H_1 blockers (diphenhydramine or hydroxyzine) and H_2 blockers (cimetidine), have been used to treat the pruritus associated with cholestasis, but they rarely provide significant relief from itching and were not found beneficial in a small controlled trial. Because H_1 blockers have a mild sedative effect, however, they can help the patient who develops insomnia due to nocturnal itching.

Cholestyramine

The nonabsorbable anion exchange resin, cholestyramine, is probably the most effective agent for the control of pruritus. Cholestyramine is available as a powder which, to be palatable, must be suspended in a liquid such as fruit juice. This resin theoretically works by binding bile acids in the small bowel, thus preventing their absorption and promoting their elimination in the feces.

Starting doses are generally 12 to 16 g per day but may be increased if the pruritus is not relieved. Because duodenal bile acid concentration is maximal shortly after a meal (particularly at breakfast which follows an overnight fast), patients with intact gallbladders are generally given a 4-g dose of cholestyramine 30 minutes before meals with a double dose (8 g) before breakfast. The therapeutic effect of cholestyramine does not occur immediately. Patients should be apprised of this and encouraged to continue taking the medication in spite of a lack of any immediate effect. Patients who respond to this treatment typically do so within 2 weeks. If after this 2-week period relief from pruritus is not achieved, the dose should either be increased or one of the alternate treatments (see below) instituted.

Side Effects. Cholestyramine has several adverse side effects, including worsening of the fat malabsorption that frequently occurs with cholestasis and aggravation of fat-soluble vitamin deficiencies (see below). Cholestyramine may bind to and impair the absorption of medications such as digoxin, phenobarbital, thyroxine, warfarin, thiazides, tetracycline, and penicillin. To avoid this problem, other medicines should be taken at least 1 hour before and/or 4 to 6 hours after the last dose of cholestyramine and their serum levels should be checked where appropriate (e.g., with digoxin). Eliminating the evening dose of cholestyramine may also provide a "window of opportunity" for administration of other oral medications. Other side effects of cholestyramine include constipation, worsening of hemorrhoidal disease, cheilosis, and hyperchloremic metabolic acidosis.

Phenobarbital

Phenobarbital has been reported to be effective in the treatment of pruritus in several uncontrolled studies, but one controlled trial reported no benefit. The mode of action of phenobarbital in alleviating the pruritus associated with cholestasis has been theorized to involve either enhancement of bile-acid-independent bile flow, induction of anion binding proteins, or increased hepatic extraction of potential pruritogens. Phenobarbital administration is usually begun at a dose of 120 mg per day (3 to 5 mg per kilogram of body weight per day in children) and may be administered as a single night-time dose to facilitate sleep. As with cholestyramine, 2 to 4 weeks of phenobarbital therapy may be required before symptomatic improvement is seen.

The major side effect of phenobarbital is drowsiness, which is most severe early in the treatment course. It is important to monitor serum levels (therapeutic range, 10 to 40 µg per milliliter) to avoid overdosage. Phenobarbital also may occasionally produce paradoxical hyperexcitability in children. As a barbiturate, phenobarbital is physically addicting and should always be tapered rather than stopped abruptly to prevent the withdrawal syndrome. Furthermore, because phenobarbital is a potent inducer of both hepatic cytochrome P-450 and drug-hydroxylating enzyme activities, all concomitantly administered medications must be closely monitored and, where appropriate, plasma concentrations of these drugs measured. If after 1 month of treatment phenobarbital does not provide significant relief from the pruritus, the drug should be tapered and another treatment instituted. Apart from its sedative effect, we have not found phenobarbital to be strikingly effective in patients with severe pruritus.

Plasma Exchange

For pruritus refractory to cholestyramine and phenobarbital, plasma perfusion through charcoal-coated beads, activated charcoal, or anion exchange resins has been used in small uncontrolled trials with reported success. Plasma perfusion lowers bile acid concentrations in the peripheral circulation, and the therapeutic responses obtained have been attributed to this. The apparent duration of relief of pruritus after these measures, however, greatly exceeds the duration of the fall in bile acid concentration. Plasma removal or plasmapheresis has also been used in the treatment of xanthomatous neuropathy in patients with primary biliary cirrhosis and hypercholesterolemia. These techniques must be viewed as experimental, and they generally require specialized equipment and/or personnel. Even after a therapeutic response has been achieved, patients will require additional treatments at varying frequencies to maintain relief of their symptoms.

Ultraviolet-B Light

Ultraviolet-B (UV-B) light (290 to 320 nm) in a dose slightly below a minimal erythemal dose has also provided relief from pruritus in patients whose cholestasis has been refractory to other forms of treatment. The exact mechanism of the therapeutic effect of UV light on pruritus is not known but may possibly involve nonspecific effects on sensory nerve endings responsible for the itch sensation. UV-B light therapy remains experimental and should only be tried in patients refractory to other measures.

FAT MALABSORPTION

Bile acids play an important role in the absorption of dietary fats and fat-soluble vitamins. In the presence of cholestasis, the ability to absorb dietary fats decreases as the intestinal concentration of bile acids falls. If cholestasis is severe or prolonged, a number of important nutritional deficiency syndromes may result. The use of cholestyramine can exacerbate malabsorption by binding directly to bile acids and further decreasing intraluminal bile acid concentrations.

Dietary Fat Manipulation

Malabsorption of dietary fat in patients with cholestasis does not usually cause clinical symptoms (Table 3). When severe, however, it can lead to steatorrhea, diarrhea, and significant loss of dietary calories. Symptomatic steatorrhea can usually be controlled by reducing dietary fat to 40 g per day or less, while antidiarrheal drugs are of little additional benefit. Dietary supplementation with medium chain triglycerides provides an important source of essential fatty acids and calories. These triglycerides are absorbed even in the absence of bile acids and should be given in a dose of 2 to 6 tablespoons (approximately 90 Kcal per tablespoon) each day. This may cause loose stools in some patients.

Vitamin K

Vitamin K deficiency occurs commonly in patients with cholestasis and fat malabsorption and can lead to hypoprothrombinemia and bleeding. It is not necessary to check serum levels of vitamin K because prolongation of the prothrombin time serves as a sensitive indicator of diminished body stores. When vitamin K deficiency is suspected, it is important to inquire about the use of cholestyramine, Coumadin, antibiotics, and aspirin. The patient with vitamin K deficiency should be treated with phytonadione (AquaMEPHYTON), 10 mg per day IM for 3 days. If the prothrombin time does not return to normal, impaired hepatic synthesis of clotting factors should be considered. Adults with chronic cholestasis may require vitamin K, 10 mg IM one to two times each month as dictated by the prothrombin time. Infants and children

TABLE 3 Nutritional Deficiencies Complicating Cholestasis

Manifestation		Diagnosis	Treatment	Adverse Effects
Dietary fat malabsorption	Steatorrhea	Sudan stain of stool	40-g fat diet	Caloric insufficiency
		24-hr stool fat collection	Dietary supplementation with medium chain triglycerides, 2–6 tablespoons per day	Loose stools
Vitamin K	Hypoprothrombinemia	Prothrombin time	Vitamin K (phytonadione), 5–10 mg IM acutely then oral/parenteral supplementation as needed	Hematoma, hemolysis (rare), anaphylaxis from IV administration
Vitamin A deficiency	Night blindness, xerophthalmia, dry skin	Retinol level (normal, 30–65 µg/dl)	Aquasol A: children, 10,000–15,000 IU per day orally; adults, 25,000–50,000 IU per day orally	Increased intracranial pressure, hepatic fibrosis, lymphadenopathy
Vitamin E deficiency	Neurologic dysfunction in children	Vitamin E level (normal, 5–20 µg/ml)	Aquasol E: 200–400 IU per day orally	None
Vitamin D deficiency	Osteomalacia	Serum 25 (OH)-vitamin D_3 (normal, 15–80 ng/ml)	Ergocalciferol: 50,000–100,000 IU per day orally	Hypercalcemia, renal stones, metastatic calcification
			Oral calcium supplementation to 1.5 g or more each day	

require only 1 to 2 mg IM at similar intervals. Water-soluble synthetic vitamin K analogs (menadiol) are available for oral administration and may be effective in children and adults at doses between 5 and 15 mg each day. Absorption of those analogs may be erratic and the prothrombin time should be monitored accordingly. Vitamin K is generally safe, but local hematoma formation, hemolytic anemia, and rare cases of anaphylaxis after intravenous injection have been reported.

Vitamin A

Vitamin A (retinol) deficiency is an important cause of night blindness, conjunctival drying, xerophthalmia, and dry skin. *Zinc* is a necessary cofactor for alcohol dehydrogenase, which converts vitamin A to its active form, retinaldehyde, in the retina. Thus, coexisting zinc deficiency may exacerbate the effects of dietary retinol deficiency or malabsorption. This is particularly common in alcoholic liver disease, which is associated with profoundly decreased hepatic levels of vitamin A, and in patients with primary biliary cirrhosis. Any patient with prolonged cholestasis who has symptoms of retinol deficiency should have serum zinc and retinol levels sent, and presumptive therapy should be begun with an oral, water-miscible form of vitamin A (*Aquasol A*), 10,000 to 20,000 U per day for children and 25,000 to 50,000 U per day for adults. *Zinc sulfate* (50 mg elemental zinc) should also be given to patients with coexistent zinc deficiency. The dose should be reduced by one-half after 2 weeks of therapy. The goals of therapy are to reverse the symptoms and to normalize the retinol level to 30 to 65 µg per deciliter.

It is important to monitor the serum levels approximately every 2 months because hypervitaminosis A is associated with a number of serious toxic effects, including increased intracranial pressure, hepatic fibrosis, and lymphadenopathy. Asymptomatic patients should have serum vitamin A levels checked once or twice each year and should be treated only if serum levels are decreased.

Vitamin E

Vitamin E (tocopherol) deficiency is not associated with any known clinical syndromes in the adult. The developing nervous system is more susceptible to vitamin E deficiency, and a progressive neurologic syndrome characterized by ataxia, peripheral neuropathy, motor weakness, and posterior column dysfunction has been described in children with cholestasis. This syndrome is usually associated with low serum vitamin E levels (normal, 5 to 20 µg per milliliter), but normal levels are seen in some patients. Because vitamin E is nontoxic, and because most children with cholestasis have vitamin E deficiency, supplemental vitamin E should be given routinely. Guidelines for the proper dosage are not yet available, but 200 to 400 U per day of an oral, water-soluble preparation (*Aquasol E*) is a reasonable starting dosage. Serum levels should be monitored to ensure adequate dosage. Adults do not generally need to be monitored or treated for vitamin E deficiency.

BONE DISEASE

Metabolic bone disease occurs with increased frequency in patients with cholestasis and is a particularly common and disturbing problem in patients with primary biliary cirrhosis. In this latter group, osteoporosis appears to be the predominant lesion, with osteomalacia also present in some individuals. The serum calcium, phosphate, and parathyroid hormone levels are typically normal in both disorders, and radiographic findings are not generally diagnostic. Consequently, bone biopsy and histologic examination are essential for an accurate diagnosis. A number of abnormalities of vitamin D metabolism have been found to account for the osteomalacia, but the etiology of the osteoporosis is not known.

Vitamin D deficiency can occur in patients with cholestasis as a result of (1) diminished production of vitamin D_3 (cholecalciferol) by the action of UV light on 7-dehydrocholesterol in the skin; (2) diminished absorption of intestinal vitamin D_2 (ergocalciferol); or, rarely, (3) defective 25-hydroxylation of circulating vitamin D by hepatic microsomes; and (4) impaired enterohepatic recirculation of vitamin D_2. Vitamin D_3 is generally the predominant form of vitamin D in the serum in the northern hemisphere. This observation suggests that the lack of exposure to UV light may be more important than malabsorption in the usual patient and helps explain the apparently higher incidence of osteomalacia reported from studies in England as compared with the United States.

Patients with chronic cholestasis should be cautioned about the use of drugs known to induce metabolic bone disease, including alcohol and phenobarbital. Exercise and exposure to sunlight have not been shown to prevent bone disease but should be recommended. In addition, dietary calcium should be maintained at 1.5 g or more each day. Serum 25-(OH)-vitamin D levels seem to reflect body stores of vitamin D and should be measured several times each year.

Vitamin D deficiency or osteomalacia should be treated with oral vitamin D_2 (ergocalciferol, 50,000 to 100,000 U each day). This is not a water-soluble preparation, so if the 25-(OH)-vitamin D levels fail to normalize, ergocalciferol therapy should be replaced by 25-(OH)-vitamin D (calcifediol, 50 to 100 μg orally every 1 or 2 days) because it may be better absorbed by patients with steatorrhea. Patients with severe malabsorption may require intramuscular injections of ergocalciferol. The goals of therapy are to maintain serum 25-(OH)-vitamin D levels in the high-normal range while also maintaining normal calcium, phosphate, and urinary calcium levels. The optimal daily dose of vitamin D must be carefully determined for each patient to ensure adequate dosage and avoid serious toxic effects, including hypercalcemia, renal stones, and metastatic calcification. Asymptomatic patients with normal 25-(OH)-vitamin D levels should not be given prophylactic vitamin D because of the potential toxicity.

SCLEROSING CHOLANGITIS

Definition

The diagnosis of sclerosing cholangitis requires compatible clinical findings and cholangiographic demonstration of multifocal annular strictures in the intra- and/or extrahepatic ducts. Liver biopsy typically demonstrates varying degrees of inflammation and obliterative fibrosis of interlobular bile ducts. Bile duct specimens, if obtained, show nonspecific inflammation and fibrosis. The diagnosis of primary sclerosing cholangitis is generally not made if there is a history of previous biliary tract surgery (apart from simple cholecystectomy) or choledocholithiasis.

General Considerations

There is no specific therapy for sclerosing cholangitis for which efficacy has been clearly established. Moreover, the rate at which the disease progresses is quite variable and the natural history of recently recognized presymptomatic disease (typical ductular abnormalities and a mildly elevated alkaline phosphatase level in an asymptomatic patient) is unknown. Consequently, the goals of therapy are to prevent the complications of cholestasis and relieve obstruction due to high-grade symptomatic strictures as they arise. It is often appropriate to do as little as possible for as long as possible, particularly when the forms of therapy under consideration have potentially serious side effects. It is also generally inappropriate to treat asymptomatic patients with radiologic abnormalities only.

Cholangiocarcinoma can mimic sclerosing cholangitis in every detail. Moreover, long-term observation of patients with apparently typical sclerosing cholangitis indicates that cholangiocarcinoma develops in 5 to 10 percent of patients, suggesting that sclerosing cholangitis may be a premalignant condition. Finally, the diagnosis of ductal cancer can be missed even after laparotomy and duct biopsy. This complicates decision-making in many patients.

Medical Therapy

Several different types of treatment have been tried in patients with sclerosing cholangitis with anecdotal reports of success. We are unaware, however, of any controlled trials demonstrating the efficacy of these approaches or even lack thereof. The types of treatment which have been tried include corticosteroids, long-term antibiotic administration, azathioprine, bile acid binding agents, and penicillamine (controlled trial in progress). We do not advocate routine administration of any of these agents, apart from appropriate antibiotics in patients with cholangitis. It is appropriate to point out, however, that most patients in whom these agents have been tried had advanced symptomatic disease. Because these patients presumably had fixed scarring of the ducts, it is not surprising that medical therapy was ineffective. The efficacy of medical therapy earlier in the course of the disease, when inflammation without fixed scarring presumably predominates, is unknown.

Nonoperative Biliary Drainage

Patients with severe symptomatic cholestasis or biliary sepsis require biliary decompression for relief of their symptoms. There are several reports of apparently successful treatment via percutaneous biliary drainage in conjunction with stenting and/or dilation of biliary strictures. This approach is reasonable in the management of such patients, particularly when symptoms are due to a readily approachable dominant stricture(s). Instrumentation of the biliary tree, however, is very likely to introduce bacteria into the previously uninfected patient, and percutaneous biliary drainage is generally unsatisfactory in the patient with multiple strictures involving the intra- as well as extrahepatic ducts. Moreover, exteriorized drainage catheters can be difficult to manage on an outpatient basis, and the situation is frequently complicated by cholangitis. In general, we view this as a temporary measure worth trying under appropriate circumstances, but with the anticipation that problems will recur following (or even prior to) removal of the catheter and that some other, more definitive treatment will be necessary in the majority of cases.

Operative Biliary Drainage

A variety of surgical procedures have been tried in patients with sclerosing cholangitis. Some groups have reported success with sphincteroplasty; however, this approach is not widely used and does not make good sense in most patients who have multiple strictures often involving the proximal ducts. Operative dilation of strictures and placement of one or more stents is a more appropriate approach, and several centers advocate a more aggressive procedure involving resection of a dominant stricture (often at the confluence of the right and left hepatic ducts, which is generally extrahepatic in location) with anastomosis of residual duct and intestine. We would favor one of the latter two approaches only in the patient with a clearly dominant and accessible biliary stricture in whom a previous attempt at percutaneous dilation has been unsuccessful. Any surgery involving the biliary tree may potentially compromise a patient's candidacy for subsequent liver transplantation and thus requires careful consideration and perhaps consultation with a transplant center. In contrast to those procedures discussed above which continue to be investigated and remain controversial, surgical management of symptomatic gallstone disease in the usual fashion is generally accepted.

Colectomy. Seventy percent or more of patients with sclerosing cholangitis have associated inflammatory bowel disease, typically ulcerative colitis. Conversely, radiologic evidence of sclerosing cholangitis is found in up to 10 percent of patients with ulcerative colitis. Early reports suggested that colectomy arrested or reversed sclerosing cholangitis in some patients especially those with "early" hepatobiliary disease. Subsequent reports, however, suggested that this was not the case; nor has colectomy been found to be beneficial in the recent experience of most observers. Particularly since sclerosing cholangitis frequently occurs in the presence of relatively mild colonic disease, we feel that the decision to perform a colectomy should be based on the severity and chronicity of the colonic disease itself and not upon an expected improvement in associated hepatobiliary disease. Colonic dysplasia has been the "justification" for colectomy in some patients with sclerosing cholangitis.

Liver Transplantation

Liver transplantation is being performed with increasing frequency and success at a variety of centers in the United States and Western Europe. A recent survey of 819 transplant procedures at eight such centers indicated that, as of August 1984, 34 patients with sclerosing cholangitis had undergone transplantation. Whereas the overall survival of 19 patients who underwent transplants prior to April 30, 1983, was only about 25 percent at 1 year, the survival of 15 patients receiving transplants more recently exceeded 75 percent at 1 year. While the follow-up of these more recently transplanted patients is relatively short, overall analysis of currently available data suggests that 80 percent of those patients who survive the first postoperative year become long-term (3- to 5-years) survivors. Thus, the recent trend toward improved survival is probably meaningful. This improvement is probably due to several factors, including the introduction of cyclosporin, improvements in operative techniques, and more stringent patient selection criteria. Given the recent improvement in survival of transplant recipients, the poor prognosis of advanced sclerosing cholangitis, and the lack of satisfactory therapeutic alternatives, liver transplantation represents an attractive option for carefully selected patients in whom biliary malignancy can be excluded.

Supported in part by NIH grants AM-26270, AM-26743, and AM-07453 and grants from the American Liver Foundation and the Bank of America Giannini Foundation.

WILSON'S DISEASE

JOHN M. WALSHE,

Wilson's disease is a genetically determined metabolic disease with a recessive mode of inheritance. The primary abnormal gene product has not been identified but the pathogenetic mechanism appears to be related to an inability to excrete the essential trace metal copper via its normal route, the bile. As a result, copper accumulates in the liver, leading to chronic or silent liver damage, and very occasionally to acute liver failure. Patients in whom the liver lesion is not fatal will eventually develop central nervous system disease involving the motor centers but sparing the sensory system. Personality and psychiatric disturbances are quite common. The incidence is about 30 per million of the population, with a carrier rate of one in a hundred.

PRINCIPAL CLINICAL FEATURES

Untreated Wilson's disease is invariably fatal. The age and presenting symptoms in some 170 cases are shown in Figure 1. These ages range from 5 to 40 years, but older patients have been reported. It can be seen that hepatic symptoms are most common before the age of 15 and neurologic (including psychiatric) symptoms after that age. Many patients can be diagnosed in the presymptomatic stage of the illness by screening of affected sibships. The hepatic illness can take almost any form but most commonly presents as subacute or chronic hepatitis; about 10 percent of patients will have an associated hemolysis. The illness may appear to be self-limiting but may present again months or years later with neurologic symptoms. Of these, the most frequent early abnormality is a speech defect with drooling, but almost any motor disturbances may occur, often with changes in personality or frank psychiatric disturbances. The sensory nervous system is never involved. Deposition of copper in Descemet's membrane of the cornea is always present once the nervous system is involved but may not be present in the hepatic stage of the illness. The biochemical disturbances that must be sought include low serum ceruloplasmin and serum copper levels, and raised urinary copper and hepatic copper concentrations; if doubt as to the diagnosis exists, the latter must be demonstrated (Table 1).

TREATMENT

Treatment is based on the hypothesis that the excess of copper found in the liver and brain destroys mitochondrial enzyme systems in the cell which are essential for normal metabolic functions. Therapy is therefore directed toward promoting the excretion of the abnormal stores of the metal and, more recently, toward reducing the absorption of the metal from the gut. "Decoppering" is achieved by the use of one of the three medical chelating agents, penicillamine, trientine, or BAL (dimercaprol). Copper absorption from the gut may be blocked by the administration of zinc sulfate or zinc acetate.

Before chelating agents are administered it is essential to document the concentrations of serum copper and ceruloplasmin; the urine copper level, the full blood count, including platelets; and to examine the urine for protein. The serum copper and ceruloplasmin levels will fall with treatment and the urine copper level should return to the normal range (less than 30 μg per 24 hours), and these changes can be used as useful markers for decrease in the abnormal body stores of the metal. Similarly the red cell, white cell, and particularly the platelet counts may all be adversely affected by penicillamine, so they should be known before treatment is started. Proteinuria may also develop as a toxic reaction to penicillamine, and for this reason the starting level of urine protein excretion also must be recorded.

Penicillamine

Once the diagnosis has been established and the necessary laboratory tests completed, treatment can be started without further delay. Penicillamine is the drug of choice. For an adolescent or adult it can be started in a dosage of 500 mg 3 times a day taken about 20 minutes before meals. The drug has its maximum cupruretic effect if it is present in the plasma as the copper is absorbed from the gut. The dosage for children is 25 mg per kilogram of body weight similarly distributed throughout the day. In presymptomatic patients and in

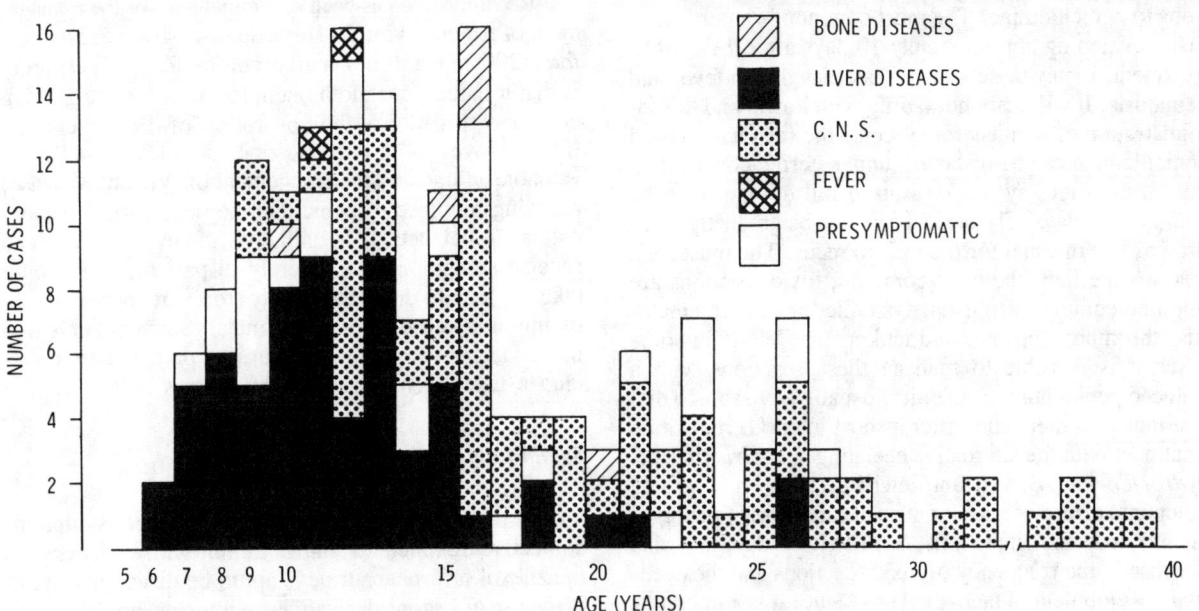

Figure 1 Distribution by age and presenting symptoms for 170 patients with Wilson's disease.

TABLE 1 Normal Values for Copper in the Body

Serum copper:	80–140 μg/dl
Serum ceruloplasmin	
Male:	33 ± 6 mg/dl
Female:	36 ± 9 mg/dl
Urine copper:	< 30 μg/24 hours
Liver copper:	< 10 μg/g wet weight– 50 μg/g dry weight

those in whom symptoms have been controlled and the body stores of copper depleted, the dose can be reduced to 750 mg or 1 g daily, taken twice a day, morning and evening, before food. The great majority of patients will recover well with this treatment, many returning to completely normal function which will be maintained as long as they persevere with therapy. If treatment is interrupted for any length of time symptoms will certainly recur. The interval before improvement of neurologic symptoms becomes apparent is very variable and, in my experience, impossible to predict. It can be as early as a few weeks, more commonly months, and occasionally years. A significant number of patients will get worse before they get better, and it is essential to warn them that this may happen. A very small percentage of patients fail to respond to treatment and follow a slowly progressive downhill course to bedridden helplessness and eventual death from secondary infection.

The liver lesions, like the neurologic lesions, will respond to treatment, but they also may need the supportive treatment given in other forms of severe hepatic disease. Once the disease is well controlled it is rare for esophageal varices to give trouble, even if they are extensive when the patient first seeks treatment, but for the first few months of treatment patients with extensive varices are obviously at risk.

Side Effects of Penicillamine. Approximately 10 percent of patients develop one of the various toxic reactions to penicillamine. The most common is an urticarial rash developing approximately 10 days after the start of treatment; it may be severe and associated with fever and hematuria. It will respond to drug withdrawal and the administration of antihistamine. Once the rash has cleared penicillamine can be restarted, under steroid cover, at 25 mg on the first day working up to full dosage over the course of 10 days. The steroid can then be gradually withdrawn. It is unusual for the rash to recur. The most serious, and perhaps the most common, toxic reactions are immune complex nephritis, systemic lupus erythematosus, thrombocytopenia, and leukopenia. While in some cases it is possible to manage these reactions with a reduced penicillamine dose, it is usually advisable to discontinue treatment and, after a short interval, reinstitute treatment with the alternative chelating agent *trientine dihydrochloride*. British anti-lewisite (BAL) has largely fallen into disuse because of the painful nature of the regular intramuscular injections, 2 ml twice a day, and also because of the frequency of toxic reactions and the eventual development of tachyphylaxis. Since it is a lipophilic compound, however, it crosses the blood-brain barrier readily and a short course of the drug may be helpful for those patients who do not appear to be responding well to penicillamine.

A variety of skin lesions are induced by penicillamine; both collagen and elastic tissue are damaged by prolonged exposure to the drug. Pyridoxine deficiency may also occur, though this requires some additional factor to precipitate it, such as a growth spurt, intercurrent infection, an inadequate diet, or pregnancy. A dose of 50 mg of pyridoxine once a week is sufficient to protect against this.

Trientine Dihydrochloride

Trientine dihydrochloride (Triethylene tetramine) is a relatively new, orally active chelating agent that has proved to be a very effective alternative treatment for patients who have developed penicillamine intolerance. It has not been officially adopted under the Orphan Drug Program and has recently been licensed in the United States and the United Kingdom for patients who need it. Like penicillamine, it should be given before meals, 600 mg 3 times a day in the early stages of the disease, reduced to twice a day once the patient has reached a maximum stage of improvement and the blood and urine copper levels have shown a significant fall from the pretreatment levels. At present there are no reports of toxicity, though these may well appear when the drug is more widely used. A particular watch should be kept for a renal lesion resulting from the development of systemic lupus erythematosus as there is some evidence that there may be cross-sensitivity here with penicillamine. It seems possible, on theoretical grounds, that long-term administration of trientine will also induce skin lesions similar to those produced by penicillamine.

Zinc

Recently zinc has been recommended for the management of patients with Wilson's disease, given as *zinc sulfate*, 200 mg 3 times a day before food. The theory is that it induces metalothionein formation in the gut mucosa and this blocks the absorption of dietary copper. If this proves to be correct, zinc sulfate may well be a valuable adjunct in the management of Wilson's disease, reducing the dose of penicillamine necessary to keep a patient in balance. It is unlikely, however, by itself to reverse symptoms in a severely ill patient, as it would take too long to deplete the body stores of copper simply by inhibiting absorption of the metal. Some patients find it produces severe epigastric burning pain and are reluctant to take it; *zinc acetate* may be less irritating.

Symptomatic Therapy

In those patients with severe neurologic symptoms subjective treatment to control tremor with such drugs as benzhexol or orphenadrine is apt to be disappointing, as is the use of L-dopa derivatives to improve bradykinesia. In my experience, attempts to reduce muscle spasm with dantrolene and baclofen have been very disappointing, and intense spasm can pull limbs into bizzare and painful positions that may eventually become fixed, requiring orthopedic correction once the disease has been brought under control.

PREGNANCY

Carefully treated patients can tolerate pregnancy and, in my own experience with 40 pregnancies in patients with Wilson's disease (33 in patients taking penicillamine and 7 in those taking trientine), there have been no problems. The children are, by definition, heterozygous for the Wilson's disease gene. The risk of such a child developing Wilson's disease itself is approximately one in 200. It is advisable, however, to screen all children with either mothers or fathers with Wilson's disease; the ceruloplasmin level should be estimated in cord blood and again when the child is between 3 months and 1 year old, by which time the ceruloplasmin should have risen from the low levels found in all neonates to the level expected when the child reaches adult years.

FAMILY SCREENING

Once Wilson's disease has been diagnosed in a family, all siblings of the propositus must be screened, whether older or younger. The theoretical risk to each sibling is one in four. The parents should also have a serum ceruloplasmin level estimated, as this will give an indication of the concentration of this protein to be expected in the heterozygotes in each particular family. It is advisable also to screen more distant relatives; I have seen two families in which first cousins were also found to be affected with the disease. If the diagnosis is confirmed in a presymptomatic relative, penicillamine therapy must be started. The dose needed is probably smaller than that required for symptomatic patients; 500 mg twice a day is probably sufficient for adults and 20 mg per kilogram daily for children.

As will all rare diseases, patients referred to specialist centers seem to do better and have fewer problems than those not so referred.

HEMOCHROMATOSIS

WILLIAM P. BALDUS, M.D.

Before considering treatment of iron-overload states, it is essential to understand certain basic concepts relevant to these conditions. The term *hemochromatosis* refers to a group of disorders characterized by a progressive increase in body iron stores. Table 1 provides a classification of iron overload states as adapted from Powell. This chapter will deal primarily with genetic hemochromatosis and, briefly, with iron overload secondary to chronic dyserythropoietic anemias.

GENETIC HEMOCHROMATOSIS

Pathogenesis

Iron overload results from increased intestinal absorption of iron which is inappropriate for the level of iron stores. This results in the deposition of iron in the parenchyma of various organs, especially the liver, heart, pancreas, and synovium of joints. The specific metabolic defect, however, remains obscure.

Clinical Features and Diagnosis

The essential feature in hemochromatosis is the magnitude of excessive iron stores. Total body iron stores in the fully established case generally exceeds 10 g and averages approximately 20 g, as compared with the normal value of less than 1 g. The frequency of clinical features observed in our series of 65 patients is noted in Table 2. The mode of presentation can vary greatly, and the underlying disease process may go unrecognized for some time. Not uncommonly, the unexpected finding of an enlarged liver or elevated serum iron concentration leads to the diagnosis when other features are absent or inapparent.

The diagnosis of hemochromatosis depends on the demonstration of markedly increased body iron stores, as reflected in biochemical tests and heavy iron deposition in the liver (Table 3). Patients with substantial elevations in percentage saturation of the iron binding capacity and serum ferritin should undergo liver biopsy. Biopsy is the definitive procedure, as it allows histochemical demonstration of heavy hepatic iron deposition (grade

TABLE 1 Classification of Iron Overload States

Genetic (Primary, Idiopathic) Hemochromatosis
  Precirrhotic stage
  Cirrhotic stage

Secondary Hemochromatosis
  Secondary to anemia due to ineffective erythropoiesis, e.g., thalassemia major, sideroblastic anemia
  Secondary to high oral intake, e.g., prolonged ingestion of medicinal iron, intake of iron with alcoholic beverages, "Bantu siderosis"
  Secondary to liver disease, e.g., alcoholic cirrhosis (infrequent); porphyria cutanea tarda; following portocaval shunt (rare)

TABLE 2 Clinical Features in Hemochromatosis

	% Before Treatment
Pigmentation	77
Hepatomegaly	72
Arthropathy	43
Hypogonadism	36
Diabetes	33
Splenomegaly	15
Cardiomyopathy	13

3–4), measurement of hepatic iron concentration, and assessment of the extent of tissue damage.

The combination of heavy iron deposition and normal hepatic architecture is referred to as "precirrhotic hemochromatosis" and represents the disease in its early stage. This is the ideal time to make the diagnosis. Hepatic iron concentrations of over 10,000 µg per gram dry weight of liver tissue are observed in overt or fully established hemochromatosis. (The significance of lesser degrees of hepatic iron concentration will be dealt with later.) Once the diagnosis of hemochromatosis is established, it is essential to screen the patient's close relatives with measurements of serum iron and iron binding capacity or serum ferritin. One can expect to find elevated values in approximately 15 percent of family members, even in the absence of clinical manifestations.

HLA Typing

Recent studies involving histocompatibility typing have confirmed the genetic basis of "idiopathic" hemochromatosis, and have shown an autosomal recessive pattern of inheritance. HLA A–3 and B–7 are considerably more prevalent in patients with hemochromatosis than in the general population. The gene frequency of a hemochromatosis-susceptibility allele in persons of Norther European ancestry is such that fully 10 percent of such populations may be heterozygote carriers of the gene. This high gene frequency, with the potential for homozygous-heterozygous marriages, accounts for the occurrence of hemochromatosis in successive generations of some families. HLA typing is of no diagnostic value in the individual patient with iron overload, but has proved useful in assessing the degree of risk among family members. Thus, siblings who are HLA-identical with the index case (proband) are at risk of developing clinically significant iron overload and should be followed closely. Approximately 25 percent of those who are heterozygous may show mild expression of the disease in the form of increased serum iron or ferritin and mildly increased hepatic iron deposition, but are not at risk of developing serious iron overload. Siblings who share neither HLA haplotype are not at risk of developing a clinically significant problem. I do not use HLA typing in routine clinical testing, as it is expensive and seldom necessary. It can be justified, however, for comparing HLA haplotypes of the proband with those of his siblings.

Role of Alcohol

The significance of hemosiderosis in alcoholic liver disease has been a matter of considerable controversy. In studies involving patients selected solely on the basis of heavy hepatic iron deposition, we concluded that patients with substantial iron overload likely have genetic hemochromatosis regardless of alcohol consumption or the presence or absence of disturbed iron metabolism in family members. Such patients should be treated with phlebotomies and advised to abstain from alcohol.

Treatment

Once the diagnosis of hemochromatosis has been established, the goal of therapy is depletion of excessive body iron stores. The simplest and most effective method to achieve this is through repeated phlebotomy, performed at weekly or twice weekly intervals. Withdrawal of 500 ml of blood will remove approximately 250 mg of iron. Since body iron stores average approximately 20 to 25 g in patients with overt hemochromatosis, weekly phlebotomies will be required for a period of about 2 years. This form of treatment is generally well tolerated, as iron is readily mobilized to form new erythrocytes.

I prefer the following protocol for phlebotomy treatment:

1. Select a "cutoff" hemoglobin value that is slightly low for the patient (e.g., 12 g per deciliter).
2. Remove 500 ml of blood by phlebotomy each week. Determine the blood hemoglobin before each phlebotomy and proceed if the value exceeds the cutoff level. If it is below that level, omit the phlebotomy on that occasion.
3. Determine serum ferritin at 6-month intervals.
4. When the hemoglobin falls below the cutoff level and remains low for three consecutive weeks without further phlebotomies, iron depletion is likely.
5. At such time, recheck the ferritin, serum iron, and iron binding capacity. If these values are subnormal, one can assume that the iron stores have been depleted. If not, continue weekly phlebotomies as above.
6. A repeat liver biopsy may be performed to confirm the absence of hepatic iron, but it is not essential.
7. Once iron stores have been depleted, the frequency of phlebotomies is reduced to one every 2 months. Most patients are maintained on five to eight phlebotomies per year with monitoring of the ferritin, serum

TABLE 3 Diagnostic Tests for Hemochromatosis

Essential	Ancillary
Serum iron and iron binding capacity	Chelation test
Serum ferritin	CT scan of liver
Stainable hepatic iron	
Hepatic iron concentration	

iron, and iron binding capacity at yearly intervals. Ideally, one would like to keep the iron parameters in the low-normal range without substantially reducing the hemoglobin.

Patients with hemochromatosis are advised to avoid ingestion of iron medication and iron-containing vitamins, but a low-iron diet is not necessary. Abstinence from alcohol should be advised.

The goals and duration of treatment should be explained to the patient at the outset, as perseverance in the treatment program is sometimes difficult. One should not expect an appreciable change in hemoglobin or serum iron concentration until late in the course of phlebotomy treatment.

Patients with mild anemia or with advanced, decompensated liver disease may require less frequent phlebotomies (e.g., biweekly) or removal of smaller amounts of blood (e.g., 250 ml).

Although certain features or complications of hemochromatosis may improve following depletion of iron stores by phlebotomy, others are not affected, including the risk of hepatocellular carcinoma (Table 4).

MILD TO MODERATE IRON OVERLOAD

Not uncommonly, screening of families or routine laboratory testing identifies an individual with mild to moderate iron overload, arbitrarily defined as transferrin saturation over 60 percent, serum ferritin over 500 ng, and hepatic iron concentration of less than 10,000 μg per gram dry weight. By contrast, patients with overt hemochromatosis have hepatic iron concentrations which characteristically exceed this arbitrary level. Individuals with mild to moderate iron overload might be heterozygotes or individuals who are homozygous but in whom the process of iron accumulation is relatively new and whose body iron stores have not yet reached their maximum. Without HLA typing of probands and siblings, this distinction may be impossible. The options are to observe such patients or to proceed with biopsy and phlebotomy treatment. In recent years, I have followed the latter course if the serum ferritin and transferrin saturation are consistently greater than the above-mentioned standards. Weekly phlebotomies are undertaken until there is evidence of depletion of iron stores, as in the patient with more overt iron overload. Since body iron stores in such patients are usually less than 10 g, iron depletion will likely be achieved more rapidly than in patients with the fully developed disease. Again, maintenance phlebotomies are appropriate to prevent the reaccumulation of iron.

TABLE 4 Response of Hemochromatosis to Phlebotomy Treatment

Improvement	Variable Response	Unchanged
Skin pigmentation	Diabetes mellitus	Arthropathy
Hepatomegaly	Cardiac abnormalities	Hypogonadism
		Underlying cirrhotic process
		Risk of hepatocellular carcinoma

IRON CHELATION THERAPY

In certain individuals with iron overload, phlebotomy treatment is not feasible because of anemia (e.g., beta thalassemia or refractory sideroblastic anemia). In such patients, chelation therapy with *deferoxamine* may be appropriate. Deferoxamine (Desferal, Ciba-Geigy Corporation, Summit, NJ) binds iron in vivo and is excreted in the urine and stool, the latter via the biliary tract. This agent removes iron from both the reticuloendothelial system and parenchymal cells. Because of poor absorption from the gut, deferoxamine must be administered parenterally. The usual dose is 1,500 to 2,000 mg per day, and the most convenient and effective route of administration is by way of continuous subcutaneous infusion using a portable injection system (Auto-Syringe, Auto-Syringe Inc., Farmingdale, NY). I recommend daily infusion over a period of 10 to 12 hours using a 27-gauge butterfly needle placed by the patient in the subcutaneous tissues of the anterior abdominal wall. Increasing the dose of Desferal or lengthening the period of infusion does not substantially increase urinary iron excretion over a 24-hour period. With this method, urinary iron excretion of 30 to 80 mg per day can be achieved. Tachyphylaxis has not been encountered. Toxicity has consisted mainly of erythema, swelling, and pain at the injection site. Addition of a small amount of hydrocortisone to the infusion generally controls such reactions. Potential systemic side effects, such as fever, tachycardia, hypertension, photophobia, and headache, have not posed a problem.

Chelation therapy must be carried out daily for at least 2 to 3 years and often indefinitely. It is expensive; the cost of Desferal alone may reach $5,000 to $10,000 a year, not including the supplies required for administration.

The use of ascorbic acid as an adjuvant to deferoxamine therapy is controversial. It has been shown that ascorbate deficiency retards mobilization of iron stores, and, in this circumstance, supplemental vitamin C enhances iron excretion following the administration of deferoxamine. There have been reports, however, of deterioration of cardiac function in some patients receiving deferoxamine and ascorbic acid in combination. For this reason, I have not administered vitamin C routinely as an adjuvant to deferoxamine therapy.

HEPATIC NEOPLASIA

PAUL H. SUGARBAKER, M.D.

Currently the only potentially curative therapy for the patient with a primary hepatic malignancy or hepatic metastases is surgical resection of the cancer. Therefore, this option should always be evaluated before other treatment alternatives are pursued. In selected patients resection can be performed with morbidity and mortality similar to that accompanying many surgical procedures that are routinely performed. Survival of patients with resected intrahepatic malignancy is far superior to that of patients whose disease runs its natural course, and 30 percent of patients are cured if complete surgical removal of the malignancy is accomplished. Unfortunately, in a majority of patients with hepatic metastases the natural course of the disease makes curative surgical intervention impossible. Sites of extrahepatic disease or diffuse involvement of the liver are the most common findings in patients with unresectable disease. In primary hepatic cancer, cirrhosis may lead to an unacceptable operative mortality with surgical resection even though the intrahepatic disease is confined to either the right or left lobe of the liver. Recently, alternative perfusion procedures have been shown to cause objective regression of intrahepatic tumor. The impact of these liver perfusion techniques on survival has not yet been established; however, their usefulness for short-term palliation in patients with symptomatic hepatic tumors has been established. Radioactively tagged antibodies directed against ferritin, a liver cancer cell constituent, have been used to deliver irradiation preferentially to hepatomas. Preliminary reports are interesting.[1]

SURGICAL TREATMENT OF METASTASES FROM COLORECTAL CANCER

Medications

Although hepatic resection is clearly of benefit to some patients, a simple calculation makes clear that it has only a small impact on the overall problem of colorectal cancer. Of 100 patients with a colorectal cancer, approximately 20 will have liver metastases at the time of operation for their primary tumor. Only five of the 20 will have resectable metastases. Of the original 100 patients another five will develop resectable metachronous hepatic metastases, for a total of ten potential resections. Three or four resected patients will survive 5 years, but one of these will develop recurrent disease. Two or three of 100 patients with primary colorectal cancer can be cured by hepatic resection. This estimate, combined with the high incidence of colorectal cancer (approximately 130,000 patients per year in the United States) would suggest that, nationwide, 13,000 liver resections must be performed annually, and that an estimated 3,900 patients would be cured by such treatment.

Traditionally, indications for resection of colorectal metastases have been extremely limited; until recently surgery was recommended only rarely. Historically, the patient considered a candidate for hepatic resection possessed a solitary metastasis to the liver, had an interval of several years between resection of a Dukes A or B primary tumor and diagnosis of the hepatic metastasis, and was relatively young. The data presented by Foster et al in the 1974 Liver Tumor Survey changed surgical thinking concerning the indications for resection of hepatic metastases from colorectal cancer (Table 1).[2] They concluded that the Dukes stage of the primary tumor and the interval between bowel and liver resection were not useful predictors of survival.

Patients with large or multiple metastases did not survive long term as often as those with similar or solitary lesions, but they did not do so poorly as to preclude consideration for resection. Additional data from August and colleagues at the National Cancer Institute revealed that patients with unilobar multiple metastases do better than those with bilobar metastases (life table analysis 2-year survival of 80% versus 34%).[3] Positive surgical margins were associated with a very poor prognosis. They also reported no difference in survival between patients with solitary and multiple (2 to 4) lesions. Fortner et al from Memorial Sloan Kettering and Adson et al from the Mayo Clinic found the Dukes classification of the primary tumor to be a significant factor in predicting survival after hepatic resection.[4,5] The usefulness of resecting a small number of lesions from both lobes should not automatically be rejected.

Data recently reported from the National Cancer Institute suggest that early detection of hepatic metastases and prompt therapeutic intervention may be important to prevent further spread from liver lesions to regional lymph nodes (cascade phenomenon).[6] This may increase the proportion of colorectal cancer patients undergoing potentially curative hepatic resections. Lymph drainage from all portions of the liver merges into several major thoracoabdominal lymphatic pathways, including the internal mammary chain via transdiaphragmatic connections, the posterior mediastinal chain through both

TABLE 1 Prognostic Factors Useful in Selecting Patients for Resection of Hepatic Metastases from Colorectal Cancer*

Clinical Factor	Prognostic Effect
Solitary metastasis	Positive
2–4 metastases	Positive
Unilobular metastases	Positive
Large size of hepatic tumor deposit	Unclear
Small size of hepatic tumor deposit	Unclear
Dukes stage B primary	Positive
Dukes stage C primary	Adverse
Bilobular metastases	Adverse
5 or more metastases	Adverse
Elevated preoperative CEA	No effect
Method of detection of metastases	No effect
Positive surgical margins	Very adverse
Margins less than 2 cm	Adverse

* Foster et al[1]

TABLE 2 Results of Surgical Treatment of Hepatic Metastases from Colorectal Cancer

Author	Period	No. of Patients	Operative Mortality (%)	Survival (%) 1	2	3	5 Yr
Liver Tumor Survey	1960-74	126	8/126 (6)				18
Attiyeh et al[7]	1950-76	25	1/25 (4)				40
Bengmark et al[8]	1971-79	39	2/39 (5)			23	
Thompson et al[9]	1955-80	22	0/22 (0)	80	42	38	31
Rajpal et al[10]	1972-81	34	4/34 (12)	85	52	40	
Iwatsuki et al[11]	1964-82	24	0/24 (0)	91	73	73	52
Fortner et al[15]	1971-82	65	6/65 (9)	89	71	57	40
Steel et al[12]	1977-83	30	2/30 (7)	90	75	65	
Adson et al[14]	1948-82	141	3/41 (2)	82	56	40	25
August et al[6]	1976-83	33	0/33 (0)	90	72	53	35

transdiaphragmatic and celiac connections, and the cisterna chyli via the portal pedicle. August et al[6] described a series of patients who underwent resection of colorectal cancers who subsequently developed hepatic metastases which proved unresectable at celiotomy because of portal or celiac lymph node metastases. This lymphatic spread likely arose via "remetastasis" from the liver metastases. Their report highlights the clinical significance of hepatic lymphatic efferents as pathways for secondary metastasis of liver metastases. Delay in diagnosis may permit secondary spread from hepatic metastases, resulting in unresectability. This hypothesis strongly suggests that careful follow-up after primary colorectal cancer resection is indicated.

Results

Table 2 summarizes the experiences of nine groups with resection of colorectal hepatic metastases. Five-year survival estimates of 30 to 40 percent are repeatedly found in these reports. The results of Iwatsuki et al showing an operative mortality of 0 percent and a 5-year actuarial survival of 52 percent are particularly impressive.[11] However, these data must be interpreted with caution because (1) 5-year survival does not necessarily mean cure, since as many as 25 percent of 5-year survivors may ultimately die from recurrent disease; (2) these data refer to crude survival and therefore death may result from causes unrelated to the malignancy; and (3) in the more recent series a number of patients received adjuvant chemotherapy or radiation therapy in addition to surgery. Nevertheless, the benefit of resection is clear, especially when these rates are contrasted with the near 0 percent 5-year survival of patients with untreated hepatic metastases. These data strongly suggest that if resection is possible it should be attempted.

SURGICAL TREATMENT OF PRIMARY LIVER CANCER

Indications

As with metastases from colorectal cancer, *hepatic resection* offers the only chance for cure in patients with hepatocellular carcinoma. Resection should be performed even if the tumor is massive, provided it is limited to a technically resectable portion of liver. Even multifocal bilobular tumor can be considered for resection. When wedge resection or anatomic lobectomy will not permit complete excision, trisegmentectomy can sometimes achieve removal of the tumor. The main obstacles to resection are cirrhosis, hepatic insufficiency, diffuse liver involvement, vascular invasion, direct invasion of extrahepatic structures, and distant metastases. If cirrhosis is present and liver function is compromised preoperatively, the regenerative capacity of the liver will be severely limited. Even if the operation is technically perfect, gradual and progressive liver failure may lead to the patient's demise if normal hepatic parenchyma must be sacrificed to resect the tumor. It should be noted, however, that some patients with large tumors completely occupying one lobe may be resected with minimal sacrifice of the normal parenchyma. In these patients, if the operation is technically flawless, rapid postoperative recovery is possible because little functioning parenchyma is sacrificed and the nutritional burden of a large tumor mass is eliminated.

Unfortunately, only a few patients are suitable candidates for operation, and of those operated upon fewer than 50 percent are found to have resectable tumors. Typically, resectability rates are 10 to 20 percent. Lin, an advocate of aggressive surgical resection of hepatocellular cancer, reported 31 percent resectability.[13] To emphasize the importance of an aggressive outlook, Lin noted that at the same institution at which the 31 percent figure was found on the surgical service, only 7 percent of patients were considered operable when treated by the medical service. Presumably this reflects disagreements on the proper selection of patients for resection on the part of the treating physician rather than differences in the patient populations.

Results

Table 3 summarizes data concerning survival of patients undergoing resection of primary hepatic malignancy, mainly hepatocellular carcinoma. Five-year survival figures of 35 to 45 percent are repeatedly observed, about the same range seen for colorectal cancer metastases. Approximately 20 percent of 5-year survivors die of recurrent cancer. Unfortunately, resected patients comprise a highly selected group; few individuals with multiple foci of cancer or with severe cirrhosis can be considered for surgical treatment. Yet the conclusion must be that resection of hepatocellular cancer can result in long-term survival in carefully selected patients.

To increase the resectability rate among a high-risk population, Chinese investigators have conducted a mass screening program using serum alpha-fetoprotein determination among nearly 1.7 million people near Shanghai. Tang[16] reported that 56 percent (417/745) of asymptomatic patients found to have hepatoma in this screening program were resectable at laparotomy.

SURGICAL TREATMENT OF OTHER METASTASES

Favorable results have been reported in the treatment of *Wilms' tumor*, where chemotherapy and radiation therapy are combined with resection, and functioning endocrine neoplasms such as *gastrinoma* and *carcinoid*. Martin et al reported a series of four complete resections of carcinoid metastases and one partial resection.[17] The palliated patient remained symptom free for 19 months; one completely resected patient died symptom free of a myocardial infarction 6 months after resection, and the other three patients were alive and asymptomatic 12 to 45 months after resection. Results following resection of hepatic metastases from other primary tumors are less encouraging.

PALLIATIVE HEPATIC RESECTION

Because of the broad range of disease left behind after so-called palliative resections and because of the subjective nature of the assessment of palliation of pain and suffering, it is impossible to make definitive statements concerning the efficacy of noncurative hepatic resections in treating malignant disease. Nevertheless, some trends emerge. There is agreement that resection of symptom-producing functional liver metastases of *carcinoid tumors* can offer excellent palliation even if a small amount of tumor remains following surgical excision. Foster and Berman reviewed a collected experience of 44 patients.[2] Palliation of all but cardiac symptoms was achieved in 35 of the 36 patients in whom follow-up information was available, with a duration of a few weeks to more than 6 years. Norton et al at the National Cancer Institute reported three cases involving hepatic resections of metastatic *gastrinoma* with favorable outcomes.[18]

Results following palliative resection of *primary liver tumors* are equivocally favorable. For hemorrhage from acutely ruptured hepatocarcinoma, resection, when feasible, is the procedure of choice, even if other foci of tumor are left behind. Long-term survivors have been reported. The benefit of partial resection of bulky disease in the face of multifocal hepatic lesions is supported by the report of Okuda and coworkers (52% 1-year survival and 22% 5-year survival) and Fortner and colleagues.[19,20] Recent results of palliative treatment with hepatic artery infusion may be more encouraging[21] (see below).

Approach to Hepatic Resection

Safe hepatic surgery is based on knowledge of vascular and ductal anatomy. Liver anatomy allows five major resections (Fig. 1): right and left lobectomy, lateral segmentectomy, and right and left trisegmentectomy. The latter terms are based on anatomic descriptions in which four liver segments are recognized, two in each lobe. Details of the optimal plane of transection are given in the figure legend. Based on Couinaud's description of eight liver segments, several operations in which one, two, or three of these segments are resected have been described.[23] They offer a theoretical advantage in patients with concomitant cirrhosis in that less normal parenchyma is resected. Small tumors or tumors at the hepatic periphery can be removed by a wedge resection. Liver transplantation as a treatment modality is of renewed interest in patients with hepatocellular carcinoma. This is discussed in the chapter *Liver Transplantation: Gastroenterologic Considerations*.

Hepatic Lobectomy

After opening the abdomen of the patient with colon cancer, the operative site of the previous primary large bowel tumor should be explored. A careful examination

TABLE 3 Results of Surgical Treatment of Primary Hepatic Malignancies

Author	Period	No. of Patients	No. (and %) with Hepatocellular Carcinoma	Operative Mortality (%)	Survival (%) 1	2	3	5 Yr
Liver Tumor Survey	1960–74	127	109 (86)	27/127 (21) (A)		67		28
Lin[13]	1954–74	118		14/118 (12) (B)	35	24	20	19
Adson and Weiland[14]		46	43 (93)	2/46 (4) (B)			65	36
Fortner et al[15]	1970–80	42	30 (71)	7/42 (17) (B)	85		50	37
		15			100		85	76
Thompson et al[9]	1955–80	26	26 (100)	7/26 (27)	70	40	38	38
Iwatsuki et al[11]	1964–82	43	29 (67)	4/43 (9) (A+B)	78	60	56	46
		32			80	60	58	40

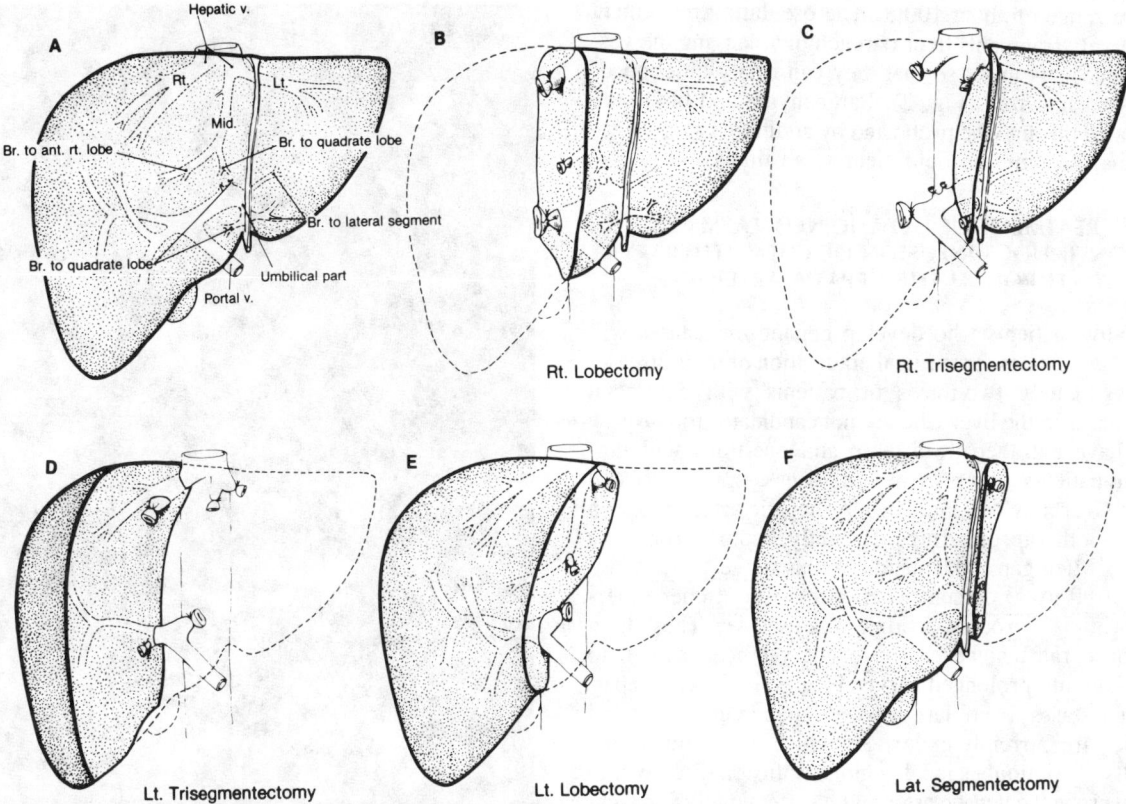

Figure 1 Hepatic resections commonly employed for metastatic or primary hepatic malignancy. The anatomic basis of major hepatic resections rests upon identification of relevant portal and hepatic venous structures and preservation of those tributaries that supply/drain liver parenchyma remaining behind. In cancer surgery, however, the primary objective is to resect the tumor with an adequate margin. Because of the rich network of interconnections within both the portal venous and hepatic venous systems, it is often acceptable to sacrifice structures connecting with tissue that will remain behind if such sacrifice is necessary to achieve adequate tumor resection. The portal vein courses in a sagittal plane in the umbilical fissure and supplies both the quadrate lobe (with its "feedback" structures) and the left lateral segment. In a left lateral segmentectomy (F) it should be spared by transecting the liver about 1 cm to the left of the umbilical fissure and falciform ligament. To spare it when performing a right trisegmentectomy (C), the parenchymal transection should be done approximately 1 cm to the right of the umbilical fissure. In a left lobectomy (E), the middle hepatic vein branch from the anterior part of the right lobe should be spared. The caudate lobe receives vessels and ducts from both the right and the left hilar structures and drains directly into the vena cava. It can be removed in conjunction with any of the major resections as tumor anatomy necessitates. From Ottow RT, Sugarbaker PH, August DA. Surgical therapy of hepatobiliary tumors. In: Bottino JC (ed). Therapy of neoplasms confined to the liver and biliary tract. Amsterdam, Martinus Nijhoff, 1985.

of the pelvis should be performed to rule out pelvic implants and peritoneal carcinomatosis. The retroperitoneum should be assessed as well as is possible from the anterior portion of the abdomen. Finally, when the surgeon is convinced that the viscera and retroperitoneum are free of tumor, the liver itself should be carefully examined by bimanual palpation. One must carefully check the hepatic and celiac lymph nodes. If any are enlarged and firm, a cryostat section must be obtained. In my experience, a frequent cause for canceling a hepatic resection intraoperatively is involvement of these node groups. If no disease is found outside of the liver, the chest may be opened, the costal cartilage divided, and diaphragm split for good exposure of the liver and its hepatic veins. To ensure low morbidity and mortality the lobe of the liver to be removed must be freely mobilized, preliminary ligation of portal structures performed, and meticulous dissection through hepatic parenchyma completed.

Technique of Metastasectomy. Prior to beginning the parenchymal dissection, the foramen of Winslow must be clearly identified. A soft rubber drain is passed around the portal structures to occlude the vascular supply to the liver intermittently while the surgeon is dissecting through it. An attempt should be made to stay approximately 1 cm from each metastasis, and they are removed with clear margins. Inflow occlusion of the liver classically is limited to 30 minutes. This period can be safely extended, possibly up to 60 minutes. Following removal of the metastasis and ligation of the vessels in the surrounding liver, a Gelfoam plug is placed within the defect to encourage blood clotting. It is especially important to check for bile leaks upon removal of the Gelfoam; if noted, they should be suture ligated.

The Ultrasonic Dissector. The Cavitron Ultrasonic Aspirator (CUSA) consists of a hollow titanium probe, oscillating longitudinally at a frequency of about 23 kHz over a range of about 100 μ. The oscillating movement selectively fragments liver parenchyma, leaving the vessels and ducts intact so that they can easily be clipped, tied, or cauterized (Fig. 2). Parenchyma and blood are aspirated through the probe and by additional suction apparatus, keeping the field clear at all times.

TREATMENT OF HEPATIC NEOPLASMS BY CONTINUOUS INFUSION OF CHEMOTHERAPY THROUGH THE HEPATIC ARTERY

Most patients who develop hepatic metastases will not be candidates for surgical eradication of their disease. Approximately two-thirds of patients with colorectal metastases to the liver who are not candidates for surgery will have extrahepatic disease and one-third will not. Those patients who present with disease spread isolated to the liver may be candidates for hepatic artery infusion of chemotherapeutic drugs. Recently, reports from Ann Arbor, Michigan and Houston, Texas suggest a response rate of 60 to 80 percent when intra-arterial chemotherapy with 5-fluorodeoxyuridine was used.[21,22] These high response rates however, have not yet been shown to translate into prolonged survival for patients with hepatic metastases from large bowel malignancy. Several studies are currently under way which will compare the results of continuous local-regional infusion directly into the liver via the hepatic artery with systemic infusion techniques into a central vein. Indeed, early results from these studies suggest no difference in survival in the two groups of patients. There is, however, a markedly increased incidence of *adverse side effects* with the *intra-arterial drug*. Problems with duodenitis and gastritis are seen in approximately 50 percent of patients given arterial infusion. Also, nearly all patients develop some chemical hepatitis in response to the direct infusion of chemotherapy. About one-third of these patients go on to develop chemotherapy-induced sclerosing cholangitis, and some deaths from this disorder have been reported.[24]

It is clear that hepatic artery infusion should not be accepted as a standard treatment for hepatic metastases from colorectal malignancy or primary hepatocellular carcinoma at this point. Further investigations comparing arterial infusion with systemic infusion and with no treatment in this population of patients are required.

TREATMENT OF HEPATIC METASTASES IN THE PRESENCE OF EXTRAHEPATIC DISEASE

A dilemma arises in all patients who develop hepatic metastases along with disseminated disease from gastrointestinal malignancy. In patients with gastric malignancy the FAM (5-fluorouracil [5-FU], adriamycin, and mitomycin-C) regimen has been shown to improve the long-term survival of those with metastatic disease. This is described in the chapter *Gastric Carcinoma*. The results in patients with other gastrointestinal malignancies are less straightforward. The results of multiple agent chemotherapy compared with 5-FU alone in patients with metastatic colorectal cancer are shown in Table 4. It should be noted that no combination of agents gives better results

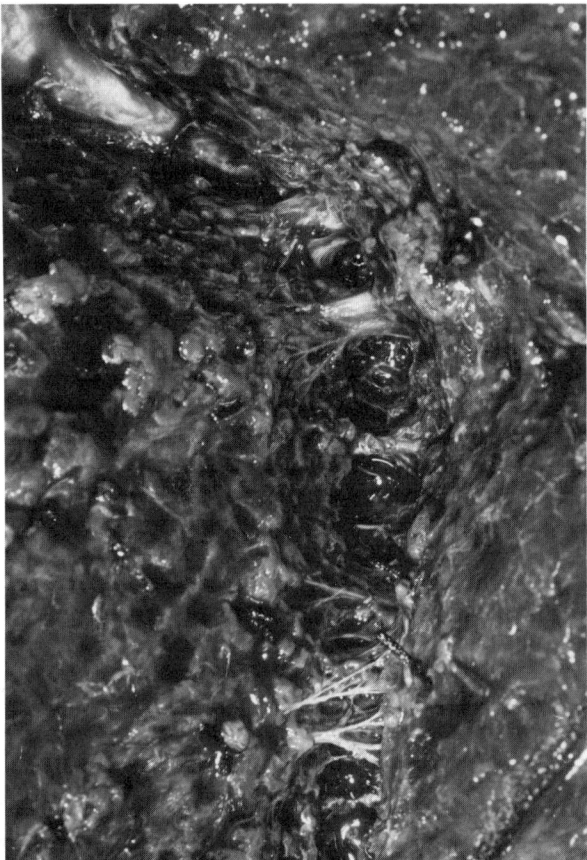

Figure 2 Proper technique using ultrasonic dissection of the liver with the Cavitron Ultrasonic Aspirator (CUSA) results in hemostasis of microvasculature and dissects the larger vessels and ducts free of parenchyma so they can be ligated in continuity before division.

than single agents such as 5-FU, mitomycin-C, or methyl-CCNU. Suggestions for treatment of patients with hepatic metastases with extrahepatic disease cannot be simply formulated. No clearly superior treatment plan exists. If patients (especially aged patients) are not anxious to be treated, no attempt at chemotherapy is required. In those patients who desire treatment, sequential single agent chemotherapy with careful monitoring of progression or regression of disease is indicated. The drug of choice to initiate therapy is usually 5-FU. Liver-spleen scans and carcinoembryonic antigen assays should be followed to assess the response. If after three to four cycles of treatment disease progression is seen, a second line agent, such as mitomycin-C, may be utilized. Again the patient is carefully followed and treatment continued if disease stabilization or regression is achieved. If there is clear progression, the treatment should be stopped. In this manner patients who respond to the drug may realize their maximal benefit from treatment. The majority of patients who fail to respond will not suffer a prolonged adverse effect on their quality of life as a result of ineffective chemotherapy treatments. Adjuvant therapy for colorectal cancer is discussed in a separate chapter.

Patients with large, symptomatic hepatic metastases from a wide variety of malignancies may be substantially

TABLE 4 5-Fluorouracil Plus Methyl-CCNU Combination Regimen in Advanced Colon Cancer

Treatment	No. of Patients	No. of Partial Responses (%)	Survival Superior To 5-FU Alone
5-FU + methyl-CCNU	489	98 (20)	No
5-FU + methyl-CCNU + vincristine	358	82 (23)	No
5-FU + methyl-CCNU + DTIC	83	14 (14)	No
5-FU + methyl-CCNU + vincristine + streptozocin	71	11 (15)	No
	54	15 (27)	Not done

5-FU = 5-fluorouracil; DTIC = Dimethyl triazeno imidazole carboxamide

Modified from Sugarbaker PH, MacDonald J, Gunderson L. Colorectal cancer. In: DeVita V, Hellman S, Rosenberg SA, eds. Principles and practice of oncology. Philadelphia: JB Lippincott Co, 1982.

palliated by radiation therapy. Success has also been achieved with angiographic embolization of tumor masses through a percutaneous route. This method of treatment has been especially effective in tumors richly vascularized by the hepatic artery, such as insulinomas, carcinoid tumors, or other metastases that show a marked blush on arteriography.

Hepatic artery perfusion by a percutaneous route is also sometimes beneficial for palliation in patients who have large, painful hepatic metastases. Shrinkage of these tumor masses is the rule rather than the exception if adequate doses of drug can be used.

Occasionally hepatic artery ligation may be utilized in patients with large and symptomatic tumors. Recent reports of intra-arterial chemotherapy following hepatic artery ligation suggest favorable responses when these two treatments are combined. Others have suggested that, following hepatic artery ligation, perfusion of 5-FU into the portal vein gives maximal tumor shrinkage. Further studies to establish the optimal means of perfusing the liver to shrink metastases are required.

ANTIBODY-DIRECTED CELLULAR IRRADIATION

Polyclonal antibodies directed against the large ferritin stores in primary liver cancer cells are being used, at some centers, to deliver irradiation to primary hepatomas. In preliminary, uncontrolled studies of 104 patients with primary hepatomas, Order et al[1] at the Johns Hopkins Oncology Center described "remission" in almost half and "total remission" in 7 percent. This interesting technique of delivering irradiation preferentially to tumor cells while sparing normal cells is also being applied to Hodgkin's disease.

REFERENCES

1. Order SE. Radioimmunoglobulin therapy of cancer. Comp Ther 1984; 10:9–18.
2. Foster JH, Berman MM. Solid liver tumors. In: Ebert P, ed. Major problems in clinical surgery. Philadelphia: WB Saunders, 1977; 1.
3. August DA, Sugarbaker PH, Gianola FJ, Ottow RT, and Schneider PD. Hepatic resection of colorectal metastases: Influence of clinical factors and adjuvant intraperitoneal 5-fluorouracil via Tenckhoff catheter on survival. Ann Surg 1985; 210:210–218.
4. Fortner JG, Silva JS, Golbey RB, et al. Multivariate analysis of a personal series of 247 consecutive patients with liver metastases from colorectal cancer. I. Treatment by hepatic resection. Ann Surg 1984; 199:306–316.
5. Adson MA, van Heerden JA. Major hepatic resections for metastatic colorectal cancer. Ann Surg 1980; 191:576–583.
6. August DA, Sugarbaker PH, and Schneider PD. Lymphatic dissemination of hepatic metastases: Implications for the follow-up and treatment of patients with colorectal cancer. Cancer 1985; 55:1490–1494.
7. Attiyeh FF, Wanebo HJ, Stearns MW. Hepatic resection for metastasis from colorectal cancer. Dis Colon Rectum 1978; 21:160–162.
8. Bengmark S, Hafstrom L, Jeppsson B, et al. Metastatic disease in the liver from colorectal cancer: an appraisal of liver surgery. World J Surg 1982; 6:61–65.
9. Thompson HH, Tompkins RK, Longmire WP. Major hepatic resection: a 25-year experience. Ann Surg 1983; 197:375–388.
10. Rajpal S, Dasmahapatra KS, Ledesma EJ, et al. Extensive resections of isolated metastasis from carcinoma of the colon and rectum. Surg Gynecol Obstet 1982; 155:813–816.
11. Iwatsuki S, Shaw BW, Starzl TE. Experience with 150 liver resections. Ann Surg 1983; 197:247–253.
12. Steele G (Jr), Osteen RT, Wilson RE, et al. Patterns of failure after surgical cure of large liver tumors. A change in the proximate cause of death and a need for effective systemic adjuvant therapy. Am J Surg 1984; 147:554.
13. Lin TY. Recent advances in techniques of hepatic lobectomy and results of surgical treatment for primary carcinoma of the liver. Prog Liver Dis 1976; 5:668.
14. Adson MA, Weiland LH. Resection of primary solid hepatic tumors. Am J Surg 1981; 141:18.
15. Fortner JG, Maclean BJ, Kim DK, Howland WS, Turnbull AD, Goldiner P, Carlon G, Beattie EJ Jr. The seventies evolution in liver surgery for cancer. Cancer 1981; 47:2162.
16. Tang, Z. Treatment of primary liver cancer with special reference to the east part of China. Ann Acad Med Singapore 1980; 9:251.
17. Martin JK, Moertel CG, Adson MA, Schutt AJ. Surgical treatment of functioning metastatic carcinoid tumors. Arch Surg 1983; 118:537.
18. Norton JA, Sugarbaker PH, Doppman JL, Wesley RA, Morton PN, Garner JD, Jensen RT. Aggressive resection of metastatic disease in selected patients with malignant gastrinoma. Ann Surg (in press).
19. Okuda K, et al, Primary liver cancers in Japan. Cancer 1980; 45:2663.
20. Fortner JG, Kim DK, Maclean BJ, Barrett MK, Iwatsuki S, Turnbull AD, Howland WS, Beattie EJ Jr. Major hepatic resection for neoplasia: personal experience in 108 patients. Ann Surg 1978; 188:363.
21. Ensminger WD, Niederhuber J, Dakhill S, Thrall J, Wheeler R. Totally implanted drug delivery system for hepatic arterial chemotherapy. Cancer Treat Rep 1981; 65:393–400.
22. Patt YZ, Mavligit GM, Chuang VP. Percutaneous hepatic arterial infusion (HAI) of mitomycin C and floxuridine (FUDR): an effective treatment for metastatic colorectal carcinoma in the liver. Cancer 1980; 46:261–265.
23. Couinaud C Le foie. Etudes anatomiques et chirurgicales. Paris: Masson, 1957.
24. Chang AE, Schneider PD, Sugarbaker PH. Hepatic arterial infusion chemotherapy with the implantable pump: status of clinical trials in colorectal hepatic metastases. In: Lokich J. Infusional chemotherapy (in press)

HIGH BILIARY STRICTURE

JAMES SITZMANN, M.D.

STRICTURE OF THE BILE DUCT

Biliary strictures may conveniently be classified as benign or malignant. Either type presents the clinician with a difficult management problem despite the advent of improved operative techniques and new developments in invasive radiologic techniques. Nevertheless, the patient with a malignant or benign stricture today faces a better prognosis than in years past owing to these advances. Patients with benign strictures now can look forward to long, productive lives and a relatively low incidence of recurrent stricture, and patients with malignant strictures also will have significant prolongation of life if the strictures are operable. The causes of death remain the same for both groups: either liver failure due to biliary cirrhosis or sepsis secondary to cholangitis. Both represent ultimately the failure to control the stricture process.

Benign Stricture

Nearly all benign strictures have traditionally been thought secondary to operative injuries to the common bile ducts; and the majority of benign strictures are, in fact, iatrogenic and result from surgical trauma. Today, however, we would also include various disease states that lead to a stricture, such as sclerosing cholangitis, oriental cholangitis (Caroli's disease), or gallstone erosion of the bile ducts, as causes of benign stricture. The treatment of a benign stricture will vary somewhat depending on the etiologic agent, and the prognosis also depends upon the underlying cause of the stricture.

Primary Benign Stricture

Stricture secondary to operative trauma follows injury to the common bile duct or to the right or left hepatic duct during the course of cholecystectomy, choledochostomy, gastrectomy, or major pancreatic procedures. Typically the injury involves transection of the bile duct, excision of a segment, or partial or complete occlusion of the duct with suture or metallic clip.

The injury usually is unnoticed at the time, but if it is recognized, it should be repaired immediately. If the duct has been severed or a small portion (less than 1 cm) excised, an end-to-end anastomosis should be performed with 4–0 or 5–0 interrupted prolene sutures. Some surgeons use an absorbable suture, which is also acceptable. The duct should be stented with a T-tube brought out through the area distal to the repair. If a large segment of the duct has been removed, the proximal segment of the duct should be anastomosed to a Roux-en-Y jejunal loop and stented with a T-tube. The T-tube can be removed in 6 weeks to 3 months if a satisfactory repair has been made.

If the biliary injury is not recognized at the time of operation, it will declare itself in the early postoperative period by excessive or prolonged biliary drainage from the abdominal drains, frequently associated with jaundice and fever.

Whenever an injury to the biliary tree is suspected, whether in the early postoperative period or after discharge from the hospital, biliary anatomy must be defined by either percutaneous transhepatic cholangiography (PTC), or by T-tube study if a T-tube is in place, or by fistulogram (injection of a fistulous tract with dye) if a fistula is present. Endoscopic retrograde cholangiography (ERCP) can also be used. Probably the single best study is the PTC, because if the bile ducts are damaged, a percutaneous catheter can be placed into the bile ducts for external drainage, thus decreasing the chance of development of sepsis as well as resolving jaundice if present.

If the stricture or injury is newly diagnosed, even if external drainage by a Ring catheter has been established, the patient will need reconstruction. Percutaneous dilation or stent placement is not appropriate in this situation because of the high incidence of recurrent stenosis and ongoing sepsis in this setting. Once the patient's biliary tree is drained adequately and antibiotics begun, any sepsis should be controlled. If there is a concurrent biliary cutaneous fistula, an intra-abdominal collection should be ruled out by computed tomography (CT) scan or sonogram and/or fistulogram. If there is an abscess (usually in the subhepatic position), this will need to be drained adequately prior to any reconstruction, either by percutaneous catheter placement through the fistulous tract or by open transabdominal drainage. For patients who are this ill, I typically commence central intravenous nutrition.

Reconstruction is attempted when sepsis is resolved and the nutritional status of the patient is optimal. The operative approach is via a bisubcostal incision. The proximal biliary tree is identified and the area of the stricture dissected free and resected, so that fresh, undamaged duct is available for anastomosis to a Roux-en-Y jejunal loop. If the stricture is too high to be resected (i.e., it involves intrahepatic right or left duct), it can be dilated with a Bakes dilator. Following resection a Stone forceps is inserted through the biliary tree and out the dome of the liver. A Silastic stent is sewn to the tip of the forceps and brought through the bile ducts. Stents are 60-mm long and have multiple side holes. The stents are 10 mm, 8 mm, and 6 mm in diameter. The largest stent possible should be placed. The bile duct is then anastomosed to a Roux-en-Y jejunal loop with the silastic tube acting as a stent. Every effort is made to approximate mucosa to mucosa. If the bifurcation is involved, or if both ducts are involved, two stents are placed. The subhepatic and subdiaphragmatic spaces should be well drained with Penrose or sump drains.

Postoperatively the stents are left open to gravity drainage until the cholangiogram demonstrates a patent anastomosis without a leak. The stent is then clamped and the drains are removed. The stents should be irrigated with

20 ml of saline each day and should be replaced every 3 or 4 months, or sooner if occluded with sludge. In benign strictures the stent usually needs to remain in place for one year.

Stent replacement can be done as an outpatient procedure by a radiologist. Under fluoroscopic control, a guidewire is passed through the stent and the stent removed. A new stent is fed over the guidewire into position. The guidewire is then removed and the stent placement is confirmed by cholangiogram.

Recurrent Benign Stricture

Once the primary iatrogenic stricture has been repaired, the prognosis is excellent. Nonetheless, recurrent stricture occurs in approximately 30 to 50 percent of patients over the course of their lifetimes following adequate repair and stenting. Most of these recurrent benign strictures occur within 2 to 3 years of the primary repair. Typically the patient presents with Charcot's triad of right upper quadrant pain, fever, and jaundice.

Diagnosis is possible only with a PTC; CT scan is particularly unhelpful and sonogram or technetium 99m disofenin scans are only marginally more senstive. The recurrent stricture is typically at the site of the biliary-enteric anastomosis; bile duct stones frequently are present. The treatment of this type of stricture is usually nonoperative, since transhepatic balloon dilation has a high degree of success. Initially the biliary anatomy should be defined by standard transhepatic cholangiography. If a stricture is present, a Ring catheter should also be inserted to drain the biliary tree, preferably traversing the area of stricture. The patient should begin to receive intravenous antibiotics and the Ring catheter is placed for external drainage until cholangitis resolves. Then the stricture can be safely dilated percutaneously. Usually I leave a catheter in place and capped at the skin level for 3 to 4 months and repeat cholangiography every 1 to 2 months to ensure that the dilated stricture remains open. If there are associated stones, these can be crushed transhepatically and will pass once the stricture is dilated.

The results following percutaneous balloon dilation of benign recurrent stricture are encouraging, although the technique is still so new that adequate long-term results are not available. One can expect to dilate anastomotic strictures three to four times over a 3-month period to ensure a stable patent anastomosis. The chapter *Percutaneous Transhepatic Biliary Drainage and Retained Biliary Stone Extraction* provides additional information.

Sclerosing Cholangitis

Sclerosing cholangitis is a chronic disease of unknown origin which results in multiple fibrotic strictures in the bile ducts. It is noted to occur in association with ulcerative colitis, Crohn's disease, chronic pancreatitis, thyroiditis, retroperitoneal fibrosis, and mediastinal fibrosis. Most patients have diffuse involvement of intra- and extrahepatic bile ducts. Many patients, however, will have their most restrictive obstruction at the bifurcation of the hepatic ducts. If this occurs, a direct surgical attack can offer hope of reasonable palliation. Therefore the indications for operative palliation of sclerosing cholangitis are (1) persistent jaundice, (2) the hepatic bifurcation lesion as the most restrictive obstruction, and (3) absence of advanced biliary cirrhosis (no evidence of portal hypertension, ascites, or encephalopathy). Liver transplantation is being employed for some of these patients. There is a separate chapter on *Liver Transplantation: Gastroenterologic Considerations*.

Transhepatic cholangiography is used to confirm the diagnosis and define the biliary anatomy. A ring catheter should be placed to decompress the biliary tree and help identify the bile ducts at the time of surgery. Preoperative antibiotics and intravenous alimentation are routinely used.

At operation, a cholecystectomy is performed and the common bile duct is identified and divided distally. The common duct is then dissected free of the portal vein and the bifurcation mobilized. The right and left ducts are divided and the duct removed. The right and left hepatic ducts are then dilated with a Bakes dilator to accommodate at least a 6-mm Silastic stent for a distance of 5 cm. A Silastic stent is then brought through the duct and exits from the dome of the liver. Occasionally three stents are needed if the right middle lobe duct enters close to the bifurcation. With the stents in position, a Roux-en-Y hepaticojejunostomy is performed.

The stents are left in position permanently, since the natural history of sclerosing cholangitis is progressive. The stents are irrigated daily with 20 ml of saline and changed every 3 to 4 months over a guidewire.

Stricture Due to Stone Disease

Strictures resulting from biliary stones are relatively rare in the western hemisphere. They occur more commonly in the Orient, with *oriental cholangitis* (Caroli's disease) being the most common cause of intrahepatic stricture. The cause of the stricture is local pressure on the bile duct associated with ongoing chronic infection. Treatment is directed at stone removal and control of infection. Occasionally the stricture is focal, but more often they are multiple.

The diagnosis rests on cholangiography in the patient with signs and symptoms of cholangitis. Either ERCP or PTC is adequate to define the biliary anatomy. In patients with oriental cholangitis the intrahepatic ducts typically are almost saccular, with multiple areas of dilatation in narrowings with stones throughout. If the stricture is due to gallstones, usually the cause is a single stone eroding from the gallbladder into the right hepatic or proximal common bile duct. The patient with oriental cholangitis should begin to receive antibiotics, and the biliary tree should be drained by formal exploration via a choledochotomy. Frequently it is technically not possible to retrieve all the stones from the saccular dilated biliary radicals. In these instances stones can be crushed by transhepatic catheters or through the T-tube, which should be left in place after such as exploration. If the saccular dilatations and stone disease are confined to one lobe, some recommend resection of the involved lobe, but it is quite rare that the disease is confined to only one lobe.

If the stricture results from a single gallstone eroding through the duct, a cholecystectomy and a primary repair should be done, if possible stented with a T-tube. If that is not possible, it is probably best to reconstruct formally with a transhepatic Silastic stent and hepaticojejunostomy.

MALIGNANT TUMORS OF THE BILE DUCT

Primary malignant tumors of the bile ducts are uncommon. Most are adenocarcinomas located near or at the hepatic bifurcation (Klatskin tumor). Occasionally a primary squamous cell carcinoma occurs in this area, but more commonly a squamous cell tumor arises from the gallbladder and locally advances to involve the proximal biliary tree.

Both squamous carcinomas and adenocarcinomas present with the gradual onset of painless jaundice. ERCP will usually show a normal common duct and possibly a collapsed or nonvisualized gallbladder with an abrupt blockage at the bifurcation. PTC is more helpful, diagnostically and therapeutically, and is the test of choice. It should delineate a near-total or total bifurcation or high ductal stricture. If possible, a Ring catheter should be placed across the obstruction to provide external drainage. Although many physicians would obtain a CT scan to access "extent" of tumor, this test is only occasionally helpful in accurately defining the extent of tumor growth. A better, less expensive test would be the sonogram to assess gallbladder involvement or local liver extension. An even more important test for preoperative staging is *splanchnic arteriography* and *venography* to assess portal venous or hepatic arterial involvement by tumor. If either of these structures is involved, the patient is not a candidate for resection. Other contraindications to resection include advanced age and general debility, or evidence of ascites or parenchymal liver disease. Most patients will also exhibit marked malnutrition and this should be improved preoperatively. The cholangiographic diagnosis of proximal bile duct tumor is considered so definite that tissue confirmation prior to resection is unnecessary.

If the preoperative arteriogram shows no portal involvement, or just isolated left or right portal involvement, an exploration to judge resectability should be performed. Initially the surgeon must dissect the portahepatic structures as completely as possible, identifying hepatic arterial supply and portal venous supply and common duct. The gallbladder should be removed at this time. Once proximal portal venous and hepatic arterial control is established, the common duct is divided distally and then dissected free of the portal vein and hepatic artery. Occasionally the hepatic artery will need to be sacrificed for adequate extirpation of the tumor, but only if the portal vein is free of involvement. If the right or left portal vein is involved, a lobectomy can be performed in addition to the resection of the birfurcation.

If the tumor extends into hepatic parenchyma, or has extended far up the right or left ducts, a clear surgical margin will be almost impossible to obtain. At this point, heroics should be avoided and the bulk of the tumor removed. Thus, the entire extrahepatic biliary tree is resected, rarely in combination with a lobectomy. One should combine extrahepatic biliary resection with a lobectomy cautiously, as this will increase the operative mortality to 20 to 25 percent. The addition of lobectomy should be considered only if a curative margin is to be established. It definitely should not be considered as part of the palliative procedure. "Chasing" a positive margin at the right or left hepatic duct far into the hepatic parenchyma also is to be avoided.

Once the extrahepatic biliary tree is resected with or without clear margins, the patient undergoes reconstruction with bilateral hepaticojejunostomies. If tumor remains, the areas should be marked with silver clips for future radiotherapy. Silastic stents (6 mm) are inserted in the right and left hepatic ducts. With the stents in place, a Roux-en-Y jejunal loop 60-cm long is brought retrocolic, and bilateral hepaticojejunostomies are constructed with 6-0 prolene interrupted sutures (Fig. 1). The internal limb of the stent is placed into the bowel and the other end is brought out the dome of the liver and then exteriorized through a flank stab wound.

If the tumor is completely unresectable due to unsuspected portal venous or hepatic parenchymal involvement, the common duct is transected below the tumor and the tumor forcibly dilated until a 6-mm Silastic stent can be placed in each duct. Then a hepaticojejunostomy is performed to the end of the duct. The anastomosis should be well drained with Penrose or Axiom sump drains.

Postoperatively the stents are left to drain by gravity until cholangiography demonstrates that all bile leaks have sealed. The stents are then clamped with stopcocks and irrigated daily with 20 ml of saline. The stents are left in place permanently whether the resection was considered curative or palliative and are replaced every 3 to 6 months. All patients receive 5,000 rads of *external radiation* during the postoperative period. An additional 2,000 rads of *local radiation* is delivered by placing iridium 192 seeds down the Silastic stent and leaving them in position for 48 hours. This is an inpatient procedure following the course of external beam radiotherapy. Overall survival is excellent with mortality being less than 4 percent.

Nonoperative Management of Malignant Strictures

While any patient with a potentially resectable lesion should be offered an operation, the alternative to definitive therapy, percutaneous stent placement, is a safe and effective short-term management. The main drawback of percutaneous stent placement is the development of sepsis if the patient survives long enough. The incidence of hepatic abscess or major episodes of hemobilia progressively increases over a 6- to 12-month period, so I do not recommend this form of therapy if the patient is expected to live longer than 12 to 18 months. The indications

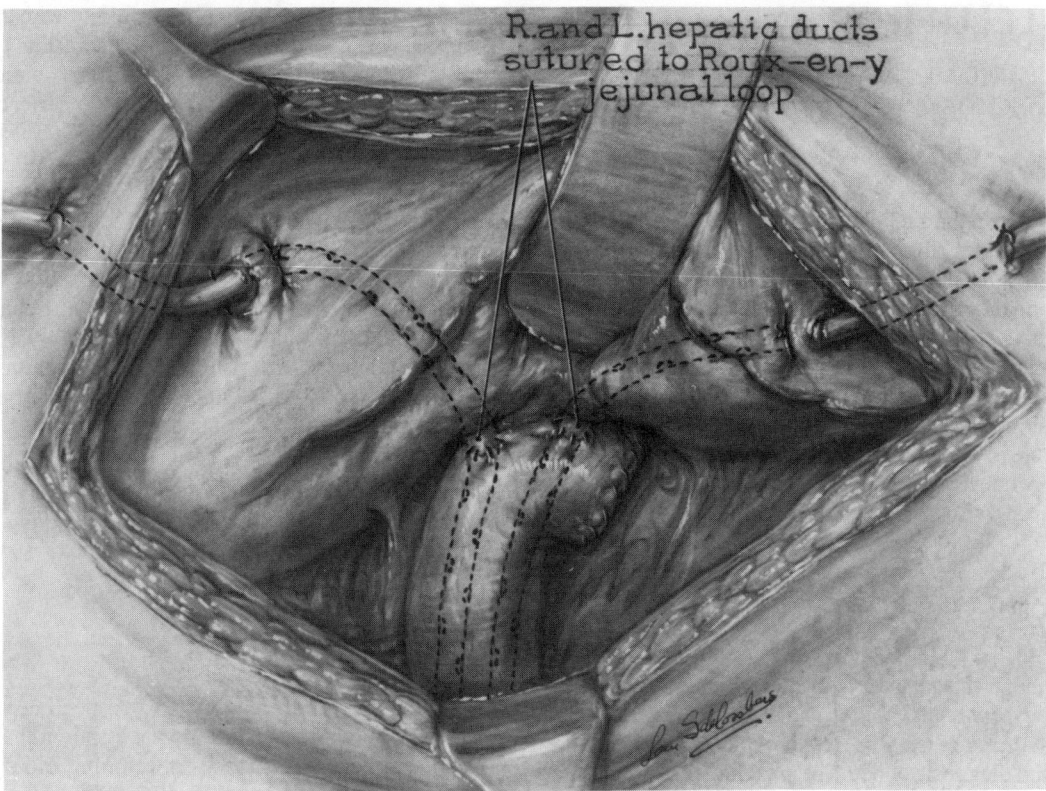

Figure 1 A Roux-en-Y jejunal loop is constructed and bilateral hepaticojejunostomies are performed. The ends of the stents are brought out onto the anterior abdominal wall and left to gravity bile bag drainage. (From Cameron JL, et al. Proximal bile duct tumors: surgical management with Silastic transhepatic biliary stents. Ann Surg 1982; 196:412.

for percutaneous management of a malignant stricture are (1) advanced disease and limited life expectancy, or (2) acute illness.

Candidates for percutaneous drainage should have antibiotics initiated the day prior to catheterization. The percutaneous entrance site is determined by PTC and the liver approached laterally. The most suitable duct is one that is of large diameter and has a straight course toward the obstruction. Once the anatomy has been defined, a large sheath type needle is inserted into the duct. A guidewire is then passed through the sheath and through the obstruction and the sheath is removed. In some patients with total biliary obstruction the guidewire will not pass through the stenotic segment. In these patients, if external drainage of the biliary tree is employed for 48 hours, the decrease in pressure and the dilation of the biliary tree above the narrowing frequently relieve the stenosis, allowing easier passage of the guidewire. A specially modified polyethylene pigtail catheter (Ring catheter) is advanced over the guidewire through the duct and down into the duodenum. The catheter has side holes in the proximal part which lie in the biliary tree and also in the distal part for drainage into the duodenum. The distal part of the catheter is angulated to facilitate positioning in the common bile duct and duodenum. It is important to position the catheter correctly to avoid obstruction of the ampulla of Vater. This occurs if the pigtail is not re-formed in the duodenum. The position of the catheter is confirmed radiologically and the catheter secured to the skin with a suture. Postdrainage cholangiography is performed daily for 2 to 3 days to confirm that the catheter has remained in position. Patency is maintained by twice daily irrigation with 25 ml of saline. Pain is a frequent accompaniment after catheter placement but usually subsides after a few days and necessitates only oral analgesia.

Occasionally patients develop bile leakage from the percutaneous placement site. In this case the catheter usually is demonstrated radiologically to be obstructed at the distal end. Leakage from the catheter is resolved by passing a guidewire through it. After the initial percutaneous drainage catheter has formed a sheath around it (approximately 1 week), the Silastic percutaneous stent can be placed forcibly through and past the stricture and this can be directed toward internal drainage and then capped at the skin, thus allowing the patient greater mobility. As mentioned previously, the most worrisome long-term complication of this form of therapy is the development of sepsis and intrahepatic abscesses or cholangitis, but nonetheless it remains a viable alternative treatment for the patient in need of short-term management. The technique, as well as follow-up and complications, is described in the chapter *Percutaneous Transhepatic Biliary Drainage and Retained Biliary Stone Extraction.*

CHOLELITHIASIS

HANS FROMM, M.D.
MAURO MALAVOLTI, M.D.

New data regarding the epidemiology and natural history of gallstones have removed much of the controversy which surrounded the indications for medical versus surgical treatment of gallstones. Although there was little disagreement as to the need for surgical intervention in acute biliary tract disease, considerable differences of opinion existed concerning the management of gallstone carriers with either no symptoms or nonspecific ones. In this chapter, the role of surgical vis-a-vis that of medical treatment will be delineated in the different clinical settings of cholelithiasis.

DIFFERENTIAL DIAGNOSTIC CONSIDERATIONS AND MANAGEMENT OF ACUTE GALLBLADDER DISEASE

Although this chapter is primarily aimed at discussing the key elements of the medical and surgical treatment of gallstone disease, a few comments regarding the differential diagnosis of acute biliary tract disease and the indications for gallbladder surgery are in order. On one hand, the diagnosis is not always easy to establish because of the variability of the clinical manifestations of gallbladder disease. On the other hand, nonspecific symptoms are frequently used as indications for a cholecystectomy, in spite of the fact that they are neither caused by, nor significantly associated with, the presence of gallstones. In most cases the clinical picture of an acute gallbladder attack is marked by a so-called biliary colic. The term "colic" is not entirely appropriate, since biliary pain is usually steady rather than "colicky." It is typically located in the epigastrium and/or right upper quadrant of the abdomen, lasting several hours with a crescendo-plateau-decrescendo sequence. A biliary colic can also begin suddenly and end abruptly; however, since gallstones are very common, they frequently coexist with other conditions such as irritable colon, peptic ulcer, reflux esophagitis, and ischemic heart disease, any of which may stimulate symptoms of a gallbladder attack. Therefore, if the presence of gallstones is documented by ultrasonography or other imaging techniques in a patient with acute abdominal pain, acute gallbladder disease represents only one of several differential diagnostic possibilities. It is thus necessary to corroborate the clinical impression of acute biliary tract disease by laboratory tests, such as the measurement of serum alanine aminotransferase, asparate aminotransferase, alkaline phosphatase, and/or amylase, which are frequently abnormal within a 24-hour period after an attack. Even if the biliary origin of the pain has been established, the decision to operate should not be an automatic one. Although an elective cholecystectomy is, in the hands of an experienced surgeon, very safe, the operation carries a significant mortality rate in elderly debilitated patients, especially if they present with cardiovascular and/or pulmonary disease in addition to biliary complications. The frequency of biliary colic attacks varies considerably, with some patients experiencing them weekly and others only once in a lifetime. It is therefore advisable to treat high-risk patients medically to determine both their chances of improving with medical treatment and the likelihood of their remaining free of symptoms and complications after improvement has taken place. If a cholecystectomy is indicated, the operation should be performed by an experienced surgeon, regardless of whether a "difficult case" or only a "routine" elective cholecystectomy is involved. It is not unusual that anatomic variations of the biliary tree and other unexpected intraoperative findings change a "routine" case into a difficult one.

MANAGEMENT OF GALLSTONE PATIENTS WITH EITHER NO SYMPTOMS OR NONSPECIFIC SYMPTOMS

Expectant Management

Several carefully conducted prospective studies in both the United States and Italy have shown that the risk of subjects with silent stones developing biliary pain is very low, i.e., approximately 1 to 2 percent per year. The risk of development of complications from gallstones is even lower. Only about 10 percent of the patients with biliary pain develop complications. Furthermore, biliary complications, such as gallbladder perforation, bile duct obstruction, and ascending cholangitis, are virtually always preceded by attacks of biliary pain. A risk-benefit analysis based on these data convincingly shows that prophylactic cholecystectomy does not increase life expectancy. Patients with silent stones who are managed expectantly and undergo cholecystectomy only if they develop biliary pain or complications live as long as those who choose prophylactic cholecystectomy. The latter mode of treatment, however, has been estimated to be almost four times as expensive as expectant management. A prophylactic cholecystectomy should therefore not be considered in patients with silent stones. The same recommendation applies to patients with gallstones who have nonspecific symptoms, such as "dyspepsia," heartburn, fat intolerance, and irritable bowel-induced pain. These symptoms bear no significant relation to the presence of gallstones and thus do not represent an indication for cholecystectomy.

Bile Acid Dissolution Treatment

General Criteria For and Features of Gallstone Dissolution Therapy. A select group of patients with gallstones, namely those with cholesterol stones, may benefit from treatment with either chenodeoxycholic acid (cheno) or its 7β-epimer, ursodeoxycholic acid (urso), or a combination of the two. Cheno and urso are bile acids that naturally occur in both man and several animal species. Ingestion of either 14 to 15 mg per kilogram of body weight per day of cheno or 10 to 13 mg per kilogram per day of urso results in the dissolution of gallbladder stones in 50 to 90 percent of the patients. The gallbladder has to be functioning, as evidenced by its adequate filling with contrast medium during an oral cholecystogram, and the gallstones have to be radiolucent. Nonvisualization of the gallbladder and calcification of the stones make it unlikely that the dissolution treatment will succeed. Small and floating stones respond best and fastest to the bile acid treatment. In contrast, stones larger than 1.5 cm in diameter dissolve poorly. The success rate of cholelitholytic therapy is thus mainly determined by the composition and size of the stones as well as by gallbladder function. The length of treatment varies from 6 to 24 months, depending upon the individual stone and gallbladder characteristics. The treatment can be considered a failure if there is no change in stone size after 1 year. The progress of gallstone dissolution is documented by follow-up oral cholecystograms after 1 and 2 years. The advantage of oral cholecystography over ultrasonography of the gallbladder lies in the ability of the radiographic technique to provide information on gallbladder function. Ultrasonography, however, is more sensitive for the detection of small stone remnants that may remain in the gallbladder as a result of incomplete dissolution. These residues may act as a nidus for the formation of new concrements, probably explaining, at least in part, the stone recurrence that is observed in approximately 10 percent of the cases per year. It is therefore our practice to follow patients after successful dissolution therapy with twice yearly ultrasonograms. If stones recur, they usually respond to a relatively short course of cholelitholytic therapy with either bile acid.

Differential Therapeutic Features of Cheno and Urso. Cheno and urso are equally efficacious. Although they both are safe for medical use, urso is safer. Cheno treatment is associated with minor to moderate elevations of serum transaminases in about 20 percent of cases. These occur during the first 3 to 6 months of treatment and are almost always transient, in spite of continued cheno administration. There is no evidence that chemo causes any permanent functional or histologic abnormalities of the liver. The changes, if any, always disappear after discontinuation of cheno, although this is, as noted above, not usually necessary.

The second side effect of cheno relates to its cathartic action, which results in the development of diarrhea in a significant number of patients. The occurrence of diarrhea is dose-dependent and therefore more common in the patients who adhere to the optimal dose of 15 mg per kilogram per day than in those who take lower doses. The diarrheal effect of cheno is less pronounced and can often be avoided if the optimal therapeutic dose is built up slowly over several weeks, allowing for an adjustment of the intestine to the secretory action of this bile acid.

The third side effect of cheno is a minor one. In the National Cooperative Gallstone Study it was observed that, during the 2-year treatment period, cheno caused an approximately 10 mg percent increase of serum cholesterol in the low-density lipoprotein fraction. There is little reason to believe that this rise poses any significant cardiovascular risk, especially since the duration of cheno treatment does not exceed 2 years.

In contrast to cheno, urso has no known side effects. Neither liver test abnormalities nor diarrhea have been observed as a result of urso treatment. There is also no evidence that urso affects serum cholesterol levels. For these reasons, urso has become the drug of choice as far as gallstone dissolution therapy is concerned. There are, however, several reasons for keeping cheno available for cholelitholytic treatment. First, the concern regarding the described side effects of cheno is most certainly exaggerated in view of the considerable experience which now exists with this compound. Cheno is safe if the patient is properly monitored with measurements of serum transaminases during the first 6 months of treatment. Second, cheno is, in contrast to urso, approved by the Food and Drug Administration (urso is currently under review for approval). Third, cheno is less expensive than urso. A fourth and important reason for continuing the use of cheno lies in the potential this compound has in combination with urso. Our preliminary experience and that of other investigators suggest that a combination of half of the optimal doses of cheno (about 7.5 mg per kilogram per day) and urso (about 6.5 mg per kilogram per day) causes no side effects and is as effective as the optimal doses of either compound alone. The reason for the apparent safety of the cheno-urso combination probably relates to both the relatively low dose of cheno and a possible hepatoprotective effect of urso.

A 1-year course of treatment with cheno at a dose of 15 mg per kilogram per day costs about $1,200. The cost for urso would be somewhat higher. A 2-year treatment with either bile acid, however, would still be significantly less expensive than a cholecystectomy.

Common Duct Stones. The presence of common duct stones in patients after cholecystectomy usually is an indication for endoscopic papillotomy (the exceptions are patients immediately after a cholecystectomy who have a biliary tube in place and are found to have retained common duct stones. The treatment of this special condition is discussed in the chapter *Percutaneous Transhepatic Biliary Drainage and Retained Biliary Stone Extraction*). In selected cases, in which the stone causes no significant obstruction of the common duct, however, bile acid treatment can be considered. It is probably safer to use urso than cheno, especially since the common duct stones can be associated with intermittent liver test abnormalities. Experience gained in studies of patients with chronic active hepatitis treated with urso indicates that this bile acid can also be safely used in the presence of abnormal liver tests.

Other Clinically Applicable Methods of Gallstone Dissolution. Current research efforts are directed at devising treatment methods which not only allow a speedier dissolution of cholesterol gallstones, but also are effective against pigmented and calcified stones. Although tangible progress has been made in regards to the first goal, no agent has yet been found which is both effective and safe for the dissolution of pigmented and calcified stones. The first progress concerning accelerated gallstone dissolution was recently reported by investigators from the Mayo Clinic. Cholesterol gallstones were dissolved in the gallbladder using *methyl tert-butyl ether*, which is instilled via a catheter placed transhepatically through the gallbladder bed. Following exposure of the stones to the ether, the gallbladder content is aspirated through the catheter. By repeating the instillation and aspiration several times, cholelitholysis can be accomplished within a few hours. The procedure has so far been tested only at the Mayo Clinic. Further experience is necessary before its utility for medical practice can be assessed. The relatively invasive nature of the procedure, however, will probably limit its application to patients with biliary pain and/or complications who either present a high surgical risk or refuse a cholecystectomy.

MANAGEMENT OF CHOLELITHIASIS IN DIABETES MELLITUS

There is only limited information regarding the natural history of gallstones in diabetic patients. Contrary to common belief, there are no solid data supporting the need for prophylactic cholecystectomy in patients with diabetes mellitus and gallstones. In the absence of convincing proof that patients with diabetic gallstones are at increased risk of developing biliary pain and/or complications, either expectant management, or cholelitholysis appears to be advisable in this condition, as long as the stones cause no symptoms.

MANAGEMENT OF PATIENTS WITH NONVISUALIZING GALLSTONES

The term "nonvisualization of the gallbladder" refers to the failure of this organ to fill with contrast medium during oral double-dose cholecystography. This may be due to either inadequate hepatic extraction of the dye (hepatic dysfunction, intrahepatic cholestasis), gallbladder dysfunction (insufficient intestinal release of cholecystokinin or inadequate contractile response of the gallbladder to this hormone), cholecystitis, or cystic duct obstruction. A cholecystectomy should certainly be considered if nonvisualization occurs because of the latter two conditions. In contrast, expectant management is probably reasonable if the patient has neither evidence of active gallstone disease nor a history of previous gallbladder attacks. Long-term studies are needed to further define the prognosis of asymptomatic gallstone patients with nonvisualizing gallbladders.

ACALCULOUS CHOLECYSTITIS

Cholecystitis seldom occurs in the absence of gallstones. Acalculous cholecystitis usually represents a complication of serious systemic illnesses, such as severe burns and sepsis. In addition, so-called cholesterolosis of the gallbladder can, although rarely, cause abdominal pain suggestive of gallbladder disease. With these rare exceptions, however, the diagnosis of acute gallbladder disease becomes most unlikely if neither gallstones nor gallbladder sludge can be found by ultrasonography.

CONCLUSION

Careful prospective studies and surveys of relatively large population groups in the United States and Western Europe have shown that the majority of gallstones are silent and never lead to complications. Expectant management is therefore advisable in both patients with silent stones and those in whom they are associated with nonspecific symptoms. A cholecystectomy should be considered only after the development of biliary pain and/or complications.

PERCUTANEOUS TRANSHEPATIC BILIARY DRAINAGE AND RETAINED BILIARY STONE EXTRACTION

STEPHEN L. KAUFMAN, M.D.

PERCUTANEOUS TRANSHEPATIC BILIARY DRAINAGE

In recent years percutaneous transhepatic biliary drainage has become an important method in the management of patients with obstructive jaundice. Benign and malignant lesions causing biliary obstruction can be managed by the placement of percutaneous stents to effect biliary decompression and internal biliary drainage. These stents may be the only means of therapy necessary for palliation of disease in patients with unresectable malignancies. The percutaneous track may be utilized for the dilation of benign biliary strictures or for removal of biliary calculi. Alternatively, percutaneous biliary drainage may be an initial temporizing measure in some patients prior to definitive surgical procedures. We have performed percutaneous biliary drainage in over 400 patients in the last 5 years at our institution. This chapter is a review of our experience.

Indications and Results

Nonsurgical Palliation of Inoperable Malignancies

The most common indication for biliary drainage is the palliation of inoperable malignancies producing biliary obstruction. The most common neoplasm in this category is carcinoma of the pancreas. Operative biliary decompression in these patients carries a mortality as high as 33 percent with a concomitant postoperative morbidity rate. Since the mean survival rate following palliation for jaundice is only from 4 to 6 months, a nonsurgical form of palliation such as percutaneous biliary drainage is attractive. Primary bile duct tumors, especially those located at the junction of the right and left hepatic ducts (Klatskin tumors), are especially difficult to manage surgically but are readily amenable to transhepatic drainage. Drainage of both the left and right hepatic ducts is indicated in most of these patients to provide complete biliary drainage and prevent development of cholangitis in the undrained segment. Transhepatic biliary drainage may also be indicated for some patients with localized metastases to the porta hepatis or peripancreatic nodes. Biliary drainage is generally ineffective in relieving jaundice in patients with peripheral hepatic metastases. The procedure should likewise be avoided in patients with advanced, widespread metastatic disease, especially those with a serum bilirubin level over 20 ml per deciliter; these patients have a high in-hospital mortality rate following biliary drainage.

Overall, approximately 85 percent of patients undergoing percutaneous biliary drainage benefit from the procedure. The severe pruritus which frequently is present is relieved dramatically, often within 24 hours. Liver function improves in the majority of patients. In most cases biliary drainage is provided by an internal/external stent. A disadvantage of this technique is the continued presence of an external limb of the tube, which may be painful in some patients and may be limiting psychologically. Therefore, in some patients with malignant biliary obstruction, large-bore internal endoprostheses may be placed through the percutaneous track within 1 week of the initial procedure. These stents obviate the need for an external catheter and the possibility of external bacterial contamination of the bile. A disadvantage of endoprostheses is the lack of easy accessibility to the biliary system in the event of obstruction of the prosthesis. Thus, even though prostheses have remained patent for up to 18 months in some patients, we limit their use to patients with limited life expectancies, such as those with pancreatic carcinoma or metastatic tumors.

Preoperative Biliary Decompression

Percutaneous biliary drainage may be performed prior to definitive biliary tract surgery in an attempt to reduce operative morbidity and mortality. The use of biliary drainage for this purpose, however, is controversial. Early retrospective studies showed a significant reduction in morbidity and mortality when preoperative percutaneous biliary drainage was performed. Recently, two randomized studies of preoperative percutaneous biliary decompression have been published.[1,2] Although one study showed a significant reduction in mortality and morbidity and a shorter hospital stay for patients drained percutaneously, the other study showed no differences. Since serum bilirubin levels above 10 ml per deciliter have been associated with increased operative mortality, we perform preoperative biliary drainage in such patients. We feel that patients with biliary obstruction and sepsis also benefit from preoperative biliary decompression.

Benign Strictures

Percutaneous drainage is an especially effective means of treating benign biliary strictures. The overwhelming majority of such strictures occur following surgery for biliary calculi. The strictures are usually located high within the biliary tree, are difficult to manage surgically, and carry a significant rate of recurrence and surgical morbidity and mortality. Percutaneous biliary drainage provides initial biliary decompression in these patients and will help relieve the sepsis which not infrequently complicates such strictures. Subsequently, benign strictures may be managed definitively by percutaneous dilation using balloon angioplasty catheters. Most patients with strictures at bilioenteric anastomoses can be treated successfully with balloon dilation alone with subsequent removal of the biliary catheter after several months. We have been successful in treating six of seven such patients, with a follow-up of up to 23 months. Patients with primary biliary strictures within the biliary tree may develop restenosis following balloon dilation. These patients require stenting with large-caliber silicone catheters (16 to 20 F) for up to 12 months before stent removal. Healing around such large stents results in correction of such strictures. We have been successful in four of sic such patients, with follow-up periods of up to 30 months after cahteter removal.

Relief of Biliary Sepsis

Percutaneous biliary drainage combined with aggressive antibiotic therapy may be life-saving in patients with sepsis associated with biliary obstruction. Since systemic antibiotics do not enter obstructed biliary systems sufficiently to reach therapeutic levels, some form of drainage is required to eradicate the source of infection. We have encountered a mortality rate of 17 percent in such patients managed with percutaneous biliary drainage, compared with a mortality rate from 50 to 75 percent with surgical decompression. It is essential to limit the amount of contrast material injected during diagnostic cholangiography in such patients and to minimize manipulation within the biliary tree in order to limit bacteremia. External biliary drainage therefore is usually initially instituted. The catheter may be manipulated through the biliary obstruction into the duodenum once sepsis has been controlled. Associated benign strictures may then be dilated and calculi, if present, may be removed through the percutaneous track.

Post-traumatic Biliary Leakage

Percutaneous biliary drainage provides a nonoperative means of biliary diversion in patients with major injuries to the bile ducts manifested by biliary leaks and fistulas. Most such patients have suffered inadvertent biliary trauma during surgery. Transhepatic biliary drainage may eliminate the need for further surgical procedures or may allow the patient's condition to improve prior to subsequent definitive surgery. Biliary leaks have completely sealed with 9 days to 2 months of drainage in our patients. Balloon dilation of associated strictures and removal of biliary calculi can then be performed through the drainage track. Patients with intra-abdominal abscesses or complete biliary obstruction require surgery after their condition has stabilized.

Bile Duct Calculi

In most cases, common duct calculi are best managed surgically or by endoscopic sphincterotomy. Calculi may be removed through the percutaneous track when they are incidentally noted following biliary drainage for other indications (sepsis, strictures, or leaks) and the patient otherwise does not require surgery. The technique is similar to that used for removing biliary calculi through T-tube tracks.

Technique

Patient Preparation

Informed consent must be obtained prior to the procedure. It should be emphasized to the patient that an external tube may be necessary depending on the cholangiographic findings. Patients who are totally uncooperative or are psychologically incapable of accepting an external tube for more than a short period should be offered alternative forms of therapy. Adequate clotting function is essential. A platelet count less than 50,000 per cubic millimeter or a prothrombin time more than 2 to 3 seconds above control values contraindicates percutaneous drainage. Vitamin K or fresh frozen plasma may be administered to patients with inadequate prothrombin times. Ascites is not a contraindication to biliary drainage although it may make the procedure more difficult.

All patients receive broad-spectrum antibiotics before the procedure is performed to reduce the incidence of septic complications. Intravenous antibiotics are started several hours prior to the procedure and continued for 24 hours afterward. For patients who are not clinically infected we use intravenous cefoxitin. Patients who are septic receive a combination of gentamicin, clindamycin, and ampicillin unless cultures and antibiotic sensitivities are available. Intravenous narcotics are administered prior to the procedure for analgesia.

Percutaneous Biliary Drainage

Diagnostic percutaneous transhepatic cholangiography is initially carried out with a 22-gauge Chiba needle. A right lateral approach is used, with care taken to avoid the right costophrenic sulcus to prevent bile contamination of the pleural space or pneumothorax. To keep the intrabiliary pressure low and to reduce the incidence of bacteremia, the smallest amount of contrast material necessary for anatomic definition is used. The anatomy of the biliary tree demonstrated by the initial cholangiogram determines the approach for percutaneous biliary drainage. An 18-gauge sheathed needle is used for a second puncture of the bile ducts for the drainage procedure. A right lateral intercostal approach is usually employed unless the left biliary tree has to be drained. The entry site into the biliary tree for drainage should be into a peripheral biliary duct to avoid trauma to the major vascular structures in the porta hepatis. An ideal duct for drainage is relatively large and has a direct course toward the point of obstruction. For drainage of the left biliary system an anterior subcostal approach into a peripheral left bile duct is used. Lateral and oblique fluoroscopy are of great help in localizing the biliary ducts in three dimensions. Once a bile duct has been entered a guidewire is placed through the sheath and manipulated through the biliary system to the point of obstruction. Special torque guidewires are helpful in this regard, and the sheath may then be advanced over the guidewire. Guidewires are used to maneuver through the biliary obstruction. This can usually be accomplished even though complete biliary obstruction is present. The sheath may then be advanced into the duodenum, and a special rigid guidewire introduced through the sheath. The sheath may then be removed and an 8.3 F pigtail catheter (Cook Inc., Bloomington, IN) with multiple side holes passed over the guidewire through the stricture and into the duodenum. Side holes must be positioned within the biliary tree above the area of obstruction as well as within the duodenum. They must not be located within the hepatic parenchyma or bleeding through the tube may occur. If passage through the area of biliary obstruction cannot be achieved, a catheter is placed above the obstruction and allowed to drain externally for approximately 48 hours. At this time, with the biliary tree decompressed, passage through the obstruction can usually be achieved. Our success rate in achieving internal biliary drainage has been approximately 90 percent. In patients presenting with sepsis or cholangitis, no attempts are made to pass through the area of obstruction until the infection has been controlled.

Follow-up

Even when internal biliary drainage is achieved, bile is allowed to drain externally from the catheter into a bile bag for 48 to 72 hours. The catheters are flushed twice daily with 10 to 20 ml of sterile saline. After 48 to 72 hours of external drainage a cholangiogram is performed, and if the catheter is patent and in good position, its external limb is closed off with a heparin lock adapter and internal drainage instituted. For patients who are candidates for long-term biliary drainage, the initial pigtail catheter may be replaced with larger, softer tubes after approximately 1 week. We are currently using silicone catheters from 10 to 12 F (Mentor Corp., Goleta, CA) for this purpose. The catheter size may be increased at 2 F increments at each subsequent catheter change. The larger silicone catheters are more comfortable for the patient and occlude less frequently than smaller catheters. Eventually, however, all biliary catheters will occlude. The external-internal stents are routinely changed on an outpatient basis every 2 to 3 months.

In patients with unresectable malignancies producing biliary obstruction, tissue diagnosis may be obtained nonoperatively. Bile samples for cytologic examination are readily obtained through the biliary catheter and may be positive in up to 40 percent of patients with various neoplasms. If cytologic studies are negative, aspiration biopsy using a 22-gauge needle can be performed under fluoroscopic or ultrasonic localization.

Percutaneous Insertion of an Endoprosthesis

Permanent internal endoprostheses have the advantage of eliminating the need for an external catheter in selected patients with malignant biliary obstruction. We have limited use of this technique to patients with localized common bile duct or common hepatic duct obstruction and life expectancies of 6 months or less. The endoprosthesis may be placed within a week after internal biliary drainage. We currently use a 12 F soft stent (Medi-Tech Inc., Watertown, MA). This stent is inserted over a guidewire through the biliary drainage track and positioned with its distal end in the duodenum and proximal side holes above the area of biliary obstruction. This system has a suture which is attached to the stent and tied subcutaneously to prevent stent migration. A drainage catheter is left proximal to the prosthesis for a short time and removed when the endoprosthesis has been shown to function adequately.

Dilation of Benign Strictures

Benign biliary strictures may be dilated using balloon angioplasty catheters via the biliary drainage track. Dilation is usually performed from 2 to 4 weeks after the initial drainage procedure on an outpatient basis. The biliary drainage catheter is exchanged over a guidewire for a balloon catheter. The balloon is inflated within the strictured segment for periods up to 20 minutes. Balloons from 6 to 12 mm in diameter when inflated are used. Dilation may be performed several times on a weekly basis as an outpatient procedure. Following each procedure a new drainage catheter is placed. Strictures at bilioenteric anastomoses tend not to recur following dilation. Primary biliary strictures may recur and require stenting with larger silicone catheters of up to 16 to 20 F for up to 12 months. In such cases catheter size is increased by 2 F increments at each subsequent procedure. For either type of stricture, after balloon dilation and an appropriate period of stenting, the dilation should be challenged by exchanging the internal stent for a catheter placed above the stricture. This tests the ability of the previously strictured segment to maintain bile flow. If the patient does well under this challenge and the stricture has not recurred, the stent may be removed.

Complications

The most common complications associated with percutaneous biliary drainage are related to infection. Episodes of cholangitis within the first 3 days following biliary drainage have occurred in approximately 11 percent of our patients. With long-term drainage, cholangitis has occurred in approximately 22 percent of patients. These late episodes of cholangitis are usually related to obstruction of the catheter by inspissated bile and are readily managed by replacement of the tube and antibiotics. Difficulty in flushing the biliary stents or leakage of bile around the stents is usually associated with impending catheter obstruction. Patients experiencing these problems are instructed to return for catheter exchange to preclude the development of cholangitis. We have had three patients develop intrahepatic abscess following chronic biliary drainage for 8 months or longer. Patients presenting with late episodes of sepsis not responding to catheter change and antibiotics should have ultrasound or computed tomography examinations to detect intrahepatic abscesses not communicating with the biliary system. Intrahepatic abscesses require prompt percutaneous or surgical drainage.

Minor degrees of hemobilia are common immediately after biliary drainage and are of little significance. Hemorrhage through the transhepatic catheter may occur if side holes are positioned within the hepatic parenchyma. This can be easily corrected by adjustment of the position of the tube. Hemobilia may occur up to several months following biliary drainage due to hepatic artery aneurysms or arterio-portal fistulas adjacent to the biliary catheter. Hepatic arteriography should be performed if intractable hemobilia through the stent occurs. Hepatic artery aneurysms or arterio-portal fistulas may be managed by transcatheter embolization using detachable balloons or other materials. We have successfully embolized nine such patients with hemobilia secondary to percutaneously placed transhepatic stents. Bile pleural effusion or pneumothorax has occurred in 1 percent of cases. This complication is usually due to technical error with failure to avoid the right costophrenic sulcus. Postoperative mortality related to biliary drainage is less than 2 percent.

RETAINED BILIARY STONE EXTRACTION THROUGH THE T-TUBE TRACT

Retained biliary calculi may be found in from 4 to 8 percent of patients following cholecystectomy and common bile duct exploration. A major advance in the nonoperative removal of such calculi was Burhenne's employment of flexible, steerable catheters for selective catheterization of the bile ducts via the T-tube track. (His experience was described in the 1984-1985 edition of this book.)[3] Nonoperative stone extraction can be performed in up to 95 percent of patients using this technique on an outpatient basis with minimal morbidity. The complication rate is approximately 5 percent, with most complications being minor.

Retrieval of retained calculi through the T-tube track is usually performed as an outpatient procedure. Hospital admission or antibiotic coverage is required only if there is a history of cholangitis or if mulitple intrahepatic calculi are present. It is necessary to wait approximately 5 weeks after surgery to perform the procedure. This allows a firm track to form around the T-tube. The procedure is facilitated by the use of a T-tube of 14 F or greater. It is also preferable that the T-tube be brought out from the right side of the anterior abdominal wall rather than from the subcostal area close to the midline. An anterior T-tube track is generally more tortuous than a lateral track, and entry into the biliary system and manipulation within it are more difficult. An anterior track also makes it difficult for the radiologist to keep his or her hands out of the primary x-ray beam.

Alternative nonoperative means of removing retained biliary calculi are endoscopic sphincterotomy and the use of solubilizing agents to dissolve calculi. Endoscopic sphincterotomy is associated with a higher morbidity rate than removal through the T-tube track, and in most cases extraction through the track should be attempted first. Endoscopic sphincterotomy should be the initial procedure if the patient's condition precludes waiting 5 weeks for the T-tube track to solidify, if there is an anteriorly located track or a small-caliber T-tube has been used, or if the calculus is impacted at the ampulla. Dissolution of retained biliary calculi is less effective than calculus removal through the T-tube track and requires many days of inpatient hospitalization. It is difficult to justify this technique in the majority of cases, if only on an economic basis.

Technique

An initial T-tube cholangiogram should be performed to document the presence and position of biliary calculi. If stones are present, the T-tube is removed. A steerable catheter (Medi-Tech Inc., Watertown, MA) is inserted through the T-tube track into the biliary system and directed toward the calculus. Both intrahepatic and extrahepatic biliary calculi are accessible with this technique. If possible, the steerable catheter is advanced beyond the calculus. A stone basket is then advanced through the steerable catheter. The stone basket consists of the basket itself and a Teflon catheter in which the closed basket is introduced through the steerable catheter system. Stone baskets come in several diameters; the diameter should approximate the diameter of the duct in which the calculus is located. The steerable catheter is then retracted while the position of the stone basket is maintained. The basket introducer catheter is then withdrawn, allowing the stone basket to open within the biliary duct beyond the calculus. The whole system is then withdrawn as a unit. If the stone is snared within the basket, it will be seen to move with the basket as the system is withdrawn through the T-tube track. In some cases it may not be possible to advance the steerable catheter or the basket assembly beyond a partially obstructing calculus. In this situation the stone basket may be removed from its introducer catheter and replaced with a J-tipped angiographic guidewire. The angiographic guidewire can usually be advanced beyond the stone and may be followed by the introducer catheter. The guidewire is then replaced with the basket, the basket is opened, and the calculus snared and removed as described. Multiple calculi may be present in approximately 25 percent of cases. It is usually possible to extract only one calculus at a time in the stone basket. With multiple calculi, the steerable catheter system is reintroduced into the biliary system as many times as necessary to remove the calculi. When multiple calculi are present, several sessions may be required, several days apart, to remove all of them. Calculi too large to remove through the T-tube track may be crushed within the basket and the fragments removed individually. Following the procedure, whether or not all stones have been removed, a straight red rubber tube is placed within the biliary tree. The patient is asked to return in 2 to 3 days, at which time repeat cholangiography may be performed and residual stones, if present, may be removed. If no calculi are present, the tube may be removed and the patient discharged.

If may be difficult to remove calculi impacted either in the intrahepatic ducts or at the ampulla. Calculi impacted in intrahepatic ducts may be dislodged using Fogarty balloon catheters. The Fogarty catheters are advanced through the steerable catheter beyond the calculi. The Fogarty balloon may then be inflated to a diameter not exceeding that of the bile duct. The catheter is then withdrawn, dislodging the calculi and retracting them to where they may be successfully snared with the stone basket. Stones impacted at the ampulla may be difficult to dislodge and are probably best removed by endoscopic sphincterotomy. There is a separate chapter on *Endoscopy in Bile Duct Obstruction and Ampullary Dysfunction*.

REFERENCES

1. Hatfield ARW, Terblanche J, Fataar S, et al. Preoperative external biliary drainage in obstructive jaundice. Lancet 1982; 2:896-899.
2. Gundry SR, Strodel WE, Knol JA, et al. Efficacy of preoperative biliary tract decompression in patients with obstructive jaundice. Arch Surg 1984; 119: 703-708.
3. Burhenne HJ. Retained biliary stone extraction: radiologic technique. In: Bayless TM, ed. Current therapy in gastroenterology and liver disease 1984-1985. Burlington, Ontario: BC Decker Inc, 1984; 461.

ENDOSCOPY IN BILE DUCT OBSTRUCTION AND AMPULLARY DYSFUNCTION

JOSEPH E. GEENEN, M.D., F.A.C.P., F.A.C.G.
RAMA P. VENU, M.D., F.A.C.P., F.A.C.G.

There are a variety of abnormalities leading to bile duct obstruction and ampullary dysfunction which can be effectively managed endoscopically. Such therapeutic procedures are made possible by the advent of endoscopic retrograde cholangiopancreatography (ERCP). The technique of ERCP has improved considerably during the past decade as a result of extensive experience on the part of endoscopists coupled with technical improvements in the lateral-viewing endoscope. More recently, the technique of sphincter of Oddi (SO) manometry using a constantly perfused polyethylene catheter has been introduced as another diagnostic tool. Though its full potential is yet to be realized, SO motility studies have already provided valuable information regarding the physiology of biliary drainage, as well as the pathophysiology of certain hitherto unknown pancreaticobiliary disorders.

INDICATIONS AND CONTRAINDICATIONS OF ENDOSCOPIC RETROGRADE CHOLANGIOPANCREATOGRAPHY

A complete diagnostic evaluation using the technique of ERCP employs three distinct but interrelated steps: (1) endoscopic evaluation of the papilla and its surrounding area, (2) radiographic evaluation of the bile duct and pancreatic duct; and (3) SO motility studies in selected cases.

A lateral-viewing endoscope, the instrument of choice for performing ERCP, is uniquely suitable for evaluation of the papilla and peripapillary area. Normal papilla appears as a pinkish mound of tissue with reticulated margins surrounding the papillary orifice. A vertical mucosal fold located caudad and a transverse mucosal fold located cephalad are two useful landmarks in locating the papilla. The size and shape of normal papillae vary from person to person. Each papilla has a face of its own.

A number of papillary and peripapillary abnormalities, such as tumors, papillitis (as a result of pancreatitis, impacted common bile duct stone, or a recently passed stone), choledochocele, duplication cyst, diverticulum, and choledochoduodenal fistula, may present a characteristic endoscopic appearance helpful in establishing a diagnosis. Following endoscopic observation, radiographic evaluation of the common bile duct and pancreatic duct is carried out. Given the anatomic proximity of the pancreatic duct and the common bile duct, both ductal systems are usually visualized simultaneously. In many clinical situations, however, either the bile duct or the pancreatic duct becomes the primary focus of interest.

One of the major indications for endoscopic retrograde cholangiopancreatography is to distinguish between jaundice due to extrahepatic biliary tract obstruction and intrahepatic jaundice (Table 1). In this situation ERCP provides useful information not only on the site and severity of obstruction, but also on the etiology of such obstruction. The technique is especially suitable in the evaluation of patients who may also have coagulation abnormalities. Endoscopic retrograde cholangiopancreatography is preferable to percutaneous transhepatic cholangiography when intrahepatic biliary ductal abnormalities are strongly suspected, i.e., primary biliary cirrhosis or sclerosing cholangitis. Additionally, ERCP permits direct visualization of the papilla of Vater. Thus biopsy and cytologic specimens may be taken from the papilla when papillary carcinoma is suspected. Rare biliary tract abnormalities, such as choledochocele, choledochal cyst, choledochoduodenal fistula, and sump syndrome, can also be diagnosed by using this technique. Furthermore, ERCP may be indicated in patients with known biliary tract obstruction when nonoperative management is contemplated.

In patients with recurrent acute pancreatitis, a surgically correctable lesion may be detected with radiography of the pancreatic duct. Pancreas divisum, a congenital malunion of the dorsal and ventral pancreatic buds, can be diagnosed only by ERCP. Endoscopic retrograde cholangiopancreatography may provide a preoperative road map for the surgeon in patients with chronic pancreatitis. A diagnosis of chronic pancreatitis also can be made in most patients using ERCP. Characteristic radiographic abnormalities may be detected in the majority of patients with carcinoma of the pancreas. Finally, in patients with recurrent abdominal pain, abnormal liver function tests, and hyperamylasemia, ERCP examination may provide information leading to the diagnosis of minute gallstones or papillary stenosis.

The contraindications for ERCP are limited and in general are similar to those for any upper gastrointestinal endoscopy. In patients with severe cardiopulmonary diseases, ERCP may be hazardous. If the patient has had a recent acute myocardial infarction, this procedure should

TABLE 1 Indications for Endoscopic Retrograde Cholangiopancreatography

Jaundice of undetermined etiology
  Extrahepatic biliary tract obstruction
    Gallstones
    Tumors (benign or malignant)
    Strictures
    Sclerosing cholangitis
    Sphincter of Oddi dysfunction
  Intrahepatic biliary tract obstruction
    Hepatitis
    Cholestatic jaundice related to drugs
    Cirrhosis (primary biliary)
    Malignancy (primary or metastatic)
Endoscopic biopsy and cytology
  Brush cytology or biopsy
  Fluid collection for cytology
Sphincter of Oddi disorders
  Papillary stenosis
  Biliary dyskinesia

TABLE 2 Complications of Endoscopic Retrograde Cholangiopancreatography

Common to upper gastrointestinal endoscopy
  Drug reaction
  Cardiorespiratory symptoms
  Esophageal perforation
Peculiar to ERCP
  Acute pancreatitis
  Cholangitis
  Pancreatic sepsis
  Instrumental injury

be avoided. Following an attack of acute pancreatitis, ERCP is generally avoided for several weeks; however, acute pancreatitis associated with common bile duct stones or gallbladder stones is an exception to this rule. Hepatitis B surface antigenemia is not a contraindication for ERCP, but caution should be exercised by all personnel who come in direct contact with the patient during the procedure.

In patients with a history of iodine sensitivity, ERCP can generally be performed with minimal risk. Intravenous administration of steroids and antihistamines prior to contrast instillation might further guard against any adverse reaction to contrast material.

Complications of ERCP can be divided into those common to any upper gastrointestinal endoscopy and those peculiar to ERCP examination (Table 2). The decrease in the partial pressure of oxygen and the resultant hypoxemia along with vagal stimulation may be responsible for the various cardiopulmonary complications. A recent report suggests that adequate premedication using valium and meperidine might decrease the incidence of such complications. Instrumental injury, pancreatitis, and infection are the major complications peculiar to ERCP. Increased injection pressure during contrast instillation into pancreatic ducts and overfilling of the lateral branches of the pancreatic duct are considered to be two major factors leading to acute pancreatitis following ERCP. A generous contrast instillation beyond the area of a stricture in the pancreatic duct or bile duct may predispose to infection. Overfilling of a pancreatic pseudocyst also might lead to severe infection. In this situation, prophylactic antibiotic treatment and early surgical consultation may be undertaken.

NONOPERATIVE MANAGEMENT OF BILIARY TRACT OPERATIONS

The major causes of extrahepatic biliary tract obstruction include biliary duct stones, malignancy, or iatrogenic strictures. Rarely, papillary tumors, papillary stenosis, choledochocele, pseudocyst of the pancreas with extrinsic compression, or sump syndrome may also cause biliary tract obstruction. During the past decade, a number of endoscopic therapeutic procedures have evolved in the management of these disorders (Table 3). Those therapeutic interventions currently in practice include endoscopic retrograde sphincterotomy (ERS), balloon dilatation, internal and external biliary stents, placement of nasobiliary catheters, percutaneous T-tube extraction, or dissolution of stones.

Common Bile Duct Stones

On average, 4 to 7 percent of patients may have retained common bile duct stones following cholecystectomy and common bile duct exploration. The therapeutic approaches currently available in this situation are: (1) infusion of a gallstone-dissolving agent through the T-tube, (2) percutaneous stone extraction via T-tube track, and (3) ERS and extraction of stone.

While infusion of dissolution agent and percutaneous removal of common bile duct stones require an intact T-tube, ERS can be performed even in patients without a T-tube. For many years, surgeons used saline or heparin lavage to flush out common bile duct stones. Most recently, mono-octanoin (Capmul), a gallstone-dissolving agent, has been used via a T-tube or nasobiliary catheter. Capmul is administered continuously at the rate of 2 to 5 ml per hour using an infusion pump. Most patients tolerate Capmul infusion well, and side effects, such as increased frequency of bowel movements and abdominal pain or fever, are rarely noted. This relatively simple procedure is effective in fewer than 50 percent of subjects with common bile duct stones, which may be due to the fact that mono-octanoin is effective only against cholesterol stones. Another gallstone dissolution agent, methyl terbutyl ether, is on the horizon and shows more encouraging results.

Percutaneous extraction of a stone is performed through the fibrous track created by a surgically placed T-tube. A steerable, flexible catheter is advanced through the track to slightly beyond, or immediately adjacent to, the stone in the bile duct under fluoroscopic control. A Dormia basket is passed through the catheter. By retracting both the catheter and the basket, the stone can be captured and removed. The major limitation of this procedure is the relatively large size of stones which may get trapped at the exit site, necessitating surgical intervention. There is a separate chapter on this technique (*Percutaneous Transhepatic Biliary Drainage and Retained Biliary Stone Extraction*).

By and large, in experienced hands, percutaneous extraction is successful in 80 to 90 percent of patients. Complications, including trauma to the bile duct mucosa leading to strictures, false passage of the catheter, pancreatitis, or sepsis, have been reported in 5 percent of pa-

TABLE 3 Endoscopic Therapeutic Modalities for Bile Duct Obstruction

Endoscopic Retrograde Sphincterotomy	Stents	Balloon Dilation
Common bile duct stones	Benign strictures	Biliary stricture
Papillary stenosis	Malignant strictures	Sclerosing cholangitis
Periampullary neoplasm	Primary	Papillary stenosis
Choledochocele	Metastatic	

tients. Besides the percutaneous radiographic technique, successful endoscopic approach using a semiflexible choledochofiberscope or bronchoscope advanced through a T-tube track has also been reported, although this is not widely used.

Endoscopic Retrograde Sphincterotomy

In the absence of a T-tube track, biliary tract obstruction resulting from common bile duct stones can be effectively managed by ERS, which is widely accepted as the procedure of choice for the treatment of choledocholithiasis in high operative risk patients who have had previous cholecystectomy. Successful therapeutic outcome of ERS has also been reported from Europe and the United States in high-risk patients with intact gallbladders with stones who also have symptomatic common bile duct stones. About 15 percent of these patients may subsequently develop acute cholecystitis requiring operative intervention.

Other indications for ERS include papillary stenosis, periampullary carcinoma, choledochocele, sump syndrome, and as a preliminary procedure prior to stent placement or balloon dilatation (Table 4). A recent American Society for Gastrointestinal Endoscopy survey on 5,790 sphincterotomies in the United States proved ERS to be successful in 87 percent of cases (Table 5). Acute complications, including bleeding, pancreatitis, perforation, cholangitis, or trapped basket, were noted in 6.8 percent of patients. The mortality rate was 0.4 percent (Table 6).

Contraindications for ERS are few and consist of coagulation disorders, long stricture of common bile duct, and inability to position the sphincterotomy properly.

The same lateral-viewing endoscope used for diagnostic ERCP is used for ERS. An electrocautery incision is made using an Erlangen-type sphincterotome, which enlarges the papillary orifice without causing significant bleeding. Following sphincterotomy, stones may be extracted using a Fogarty balloon catheter or a Dormia basket. Stone size seems to be the single limiting factor for a successful extraction following endoscopic sphincterotomy. Recently, lithotripsy using a basket with steel wires that can exert pressure on the stone caught inside (thus fragmenting the stone) has been successfully used at many centers. Additionally, lithotripsy using a laser beam for large stones is being studied in Japan. In the

TABLE 4 Indications for Endoscopic Sphincterotomy

Residual or recurrent common bile duct stones following cholecystectomy

Common bile duct stones in high surgical risk patients with gallbladder in situ

Papillary stenosis

Periampullary carcinoma

Sump syndrome

Choledochocele

Gallstone pancreatitis

As a preliminary step for stent placement or balloon dilation

TABLE 5 Endoscopic Retrograde Sphincterotomy Results

		Percentage
Procedures attempted	5,790	100
Procedures successful	5,059	87.3
Acute complications	393	6.7
Late complications	62	1.1
Mortality	22	0.37
Physicians reporting	75	

From American Society for Gastrointestinal Endoscopy survey by Dr. Jack Vennes, 1983.

minority of high operative risk patients with a history of recurrent cholangitis, internal biliary stent placement may be a reasonable alternative when stone extraction is unsuccessful.

Stents and Drains for Biliary Duct Strictures

Strictures involving the bile duct may result from primary or metastatic cancer, inflammation secondary to pancreatitis, instrumental injury leading to postoperative strictures, and sclerosing cholangitis (Table 7). Operative management of unselected biliary duct strictures is associated with a mortality rate of 13 percent and a complication rate of 25 percent. Recurrence rate following operative management may be as high as 25 to 33 percent. This unacceptably high incidence of morbidity and mortality led to the emergence of a variety of nonoperative modalities of therapy.

Transhepatic stent placement with either internal or external drainage was one of the earliest procedures attempted. The technique of percutaneous biliary drainage involves transhepatic insertion of a drainage catheter into the biliary duct. The catheter may be advanced through areas of bile duct stricture into the duodenum. Multiple side holes in the catheter help drainage and decompression. The catheter also provides access to the biliary ducts for a variety of secondary therapeutic intervention procedures, such as placement of an indwelling endoprosthesis, balloon dilation of biliary strictures, basket extraction of stone, or biopsy of a tumor mass. The percutaneous approach might be desirable for strictures involving intrahepatic ducts or multiple strictures at the porta hepatis. A permanently protruding biliary drainage catheter may have several drawbacks, however, including malfunction due to occlusion, migration, bacterial colonization leading to cholangitis, local pain, and the adverse psychological impact of a catheter protruding through the skin.

In this context, an endoscopically placed internal biliary stent seems to be more attractive, particularly in patients with malignant strictures involving the extrahepatic biliary tract. Most stents are polyethylene tubes with an outer diameter of 7 to 12 F and 10 to 15 cm in length, with multiple side holes at both ends. Stents are fashioned with a single pigtail curl at one end or a double pigtail curl, one at each end, or with flaps or barbs at each

TABLE 6 Acute Complications of Endoscopic Retrograde Sphincterotomy

	Number	Surgery	Death
Bleeding, nontransfused	38	0	0
Bleeding, transfused	85	18	11
Pancreatitis	122	5	6
Perforation	57	28	1
Cholangitis	78	26	2
Trapped basket	13	9	2
Total	393 (6.8%)	86 (22%)	22 (0.37%)

From American Society for Gastrointestinal Endoscopy survey by Dr. Jack Vennes, 1983.

end. The flap, barb, or pigtail prevents the displacement of the stent.

For placement of these stents, a small endoscopic sphincterotomy incision is made initially to enlarge the papillary orifice. A long guidewire is then advanced into the bile duct beyond the strictured segment, and an appropriate stent is threaded over the guidewire. The stent is pushed into the bile duct using a pusher tube under fluoroscopic and endoscopic guidance. Once the stent is in position, guidewire and pusher tube are taken out. This procedure is successful in 60 to 70 percent of patients and is rarely associated with infection, bleeding, bile leak, or plugging of stent.

Transpapillary Nasobiliary Catheter

For temporary decompression or drainage of the bile duct in patients with fulminant ascending cholangitis or an impacted common bile duct stone following an endoscopic sphincterotomy, and to decrease the morbidity associated with surgery in patients with periampullary tumors, a transpapillary nasobiliary catheter seems to be an ideal therapeutic endeavor. The nasobiliary catheter can function just like a T-tube, allowing biliary drainage into a bag attached to the other end of the catheter. Multiple perforations near the tip of the catheter, which is fashioned like a pigtail and placed high up in the bile duct beyond the area of obstruction, facilitate the flow of bile into the catheter. This same catheter also can be used for perfusing antibiotics or gallstone dissolving agents such as Capmul. The technique is simple. Following endoscopic sphincterotomy, the catheter, 300 cm long, and 5 to 7-F diameter, is advanced through the biopsy channel. A long guidewire is used to help manipulate the catheter under fluoroscopy. The catheter with the guidewire is advanced to the bile duct under constant fluoroscopic monitoring. When the curled end of the catheter is in the desired position, the guidewire is removed, followed by slow withdrawal of the endoscope. The proximal end of the catheter is then transposed to the nose. An 18 F nasogastric tube is passed through the nose to the pharynx and grasped with a forceps introduced into the mouth. The nasogastric tube is then brought out. The proximal end of the biliary catheter is threaded into the nasogastric tube, which is slowly withdrawn. The nasobiliary catheter may also be used for antibiotic infusion into the bile duct, the efficacy of which is not yet proven.

Balloon Dilation

While stent placement offers a permanent solution for most neoplastic strictures, it seems less desirable in benign strictures, especially in young patients. In this situation, balloon dilation may be more appropriate. A balloon catheter (similar to the one used for angioplasty) is used for dilation of biliary duct strictures. When the inflated balloon is stationed at the stricture segment, it exerts a radial force, thus achieving dilation. The procedure may be repeated periodically for progressive dilation of the strictured segment. In addition to dilation of biliary duct strictures, balloon dilation may also be useful for widening a stenosed biliary enterostomy anastomosis or stenosis at the choledochoduodenostomy site. In certain cases of malignant strictures with significant narrowing, balloon dilation facilitates subsequent internal biliary stent placement.

The technique of advancing the balloon catheter into the strictured segment of the bile duct is similar to nasobiliary catheter placement. A guidewire is initially passed into the bile duct and advanced through the stricture. The balloon catheter is threaded over the guidewire into the desired position of the biliary duct. The radiographic markers located at the proximal and distal end of the balloon help to ensure the proper position of the balloon under fluoroscopy. The balloon is then inflated to a pressure of 4 to 6 ATU for 30-second increments. The procedure may be repeated two or three times.

MANOMETRIC EVALUATION AND TREATMENT OF AMPULLARY DYSFUNCTION

Papillary dysfunction may result from a structural abnormality involving the intramural portion of the common bile duct or a functional disorder of the smooth muscle constituting the sphincter of Oddi. The former is usually designated as papillary stenosis; the latter as sphincter of Oddi dyskinesia. Papillary stenosis may be etiologically related to irritation of the ampullary segment by gallstones, mechanical trauma during surgery, or benign or malignant tumors involving the ampulla. Sphinc-

TABLE 7 Origin of Biliary Tract Strictures

Iatrogenic (postoperative)
Neoplasm, primary or metastatic
Acute pancreatitis with phlegmon
Pseudocyst of the pancreas
Chronic pancreatitis
Sclerosing cholangitis
Papillary stenosis

ter of Oddi dyskinesia is a poorly defined disorder variously known as dystonia, dysenergia, spastic or atonic distention, postcholecystectomy syndrome, and sphincterismus, among other things.

We have used a high fidelity manometric pressure recording system to evaluate the motility characteristics of the sphincter of Oddi. This triple lumen polyethylene catheter can be advanced through the biopsy channel of a lateral-viewing scope during ERCP. The pressure characteristic can be recorded by a pull-through technique. The SO demonstrates a basal pressure that averages 8 mm above the common bile duct pressure. Superimposed on the basal pressure are high-amplitude phasic wave contractions which occur at the mean frequency of 4 ± 0.5 per minute. The phasic wave contraction measures 130 ± 16 mm Hg in amplitude and 4.3 ± 1.5 seconds in duration. Phasic wave activity can be recorded over a 4- to 6-mm segment of the distal choledochus (i.e., the sphincter zone). Contraction waves are antegrade, or directed toward the duodenum, in 61 percent of patients. A number of recent studies indicate that SO manometry may be a suitable diagnostic tool to evaluate patients with possible sphincter of Oddi dysfunction. These patients might present with biliary colic, abnormal liver function tests, or recurrent acute pancreatitis. The common bile duct may be dilated (>12 mm) and there may be delayed drainage of contrast material (>45 minutes). At least four characteristic motility abnormalities have been reported thus far in patients with ampullary dysfunction: (1) elevated SO basal pressure (>30 mm Hg), (2) retrograde propagation of phasic wave contractions, (3) paradoxic increase in basal pressure following intravenously administered CCK-octapeptide, and (4) increase in the frequency of phasic wave contractions (>8 per minute) or tachyoddia.

A prospective randomized study was conducted in 45 patients with presumptive SO dysfunction. All patients had prior cholecystectomy and biliary-like pain along with abnormal liver function tests or a dilated common bile duct or delayed drainage. Following ERCP, patients were selected for ERS or sham ERS. Sphincter of Oddi pressures were taken in all patients. Significant improvement was noted in 91 percent of patients who had elevated basal pressure, whereas only 45 percent of the group who had normal SO basal pressure showed improvement, thereby supporting the importance of proper selection of patients for endoscopic sphincterotomy by performing SO manometry studies.

Endoscopic sphincterotomy produces characteristic changes in the motor function of the SO. While the basal sphincter tone is completely abolished for at least 2 years, phasic wave contractions reappear 2 years following ERS. One year after ERS the incision has shortened by 30 percent, with no further reduction in the incision length at 2 years.

ACUTE CHOLECYSTITIS

JOEL J. ROSLYN, M.D.
HENRY A. PITT, M.D.

Acute cholecystitis has traditionally been associated with cystic duct obstruction, which usually results from impaction of a gallstone either in the cystic duct or in Hartmann's pouch. In addition, cholecystitis can develop in the absence of gallstones (acalculous cholecystitis) as a result of cystic duct obstruction secondary to edema, fibrosis, or the congenital presence of a long, tortuous cystic duct of small diameter. Although numerous theories have been proposed and countless experiments performed, the mechanisms by which cholecystitis develops in patients, with or without gallstones, remain unclear. It would seem, however, that both disease entities are in fact related and that their causes are multifactorial. Cystic duct occlusion, either mechanical or functional, in combination with alterations in gallbladder biliary lipid composition, would seem to initiate a series of events that culminate in the local release of inflammatory agents resulting in acute cholecystitis.

The clinical hallmark of acute cholecystitis is persistent right upper quadrant pain. The onset and character of this pain are similar to those occurring in patients with biliary colic; however, in contrast to the case with biliary colic, the pain of acute cholecystitis persists and is generally unremitting for several days. With time and progression of the inflammatory process, the gallbladder becomes more distended, inflammation develops in the contiguous parietal peritoneum, and the patient complains of more localized right upper quadrant pain. This sometimes subtle change in pain patterns reflects the shift from visceral to parietal pain. Many of these patients will have anorexia, nausea, and vomiting associated with a low-grade temperature.

During physical examination, the patient is usually reluctant to move, reflecting the peritoneal component of the discomfort. Palpation will elicit localized tenderness in the right upper quadrant associated with guarding and rebound. The classic finding of acute cholecystitis is a positive Murphy's sign, which refers to inspiratory arrest during deep palpation in the right upper quadrant. The complaints and physical findings of patients with acute cholecystitis, however, vary considerably, and therefore the persistence of right upper quadrant discomfort for a prolonged period may be an important clue to the diagnosis of acute cholecystitis. Most patients with uncomplicated acute cholecystitis have a mild leukocytosis in the range of 12,000 to 15,000 per cubic millimeter. Mild jaundice may be present in up to 30 percent of patients and is often due to contiguous inflammation rather than acute obstruction by common duct stones. Elevated alkaline phosphatase and transaminase levels may also be found.

DIFFERENTIAL DIAGNOSIS

The differential diagnosis of acute cholecystitis includes other common causes of an acute abdomen, such as appendicitis or perforated ulcer. In addition, pancreatitis, pyelonephritis, right lower lobe pneumonitis, and myocardial infarction must all be considered. One of the most difficult problems in differential diagnosis is distinguishing acute cholecystitis from acute cholangitis. The latter problem results from obstruction of the extrahepatic or intrahepatic bile ducts, whereas acute cholecystitis is generally associated with cystic duct obstruction.

The median age of patients with acute cholecystitis is in the 50s, compared with the 60s for patients with acute cholangitis. Acute cholecystitis is seen slightly more often in women (female:male ratio of 3:2), whereas acute cholangitis is seen with equal frequency in men and women. Patients with acute cholecystitis are more likely to have right upper quadrant pain and tenderness, and patients with acute cholangitis are more likely to have chills and jaundice. While leukocytosis is common to both entities, a white blood cell count above 20,000 per cubic millimeter occurs more frequently with cholangitis. Similarly, a bilirubin concentration greater than 5.0 mg per deciliter and other liver function test abnormalities occur more often in patients with cholangitis.

DIAGNOSIS

During the past fifteen years, new diagnostic modalities, such as ultrasound and cholescintigraphy, have been introduced and have revolutionized our approach to the patient with suspected cholecystitis. Before discussing these tests, however, the value of plain roentgenograms and of oral and intravenous cholangiography will be discussed. Supine and upright radiographs of the abdomen may be useful in the overall evaluation of patients with abdominal pain but are rarely diagnostic in patients with cholecystitis. Visualization of gallstones on a plain abdominal radiograph is possible in the 15 to 20 percent of patients whose stones are partially calcified. Plain radiographs of the abdomen may also demonstrate air in the wall or lumen of the gallbladder or in the biliary tree of those rare patients with emphysematous cholecystitis or cholecystoenteric fistula.

While oral cholecystography (OCG) has been the gold standard for the diagnostic evaluation of patients with chronic cholecystitis since its introduction more than 50 years ago, its value is severely limited in the patient with suspected acute cholecystitis. Similarly, intravenous cholangiography, which had once been the test of choice for acute cholecystitis, is now rarely used because of poor imaging associated with jaundice, severe allergic reactions, and less accuracy than newer tests.

During the past several years, abdominal ultrasonography has become a mainstay in the evaluation of patients with suspected cholelithiasis or cholecystitis. Numerous studies have confirmed that ultrasonography is more than 90 percent accurate for diagnosing cholelithiasis, and it is being used with increasing frequency to diagnose cholecystitis. Specific criteria for identifying acute inflammation of the gallbladder based on ultrasonography include the size and shape of the gallbladder, gallbladder wall thickness, and the presence of pericholecystic fluid collections. The overall accuracy of ultrasonography in diagnosing acute cholecystitis is probably somewhere between 80 and 85 percent, because some patients are "gassed out" and others have a single small stone obstructing the cystic duct which is missed by ultrasound.

Currently, the most accurate means of diagnosing acute cholecystitis, and our test of choice, is hepatobiliary scintigraphy. Cholescintigraphy had a rather limited role in the evaluation of patients with cholecystitis until 1975, when Harvey introduced the technetium 99 labeled and substituted iminodiacetic acid derivatives as new and improved agents to facilitate hepatobiliary scanning. A group of related analogues of technetium 99 iminodiacetic acid are now being used. These radionuclide substances are administered intravenously, taken up by the liver, and then excreted unconjugated and unchanged by the hepatocytes. While this imaging technique is not a suitable diagnostic test for cholelithiasis, cholescintigraphy is a very accurate means of diagnosing cystic duct obstruction, which is the sine qua non of acute cholecystitis.

Failure to opacify the gallbladder by cholescintigraphy after 60 minutes is diagnostic of cystic duct obstruction and, in the right clinical setting, is highly suggestive of acute cholecystitis. Delayed visualization of the cystic duct and gallbladder after 4 hours, even in patients with altered hepatocellular function, is diagnostic of cholecystitis except in those patients receiving total parenteral nutrition or in those who are on a prolonged fast. Extreme caution must be exercised in the interpretation of a scan in which imaging of the liver is obtained without any evidence of radionuclide in any portion of the extrahepatic biliary system. While this situation occasionally may be due to complete extrahepatic obstruction, more frequently it indicates diffuse parenchymal disease.

TREATMENT

Supportive Measures

Almost without exception, patients with suspected cholecystitis should be admitted to the hospital for diagnostic evaluation and management. The diagnosis of acute cholecystitis is based largely on clinical criteria as outlined above. Confirmation of the diagnosis can generally be made with either biliary scintigraphy or ultrasonography. In view of the fact that most cases of cholecystitis are self-limited, the early management of this disease focuses on patient comfort, restoration of homeostasis, and prevention of disease progression. In recent years, we have become less rigid in employing nasogastric tubes for gastric decompression, and generally reserve this intervention for the patient who is extremely nauseated or who has been vomiting.

Nevertheless, oral intake should be restricted in all patients to avoid further gallbladder contraction and increased intragallbladder pressure. Intravenous fluid therapy will therefore be necessary to restore fluid and electrolyte balance in patients who have been vomiting and to maintain normal intravascular volume. Traditionally, relief of pain by the parenteral administration of *meperidine* has been a priority. We generally attempt to avoid the use of morphine in patients with acute cholecystitis because of its deleterious effects on sphincter of Oddi motor activity. Meperidine also has this problem but to a lesser degree. Thus, the recent report suggesting that *indomethacin* is excellent for pain relief in acute cholecystitis may have some merit, but this study needs confirmation.

Antimicrobial Therapy

Septic complications continue to be a source of significant morbidity following cholecystectomy in patients with acute cholecystitis. Several studies have demonstrated a direct correlation between the presence of bacteria in bile at the time of surgery and postoperative infective complications. In most cases the organisms leading to wound infection and other septic complications are similar to those found in the patient's bile. In normal healthy subjects without gallstones, the incidence of positive bile cultures is essentially zero. In contrast, the incidence of positive bile cultures in patients with acute cholecystitis ranges between 30 and 70 percent. Several studies have demonstrated that the incidence of positive bile cultures increases significantly with age. Moreover, a recent study suggests that the incidence of positive cultures also correlates with the duration of the patient's illness. This observation supports the concept that bacterial infection is not a primary pathogenic mechanism in acute cholecystitis but is a secondary complication.

The most common organism cultured from the gallbladder bile in patients with acute cholecystitis is *Escherichia coli*. Other common bacteria include *Klebsiella pneumoniae* and *Streptococcus faecalis* (enterococcus), which are also of enteric origin. Although anaerobes, including *Bacteroides fragilis*, have been reported to occur in as many as 20 to 40 percent of patients undergoing biliary surgery, anaerobes are most likely to be recovered from elderly patients, those with complex biliary problems, and those presenting with cholangitis. The incidence of anaerobic infection in patients with "routine" acute cholecystitis is less than 10 percent. Those subgroups of patients with acute cholecystitis most likely to harbor anaerobes include patients with emphysematous cholecystitis and those with empyema of the gallbladder.

Although some authors have questioned the routine use of antibiotics in patients with acute cholecystitis, we feel that appropriate antimicrobial therapy is advisable in the management of most of these patients. A common argument against routine use of antibiotics in this situation is that therapeutic levels of antibiotics in the biliary system are not achieved if there is obstruction of the cystic or common duct. The goal of antimicrobial therapy in this clinical situation, however, is not to sterilize an infected biliary tree but rather to obtain adequate tissue levels so as to reduce the incidence of wound and intra-abdominal infections.

Antibiotics are begun immediately in patients who present with fever, leukocytosis, leukopenia, or septic shock. If the patient has no fever and minimal or no leukocytosis, however, antibiotics are withheld until the diagnosis is established and the patient is about to undergo surgery. In this subset of patients with "mild" cholecystitis, the incidence of positive bile cultures is low, and antibiotic administration may be limited to a short perioperative course. In patients with more severe cholecystitis, antibiotics are continued postoperatively until the patient has become afebrile and his leukocytosis has resolved for at least 24 hours. In most patients these criteria are met by the fifth postoperative day.

With the recent proliferation of newer antibiotics the choice of specific agents has become a matter of considerable debate. For many years, most experts recommended the combination of a *penicillin* and an *aminoglycoside* for patients with biliary infections. This combination provides excellent coverage for the gram-negative aerobes and synergistic action against enterococci. The one problem with this choice is the toxicity of the aminoglycosides, especially in elderly patients, in those with pre-existing renal disease, and in those who present with jaundice or septic shock. Thus, newer, potentially less toxic antibiotics, such as *piperacillin, mezlocillin,* and *cefoperazone*, which have broad spectra against biliary organisms and high biliary excretion, are now being suggested. Whether these agents truly are less toxic and equally efficacious, however, must await the results of ongoing randomized trials. In patients with empyema or emphysematous cholecystitis coverage for *Clostridium perfringins* and *B. fragilis* should be part of the antibiotic regimen.

Timing of Cholecystectomy

In most cases, cholecystectomy, either early or delayed, is mandated in patients with acute cholecystitis. The optimal timing for cholecystectomy in such patients has been another area of controversy. For many years, the standard of practice was to admit patients with acute cholecystitis to the hospital for a period of intense medical management. These patients would be allowed to "cool down" and then would be discharged home. They would return in approximately 6 to 10 weeks for an elective cholecystectomy. The rationale for this mode of therapy was to allow resolution of the acute inflammatory process and to facilitate the operative procedure.

A series of studies, however, has questioned this rationale and demonstrated that the morbidity and mortality rates are similar for patients undergoing either early or delayed cholecystectomy. In addition, these prospective trials have identifed a recurrence rate of 15 to 20 percent for patients undergoing delayed cholecystectomy and have documented increased cost for the delayed procedure. Moreover, it was the impression of these authors that the operation, when performed early in the course of the clinical disease, is technically easier than when performed electively 6 to 10 weeks later. Further support for early cholecystectomy for patients with acute cholecystitis is provided by the finding of significantly increased morbidity and mortality for those patients who fail to improve after a trial of conservative medical management and require emergency cholecystectomy 5 to 10 days following the onset of their symptoms.

Currently, we perform *urgent cholecystectomy* on most patients with acute cholecystitis within 2 to 4 days after the onset of their symptoms. Following a diagnosis of acute cholecystitis, which is usually a rapid process, these patients are managed with intravenous hydration, nasogastric decompression, and broad-spectrum antibiotics as outlined above. If they demonstrate signs of clinical improvement, we perform an urgent cholecystectomy during the next operating day. If there is no initial improvement, however, or if there are signs of clinical deterioration, we will proceed with *emergency cholecystectomy*. Occasionally, cholecystectomy may be ill advised in extremely high-risk patients. In this clinical setting we will not hesitate to perform a *cholecystostomy*, under local anesthesia if necessary. In our opinion, percutaneous cholecystostomy is almost never indicated because it does not allow observation of a gangrenous gallbladder that must be resected.

Another consideration for the surgeon performing cholecystectomy in patients with acute cholecystitis is whether to perform operative cholangiography or common duct exploration. Because of acute inflammation, cystic duct cholangiography may be more difficult to perform than in patients undergoing cholecystectomy for chronic cholecystitis. Nevertheless, we recommend that every attempt be made to perform *cholangiography* either via the cystic duct or by direct, fine-needle puncture of the common bile duct.

Approximately 15 to 20 percent of patients with acute cholecystitis will also have common duct stones. Moreover, the incidence of choledocholithiasis is higher in patients with a preoperative bilirubin concentration above 5.0 mg per deciliter. Thus, *common duct exploration* in patients with acute cholecystitis is indicated when operative cholangiography is positive and when patients have severe jaundice. In this latter group, we usually perform either percutaneous or endoscopic cholangiography preoperatively.

COMPLICATIONS OF CHOLECYSTITIS

Gallbladder Perforation

Gallbladder perforation, either acute free perforation with bile-stained peritoneal fluid, subacute perforation with pericholecystic right upper quadrant abscess, or chronic perforation with formation of either cholecystoenteric or cholecystocutaneous fistula occurs in less than 5 percent of patients with acute cholecystitis. The preoperative diagnosis of gallbladder perforation is difficult in that the symptoms are frequently comparable to those of patients with uncomplicated cholecystitis. The successful management of gallbladder perforation is based on early recognition. A recent study from UCLA has suggested that acute free perforations tend to occur in patients who are immunocompromised without any antecedent history of gallstone disease. In contrast, a chronic perforation with fistula formation tends to develop in elderly patients who have a longstanding history of chronic gallstone disease. The clinical suspicion of gallbladder perforation should prompt early evaluation with cholescintigraphy or ultrasonography. Aggressive treatment with fluid resuscitation, nasogastric decompression, and intravenous broad-spectrum antibiotic therapy should be instituted, followed by an expeditious laparotomy, especially for patients with free perforations. The management of cholecystoenteric fistulas is beyond the scope of this chapter.

Emphysematous Cholecystitis

Emphysematous cholecystitis, defined by the radiographic demonstration of gas within either the gallbladder wall or lumen, is associated with a significant morbidity and mortality rate. Emphysematous cholecystitis is more common in elderly men and is associated with gangrene and perforation of the gallbladder. Clostridial organisms are present in almost 50 percent of these patients and frequently account for the remarkable radiographic features of this disorder. Despite the severity of this problem and the magnitude of the associated complications, many patients with emphysematous cholecystitis do not appear overtly septic. In any event, the potential for serious morbidity and mortality is so great that prompt cholecystectomy is indicated.

Empyema of the Gallbladder

Another complication of untreated cholecystitis is empyema of the gallbladder. Empyema also occurs more commonly in the elderly population and in the compromised host. Empyema is usually found unexpectedly at laparotomy for acute cholecystitis. Antibiotic coverage for anaerobes should be added when empyema is encountered. Even though many of these patients are elderly and extremely ill, every effort should be made to perform a cholecystectomy as opposed to cholecystostomy. To leave the infected gallbladder wall by performing cholecystostomy may delay or prevent recovery. This principle also applies to emphysematous and gangrenous cholecystitis.

CONCLUSIONS

Acute cholecystitis is the most common complication of gallstone disease. The diagnosis of this entity is based largely on clinical criteria, and confirmatory evidence is generally available either by biliary scintigraphy or abdominal ultrasonography. In most instances, early cholecystectomy performed within the first 3 to 4 days after the onset of symptoms is our preferred choice for definitive treatment. Survival for patients with acute cholecystitis is related to age, extent of disease, and the host's immune status. Nearly all patients who expire are either over 60 years of age or are immunocompromised.

ACUTE PANCREATITIS: MEDICAL CONSIDERATIONS

PETER A BANKS, M.D.

Acute pancreatitis is an inflammatory process triggered by activated pancreatic enzymes. The factors that mediate this activation are poorly understood. The factors that govern its intensity once inflammation occurs are also poorly understood. In mild pancreatitis, the inflammatory response is characterized mainly by edema and is confined predominantly to the pancreas. In severe pancreatitis, the response is more injurious and includes pancreatic necrosis and hemorrhage. In addition, pancreatic exudate containing activated pancreatic enzymes, toxins, and vasoactive material spills out of the pancreas into retroperitoneal spaces, into the lesser sac, and at times into the peritoneal cavity. This exudate produces an extensive chemical burn that permits the loss of protein-rich fluid into these third spaces. If activated enzymes and materials are then reabsorbed into the systemic circulation, they may produce additional harmful effects: first, they increase capillary permeability and induce systemic vasodilation, thereby intensifying hypovolemia and hypotension; second, they may damage end organs directly, causing respiratory failure, renal failure, congestive heart failure, and coma.

There is no treatment at present either to inhibit the activation of enzymes or to modify the intensity of the inflammatory response. Treatment is therefore supportive: during the first few days of severe pancreatitis, when events are dominated by harmful effects of enzymes and toxins both locally and systemically, the goals of therapy are correction of hypovolemia and prevention (or treatment) of organ failure; later, after 5 to 7 days, additional treatment may be required for complications of pancreatic necrosis, including pancreatic abscess and pancreatic pseudocyst.

This chapter will outline first the criteria for determining the severity of pancreatitis and then fundamentals of medical treatment of mild and severe pancreatitis.

DETERMINATION OF SEVERITY OF PANCREATITIS

In mild pancreatitis, mortality is usually less than 5 percent; in severe pancreatitis, it is approximately 30 percent. Approximately one-half of all deaths occur during the first several days as a result of cardiovascular instability, respiratory failure, and renal failure; the remaining deaths occur after the first week as a consequence of pancreatic abscess and other complications.

During the first several days, the distinction between mild and severe pancreatitis is at times difficult. Clinical clues suggestive of severe pancreatitis include tachycardia, hypotension, dyspnea, and oliguria. Additional help is provided by etiology and circumstances. For example, idiopathic and postoperative pancreatitis have a far higher mortality (approximately 15% to 50%) than alcohol-related or gallstone-related pancreatitis (each approximately 5%). Also, the likelihood of a fatal outcome is greatest during the first or second episode, far less during a subsequent one.

More objective criteria of severity of pancreatitis are provided by Ranson's 11 prognostic signs (Table 1). If fewer than three of these 11 signs are positive, pancreatitis is usually mild and rarely fatal; if three or four are positive, pancreatitis is usually more severe and fatal in approximately 15 to 20 percent of patients; as the number of positive signs increases, mortality also increases. Since all 11 prognostic signs are measured within 48 hours of admission (5 at the time of admission and 6 during the next 2 days), the clinician can rapidly assess the severity of disease and prognosis. This assessment need not consume a full 48 hours. Of the six signs that are documented within 48 hours, only the criterion of fluid sequestration requires this entire time interval; the remaining five criteria are valid at any time during the 48-hour interval. For example, whenever the serum calcium level falls below 8 mg per 100 ml during the initial 48 hours (even if this occurs at the time of admission), this prognostic sign is recorded as positive.

Other criteria have been proposed to gauge severity of pancreatitis. One method utilizes three characteristics of peritoneal fluid recovered by diagnostic aspiration: the

TABLE 1 Prognostic Signs in Acute Pancreatitis

At Admission or Diagnosis
    Age over 55 years
    White blood cell count over 16,000/mm^3
    Blood glucose over 200 mg/100 ml
    Serum lactic dehydrogenase over 350 IU/100 ml
    Serum glutamic oxaloacetic transaminase over 250 IU/100 ml

During Initial 48 Hours
    Hematocrit fall greater than 10 percentage points
    Blood urea nitrogen rise more than 5 mg/100 ml
    Serum calcium level below 8 mg/100 ml
    Arterial PO$_2$ below 60 mm Hg
    Base deficit greater than 4 mEq/L
    Estimated fluid sequestration more than 6 L

ability to aspirate more than 10 ml of free peritoneal fluid of any color, the aspiration of any quantity of free fluid that is brown in color, or the recovery following saline lavage of any amount of mid-straw-colored or darker fluid have all been considered valid markers of severe pancreatitis. Finally, a poor prognosis may be indicated by a computed tomographic (CT) scan that shows an intense and severe pancreatic and peripancreatic inflammatory response.

Once the clinician has determined whether pancreatitis is mild or severe, appropriate therapeutic strategy can be structured as outlined below.

TREATMENT OF MILD PANCREATITIS

Intravenous Rehydration

Although third space losses of fluid are not severe in mild pancreatitis, significant hypovolemia may occur because of inadequate fluid intake, severe vomiting, and diaphoresis. Unless hypovolemia is treated vigorously, splanchnic vasoconstriction may ensue, and the arterial circulation of the pancreas may be compromised. If pancreatic ischemia is thereby allowed to occur, the inflammatory response intensifies, and an episode of mild pancreatitis is converted into severe pancreatitis.

For these reasons, the most important requirement of therapy in patients with mild pancreatitis is vigorous intravenous rehydration. A reasonable mixture is 5 percent dextrose in half-strength saline containing appropriate amounts of potassium. A *metabolic flow sheet* is strongly advised during the first several days to plan the rate of fluid replacement. Measurements that help in this assessment include postural vital signs, accurate charting of intake and output every 8 hours, urine specific gravity, daily weight, and daily measurement of hematocrit, blood urea nitrogen, and electrolytes. It is strongly recommended that instructions pertaining to intravenous hydration be reevaluated by a physician at least every 8 hours to ensure adequacy of fluid replacement and thereby avoid hypovolemia. This advice is particularly applicable during weekends, where there may be a tendency to anticipate fluid needs for a 24-hour interval (or longer).

Nasogastric Suction

A nasogastric tube is not required in all cases of mild pancreatitis. The need to "put the pancreas to rest" by preventing gastric acid from reaching the duodenum and stimulating basal pancreatic secretion (by liberation of the hormone secretin) has been overstated. Available evidence now indicates that basal acid is not harmful in acute pancreatitis. Therefore it is not necessary either to aspirate gastric acid or to reduce secretion of acid (by the use of a histamine$_2$ (H$_2$) receptor blocker, anticholinergic agent, or glucagon). A nasogastric tube should be inserted if there is gastric or intestinal ileus or if nausea and vomiting are intractable.

Pain Control and Antibiotics

Control of abdominal pain can usually be achieved by *meperidine* in conventional dosages. Morphine is generally not recommended because it may cause spasm of the sphincter of Oddi and thereby impair the outflow of biliary and pancreatic secretions into the duodenum. Available evidence indicates that antibiotic therapy is not helpful in mild pancreatitis. Accordingly, I prescribe an antibiotic only if a source of infection is documented, such as in the urinary tract or biliary system.

Reintroduction of Oral Feedings

Once abdominal pain and tenderness have subsided, serum amylase has returned to normal, and the patient is once again hungry, it is reasonable to initiate nourishment by mouth (usually by the fourth to seventh day). During the first several days of oral intake, it would appear prudent to reduce the delivery of acid stimulated by food into the duodenum and also to reduce the stimulation of pancreatic enzyme secretion. These goals are sensible in view of the experience that excessive food intake on occasion leads to a significant exacerbation of pancreatitis. The delivery of acid into the duodenum following oral intake can be reduced by a *liquid antacid* prescribed 1 hour after meals and at bedtime and at times by an H$_2$ receptor blocker as well. Pancreatic enzyme secretion can be reduced first by providing food in *six small feedings*, next by emphasizing foods that are rich in *carbohydrate* rather than fat and protein, and finally by providing calories as *liquids* (which stimulate less pancreatic secretion than solid food).

TREATMENT OF SEVERE PANCREATITIS

Strategy During the First Few Days

Transfer to Intensive Care Unit

Severe pancreatitis requires very close supervision which is best provided in an intensive care unit. A variety of measurements and requirements during the first several days are listed in Table 2. Measurement of central venous pressure is required in almost all patients to gauge adequacy of fluid replacement. A low central venous pressure (e.g., 0 to 2 mm Hg) clearly demonstrates a need for additional vigorous rehydration. Even if the central venous pressure is in a normal range, vigorous rehydration may still be required. In this circumstance, measurements provided by a Swan-Ganz catheter inserted into the pulmonary artery help enormously in the assessment of fluid needs and the capacity of the heart to tolerate additional rehydration. A Swan-Ganz catheter is of particular help when fluid requirements are massive, respiratory function is deteriorating, and cardiovascular status is unstable. This type of catheter provides a wide variety of important measurements, including pulmonary artery

TABLE 2 Appropriate Measurements and Bedside Care in Severe Pancreatitis

Vital signs, at least hourly
Central venous pressure, at least hourly
Pulmonary artery pressures (from Swan-Ganz catheter), if indicated
Arterial blood gas analysis, at least every 12 hours and at times every 1 to 3 hours
Measurement of intake and output, at least every 8 hours
Foley catheter to gravity drainage, measure urine output every hour
Nasogastric tube to low intermittent suction, maintain intragastric pH at 7 by instilling liquid antacid every 2 hours
Humidified oxygen at 2 L/min via nasal prongs or mask
For pain, Demerol 100 mg and Vistaril 25 mg every 3 to 6 hours IM
Daily weight
Daily electrocardiogram
Blood tests, one or more times daily, CBC, blood sugar, electrolytes, BUN, creatinine, calcium, magnesium, prothrombin time, platelet count, total protein with albumin, and lipase (or amylase)
Blood tests, every 2 to 4 days, liver function tests

pressure, central venous pressure, and cardiac output. Whenever necessary, pulmonary artery wedge pressure (indicative of left atrial pressure) can also be measured and compared with pulmonary artery diastolic pressure: if wedge pressure is normal, an increased pulmonary artery diastolic pressure is caused by pulmonary complications of pancreatitis; if elevated, it is caused by congestive heart failure.

In most intensive care units, a bedside console provides a visual recording of the electrocardiogram, the pulmonary artery wave form of systolic and diastolic pressure, and a radial artery pressure wave form (if a transducer is placed in the patient's radial artery). In additon, there is a continuous digital print-out of pulse, pulmonary artery systolic and diastolic pressure, and radial artery systolic and diastolic pressure. Only in an intensive care unit setting can sophisticated equipment such as this be utilized to best advantage and appropriate measurements made often enough for optimal patient care.

Fluid Resuscitation

The important word is *resuscitation*. The amount of fluid required each 24 hours to compensate for excessive third space losses and to prevent hypovolemia is at times enormous. Measurements provided by a central venous pressure catheter or a Swan-Ganz catheter are required to gauge adequacy of fluid resuscitation. During the first several days, daily replacement is often in excess of 5 to 6 L. When there is substantial loss of albumin and significant hypotension, fluid replacement should include colloid. If there is retroperitoneal hemorrhage, whole blood or packed red blood cells is required.

Nasogastric Tube

A nasogastric tube is a definite help in cases of severe pancreatitis. Aspiration of gastric contents counteracts intractable nausea and vomiting, thereby reducing the threat of aspiration, and helps in the treatment of gastric and intestinal ileus. In addition, a nasogastric tube serves as a conduit to instill liquid antacids to maintain the intragastric pH as close to 7 as possible and thereby prevent stress ulcerations. The parenteral use of an H_2 receptor blocker may also be helpful in maintaining intragastric pH at 7.

A variety of measures that reduce pancreatic flow of fluid, including glucagon, anticholinergic agents, calcitonin, and somatostatin do not improve mortality and morbidity in severe pancreatitis. The concept of "resting the pancreas" in patients with acute pancreatitis really means the avoidance of oral alimentation until pancreatic inflammation has subsided.

Respiratory Care

Hypoxemia may occur for many reasons, including atelectasis, pneumonia, pleural effusions, fatigue, congestive heart failure, and—after the first 2 or 3 days—adult respiratory distress syndrome. Humidified oxygen should be provided by mask or nasal prongs. If hypoxemia persists, endotracheal intubation and assisted ventilation may become necessary. It is essential to determine whether hypoxemia is caused by congestive heart failure (characterized by an increased pulmonary artery wedge pressure) or by adult respiratory distress syndrome (characterized by a normal pulmonary artery wedge pressure). If there is evidence of adult respiratory distress syndrome, positive end expiratory pressure is also required.

Cardiovascular Care

Congestive heart failure should be treated by parenteral digitalization and diuretic therapy. Cardiac arrhythmias, myocardial infarction, and cardiogenic shock are treated by conventional pharmacologic strategy.

Renal function may deteriorate despite adequate fluid resuscitation. If there is evidence of acute tubular necrosis, an intravenous diuretic at a high dosage (or intravenous mannitol) and at times peritoneal dialysis are required. Since furosemide increases pancreatic volume flow, an alternate diuretic should be utilized.

Pain Relief

Severe pain should be treated with an effective medication such as meperidine, 75 to 100 mg IM or IV as required every 3 to 4 hours. At times, meperidine is needed every 2 to 3 hours to relieve agonizing pain. The effects of meperidine can be enhanced with medications such as Vistaril. Instructions for narcotic medications should be reevaluated several times each day to titrate this requirement. The source of pain should also be reevaluated to exclude a complication such as myocardial infarction, infarction of small or large bowel, or acute gastric dilation caused by a poorly functioning nasogastric tube.

Treatment of Infection

There is no evidence that the prophylactic use of antibiotics improves morbidity or prevents the development of a pancreatic abscess. Accordingly, I refrain from using antibiotic therapy until a specific infection is documented, such as biliary tract sepsis, urinary sepsis, or pneumonia. Some clinicians advise antibiotic use if a large phlegmon is seen on CT, hoping to prevent abscess formation.

If a pancreatic abscess is documented, appropriate antibiotic therapy should be instituted and surgical debridement of infected retroperitoneal tissue should be performed. A reasonable combination of antibiotics includes gentamicin, ampicillin, and either Flagyl or clindamycin. Antibiotic therapy by itself cannot cure a pancreatic abscess, and mortality is virtually 100 percent without surgical debridement.

The distinction between a pancreatic abscess and an infected pancreatic pseudocyst should be clearly understood. An abscess is a spreading infection involving necrotic tissue in the retroperitoneum that requires extensive surgical debridement. An infected pseudocyst is an infection of fluid contained within this structure. The latter also requires antibiotic therapy as well as either surgical drainage or percutaneous drainage using a pigtail catheter (if a safe route of entry can be confirmed by CT scan). Serial CT determinations may prove helpful during this critical phase of management.

Treatment of Metabolic Complications

Hyperglycemia may occur early in the course of severe pancreatitis, but blood sugar levels then normalize as the inflammatory process subsides. Because an elevated blood sugar level may spontaneously return to normal, insulin should be administered with great caution and usually at intervals of at least 6 to 8 hours. A determination of blood sugar level should be obtained just prior to each dose to avoid hypoglycemia. In general, a blood sugar less than 250 mg per 100 ml does not require insulin therapy. Blood sugar levels that continue to be higher than 250 mg per 100 ml (and particularly 300 mg per 100 ml) should be treated cautiously with subcutaneous or intravenous regular insulin.

Hypocalcemia may occur either because of a decrease in unionized or ionized calcium. Reduction in serum unionized calcium is usually caused by the loss of calcium bound to albumin into third spaces. This decrease has no physiologic importance and does not require intravenous calcium administration. Infusion of fluids that contain albumin usually restores unionized serum calcium to normal levels.

Signs of neuromuscular irritability may occur when serum ionized calcium levels are decreased. A reduction in ionized calcium could occur through several potential mechanisms, including deposition of ionized calcium within areas of fat necrosis and the development of hypomagnesemia. A reduction in ionized calcium not associated with a reduction in magnesium levels can be treated with calcium gluconate. A 10-ml ampule of 10 percent calcium gluconate can be administered intravenously in 1,000 ml of replacement fluid over 4 to 6 hours. Additional calcium can be infused over a similar interval until there is clinical improvement. The clinician should bear in mind that a 10-ml ampule contains 1 g of calcium gluconate but only 93 mg of calcium. Since 400 mg of dietary calcium are absorbed daily, calcium replacement provided by this protocol is not excessive. In an emergency, two 10-ml ampules of 10 percent calcium gluconate can be safely administered intravenously over a 10- to 15-minute period. Before initiating calcium replacement at a rapid rate, the clinician must be sure that the patient is not hypokalemic and is not receiving treatment with digitalis. In either situation, a rapid infusion of calcium may induce a fatal arrhythmia because infused calcium binds to myocardial receptors and may intensify harmful effects of hypokalemia on the heart.

If a reduction in ionized calcium is caused by coexisting hypomagnesemia, a 2-ml ampule of 50 percent magnesium sulfate can be diluted in 1,000 ml of replacement fluid and infused over 4 to 6 hours. One ampule contains only 8 mEq of magnesium, which is slightly less than the amount of dietary magnesium absorbed daily by the small intestine. Accordingly, if magnesium deficiency is more severe, 2 ampules can be safely administered as above. If magnesium deficiency is extreme and renal function is normal, it is safe to dilute 5 ampules (40 mEq) of 50 percent magnesium sulfate in 500 ml of replacement fluid and infuse it slowly over a 6-hour period. The adequacy of magnesium replacement can be gauged by increases in serum calcium and magnesium. In addition, when serum magnesium levels are restored, urinary magnesium levels increase.

Removal of Activated Pancreatic Enzymes

Currently available protease inhibitors are ineffective when administered intravenously. Hemodialysis is also ineffective in improving survival. In recent years, there has been increased interest in the efficacy of *peritoneal lavage* to remove activated pancreatic enzymes and toxins contained in ascitic fluid before they can be reabsorbed into the circulation. While there have been anecdotal reports of improvement following peritoneal lavage and one earlier prospective study that suggested an improved survival, a recent multicenter prospective randomized study did not demonstrate any improvement in survival among patients who underwent peritoneal lavage compared with those who did not. Nonetheless, it is possible that additional studies will demonstrate that a subset of patients benefits from peritoneal lavage. For example, variables that were not considered in this recent study were the volume of ascites and the quantity of toxic materials in the ascitic fluid. Until further studies are performed, I am willing to attempt peritoneal lavage as a potentially life-saving strategy if there is *considerable ascitic fluid* and if a patient with severe pancreatitis is *deteriorating rapidly* because of refractory *hypotension*, progressive *respiratory or renal failure*, or deepening *coma.* A similar view is expressed in the chapter *Pancreatitis: Surgical Considerations.*

If there is little or no ascitic fluid, peritoneal lavage cannot be expected to be beneficial, since this technique does not dialyze enzymes or toxins from the systemic circulation. Faced with a severely ill and failing patient, the clinician now has only two options. One is an emergency laparotomy in the hope of preventing a fatal outcome. Before considering this option, I would suggest an emergency CT scan in an effort to find a treatable condition. For example, if an early pancreatic abscess is confirmed by the presence of retroperitoneal air bubbles, a surgical approach has a reasonable expectation of being beneficial. If a large pancreatic fluid collection is discovered within the lesser sac, the anterior pararenal space, or the posterior pararenal space, an experienced radiologist can aspirate this fluid via a safe percutaneous route guided by CT scan. The purpose of this aspiration—much like the theory of peritoneal lavage—is to remove as much fluid containing enzymes and toxins as possible before they gain access to the circulation. Although this strategy has not as yet been subjected to a prospective trial, it is a reasonable effort in my view to stabilize blood pressure and improve organ function in a patient who is failing rapidly. If CT scan does not show an abscess or a significant fluid collection, an emergency laparotomy can still be considered, with goals and expectations that are described in the chapter *Pancreatitis: Surgical Considerations.*

Nutritional Support

Patients seriously ill with pancreatitis cannot be fed orally for several weeks. Some patients require nutritional support for several months. Nutrition is best achieved by instituting total parenteral nutrition within a few days of hospitalization. Intravenous fat emulsions have not caused an exacerbation of pancreatitis among patients with normal triglyceride levels. If serum triglyceride levels are markedly increased, fat emulsions should not be utilized.

Once pancreatitis has improved clinically, a final CT scan should be performed. If a large phlegmon is still demonstrated, and especially if there is residual abdominal tenderness or hyperamylasemia, total parenteral nutrition should be continued until there is complete clinical improvement and additional radiologic improvement. Oral feedings can then be initiated very cautiously. This strategy is outlined in the section on mild pancreatitis.

Miscellaneous

Disseminated intravascular coagulation is an infrequent but serious complication of acute pancreatitis. The use of intravenous heparin is controversial. Initial strategy should be directed toward intravenous replacement of coagulation factors (fresh frozen plasma and platelets as needed).

Gastrointestinal bleeding may occur for a variety of reasons including stress ulcerations and esophageal varices. Maintenance of intragastric pH in an alkaline range helps prevent stress ulcerations. *Intestinal obstruction* caused by an extension of inflammatory exudate into the mesentery of the small intestine may require surgical treatment if either a nasogastric tube or long tube is not helpful. *Bowel infarction* may occur because of thrombosis of blood vessels or encroachment by inflammatory exudate, and requires surgical treatment. Occasionally ischemic colitis of the splenic flexure or proximal descending colon may cause rectal bleeding.

Metabolic acidosis occurs for a variety of reasons, including renal insufficiency, lactic acidosis, ketoacidosis (either diabetic or alcoholic), and drug intoxification (such as with salicylates, methanol, or ethylene glycol). All are characterized by an increased serum anion gap. Lactic acidosis occurs in acute pancreatitis on the basis of severe hypotension and occasionally on the basis of metabolism of alcohol. Treatment includes copious intravenous fluid replacement, colloid therapy, and the administration of sufficient amounts of bicarbonate intravenously to maintain an arterial pH greater than 7.1. The treatment of alcoholic ketoacidosis includes the administration of intravenous fluids that contain glucose and sodium chloride and the infusion of sodium bicarbonate to maintain the arterial pH greater than 7.1.

Pancreatic encephalopathy may be manifested by a wide variety of neurologic and psychiatric signs and symptoms. Various mechanisms include high fever, hypotension, respiratory failure, electrolyte derangement, hypocalcemia, alcohol withdrawal, metabolic acidosis, and coagulopathy. Pancreatic enzymes may also be responsible by either inducing brain damage directly or causing a toxic state. There are anecdotal reports of improvement in pancreatic encephalopathy following initiation of peritoneal lavage.

Obstructive jaundice has several explanations, including edema of the head of the pancreas compressing the distal common bile duct and the presence of retained stones. Pancreatic edema usually recedes following several days of medical treatment of pancreatitis. Retained common bile duct stones pose a more serious problem. If there is ascending cholangitis, surgical decompression of the common bile duct is usually required. In the absence of sepsis, a cautious interval of medical management of pancreatitis is warranted until a more elective operation can be performed during the same admission after severe pancreatitis has subsided. The role of endoscopic papillotomy for retained stones in acute pancreatitis has not as yet been defined. The risks and benefits of endoscopic papillotomy compared with conventional surgical treatment have not been studied in a prospective, randomized, controlled trial. A firm recommendation can therefore not be made. If an extremely poor risk patient requires emergency surgical decompression of the common bile duct, it is reasonable to consider endoscopic papillotomy as an alternative if an endoscopist is available with skill and experience in this procedure.

Strategy After the First Week

A pancreatic abscess usually does not occur until after the first week. Even if appropriate antibiotics are utilized, mortality is virtually 100 percent unless aggressive surgical debridement is performed.

A sterile pancreatic pseudocyst requires urgent treatment if it is expanding rapidly, becomes secondarily infected, or causes significant bleeding. The role of pigtail catheter drainage of a sterile pancreatic pseudocyst has not yet been defined. A rapidly expanding pseudocyst can be decompressed at least temporarily by percutaneous aspiration. An infected pancreatic pseudocyst can be treated by surgical drainage or by an indwelling pigtail catheter if a safe portal of entry can be found to insert the catheter. A pseudocyst associated with bleeding is best treated by surgical ligation of bleeding vessels and at times by a limited pancreatic resection once the site of bleeding has been localized by arteriography.

An uncomplicated pancreatic pseudocyst is usually treated medically for 4 to 6 weeks. It would seem reasonable to curtail or avoid oral intake in an effort to reduce pancreatic secretion and thereby prevent further accumulation of pancreatic fluid within the pseudocyst. If total parenteral nutrition is required during this interval because of the severity of pancreatitis, the advisability of oral intake is not an issue. If pancreatitis has subsided, however, and the patient would otherwise be receiving oral intake, it is not known whether the institution of total parenteral nutrition is more helpful than oral nutritional strategy, such as an elemental diet, in promoting shrinkage of a pseudocyst. If a pancreatic pseudocyst has not resolved spontaneously after 4 to 6 weeks, surgical decompression is usually required if it is causing symptoms or is more than 6 cm in diameter. The chapter *Pancreatitis: Surgical Considerations* also discusses this issue.

TREATMENT OF RECURRENT PANCREATITIS

Recurrent pancreatitis caused by biliary calculi is best treated by a cholecystectomy. It is much more difficult to prevent recurrent episodes of pancreatitis caused by alcohol, and the patient should be strongly urged to discontinue the use of alcohol. Recurrent pain severe enough to cause narcotic addiction requires serious consideration of surgery, especially if the main pancreatic duct is dilated. Recurrent pancreatitis caused by metabolic abnormalities such as hypertriglyceridemia or hypercalcemia is treated by conventional methods to lower the serum values.

Recurrent pancreatitis secondary to sphincter of Oddi stenosis or dysfunction is best diagnosed by endoscopic manometry and treated by either endoscopic papillotomy or surgical sphincteroplasty.

The discovery of pancreas divisum on endoscopic retrograde cholangiopancreatography raises the possibility that this anatomic variant is the cause of recurrent pancreatitis. It is important to exclude other causes of pancreatitis. Endoscopic manometric evaluation of the sphincter of Oddi and cholecystectomy are important steps in this evaluation. Therapeutic approaches directed toward the accessory papilla in an effort to improve drainage of the dorsal duct include endoscopic dilation, endoscopic stinting, and surgical sphincteroplasty. These various procedures have not yet been subjected to a prospective clinical trial, and no firm recommendation can be made among them at present. In addition, criteria that would enable the clinician to determine which patients with pancreas divisum are likely to benefit from one of these approaches have not yet been rigorously defined.

PANCREATITIS: SURGICAL CONSIDERATIONS

ANDREW L. WARSHAW, M.D.

Recent convocations in Cambridge and Marseille to classify pancreatitis have agreed that it is possible to distinguish three types: *acute, chronic,* and *obstructive.* Although there is overlap in the clinical manifestations, these are in fact three different diseases. The role of surgical treatment differs in each. In general, surgery can respond only to the complications of pancreatitis and their symptoms. It cannot effect a cure or improve pancreatic function, and may fail even to halt the progression of the disease. When a specific cause for recurrent acute pancreatitis can be identified, surgical correction can end the succession of attacks, but the natural history of chronic pancreatitis is comparatively inexorable.

ACUTE PANCREATITIS

The clinical course of acute pancreatitis can be separated into three phases, each with its own characteristics and appropriate treatment. The early phase is one of inflammation and vascular instability, generally lasting one to several days. The phenomena during this period may be life-threatening but are nonetheless reversible. It is during the middle phase, beginning about the fourth day and lasting from 1 to several weeks, that tissue destruction becomes recognizable. Phlegmon, or swelling, of the pancreas, recognizable on computed tomography (CT) scan in up to 50 percent of patients, may also harbor areas of pancreatic and peri-pancreatic necrosis. Thrombosis and erosion of local blood vessels may produce further visceral infarction, fistulas, and hemorrhage. In the late phase, beginning about 2 weeks after onset, there is risk of infection of the necrotic tissues.

Early Phase

Surgery for Diagnosis

Even today, the diagnosis of acute pancreatitis is often uncertain. All current laboratory and radiographic tests give both false-positive and false-negative results, and the clinical picture may overlap with a number of other diseases, most notably perforated ulcers, acute cholecystitis, intestinal ischemia, and closed-loop obstruction or perforation. The serum amylase level may increase in any of these entities. When in doubt, especially if a patient has impressive signs of peritoneal irritation, it is safer to explore than to miss a potentially lethal but surgically correctible lesion. It should not be an embarrassment to find "only pancreatitis" in these circumstances, nor should a simple exploration cause harm or aggravate the pancreatitis. There is no indication to place any drains or tubes in viscera under these circumstances unless there is abundant toxic ascites (see below) or reason to believe that the patient needs biliary decompression for cholangitis.

Surgery for Organ Dysfunction

Profound impairment of circulatory, renal, and pulmonary function may not respond to volume replacement and other supportive therapy. There is evidence that the body-wide effects on function of many organs may be mediated by toxic and vasoactive substances that are absorbed from the brownish peritoneal exudate (toxic ascites) that is present in fulminant cases. Removal of this ascitic fluid should therefore be beneficial. Many surgeons, including myself, have the impression that *peritoneal lavage* is effective, but a definitive study has not been performed. The best and most recent one showed no benefit of lavage in severe pancreatitis, but did not address specifically those patients with circulatory dysfunction (shock).

I continue to use peritoneal lavage in patients who show signs of shock, tachycardia (>130), ongoing major volume requirements, and progressive renal or pulmonary failure despite 24 hours of vigorous medical treatment. There is no evidence that lavage benefits any other category of patient, and it is not indicated, for example, for treatment of pain or purely on the basis of Ranson's signs of severity.

Catheters for peritoneal lavage may be placed percutaneously or surgically. The percutaneous technique will suffice in most cases. With local anesthesia a Tenckhoff catheter, as used for renal dialysis, is placed under direct vision through a short midline subumbilical incision. Standard peritoneal dialysis fluids, containing 500 U of heparin and a broad-spectrum antibiotic with enteric coverage, will suffice in most cases. Because of the glucose in the dialysis solution, care should be taken to monitor blood sugar. It is advisable to use only 1 L per lavage to reduce the risk of precipitating the need for intubation and assisted ventilation. Also, the lavage fluid need not equilibrate in the peritoneal cavity, but can be introduced and drained continuously. If the lavage is working, its effects will be apparent almost immediately. Within a few hours, the heart rate will fall dramatically toward 100, the blood pressure will rise, and the volume requirements will fall. The lavage need not be continued for more than a day or two once improvement has occurred.

If the percutaneous lavage is ineffective after several hours, laparotomy is recommended to ensure that the diagnosis is correct and to place the lavage catheters directly into the lesser sac. On occasion the toxic ascites is loculated there and has not been effectively removed by the percutaneous catheter in the greater peritoneal cavity. Of course, some patients with overwhelming pancreatitis will respond to nothing.

Surgery to Excise the Disease

Major pancreatic resection and even total pancreatectomy during the early phase of pancreatitis has its advocates, particularly in France; however, there are no objective criteria either for selecting patients for excision or for deciding how much pancreas to remove. Much recoverable pancreas is wasted, and the results with regard to preventing death or abscess are no better than with the more conservative approach being outlined here. Early pancreatic resection is not recommended.

Surgery to Prevent Progression of Pancreatitis

Gallstone pancreatitis is caused by passage through or lodging of a stone at the ampulla of Vater. A common duct stone can be demonstrated in about 70 percent of patients during the first 24 hours of gallstone pancreatitis. This has led some to advocate early common duct exploration (within 48 hours) to remove that stone, with the claim that the progression from edematous to necrotizing pancreatitis will be aborted. The idea has several weaknesses and limitations. First, the differentiation of gallstone from other forms of pancreatitis is often difficult. Biochemical criteria, such as an elevated SGOT, are helpful, but direct cholangiography (transhepatic or endoscopic) is needed to be sure. Second, many of the patients studied have undoubtedly had only chemical hyperamylasemia ("pseudopancreatitis") induced by the obstructing stone, not true pancreatic inflammation. Third, other investigators have found higher complication and mortality rates among patients subjected to early biliary surgery. Because 95 percent of cases of gallstone pancreatitis will quiet down on medical management without progression to a fulminant form, and 95 percent of stones will pass spontaneously in the first week, surgical intervention to remove the stone within 48 hours does not at present seem justifiable. Cholecystectomy and, if still necessary, common duct exploration can be safely and effectively delayed until the pancreatitis subsides. I perform the operative procedure at a quiescent time later during the same hospital admission.

Endoscopic techniques using endoscopic retrograde cholangiopancreatography (ERCP) and sphincterotomy to remove the common duct stone early in gallstone pancreatitis are also undergoing trials. Several preliminary reports suggest that sphincterotomy and clearing of stones can be accomplished safely. Many of the same hesitations stated above are applicable to this approach as well. There is also the concern about aggravating the pancreatitis if contrast is injected into the pancreatic duct during ERCP. Final judgment about the role of this technique awaits greater experience.

Middle Phase

The middle phase of pancreatitis, beginning toward the end of the first week, is characterized by inflammatory swelling or phlegmon of the pancreas and peripancreatic tissues. Areas of ischemic and enzymatic necrosis may develop within the phlegmon, occupying small patches or large confluent areas of the pancreas and surrounding tissues. If the necrotic areas are small, natural repair processes may be successful in healing them. Dead tissue that cannot be cleared will sooner or later manifest itself by signs of inflammation and still later by superinfection.

Phlegmon

The pancreatic inflammatory mass is treated by withholding feedings until pain, fever, hyperamylasemia, and leukocytosis have subsided. There is evidence that premature feeding may promote the progression to tissue necrosis and abscess. The phlegmon should be followed by weekly CT scan, if available, to document resolution or to detect the appearance of liquefaction necrosis.

Gastric outlet obstruction by the phlegmon may persist for weeks and on occasion has necessitated a gastrojejunostomy. Compression and partial obstruction of the intrapancreatic portion of the common bile duct is common, but always resolves and virtually never requires tube drainage unless there are also gallstones and cholangitis.

Necrosis

Large areas of necrosis of pancreatic and peripancreatic tissue may advertise their presence by signs of inflammation, pain, and tenderness but often remain clinically silent. The best available means of demonstrating the lucent, liquefying regional necrosis is CT scan. Large areas of necrosis should be debrided before infection gets established. Smaller areas can be followed unless signs of inflammation appear. When in doubt, needle aspiration under CT or ultrasound guidance can be helpful to search for evidence of infection.

Acute Pseudocyst

Fluid collections around the pancreas and in the lesser sac at this stage often represent pancreatic secretions that have leaked from the damaged gland. They are frequently associated with ongoing necrotizing pancreatitis, hemorrhage, visceral injury, and eventually abscess, and are therefore associated with a high mortality rate (on the order of 20%). On the other hand, acute pseudocysts also have the potential to resolve spontaneously or to evolve by encapsulation into mature chronic pseudocysts. If the patient is stable and not exceedingly ill, it may be safe to watch acute pseudocysts in the hope of spontaneous resolution. If there are any signs of deterioration (increased tenderness, fever, tachycardia, fluid requirements, or leukocytosis), it becomes safer to operate for external drainage of the collection and debridement of necrotic tissues. The presence of semi-solid necrotic tissues generally means that attempted percutaneous drainage of the fluid collection will be inadequate.

Hemorrhage

Erosion of major arterial vessels by proteolytic enzymes may produce exsanguinating hemorrhage. We have used arteriography to locate the site and to control the bleeding by embolization with considerable success in a small series of patients. The angiographic control, even if only partial or temporary, appears to provide the benefits of time and reduced blood loss that allow a more orderly and effective operation for debridement of the damaged area.

Thrombosis

Vessels exposed directly to the inflammatory process are at risk of thrombosis, perhaps because of the same enzymatic injury that causes bleeding if the vessel wall is penetrated. The resulting ischemia of bowel segments served by these arteries—most often the transverse colon and duodenum—can be manifested by gastrointestinal bleeding from sloughed mucosa, full-thickness bowel infarction, enteric fistulas, or later strictures. The value of arteriography in the detection of thrombosed visceral vessels in such a patient is not established. If bowel infarction occurs, the involved segment must be resected. It is safer under these circumstances to bring out both ends of the remaining bowel as stomas rather than to risk breakdown of an anastomosis. When the duodenum perforates, a pancreaticoduodenectomy may very rarely be necessary, but limited resection of the compromised duodenal wall and reconstruction with intraluminal decompression by tube are preferable when possible. Colonic and duodenal fistulas are managed by external drainage and reconstruction at a later date.

Late Phase

The transition from sterile necrosis to infected necrosis to abscess is often blurred. Infection of the necrotic tissues of the middle phase of pancreatitis can be detected as early as the second week after onset; however, it is unusual for fever and other clinical signs heralding a pancreatic abscess to be apparent before the third week. The best means of demonstrating pancreatic abscesses is the CT scan.

Antibiotic therapy is inadequate to prevent many pancreatic abscesses and never produces a cure. Drainage is the sine qua non of treatment. Percutaneous catheter drainage has a high rate of failure (40%), probably because of the associated necrotic tissues in the abscess, and therefore surgical drainage is preferred. Because pancreatic abscesses extend in unpredictable directions and are often separated, loculated, and multiple, a full transabdominal exploration is warranted, rather than a limited flank approach. Aggressive debridement and drainage should salvage 95 percent of patients, but further abscess formation necessitates reoperation or percutaneous catheter drainage in up to 30 percent. Enteric fistulas and hemorrhage from the abscess cavity are common and are treated as described in the section on pancreatic necrosis.

Persisting Pancreatitis

A few patients continue to have low-grade signs of pancreatic inflammation for many weeks or even several months, without focal collections or areas of necrosis demonstrable by CT scan to target for debridement or drainage. ERCP may identify irreversible injury to the pancreatic duct or underlying anomalies that do not allow the pancreatitis to subside. In other patients there may be microabscesses or unrecognized duodenal wall injury. Resection of the pertinent area, even if it requires pancreaticoduodenectomy, however radical that may seem, may be the only option left. Distal pancreatectomy is indicated when the pancreatic duct becomes obstructed by the necrotizing process and its healing by scar.

After the Attack

Once the patient has recovered, it is time to look with ultrasound and ERCP for remediable causes in order to prevent recurrence. Surgically treatable factors include gallstones, pancreatic cancer, ampullary stenosis, accessory papilla stenosis associated with pancreas divisum, and anomalies of the pancreaticobiliary systems (e.g., enteric duplication cysts, choledochal cysts, duodenal diverticula).

CHRONIC PANCREATITIS

Far and away the most common indication for operation in cases of chronic pancreatitis is pain. Other complications, such as pseudocysts or obstruction of the common bile duct or duodenum, are present in about 40 percent of patients presenting for surgical treatment and occasionally occur without pain. Although the pain may "burn out" as the gland deteriorates over the years, it is unreasonable to require that a patient wait years for possible spontaneous relief if an effective, immediate, and safe surgical solution exists. The purpose of surgery in chronic pancreatitis is only to remedy specific problems. No operation can improve or stabilize pancreatic function.

Pain

The tactics of the two major surgical alternatives for reducing pancreatic pain are improvement of drainage of the pancreatic duct or resection of pancreatic tissue. Drainage (decompressive) procedures are preferable because they are safer, relatively simple, and conserve pancreatic tissue and residual function; however, they require the presence of a dilated pancreatic duct, usually more than 7 mm. ERCP has thus become the central tool for planning the best surgical approach.

In perhaps 60 percent of patients failing to improve with medical therapy, the main pancreatic duct will be dilated, sometimes three to four times normal size. Functionally significant strictures occur in a minority. Recent measurements have confirmed the hypothesis that the pressure in these dilated ducts is high in patients with pain. The optimal treatment is a *modified Puestow operation*—a long side-to-side anastomosis of the pancreatic duct to a Roux-en-Y loop of jejunum. In my experience of 45 cases, this operation provides good pain relief in more than 80 percent of patients, with one surgical death and no other complications in the series. Other forms of operation for duct decompression, such as transduodenal sphincteroplasty or caudal pancreaticojejunostomy (distal drainage), have been ineffective and should not be considered.

Patients whose main pancreatic duct is not dilated are not candidates for pancreaticojejunostomy. Resection of the distal 50 to 60 percent of the pancreas is rarely successful. The principal indication for that operation is the treatment of patients with obstructing lesions of the midpancreatic duct (see below). *Distal subtotal (95%) pancreatectomy* (Child procedure) has had somewhat greater success. Some say it is effective in 60 percent of cases, though virtually all patients become diabetic. Especially if the pancreatitis appears to be disproportionately localized to the head of the gland, perhaps with a mass, resection of the head (pancreaticoduodenectomy, Whipple procedure) may be the best alternative. *Pancreaticoduodenectomy* is a complicated operation, more difficult for chronic pancreatitis than for cancer, but in appropriately selected patients the rate of satisfactory pain relief exceeds 70 percent. Enough pancreas is preserved that many patients do not immediately develop diabetes. I favor preservation of the antrum and pylorus, as described by Longmire.[1] Total pancreatectomy, especially in the alcoholic patient, can and should almost always be avoided.

Pseudocysts

Pancreatic pseudocysts associated with chronic pancreatitis should be treated surgically if they are symptomatic, larger than 4 cm, or persist for more than 6 weeks. In the absence of a recent identifiable attack of acute pancreatitis, it may safely be assumed that all pseudocysts in patients with chronic fibrotic pancreatitis have a thick, mature wall at the time of presentation. There is therefore no need to observe them either to let the wall mature or in the futile hope of spontaneous resolution. Percutaneous drainage by needle or catheter has uniformly failed in my experience because of either recurrence, infection, or persistent fistula. The worldwide experience thus far is not much more encouraging.

The preferred surgical treatment is internal drainage to the stomach, duodenum, or jejunum. Results of the three methods have been similar: less than 5 percent postoperative complications and less than 5 percent recurrence. The choice is most simply based on proximity—the hollow viscus (excluding the colon) nearest the pseudocyst can be used for the anastomosis. In practice, large pseudocysts are most frequently drained into the stomach and smaller ones into the intestine.

Bile Duct Stenosis

Stenosis of the intrapancreatic portion of the common bile duct develops as a consequence of extrinsic compression and constriction by pancreatic fibrosis. Differentiation of chronic pancreatitis from pancreatic cancer may be difficult in some cases. The first sign of functional significance of the stenosis is a raised serum alkaline phosphatase level. Later jaundice and eventually secondary biliary cirrhosis may develop. Decompression of the bile duct by choledochoduodenostomy or choledochojejunostomy is indicated when the alkaline phosphatase elevation persists, hyperbilirubinemia supervenes, or liver biopsy shows evolution toward cirrhosis. I have abandoned anastomoses using the gallbladder instead of the common duct as the conduit because of later complications related to chronic biliary stasis and stone formation.

Duodenal Obstruction

Duodenal obstruction is the consequence of progressive and unremitting fibrotic narrowing, rather than transitory edema (as in acute pancreatitis). It is treated by bypass with a gastrojejunostomy. We have not felt it necessary to perform a complementary vagotomy in the absence of peptic ulcer disease.

Venous Obstruction

The splenic vein (commonly) and the portal-superior mesenteric veins (occasionally) are occluded in the course of chronic pancreatitis. This phenomenon has no relation to liver disease. Its clinical consequences range from nil to bleeding varices, but the enlarged veins may make surgery in the region of the pancreas bloody and difficult. The treatment of splenic vein obstruction is splenectomy, and the surgeon should be prepared to do this first if "left-sided" portal hypertension is encountered during pancreatic surgery. Portal-superior mesenteric vein obstruction allows for no easy remedy, by shunt or otherwise. Splenectomy may confer some benefit in these patients, in part because the splenic vein is usually occluded as well. Gastrointestinal bleeding from varices may have to be controlled by endoscopic sclerotherapy.

TABLE 1 Indications for Surgical Treatment in 60 Consecutive Patients with Chronic Pancreatitis

Indication	No. of Patients
With dilated pancreatic duct (>7 min)	(40)
pain	39
+ bile duct obstruction	22
+ duodenal obstruction	1
+ biliary and duodenal obstruction	3
+ pseudocyst	10
Bile duct obstruction (painless)	1
Without dilated pancreatic duct	(20)
pain	20
+ bile duct obstruction	1
+ duodenal obstruction	0
+ pseudocyst	5

Seven patients also had splenic vein and three had portal-superior mesenteric vein obstruction.

Pancreatic Ascites and Pleural Effusions

These chronic fluid collections are caused by an internal fistula from the pancreas to the peritoneum or pleural space. The point of origin, usually from a ruptured pseudocyst, can be demonstrated by ERCP in more than 80 percent of cases. While occasional cases will respond to conservative therapy using repeated withdrawal of the fluid and pharmacologic inhibition of the pancreas, most will require surgical treatment. The most common surgical tactic is to anastomose a Roux-en-Y loop of jejunum to the site of the leak to channel the secretions back into the gut. When the disruption is in the tail of the pancreas, distal pancreatectomy is effective and simple. In patients whose effusions collect in the pleural space, the retroperitoneal fistula into the chest can be identified and interrupted below the diaphragm. Once the origin of the fistula has been dealt with by pancreaticojejunostomy or resection, the pleural end of the fistula will heal and the effusion will not reaccumulate.

Multiple Problems

Many patients with chronic pancreatitis have more than one reason for needing an operation, either synchronously or metachronously (Table 1). Planning appropriate surgery requires specific evaluation of each of the potential trouble spots in advance.

OBSTRUCTIVE PANCREATITIS

Obstructive pancreatitis by definition is secondary to a specific obstructing lesion. The treatment is therefore directed toward defining the nature of the obstruction, and then removing it, with or without the damaged pancreas distal to the point of obstruction. This is the form of pancreatic injury that is found behind tumors of the head of the pancreas or high-grade ampullary obstruction from any cause. A pure obstructive component may be added to the basic lesion of chronic pancreatitis if complete main duct occlusion by stricture or stone develops. Less well appreciated is the phenomenon of main duct occlusion in acute pancreatitis, caused by necrosis of a segment of the pancreas and subsequent healing and fibrosis. If this process results in loss of a section of the main pancreatic duct, the duct may end blindly in scar. The obstructed distal pancreas will give rise to pain and perhaps recurrent inflammatory signs unless and until it atrophies.

Removing the isolated tail of the pancreas is curative. The same sequence and solution may apply in some patients after drainage of a pseudocyst; the pseudocyst was the visible indicator of pancreatic injury, and, following its drainage, the tail of the pancreas may become symptomatic at a later date as the outflow of its secretions becomes restricted. Pancreatography once again is the key to elucidating the problem and formulating a solution.

REFERENCE

1. Traverso LW, Longmire WP Jr. Preservation of the pylorus in pancreatico-duodenectomy. A follow-up evaluation. Ann Surg 1980; 192:302.

CHRONIC PANCREATITIS: EXOCRINE AND ENDOCRINE INSUFFICIENCIES

PHILLIP P. TOSKES, M.D.

Patients with chronic impairment of pancreatic exocrine function usually present with abdominal pain or diarrhea, steatorrhea, and weight loss. Those patients who have abdominal pain as their chief complaint may develop diarrhea, steatorrhea, and weight loss or always have abdominal pain as their major symptom and never evolve into frank exocrine insufficiency. Approximately 15 percent of patients with chronic pancreatitis will never manifest abdominal pain and will present initially with diarrhea, steatorrhea, and weight loss.

In adults the usual causes of pancreatic exocrine impairment are alcohol-induced chronic pancreatitis, pancreatic resection, pancreatic cancer, and idiopathic chronic pancreatitis. In children the usual cause is cystic fibrosis.

The diagnosis of chronic pancreatitis in general is difficult to make and is often done by exclusion. This is especially true of those patients whose main manifestation is pain, since they often have just mild to moderate impairment of exocrine function, while those with steatorrhea have severe impairment of exocrine function. Often the diagnosis of chronic pancreatitis has necessitated the use of invasive tests that are uncomfortable for the patient, time-consuming for both patient and physician, and expensive; consequently, the diagnosis is often not made. Now, however, a group of pancreatic function tests (bentiromide, trypsin-like immunoreactivity) are emerging that are simple to perform and that provide the clinician with very good sensitivity and specificity, especially in those patients with pancreatic steatorrhea. Such tests may also be valuable in assessing the response to therapy, e.g., an improvement in the bentiromide test after administration of pancreatic extract. These tests of pancreatic function are characterized by their ease of performance and excellent acceptance by patients. They are noninvasive, inexpensive, and can be performed in an office or clinic setting. For those patients with mild to moderate impairment of exocrine function, i.e., the patients with chronic abdominal pain and no steatorrhea, direct tube tests, such as the secretin test or endoscopic retrograde cholangiopancreatography (ERCP), remain the most consistent way to make the diagnosis of chronic pancreatitis.

PANCREATIC EXTRACT THERAPY

The cornerstone of the therapeutic approach to patients with chronic pancreatitis is the use of pancreatic extracts. This is true whether one is treating steatorrhea or pain, since the principles of therapy are similar. A potent pancreatic enzyme formulation must be employed to ensure that the relevant enzymes (lipase for steatorrhea, proteases for pain) escape destruction by gastric acid and reach the duodenum.

Treatment of Steatorrhea

Since pancreatic extract traditionally has been used to decrease steatorrhea in patients with pancreatic insufficiency, the treatment of pancreatic steatorrhea will be discussed first. Steatorrhea does not occur until lipase output is less than 10 percent of normal. I direct therapeutic efforts toward administering exogenously to the patient a source of lipase that will replace the endogenous lipase that the damaged pancreas cannot secrete. The goals of therapy are to decrease diarrhea and steatorrhea, enable the patient to gain weight, and increase the patient's sense of well-being. These goals are quite readily achieved, despite the fact that steatorrhea can rarely be completely corrected.

Selection of the Best Pancreatic Extract

The ideal pancreatic extract preparation does not yet exist. A preparation is needed with ten times the amount of lipase that is currently available. This would allow the patient to take fewer tablets or capsules—an important practical point, since therapy is lifelong. Thus the lipase content of the preparation is a critical factor. Of the many preparations available, only the following, listed in order of decreasing lipase content, have enough lipase to consider their use: Ilozyme, Ku-Zyme HP, Festal, Cotazym, Pancrease, Cotazym-S, and Viokase. Therapy should be initiated with an appropriate dose of pancreatic extract, as detailed in Table 1. If the patient does not respond adequately, the following should be considered: (1) Is the diagnosis correct? (2) Is there concomitant disease, such as bacterial overgrowth or sprue? (3) Is there a need for adjuvant therapy? My experience indicates that as many as 25 percent of patients with chronic pancreatitis may have concomitant small intestine bacterial overgrowth due to previous gastrointestinal surgery or perhaps hypomotility of the intestine from chronic abdominal pain or frequent usage of narcotics. These patients may need both pancreatic extract and antimicrobial therapy before diarrhea and steatorrhea can be effectively treated.

Adjuvant Therapy

Probably the most important factor leading to less than satisfactory treatment of steatorrhea following the administration of a potent pancreatic extract preparation is the destruction of lipase within the acid environment of the stomach. Pancreatic lipase is irreversibly inactivated below a pH of 4. Thus, the goal is to maintain the intragastric pH above 4 for as long as possible after the ingestion of the pancreatic extract preparation. In my opinion this is best achieved with the use of sodium bicarbonate. This is an effective, inexpensive therapy which, in the doses detailed in Table 1, has not led to any significant complications. My extensive experience has demonstrated that histamine$_2$ receptor antagonists (cimetidine, ranitidine) and other antacids (calcium carbonate, magnesium-aluminum hydroxide) are not very effective. The latter antacids may actually make steatorrhea worse by the formation of calcium or magnesium soaps.

Theoretically the use of enteric-coated microspheres (Pancrease or Cotazym-S) should obviate the need for adjuvant therapy, since these preparations will not release their contents until a pH of approximately 5.5 exists. Although these preparations are effective in some patients, other patients respond best to conventional preparations with sodium bicarbonate. Some of the problems with the microsphere preparations are that they do not contain enough lipase, they are large, and may empty slowly from the stomach. It is important to consider adjuvant therapy if the approach suggested in Table 1 fails, because increasing the dose above that listed in the table does not achieve much more reduction in steatorrhea, yet leads to a marked increase in bloating and cramps.

TABLE 1 Approach to Treatment of Pancreatic Maldigestion

Pancreatic Extract

Schedule: Before meals (and at bedtime if the patient experiences pain)

Dose: Viokase, 8 tablets each time *or*
Cotazym, 6 capsules each time *or*
Ilozyme, 4 capsules each time *or*
Pancrease, 3 capsules each time (enteric coated)

If no significant improvement occurs with extract alone add:

Sodium Bicarbonate*†

Schedule: Before and after each meal (and at bedtime if the patient experiences pain)

Dose: Sodium bicarbonate, 650 mg before and after meals (and 1,300 mg at bedtime if needed)

* I have not noted hypercalcemia or milk-alkali syndrome with this dose of sodium bicarbonate.
† I do not recommend concomitant treatment with sodium bicarbonate and enteric-coated enzyme preparations, since increased gastric pH may cause premature release and inactivation of enzymes.

Treatment of Pain

The treatment of the pain associated with chronic pancreatitis follows the same approach with respect to pancreatic extract preparations and adjuvant therapy as the treatment of steatorrhea outlined in Table 1. The pathogenesis of the pain associated with chronic pancreatitis is not understood, with the exception of the pain related to a pseudocyst. Drainage of a pseudocyst often will bring dramatic relief of pain. If no pseudocyst is found, two patterns emerge: (1) some patients have minimal or no abnormalities on ERCP and an abnormal secretin test, and (2) others will have dilated ducts or strictures or both detected by ERCP. Traditionally, the abnormalities of the latter group have been thought to be amenable to surgery. The findings at ERCP largely dictate the surgical approach, but the surgical procedure of choice has been pancreatic duct drainage.

Rationale

Treatment of the former group, i.e., those with normal ducts at ERCP, has been completely unsatisfactory, but recent data suggest that large doses of pancreatic extract may relieve the pain in these patients. It appears that pharmacologic doses of proteases may inhibit pancreatic exocrine secretion, thus putting the pancreas at rest and affording relief of pain. These clinical observations fit with a large amount of data in experimental animals which indicates that the amount of trypsin and chymotrypsin within the lumen of the proximal duodenum exerts a controlling influence on pancreatic exocrine secretion.

It would thus seem reasonable to approach the patient with chronic pancreatitis and pain in the following manner (Fig. 1). After other causes of abdominal pain have been appropriately excluded, an ultrasound or computed tomography scan of the pancreas should be performed. If no abnormality is found, a secretin test should

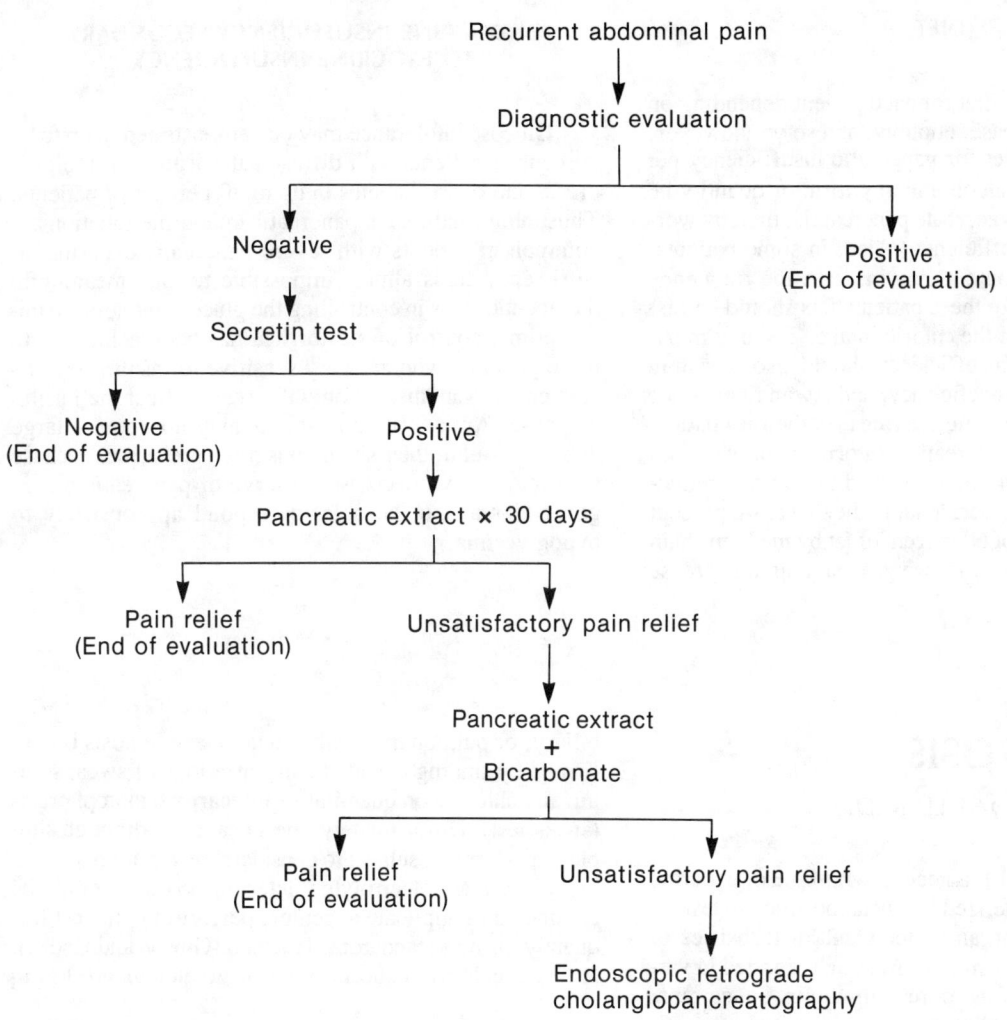

Figure 1 Algorithm for evaluating patients with recurrent abdominal pain.

be done. Invariably, if the pain is related to chronic pancreatitis, the secretin test will be abnormal. If the secretin test confirms the clinical impression of chronic pancreatitis, a trial of pancreatic extract therapy is indicated (e.g., Viokase, 8 tablets with meals and at bedtime) for 30 days. If relief from pain is achieved, no further steps need to be taken. If the result is unsatisfactory, the pancreatic extract should be enhanced with sodium bicarbonate (650 mg before and after each meal and 1300 mg at bedtime). If the results still are unsatisfactory, ERCP should be performed, looking for an inflammatory stricture or other lesion that might be corrected with surgery. It is noteworthy that few patients progress all the way to ERCP. The clinical course of patients receiving pancreatic extract for pain has not been fully defined as yet. I have had some patients receiving this therapy for 4 years who suffer a relapse when the therapy is stopped. Others have had the pancreatic extract stopped after shorter periods of treatment with no relapse.

Pharmacologic suppression of pancreatic exocrine secretion with proteases has been demonstrated in patients with chronic pancreatitis and in healthy subjects. Pancreatic proteases in the proximal small intestine apparently modulate pancreatic exocrine secretion in humans. The clinical implications of pharmacologic suppression of pancreatic output are exciting. By increasing the intraluminal concentration of pancreatic enzymes with orally administered exogenous enzymes, endogenous production of pancreatic enzymes is either directly or indirectly decreased. In patients with chronic pancreatitis, pancreatic extract reduces secretion and alleviates pain. Pancreatic extract should be considered the treatment of choice for most patients with chronic pancreatitis and recurrent abdominal pain.

DIET

I individualize the diet for each patient depending on the severity of the disease, etiology, and so on; however, there is no specific diet for pancreatic insufficiency per se. I recommend that alcohol in any form or quantity be avoided, since it can exacerbate pancreatitis, thereby worsening pancreatic insufficiency. Also, in some patients, meals with high fat content may increase the frequency and intensity of pain. In these patients fats should be restricted to 25 percent of the caloric intake. The diet in patients with pancreatic insufficiency should also be rich in protein to avoid protein deficiency, and low in fiber, since fiber may inhibit pancreatic enzymes. In the rare patient who has documented pancreatic steatorrhea but who does not respond to the program suggested in Table 1, reduction of long chain triglyceride fat in the diet to 40 percent of fat and substitution of 60 percent of fat by medium chain triglycerides may increase weight gain and decrease steatorrhea.

ENDOCRINE INSUFFICIENCY SECONDARY TO EXOCRINE INSUFFICIENCY

Glucose intolerance may be demonstrated in up to 90 percent of patients with diffuse calcification of the pancreas, and overt diabetes in up to 70 percent of patients. Thus, abnormalities in pancreatic endocrine function are common in patients with severe pancreatic exocrine insufficiency. It is almost impossible to take meaningful therapeutic steps in controlling the glucose intolerance until optimal control of steatorrhea has been achieved. In these patients, who are very sensitive to insulin, significant changes in absorption will greatly affect the insulin response. Although such patients may not require large doses of insulin, their situation is often precarious because they may have a decreased reserve of pancreatic glucagon and may not be able to respond appropriately to hypoglycemia.

CYSTIC FIBROSIS

JOHN D. LLOYD-STILL, M.D.

Cystic fibrosis (CF), a genetic syndrome of exocrine dysfunction, is characterized by ductal obstructive lesions throughout multiple organ systems and disturbances of mucus and electrolyte secretion. Although reported in various racial groups, CF is more common in Caucasians, occurring in one in 2,000 births. It is inherited in an autosomal recessive fashion with a gene frequency of 5 percent, making it the most common lethal genetic defect of Caucasian populations.

The specific genetic defect remains obscure. The heterozygote cannot be positively identified. Elevated concentration of sweat sodium and chloride are diagnostic features of the disease. More than 95 percent of new diagnoses of CF are made in children; however, among those who reach age 18, more than one-fifth were diagnosed after the age of 15. The majority of patients survive into adolescence, and 50 percent live beyond their twentieth birthday.

Many symptoms are produced. Cystic fibrosis is a major cause of malabsorption in infants and children in the United States. Chronic obstructive pulmonary disease is eventually present in the majority of patients and accounts for much of the morbidity and almost all of the mortality associated with the disease beyond the neonatal period. Gastrointestinal symptoms occur in 85 to 90 percent of patients with the disease (Table 1).

DIAGNOSIS

The diagnosis of CF is based on a suspicion of the disorder and a history of pancreatic, intestinal, hepatic, biliary, or pulmonary involvement. The diagnosis is confirmed by finding elevated concentrations of sweat sodium and chloride on quantitative pilocarpine iontophoresis (sweat test). Unfortunately, the sweat test, although simple to perform, is subject to considerable variation in reliability. Sweat electrolyte determinations should be conducted in duplicate at centers performing the test frequently, using a standardized method (Gibson and Cooke). A sweat chloride concentration of greater than 60 mEq

TABLE 1 Incidence of Gastrointestinal Manifestations in Cystic Fibrosis

Organ	Complication	Approximate Frequency
Pancreas	Total achylia	85–90%
	Partial or normal function	15–20
	Pancreatitis	
	Abnormal glucose tolerance	20–30
	Diabetes	1–2
Intestine	Meconium ileus	10–15
	Rectal prolapse	20
	Distal intestinal obstruction syndrome (meconium ileus equivalent)	10–20
	Intussusception	1–5
	Pneumatosis intestinalis	
	? Mucosal function impaired	
Liver	Fatty liver	15–30
	Focal biliary fibrosis	25
	Cirrhosis with portal hypertension	2–5
Biliary	Gallbladder abnormal, nonfunctional, or small	45
	Gallstones	4–12
	Cholecystitis	

per liter has been considered diagnostic of CF when clinical findings or family history are supportive. With a confidence level of 99 percent, patients with CF will have sweat chloride and sodium concentrations greater than 72 mEq per liter. The diagnosis may be more difficult in adults because sweat electrolyte concentrations increase with age. Borderline values (55 to 65 mEq per liter) remain a difficult problem, requiring careful clinical correlation including family history, pulmonary findings, and analysis of pancreatic secretion after stimulation with pancreozymin-secretin.

PANCREATIC INSUFFICIENCY

Pancreatic Extracts

In patients with exocrine pancreatic deficiency, protein and fat maldigestion and fecal loss are the primary clinical manifestations, although there may be considerable variation in severity from one patient to another. The usual CF patient with malabsorption must take pancreatic enzyme supplements with each meal to enhance (but, unfortunately, not normalize) the intestinal uptake of fat and protein. Stomach acid inactivates pancreatic enzymes, and a major advance in the past decade has been the development of coated, pH-sensitive microspheres available in capsule form, which are much more effective than previous products (Table 2). My initial preference is to use one of the enteric-coated microspheres; the exact dosage depends on the individual's age, degree of pancreatic insufficiency, quantity of fat ingested, and the commercial preparation chosen. Dosage is determined by improvement in symptoms, decrease in number of bowel movements, and weight gain confirmed if necessary by measuring coefficient of fat absorption. For infants during the first year of life, the powder form of Viokase is advantageous. Overdosage results in constipation and perianal excoriation.

Patients with CF have increased gastric acidity and lowered duodenal pH secondary to depressed HCO_3 secretion. If oral pancreatic enzymes do not lead to marked improvement in fat absorption, efforts to overcome the acid pepsin inactivation should include the concomitant administration of pancreatic enzyme with either antacids or cimetidine; either regimen improves fat digestion and decreases steatorrhea, but high doses of sodium bicarbonate (1 to 4 g with each meal) are sometimes unpalatable. The long-term effects of cimetidine (5 mg per kilogram of body weight one-half hour before meals) are unknown, and therefore it cannot be recommended for lifelong usage. An ideal way to alkalinize the upper gastrointestinal tract in patients with CF remains to be found.

Nutritional Therapy

In addition to the use of pancreatic supplements, careful nutritional management is mandatory. The nutritional care of patients with CF is based on an assessment of requirements, taking into consideration age, height, weight, anthropometrics, severity of lung disease, anorexia, pancreatic insufficiency, and other intraluminal phase abnormalities or mucosal dysfunction.

The complicating factors involved in our approach to the nutritional management of cystic fibrosis patients are shown in Figure 1. A number of dietary surveys have shown that, except for a few infants who have a voracious appetite, CF patients eat less than normal, with an average consumption of 80 percent of required daily allowance (RDA). Although an increase of 50 to 100 percent of caloric intake is recommended for the child with CF, in practice it is rarely possible to achieve an intake of more than 130 percent of RDA. Several of these recommendations are shown in Table 3. Some authorities recommend calculating energy intake per kilogram ideal rather than actual body weight, and calculated on this basis a target of 125 percent of dietary recommendations is a realistic goal that takes the patient's stature into account. Fats can supply 40 to 50 percent of total daily caloric requirements as long as the patient can tolerate this amount. Fat intakes over 100 g per day often cause gastrointestinal symptoms such as crampy abdominal pain. The es-

TABLE 2 Enzyme Content of Commercial Pancreatic Extracts

	Trade Name	Generic Name	Enzyme Activity (NFU)*			Suggested Starting Dose
			Lipase	Amylase	Protease	
			Per Capsule			
Enteric-coated microspheres	Pancrease	Pancrelipase	4,000	20,000	25,000	1–3 capsules
	Cotazym-S	Pancrelipase	5,000	20,000	20,000	1–3 capsules
			Per Tablet			
Nonenteric-coated	Viokase	Pancreatin	8,000	30,000	30,000	3–6 tablets
			Per ¼ Teaspoon Powder			
			16,800	70,000	70,000	1–2 teaspoons

NFU = National Formulary Units

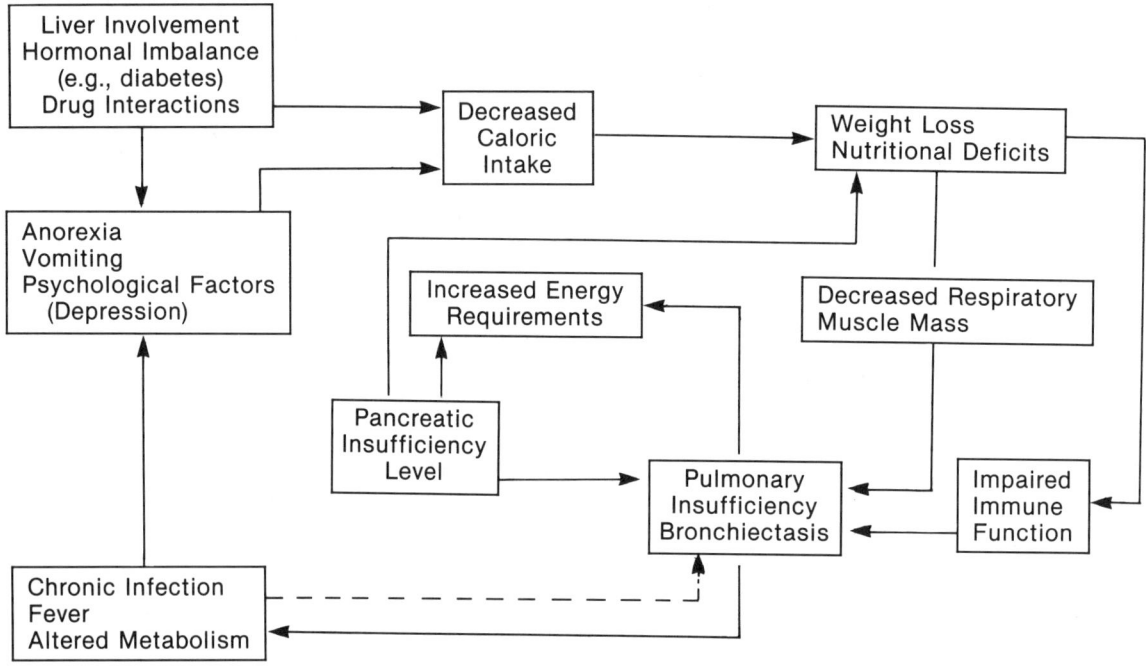

Figure 1 Some of the factors modifying our approach to dietary supplementation and other treatments in cystic fibrosis.

sential fatty acid composition of blood and tissues is altered in CF and resembles that found in protein-calorie malnutrition. Attempts to provide fatty acid supplementation have yielded variable results. A triglyceride emulsion (Microlipid), containing 74 percent linoleate and given daily in a volume that supplied 7 percent of calories as essential fatty acids, normalized plasma levels of fatty acids in compliant patients. Many patients, however, find this preparation unpalatable.

It is appropriate initially to try dietary manipulations, such as the use of fortified milk, milkshakes, eggnog, instant puddings, or Instant Breakfast, and the addition of granola. Commercial glucose polymer (Polycose) is also available. There are various commercially available liquid formulas for oral supplementation (e.g., Ensure, Sustacal, and so on). Vivonex is contraindicated because it is low in fat content and worsens the essential fatty acid deficiency. Medium chain triglycerides (MCTs) constitute appropriate energy supplements for CF patients, but tolerance is not always satisfactory. They are deficient in essential fatty acids and growth rate may remain unchanged. Although MCTs are less dependent than long chain triglycerides on intraluminal lipolysis and micellar solubilization before their absorption and transport by the

TABLE 3 Recommended Daily Energy and Protein Intake In Normal Individuals and Patients With Cystic Fibrosis

Age (yr)	Energy Needs (Kcal)		Protein Intake (g/kg)	
	Normal (100% of RDA)	CF (130% of RDA)	Normal	CF
0.0–0.6	kg × 115 (95–145)*	kg × 150	2.2	4
0.6–1.0	kg × 105 (80–135)	kg × 137	2.0	4
1–3	1,300 (900–1,800)	1,690	1.8	3
4–6	1,700 (1,300–2,300)	2,210	1.5	3
7–10	2,400 (1,650–3,300)	3,120	1.2	3
Male				
11–14	2,700 (2,000–3,700)	3,510	1.0	3
15–18	2,800 (2,100–3,900)	3,640	0.85	3
Female				
11–14	2,200 (1,500–3,000)	2,860	0.8	3
15–18	2,100 (1,200–3,000)	2,730	0.84	3

* Numbers in parentheses are ranges.

CF = cystic fibrosis; RDA = required daily allowance

portal vein, pancreatic supplements should be used in infants with CF who are consuming formulas containing 40 percent MCT (e.g., Pregestimil).

When all these supplementations are unsuccessful, attempts are made to provide caloric supplementation in a manner that does not depend on voluntary ingestion. This may be done by nasogastric infusions, gastrostomy, jejunostomy feedings, or parenteral alimentation, either peripheral or central. Unfortunately, most patients are reluctant to undertake these forms of supplemental nutritional therapy until their disease is far advanced. When the pulse rate is greater than 100 beats/min or lung function is under 30 percent of predicted, constant nutritional supplementation is usually ineffective.

Nasogastric infusions used either continuously or intermittently at night have been shown to reverse metabolic imbalance in patients with CF. Unfortunately, the presence of the tube in the oropharynx increases cough, and few patients (except infants) tolerate long-term use of a nasogastric tube. Recently, evaluation of incisionless gastrostomy feedings, rather than a formal gastrostomy, has been undertaken in patients with CF. Despite initial enthusiasm, long-term use of this form of treatment is unsatisfactory owing to intolerance of the volume required, lack of appetite, associated infections, and other problems with gastroesophageal reflux. In an attempt to circumvent these problems, permanent placement of a jejunostomy is currently undergoing trial and is said to obviate many of the disadvantages of gastrostomy.

Parenteral alimentation with a central venous catheter results in temporary improvement in nutritional deficiencies, but most of these benefits are lost as soon as the catheter is removed. Since these patients are usually treated with intravenous antibiotics, nutritional supplementation by the peripheral route becomes more difficult. Attempts to correct the essential fatty acid abnormalities by the intravenous route are not practical for long-term supplementation.

Additional nutritional treatments are shown in Table 4. Multivitamins are given twice daily. Vitamin A requirements are 5,000 to 10,000 IU per day, and the vitamin D intake should be around 800 U per day. Vitamin K is recommended in all infants and is given to patients with chronic liver disease or complications of hemoptysis. Angular stomatitis secondary to riboflavin deficiency is sometimes seen with antibiotic administration; riboflavin may be supplemented at a dose of 10 to 30 mg daily. Water-miscible vitamin E is given in dosages ranging from 50 IU per day for infants to 200 IU per day for adults. Trace minerals should be provided at least at the RDA, and in patients with severe malnutrition and growth failure, added zinc is advisable. Salt loss may be of concern in patients with CF because of excess sweating. In hot climates salt depletion can be catastrophic, leading to hyponatremic dehydration and shock. Although the American diet contains an excess of sodium, the recent reduction in the salt content of many baby foods has rendered infants with CF more vulnerable to the effects of salt loss than previously. With vigorous exercise and heat stress, added sodium chloride is recommended. Patients with abnormal glucose tolerance and frank diabetes mellitus are managed by standard techniques.

INTESTINAL COMPLICATIONS

Meconium Ileus

Meconium ileus, which occurs in 10 to 15 percent of patients with CF, is the second most common cause of intestinal obstruction in the newborn period. The mortality has been reduced from over 60 percent to almost zero by a combination of early recognition and nonoperative treatment with Gastrografin enemas. Gastrografin is a radiopaque aqueous solution that contains a small amount of Tween 80 (polysorbate 80), and has an osmolality of 1,900 mOsm. It is usually diluted 2:1 or 3:1 with normal saline. Hypertonic enemas may cause dangerous fluid and electrolyte shifts, especially when administered to small infants, and appropriate intravenous therapy must be undertaken to prevent circulatory failure. Multiple Gastrografin enemas may be tried. In one-third of patients with meconium ileus there is associated atresia, stenosis, or volvulus and surgery will be required. If surgery is necessary, irrigating solutions can be used during the operation and postoperatively to dissolve and dislodge the ab-

TABLE 4 Nutritional Management of Cystic Fibrosis

High-calorie (130% RDA calorie needs), high-protein diet

Pancreatic supplements (Pancrease, Cotazym-S, Viokase, etc.)
    With bicarbonate
    With cimetidine, Ranitidine

Multivitamins twice daily to supply*:

Vitamin A,	5,000–10,000 IU
Vitamin D,	800 U
Vitamin B,	RDA
Vitamin C,	RDA

Added:
Vitamin E (water miscible)	200 IU
?Vitamin K	5 mg/3 days per week

Added:
?Sodium	2–4 g NaCl
Trace minerals	RDA

Nutritional supplements
    Medium chain triglycerides (formulas—Portagen, Pregestimil; MCT oil)
    Glucose polymers (Polycose, etc.)
    "Meal replacement products"—Ensure, Magnacal, Sustacal, etc.
    Calorie and protein boosters—Instant Breakfast, Citrolein, high-protein jello, microlipid, etc.

"Force" feeding regimens
    Enteral—nasogastric tube, gastrostomy, jejunostomy
    Intravenous—peripheral or central alimentation

Vitamin therapy for drug–nutrient interactions*
    Riboflavin   10–30 mg daily

* Dosages are for adolescents and adults
RDA = required daily allowance

normal meconium. N-acetyl-cysteine (Mucomyst), which reduces the viscosity of mucoprotein by cleaving disulfide bonds in the mucoprotein molecule, and polysorbate 80, a mild industrial detergent and preservative, are now generally recognized as safe and effective. Pancreatic enzymes (Viokase powder) can also be instilled through an indwelling enterostomy tube to help dissolve the meconium concretions. Parenteral hyperalimentation is usually administered to infants who are operated on for meconium ileus. Cholestatic jaundice is present in at least 50 percent of these infants. Long-term complications are the same as with any other form of intestinal surgery or resection.

Distal Intestinal Obstruction Syndrome

This disorder is sometimes called meconium ileus equivalent. Sticky intestinal secretions mixed with only partially digested food may lead to partial or complete bowel obstruction. Diagnosis is suggested by a history of recurrent bouts of abdominal pain, and on examination an abdominal mass is usually felt in the right lower quadrant. Vigorous medical treatment is recommended. Large doses of mineral oil (several tablespoons per day) are usually effective. If the patient has been noncompliant with a regimen of pancreatic enzymes they are increased, but in other patients this syndrome can be precipitated by an excess of pancreatic enzymes. If there is abdominal tenderness or signs of intestinal obstruction, one or more Gastrografin enemas diluted 2:1 with water or saline is usually successful if the diagnosis is not delayed. On rare occasions there is an associated ileocolic intussusception that may require reduction by standard barium enema technique. When disimpaction is impossible, surgery must be undertaken. Appendicitis must be considered in the differential diagnosis.

Rectal Prolapse

The incidence of rectal prolapse is less than the 20 percent originally reported. This complication is usually a presenting symptom in the toddler age group, and there may be no other symptoms of the disease. Medical management with pancreatic enzymes is almost always successful, and surgery should not be undertaken.

Hepatobiliary System

The bile is lithogenic in CF, and infants with meconium ileus undergoing surgery frequently develop prolonged cholestasis that is aggravated by intravenous hyperalimentation. An enlarged liver secondary to fatty infiltration is seen in malnourished, hypoproteinemic infants at diagnosis and responds to treatment with pancreatic enzymes and nutritional therapy. There is some evidence that these infants are more likely to develop complications secondary to biliary cirrhosis and portal hypertension. Abnormalities in liver function are common and most often involve elevations in alkaline phosphatase. Fecal bile acids are increased and are normalized by pancreatic enzyme replacement. Clinically significant cirrhosis and portal hypertension occur in 2 to 5 percent of patients, and the incidence increases with age. The treatment of symptomatic liver disease in patients with CF is similar to that of other conditions associated with hepatic failure. Particular attention should be paid to blood sugar, ammonia, electrolytes, prothrombin time, and nutritional status, including protein intake.

The treatment of bleeding esophageal varices is controversial. Some authorities advocate sclerotherapy as the initial treatment of choice. Portosystemic shunts have been successfully performed in patients with CF, provided their pulmonary status is adequate. Surgery in patients with a clinical (Shwachman) score less than 50 carries a high mortality rate. Prophylactic shunting and splenectomy for leukopenia or thrombocytopenia are best avoided. Currently liver transplantation is being evaluated in these patients.

Abnormalities of the biliary tree are common, and ultrasound may show a microgallbladder and/or gallstones. Cholecystectomy is best avoided unless clinically indicated. Computerized tomography and ERCP occasionally demonstrate obstructive lesions of the biliary tree secondary to pancreatic fibrosis.

TABLE 5 Pulmonary Therapy in CF

Antibiotics (continuous or intermittent)
  Outpatient (obtain sensitivities)
    Dicloxacillin
    Cephalosporin
    ? Co-trimoxazole
    ? Tetracycline
  Inpatient (obtain sensitivities)
    Aminoglycoside and broad-spectrum penicillin
  Aerosol
    Tobramycin

Postural drainage, vibration, chest physiotherapy, exercise programs

Bronchodilators
  Theophylline*
  Adrenergic agents*

Prophylaxis
  Influenza vaccination

* Response measured by pulmonary function testing

PULMONARY DISEASE

Pulmonary complications account for most of the morbidity and almost all the mortality from CF. Bacteriologic studies of the sputum show a predominance of mucoid *Pseudomonas aeruginosa* in more than 70 percent of patients. *Staphylococcus aureus, Hemophilus influenzae, P. cepacia,* and other gram-negative organisms account for fewer cases. Viral infections are at least as common as in the general population. The general principles of therapy are shown in Table 5. The role of antibiotics in this disease is controversial. In some centers antibiotics are administered intermittently, depending on clinical manifestations and the sensitivity of the sputum microorganisms. In other centers a continuous regimen is used. Outpatient management of gram-negative flora is difficult because the microorganisms are usually resistant to orally administered antibiotics. Hospitalized patients are given a combination of an intravenous aminoglycoside and a broad-spectrum penicillin. Pharmacokinetics are frequently abnormal in CF. Tobramycin given by aerosol has been shown to be effective in patients with well-established bronchiectasis.

A prophylactic regimen of vibration and postural drainage is the mainstay of treatment aimed at preventing the accumulation of secretions and secondary infection. When bronchospasm is present, antispasmodics such as slow acting theophylline may be given. Blood levels should be followed, as there is wide variation in absorption and metabolism. Exercise programs should be encouraged. Mucolytic agents such as N-acetyl-cysteine are sometimes given. Allergic bronchopulmonary aspergillosis occurs in 5 percent of patients and is treated with corticosteroids. Complications such as pneumothorax and hemoptysis require specialized techniques for therapy. Pneumothorax is treated with chest tube and underwater suction; recurrent episodes are indications for chemical sclerosis or parietal pleurectomy. Hemoptysis is treated conservatively with correction of underlying clotting dysfunction, blood transfusions, temporary cessation of chest physical therapy, and intravenous antibiotics. Recurrent major hemoptysis is treated by either endobronchial tamponade or bronchial artery embolization. Cystic fibrosis causes pulmonary artery hypertension and cor pulmonale. Oxygen is markedly beneficial, but diuretics and digoxin are less important than treatment of the pulmonary infection. Various methods of home care, such as long-term administration of intravenous antibiotics, may be helpful.

Cystic fibrosis is a multisystem disorder requiring a coordinated care plan for optimal management. With an integrated approach, major manifestations can be treated early and many complications avoided. Much additional information and support can be obtained from the Cystic Fibrosis Foundation, 6000 Executive Boulevard, Suite 309, Rockville, MD 20852. The Cystic Fibrosis Foundation publishes numerous informational booklets on genetics, symptoms, diagnosis, job training, cystic fibrosis and pregnancy, living with cystic fibrosis, guides for young adults, adolescents, teachers, and others. The Foundation chapters can be a major source of psychological support, as well as fulfilling their primary goal of fund raising to support research into the basic cause of the disease.

PANCREATIC AND PERIAMPULLARY NEOPLASIA

JON vanHEERDEN, M.B., Ch.B., F.R.C.S.(C), F.A.C.S., M.S.(Surg)(Minn)

Adenocarcinoma of the pancreas is currently the fourth leading cause of cancer death in the United States. Prevalence of this malignancy is steadily increasing and may be reaching epidemic proportions. This increased prevalence is etiologically intriguing; theoretically, it should be related to the increased ingestion or inhalation of some carcinogenic agent. As expected, therefore, both tobacco and caffeine have lately been incriminated, but supporting evidence for either is suppositional at best.

Malignant growths in the pancreatoduodenal region often elude early diagnosis. Recesses of the lesser sac often lead to diagnosis at the time of advanced tumor growth. Despite this unfortunate fact, there is something inherently different about the biologic behavior of adenocarcinoma of the pancreas in particular, which appears to transcend the boundaries of either surgical, chemotherapeutic, or radiotherapeutic intervention. I have often witnessed death due to widespread metastases months after resection of a tumor less than 1 cm in size with no evidence of either regional or local extension; this behavior is distinctly unusual for most other malignancies.

The key issue is not to think of carcinoma of the pancreas collectively. There are many different cancers occurring in this region, all of which may present in an identical fashion, yet each has its own inherent biologic behavior. Every attempt should be made to separate the following tumors occurring in the pancreatoduodenal region; this usually entails histologic interpretation: (1) Pancreas ductal adenocarcinoma, islet cell adenoma—functioning and nonfunctioning, islet cell carcinoma—functioning and nonfunctioning, cystadenocarcinoma; (2) common bile duct carcinoma; (3) ampullary carcinoma; and (4) duodenal carcinoma. An idea of the variability in biologic behavior is evident if one looks at the resectability rates of different histologic types noted in Table 1.

TABLE 1 Resectability Rates of Histologic Types of Pancreatic Tumors

Histologic Types	Resectability Rate (%)
Pancreas (adenocarcinoma)	10
Ampulla	95
Duodenal	50
Cystadenocarcinoma	90
Islet cell carcinoma (pancreas)	65
Islet cell adenoma (pancreas)	100

DIAGNOSTIC ASPECTS

The classic approach to treatment of any condition is to subdivide the therapeutic "attack" into four phases: (1) preventive treatment, (2) treatment of the condition, (3) treatment of the complications, and (4) follow-up and advice. Since we are, as yet, in the dark regarding preventive treatment, options today combine treatment of the condition, treatment of the complications, and follow-up care. To many clinicians, this area (work-up and therapy) is a morass. Few patients are more "overinvestigated" than those with obstructive jaundice, and few diseases exist in which there are so many different and controversial therapeutic options.

The diagnosis is fairly straightforward in the patient who presents with the classic symptom complex of unrelenting midepigastric pain that radiates straight through to the back, accompanied by weight loss, general malaise, and anorexia. In this instance, with the exception of the routine electrolyte and hematologic investigation, computerized tomography (CT) is the only preoperative investigation worth obtaining. This investigation will clearly confirm the diagnosis, suggest the extent of the condition, and help determine whether operative intervention is indicated with the possibility of resection or not. Little is gained by obtaining an upper gastrointestinal series. If a CT scan clearly shows metastases or signs of nonresectability, such as small bowel mesenteric involvement and/or superior mesenteric vessel or portal vein encasement, a percutaneous fine needle aspiration should be considered to confirm the presence of a ductal adenocarcinoma. The decision should then be made whether radiologic decompression will suffice, or whether the patient should be offered surgical intervention for duodenal and biliary bypass.

The diagnosis is often less clear in the patient with duodenal and ampullary lesions. Symptoms are characteristically nonspecific and mild. A mild hypochromic, microcytic anemia is fairly common, and may be the clue. Familial history of Gardner's syndrome should alert the clinician to the possibility of ampullary and/or duodenal tumors. In this type of patient, both upper gastrointestinal roentgenography and upper gastrointestinal endoscopy are most valuable. Computerized tomography is much less helpful in the patient with both ampullary and duodenal malignancies. Although endoscopic retrograde cholangiopancreatography can be clearly diagnostic in some instances, its use is somewhat limited since the advent of CT. Its principal use is in the patient who has a normal CT scan and in whom the clinical suspicion is strong. This is seldom the case.

Regardless of the individual therapeutic modality decided upon, histologic confirmation is mandatory in every patient. It is crucial to differentiate between the highly lethal carcinoma of the pancreas and the biologically benign chronic pancreatitis which so often may exactly mimic a pancreatic malignancy. Whether this histologic confirmation is accomplished by open biopsy, of a distant node, or by percutaneous computerized tomographically guided fine needle aspiration is dictated by the individual circumstances encountered.

THERAPEUTIC OPTIONS

The therapeutic options available are:

1. No treatment
2. Needle biopsy followed by adjuvant chemotherapy and/or radiotherapy
3. Percutaneous transhepatic biliary decompression alone
4. Percutaneous transhepatic biliary decompression and needle biopsy followed by adjuvant therapy
5. Surgical exploration with biopsy and biliary and/or duodenal bypass*
6. Surgical exploration and total pancreatectomy*
7. Surgical exploration and subtotal pancreatectomy*
8. Surgical exploration and extended regional pancreatoduodenectomy*
9. Surgical exploration, biopsy, and intraoperative therapy
10. Therapeutic splanchnic block in nonresectable situations

PREOPERATIVE PHASE

Three vital questions need to be asked and answered during the preoperative phase: First, has malignancy spread beyond the confines of resectability? Second, is either biliary or duodenal bypass indicated? Third, if operation, especially with intent of "cure" is planned, is the patient in optimal condition?

To answer these questions, I urge examination of the supraclavicular fossae (Virchow's node) in all patients. Look carefully at the CT scan with the radiologist, take a careful history regarding both cholangitis and duodenal obstruction, quantitate (on a scale of 1 to 10) back pain when present, assess clotting parameters (prothrombin time and accelerated partial thromboplastin time), as well as nutritional status (percentage weight loss and serum albumin). Although vitamin K is often required, I do not believe that either preoperative hyperalimentation or transhepatic biliary decompression is indicated. Prospective randomised studies have clearly demonstrated the lack of benefit from preoperative percutaneous biliary decompression and have equally clearly demonstrated the increased incidence of sepsis which accompanies catheter placement. I have never used either, and have no reason to regret this "omission." There is, to my mind, no indication for preoperative hyperalimentation in patients with these types of malignancies. To be efficacious, such hyperalimentation should be for a minimum of 2 to 3 weeks; I believe it is better for these patients to be bypassed, which allows them to commence oral intake within days of an operation, be it resection or bypass.

---

*With or without adjunctive chemotherapy and/or radiotherapy

Severe, unrelenting intrascapular pain is a common symptom. I have been impressed with the pain relief obtained by percutaneous injection of absolute alcohol through paravertebral needles placed by x-ray guidance (performed by our anesthesiologists). This is usually done at the end of a palliative operative procedure by rolling the patient onto a stretcher in the prone position, or with the patient awake when operation is not contemplated. If surgical intervention is not indicated (extent of disease, associated diseases, no duodenal obstruction, and so on) and if pruritus (often with a high serum bilirubin concentration) is present, I usually place a permanent percutaneous transhepatic catheter with either external, or preferably internal, drainage of bile. Electrolyte and acid-base disturbances are overrated in these diseases and are of little, if any, practical importance. Anemia (hypochromic and microcytic) is common, especially in ampullary and duodenal lesions, and should be corrected by appropriate preoperative transfusions.

OPERATIVE PHASE

Operation is usually performed for one of two reasons: to afford biliary and/or duodenal decompression in the obviously nonresectable patient, or to assess resectability and thus possibly to offer a cure.

Decompression Surgery

If biliary decompression is the aim, I prefer a simple side-to-side cholecystojejunostomy. There is no need for a complementary jejunojejunostomy. I try to avoid using the duodenum for the biliary-enteric anastomosis, fearing future obstruction, but do not hesitate to use same when the gallbladder is absent or when the tumor is situated mainly in the neck of the gland. Roux-en-Y choledochojejunostomies, in my experience, are seldom indicated, and have been technically difficult because of "cramped quarters." If no form of biliary decompression is possible, it is best to close and place a percutaneous transhepatic biliary catheter postoperatively. I routinely like to add a concomitant gastrojejunostomy. Roughly 15 percent of patients will develop duodenal obstruction prior to demise following biliary diversion alone, which is unacceptable. The addition of this simple anastomosis has not increased the postoperative morbidity, in my experience, although some patients (approximately 5% to 10%) might exhibit delay in gastric emptying for 10 to 20 days following duodenal bypass.

Resection

If resection is contemplated, a logical sequence should be followed, as outlined below.

Biopsy

Biopsy is done transduodenally whenever possible, using either a Tru-cut or Vim-Silverman needle. Complications as a result of this technique are exceptionally rare, since all "fistulas" are internal. When the opportunity arises (usually with larger exophytic tumors) a simple "shave biopsy" can be performed easily and safely. Fine needle aspiration is being evaluated and may become the biopsy technique of choice.

Assessment of Resectability and Resection

Part of the assessment of resectability occurs preoperatively when the factors of associated disease, nutritional status, age (When is a patient too old to have a pancreatic resection? I don't know.), sex (females do better), surgical experience (Have I done this operation? Can I do it well?), and extent of disease are considered.

Having made the decision to proceed with operation, we now need to assess resectability of this biopsy-proven malignancy. First, look for distant spread to the liver, diaphragm, pelvis and peritoneal surfaces. Pay particular attention to the ligament of Treitz area and the base of small bowel mesentery. Second, look for regional extension to the celiac axis, hepatoduodenal ligament, and paraduodenal and retroduodenal areas. If these are clear, assess superior mesenteric and portal vein invasion by clearly digitally separating the pancreas from the superior mesenteric vein and its junction with the splenic vein. Once each of these sequences has been completed, resection becomes a technical feasibility. I have not been convinced that the operation of extended regional pancreatoduodenectomy with resection of the portal vein is indicated. The low yield appears outweighed by its attending high operative morbidity and mortality.

I prefer the subtotal pancreatoduodenectomy (Whipple procedure) to total pancreatectomy. It has been clearly shown, to my satisfaction, that there is no difference in operative mortality or morbidity or in the percentage of long-term survival when these two operations are compared. The current indications for total pancreatectomy in my practice are (1) friable texture of the pancreas resulting in a tenuous anastomosis, (2) tumor at the line of resection, and (3) presence of diabetes mellitus (a relative indication). In addition, there are vigorous arguments for and against total pancreatectomy. In its favor are the following factors: no pancreatojejunal anastomosis, no postoperative pancreatitis, better cancer operation, wider margin of tissue, no transection (thus spillage) of pancreas, better lymphadenectomy, and eradication of multicentric intrapancreatic malignancy. Militating against its use are loss of endocrine function, loss of exocrine function, and increased risk of peptic ulcer disease.

The pancreatojejunal anastomosis is crucial to a favorable outcome. The pancreatic duct is seldom of a sufficient size to enable a mucosa-to-mucosa anastomosis. I therefore prefer to stent the main pancreatic duct with a small (PE-190) but long (5 to 6 inches) Silastic catheter that subsequently passes spontaneously, and to utilize two layers of running 2-0 or 3-0 silk. It is also advisable to place a size 12 T-tube in the common duct with the distal limb in the jejunum and to drain the area with two suction drains (Jackson-Pratt type) for at least 7 days.

Intraoperative radiotherapy utilizing high-dose "boost" electrons delivered during laparotomy in nonresectable patients is currently under investigation. A cone is placed encompassing the entire malignancy, and a total dose of 2,000 rads is given. This is followed by 5,000 rads via external beam. It is too early to draw any conclusions, but preliminary results in about 24 patients are encouraging. I believe that the next logical step might be to utilize this modality or some modification thereof in patients in whom a "curative" resection has been performed.

Longmire and Traverso recently popularized the so-called pylorus-preserving variation of the Whipple procedure. I am using this more often and find it appealing and acceptable. In this variation the entire stomach, pylorus, and about 2.5 cm of duodenum are preserved; the procedure is completed by performing an end-to-side duodenojejunostomy which is distal to the initially constructed end-to-end pancreatojejunostomy and end-to-side choledochojejunostomy.

Islet Cell Tumors

The two most common functioning islet cell tumors encountered in this region, insulinomas and gastrinomas, are also worthy of note. In my experience, roughly 10 percent of insulinomas and 20 percent of gastrinomas are malignant and should be treated surgically, as one would any islet cell malignancy, by following the aforementioned guidelines.

The nonmalignant remainders in both these tumors are due to adenomas that are usually single, unless they occur as one manifestation of the multiple endocrine neoplasia type I syndrome (pituitary adenomas, parathyroid disease, pancreatic islet cell tumors), in which case they are usually multiple. These adenomas are usually accurately localized for the surgeon preoperatively and can be detected intraoperatively by gentle palpation of the gland in its entirety. Insulinomas are usually less than 1 to 5 cm in diameter. Gastrinomas are more elusive, and, in my experience, the majority of those resected for subsequent cure are small (3 to 4 mm) and are situated in the lateral wall of the duodenum (duodenal carcinoid). The majority of these adenomas can be simply enucleated.

In the pancreas, I prefer to use the coagulating electrocautery, remaining close to the tumor surface. Care must be taken to avoid damage to the main pancreatic duct, which is best done by being extremely fastidious in the dissection. If there is any question of injury, it is advisable to administer 1 mg of secretin intravenously, watching for an excessive outpouring of clear pancreatic juice. If a leak is demonstrated, I like to attempt a direct repair with 5-0 silk, close to the pancreas, over the "divot," and drain well. Occasionally, the more "conservative" approach is favorable and one proceeds with a distal pancreatectomy.

POSTOPERATIVE PHASE

The major postoperative complications are hemorrhage, fistula formation, and sepsis, which are the result of a leaking pancreatojejunal anastomosis. These must be suspected if a fever spike or an increase in drainage occurs, and therefore it is quite helpful to assay the amylase content of the drainage daily. Most leaks, in my experience, have been minor and are controlled by prolonged drainage. If the leak increases, hemoglobin drops, or if sepsis is evident or impending, early reoperation with conversion to a total pancreatectomy is indicated if a Whipple procedure had been performed previously. A leaking pancreatojejunal anastomosis is the single-most important cause of early death following a Whipple procedure. The most common and most lethal late complication is tumor recurrence. In addition, during the postoperative period, there is no need for either hyperalimentation or systemic antibiotics in most patients.

Adjuvant Therapy

Since approximately 90 percent of pancreatic adenocarcinomas are nonresectable, the question of adjuvant chemotherapy and/or radiotherapy always comes up. Although chemotherapy is so commonly administered, there is little evidence to support its use. Polychemotherapy appears to be no better than single agent therapy. For now, I continue to enter patients into investigative protocols "seeking the truth," but find myself "avoiding" chemotherapy in more and more patients. There certainly is minimal justification for treatment of a patient with adenocarcinoma of the pancreas in an off-protocol noninvestigational setting. Exceptions to this philosophy are patients with nonresectable islet cell malignancies, in whom prolonged survival and a response rate of about 60 percent may be obtained with the use of streptozocin. Adjuvant radiotherapy for adenocarcinoma has an equally unimpressive record thus far.

THERAPEUTIC OUTCOME

Outcome depends on the pathological type of the malignancy encountered, coupled with the experience of the surgeon. Other influences include age, sex, host resistance, multicentricity, nodal status, and tumor dedifferentiation. The most tangible results pertain to operative mortality (30 days following operation) and 5-year survival rates. These are summarized in Table 2.

Three quotations summarize best my personal philosophy regarding adenocarcinoma of the pancreas:

"With a radical procedure, it is quite clear that more life is lost than gained. It is not the aim of our treatment

TABLE 2 Outcome After Periampullary Tumor Operations

Tumor	Operative Mortality	Five-Year Survival (%)
Duodenal		45
Ampullary		40
Bile duct		20
Islet cell	10 to 30%	35
Adenocarcinoma of the pancreas		5
Cystadenocarcinoma		40

to achieve an occasional 5-year survival at any cost, but to do what is best for the large majority of patients." (Hertzog)

"The reflective surgeon must ask himself whether or not more months of life are not lost through resection than through bypass." (Esselstyn)

"Although the average long-term results of pancreatoduodenectomy for cancer are very poor, no man is an average, and resection does provide the only chance of cure. Individually, many patients might very well opt for a considerable operative hazard with a small chance of cure rather than an inconsiderable hazard and no chance for cure." (Lord Smith of Marlow)

CONCLUSION

Any cancer left in situ will continue to grow, probably metastasize, and in all likelihood be the cause of death. It is painfully obvious that resection offers the patient the only possibility of cure, albeit rare. This idea must be carefully tempered and weighed by each of us. I encourage everyone to reevaluate his or her personal experience, especially with resective procedures of the pancreas. What has been your operative mortality and morbidity rate, and how many patients have survived 3 or 5 years? With the exceptionally low long-term survival, operative mortality has to be kept to a minimum. Some reputable centers have, as a matter of routine, abandoned resective procedures for adenocarcinoma of the pancreas—certainly food for contemplative thought.

For now, having reviewed my own experience, and that of our institution, I believe patients with ampullary, duodenal, and common bile duct adenocarcinomas should be considered for resection. Patients with pancreatic islet cell tumors, both benign and malignant, and pancreatic cystadenocarcinomas should similarly be offered resection. Pancreatic adenocarcinoma is the "burr under the saddle." Selective resection should be offered after careful, mature, and experienced surgical deliberation. The resection of choice is the Whipple procedure.

Adjunctive chemotherapy and/or radiotherapy either postoperatively or intraoperatively is highly investigational at this time but should be pursued in a prospective investigative fashion. Finally, since early diagnosis does not appear to influence surivival, the onus is on prevention.

INDEX

The letter *f* following a page number indicates a figure; the letter *t* following a page number indicates a table.

A

Abdominal abscess, 237
Abdominal cavity sepsis. *See* Sepsis, intra-abdominal
Abdominal epilepsy, 105–106
Abdominal pain
  in children, 349–353
    clinical classification of, 350t
    clinical strategy in, 351–353
      rationale for, 349–350
    dysfunctional, 350
    organic, 350
    prognosis for, 353
    psychogenic, 350
  chronic
    analgesic block for, 148–149
    approach to patient with, 148
    behavioral treatment approach to, 141–145
    biofeedback and relaxation training in, 144
    case report, 144–145
    cognitive psychotherapy for, 143–144
    de novo reassessment of, 146
    definitions of, 146
    family therapy for, 143
    inappropriate drug use in, 148
    interaction with patient with, 142
    intractable, 145–149
    localization of, 147
    mechanisms of, 146–147
    referral in, 145
    self-control strategies in, 144
    somatic, 147
    transcutaneous electrical nerve stimulation for, 149
    visceral, 147
  with intestinal gas, 340–341
Abscess
  abdominal, 237
  anorectal, 302–303, 302f
  intra-abdominal, 274–275
  of liver, 275–276
  of pancreas, 275
  pericolic, 348
  of spleen, 276
  tubo-ovarian, 276
Acetaminophen hepatotoxicity, 393
  clinical course of, 393t
Achalasia, 37–39
  clinical manifestations of, 37
  diagnosis of, 37–38
  dilation vs. surgical therapy in, 39
  esophagomyotomy in, 38–39
  pharmacologic approaches to, 39
  pneumatic dilation in, 38
  treatment of, 38–39
Acidosis, in intestinal ischemia, 240
Acquired immune deficiency syndrome (AIDS), 186–187, 268–270
  candidiasis and, 2
  cryptosporidia in, 168
  secretory diarrhea with, 244
Acyclovir
  for anorectal herpetic infection, 266
  for herpes esophagitis, 64–65
  for herpetic gingivostomatitis, 1
  for mucositis, 6
Adenocarcinoma, esophageal, in Barrett's esophagus, 18–19
Adenomatosis, hereditary, 330–333
Adhesions, 236
Adolescents
  abdominal pain in, 349–353
  with Crohn's disease, 227
Adrenocorticotropic hormone (ACTH)
  for Crohn's disease, 293
  for fulminant colitis, 287
  for inflammatory bowel disease, 225, 225t
Agammaglobulinemia, 184–185
Aganglionosis, 250
Albendazole, 263
Alcoholics Anonymous, 372
Alcoholism, 369–373
  Alcoholics Anonymous for, 372
  delirium tremens with, 371
  disulfiram for, 372–373
  hallucinations with, 370
  hyperglycemia with, 371
  and liver disease, 374–376
  long-term management of, 372
  nutritional therapy, 371
  office management of, 371t
  patient-physician relationship, 369
  recognition of, 370
  seizures with, 370–371
  treatment of, 370–373
  vs. complications of alcoholism, 369t
  withdrawal syndrome, 370–371
Alkaline reflux esophagitis, 93
Alkaline reflux gastritis, 93–94
  consideration of, prior to antireflux surgery, 13
  diagnosis of, 93–94
  medical treatment of, 94
  surgical treatment of, 94
Allergic gastroenteropathy, 193–197
Allergy, cow's milk, substitute formulas for, 194t
Alpha-adrenergic agents, 246, 246t
Alpha$_1$-antitrypsin, 198
Alpha$_2$-agonists, 181
Amebiasis
  asymptomatic carrier, 262
  hepatic, 263
  intestinal, 262–263, 268
Amebic abscess, 275
Amino acid therapy, 368
Amitriptyline (Elavil)
  for depression, 137
  in irritable bowel syndrome, 345
  for glossitis, 2
Amoxicillin, 278t
Amphotericin B
  for bacterial infections, 192
  for *Candida* esophagitis, 68, 270
  for *Candida* peritonitis, 274
Ampicillin
  for endocarditis, 278t
  for fulminant colitis, 285
  for pyogenic liver abscess, 276
  for *Salmonella* infection, 268
  for shigellosis, 267
Ampullary dysfunction, 432–433
Analgesics
  inappropriate use of, 148
  for irritable bowel syndrome, 344
Ancylostoma duodenale infection, 169
Anemia, pernicious, 125–126
Angelchik prosthesis, 14–15
Angiodysplasia, 348
  nonbleeding, laser treatment of, 31
Angiography, for bleeding vascular ectasia, 337
Angiotherapy, for gastrointestinal bleeding, 82
Anion binding agents, 178
Anisakiasis, 170–171
Anorectal disorders, 301–307
Anorectal syphilis, 266–267
Anorexia nervosa, 116–120
  complications of, 119t, 120
  diagnosis of, 117
  in-hospital treatment program for, 117–118
  medication for, 118–119
  treatment of, 117
    outpatient, 119–120
Anoscopy, in gastrointestinal bleeding, 334
Antacids
  for alkaline reflux gastritis, 94
  for duodenal ulcer, 66–67, 67t
    side effects of, 68
  for esophageal reflux, 7
  for gastric ulcer, 70
  for gastrointestinal bleeding, 82
  for peptic disease, in chidren, 88
  for reflux esophagitis, 19t
  for stress ulcer, 92
Anti-inflammatory agents, toxicity with, 392
Antiarrhythmic agents, toxicity with, 392
Antibiotics. *See also specific drugs*
  for acute cholecystitis, 435
  for appendicitis, 275
  for bacterial overgrowth syndrome, 157
  for Crohn's disease, 218–219, 294
  for diarrhea, 255–257, 256t
  for esophageal caustic injury, 23–24
  for intra-abdominal sepsis
    failure to respond, 272
    selection of, 271
    timing of, 271
  for pancreatic abscess, 275
  for portosystemic encephalopathy, 369
  for pyogenic liver abscess, 276
  for traveler's diarrhea, 258t, 259, 261
  for tropical enteropathy, 159–160

for ulcerative colitis, 283-284
for Whipple's disease, 160-161, 161t
Anticholinergic agents
 for Crohn's disease, 217
 for diarrhea, 354
 for esophageal spasm, 34
 for gastrinoma, 78
 for peptic disease, in children, 88-89
 for postprandial hypoglycemia, 156
Antidepressants
 toxicity with, 392
 use of, 137
Antidiarrheal agents, 255
 for irritable bowel syndrome, 344
 for ulcerative colitis, 284
Antiemetic agents, 104t
 for gastroparesis, 98
Antiflatulents, 344
Antihistamines, 402
Antimitochondrial antibody, 398
Antinauseant agents, 104t
Antireflux procedures
 choice of repair, 13-15, 13t, 15t
 pathophysiologic indications for, 9t
 patient evaluation in, 9
 patient selection and clinical indications for, 10-13, 10t
 primary, results of, 13t
 repeat, vs. colon interposition, 15-16
Antireflux therapy for Barrett's esophagus, 18, 18t, 19t
Antispasmodic agents, 244
Antiviral therapy, 389
Anus
 fissure of, 302
 in infants, 90
 imperforate, 310
 pain, 250
Anxiety, and irritable bowel syndrome, 345
Anxiolytic agents, 354
Aperistalis, antireflux procedure for, 12
Aphthous ulcer, 1
Appendicitis, 275
 with Crohn's disease, 231
Appetite suppressants, 115
Aquasol A, 404
Aquasol E, 404
Argon laser
 characteristics of, 30, 30t
 efficacy and safety of, 31
Arteriography
 in diverticular disease, 348
 in gastrointestinal bleeding, 334, 336
Arteriovenous malformation, in gastrointestinal bleeding, 87
Arthritis, and Crohn's disease, 222
Ascariasis, 169
Ascaris lumbricoides, 169
Ascites, 361-364
 aggravating factors, 362, 363t
 and bacterial peritonitis, 362
 causes of, 362, 363t
 with chronic pancreatitis, 446
 with liver disease, 362
 peritoneovenous shunts for, 364
 reinfusion, 364
 treatment of, 362-364, 363t
Aspirin, and gastric ulcer, 69
Ataxia telangiectasia, 183
Atropine (Lomotil)
 for diarrhea, 354
 for duodenal ulcer, 67
 for irritable bowel syndrome, 344

for postprandial hypoglycemia, 156
Azathioprine
 for Crohn's disease, 220
 for idiopathic chronic active hepatitis, 390
 for inflammatory bowel disease, 225t, 226
 for ulcerative colitis, 283

B

Bacillus cereus infection, 253, 254t
Bacitracin, 192
Bacteremia, with gastrointestinal procedures, 277t, 278-279, 278t
Bacterial infections, following bone marrow transplant, 192
Bacterial overgrowth syndrome, 156-160
 antibiotic management of, 157
 causes of, 157
 and diabetic diarrhea, 180
 nutritional considerations in, 157-158, 158t
 surgical management of, 159
 therapeutic approach to, 157
Bacterial peritonitis, 272
Balantidium coli infection, 264
Balloon tamponade
 in esophageal varices, 378
 in children, 89
 in gastrointestinal bleeding, 83
Barrett's esophagus, 16-20
 adenocarcinoma in, 18-19
 antireflux procedure for, 11
 colonic neoplasms and, 19-20
 diagnosis of, 16-17
 endoscopic evaluation of, 16-17, 17f
 histologic evaluation of, 17
 potential difference profile of, 17, 17f
 radiologic evaluation of, 16
 surveillance of, 18-20
 treatment of, 18
B-cell disorders, 182-187
Belching, excessive, 340
Belsey partial fundoplication, 14
Benzimidazole, 71
Bethanechol
 chemical structure of, 99f
 for dysuria, 253
 for esophageal reflux, 7, 8
 for gastroparesis, 99
 for reflux esophagitis, 19t
Bile duct obstruction
 endoscopic management of, 429-432
 ERCP in, 429-430, 429t, 430t
 nonoperative management of, 430-432, 430t, 431t, 432t
Bile duct stenosis, with chronic pancreatitis, 446
Bile gastritis, *See* Alkaline reflux gastritis
Bile salt malabsorption, in short bowel syndrome, 174
Biliary cirrhosis, primary, 397-400
Biliary drainage, percutaneous transhepatic, 424-427
 complications of, 427
 indications for, 425-426
 technique of, 426-427
Biliary duct cancer
 failure patterns in, 132-133
 treatment alternatives in, 132, 132t, 133t
Biliary obstruction, treatment of, 401
Biliary stone extraction, 428
Biliary tract stricture, high, 418-421
 benign, 418-419
 due to stone disease, 419-420

 irradiation of, 420
 malignant, 420-421
 nonoperative management of, 420-421
 percutaneous drainage for, 425
 sclerosing cholangitis and, 419
 stents and drains for, 431-432, 432t
 surgery for, 418, 420, 421f
Biofeedback, for diarrhea, 355
Bismuth subsalicylate
 for diarrhea, 255, 258-259, 258t
Bleeding. *See* Hemorrhage
Bloating, 103-105, 340-341
Bone disease, with cholestasis, 404-405
Bone marrow transplant
 effects of conditioning, 188
 gastrointestinal problems in, 188-192
 graft vs. host disease, 188-191
 intestinal infections following, 192
Brachytherapy, for esophageal cancer, 59-60
Bromocriptine, 368
Budd-Chiari syndrome, 386, 394
Bulimia, 116-117
 complications of, 119t, 120
 diagnosis of, 117
 medication for, 118
 treatment of, 117
Burns, esophageal. *See* Esophagus, caustic injury of

C

Calcium, for primary biliary cirrhosis, 399
Calcium-channel blockers, for esophageal spasms, 36
Calcium malabsorption, in short bowel syndrome, 174
Calcium oxalate calculus, 176
Calcium oxalate nephrolithiasis, 177-179
Calcium polycarbophil, for diarrhea, 255
Calories
 daily intake of, 113t
 used in exercise, 114t
Cambendazole, 263
Campylobacter jejunii infection, 184, 268
Campylobacter pyloridis infection, 100
Cancer. *See specific diagnosis*
Candida esophagitis, 61-64, 64f
Candida tropicalis, 183
Candidiasis, 2
 chronic mucocutaneous, 186
 in peritonitis, 273-274
Canker sore, 1
Capillaria philippinensis, 170
Capillariasis, 170
Carbenoxolone, 68
Carbohydrate, in parenteral nutrition, 202
Carbohydrate malabsorption, 149-153
 for lactose, 150-152, 150t, 151t
 for monosaccharide, 152-153, 152t
 for sorbitol, 153, 153t
 for sucrose, 152, 152t
Carbon dioxide laser, characteristics of, 30t
Carbon tetrachloride, liver disease associated with, 394
Carcinoid syndrome, malignant, 247-248
Carcinomatosis, 237
Cardia
 mechanically defective, 9-10
 tumors of, 54-57
Caries, 2, 5
Caroli's disease, 419
Cartilage hair hypoplasia, 186
Catheter

balloon, coaxial, 26
    transpapillary nasobiliary, 432
Cefamandole, 273
Cefotaxime, 273
Cefoxitin
    for pyogenic liver abscess, 276
    for tubo-ovarian complex, 276
Ceftriaxone, 266
Celiac sprue
    and diabetic diarrhea, 180
    dietary treatment of, 162-164, 163t, 164t
    and related diseases, 162-166
    symptomatic therapy for, 164-165
Cephalosporin, preoperative, in Crohn's disease, 230
Cestodes, 171-172
Charcoal
    for excessive flatus, 342
    for liver disease, 393
Chemotherapy. *See also specific drugs*
    causing nausea and vomiting, 102-103
    for esophageal cancer, 57, 60
    for gastric cancer, 122, 123, 123t
    for liver cancer, 416-417
    for rectal cancer, 318
Cheno, features of, 423
Chest pain, 34
    esophageal causes of, therapy for, 36t
    evaluation of, 35f
Chest symptoms, antireflux procedure for, 12
Children
    abdominal pain in, 349-353
    esophageal varices in, 89-90
    gastrointestinal bleeding in, 88-91
    inflammatory bowel disease in, 223-227
    peptic disease in, 88-89
    postprandial hypoglycemia in, 155
    reflux in, antireflux procedure for, 12
Chlamydia trachomatis infection, 266
Chlamydial proctitis, 306
Chloramphenicol, 159
Chlordiazepoxide
    for alcohol withdrawal symptoms, 371
    for glossitis, 2
Chloroquine
    for amebiasis, 263
    for amebic abscess, 275
Chlorpheniramine, 196
Chlorpromazine
    for anorexia nervosa, 118
    for diarrhea, 246t, 247
    for hiccups, 103
Cholangiopancreatography, endoscopic retrograde (ERCP), 429-430
    complications of, 430, 430t
    indications for, 429, 429t
Cholangitis
    oriental, 419
    sclerosing, 405-406, 419
        diagnosis of, 405
        liver transplantation in, 406
        medical treatment of, 405-406
        surgical treatment of, 406
Cholecystectomy, 435-436
Cholecystitis
    acalculous, 424
    acute, 433-437
        antibiotics for, 435
        cholecystectomy for, 435-436
        complications of, 436
        diagnosis of, 434
        differential diagnosis of, 434
        Murphy's sign in, 433

    treatment of, 434-436
    emphysematous, 436
Cholelithiasis, 422-424
    bile acid dissolution treatment of, 422-424
    in diabetes mellitus, 424
    expectant management of, 422
    nonvisualizing, 424
Cholestasis, 400-405
    biliary obstruction with, 401
    bone disease with, 404-405
    causes of, 401t
    fat malabsorption with, 403-404
    intrahepatic, 394
    nutritional deficiencies complicating, 404t
    pruritus with, 401-403
Cholestyramine
    for alkaline reflux gastritis, 94
    for Crohn's disease, 217-218
    for diarrhea, 256, 256t, 354
    for pruritus, 399, 402, 402t
    for small bowel syndrome, 174
Cholinergic (muscarinic) receptor antagonists, 71
Chromoendoscopy, in gastric carcinoma, 125
Cimetidine
    for duodenal ulcer, 68
    for esophageal reflux, 8
    for gastric ulcer, 70-71, 71f
    for gastrinoma, 77, 78
    for gastrointestinal bleeding, 82
    for peptic disease, in children, 88
    for pruritus, 402, 402t
    for reflux esophagitis, 19t
    for stress ulcer, 92
Cirrhosis
    alcoholic, 375-376
    primary biliary, 397-400
        antimitochondrial antibody in, 398
        clinical features of, 397-398
        diagnosis of, 398
        diseases associated with, 398-399
        epidemiology and etiology of, 397
        fat malabsorption with, 400
        hepatic osteodystrophy with, 399
        prognosis of, 399
        pruritus with, 399
        treatment of, 399-400
        vitamin deficiency with, 400
Cisplatin, 123, 123t
Clindamycin
    for mucositis, 6
    for pyogenic liver abscess, 276
    for tubo-ovarian complex, 276
Clonidine
    for diarrhea, 181, 246
    for pancreatic cholera syndrome, 247
Clostridium difficile infection, 182, 221
Clostridium perfringens infection, 253, 254t
Clotrimazole
    for candidal esophagitis, 62
    for candidiasis, 2
Coating agents
    for duodenal ulcer, 67, 67f
    for gastric ulcer, 71
Cobalamin, 159
Coccidian parasites, 168
Codeine
    for caries, 5
    for diarrhea, 159, 181, 354
    for diverticular disease, 345
    for irritable bowel syndrome, 344
Cold sore, 1
Colectomy

    prophylactic, 297-298
    in sclerosing cholangitis, 406
Colitis
    Crohn's, 285-290
    ischemic, 243
    radiation, 339
    ulcerative. *See* Ulcerative colitis
Colloids, hydrophilic, in irritable bowel syndrome, 343-344
Colon
    adenomatous polyps of, 299
    complete obstruction of, 238-239
    Crohn's disease of, 291-296
    diverticular disease of, 345-349
    parasitic disease of, 262-264
    partial obstruction of, 239
    structural disease of, 250
Colon cancer, 321-323
    and Crohn's disease, 292
    genetic factor, 328-330
Colon polyps, 325-328
    adenomatous, 325-326
    on barium enema x-ray, 325
    malignant, 327-328
    pedunculated, 328
    polypectomy for, 326-327
        follow-up after, 328
    sessile, 327-328
Colonic neoplasms, and Barrett's esophagus 19-20
Colonic ulcer, bleeding of, 338
Colonic varices, bleeding of, 338
Colonoscopy
    in diverticular disease, 348
    in gastrointestinal bleeding, 336
Colorectal cancer
    adjuvant therapy for, 320-325
    failure after conventional treatment of, 133
    hepatic metastasis from, surgical treatment of, 412-413, 412t, 413t
    intraoperative and external irradiation of, 133
    staging systems, 320-321, 321t
Colostomy
    complications of, 313-314
    indications for, 313
    ostomy care, 313-314
    surgical techniques, 313
Coma, clinical profile, 386t
Combined immunodeficiency disease, 185-186
Condyloma acuminatum, 267, 305-306
Condyloma latum, 267
Constipation, 248-250
    clinical considerations, 250
    control mechanisms, 249-250
    incontinence with, 309
    irritable colon syndrome with, 250
    myogenic factors, 249
    neuro-endocrine factors, 249-250
    with no structural abnormalities identified, 250
    physiology of, 249
    with structural disease of colon, 250
    transit-pressure alterations, 250
    water absorption, 250
Contraceptive toxicity, oral, 393-394
Corrosives, household, 20t
Corticosteroids
    for alcoholic hepatitis, 375
    for bacterial peritonitis, 272
    for Crohn's disease, 219, 292-293
    for esophageal caustic injury, 23

for fulminant colitis, 287
for ulcerative colitis, 282-283
Cow's milk allergy, substitute formulas for, 194t
Cricopharyngeal myotomy, 42
Cricopharyngeus, foreign bodies in, 47, 47f
Crohn's disease, 216-223. *See also* Inflammatory bowel disease
  abscess with, 232
  acute, 220-221
  adjunctive medications for, 217-218
  in adolescents, 227
  age of inset of, 296
  anal and perianal, 306-307
  antibiotics for, 218-219, 294
  appendicitis with, 231
  arthritis and, 222
  cancer with, 300
    early diagnosis of, 298
  in children, 223-227
  chronic, 221
  with colitis, 285-290
  of colon, 291-296
  colon cancer with, 292
  complications of, 222-223
  corticosteroids for, 219, 292-293
  cutaneous manifestations of, 222
  definition of, 291
  diagnosis of, 216
  differential diagnosis of, 291
  emergency situations in, 231-232
  fistula with, 222
    management of, 231
  gastric involvement and, 222
  gastroduodenal involvement and, 222, 231
  growth failure in, 223, 224f
    surgical treatment of, 226, 226t
  histologic features of, 292
  immunosuppressive therapy for, 219-220, 293-294
  intestinal obstruction and, 237
  intraoperative management of, 230-231
  malabsorption in, 224, 224t
  medical management of, 216-220, 292-294
  metronidazole for, 294
  mucosal dysplasia with, 297
    colonic biopsies for, 300
    interpretation of, 299
    surveillance for, 298-299
  nutritional management in, 217, 221
  occular manifestations and, 222
  perforation with, 232
  postoperative management of, 232
  pregnancy and, 222
  pregnancy and fertility in, 292
  preoperative preparation, 229-230
  in protein-losing enteropathy, 199-200
    monitoring protein response in, 200
  recurrent, 221-222, 232
  strictureplasty and, 231
  sulfasalazine for, 218, 293
  surgery for, 229-232, 294-295
    prognosis and indications for, 295-296
  toxic megacolon with, 232
Cryptosporidium infection, 168, 264
Cystic fibrosis, 450-455
  diagnosis of, 450-451
  distal intestinal obstruction syndrome in, 454
  gatrointestinal manifestations in, 450t
  hepatobiliary system in, 454
  intestinal complications in, 453-454
  meconium ileus with, 453-454

nutritional therapy in, 451-453, 452f, 452t, 453t
  pancreatic extracts in, 451, 451t
  pancreatic insufficiency with, 451-453
  pulmonary disease with, 454-455, 454t
  rectal prolapse with, 454
Cysticercosis, 172
Cystitis, in intestinal pseudo-obstruction, 253

D

Decompression, tube, in intestinal obstruction, 235-236
Defecation habits, poor, 250
Deferoxamine, 411
Dehydroemetine, 263
Delirium tremens, 371
Delta agent, 382
Dental decay, 2, 5
Depression, 136-137
  and irritable bowel syndrome, 345
  medication for, 137
Desipramine
  for anorexia nervosa and bulimia, 118
  for depression, 137
  for diarrhea, 354
Dexamethasone, 103
Di George syndrome, 185
Diabetes mellitus
  cholelithiasis in, 424
  diarrhea in, 179-181
  hypoglycemia in, 154-155
    treatment of, 156
  incontinence with, 309
Dialysis
  in hepatorenal syndrome, 365
  peritonitis associated with, 273
Diarrhea
  in acute graft vs. host disease, 190
  acute infectious, 253-257
    antibiotics for, 255-257, 256t
    antidiarrheal agents for, 255
    diagnosis of, 253, 254t
    dietary modification for, 254
    fluid therapy for, 254-255, 255t
    hospitalization for, 257
    treatment of, 253-257
  bloody, 253
  Campylobacter, 256
  choleretic, 172
  diabetic, 179-181
    conditions associated with, 180
    decision to treat, 179-180
    treatment of, 180-181
  functional, 353-355
    diagnosis of, 353
    treatment of, 354-355
  incontinence with and without, 308
  secretory, 244-248
    AIDS with, 244
    alpha-adrenergic agents in, 246, 246t
    carcinoid syndrome with, 247-248
    chloropromazine in, 246t, 247
    chronic, 248
    fluid and electrolyte replacement in, 245
    glucocorticoids in, 246t, 247
    opiates in, 245-246, 246t
    pancreatic cholera syndrome with, 247
    pharmacologic intervention in, 245-247, 246t
    prostaglandin synthetase inhibitors in, 246, 246t
    somatostatin in, 246t, 247

    thyroid carcinoma with, 248
    verapamil in, 246t, 247
    Zollinger-Ellison syndrome with, 248
  symptomatic therapy for, 158-159
  traveler's, 257-262
    antibiotics for, 259, 261
    dietary discretion in, 258
    maintenance of hydration in, 260-261
    nonantimicrobial drugs for, 258-259
    prevention of, 258-260, 258t
    treatment of, 260-261, 260t
    vaccines for, 259-261
  watery, 253
Dicyclomine hydrochloride (Bentyl)
  for esophageal spasm, 34, 36
  for intestinal gas, 341
  for irritable bowel syndrome, 344
Dientamoeb fragalis infection, 263
Diet. *See also* Nutrition
  in acute hepatitis, 381
  alternative, 214-215
  in anorexia nervosa, 118
  balanced low calorie, 110, 112t
  in chronic pancreatitis, 450
  in Crohn's disease, 217
  in cystic fibrosis, 451-453, 452f, 452t
  diary, 111-112
  elemental, 210, 211t
  and excessive flatus, 341-342
  fad, 213-214
  in gastroparesis, 97-98
  high-fiber
    for abdominal pain, 352
    for diarrhea, 354
    for diverticular disease, 345
  in infectious diarrhea, 254
  in irritable bowel syndrome, 343-344
  lactose-free, 150t
  lamb and rice, 195t
  liquid formula, 206-212
  low calorie ketogenic, 109, 111t
  low oxalate, 177t, 178
  macrobiotic, 213-214
  nutritional supplementation of, 214-215, 215t
  in obesity, 108-110
  in peptic disease, in children, 89
  polymeric, 209-210, 210t
  in postprandial hypoglycemia, 155-156
  reducing, 214
  semistarvation, 109, 110t
  in short bowel syndrome, 173, 173t
  sucrose-restricted, 151t, 152
  and traveler's diarrhea, 258, 258t
  vegetarian, 213
Diiodohydroxyquin
  for amebiasis, 262, 263
  for *Balantidium coli* infection, 264
  for *Dientamoeba fragalis* infection, 263
Dilation
  of biliary strictures, 427, 432
  esophageal, 24
    for chest pains, 37
    instruments for, 26
    patient preparation for, 26-27
    techniques of, 27-28
  pneumatic, for achalasia, 38
Diloxanide furoate, 262, 268
Diltiazem, 36
Diphenhydramine hydrochloride, 197
Diphenhydrazine, 402, 402t
Diphenoxylate/atropine (Lomotil)
  for diarrhea, 181, 245, 344, 354

for irritable bowel syndrome, 344
Diphyllobothrium latum infection, 171
Distention, in acute graft vs. host disease, 190
Disulfiram (Antabuse), for alcoholism, 372–373
Diuretics, in ascites, 362–364, 363t
Diverticular disease
  of colon, 345–349
  fistula with, 347–348
  hemorrhage with, 348
  inflammatory complications of, 346–347
  medical treatment of, 345–346
  obstruction with, 348
  pseudotumor with, 348
  and related conditions, 348–349
  surgical management of, 346–348
Diverticular hemorrhage, 336–337
Domperidone
  for anorexia nervosa and bulimia, 118
  chemical structure of, 99f
  for nausea and vomiting, 103
  for nonulcer dyspepsia, 101
Dopamine, 99
Doxorubicin, 123, 123t
Doxycycline
  for *Chlamydia trachomatis* infection, 266
  for traveler's diarrhea, 258t, 261
D-penicillamine, for alcoholic hepatitis, 375
Dukes staging system, for colorectal cancer, 320–321, 321t
Dumping syndrome, 95
Duodenal obstruction, with chronic pancreatitis, 446
Duodenal ulcer, 66–69
  acid reduction for, 66–68
  acute, surgery for, 75
  bleeding, 68
    treatment of, 75
  cellular mechanisms in, 68
  chronic, surgery for, 72–75
  coating agents for, 67, 67f
  diagnosis and evaluation of, 66
  incidence of, 72
  neurohormonal alteration in, 67–68
  non-acid active drugs for, 68
  obstructive, 74–75
  perforated, 75
  postsecretory therapy for, 66–67, 67t
  recurrent, 75–76
  relapses, 68–69
  treatment of
    bases for, 66
    side effects of, 68
    special cases and, 68–69
    suggested method of, 69
    treatment strategies, 66–68
Duodenogastric dyssynchrony, role of, 100
Dwarfism, short-limbed, 186
Dyskinesia, gastroduodenopyloric, 95
Dyspepsia, nonulcer, 100–101, 101f
Dysphagia, 25, 33–34
  antireflux procedure for, 12
  pharyngeal, 39–44
  psychogenic, presumed, 43–44
Dysplasia
  colonoscopic biopsies for, 300
  interpretation of, 299
  mucosal, 297
  surveillance for, 298–299
Dysrhythmias, electrical, of stomach and bowel, 100
Dysuria, in intestinal pseudo-obstruction, 253

E

Electrocoagulation, for rectal cancer, 318–319
Electrolytes
  for parenteral nutrition, 202
  for secretory diarrhea, 245
  for short bowel syndrome, 174
  for tropical enteropathy, 159
Elemental diets, 210, 211t
Embolus, mesenteric arterial, 242
Emetine
  for amebiasis, 263
  for amebic abscess, 275
Emotional factor, in ulcerative colitis, 281
Empyema, of gallbladder, 436
Encephalopathy, portosystemic, 366–369
  acute, 366–368
    diagnosis of, 366
    treatment of, 366–368, 368t
  causes of, 366, 367t
  chronic, 368–369
    diagnosis of, 368
    treatment of, 368–369
  subclinical, 369
Encopresis, 309–310
Endocarditis
  prevention of, 277–278
  prophylaxis for, 277–279
  risk of, 277, 277t
Endoscopy
  bacteremia associated with, 278
  in Barrett's esophagus, 16–17, 17f
  in bleeding vascular ectasia, 337–338
  in esophageal caustic injury, 22, 22t
  in gastric polyps, 126, 127f
  in gastrointestinal bleeding, 31, 31t, 82–83
Entamoeba histolytica infection, 262–263, 268
Enteritis, radiation, management of, 237
  parenteral nutrition for, 204
Enterobius vermicularis infection, 263
Enteroclysis study, of intestinal obstruction, 238
Enterocolitis, protein-sensitive, in infants, 90
Enteropathy
  gluten-sensitive
    dietary treatment of, 162–164, 163t, 164t
    symptomatic therapy for, 164–165
  protein-losing, 197–201
  tropical, 159–160
Epilepsy, abdominal, 105–106
Ergocalciferol, for vitamin D deficiency, 405
Eructation, 103–105
Erythema nodosum, and Crohn's disease, 222
Erythrityl tetranitrate (Cardilate), 36
Erythromycin
  for *Campylobacter* infection, 268
  for caries, 5
  for *Chlamydia trachomatis* infection, 266
  for chlamydial proctitis, 306
  for diarrhea, 256, 256t
  for fulminant colitis, 285
  for gingivitis, 2
  preoperative, in Crohn's disease, 230
Esophageal cancer
  anatomy and patterns of spread of, 57–58
  chemotherapy for, 57, 60
  distribution of, 55t
  radiation therapy for, 56, 57–60
    curative, 58
    dose and administration method in, 59–60
    palliative, 59
    postoperative, 59
    side effects of, 60
    treatment volume used in, 59
  TNM staging of, 58t
  treatment guidelines for, 58
  treatment modalities for, 55t
Esophageal exclusion, for nonresectable tumors, 56
Esophageal reflux. *See also* Barrett's esophagus
  antacids for, 7–8
  bed elevation for, 7
  decreasing frequency and duration of, 7
  decreasing irritant and gastric juice in, 7–8
  diet and, 7
  in infants and children, 12
  medical management of, 6–8
    treatment modalities, 6–8
    treatment strategies, 8
  nocturnal, 6
  obesity and, 7
  postprandial, 6
  surgical treatment of, 9–16. *See also* Antireflux procedures
Esophageal ring, treatment of, 28
Esophageal sclerotherapy
  for active variceal hemorrhage, 52–53
  in children, 89–90
  complications of, 53–54
  end point of, 49, 52
  in esophageal varices, 378, 379
  indications for, 48–50
  injection technique, 50–51
  patient selection for, 49–50
  procedure schedule in, 51–52
  results of, 53
  sclerosing agent, 50
  technique of, 50–53
  variceal compression during, 51
  vs. surgery, 49
Esophageal spasm
  clinical manifestations of, 33–34, 34t
  and related disorders, 33–37
  treatment of, 34, 36–37
    surgical, 37
Esophageal sphincter, improving function of, 7
Esophageal stricture, 25–29
  antireflux procedure for, 11
  peroral dilation in, 26–28
    instruments for, 26
    patient preparation for, 26–27
    techniques of, 27–28
    treatment of specific lesions, 28–29
Esophageal varices
  bleeding
    acute, defining, 48–49
    laser therapy for, 31–32
  in children, 89–90
  portal hypertension with, 376–380
  sclerotherapy of, 48–54
    for active hemorrhage, 53–54
Esophageal web, treatment of, 28
Esophagectomy, postoperative complications following, 56t
Esophagitis
  alkaline reflux, 93
  antireflux procedure for, 11
  in Crohn's disease, 222
  infectious, 61–65
    candidal, 61–64, 64f
    clinical setting in, 61
    diagnosis of, 61
    herpetic, 64–65

treatment of, 61–65
radiation-induced, 60
Esophagomyotomy, for achalasia, 38–39
Esophagus, 1–65
   Barrett's. *See* Barrett's esophagus
   caustic injury of, 20–25
      antibiotics and corticosteroids for, 23–24
      clinical presentation of, 21
      complications of, 25
      diagnosis and initial therapy of, 21–22
      endoscopic evaluation of, 22, 22t
      esophageal stents in, 24
      management of, 22–25
      nasogastric intubation in, 23
      natural history of, 20–21, 21t
      pathology of, 20
      peroral dilation in, 24
      radiographic evaluation of, 21–22
      surgery in, 24–25
      total parenteral nutrition in, 23
   clearing of refluxed acid from, 7
   columnar epithelium-lined. *See* Barrett's esophagus
   propulsive force of, antireflux surgery and, 13
   tumors of, 54–57. *See also* Esophageal cancer
      benign, 57, 57t
      chemotherapy for, 57, 60
      evaluation of, 54–55, 55t
      intubation for palliation of, 56
      postoperative considerations in, 56, 56t
      radiation therapy for, 56, 57–60
      surgical reconstruction for, 55–56
      surgical resection for, 55, 55t
      survival and, 56
      unresectable, 56
Excretion
   urinary citrate, 178–179
   urinary magnesium, 178
Exercise, and obesity, 112–113
Exocrine insufficiency, pancreatic, and diabetic diarrhea, 180

F

Fad diets. *See also* Diet
   macrobiotic, 213–214
   recognition, assessment, and intervention in, 215–216
   reducing, 214
   vegetarianism, 213
Familial colon cancer syndrome, 328–330
Familial polyposis coli, 330–333
   colectomy/ileoanal pouch for, 333
   colectomy/ileorectal anastomosis for, 333
   extracolonic manifestations of, 330–332, 331t
   proctocolectomy/ileostomy for, 332–333
   surgical options for, 332
   treatment of, 332
Famotidine, 78
Fat intake
   in parenteral nutrition, 202
   in small bowel syndrome, 174
Fat metabolism
   with cholestasis, 403–404
   with primary biliary cirrhosis, 400
Fatty liver, alcoholic, 374
Fecal incontinence, 307–310
Feeding. *See also* Nutrition
   alternative means of, 44
   continuous, advantages of, 211

intermittent, 210–211
Fertility, and Crohn's disease, 292
Fistula-in-ano, 303
Fistulas
   with Crohn's disease, 222
      management of, 231
   in diverticular disease, 292
   parenteral nutrition for, 204
Flatus, excessive, 341–342
Flubendazole, 263
5-Flucytosine, for candidal esophagitis, 63
Fluid therapy
   for functional diarrhea, 354
   for infectious diarrhea, 254–255, 255t
   for pancreatitis, 438, 439
   for secretory diarrhea, 245
   for tropical enteropathy, 159
Fluorescein dye injection, in intestinal ischemia, 244
5-Fluorocytosine, for bacterial infections, 192
5-Fluorouracil
   for colon cancer, 321–322, 322t
   for esophageal cancer, 60
   for gastric cancer, 123, 123t
Folate, for tropical enteropathy, 159
Folic acid, for alcoholic cirrhosis, 375
Food
   adverse reactions to, 193t
   common, gas-forming potential of, 341t
   fructose content of, 152t
   high oxalate, 175t
   organic and natural, 214
   oxalate content of, 177t
   sorbitol content of, 153t
Food fads, and alternatives, 213–216
Food groupings, common, 196t
Food hypersensitivity, differential diagnosis of, 194t
Food poisoning, acute bacterial, 253, 254t
Foreign body
   in gastrointestinal tract, 44, 45f, 46–47, 47f
      radiolucent, 47
      sharp and pointed, 46–47
   in pharynx or cricopharyngeus, 47, 47f
Functional illness, 137–141
   common sense support, 139
   diagnostic evaluation of, 139
   discussion of interpersonal factors, 140
   explanation of, 139–140
   inappropriate psychiatric referral, 138–139
   patient management steps in, 139–141
   physician attitude, 137–138
   practical measures, 141
   review of study results, 139
   self-treatment measures, 140–141
Fungal infections, following bone marrow transplant, 192

G

Gallbladder
   disease of, acute, 422
   empyema of, 436
   perforation of, 436
Gallstones. *See* Cholelithiasis
Gardner's syndrome, 330–333
Gas, intestinal, 340–342
Gastrectomy
   for gastric cancer, 121
   total, for gastrinoma, 79
Gastric acid, hypersecretion of, medical treatment of, 77–78
   surgical treatment of, 78–79

Gastric cancer, 120–123
   adjuvant therapy for, 122
   advanced disease
      chemotherapy for, 122t, 123, 123t
      laser palliation for, 123
      radiation therapy for, 123
   changing death rate from, 120t
   chemotherapy for, 122
   classification and etiology of, 124
   diagnostic considerations in, 120–121
   failure patterns in, 130
   gender specific mortality from, 121t
   perspectives on, 124
   postoperative and supportive care for, 122–123, 122t
   precursors of, 124–125, 125t
   preoperative management of, 121
   radiation therapy for, 122, 122t
   surgery for, 121–122, 121t
   treatment alternatives in, 130, 130t
Gastric carcinoids, 125
Gastric disorder, antireflux procedure following, 12–13
Gastric emptying
   disorders of, 95–99
      pathophysiology of, 95–96
   measurement of, 97, 97f, 98f
   physiology of, 95
Gastric lavage, for gastrointestinal bleeding, 82
Gastric polyps, 126–127, 127f
Gastric stumps, 127–128
Gastric ulcer, 69–72
   acute vs. chronic, 69
   assessment of therapeutic response, 72
   classification of, 73t
   clinical features of, 69–70
   coating agents for, 71
   diagnosis of, 70
   healing promotion of, 70–71
   malignancy and, 128
   mucosal resistance in, 71–72
   pathogenesis of, 69
   prevention of recurrence of, 72
   surgery for, 72, 76, 76t
   treatment of, 70–72
Gastrinoma, 77–80. *See also* Zollinger-Ellison syndrome
   gastrectomy for, 79
   gastric hypersecretion in
      medical treatment of, 77–78
      surgical treatment of, 78–79
   intravenous therapy for, 77–78
   long-term follow-up in, 80
   metastatic, approach to, 80
   new drug therapy for, 78
   nonmetastatic, approach to, 79–80
   oral therapy for, 78
   parathyroidectomy for, 79
   parietal cell vagotomy for, 78
   treatment of, 77, 79–80
Gastritis, 72
   acute erosive, 91–93
   alkaline reflux (bile). *See* Alkaline reflux gastritis
   chronic atrophic, 125–126
Gastroduodenal disease, in Crohn's disease, 231
Gastroduodenopyloric dyskinesia, 95
Gastroenteropathy, allergic, 193–197
   diagnosis of, 193–194, 194t, 195t
   treatment of, 195–197, 196t
Gastroesophageal reflux. *See* Esophageal

reflux
Gastrointestinal disease, laser therapy for, 30–33
Gastrointestinal neoplasms, laser therapy for, 32–33
Gastrointestinal toxicity, in bone marrow recipients, 188
Gastrointestinal tract
 bleeding of, 90–91, 333–339
  acute, 80–87
   acid neutralization in, 82
   angiotherapy for, 82
   arteriovenous malformations in, 87
   balloon tamponade in, 83
   endoscopy in, 82–83
   evaluation and management of, 81–82
   gastric lavage in, 82
   medical treatment of, 83, 87
   secretory inhibition in, 82
   surgery for, 87
   therapeutic alternatives for, 82–83, 87
   transhepatic obliteration of varices in, 83
   treatment of specific causes of, 84f–86f, 87
   vasopressin in, 83
  causes of, 334t
  in children, 88–91
  diagnostic approach to, 333–336
  endoscopic therapy for, 31, 31t
  laser treatment of, 30–31
 disorders of, in immunodeficiency states, 181–187
 foreign bodies in, 44, 45f, 46–47, 47f
  extraction of, 44–48, 45t
  guidelines for management of, 45t
 functional disorders of, 100–106
 malignancies of, intraoperative irradiation of, 130–133
Gastrokinetic agents, 98–99, 99f
Gastroparesis, 102
 causes of, 95–96, 96t, 97
 diagnosis and management of, 96–97, 98t
 therapy for, 97–99, 98t
Gaviscon, for reflux esophagitis, 19t
Gentamicin
 for appendicitis, 275
 for endocarditis, 278t
 for pancreatic abscess, 275
 for pyogenic liver abscess, 276
 for spontaneous peritonitis, 273
Giardia lamblia, 166–167, 184, 268
Giardiasis, 166–168
Gingivitis, 2
Gingivostomatitis, herpetic, 1
Glossitis, 2
Glucocorticoids, 246t, 247
Gluten-sensitive enteropathy
 dietary treatment of, 162–164, 163t, 164t
 symptomatic therapy for, 164–165
Glycemic index, 156
Gonococcal proctitis, 306
Gonorrhea, 266
Graft-versus-host disease, 188–191
 acute, 188–191, 189t
  management of, 190–191
  prophylaxis in, 189–190
  treatment of, 189
 chronic, 191
Growth failure
 in Crohn's disease, 223, 224f
  surgical treatment of, 226, 226t
  etiology of malnutrition and, 224, 224–225,

224t
 in inflammatory bowel disease, 223–229
 medical treatment of, 225–226, 225t

H

Hallucinations, alcoholic, 370
Heller myotomy, 38–39
Hematopoietic hypoplasia, 185
Hemochromatosis, 409–411
 classification of, 409t
 clinical features of, 409, 410t
 diagnosis of, 409–410, 410t
 genetic, 409–411
 HLA typing in, 410
 mild to moderate, 411
 pathogenesis of, 409
 precirrhotic, 410
 role of alcohol in, 410
 treatment of, 410–411, 411t
Hemolytic-uremic syndrome, 90
Hemophilus influenzae infection, 184
Hemorrhage
 acute, in gastrointestinal tract, 333–336
 in acute graft vs. host disease, 190
 chronic or occult, 339
 diverticular, 336–337
 in diverticular disease, 348
 in pancreatitis, 444
 of specific lesions, 336–339
 of vascular ectasia, 337–338
Hemorrhoids, 301–302, 301f–302f, 338–339
 in children, 91
Hemosiderosis, in alcoholic liver disease, 410
Henoch-Schonlein purpura, 90
Hepatic clearance, of drugs, 356–357
Heptatic lobectomy, 415–416, 416f
Hepatic neoplasms, 412–417
Hepatic resection
 approach to, 414–415, 415f
 palliative, 414–416
Hepatitis
 acute, 380–383
  active treatment for, 381–382
  biochemical tests for, 380–381
  diagnosis of, 380
  evaluation of, 380–381
  management of, 381–383
  prevention of, 382
  prophylaxis for, 382–383
  serologic tests for, 381
 alcoholic, 374–375
 chronic, 387–390
  active, 388–390
  antiviral therapy for, 389
  idiopathic active, 390
  immunosuppressive therapy for, 389
  lobular, 388
  persistent, 387–388
Hepatitis A
 prevention, 382
 prophylaxis, 382
Hepatitis B
 prevention, 382
 prophylaxis, 383
Hepatitis-HBV, chronic active, 388–389
Hepatitis non A, non B, chronic, 389–390
Hepatobiliary system, in cystic fibrosis, 454
Hepatorenal syndrome, 364–365
Hereditary adenomatosis, 330–333
Hernia
 incarcerated, management of, 236–237
 incarcerated inguinal, 241

 parastomal, 312, 313
Herpes esophagitis, 64–65
Herpes infections, 1
Herpes simplex infection, anorectal, 266, 306
Hiccups, 103
Hill procedure, 14
Hirschsprung's disease, 90
Histamine$_2$ receptor antagonists
 for Crohn's disease, 217
 for duodenal ulcer, 68
 for esophageal reflux, 8
 for gastric ulcer, 70–71, 71f
 for gastrointestinal bleeding, 82
 for peptic disease, in children, 88
 for reflux esophagitis, 19t
HLA typing, in hemochromatosis, 410
Hookworm, 169
Household corrosives, 20t
HTLV-III virus, 269
Hurst dilator, 26
Hydatid cyst, 276
Hydralazine, 36–37
Hydration, and traveler's diarrhea, 260–261
Hydrocortisone
 for Crohn's disease, 219
 for fulminant colitis, 28, 290
 preoperative, in Crohn's disease, 230
 for ulcerative colitis, 283
Hydroxyzine, 402f, 402t
Hymenolepis, 172
Hymenolepis nana, 172
Hyper-IgM, X-linked immunodeficiency with, 183
Hyperglycemia, 371
Hyperimmunoglobulinemia, immunodeficiency with, 183
Hyperoxaluria, enteric, 176, 176t
Hyperparathyroidism, correction of, 79
Hyperphosphatemia, in intestinal ischemia, 240
Hypersecretion, of gastric acid, medical treatment of, 77–78
 surgical treatment of, 78–79
Hypertension, portal. *See* Portal hypertension
Hypnosis, for diarrhea, 355
Hypochondriasis, 134–135
Hypocitraturia, 176–177
Hypogammaglobulinemia
 of infancy, 183–184
 infantile, X-linked, 182
Hypoglycemia
 diabetic, 154–155
  treatment of, 156
 idiopathic, 155
 postprandial, 153–156
  in children, 155
  diagnostic approach to, 153–155, 154f
  "nonhypoglycemia" symptoms, 156
  treatment of, 155–156, 155f
Hypomagnesuria, 177
Hypoplasia
 cartilage hair, 186
 hematopoietic, 185
 thymic, 185
Hypovolemia, in intestinal ischemia, 240
Hysteria, 135–136

I

Idiopathic (slow transit) constipation, in women, 250
IgA deficiency, 182–183
IgG subclass deficiency, 184

Ileal pouch, 320
Ileal pouch-anal anastomosis, 314–315
Ileorectostomy, 317–318
Ileostomy
  alternatives, 314–318
  complications of, 311–313
  indications for, 310–311
  Koch pouch, 315–316
  occluding device, 316–317
  ostomy care, 310–313
  surgical techniques, 311
Ileus
  in acute graft vs. host disease, 190
  meconium, in cystic fibrosis, 453–454
Illness, functional, 137–141
Imipramine, 137
Immunodeficiency
  agammaglobulinemia, 184–185
  AIDS, 2, 186–187
  ataxia telangiectasia, 183
  B-cell disorders, 182–187
  cartilage hair hypoplasia, 186
  chronic mucocutaneous candidiasis, 186
  classification of, 181
  Di George syndrome, 185
  gastrointestinal disorders and, 181–187
  hematopoietic hypoplasia, 185
  hyperimmunoglobulinemia, 183
  IgA deficiency, 182–183
  IgG subclass deficiency, 184
  malignancy and, 128
  phagocyte function disorders, 187
  short-limbed dwarfism, 186
  T and B cell disorders, 185–186
  transcobalamin II deficiency, 185
  transient hypogammaglobulinemia, 183–184
  white blood cell disorders, 187
  Wiskott-Aldrich syndrome, 186
  X-linked immunodeficiency with hyper-IgM, 183
  X-linked infantile hypogammaglobulinemia, 182
Immunosuppressive therapy, 293–294
  in chronic hepatitis, 389
  in Crohn's disease, 219–220
  in idiopathic chronic active hepatitis, 390
  in ulcerative colitis, 283
Imuran, 2
Incontinence
  fecal, 307–310
    with constipation, 309
    diabetes-associated, 309
    without diarrhea, 308
    with diarrhea, 308
    with impaired reservoir capacity, 309
    with rectosphincteric abnormalities, 307, 308t
    treatment of adults with, 307–309
    treatment of children with, 309–310
  neurogenic, 309
Indomethacin, 158
Infantile hypogammaglobulinemia, X-linked, 182
Infants. *See also* Children
  gastrointestinal bleeding in, 90
  hypogammaglobulinemia in, 183–184
  reflux in, antireflux procedure for, 12
Infection. *See also specific types*
  cestode, 171–172
  following bone marrow transplant, 192
  nematode, 169–171
  protozoan, 166–169

Vincent's, 2
Infectious esophagitis, 61–65
Inflammation, in diverticular disease, 346–347
Inflammatory bowel disease. *See also* Crohn's disease
  in children, 91
  etiology of malnutrition in, 224, 224t
  growth failure in, 223–229
  hemorrhage and, 339
  idiopathic, and neoplasia, 296–301
  medical treatment of, 225–226, 225t
  nutritional assessment in, 225, 225t
  nutritional therapy in, 226–227, 226t, 227t
    goals of, 227–229, 228t
    parenteral, 204–205
  surgical treatment of, 226, 226t
Injury, caustic, esophageal, 20–25
Intestinal disease, urinary constituents in, 176, 176t
Intestinal gas, 340–342
  abdominal pain and, 340–341
  belching and, 340
  bloating and, 340–341
  dietary factors and, 340–341, 341t
  flatus with, 341–342
  pharmacologic agents for, 341
  simethicone for, 341
Intestinal ischemia, 239–244
  determination of viability, 243–244
  fluorescein dye injection in, 244
  incarcerated inguinal hernia with, 241
  intestinal obstruction with, 241–242
  ischemic colitis with, 243
  laboratory diagnosis of, 240
  mesenteric arterial occlusion with, 242
  mesenteric venous occlusion with, 242–243
  nonocclusive mesenteric, 242
  patient preparation for surgery, 240
  radiologic evaluation of, 240
  second-look laparotomy, 244
  ultrasound in, 243–244
  volvulus with, 241–242
Intestinal lymphangiectasia, 200–201
Intestinal obstruction, 232–239
  acute postoperative, 238
  causes of, 233t
  diagnosis of, 232–235
  in diverticular disease, 348
  enteroclysis study, 238
  ischemia with, 241–242
  large bowel lesions, management of, 238–239
  mechanical, recognition of, 232–233
  operative vs. nonoperative management of, 236
  partial or complete, distinguishing, 233–234
  primary lesion, identification of, 235
  recognition of vascular compromise, 234–235
  small bowel lesions, management of, 236–238
  systemic factors, 235
  treatment of, 235–239
  tube decompression, 235–236
Intestinal obstruction syndrome, in cystic fibrosis, 454
Intestinal pseudo-obstruction, chronic, 251–253
  causes of, 251t
  urinary problems in, 253
Intussusception
  in children, 91
  in infants, 90

Iron chelation therapy, 411
Iron overload. *See* Hemochromatosis
Irritable bowel syndrome, 342–345
  dietary managment of, 343–344
  drug therapy for, 344
  education and reassurance in, 343
  establishing confidence in, 342–343
  managing fears and misconceptions in, 343
  psychologic factors in, 345
  treatment of, 101, 342–343, 342t
Irritable colon syndrome, with constipation, 250
Ischemia, intestinal, 239–244
Islet cell tumors, 458
Isoniazid
  toxicity, 392
  for tuberculous peritonitis, 274
Isopropamide, 78
Isosorbide dinitrate (Isordil), 36
Isospora belli infection, 168
Isospora hominis infection, 168
Isosporiasis, 168

J

Jaundice, in acute graft vs. host disease, 190–191
Juvenile polyps, 90

K

Kaopectate, 255
Kaposi's sarcoma, 270
Ketoconazole (Nizoral)
  for candidal esophagitis, 62
  for candidiasis, 2
Klatskin tumor, 420, 425
Kock pouch, 315–316

L

Lactose intolerance
  abdominal pain and, 352
  in excessive flatus, 341
  in irritable bowel syndrome, 343
Lactose malabsorption, 150–152, 150t, 151t
  in Crohn's disease, 217
  in short bowel syndrome, 175
Lactulose, for portosystemic encephalopathy, 368
Lamb and rice diet, 195t
Large bowel lesions, management of, 238–239
Laser therapy
  applications of, 30–33
  future developments of, 33
  for gastric cancer, 123
  for gastrointestinal disorders, 30–33
  for malignant stricture, 29
  physical principles of, 30, 30t
Laxatives
  for chronic secretory diarrhea, 248
  for irritable bowel syndrome, 344
L-dopa, for portosystemic encephalopathy, 368
Leiomyomas, of esophagus, 57
Letterer-Siwe disease, 185
Leukoplakia, 5–6
Levator syndrome, 305
Levophed, 91
Lidamidine, for diarrhea, 181, 246, 355
Lidex in orabase, 1
Liquid formula diets, enteral feeding with,

206-212
Lithium
  for diarrhea, 246t, 247
  for pancreatic cholera syndrome, 247
Liver. *See also* Hepatic *entries*
  characterization of drugs eliminated by, 358t
  echinococcal cysts of, 276
  highly extracted drugs by, 357
  poorly extracted drugs by, 357-358
Liver abscess, 275-276
Liver cancer, 412-417
  antibody-directed irradiation of, 417
  chemotherapy for, 416-417
  metastasis from colorectal cancer, 412-413, 412t, 413t
  primary, 413-414, 414t
  transplant in, 395
Liver disease
  alcoholic, 374-376
    cirrhosis with, 375-376
    fatty liver with, 374
    hemosiderosis in, 410
    hepatitis with, 374-375
  altered drug metabolism in, 356-361
  chronic, transplant in, 395
  drug-induced, 391-394
    acute, 392
    chronic, 392
    classification of, 391-392, 391t, 392t
    idiosyncratic, 392-393
    monitoring of, 392
    occupational, 394
    treatment of, 392-394
    vascular lesions with, 394
  influence on drug disposition, 359-360, 360f
  influence on protein binding, 360-361
  pharmacokinetic concepts in, 356-357
  safe prescription of drugs with, 361
Liver failure, fulminant, 383-387
  complications of, 384t
  considerations in, 386-387
  supportive care in, 383-385, 384t
  transplant in, 395-396
  treatment of, 385-386
    response to, 386
Liver toxicity, in bone marrow recipients, 188
Liver transplantation, 394-397
  candidates for, 394-396
  in chronic liver disease, 395
  follow-up period, 397
  in fulminant hepatic failure, 395-396
  in hepatobiliary malignancy, 395
  perioperative period following, 396-397
  rejection following, 396
  renal dysfunction following, 396
  in sclerosingcholangitis, 406
Loffler's syndrome, 169
Long segment stricture, treatment of, 28
Loperamide (Imodium)
  for diarrhea, 158-159, 181, 246, 354
  for irritable bowel syndrome, 344
  for pancreatic cholera syndrome, 247
  for *Trichuris trichiura* infection, 263
Lorazepam, for anorexia nervosa, 118
Lymphangiectasia, intestinal, diagnosis of, 200-201
  treatment of, 201
Lymphoma, 165-166

M

Macrobiotic diets, 213-214
Magaldrate, 94
Malabsorption syndrome
  and carbohydrates, 149-153
  in Crohn's disease, 224, 224t
  and diabetic diarrhea, 180
  IgA deficiency in, 182
  in short bowel syndrome, 174-175
  tropical, 159-160
  unresponsive, 165
Malnutrition, in inflammatory bowel disease, 224, 224t
Maloney dilator, 26
Maloplakia, of colon, 182
Mannitol, for increased intracranial pressure, 384
Maprotiline (Ludiomil), for depression, in irritable bowel syndrome, 345
Mebendazole (Vermox)
  for ascariasis, 169
  for *Enterobius vermicularis* infection, 263
  for hookworm infection, 169
  for hydatid cyst, 276
  for *Trichuris trichiura* infection, 263
Mebeverine hydrochloride
  for diarrhea, 355
  for diverticular disease, 345
Meckel's diverticulum, 90
  bleeding of, 338
Meconium ileus, in cystic fibrosis, 453-454
Megacolon, toxic, 288-289
  in Crohn's disease, 232
Menadiol, 404
Menetrier's disease, 128
6-Mercaptopurine
  for Crohn's disease, 220, 293
  for ulcerative colitis, 283
Mercury, in gastrointestinal tract, 47
Mesenteric arterial occlusion, 242
Mesenteric ischemia, nonocclusive, 242
Mesenteric venous occlusion, 242-243
Metal dilator, with guide wires, 26
Methylprednisolone
  for acute graft vs. host disease, 189
  for alcoholic hepatitis, 375
  for inflammatory bowel disease, 225
  for ulcerative colitis, 283
Methylprednisone
  for bacterial peritonitis, 272
  for Crohn's disease, 219
Metoclopramide
  for alkaline reflux gastritis, 94
  chemical structure of, 99f
  for gastroparesis, 99
  for hiccups, 103
  for intestinal gas, 341
  for intestinal pseudo-obstruction, 158
  for nausea and vomiting, 103
  for nonulcer dyspepsia, 101
  for reflux esophagitis, 19t
Metrifonate, 264
Metronidazole (Flagyl)
  for amebiasis, 262, 263, 268
  for amebic abscess, 275
  for bacterial infections, 192
  for *Balantidium coli* infection, 264
  for Crohn's disease, 218, 294
  for fulminant colitis, 285
  for *Giardia* infections, 167, 268
  for inflammatory bowel disease, 225t
  for portosystemic encephalopathy, 369
  for pyogenic liver abscess, 276
Miconazole, for candidal esophagitis, 62-63
Milk products, lactose content of, 151t
Minerals, for bacterial overgrowth syndrome, 157-158, 158t
Mitomycin
  for advanced gastric cancer, 123, 123t
  for esophageal cancer, 60
Monosaccharide malabsorption, 152-153, 152t
Morbidity, after proximal gastric vagotomy, 73
Mortality, after proximal gastric vagotomy, 73
Motility disorders, diffuse, parenteral nutrition for, 204
Mouth, painful, 1-6
Mucilaginous agents, for diarrhea, 354
Mucosal resistance, drugs improving, 71-72
Mucositis, 6
Multiple enzyme neoplasia (MEN), 77
Muscle relaxants, for esophageal spasms, 36-37
Myogenic disease, treatable, 42
Myogenic factors, and constipation, 249
Myotomy
  bidirectional, 312f
  cricopharyngeal, 42
  for esophageal spasm, 37

N

N-acetylcysteine (Mucomyst), 393
Naloxone
  for bacterial peritonitis, 272
  in gastric emptying, 103
Nasobiliary catheter, transpapillary, 432
Nasogastric intubation
  in esophageal caustic injury, 23
  in pancreatitis, 438, 439
Natural foods, 214
Nausea and vomiting, 101-103
  in acute graft vs. host disease, 190
  behavioral strategies for, 103
  central control of, 102f
  chemotherapy causing, 102-103
  differential diagnosis of, 102t
  drug therapy for, 102-103
Necator americanus infection, 169
Neisseria gonorrhoeae infection, 266
Nematode infections, 169-171
Neodymium: yttrium aluminum garnet (Nd:YAG) laser
  characteristics of, 30, 30t
  efficacy and safety of, 31
Neomycin, preoperative, in Crohn's disease, 230
Neoplasia, inflammatory bowel disease and, 296-301
Nephrolithiasis, 175
  treatment of, 177-179, 178t
Nerve blocks, for abdominal visceral pain, 148-149
Neuro-endocrine factors, and constipation, 249
Neurogenic disease, treatable, 42
Neurogenic incontinence, 309
Neurohormones, alteration of, in duodenal ulcer, 67-68

Neutropenia, 183
Niacin, side effects of megadoses of, 215t
Niclosamide
  for *Diphyllobothrium latum* infection, 171
  for taeniasis, 171
Nifedipine
  for achalasia, 39
  for esophageal spasms, 36
Niridazole (Ambilhar), 264
Nissen fundoplication, 13-14, 14f
Nitrates, for esophageal spasm, 34, 36
Nonantimicrobial drugs, for traveler's diarrhea, 258-259, 258t
Nortriptyline, for depression, 137
Nutrients, daily intake of, 113t
Nutrition. *See also* Diet
  in alcoholics, 371
  in bacterial overgrowth syndrome, 157-158, 158t
  enteral
    complications of, 211-212
    delivery methods, 210-211
    elemental diets, 210, 211t
    indications for, 207, 207t
    with liquid formula diets, 206-212, 210t, 211t
    monitoring techniques, 211
    polymeric diets, 209-210, 210t
    rationale for, 207
    routes of access, 207-208, 209f
  in inflammatory bowel disease, 225, 225t
  parenteral, 201-206
    central vein, 203-204
    complications of, 205-206, 205t
    in Crohn's disease, 217, 221
    in esophageal caustic injury, 23
    in fulminant colitis, 286
    home, 206
    indications for, 204-205, 204t
    nutrients in, 202-203
    peripheral vein, 203
    quality control in, 201-202
    in short bowel syndrome, 173
    types of, 203-206
  in ulcerative colitis, 280-281
Nystatin
  for candidal esophagitis, 61-62
  for candidiasis, 2
  for oral thrush, 270

O

Obesity, 106-116
  appetite suppressants, 115
  body measurements, 110-111
  diet diary, 111-112
  dietary management, 108-109, 110t, 111t, 112t
  evaluation of, 106, 107t
  exercise and, 112-113, 114t
  first return visit, 107-111
  follow-up visit, 111-113
  psychologically oriented therapy for, 114-115
  supportive measures, 114-115
  surgery for, 116
  weight goals, 108, 108t
  weight maintenance, 115-116
Omeprazole
  for duodenal ulcer, 68
  for gastrinoma, 78
Opiates, for diarrhea, 245-246, 246t, 354
Opioids, for diabetic diarrhea, 180-181

Oral contraceptive toxicity, 393-394
Oral pain, 1-6
Oral ulcerations, in Crohn's disease, 222
Organic foods, 214
Osteodystrophy, with primary biliary cirrhosis, 399
Ostomy, care of, 310-314
Oxamniquine (Vansil), 264

P

Pain
  abdominal. *See* Abdominal pain
  anal, 250
  chest, 34, 35f, 36t
  in pancreatitis, 438, 439, 445
    treatment of, 448, 448t
  oral, 1-6
  umbilical, 147
  visceral, 147
Pancreatic abscess, 275
Pancreatic cancer, 455-459
  adjuvant therapy for, 458
  decompression surgery for, 457
  diagnostic aspects of, 456
  failure patterns in, 132
  operative phase, 457-458
  postoperative phase, 458
  preoperative phase, 456-457
  resection of, 457-458
  therapeutic options in, 456
  therapeutic outcome, 458-459
  treatment alternatives in, 131, 131t
Pancreatic cholera syndrome, 247
Pancreatic enzymes, in cystic fibrosis, 451, 451t
Pancreatic exocrine insufficiency, and diabetic diarrhea, 180
Pancreatitis
  acute
    early phase of, 442-443
    fluid resuscitation in, 438, 439
    late phase of, 444-445
    medical treatment of, 437-442
    middle phase of, 444
    nasogastric suction in, 438, 439
    nutritional support in, 441
    pain management in, 438, 439-440
    peritoneal lavage for, 443
    prognostic signs in, 437t
    pseudocyst with, 444
    removal of pancreatic enzymes in, 440-441
    respiratory care in, 439
    surgical considerations in, 442-445
    treatment of metabolic complications in, 440
  chronic, 445-446
    adjuvant therapy for, 448
    ascites with, 446
    bile duct stenosis with, 446
    diet in, 450
    duodenal obstruction with, 446
    endocrine insufficiencies with, 447-450
    exocrine insufficiencies with, 447-450
    pain treatment in, 448, 448t
    pain with, 445
    pleural effusion with, 446
    pseudocyst with, 445-446
    steatorrhea with, 447
  determination of severity of, 437-438, 437t
  mild, treatment of, 438
  persisting, 445

  recurrent, 442
  severe, 438-442
  unresolving, parenteral nutrition for, 204
Papaverine, 242
Parasites
  colon, 262-264
  of small intestine, 166-172
    treatment of, 167t
Parasitic infections, following bone marrow transplant, 192
Parastomal hernia, 312, 313
Parastomal skin damage, 313
Parastomal ulcer, 312
Parathyroidectomy, for gastrinoma, 79
Paromomycin (Humatin)
  for amebiasis, 262, 268
  for giardiasis, 167
  for hymenolepis, 172
  for taeniasis, 171
Peliosis hepatis, 394
Penicillamine
  for alcoholic hepatitis, 375
  side effects of, 408
  for Wilson's disease, 407-408
Penicillin
  for caries, 5
  for gingivitis, 2
  for syphilis, 267
Pentazocine (Talwin), for irritable bowel syndrome, 344
Peppermint oil, for diarrhea, 355
Peptic stricture, treatment of, 28
Peptic ulcer. *See also* Duodenal ulcer; Gastric ulcer
  in children, 88-89
  surgery for, 72-76
Perforation, of gastrointestinal tract, 47-48
Perianal abscess, 302-303, 302f-303f
Pericolic abscess, 348
Peridiverticulitis, 348
Periodontal disease, 2
Peritoneovenous shunt, for ascites, 364
Peritonitis, 272-274
  Candida, 273-274
  with peritoneal dialysis, 273
  secondary bacterial, 272
  with shunts, 273
  spontaneous (primary), 273
  tuberculosis, 274
Pernicious anemia, 125-126
Peroxide-saline mouth rinse, 2
Phagocyte function disorders, 187
Pharyngeal dysphagia, 39-44
  analysis of dysfunction, 40-41
  basic principles of, 40
  clinical analysis of, 40-41
  prosthodontics in, 41
  radiographic examination of, 41
  rehabilitation approach to, 42-43
  special problems in, 43-44
  therapeutic approaches to, 41-43
Pharyngeal surgery, role of, 42
Pharynx, foreign bodies in, 47, 47f
Phenobarbital, for pruritus, 399, 402t, 403
Phenobarbitol, for abdominal epilepsy, 106
Phenytoin (Dilantin)
  for abdominal epilepsy, 106
  toxicity of, 392
Phlebotomy, in hemochromatosis, 410-411, 411t
Phlegmon, 444
Phytonadione, 403
Piperazine citrate (Antepar)

for ascariasis, 169
for *Enterobius vermicularis* infection, 263
for gastric ulcer, 71
for nonulcer dyspepsia, 100
Plasma exchange, for pruritus, 402t, 403
Pleural effusion, with chronic pancreatitis, 446
Pneumocystis carinii infection, 185, 268
Pneumonia, aspiration, antireflux procedure for, 11
Podophyllin, 267
Polymeric diets, 209–210, 210t
Polypectomy
　colon, 326–327
　for gastric polyps, 126–127
　hemorrhage following, 338
Polyps
　of colon, 325–328
　gastric, 126–127, 127f
　juvenile, 90
Portacaval shunt, for esophageal varices, 379
Portal hypertension, 376–380
　in children, 89
　complication of, 379–380
　confirmation of, 376–377
　esophageal varices with, 376–380
　　prevention of hemorrhage, 378–379
　　treatment of hemorrhage, 377–378
　extrahepatic, 49
Portosystemic encephalopathy, 366–369
Portosystemic shunts, for portal hypertension, in children, 90
Potassium chloride, for alcoholic cirrhosis, 375
Potential difference profile, of Barrett's esophagus, 17, 17f
Praziquantel
　for *Diphyllobothrium latum* infection, 171
　for hymenolepis, 172
　for *Schistosoma* species, 264
　for taeniasis, 171
Prednisolone, 283
Prednisone
　for aphthous ulcers, 1
　for Crohn's disease, 219, 220, 292
　for fulminant colitis, 290
　for idiopathic chronic active hepatitis, 390
　for inflammatory bowel disease, 225, 225t
　for laryngeal edema with respiratory stridor, 23
　for malabsorption syndrome, 165
　for ulcerative colitis, 283
　for vesiculoerosive disorders, 2
Pregnancy
　and Crohn's disease, 222, 292
　and Wilson's disease, 409
Pro-Banthine
　for gastrinoma, 78
　for postprandial hypoglycemia, 156
Proctalgia fugax, 305
Proctitis, 266, 279–284
　chlamydial, 306
　gonococcal, 306
Proctopexy, transabdominal, 304
Proctosigmoidoscopy, in gastrointestinal bleeding, 334
Propantheline bromide, for diverticular disease, 345
Propranolol, 90
Propylthiouracil, 375
Prostaglandin synthetase inhibitors, 246, 246t
Prostaglandins
　for alkaline reflux gastritis, 94

for duodenal ulcer, 68
for gastric ulcer, 71
Prosthesis
　Angelchik, 14–15
　for malignant stricture, 28–29, 29f
Prosthodontics, in pharyngeal dysphagia, 41
Prostigmine, 158
Protein
　in parenteral nutrition, 202
　reduction of, for portosystemic encephalopathy, 369
Protein-losing enteropathy, 197–201
　causes and mechanisms of, 197t
　Crohn's disease and, 199–200
　diagnosis of, 198
　intestinal lymphangiectasia and, 200–201
　management of, 199
　recognition of, 197–199
Protozoan infection, 166–169
Pruritus
　with cholestasis, 401–403
　with primary biliary cirrhosis, 399
Pruritus ani, 304–305
Pseudocyst
　with acute pancreatitis, 444
　with chronic pancreatitis, 445–446
Pseudotumor, in diverticular disease, 348
Psychologic factors, in irritable bowel syndrome, 345
Psychotherapy
　for depression, 137
　for diarrhea, 354–355
　for obesity, 114–115
Pulmonary therapy, in cystic fibrosis, 454–455
Pylorus, incomplete relaxation of, 95
Pyoderma gangrenosum, and Crohn's disease, 222
Pyrantel pamoate (Antiminth)
　for ascariasis, 169
　for *Enterobius vermicularis* infection, 263
　for hookworm infection, 169
　for trichostrongylus, 170
Pyridoxine, side effects of megadoses of, 215t
Pyrvinium pamoate, 263

Q

Quinacrine hydrochloride, 167

R

Radiation colitis, hemorrhage from, 339
Radiation enteritis
　management of, 237
　parenteral nutrition for, 204
Radiation therapy
　for biliary tract stricture, 420
　for colon cancer, 323–324, 324t
　for esophageal cancer, 56, 57–60
　for gastric cancer, 122, 123
　intraoperative, 129–133
　for liver cancer, 417
　for rectal cancer, 318, 323–324, 324t
Radiography
　in Barrett's esophagus, 16
　in cholecystitis, 434
　in esophageal caustic injury, 21–22
　in intestinal ischemia, 240
　in pharyngeal dysphagia, 41
Radionuclide scintigraphy
　in gastrointestinal bleeding, 334
　in gastroparesis, 97, 97f

Ranitidine
　for duodenal ulcer, 68
　for esophageal reflux, 8
　for gastric ulcer, 70–71
　for gastrinoma, 77, 78
　for peptic disease, in children, 88
　for reflux esophagitis, 19t
Rectal cancer, 323
　chemotherapy and radiation for, 318
　electrocoagulation in, 318–319
　intracavitary irradiation for, 318
　sphincter sparing procedures, 318–320
　surgical resection techniques in, 319–320
Rectal prolapse, 303–304, 304f, 305f
　in cystic fibrosis, 454
　treatment of, 304, 304f, 305f
Rectosigmoidectomy, perineal, 304, 305f
Rectosphincteric abnormalities, fecal incontinence with, 307, 308t
Reducing diets, 214
Reflux, alkaline. See Alkaline reflux gastritis
Reflux symptoms, persistent, antireflux procedure for, 11–12
Resection
　for diverticular bleeding, 337
　subtotal gastric, for duodenal ulcer, 74
Rifampin, for tuberculous peritonitis, 274
Roux-en-Y anastomosis
　in alkaline reflux gastritis, 94
　in biliary tract stricture, 418, 420, 421f
　in gastric cancer, 121
Rubber mercury-filled dilator, 26
Rumination, 105

S

Salmonella infection, 253, 254t, 268
　in infants, 90
Salt repletion, in functional diarrhea, 354
Sarcocystis, 168–169
Savory dilator, 26
Schatzki's ring, treatment of, 28
Schistosoma infection, 264
Scintigraphy
　hepatobiliary, for cholecystitis, 434
　radionuclide
　　in gastrointestinal bleeding, 334
　　in gastroparesis, 97, 97f
Sclerotherapy
　bacteremia associated with, 278
　equipment for, 50
　of esophageal varices, 48–54. See also Esophageal sclerotherapy
　in gastrointestinal bleeding, 83
　solutions for, 50
Seizures, alcoholic, 370–371
Sepsis
　biliary, percutaneous drainage for, 425–426
　in intestinal ischemia, 240
　intra-abdominal
　　antibiotic selection in, 271
　　associated with specific sites, 275–276
　　failure of antibiotics in, 272
　　microbiology of, 270
　　timing of antibiotics in, 271
　parastomal, 314
Sexually transmitted intestinal disease, 264–270
　clinical approach to, 264–267
　enteric pathogens in, 267–268
　physical examination in, 265
　syndromes of, 265t
　treatment of, 265, 269t
Shigellosis, 267–268

Short bowel syndrome, 172–175
  bile sale malabsorption in, 174
  calcium malabsorption in, 174, 175t
  after ileum resection, 173–174
  lactose intolerance and, 175
  after massive bowel resection, 175
  parenteral nutrition in, 173
  after proximal small bowel resection, 175
  steatorrhea with, 174
  treatment of, 173, 173t
  vitamin B_{12} therapy in, 173
  water and electrolyte balance in, 174
Shunts
  peritoneovenous, for ascites, 364
    peritonitis associated with, 273
  portacaval, for esophageal varices, 379
Sigmoidoscopy, bacteremia associated with, 278
Simethicone
  for eructation, 105
  for intestinal gas, 341
Skin damage, parastomal, 313
Small bowel dysfunction
  long segmental, 252–253
  short segmental, 251
Small bowel lesions, management of, 236–238
Small intestine
  abnormal proliferation of microflora in. *See* Bacterial overgrowth syndrome
  electrical dysrhythmias of, 100
  lesions of, management of, 236–238
  parasites of, 166–172
    treatment of, 167t
Sodium valproate toxicity, 392
Somatic pain, 147
Somatostatin, 246t, 247
Sorbitol malabsorption, 153, 153t
Spectinomycin, 266
Sphincterotomy, endoscopic retrograde, 431, 431t, 432t
Spina bifida, 310
Spiramycin, 192
Splenic abscess, 276
Sprue
  celiac, and related diseases, 162–166
  tropical, 159–160
Squamous carcinoma, esophageal, 55
Staphylococcus aureus infection, 253, 254t
Steatorrhea, 178
  with chronic pancreatitis, 447
  in Crohn's disease, 221
  in short bowel syndrome, 174
Stents, in esophageal caustic injury, 24
Steroids
  in Crohn's disease, 220–221
  liver disease associated with, 394
Stomach. *See also* Gastric *entries*
  electrical dysrhythmias of, 100
  premalignant conditions of, 124–129
    clinical evaluation of, 125
    management of, 125–128
Stomatitis, 6
Stone formation, urinary constituents in, 176, 176t
Stool retention, abdominal pain and, 352
Strangulation, of small bowel, management of, 236
  recognition of, 234–235
Stress ulcer, and erosive gastritis, 91–93
  medical treatment of, 91–92
  prophylaxis for, 92–93
  surgical treatment of, 92
Strictureplasty, in Crohn's disease, 231

Strongyloides stercoralis, 169, 263
Strongyloidiasis, 169–170
Sucralfate
  for alkaline reflux gastritis, 94
  for duodenal ulcer, 67
  for peptic disease, in children, 89
  for reflux esophagitis, 19t
Sucrose malabsorption, lactose content of, 151t, 152
Sugar-free products, sorbitol content of, 153t
Suicide, 136
Sulfamethazine, 159
Sulfasalazine
  for Crohn's disease, 218, 220, 293
  for fulminant colitis, 287
  for inflammatory bowel disease, 225, 225t
  for ulcerative colitis, 281–282
Swallowing, pharyngeal, habitual, 10
Syphilis, anorectal, 266–267

T

Tachygastria, 96
Taenia saginata, 171
Taenia solium, 171–121
Taeniasis, 171–172
Tamponade, balloon, in esophageal varices, 37, 38
  in children, 89
  in gastrointestinal bleeding, 83
Tapeworms, 171–172
TES solution, for injection sclerotherapy, 83
Tetracycline
  for amebiasis, 262
  for *Balantidium coli* infection, 264
  for chlamydial proctitis, 306
  for *Chlamydia trachomatis* infection, 266
  for *Dientamoeba fragilis* infection, 263
  for syphilis, 267
  for tropical enteropathy, 159
Tetrahydrocannabinol, 103
Thiabendazole (Mintezol)
  for capillariasis, 170
  for strongyloidiasis, 170, 263
  for trichostrongylus, 170
Thrombosis
  mesenteric arterial, 242
  mesenteric venous, 242–243
  in pancreatitis, 444
Thymic hypoplasia, 185
Thyroid cancer, diarrhea with, 248
Tincture of belladonna
  for irritable bowel syndrome, 344
  for postprandial hypoglycemia, 156
Tinidazole, for *Giardia* infections, 268
TNM staging, of esophageal cancer, 58t
Tobramycin
  for appendicitis, 275
  for pancreatic abscess, 275
  for pyogenic liver abscess, 276
Topical agents, for pruritus, 401–402
Trace elements, in parenteral nutrition, 202–203
Transcobalamin II deficiency, 185
Transcutaneous electrical nerve stimulation, 149
Transit-pressure alterations, and constipation, 250
Transpapillary nasobiliary catheter, 432
Transplant
  bone marrow, gastrointestinal problems in, 188–192
  liver, 394–397
Triaditis, 182

Trichostrongylus, 170
Trichuris trichiura infection, 263
Trientine dihydrochloride, 408
Trifluoperazine
  for diarrhea, 246t, 247
  for pancreatic cholera syndrome, 247
Trimethoprim, for traveler's diarrhea, 258t, 261
Trimethoprim-sulfamethoxazole
  for gonorrhea, 266
  for *Salmonella* infection, 268
  for shigellosis, 267
Trimipramine, for duodenal ulcer, 68
Tropical enteropathy, 159–160
Tube decompression, in intestinal obstruction, 235–236
Tuberculous peritonitis, 274
Tubo-ovarian complex, 276
Tumors
  of esophagus and cardia, 54–57
  islet cell, 458
  Klatskin, 420, 425

U

Ulcer
  aphthous, 1
  duodenal, 66–69
  gastric, 69–72
  laser treatment of, 30–31
  parastomal, 312
  peptic, surgery for, 72–76
  stress, 91–93
Ulcerative colitis, 279–284
  antibiotics for, 283–284
  antidiarrheal agents for, 284
  cancer with, 296–300
  corticosteroids for, 282–283
  emotional factors, 281
  extent of disease, 280
  fulminating, 284–291
    antibiotics for, 287
    blood studies in, 285
    corticosteroids for, 287
    hospital management of, 285–286
      monitoring, 287–288
    medical management of, 286–287
      response to, 290–291
    physical examination in, 285
    presentation and differential diagnosis of, 284–285
    surgery for, 289–290
  immunosuppressive agents for, 283
  nutrition in, 280–281
  severity of symptoms in, 280
  sulfasalazine for, 281–282
  surgical considerations in, 284
  therapeutic alternatives, 279–281
  use of drugs in, 281–284
Ultrasonography
  in cholecystitis, 434
  in intestinal ischemia, 243–244
Ultraviolet-B light, for pruritus, 402t, 403
Umbilical pain, 147
Urate nephrolithiasis, 179
Urinary citrate excretion, 178–179
Urinary magnesium excretion, 178
Urine volume, in nephrolithiasis, 177–178
Urso, features of, 423

V

Vaccines, for traveler's diarrhea, 259–260

Vagotomy
  antireflux procedure following, 12–13
  for duodenal ulcer
    parietal cell, 72–73
    proximal gastric, 72–73
    selective gastric, 74, 74t, 75t
    truncal, 73–74
  for gastric ulcer, 76
  for gastrinoma, parietal cell, 78
  for stress ulcer, 92
Vancomycin
  for bacterial infections, 192
  for endocarditis, 278t
  for peritonitis, 273
Varices, esophageal. See Esophageal varices
Vascular ectasia, bleeding, 337–338
Vasopressin
  for diverticular bleeding, 336–337
  for esophageal varices, in children, 89
  for gastrointestinal bleeding, 83
  for stress ulcer, 92
  for variceal hemorrhage, 377–378
Vegetarian diets, 213
Verapamil
  for diarrhea, 246t, 247
  for esophageal spasms, 36
  for pancreatic cholera syndrome, 247
Vesiculoerosive disorders, 1–2
Viadent, for gingivitis, 2
Vibrio parahemolyticus infection, 253, 254t
Vincent's infection, 2
Viral hepatitis. See Hepatitis

Viral infection, following bone marrow transplant, 192
Visceral pain, 147
Vitamin A
  in fat malabsorption, 404
  side effects of megadoses of, 215t
Vitamin B_{12}, in short bowel syndrome, 173
Vitamin C, side effects of megadoses of, 215t
Vitamin D
  for primary biliary cirrhosis, 399–400
  side effects of megadoses of, 215t
Vitamin E, in fat malabsorption, 404
Vitamin K
  for alcoholic cirrhosis, 375
  in fat malabsorption, 403–404
Vitamins
  for bacterial overgrowth syndrome, 157–158, 158t
  deficiency of, in primary biliary cirrhosis, 400
  megadoses of, toxic effects of, 214–215, 215t
  in parenteral nutrition, 203
Volvulus, 241–242
  midget, in infants, 90
Vomiting. See Nausea and vomiting

W

Warts, rectal, 267, 305–306
Water absorption, and constipation, 250

Water balance, in short bowel syndrome, 174
Weight goals, 108, 108t
Weight loss, in esophageal reflux, 7
Weight maintenance, 115–116
Whipple's disease, 160–162
  antibiotics for, 160–161, 161t
  central nervous system relapse in, 161
    neurologic features of, 161t
    treatment of, 161–162
  clinical and diagnostic features of, 160
  treatment of, 160–161, 161t
White blood cell disorders, 187
Wilm's tumor, treatment of, 414
Wilson's disease, 386–387, 406–409
  clinical features of, 407
  family screening for, 409
  penicillamine therapy for, 407–408
  pregnancy and, 409
  treatment of, 407–409
  trientine dihydrochloride for, 408
  zinc therapy for, 408
Wiskott-Aldrich syndrome, 186
Withdrawal syndrome, alcoholism and, 370–371

Z

Zinc therapy, for Wilson's disease, 408
Zollinger-Ellison syndrome, 75, 77
  diarrhea with, 248